Diagnosis and Management
of
GLAUCOMA

Diagnosis and Management of
GLAUCOMA

Editors

R Ramakrishnan MS DO

Chief Medical Officer and Professor
Glaucoma Services
Aravind Eye Hospital, Tirunelveli, Tamil Nadu, India

SR Krishnadas DO DNB

Director-HRD and Professor
Glaucoma Services
Aravind Eye Hospital, Madurai, Tamil Nadu, India

Mona Khurana MS

Consultant
Glaucoma Services
Aravind Eye Hospital
Tirunelveli, Tamil Nadu, India

Alan L Robin MD

Associate Professor of Ophthalmology and International Health
Johns Hopkins University
Baltimore, USA

Foreword

P Namperumalsamy

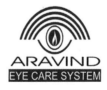

ARAVIND
EYE CARE SYSTEM

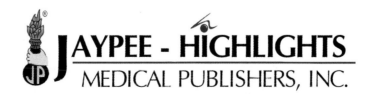

JAYPEE - HIGHLIGHTS
MEDICAL PUBLISHERS, INC.

Jaypee Brothers Medical Publishers (P) Ltd.

Headquarters

Jaypee Brothers Medical Publishers (P) Ltd.
4838/24, Ansari Road, Daryaganj
New Delhi 110 002, India
Phone: +91-11-43574357
Fax: +91-11-43574314
Email: jaypee@jaypeebrothers.com

Overseas Offices

J.P. Medical Ltd.
83, Victoria Street, London
SW1H 0HW (UK)
Phone: +44-2031708910
Fax: +02-03-0086180
Email: info@jpmedpub.com

Jaypee-Highlights Medical Publishers Inc.
City of Knowledge, Bld. 237, Clayton
Panama City, Panama
Phone: + 507-301-0496
Fax: + 507-301-0499
Email: cservice@jphmedical.com

Jaypee Brothers Medical Publishers (P) Ltd.
17/1-B Babar Road, Block-B, Shaymali
Mohammadpur, Dhaka-1207
Bangladesh
Mobile: +08801912003485
Email: jaypeedhaka@gmail.com

Jaypee Brothers Medical Publishers (P) Ltd.
Shorakhute, Kathmandu
Nepal
Phone: +00977-9841528578
Email: jaypee.nepal@gmail.com

Website: www.jaypeebrothers.com
Website: www.jaypeedigital.com

Inquiries for bulk sales may be solicited at: jaypee@jaypeebrothers.com

This book has been published in good faith that the contents provided by the contributors contained herein are original, and is intended for educational purposes only. While every effort is made to ensure accuracy of information, the publisher and the editors specifically disclaim any damage, liability, or loss incurred, directly or indirectly, from the use or application of any of the contents of this work. If not specifically stated, all figures and tables are courtesy of the editors. Where appropriate, the readers should consult with a specialist or contact the manufacturer of the drug or device.

Diagnosis and Management of Glaucoma

First Edition: **2013**

ISBN 978-93-5025-578-0

Printed at Ajanta Offset & Packagings Ltd., New Delhi.

Dedicated to

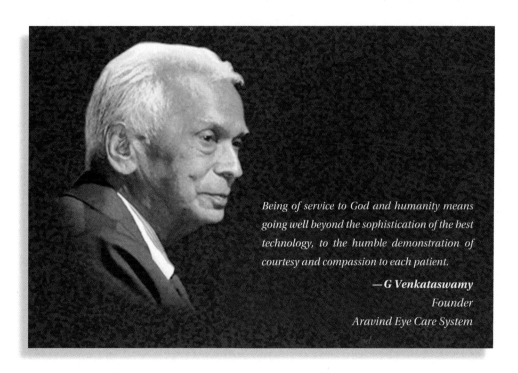

Being of service to God and humanity means going well beyond the sophistication of the best technology, to the humble demonstration of courtesy and compassion to each patient.

—G Venkataswamy
Founder
Aravind Eye Care System

Contributors

A Jayaprakash Patil MS
Specialist Registrar
Guy's and St Thomas' NHS Foundation
Trust, London, UK

Aditya Neog DO DNB
Consultant
Glaucoma Services
Medical Research Foundation
Sankara Nethralaya
Chennai, Tamil Nadu, India

Alan L Robin MD
Associate Professor of
Ophthalmology and International Health
Johns Hopkins University
Baltimore, USA

Amy Parminder MD FRCSC
Assistant Professor of Ophthalmology
Tufts University School of Medicine
Boston, USA

Anil Kumar Mandal MD DNB FNAMS
Head
Jasti V Ramanamma Children's
Eye Care Centre
LV Prasad Eye Institute, LV Prasad Marg
Banjara Hills, Hyderabad
Andhra Pradesh, India

Ankit Gupta MS
Glaucoma Fellow
Aravind Eye Hospital
Tirunelveli, Tamil Nadu, India

Anup Das MS
Glaucoma Fellow
Aravind Eye Hospital
Tirunelveli, Tamil Nadu, India

Arijit Mitra DO DNB
Medical Officer
Aravind Eye Hospital
Tirunelveli, Tamil Nadu, India

Arun Rajan MS
Glaucoma Fellow
Aravind Eye Hospital
Tirunelveli, Tamil Nadu, India

Ashish Bacchav DNB
Medical Officer, Cornea Department
Aravind Eye Hospital
Tirunelveli, Tamil Nadu, India

Ashish Kumar MS
Glaucoma Fellow
Aravind Eye Hospital
Tirunelveli, Tamil Nadu, India

Bradford Shingleton MD
Clinical Professor of Ophthalmology
Harvard Medical School
Clinical Instructor
Tufts University School of Medicine
Boston, USA

Debasis Chakrabarti MS
Consultant
Calcutta Medical Research Foundation
and Narayana Nethralaya
Kolkata, West Bengal, India

Deepak P Edward MD FACS
Professor and Chair
Department of Ophthalmology
Summa Health System, Akron
Northeastern Ohio Universities
Colleges of Medicine and Pharmacy
Rootstown, OH,USA

Devendra Maheshwari MS
Consultant
Glaucoma Services
Aravind Eye Hospital
Tirunelveli, Tamil Nadu, India

Gabor B Scharioth MD PhD
Senior Consultant
Recklinghausen Eye Centre
Recklinghausen, Germany

George V Puthuran MS
Chief Medical Officer and Professor
Glaucoma Services
Aravind Eye Hospital
Madurai, Tamil Nadu, India

GR Reddy MS
Director
Sri Venkateshwara Nethralaya
Tadepalligudem
Andhra Pradesh, India

Gus Gazzard MD
Glaucoma Specialist
Moorfields Eye Hospital
London, UK

Joshua Priluck MD
Consultant
Ophthalmology Department
Summa Health System
Akron, OH, USA

K Rangachari
Research Scholar
Centre of Excellence in Bioinformatics
School of Biotechnology
Madurai Kamaraj University
Madurai, Tamil Nadu, India

Kavitha Palanisamy MS
Consultant
Glaucoma Services
Aravind Eye Hospital
Puducherry, India

Keith Barton MD
Glaucoma Specialist
Moorfields Eye Hospital
London, UK

Kundan Karan MS
Consultant
Glaucoma Services
Aravind Eye Hospital
Madurai, Tamil Nadu, India

L Vijaya DO MS
Director
Glaucoma Services
Medical Research Foundation
Sankara Nethralaya
Chennai, Tamil Nadu, India

Mani Bhaskaran DO DNB
Assistant Professor
Clinical Sciences
Singapore Eye Research
Institute, Singapore

Manish Shah MD
Director
Foresight Eye Centre
Mumbai, Maharashtra, India

Manju Pillai DO DNB
Professor
Glaucoma Services
Aravind Eye Hospital
Madurai, Tamil Nadu, India

Matthew C Willett MD
Consultant
Department of Ophthalmology
Summa Health System
Akron OH, Northeastern Ohio University
College of Medicine and Pharmacy
Rootstown, OH, USA

Mohan Kumar MS
Glaucoma Fellow
Aravind Eye Hospital
Tirunelveli, Tamil Nadu, India

Mohideen Abdul Kader DNB
Professor
Glaucoma Services
Aravind Eye Hospital
Tirunelveli, Tamil Nadu, India

Mona Khurana MS
Consultant
Glaucoma Services
Aravind Eye Hospital
Tirunelveli, Tamil Nadu, India

MS Sunil MS DNB FRCS
Associate Professor
Regional Institute of Ophthalmology
Trivandrum, Kerala, India

Munish Dhawan MD
Consultant
RP Centre for Ophthalmic Sciences
All India Institute of Medical Sciences
New Delhi, India

Murali Ariga MS DNB
Director
Sundaram Medical Foundation
Anna Nagar, Chennai
Tamil Nadu, India

N Prasanthi MSc PhD
Senior Research Fellow
Department of Genetics
Aravind Medical Research Foundation
Aravind Eye Hospital, Madurai
Tamil Nadu, India

Nidhi Gupta MS
Glaucoma Fellow
Aravind Eye Hospital
Madurai, Tamil Nadu, India

Nikhil S Choudhari DNB
Consultant, Glaucoma Services

Medical Research Foundation
Sankara Nethralaya
Chennai, Tamil Nadu, India

NR Rangaraj MS
Senior Consultant
Premier Eye Care and
Sundaram Medical Foundation
Chennai, Tamil Nadu, India

Oswald Rondon MD
Consultant
Mass Eye and Ear Infirmary
Boston, USA

P Sathyan DO DNB
Chief and Professor
Glaucoma Services
Aravind Eye Hospital
Coimbatore, Tamil Nadu, India

P Sundaresan MSc PhD
Senior Scientist
Department of Molecular Genetics
Aravind Eye Hospital
Madurai, Tamil Nadu, India

Paul Foster MD
Glaucoma Specialist
Moorfields Eye Hospital
London, UK

Pradeep Ramulu MD PhD
Associate Professor
Wilmer Eye Institute
Johns Hopkins Hospitals
Baltimore, Maryland, USA

R Ramakrishnan MS DO
Chief Medical Officer and Professor
Glaucoma Services
Aravind Eye Hospital
Tirunelveli, Tamil Nadu, India

R Venkatesh DO DNB
Chief Medical Officer and Professor
Aravind Eye Hospital
Puducherry, India

Raka (Chatterjee) Chakrabarti MD
Consultant and Glaucoma Specialist
Susrut Eye Hospital and Research Centre
Kolkata, West Bengal, India

Ronald SH Chung MD
Consultant
Singapore National Eye Centre
Singapore
Yong Loo Lin School of Medicine
National University of Singapore
Singapore

Ronnie George MS
Senior Consultant
Glaucoma Services
Medical Research Foundation
Sankara Nethralaya
Chennai, Tamil Nadu, India

Sandeep Bachu DNB
Retina Fellow
Aravind Eye Hospital
Coimbatore, Tamil Nadu, India

Sandhya Reddy DO
Intraocular Lens Surgery Fellow
Aravind Eye Hospital
Tirunelveli, Tamil Nadu, India

Shalini Mohan MD
Consultant
RP Centre for Ophthalmic Sciences
All India Institute of Medical Sciences
New Delhi, India

Shalmali Ranaut DNB
Resident
Aravind Eye Hospital
Tirunelveli, Tamil Nadu, India

Shamira A Perera MBBS BSc FRCOphth
Consultant
Singapore National Eye Centre
Singapore

SR Krishnadas DO DNB
Director-HRD and Professor
Glaucoma Services
Aravind Eye Hospital
Madurai
Tamil Nadu, India

SR Rathinam DO DNB PhD
Consultant
Uvea Clinic
Aravind Eye Hospital and
Postgraduate Institute of
Ophthalmology
Madurai, Tamil Nadu, India

Suresh Puthalath DNB MNAMS
Chief Medical Officer
Cumtrust Eye Hospital
Calicut, Kerala, India

Tanuj Dada MD
Additional Professor
RP Centre for Ophthalmic Sciences
All India Institute of Medical Sciences
New Delhi, India

Timothea Ryan MD
Consultant
Weill Medical College of Cornell University
New York, USA

Ting Aung FRCS(Ed) FRCOphth (UK)
MMed (Ophth) FAMS PhD
Professor and Senior Consultant
Singapore National Eye Centre
Singapore

Todd E Woodruff MD
Consultant
Department of Ophthalmology
Summa Health System
Akron OH, Northeastern Ohio University
College of Medicine and Pharmacy
Rootstown, OH, USA

Valliammai Muthappan MD
Consultant
Department of Ophthalmology and
Visual Science
Washington University
St Louis, Missouri, USA

Venkat Reddy DO DNB
Senior Resident
Aravind Eye Hospital
Tirunelveli, Tamil Nadu, India

Vinay Nangia MS FRCS
Director
Suraj Eye Institute
Nagpur, Maharashtra, India

Foreword

Glaucoma is the second most common cause of glaucoma worldwide and close to 80 million will be diagnosed with glaucoma by the year 2020. With the changing demographic profile and an increasing number of aging population, Asia will have disproportionately large number of persons with glaucoma, mostly with angle-closure disease. Bilateral blindness is projected in 11 millions of those with glaucoma and effective opportunistic screening, early detection and appropriate treatment measures will remain the key-to-combat glaucoma blindness.

Widely-tipped as *silent thief of sight* owing to its largely asymptomatic nature, population-based studies have revealed that more than 90 percent of glaucoma in the developing world remains undetected. Residency and postgraduate training programs need to be well equipped to train the graduating ophthalmologists to increasingly focus on *case detection* of glaucoma by the opportunistic screening, which remains the single most effective means of early detection of glaucoma for instituting an appropriate management.

In recent years, there has been virtually an explosion of knowledge with accumulation of new information on the inheritance and pathophysiology of glaucoma. Apart from better drugs and newer surgeries that are designed to enhance the natural outflow pathways, there is a distinct possibility of gene replacement therapy and stem cell treatment for glaucoma in the not too distant future. As innovative modalities of management of glaucoma continue to evolve, better treatment outcomes are bound to provide preservation of vision and improved quality-of-life to patients with glaucoma. Ongoing studies in proteomics of glaucoma are likely to lead to diagnostic biomarkers in plasma to detect and treat the disease earlier. The evolving discipline of pharmacogenomics is also likely to individualize management of glaucoma in an attempt to improve treatment outcomes.

The text on glaucoma has been written by practitioners of glaucoma of national and international repute and the authors have made a sincere attempt to present the most complex information available on glaucoma in a very simple and lucid style. Pathophysiologic mechanisms, recent advances in glaucoma diagnostics, pharmacotherapeutics, recent improvements in surgical techniques including drainage devices and natural outflow enhancing techniques have been sufficiently covered by experts with wide experience in the respective domain of knowledge. Although exhaustive, well-written textbooks in glaucoma are already available in the world literature, my belief is that the book will serve as a comprehensive reference source for postgraduates, ophthalmologists and for those taking up fellowship programs in glaucoma. I congratulate all the editors and contributors who have assisted in getting the text published and I would like to express my special appreciation for the editorial team led by Dr R Ramakrishnan. I earnestly believe that the book will be a valuable resource addition to any library.

P Namperumalsamy
President
Aravind Medical Research Foundation
Madurai, Tamil Nadu, India
Professor and Chairman Emeritus
Aravind Eye Care System and
Postgraduate Institute of Ophthalmology

Preface

Glaucoma is a challenging yet fascinating disease. In the recent years, there have been innovative developments and improvements in the field of glaucoma. This has led to a better understanding of the pathogenesis of the disease. Definitions and classifications have been revised and changed with time. With the new and improved diagnostic instruments, simple clinical observations can be quantified and followed up. Newer and safer surgical procedures are being designed. Clinical trials and epidemiological research has shifted the trend to a more evidence-based approach in patient care. Each new discovery adds more to the understanding of the disease and its management. At the same time, it also poses a new set of unanswered questions.

Progress never stops and learning is never complete. Glaucoma has become a subspecialty in itself. Thus we decided to come out with the book on glaucoma to share our experience especially in context with the current scenario. It is a multiauthored book and each author has provided their valuable thoughts and experiences in their own writing style. Each contributor is renowned in the field of glaucoma with indispensable clinical and surgical experiences with a passion for teaching. We have tried to make the uniformity in formatting without compromising the style of each author and also added our own humble experience.

It will be useful for residents, glaucoma fellows and ophthalmologists with an interest in glaucoma. The readers will be given a clear and concise update in context with the present practice patterns. The book covers the basic examination methods, diagnostic techniques and the latest advances. The important clinical disorders and their management have been discussed. Points which can be applied to routine clinical practice are highlighted.

A text cannot say everything. It can only tell as far as all words can go. It has been rightly said that *a picture is worth a thousand words* and clinical photographs form an important part of the book. We have attempted to create an effective combination of pictures and words that we hope that it will engage the readers' interest.

Eyes see the truth and then you realize it...but first you see it through the eyes of the master.

Our *first steps* or rather *first sights* in the field of glaucoma were through the eyes of our mentors and their vision still continues to guide us. We hope that the book is informative, enjoyable, stimulates thought and translates to better patient care.

R Ramakrishnan
SR Krishnadas
Mona Khurana
Alan L Robin

Acknowledgments

The book has been possible through the inspiration and support of our mentors. Dr G Venkatasamy's vision and principles have always been a guiding light. We warmly thank Dr P Namperumalsamy and Dr Natchiar G for their support. The contributing authors are good friends and we thank them for sharing their expertise, knowledge and experience. We owe special thanks to our residents and fellows for their support. Their thoughts and inquisitiveness have been a constant source of inspiration. We appreciate the staff at glaucoma clinic for their cooperation. We gratefully acknowledge the efforts of Ms Seetha R (Administrative Assistant) who worked diligently typing and formatting the text and coordinating the material submitted by the contributors. We thank Mr Perumalsamy E and Ms Usha G (Library Staff) for their contribution in the project. We wish to thank Ms Devi Kayalvizhi K (Videographer and Clinical Photographer) and Ms Stella B, for their contribution to the clinical photographs. We appreciate the contributions of Mrs Muthulakshmi R and Mr Brem Kumar CV for the fundus photographs and OCT images. We thank the publishers M/s Jaypee Brothers Medical Publishers (P) Ltd, New Delhi, India, for making this project possible with their constant support. We appreciate the efforts and hard work put in by the editors and the kind support and patience of their families.

Contents

PART 2: GLAUCOMA—DIAGNOSTICS

PART 4: GLAUCOMA—THERAPEUTICS

PART 5: GLAUCOMA—FUTURE

PART 1

Glaucoma—Basics

Glaucoma in Developing Countries

R Ramakrishnan

BACKGROUND AND CURRENT SITUATIONS

India was the first country to launch the National Programme for Control of Blindness in 1976 with the goal of reducing the prevalence of blindness. Of the total estimated 45 million blind persons (Va < 3/60) in the world, 7 million are in India. As per information available from various studies, there are an estimated 12 million bilateral blind persons in India with visual acuity < 6/60 in better eye of which nearly 7 million are with visual acuity < 3/60 in better eye. Recent survey (1999–2001) in 15 district of country, indicated that, 2.5 million of 50 plus population is blind (visual acuity < 6/60).[1,2] Main causes of blindness in the age group of 50 plus population are as follows:[1]

1. Cataract: 62.6%
2. Refractive errors: 19.7%
3. Glaucoma: 5.0%
4. Others: 5%
5. Postsegment disorders: 4.7%
6. Surgical complications: 1.2%
7. Corneal blindness: 0.9%

Among the emerging causes of blindness, Glaucoma needs special attention. Prevalence of glaucoma is estimated to be 4 percent in population aged 30 years and above while childhood blindness due to glaucoma is 3 percent.

Two studies from South India, the Andhra Pradesh Eye Disease Study and Vellore Eye Study (VES) from an urban population of Vellore report the prevalence of primary open angle glaucoma, to be 2.56 percent at Hyderabad and 0.41 percent at Vellore respectively while prevalence of angle closure glaucoma in Andhra Pradesh eye study was 1.1 percent and in VES 4.32 percent.[3-5] According to the Aravind Comprehensive Eye Survey (ACES) prevalence of any glaucoma in rural population of South India was 2.6 percent.[6]

The prevalence percentages in different types of glaucoma according to Aravind Comprehensive Eye Survey are given in the Box.

Also, data from this study, suggests that there is no particular cut off point for IOP, beyond which glaucoma

1. Overall prevalence of primary open angle glaucoma was 1.7%
2. Prevalence of POAG among aged 40 to 60 years was 0.7%. One fifth of those with POAG had blindness in one or both eyes from glaucoma
3. PACG—0.5%
4. Secondary glaucoma (excluding Pseudoexfoliative Glaucoma)—0.3%

develops, although, increasing IOP is a significant risk factor for glaucoma.

The National Programme for Control of Blindness, though, being implemented since last 25 years has not been developed as comprehensive eye care program and this has lead to a delay in the detection and management of patients with glaucoma.[7] Major constraints in developing a comprehensive eye care program are:

1. Lack of political backing
2. ***Overemphasis on cataract:*** Skills required in diagnosing and managing glaucoma need to be acquired during residency. These facilities are available at few tertiary level institutes only. Training of eye

surgery in this field has been inadequate. It is imperative to train all ophthalmologists in this field.

3. *Inequitable distribution of eye surgeons:* There are 8500 ophthalmologist in India but there is wide disparity between urban and rural areas. Eye surgeon population ratio varies from 1:20,000 in urban area to 1 in 2,50,000 in rural area. This disparity has lead to significant differences in services offered/sought by the public.

4. *Suboptimal utilization of human resources:* It is estimated that, 50 percent qualified eye surgeons are nonoperating surgeons.

5. *Inadequate number of paramedical eye care personnel:* While, desired eye surgeon—paramedic ratio should be 1:3 to 1:4, this ratio is less.

6. *Suboptimal coverage:* Since, advanced ophthalmic services for early diagnosis of glaucoma and its management is mainly restricted to urban/semiurban areas, the geophysically remote and socioeconomically backward population remains underserved.

7. *Lack of public awareness:* *Prevention is always better than cure* and prevention can only be done if the general public is aware of the early symptoms and signs of glaucoma. The fact, that population doubling is expected every 35 years, it is estimated that approximately 19.5 million of our population will have glaucoma in urban India till 2020[8] (This does not take into account the effect of increasing life expectancy). The magnitude of the problem by year 2020, along with all the present constraints forces us to formulate adequate strategies for early diagnosis and management of glaucoma. Because of the asymptomatic nature and lack of awareness

about the disease, many individuals with the problem are not diagnosed earlier leading to a delay in its management.

GLAUCOMA IN DEVELOPING COUNTRIES LIKE INDIA

Burning Issues

1. Lack of awareness.
2. Silent and asymptomatic nature of the disease.
3. No permanent cure as it can only be controlled.
4. Life long treatment and follow-up.
5. Treatment is expensive.
6. Whatever is lost is permanent and irreversible.
7. Inadequate infrastructure and manpower.
8. Unequal distribution of ophthalmologists.

Strategies

Future Plan of Action

1. *Revamping medical education:* Upgrading the undergraduate and postgraduate courses to keep pace with diagnosis and management of glaucoma. Apart from upgrading the medical education, existing ophthalmologists should also be trained in this field.
2. Ensuring optimal utilization of human resources.
3. Improving quality of services by adopting and enforcing standard ophthalmic procedures and maintain high quality of preoperative, operative and postoperative services.
4. Opportunistic screening programmes at eye care institutions for all persons more than 35 years and those with family history of glaucoma.
5. Community-based referral by multipurpose workers of all persons with symptoms and signs of glaucoma (All individuals with diminution of vision, haloes, frequent change

of glasses, night blindness, ocular pain, family history of glaucoma).

6. Tonometry and fundus examination at eye camps.
7. Most important of all, increasing public awareness about glaucoma especially periodical ophthalmic examination which includes tonometry, gonioscopy and fundus examination of patient more than 35 years, family history of glaucoma on similar lines as regular blood pressure and blood sugar check-up.

Objectives and Targets

- Early diagnosis and management of glaucoma
- To screen all patients above 35 years who attend eye clinics
- Screening eye camps for glaucoma.

Areas which Need More Emphasis in Action Plan

1. Glaucoma should be given due importance in the program.
2. Eye care services need to be strengthened in difficult, underserved and backward areas.
3. NPCB should keep pace with latest technological advances within available resources keeping in mind, the cost effectiveness of new interventions.
4. *Equipment and supplies:* Frequency doubling perimetry and Nd:YAG laser should be provided at district hospitals and automated perimetry, Nd:YAG and argon laser at medical colleges.

Advocacy and Public Awareness

To strengthen advocacy and generate public awareness, following activities are proposed under vision 2020 initiative.[9]

National and State Level

1. Political commitment
2. Putting up blindness control (due to various causes which includes glaucoma) on the agenda of Central

Council of Health and Family Welfare where Union and State Health Ministers pass resolution on health care.

3. Constitution of a working group at national level with members from government, NGOs and other funding agencies.

4. Frequent press releases and articles in leading newspapers of the country.

5. Increased frequency of broadcast and telecast of messages on eye care to generate public awareness.

6. *Print media:* Quarterly newsletters, articles in scientific journals and development of prototype print materials.

7. Introduction of topics on eye care in school curricula.

8. Distance education modules for children as well as for para-professionals.

9. Involvement of professional organization like AIOS, IMA, etc.

District Level

1. Strengthen District Society's functioning and representation from NGOs and the community.

2. Public awareness activities to meet local needs.

3. Strong interpersonnel communication through village based link workers and community workers.

4. Motivation and involvement of village level committees, locally elected bodies, grass root NGOs, women groups, formal and non-formal leaders and other active community leaders would be necessary for enhancing coverage in the underserved areas.

5. Multisectoral approach particularly involving department of education, social welfare and media. Regular CMEs should be organized for Practicing Ophthalmologists, Family Physicians, Voluntary organization like Rotary, Lions club, etc.

Development Issues

Unlike most of the other disease states, glaucoma is not one disease entity, but a composite mixture of different pathologies: POAG, angle-closure glaucoma (ACG), secondary glaucoma, as well as congenital glaucoma. Thus, establishing a uniform case definition is not possible. Therefore it becomes necessary to decide which condition needs to be screened.

The next problem relates to actual diagnostic criteria for diagnosis of any of the glaucomas. Though, increased IOP is a major risk factor for development of glaucoma it is seen, that glaucomatous damage occurs even at lower IOP values. On the other hand, increased IOP may not cause any damage in certain individuals. So, taking a single IOP measurement may not be of very helpful in actually labeling an individual to be having glaucoma.

Next, direct ophthalmoscopy can also give rise to high percentage of false positive and negative results.

Mass visual field testing has been shown to be a potentially accurate and efficient means for screening by some authorities, but 40 percent nerve fibers may already be lost by the time, a functional field defect is detected. This means, that, the disease would not be actually detected in the early presymptomatic phase at which damage may be reversible.

All these aspects point towards a pessimistic view of instituting a glaucoma screening program. So, to screen for glaucoma, one should include the above three tests for the screening. However not only, is this a costly venture, it has resource implications. Available personnel to undertake such testing are limited. Moreover, to screen for angle closure glaucoma, Gonioscopy facilities should be available at secondary level at least.

Treatment Modalities

Apart from basic diagnostic methods, clear guidelines on treatment policies will have to be established. Compliance and cost of treatment also need to be considered for this purpose. It is seen that medical treatment may not be a feasible alternative for most populations in developing countries like ours, especially for those residing in rural area, keeping in mind, the high possibility of non compliance among them. Certain studies have been done to compare efficacy of different treatment modalities including Medical treatment, Laser Trabeculoplasty and primary Trabeculectomy. These studies, showed, that primary trabeculectomy had the best results. So, it may be best to provide primary trabeculectomy as the treatment of choice especially in developing countries like India.

To summarize, for effective screening, it is necessary to perform tonometry and fundus examination in eye camps. If required, visual fields screening can be done by using the frequency doubling perimetry. Depending on the clinical assessment, either medical or surgical treatment can be considered as the treatment of choice keeping in mind, the high rate of noncompliance.

MONITORING MECHANISM AND LATEST TECHNOLOGY

Clinical evaluation of optic disc and visual field are critical in glaucoma diagnosis and both should be monitored to determine whether glaucoma is stable or progressing.

Examination of Optic Disc

Following points should be considered while examining optic disc: Optic nerve head examination should include determination of optic disc size. One of the ways it can be done is using 5° aperture of a direct ophthalmoscope.

1. Vertical and horizontal diameter of optic nerve head and horizontal

and vertical cup disc ratio should be determined with a slit lamp using 90D lens or 78D lens.

2. When examining the optic nerve head, physicians should consider the "ISNT" rule, which means that, thickest part of a healthy neuroretinal rim (NRR) is located in inferior quadrant, followed by superior, nasal and temporal quadrants. If NRR thickness does not follow ISNT rule, then, optic nerve head must be damaged by glaucoma. The ISNT rule is independent of optic disc size so it applies to small, normal and large optic disc.

3. Color and contour of neural rim tissue should be examined.

4. Pallor of neural rim tissue exceeding the degree of cupping indicates that a nonglaucomatous optic neuropathy must be present.

5. Presence or absence of an optic disc hemorrhage, should also be assessed, because, presence of disc hemorrhage is a negative prognostic factor for patients with glaucoma.

6. Finally, reproducible and quantitative assessments of retinal nerve fiber layer (RNFL) and Optic disc could be obtained with the GDx–VCC, OCT or HRT at least in tertiary care centers.

Central Corneal Thickness Measurement

Central corneal thickness measurement (CCT) with pachymeter is also important in diagnosis of glaucoma. A high CCT (>580 μ) results in an overestimation of actual IOP, whereas a low CCT (<500 μ) results in underestimation of actual IOP. Patients with thin corneal and high IOPs have a higher risk of developing glaucoma than patients with thicker corneas.

Visual Field Testing

Standard automated perimetry (SAP) has been used to evaluate visual field in glaucoma. The Swedish interactive threshold algorithm (SITA) is the most recent advance in SAP. It reduces test duration, which in turn reduces patient's fatigue. This may improve the accuracy of clinical perimetry.

Two newer perimetry techniques include frequency doubling perimetry (FDP) and short wavelength automated perimetry (SWAP). FDP may detect glaucomatous visual field defect earlier than SAP. The Humphrey matrix (Carl Zeiss Meditec) is a new FDP instrument that allows for a more detailed evaluation of visual field. Also, it may be used to monitor for visual field progression. One time SWAP can detect the onset of glaucomatous visual field loss earlier that SAP in patients with ocular hypertension. However, SWAP test duration is long and interpreting test results is difficult due to flaw in normative database. Also, cataracts may affect results of SWAP. SITA-SWAP has a shorter test duration and may be helpful in early glaucoma diagnosis.

RESEARCH AREAS

Apart from the various diagnostic methods available, as mentioned earlier, there are certain ongoing advances in the early diagnosis and management of glaucoma.

While IOP lowering remains the only proven strategy for preventing visual loss in glaucoma, scientific advances are anticipated over the next 5 to 10 years that may lead to use of neuroprotective agents in the near future.

The oral NMDA antagonist memantine is the first neuroprotection drug to treat Alzheimer's disease. Various interventions tested in preclinical and clinical studies of glaucoma are yielding some encouraging results.

The development of neuroprotective glaucoma drugs that are able to protect the optic nerve independent of IOP lowering is an important goal because recent national institutes of health sponsored glaucoma clinical trails show that some patients experience disease progression despite seemingly adequate IOP reduction. A series of second generation memantine derivatives called nitromemantines are also currently in development and may prove to have even greater neuroprotective properties than does memantine.

Low Visual Aids

Provision of low visual aids to individuals who have already suffered severe glaucomatous damage can rehabilitate them socially and to some extent, financially.

CONCLUSION

For an effective screening, diagnosis and management of glaucoma, following facts should be considered:

1. Glaucoma being an important cause of irreversible blindness, can be taken care of, to some extent if, we as a clinician or field worker, are well trained in recognizing early symptoms and signs of glaucoma. For this, certain strict measures have to be taken to train individuals involved in community's health.

2. Also, in present scenario, it is imperative that our medical curriculum should include intensive training in this field both medical as well as surgical.

3. A strong political commitment.

4. Provision of adequate equipment at district hospitals and medical colleges.

5. Screening of all patients > 35 years, patients with diabetic retinopathy and patients with family history of glaucoma, in eye camps.

6. Also, mandatory fundus examination and tonometry at eye

camps and if required, visual field examination.

7. Strengthening our research division especially in areas of neuroprotection, early diagnosis with better visual field analysis and most importantly, in areas of low visual aids.

8. Most important of all, creating public awareness about the disease.

The above factors along with a combined effort and strong will power can certainly tackle this problem to a large extent and prevent needless blindness.

REFERENCES

1. Murthy GV, Gupta SK, Bachani D, Jose R, John N. Current estimates of blindness in India. Br J Ophthalmol 2005;89:257-60.

2. Jose R. Present status of the national programme for control of blindness in India. Community Eye Health J 2008;21:s103-4.

3. Dandona L, Dandona R, Mandal P, et al. ACG in an Urban population in Southern India: APEDS. Ophthalmology 2000;107:1702-9.

4. Dandona L, Dandona R, Srinivas M, et al. OAG in an Urban population in Southern India. Ophthalmology 2000;107:1710-6.

5. Jacob A, Thomas R, Koshi SP, et al. Prevalence of POAG in an Urban South Indian population. IJO 1998; 46: 81-6.

6. Ramakrishnan R, Nirmalan PK, Krishnadas R, Thulasiraj RD, Tielsch JM, Katz J, Friedman D, Robin AL. Aravind Comprehensive Eye Survey. Ophthalmology 2003;110:1484-90.

7. National Programme for Control of Blindness in India. Achievements. Ophthalmology Section, Directorate General of Health Services, Ministry of Health and Family Welfare, Government of India. New Delhi: Nirman Bhavan; 2004. p. 23.

8. Quigley HA, Broman AT. The number of people with glaucoma worldwide in 2010 and 2020. Br J Ophthalmol 2006;90:262-7.

9. Foster A. Cataract and "Vision 2020: the right to sight" initiative. Br J Ophthalmol 2001;85:635-9.

2 | Epidemiology of Glaucoma and the Role of Glaucoma Screening in Diagnosis

— Ronnie George —

INTRODUCTION

Epidemiological studies in glaucoma have provided us with insights into the amount of disease and its risk factors. Since racial and ethnic differences in disease type and prevalence exist, multiple studies have to be carried out in different ethnicities and regions. A large number of studies have been carried out in the past few decades. They have contributed significantly to improving our understanding of the prevalence and risk factors for glaucoma.

From these studies global estimates for disease prevalence have been derived by Broman and Quigley.[1] By the year 2010, an estimated 60.5 million persons will suffer from glaucoma (44.7 million POAG and 15.7 million PACG).

In this chapter, we attempt to summarize prevalence estimates from different populations and risk factors in these populations. The emphasis will be on adult onset primary open angle and angle closure glaucoma and on studies from the Indian subcontinent.

The prevalence of disease refers to the number of persons with disease in a specified population in a specified time period. It is dependent on the duration of disease and the number of new cases of disease (or incidence). Another factor that influences disease prevalence are the diagnostic criteria.

GLAUCOMA DEFINITIONS

Initial studies on glaucoma used the applicable definitions of glaucoma, namely that of an intraocular pressure greater than 21 mm Hg along with optic disc and/or visual field changes. Since then changes in disease definitions have emphasized optic disc or visual field changes irrespective of intraocular pressure. One of the problems with this approach in population based studies is the definition of abnormal optic discs. There was an element of subjectivity as not all studies used the same optic disc criteria for diagnosis or for the visual field testing. This further biased the selection of those with glaucoma in population based studies. This variability in definitions used in prevalence studies lead to the development of the International Society for Geographic and Epidemiological Ophthalmology (ISGEO) classification system for glaucoma for use in epidemiology studies.[2]

The ISGEO attempt to standardize definitions for glaucoma. Such standardization will greatly help increase comparability between studies in different regions and those performed by different groups. The system bases diagnosis of glaucoma on the presence of structural (optic disc) changes and functional (visual field) damage. The 97.5 percent confidence limits for the cup to disc ratios in a perimetrically normal population are used to generate the expected range of cup to disc ratios in normal persons. All those with vertical cup to disc ratios outside these limits, or specified glaucomatous optic disc changes, with abnormal visual fields are considered to have glaucoma.

Visual field testing for the entire population, in a population based setting is not always conclusive or possible in all persons because of the presence of other visually significant disorders that prevent visual field testing or the learning curve associated with perimetry. The ISGEO definitions state that any eye with a vertical cup to disc ratio larger than that seen in 97.5 percent of a perimetrically normal population which has a visual field defect would be considered to have glaucoma. If visual field testing was not possible or unreliable, stricter optic disc criteria are required to diagnose glaucoma, i.e. a vertical cup to disc ratio seen in less than 0.5 percent of the normal population.

If the optic disc could not be visualized a provisional diagnosis of glaucoma was made only if the IOP was at a level higher than that seen in 99.5 percent of the normal population.

Table 1 summarizes the reported prevalence of POAG (and the diagnostic criteria used) from a selection of population based studies from across the world.

> **Note** It is apparent that there are wide variations in the reported prevalence of POAG. Some of these differences are related to differences in the definitions used.

RISK FACTORS FOR POAG

1. *Race:* Based on a meta-analysis by Rudnicka et al[22] where 46 population based studies were analyzed to assess the effect of race on POAG prevalence, the pooled prevalence estimate for OAG was 1.4 percent (1.0–2.0%) in Asian populations, 4.2% in black populations (95% CI, 3.1–5.8%) and 2.1 percent (95% CI, 1.6–2.7%) in white populations.

2. *Age:* All population based studies show that the risk of disease increases with increasing age. This is expected since POAG is an adult onset disease. The prevalence increases with age as the cumulative number of persons affected increases. This increase appears to be exponential in Western populations. In the Chennai Glaucoma Study (Urban) the risk of disease in those above the age of 70 years was 5 times that of the 40 to 49 age group.

3. *Myopia:* Myopia has been reported to be a risk factor for POAG by only a few studies. Most studies do not report an association.

4. *Central corneal thickness:* POAG patients in the Rotterdam Study were reported to have thinner central corneal thickness (CCT) than normal. The Barbados Eye Studies, participants with POAG had thinner corneas (520.6 ± 37.7 microns) than those classified as nonglaucomatous (530.0 ± 37.7 microns). This association was not reported in all studies. In the Chennai Glaucoma Study, the only study from India that reported CCT data, the mean CCT in POAG subjects was not significantly different from that of the normal study population

5. *Diabetes mellitus:* The Blue Mountains[12] and Beaver Dam[11] studies reported that diabetes mellitus was a risk factor for POAG. However, the Baltimore Eye survey[9] did not find any relationship.

6. *Hypertension:* The relationship between systemic hypertension

Table 1 Prevalence of primary open angle glaucoma in different population based studies

Study	Study period country	Ethnicity	Age group	Number examined	POAG prevalence
Vellore eye survery (VES)[3]	1994 India	Asian	30–60	972	0.41
Andhra Pradesh eye disease survey (APEDS)[4]	1996-2000 India	Asian	40+	934	2.56
Aravind comprehensive eye survery (ACES)[5]	1995-97 India	Asian	40+	5150	1.7
Chennai glaucoma study (rural) CGS[6]	2001-03 India	Asian	40+	3924	1.62
Chennai glaucoma study (urban) CGS[7]	2001-03 India	Asian	40+	3850	3.51
West Bengal glaucoma study (WBGS)[8]	1998-99 India	Asian	50+	1324	2.99
Baltimore eye survey (BES)[9]	1985-88 US	45% Black, 55% White	40+	5308	2.49
Barbados eye study[10]	1988-92 Barbados	Black	40+	4314	7.00
Beaver dam eye study[11] (BDES)	1988-90 US	White	40+	4585	2.07
Blue mountains eye study[12] (BMES)	1992-94 Australia	White	50+	3632	2.97
Proyecto vision and eye research project[13]	1999-2000 US	Hispanic	40+	4773	1.97
Rotterdam study[14]	1990-93 Netherlands	White	55+	6774	0.80
Kongwa[15]	1996 Tanzania	Black	40+	3268	3.1
Melbourne visual impairment project (VIP)[16]	1991-98 Australia	White	40+	4652	1.83
Egna neumarkt[17]	1998 Italy	White	40+	4297	2.0
Liwan eye study[18]	2003-04	Chinese	50+	1504	2.1
Tanjong pagar[19]	1997-98 Singapore	Asian	40+	1232	1.79
Mongolia[20]	1996 Mongolia	Asian	40+	942	0.5
Mektila eye study[21]	2005 Myanmar	Asian		2076	2.0

and POAG has been reported in some studies (Baltimore,[9] Rotterdam[14]) with hypertensives being at greater risk of POAG. However, this is again not consistently seen in all reports.

7. *Family history:* Since only 10 to 60 percent of those with glaucoma have been diagnosed; a family history of no glaucoma may be inaccurate. When all first degree relatives of those diagnosed to have POAG from the Rotterdam study were examined 22.4 percent of them were found to have POAG.[23] This is nearly 10 times greater than the risk in the general population.

Risk Factors for POAG
- Race
- Age
- Myopia
- Central corneal thickness
- Diabetes+/–
- Hypertension+/–
- Family history

One of the reasons for the variations in association reported by different studies is that the number of persons with POAG and the risk factor (e.g. diabetes) is relatively small in each individual study. As a result, the power to detect a difference in the studies is relatively low.

PRIMARY ANGLE-CLOSURE GLAUCOMA

The **ISGEO** divided angle-closure into three groups namely primary angle-closure suspects (PACS), primary angle-closure (PAC) and primary angle—closure glaucoma (PACG).[2]

PACS was defined as those eyes where the pigmented trabecular meshwork was not visible for 270 degree of the circumference of the angle on gonioscopy under standard testing conditions.

Primary angle-closure was defined as PACS with an IOP level less than 97.5 percent of perimetrically normal individuals and/or the presence of peripheral anterior synechiae in such an angle, with a normal optic disc and visual fields.

The definition of **PACG** is similar to that of POAG, in those eyes which meet the gonioscopic criteria for PACS.

The reported prevalence of angle-closure glaucoma is summarized in **Table 2**.

Note Some of these differences are related to differences in the definitions used but the disparity between Asian and White populations is apparent.

RISK FACTORS FOR PACG

1. *Age:* Increasing age is a risk factor for PACG too.
2. *Biometry:* Eyes with angle-closure disease appear to have shorter axial length, a shallower anterior chamber and a thicker lens than the normal population.[24,27,28]
3. *Gender:* Female gender has been reported to be an independent risk factor for angle-closure glaucoma by most studies. This could be related to biometric differences between genders since women appear to have shorter eyes and a shallower anterior chamber depth than men.
4. *Ethnicity:* Widely varying rates of angle-closure glaucoma have

Table 2 Prevalence of angle-closure glaucoma in different population-based studies

Study	Study period	Ethnicity	Age group	Number examined	PACG prevalence
Vellore eye survey (VES)[3]	1994 India	Asian	30-60	972	4.32
Andhra Pradesh eye disease survey (APEDS)[24]	1996-2000 India	Asian	40+	934	1.08
Aravind comprehensive eye survey (ACES)[5]	1995-7 India	Asian	40+	5150	0.5
Chennai glaucoma study (rural) CGS[25]	2001-03 India	Asian	40+	3924	0.87
Chennai glaucoma study (urban) CGS[26]	2001-03 India	Asian	40+	3850	0.88
West Bengal glaucoma study (WBGS)[8]	1998-99 India	Asian	50+	1324	0.24
Baltimore eye surgery (BES)[9]	1985-88 US	45% Black, 55% White	40+	5308	0.4
Beaver dam eye study (BDES)[11]	1988-90 US	White	40+	4585	0.04
Proyecto vision and eye research project[13]	1999-2000 US	Hispanic	40+	4773	0.10
Knogwa[15]	1996 Tanzania	Black	40+	3261	0.49
Melbourne visual impairment project (VIP)[16]	1991-98 Australia	White	40+	4652	0.06
Egna neumark[17]	1998 Italy	White	40+	4297	0.6
Liwan eye study[18]	2003-04 China	Chinese	50+	1504	1.5
Tanjong Pagar[19]	1997-98 Singapore	Asian	40+	1232	1.14
Mongolia[20]	1996 Mongolia	Asian	40+	942	1.4
Mektila eye study[21]	2005 Myanmar	Asian		2076	2.5

been reported from across the world. The highest rates have been reported among Eskimos (Inuits). High prevalence have also been reported from China, Mongolia, Southeast Asia and India.[3,4,18,19,20,21,25,28]

Risk factors for PACG
- Age
- Gender
- Biometry
- Ethnicity

BLINDNESS AND GLAUCOMA

While glaucoma is a slowly progressive disease, untreated glaucoma can lead to blindness. Current estimates of the number of persons who are blind worldwide because of primary glaucoma is 8.4 million (4.5 million due to POAG and 3.9 million because of PACG). Even though the number of persons with PACG are less than the number with POAG (44.7 million POAG and 15.7 million PACG), based on estimates from China[29] the proportion of those blind with PACG (25%) is greater than with POAG (10%).

Glaucoma affects a substantial proportion of the adult population worldwide. PACG is a major cause of glaucoma in some populations. Increasing age is a consistent risk factor for the disease as improvements in socioeconomic and medical care worldwide have seen steady increases in life expectancy over the past few decades. As life expectancy increases we can expect a significant increase in glaucoma prevalence worldwide. As per Broman and Quigleys estimates,[1] by the year 2020 these figures are likely to rise from 60.5 to 79.6 million (58.6 million and 21 million POAG and PACG respectively). This is an almost 30 percent increase over a 10 years period. Approximately 40 to 60 percent of glaucoma in the community has been identified in Western populations. From India less than 10 percent of the population with glaucoma have been identified.

SCREENING FOR GLAUCOMA

There is a lot of interest in screening for glaucoma in the community because of the large number of undiagnosed cases. The rationale is that once diagnosed IOP reduction can be initiated or a YAG PI performed for angle closure disease thereby improving diagnosis rates and preventing or delaying progression.

Candidate Tests for Screening

If we assess the possible candidate tests for screening for POAG: intraocular pressure, perimetry and optic disc evaluation come to mind.

The tests used for POAG will not be able to specifically identify angle closure glaucoma. The gold standard for assessment of the filtering angle is gonioscopy in appropriate testing conditions. Other tests that have been employed for detecting a shallow anterior chamber include the oblique flashlight test, limbal and central anterior chamber depth, scanning peripheral anterior chamber depth analyzer (SPAC) and the anterior segment OCT (AS OCT).

Before population based screening using any test is considered, there are certain criteria that must be fulfilled. The WHO recommendations in order to consider a test suitable for use in a screening programme were published by Wilson and Jungner[30] for the World Health Organization (WHO) are:
1. The test should have acceptable validity (sensitivity and specificity).
2. The distribution of test values in the target population should be known and a suitable cut-off level defined and agreed.

3. The test should be reliable, i.e. variation between instruments and observers should be minimal.
4. The test should be noninvasive, safe and acceptable to the population being screened. This is important for maximum uptake of a screening program by the population. Any risk to which the subject is being put by the test should be outweighed by the benefits.
5. The test should be simple and inexpensive with the capability of being performed by trained non-medical personnel with robust equipment.
6. There must be an agreed policy on the management and further diagnostic investigation of test positive cases.

Criteria for a Screening Test

SENSITIVITY AND SPECIFICITY

1. ***The test should have acceptable validity (Sensitivity and specificity):*** Assessment of the validity of a test is in terms of its sensitivity and specificity. The **sensitivity** is the proportion of people with the disease that the test correctly identifies. The **specificity** is the proportion of normal individuals that the test correctly identifies as normal.

Table 3 is a 2 × 2 table that illustrates how these values are calculated. ***Sensitivity and specificity:*** There is an inverse relationship between the two measures. Increasing the sensitivity of the test by changing the test cut-off value (e.g.

Table 3 2 × 2 table illustrating how sensitivity, specificity, positive and negative predictive values are calculated

	Disease positive	*Disease negative*	*Total*
Test positive	A	B	A+B
Test negative	C	D	C+D
Total	A+C	B+D	A+B+C+D

Sensitivity = A/A+C, Specificity = D/B+D

Positive Predictive Value: A/A+B; *Negative predictive Value:* D/C+D using an IOP> 18 mm Hg to diagnose glaucoma instead of an IOP> 21 mm Hg) we will identify more people with the disease but also falsely identify a larger number of normal persons as having disease, i.e. a decrease in specificity.

> **Sensitivity:** The proportion of people with the disease that the test correctly identifies
> **Specificity** is the proportion of normal individuals that the test correctly identifies as normal
> **Positive predictive values:** The proportion of persons with a positive test who have disease
> **Negative predictive value** proportion of persons with a negative test who are normal

PREDICTIVE VALUE

The other factor to be considered is the predictive value of the test. Once we order a test we only know whether it is beyond our set cut off value for "normal" or not. The **positive predictive values** tell us the proportion of persons with a positive test who have disease, the **negative predictive value** tells us proportion of persons with a negative test who are normal. **The predictive values are influenced by the prevalence of disease** (the number of persons with disease in the population being tested).

Table 4A illustrates an example, where we study 1000 persons assuming the prevalence of POAG in the population is similar to that found in the community, i.e. about 5 percent (50 persons) and that the sensitivity and specificity of an IOP > 21 mm Hg by applanation tonometry is 50 percent and 90 percent respectively. The positive predictive value of an IOP > 21 mm is 21 percent, this means that only 1 in 5 persons (20%) who have an IOP > 21 mm Hg will actually have POAG. On the other hand, if the test is negative only 3 percent of those with a negative test will have glaucoma (negative predictive value of 97%).

If we test using the same criteria in persons visiting an eye hospital the prevalence of POAG is likely to be higher, lets assume 30 percent, the predictive values would change **(Table 4B)**. The positive and negative predictive values become 68 percent and 81 percent respectively. This means that 2 of 3 (68%) people with an IOP > 21 mm Hg will actually have glaucoma and 4 of 5 people with an IOP less than 22 mm Hg will be normal. As is apparent from this example, the positive and negative predictive values also show an inverse relationship.

If we use IOP to screen in the community for every person with glaucoma who we detect, we would have advised four other people to have a detailed eye examination. Not many countries have the infrastructure to deal with the large number of false-positive referrals. Since the majority of those referred will not have the disease the public perception of the screening program would also suffer.

To put these figures in perspective if, hypothetically, we were to do IOP screening in all 300 million adults in India who are over 40 years of age approximately 12 percent or 36 million persons would have elevated IOP, of whom only 7 million would have POAG. To accurately diagnose these 7 million people we would have examined 29 million persons without glaucoma. This is obviously impossible.

Glaucoma prevalence in the community is close to five percent. **Unless the test used has high sensitivity 85 percent and even higher**

Table 4A Illustrative example for calculation of predictive value

	Disease positive	Disease negative	Total
Test positive (IOP > 21 mm Hg)	A = 25	B = 95	A+B = 120
Test negative (IOP ≤ 21 mm Hg)	C = 25	D = 855	C+D = 880
Total	A+C = 50	B+D = 950	A+B+C+D = 1000

Positive Predictive Value: A/A + B = **25/120 or 21%**
Negative Predictive Value: D/C + D = **855/880 or 97%**

Table 4B Illustrative example for calculation of predictive value

	Disease positive	Disease negative	Total
Test positive (IOP > 21 mm Hg)	A = 150	B = 70	A+B = 220
Test negative (IOP ≤ 21 mm Hg)	C = 150	D = 630	C+D = 780
Total	A+C = 300	B+D = 700	A+B+C+D = 1000

Positive Predictive Value: A/A + B = **150/220 or 68%**
Negative Predictive Value: D/C + D = **630/780 or 81%**

specificity (95–98%) the proportion of false positives and negatives would be unacceptably high.

2. *The distribution of test values in the target population should be known and a suitable cut-off level defined and agreed:* Tables **5 and 6** provide the reported sensitivity and specificity of some tests for POAG and PACG.

CONCLUSION

While some of the tests meet Wilson and Junger's criteria 3, 4 and 5 for screening, it is apparent that no single test appears to have adequate diagnostic accuracy in detecting glaucoma.

Table 5 Sensitivity and specificity of diagnostic tests for POAG

Test	Sensitivity	Specificity
Tonometry (At cut off IOP > 21 mm Hg)[31,32]	25.1–47.1%	92.4–95.3%
Optic disc examination (CDR ≥ 0.55)[31]	59%	73%
Automated perimetry[33]	97%	84%
Frequency doubling technology[34,35]	90–94%	91–96%
Stereophotographs[6]	94%	87%
HRT 2[36,37]	73–84%	77–90%
OCT, RNFL[36,37]	86–82%	84–84%
GDx VCC[37]	84%	84%

Table 6 Sensitivity and specificity of diagnostic tests for primary angle closure disease

Test	Sensitivity	Specificity
Oblique flashlight test[38,39]	80–86%	69–70%
VH grade ≤ 2[38-41]	62–80%	89.3–92%
AS-OCT[42]	94.1%	55.3%
SPAC[43]	84.9%[31]	73.1%[31]

REFERENCES

1. Quigley HA, Broman AT. The number of people with glaucoma worldwide in 2010 and 2020. Br J Ophthalmol 2006; 90(3):262-7.

2. Foster PJ, Buhrmann R, Quigley HA, Johnson GJ. The definition and classification of glaucoma in prevalence surveys. Br J Ophthalmol 2002; 86(2):238-42.

3. Jacob A, Thomas R, Koshi SP, et al. Prevalence of primary glaucoma in an urban south Indian population. Indian J Ophthalmol 1998;46:81-6.

4. Dandona L, Dandona R, Srinivas M, et al. Open angle glaucoma in an urban population in southern India. The Andhra Pradesh Eye Disease Study. Ophthalmology 2000;107:1702-9.

5. Ramakrishnan R, Nirmalan PK, Krishnadas R, et al. Glaucoma in a rural population of southern India: the Aravind Comprehensive Eye Survey. Ophthalmology 2003;110:1484-90.

6. Vijaya L, George R, Baskaran M, Arvind H, Raju P, Ramesh SV, Kumaramanickavel G, McCarty C. Prevalence of primary open-angle glaucoma in an urban south Indian population and comparison with a rural population. The Chennai Glaucoma Study. Ophthalmology 2008;115(4):648-54.

7. Vijaya L, George R, Paul PG, Baskaran M, Arvind H, Raju P, Ramesh SV, Kumaramanickavel G, McCarty C. Prevalence of open-angle glaucoma in a rural south Indian population. Invest Ophthalmol Vis Sci 2005;46(12):4461-7.

8. Raychaudhuri A, Lahiri SK, Bandyopadhyay M, Foster PJ, Reeves BC, Johnson GJ. A population based survey of the prevalence and types of glaucoma in rural West Bengal: the West Bengal Glaucoma Study. Br J Ophthalmol 2005;89(12):1559-64.

9. Tielsh JM, Sommer A, Katz J, et al. Racial variations in the prevalence of primary open-angle glaucoma. The Baltimore Eye Survey. JAMA 1991; 266:369-74.

10. Leske MC, Connell AM, Schachat AP, Hyman L. The Barbados Eye Study. Prevalence of open angle glaucoma. Arch Ophthalmol 1994;112:821-9.

11. Klein BE, Klein R, Sponsel WE, et al. Prevalence of glaucoma. The Beaver Dam Eye Study. Ophthalmology 1992; 99:1499-504.

12. Mitchell P, Smith W, Attebo K, Healey RR. Prevalence of open-angle glaucoma in Australia. The Blue Mountains Eye Study. Ophthalmology 1996;103:1661-9.

13. Quigley HA, West SK, Rodriguez J, Munoz B, Klein R, Snyder R. The prevalence of glaucoma in a population-based study of Hispanic subjects: Proyecto VER. Arch Ophthalmol 2001; 119:1819-26.

14. Dielemans I, Vingerling JR, Wolfs RC, et al. The prevalence of primary open-angle glaucoma in a population based study in the Netherlands. The Rotterdam Study. Ophthalmology 1994;101:1851-5.

15. Buhrmann RR, Quigley HA, Barron Y, West SK, Oliva MS, Mmbaga BB. Prevalence of glaucoma in a rural East African population. Invest Ophthalmol Vis Sci 2000;41(1):40-8.

16. Weih LM, Nanjan M, McCarty CA, Taylor HR. Prevalence and predictors of open-angle glaucoma, results from the visual impairment project. Ophthalmology 2001;108:1966-72.

17. Bonomi L, Marchini G, Marraffa M, et al. Prevalence of glaucoma and intraocular pressure distribution in a defined population: the Egna-Neumarkt Study Ophthalmology 1998;105:209-15.

18. He M, Foster PJ, Ge J, Huang W, Zheng Y, Friedman DS, Lee PS, Khaw PT. Prevalence and clinical characteristics of glaucoma in adult Chinese: a population-based study in Liwan District, Guangzhou. Invest Ophthalmol Vis Sci 2006;47(7):2782-8.

19. Foster PJ, Oen FTS, Machin D, et al. The prevalence of glaucoma in Chinese residents of Singapore: a cross-sectional population survey of the Tanjong Pagar district. Arch Ophthalmol 2000; 118:1105-11.

20. Foster PJ, Baasanhu J, Alsbrik PH, et al. Glaucoma in Mongolia. A population based survey in Hovsgol province, Northern Mongolia. Arch Ophthalmol 1996;114:1235-41.

21. Casson RJ, Newland HS, Muecke J, McGovern S, Abraham L, Shein WK, Selva D, Aung T. Prevalence of glaucoma in rural: the Meiktila Eye Study. Br J Ophthalmol 2007;91:710-4.

22. Rudnicka AR, Shahrul Mt-Isa, Owen CG, Cook DG, Ashby D. Variations in Primary Open-Angle Glaucoma Prevalence by Age, Gender and Race: A Bayesian Meta-analysis. Invest Ophthalmol Vis Sci 2006;47:4254-61.

23. Wolfs RCW, Klaver CCW, Ramrattan RS, van Duijn CM, Hofman A, de Jong PTVM. Genetic Risk of Primary Open-angle Glaucoma Population-Based Familial Aggregation Study Arch Ophthalmol 1998;116:1640-5.

24. Dandona L, Dandona R, Mandal P, Srinivas M, John RK, McCarty CA, Rao GN. Angle-closure glaucoma in an urban population in southern India. The Andhra Pradesh eye disease study. Ophthalmology 2000;107(9):1710-6.

25. Vijaya L, George R, Arvind H, Baskaran M, Paul PG, Ramesh SV, Raju P, Kumaramanickavel G, McCarty C. Prevalence of angle-closure disease in a rural southern Indian population. Arch Ophthalmol 2006;124(3):403-9.

26. Vijaya L, George R, Arvind H, Baskaran M, Ve Ramesh S, Raju P, Kumaramanickavel G, McCarty C. Prevalence of primary angle-closure disease in an urban south Indian population and comparison with a rural population. The Chennai Glaucoma Study. Ophthalmology 2008;115(4): 655-60.

27. George R, Paul PG, Baskaran M, Ramesh SV, Raju P, Arvind H, McCarty C, Vijaya L. Ocular biometry in occludable angles and angle closure glaucoma: a population based survey. Br J Ophthalmol 2003;87(4):399-402.

28. Alsbirk PH. Primary angle-closure glaucoma. Oculometry, epidemiology and genetics in a high-risk population. Acta Ophthalmol Suppl 1976;127: 5-31.

29. Foster PJ, Johnson GJ. Glaucoma in China: How big is the problem? Br J Ophthalmol 2001;85:1277-82.

30. Wilson JMG, Jungner G. Principles and Practice of screening for disease. WHO: Geneva, (Public Health Papers No 34) 1968.

31. Teilsch JM, Katz J, Singh K, et al. A population based evaluation of glaucoma screening: the Baltimore Eye Survey. Am J Epidemiol 1991;134:1102-10.

32. Vijaya L, George R. Chennai Glaucoma Study data, Personal communication.

33. Katz J, Sommer A, Gaasterland DE, Anderson DR. Comparison of analytic algorithms for detecting glaucomatous visual field loss. Arch Ophthalmol 1991;109(12):1684-9.

34. Quigley HA. Identification of Glaucoma-related Visual Field Abnormality with the Screening Protocol of Frequency Doubling Technology. Am J Ophthalmology 1998;125:819-29.

35. Robin AL, Patel S, Friedman DS, et al. Algorithm for interpreting the results of the frequency doubling perimeter; Am J Ophthalmol 2000;129:323-7.

36. Greaney MJ, Hoffman DC, Garway-Heath DF, Nakla M, Coleman AL, Caprioli J. Comparison of optic nerve imaging methods to distinguish normal eyes from those with glaucoma. Invest Ophthalmol Vis Sci 2002; 43(1):140-5.

37. Medeiros FA, Zangwill LM, Bowd C, Weinreb RN. Comparison of the GDx VCC scanning laser polarimeter, HRT II confocal scanning laser ophthalmoscope and stratus OCT optical coherence tomograph for the detection of glaucoma. Arch Ophthalmol 2004; 122(6):827-37.

38. Congdon N, Quigley HA, Hung PT, et al. Screening techniques for angle-closure glaucoma in rural Taiwan. Acta Ophthalmol Scand 1996;74:113.

39. Thomas R, George T, Braganza A, et al. The flashlight test and van Herick's test are poor predictors for occludable angles. Aust NZ J Ophthalmol 1996;24(3):251-6.

40. Devereux JG, Foster PJ, Baasanhu J, Uranchimeg D, Lee PS, Erdenbeleig T, Machin D, Johnson GJ, Alsbirk PH. Anterior chamber depth measurement as a screening tool for primary angle-closure glaucoma in an East Asian population. Arch Ophthalmol 2000;118(2):257-63.

41. Foster PJ, Devereux JG, Alsbirk PH, Lee PS, Uranchimeg D, Machin D, Johnson GJ, Baasanhu J. Detection of gonioscopically occludable angles and primary angle-closure glaucoma by estimation of limbal chamber depth in Asians: modified grading scheme. Br J Ophthalmol 2000;84(2):186-92.

42. Nolan WP, See JL, Chew PT, Friedman DS, Smith SD, Radhakrishnan S, Zheng C, Foster PJ, Aung T. Detection of primary angle closure using anterior segment optical coherence tomography in Asian eyes. Ophthalmology 2007;114(14):33-9.

43. Baskaran M, Oen FT, Chan YH, Hoh ST, et al. Comparison of the scanning peripheral anterior chamber depth analyzer and the modified van Herick grading system in the assessment of angle closure. Ophthalmology 2007;114;501-6.

3

Natural History of Glaucoma

Ronnie George

INTRODUCTION

While it is known that primary open angle glaucoma is a slowly progressive disease, there is little data available on the rates of disease progression in a population. There are multiple reasons for this. Since the disease is slowly progressive, even long (5–7 years) clinical trials do not actually follow-up a patient from disease onset to blindness, the study duration comprises a small portion of the course of the disease. Another problem with assessing progression is the change in technology every decade or so. Elderly glaucoma patients who have had the disease for a few decades would have undergone visual field testing on the Goldmann perimeter, early versions of automated parameter such as HFA 1, full threshold testing and SITA. These methods are not directly comparable and difficulties exist in estimating progression since all of them measure disease severity differently.

However, even with these limitations we do have some published evidence on how primary open angle glaucoma progresses. From the untreated arms of the Ocular Hypertension Treatment Study (OHTS)[1] and the Early Manifest Glaucoma Trial (EMGT)[2] we have progression rates for untreated ocular hypertension and early glaucoma. We have progression data on a cohort of untreated glaucoma patients from the St Lucia Study[3] and from a cohort of untreated ocular hypertensives from the Vellore Eye Survey.[4] The St Lucia Study was a population-based study carried out on an island population, for various reasons glaucoma treatment was not available for almost a decade to those diagnosed to have POAG in the study. Data from these patients provide valuable information on the natural history of untreated POAG.

OCULAR HYPERTENSION TREATMENT STUDY (OHTS)

In the OHTS study, persons with ocular hypertension were randomized to receive either treatment to reduce IOP or were followed up without treatment.

Both groups underwent serial optic disc photography and visual fields. In the untreated group 9.5 percent of persons progressed to develop POAG over a 5 years period compared to 4.4 percent for the treated group.[1]

EARLY MANIFEST GLAUCOMA TRIAL (EMGT)

In the EMGT those with newly diagnosed early glaucoma were randomized to IOP reduction using a combination of trabeculoplasty and topical medication. The control group was followed up without treatment. At 5 years, 62 percent of those followed up without treatment progressed compared to 45 percent of those who received treatment.[2]

ST LUCIA STUDY

The St Lucia study examined a cohort of glaucoma patients and glaucoma suspects re-examined 10 years after the baseline visit. These subjects had all stopped medication if it had been started at the baseline examination. Between 52 and 55 percent of these eyes progressed over the 10 years untreated period.[3] Sixteen percent of eyes progressed to end stage glaucoma as defined by their visual field criteria.

THE VELLORE EYE SURVEY

The Vellore Eye Survey was the first population based glaucoma prevalence study carried out in India. Twenty-five of the twenty-nine ocular hypertensives diagnosed at baseline were re-examined. After correction for CCT they were reclassified as ocular hypertensive if the corrected IOP was above 21 mm Hg. Among untreated ocular hypertensives 17.4 percent (95% CI: 1.95 to 32.75%) progressed to develop POAG (optic disc and visual field changes) over a 5 years period. One of the normals controls had progressed to develop POAG.[4]

METHODS OF ASSESSMENT OF PROGRESSION IN A POPULATION AND PROBLEMS ENCOUNTERED

All these studies illustrate that glaucoma is a slowly progressive disease. However, even the 5 years follow-up is inadequate to assess lifetime risk.

The other problems with assessing progression are the loss to follow-up during the long study period. Mortality is also a factor since glaucoma affects an elderly patient cohort.

These are also ethnic differences in disease severity that require different estimates for different population subgroups.

Problems in assessing rate of progression in the population
• Slowly progressive disease
• Smaller study duration
• Change in technology
• Ethnic differences in disease severity
• Mortality
• Drop out

The other method of assessing progression, from a recent report by Broman, Quigley and co-authors, employs an elegant technique of gathering this information from existing population based studies. Data from multiple population based studies from across the world were used to derive these estimates.[5] This approach uses two sets of information, one that once POAG is established it does not reverse and second that mortality rates among those with POAG do not differ significantly from the general population. If these two are true, and the prevalence of disease in different age groups of a population is known, one can assume that the increase in prevalence of glaucoma with increasing age is attributable to the new cases developing glaucoma with time or the incidence of disease after making corrections for the expected mortality rates for the population. This method of assessing incidence was described by Leske et al[6] and has been confirmed by incidence studies.

From population-based studies we know the baseline mean deviation (MD) values at the time of diagnosis for different ages. It is also possible to assess the incidence of disease at each age as described earlier. From these two parameters it is possible to estimate the estimated duration of disease. Once the duration of disease has been calculated for individuals, the rate of progress in mean duration change/year can be calculated. Since a MD of less than approximately – 30 dB corresponds to blindness it is possible to then estimate the duration of untreated POAG from onset to blindness. Based on these estimates, the mean rate of progression for POAG is 1.12 dB/year for Caucasians. The rates are somewhat higher for the Chinese (–1.56 dB/yr) and African Americans (–1.33 dB/yr). From these data, it is possible to extrapolate that POAG takes 25 to 27 years to progress to blindness on an average. There are, of course, those in whom the disease progresses more rapidly and others where it is slower. Based on these estimates, the average duration of disease in the population at the time of diagnosis was 14 years. This is similar to data reported from other sources. These estimates are for the worse eye of a glaucoma patient. Since most patients with POAG have somewhat asymmetric disease the estimated duration of disease at the time of diagnosis in the better eye is less. As a result the risk of bilateral blindness is lower and hence relatively few persons have bilateral blindness as compared to unilateral blindness.

PRIMARY ANGLE CLOSURE DISEASE

Even less is known about the natural history of primary angle closure disease partly because it more prevalent in only a few populations. These populations generally reside in less developed areas of the globe from where less population based data is available.

Clinic-based studies from a white Caucasian population reported that 19% of those with untreated PACS or PAC progressed to PACG over a mean follow-up period of 2.5 years. Most (68%) presented with nonacute angle closure.[7]

There is very little population based data available on the natural history of primary angle closure disease, mostly from India. Those diagnosed to have PACS and PAC in the Vellore Eye Survey were followed up untreated over a 5 years period.[8]

Eleven 22 percent (95% CI: 9.8 to 34.2) of 50 persons with PACS progressed to develop PAC over a 5 years period, none progressed to PACG. All those who progressed had bilateral PACS at baseline. One previously normal person progressed to PAC with time, the relative risk for progression among those with PACS to PAC was 24.2 (95%CI: 3.2 to 182.4). Eight (28.5%, 95% CI: 12-45%) of 28 persons diagnosed to have PAC at baseline progressed to PACG over similar time frame. Of these, 9 had undergone

YAG PI, of whom one (11.1%) progressed. Seven (36.8%) of the 19 who refused YAG PI at the baseline progressed. None became blind because of glaucoma.

In both groups no patients suffered from an acute angle closure attack during the 5 years period. In the same study cohort those with primary angle closure were also re-examined without treatment. 27.8 percent progressed to primary angle closure glaucoma with optic disc and visual field changes.[9] The progression rate among those who had undergone a YAG iridotomy at the baseline visit was 11 percent. None of the cases in this study presented with an acute angle closure attack during the study period.

CONCLUSION

The mean rate of progression of POAG is little over 1dB loss per year. However, it is important to remember that this is the mean rate of progression and there are eyes that progress at much faster rates, one in six untreated cases from the St Lucia study progressed to end stage glaucoma over a 10 years period.

REFERENCES

1. Kass MA, Heuer DK, Higginbotham EJ, Johnson CA, Keltner JL, Miller JP, Parrish RK 2nd, Wilson MR, Gordon MO. The Ocular Hypertension Treatment Study: a randomized trial determines that topical ocular hypotensive medication delays or prevents the onset of primary open-angle glaucoma. Arch Ophthalmol 2002; 12:701-13.

2. Leske MC, Heijl A, Hussein M, Bengtsson B, Hyman L, Komaroff E. Early Manifest Glaucoma Trial Group. Factors for glaucoma progression and the effect of treatment: the early manifest glaucoma trial. Arch Ophthalmol 2003;121:48-56.

3. Mason RP, Kosoko O, Wilson MR, et al. National survey of the prevalence and risk factors of glaucoma in St. Lucia, West Indies, I: prevalence findings Ophthalmol 1989;96:1363-8.

4. Thomas R, Parikh R, George R, Kumar RS, Muliyil J. Five-year risk of progression of ocular hypertension to primary open angle glaucoma. A population-based study. Indian J Ophthalmol 2003;51:329-33.

5. Broman AT, Quigley HA, West SK, Katz J, Munoz B, Bandeen-Roche K, Tielsch JM, Friedman DS, Crowston J, Taylor HR, Varma R, Leske MC, Bengtsson B, Heijl A, He M, Foster PJ. Estimating the rate of progressive visual field damage in those with open-angle glaucoma, from cross-sectional data. Invest Ophthalmol Vis Sci 2008;49:66-76.

6. Leske MC, Ederer F, Podgor M. Estimating incidence from age-specific prevalence in glaucoma. Am J Epidemiol 1981;113:606-13.

7. Wilensky JT, Kaufman PL, Frolichstein D, et al. Follow-up of angle-closure glaucoma suspects. Am J Ophthalmol 1993;115:338-46.

8. Thomas R, Parikh R, Muliyil J, Kumar RS. Five-year risk of progression of primary angle closure to primary angle closure glaucoma: a population-based study. Acta Ophthalmol Scand 2003;81:480-5.

9. Thomas R, George R, Parikh R, Muliyil J, Jacob A. Five-year risk of progression of primary angle closure suspects to primary angle closure: a population based study. Br J Ophthalmol 2003;87:450-4.

4 | Genetics of Glaucoma and Its Future

N Prasanthi, K Rangachari, SR Krishnadas, P Sundaresan

CHAPTER OUTLINE

- ❖ Overview
- ❖ Primary Open Angle Glaucoma (POAG)
- ❖ Basic Genetics
- ❖ Research Methods to Identify the Candidate Gene
- ❖ Methodology to Identify Nucleotide Variations in the Candidate Genes
- ❖ Genetic Loci Linked to Primary Open Angle Glaucoma and Congenital Glaucoma
- ❖ Genetic Loci Associated with Primary Angle-Closure Glaucoma
- ❖ Genetic Loci Associated with Exfoliation Glaucoma
- ❖ Genetic Loci Associated with Anterior Segment Dysgenesis Syndromes
- ❖ Role of Mitochondrial DNA in Pathogenesis of Glaucoma

OVERVIEW

Glaucoma is the second leading cause of blindness worldwide after cataract. As the world's population continues to age, the number of persons with glaucoma will continue to rise. Due to the late onset of the disease, asymptomatic nature and poor sensitivity and specificity of many screening tools available to diagnose glaucoma, it is very difficult to diagnose the disease in early stage. With the help of recent genetic and molecular biology techniques, we can prediagnose the risk for glaucoma to some extent. Screening for mutations in the candidate genes of the patients and the family members will helps to predict and diagnose the disease in their offsprings (by routine clinical check-up) followed by genetic counseling. Though there are reports suggesting the role of environmental factors in causing the disease, genetic predisposition due to the presence of nucleotide variations have been reported extensively. A brief description of genes associated with different forms of glaucoma follows.

INTRODUCTION

Glaucoma is a complex and genetically heterogeneous disease characterized by the progressive apoptotic death of retinal ganglion cells that leads to excavation of the optic nerve head and to visual field loss, eventually producing blindness. It is estimated that 70 to 80 million people will have glaucoma by the year 2020 worldwide.[1] Increasing age, African ancestry, family history and elevated intraocular pressure (IOP) are leading risk factors for the disease. High IOP is the only proven treatable factor known to date. Glaucoma is usually associated with elevated IOP but nevertheless, a variant of primary open angle glaucoma has been reported wherein the intraocular pressure is always reported to be within normal range (Normal Pressure Glaucoma). The exact cause of elevation in IOP is unknown. However, increase in resistance to aqueous outflow by obstruction of the trabecular meshwork (TM)—the aqueous humor outflow pathway is thought to be the major cause of increase in IOP in open angle glaucoma. Most individuals with glaucomas are asymptomatic in its initial phase but patients experience visual field loss progressively at later stages associated with elevations in IOP. Continued research efforts are attempting to identify the site of resistance within the trabecular meshwork and the mechanism that changes the overall resistance resulting in elevated IOP.

PRIMARY OPEN ANGLE GLAUCOMA (POAG)

Among the various subtypes of glaucoma, POAG is the most common form of the glaucoma.[2] It affects one to two percent of all individuals over the age of 40 years and eight to ten percent in the above 65 age group.[3] POAG is frequently associated with elevated

IOP, although a proportion of individuals do not demonstrate increased intraocular pressures on tonometry in the course of their disease. POAG tends to occur in families and the pattern of inheritance is very difficult to identify due to relatively late onset of the disease. First degree relatives of affected individuals have three to nine fold higher risk than control family members.[4] This strongly indicates that specific genetic defects contribute to the pathogenesis of the disease. Juvenile onset open angle glaucoma (JOAG) is a form of POAG that manifests clinically between the age of 3 and 30.[5,6] The late onset form of this condition is POAG which usually manifests clinically in adults over the age of forty is the most prevalent type.[7,8]

Most of the studies propose that the mode of disease inheritance is autosomal dominant with incomplete penetrance. Interaction of multiple genes and effects of environmental stimuli seems to play a significant role in causing the disease.[9]

BASIC GENETICS

The human traits and characteristics are determined by 23 pairs of chromosomes. Each individual cell (except the gametes-ovum and the sperm cell) has 22 autosomal pairs and one sex pair which contains either two X type chromosomes in a female or an X and Y type chromosomes in males. Each pair of chromosome contains a DNA molecule from each parent. The DNA is made of nucleotides and each nucleotide is formed by a varying sequence of one of the four nucleic acids; cytosine, thymine, adenine and guanine. A codon is a series of three nucleic acid base pairs. The sequence of the base pairs and codons determine the nature of amino acids and ultimately the protein synthesis directed by the DNA nucleotide sequence. The DNA is the template from which a

complementary RNA is made and the latter molecule governs the synthesis of proteins within a cell. Groups of DNA bases that are ultimately transcribed into messenger (m)RNA that translates into a protein are referred to as exons. The DNA strands that result in inactive mRNA in between strands of exons are called introns. During the process of protein synthesis within a cell, introns are stripped away and only the active mRNA composed of exons drive protein synthesis. The RNA bases dictates sequence of amino acids that make a protein. Even if the amino acid sequence is altered by a single amino acid, it could result in a lethal effect to the organism or its functioning (these changes are usually at a molecular level and are referred to as mutations).

RESEARCH METHODS TO IDENTIFY THE CANDIDATE GENE

Several methods have been used to identify the disease-causing genes. Candidate gene approach, positional cloning and linkage analysis are important amongst them.

- Candidate gene approach can be used when the function of a known gene could be suspected in causing the disease.
- Potential disease-causing genes can be identified and evaluated using positional cloning based on chromosomal location, deletions and translocations in the patients.
- Using linkage analysis one can study the disorders like glaucoma with poorly understood disease pathways. Linkage analysis can be used when there are no clues to identify the location of disease-causing genes. This can be done based on the availability of large families in which the disease is transmitted in a Mendelian fashion. All the family members are typed with large number of genetic markers

with known chromosomal locations to identify markers closely linked to the disease-causing gene. Because the likelihood of a recombination event between a gene and a genetic marker is proportional to the intervening distance, a disease gene and markers that are close to it are almost always inherited together. Such linked markers are easily identified as they are inherited with the disease phenotype more often than can be explained by chance. The known position of a linked marker indicates the approximate chromosomal location of the disease-causing gene.[8]

METHODOLOGY TO IDENTIFY NUCLEOTIDE VARIATIONS IN THE CANDIDATE GENES

Many techniques have been followed by different research groups but the most commonly used techniques are as follows (**Figure 1**):

- Genomic DNA is isolated from the patients whole blood.
- Polymerase chain reaction (PCR) is performed using a set of primers that covers the target region.
- Nucleotide changes are observed based on the band shift in single strand confirmation polymorphism (SSCP) analysis.
- Confirmation of nucleotide changes is done by performing Bidirectional sequencing using dye termination chemistry.

GENETIC LOCI LINKED TO GLAUCOMA

Using linkage analysis of a single large family, Sheffield et al mapped the location of a gene which causes JOAG to a region on chromosome one. This linkage site was designated as GLC1A.[10] The term GLC1A comes from "GLC" stands for glaucoma, "1" stands for primary open-angle and "A"

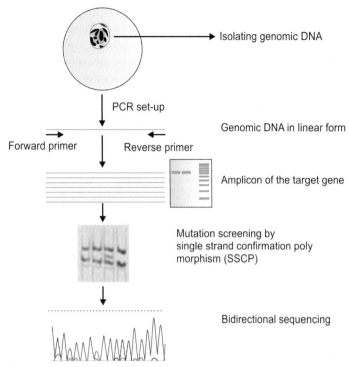

Isolating genomic DNA

PCR set-up

Genomic DNA in linear form

Forward primer   Reverse primer

Amplicon of the target gene

Mutation screening by
single strand confirmation poly
morphism (SSCP)

Bidirectional sequencing

Fig. 1 Methodology to identify nucleotide variations in candidate genes

stands for first linkage for this disease. The inheritance of several markers in the chromosomal region 1q21-31 was found nearly identical to the pattern of transmission of JOAG through the family. Subsequent linkage studies of additional JOAG families confirmed that a *JOAG* gene was located on chromosome one .[11-13] Following this discovery, the *GLC1A* locus was intensively studied as the gene responsible for *JOAG* and POAG.

Till date, 25 loci have been found to be linked with POAG **(Table 1)**[14] but only three genes viz Myocilin,[15] Optineurin[16] and WDR36[17] have been identified to be associated with POAG so far.

MYOCILIN GENE (MYOC/TIGR)
Identification of Myocilin as a Candidate Gene

Through recruitment of more families and study of additional genetic markers, the region of interest was narrowed to an area small enough to consider individual genes.[34] By yeast artificial chromosome (YAC) sequenced tagged site (STS) content and radiation hybrid mapping, three genes namely *APT1LG1, TXGP1* and *TIGR* were found to map within the GLC1A region.[35]

Polansky et al hypothesized that steroid-induced ocular hypertension (OHT) and possibly POAG might be mediated through glucocorticoid induction of specific genes in the trabecular meshwork.[36] Changes in the gene expression of trabecular meshwork cells were determined by comparing corticosteroid treated cells with control cells and a protein was discovered which markedly increased when the trabecular meshwork cells were exposed to corticosteroids. The protein was named as trabecular meshwork-inducible glucocorticoid response protein (*TIGR*). The cDNA encoding the TIGR protein was independently cloned from several human tissues (TM cells,[36-38] ciliary body,[39] retina[40]) and was subsequently mapped within

the chromosome 1q GLC1A locus.[15] Many names for this gene have been coined as a consequence of its independent discovery by several laboratories. These include *TIGR, GLC1A,* myocilin, and TIGR/myocilin. In 1998, HUGO assigned the gene name myocilin and it is now referred to as *MYOC.*[41]

Myocilin was evaluated by screening for disease-causing mutations in JOAG and POAG pedigrees.[15]

Myocilin Structure

The Myocilin gene spans about 17kb genomic region containing 3 exons which encodes for 55 to 57KDa protein (504 amino acids) and maps to chromosome 1q24.3–1q25.2.[37,40] The aminoterminal region of myocilin, encoded by exon 1, contains a peptide signal sequence (amino acids 1–32) and a leucine zipper-like motif composed of about 50 amino acid residues with periodic arginine and leucine repeats arranged along an α-helix. The central region of the protein (amino acids 203–245) is encoded by exon 2 and neither structural nor functional domains have been described in this location so far. The carboxyl-terminal half of myocilin, encoded by exon 3, is homologous to olfactomedin, an extracellular matrix protein of unknown role which is abundant in the olfactory neuroepithelium. This domain contains a single disulfide bond connecting cysteine residues 245 and 433. Interestingly enough, most mutations (missense) reported so far in the *MYOC* gene in glaucoma patients are heterozygous and are confined to exon 3.[42]

Upstream of the coding sequence (exon) is the promoter region, which contains DNA sequences that regulate myocilin expression at the level of transcription. These regions include the following promoter elements: TATA box, Sac box, AP-1 like sequence, AP-2 site, NF-κB-related site and E-box.

Table 1 Genetic loci linked to glaucoma

Locus	Chromosomal location	Gene	Phenotype	Reference
GLC1A(JOAG1)	1q21-31	Myocilin	JOAG, POAG	(Sheffield et al. 1993)[10]
GLC1B	2cen-q31	–	POAG	(Stoilova et al. 1996)[18]
GLC1C	3q21-24	–	POAG	(Wirtz et al. 1997)[19]
GLC1D	8p23	–	POAG	(Trifan et al. 1998)[20]
GLC1E	10p14-15	Optineurin	NTG, POAG	(Sarfarazi et al. 1998)[21]
GLC1F	7q 35-36	–	POAG	(Wirtz et al. 1999)[22]
GLC1G	5q 22.1	WDR36	POAG	(Monemi et al. 2005)[23]
GLC1H	14q 11-q13	–	–	(Suriyapperuma et al. 2007)[24]
GLC1I	15q 11-13	–	POAG	(Allingham et al. 2005)[25]
GLC1J (JOAG2)	9q 22	–	JOAG	(Wiggs et al. 2004)[26]
GLC1K (JOAG3)	20p 12	–	JOAG	(Wiggs et al. 2004)[26]
GLC1L (JOAG4)	3p 21-22	–	–	(Baird et al. 2005)[27]
GLC1M (JOAG5)	5q 22.1-q32	–	–	(Pang et al. 2006)[28]
GLC1N (JOAG6)	15q 22-q24	–	–	(Wang et al. 2006)[29]
–	19q 12	–	–	(Wiggs et al. 2000)[30]
–	17q 25.1-17q25.3-	–	–	(Wiggs et al. 2000)[30]
–	14q 11.1-14q11.2-	–	–	(Wiggs et al. 2000)[30]
–	14q 21.1-q21.3	–	–	(Wiggs et al. 2000)[30]
–	17p 13	–	–	(Wiggs et al. 2000)[30]
–	10p12.33-p12.1	–	–	(Nemesure et al. 2003)[31]
–	2q 33.1-q33.3	–	–	(Nemesure et al. 2003)[31]
–	2p14	–	–	(Wiggs et al. 2000)[30]
–	2p15-16-	–	–	(Lin et al. 2008)[32]
–	1p32	–	–	(Charlesworth et al. 2005)[33]

The structure of Myocilin is conserved through evolution and is 80 percent homologous with mouse Myocilin.[43,44]

Myocilin is a glycoprotein abundantly expressed in many ocular tissues such as the iris, ciliary body and TM.[45] It is also expressed in many non-ocular tissues, including the heart and skeletal muscles.[46] Report says that the increase in IOP is due to the blockage of TM which takes place by the increase in the production of myocilin protein.[37] Studies on recombinant myocilin in the anterior segments of cadaveric human eyes demonstrated the decrease in outflow facility.[47] On the other hand, the adenoviral overexpression of myocilin by transfecting the TM of perfused anterior segments demonstrated an increase in outflow facility.[48] One of the study carried out on null mice (that lack myocilin protein) showed, overexpression of mutant myocilin protein failed to induce glaucoma.[49,50] Whereas another study reported increase in IOP and retinal ganglion cell death after overexpression of same point mutation on transgenic mice.[51] More studies are required to understand the relation between myocilin and the outflow facility.

Myocilin has been found in many of the organelles (including endoplasmic reticulum and golgi apparatus) which are involved in secretary pathway. It is also associated with mitochondria. Investigators observed that the mutant myocilin causes depolarization of mitochondrial membrane, decreased generation of ATP and reactive oxygen species. As a result, both mitochondria-independent apoptosis and mitochondria-mediated apoptosis cannot be ruled out.[52,53] Mitochondrial abnormalities in patients with POAG suggested mitochondria dysfunction could be a risk factor for POAG.[54] Pro370Leu mutant myocilin causes mitochondrial defects, which may lead to TM cell dysfunction and even cell death.[55]

Over180 variants have been identified within the exons and surrounding noncoding regions of the MYOC gene. Approximately 40 percent of the identified variants have been characterized as disease causing, of which the majority (~85%) being missense mutations.[56] Myocilin mutations have been found in two to four percent of POAG cases.[57] Most of the diseases causing mutations were found in exon-3 of MYOC gene, few in exon-1 but none in the exon-2. As most of the mutations were identified in the olfactomedin domain which is mostly encoded by exon-3, it becomes important to study this region.

The mutations in the transcription regulatory region (promoter and enhancer region) can change the expression level of myocilin mRNA transcript. The altered protein coding sequence has the ability to alter the three dimensional structure, effectively burying important charges that regulate cleavage sites and presumably normal function.[58] One of the hypothesis says that the pathogenic mutations of myocilin has the ability to misfold the protein and forms aggregates (called Russell bodies). The misfolded or unfolded protein can activate mitochondria-independent apoptosis pathway via unfolded protein response which leads to cell death and breakdown of TM cell structure. This leads to the obstruction of aqueous humor out flow which results in elevation of IOP.[59-63]

Myocilin—Clinical Significance

Mutations in the *MYOC* gene account for three to five percent of adult onset primary open angle glaucoma and a significant proportion of juvenile open angle glaucoma. Variations in the mutations in the gene may result in variations in the course and progression of the disease. It is likely that mutant myocilin or myocilin overexpression affects outflow facility and function of the trabecular meshwork. Trabecular meshwork cells lose adhesiveness and contractility when myocilin protein is overexpressed. It has been hypothesized that mutations in myocilin causes accumulation of deleterious products in the endoplasmic reticulum of trabecular cells which predisposes to apoptosis. Mutated myocilin may also assume abnormal shape and may accumulate in cells causing premature cell death or may directly cause obstruction of aqueous outflow facility. Several mutations in the exon–3 region and polymorphisms in the promoter region of the myocilin gene have been reported and in spite of different loci, the phenotypic characteristics are mostly similar: early onset and generally progressive open angle glaucoma. In a family study from Tasmania, a specific type of Thr 377 Met mutation was associated with a younger age of onset, higher IOPs and higher likelihood of progressing to glaucoma filtering surgery. The summary of findings from several investigators on myocilin is that the presence of mutations in this gene somehow deleteriously affect the function of the trabecular meshwork and causes glaucoma in a significant number of persons with juvenile open angle glaucoma and a minority of those with adult onset open angle glaucoma. Mutations in the gene encoding myocilin have a significant role in pathogenesis of glaucoma in a minority of patients, although it requires some aggravating factors, probably environmental, to cause glaucoma. Since mutations have been reported in only a fraction of patients with clinically evident glaucoma, routine screening of the populations for mutations in myocilin has not become routine clinical practice.

OPTINEURIN GENE (OPTN)

The optineurin or the *OPTN* gene was observed as the second gene implicated in the pathogenesis of glaucoma.[16] The locus was identified by linkage analysis in a large British family with adult onset normal tension glaucoma (NTG) phenotype on chromosome 10p14 (GLC1E).[21] *OPTN* spans ~37 kb genomic region containing 16 exons (13-coding exons, 3-noncoding exons at 5^1 region) and encodes a 577-amino acid secretary protein.[16] Alternative splicing yields at least three different isoforms.

Optineurin was previously known as *FIP-2* and its expression has been localized to several ocular (TM, retina and nonpigmented ciliary epithelium)[16] and nonocular tissues.[64] Optineurin was found to be localized in the golgi apparatus and upon apoptotic stimuli it translocates to the nucleus, mediated via a GTPase rab8, an interactor of optineurin.[65] Optineurin expression protects cells from oxidative stress, where as the optineurin mutation, E50K, can cause oxidative stress to the cells which can lead to cell death.[65]

In a Caucasian population, it has been reported that sequence variations in *OPTN* gene are responsible for 16.7 percent of normal tension glaucoma cases.[16] The missense mutation Glu50Lys was identified as a most common *OPTN* mutation in families (13.5%), mostly with normal tension glaucoma. Furthermore, the Met98Lys variation was identified as a risk associated variation in 13.6 percent of familial and sporadic cases and 2.1 percent of controls. Though few mutations have been reported, recent genetic studies suggest that the *OPTN* gene may not have any major role towards POAG causation.

Clinical significance: *OPTN* mutations are important in a small subset of patients with normal pressure and primary open angle glaucoma, but the prevalence of mutations in these glaucoma populations are rather small that screening the general populations for these mutations is not a useful exercise.

WD REPEAT DOMAIN 36 GENE (WDR36)

WDR36 is another gene associated with *POAG*, linked to the *GLC1G* locus in chromosome 5q22.1.[17] The WDR36 gene spans about 34.7 kb genomic region containing 23 exons which encodes a 105KDa protein (950 amino acids). It has four conserved domains: (i) nine WD40 repeat domain; (ii) Utp21 domain; (iii) AMP-dependent synthetase and ligase domain and (iv) cytochrome cd1-nitrite reductase-like domain. Expression of *WDR36* has been identified in human ocular and nonocular tissues. Reports suggest that the protein encoded by *WDR36* gene might be involved in T-cell activation and proliferation.[66] Recently, it has been shown that this gene is required for ribosomal RNA processing and maintaining the proper nuclear morphology. The loss of function of this gene activates the p53 stress-response pathway.[67] It has been observed that the mutations in this gene can alter the cellular phenotype, when present in a permissible genetic background and support the role of WDR36 as a modifier locus in polygenic POAG.[68]

Four sequence variations in WDR36 gene were identified as disease associated variations in a total of 5 percent POAG families.[17] Few reports state that WDR36 gene has low[69,70] or no association with open angle glaucoma (OAG).[71,72] Though the probable disease causing variants were reported in 17 percent of the patients, the distribution of variants did not show consistent segregation in the pedigrees of the glaucoma patients. As the sequence variants seem to be associated with increased severity of the POAG, they concluded that WDR36 may be a modifier gene for POAG.[73] Further studies have to be carried out to understand the exact role of WDR36 gene in the pathogenesis of POAG and NTG.

CYTOCHROME P450 FAMILY 1 SUBFAMILY B POLYPEPTIDE 1 (CYP1B1)

The CYP1B1 gene was identified to cause primary congenital glaucoma (PCG) in an autosomal recessive mode of inheritance.[74,75] Later, it was observed that the mutations in this gene also causes early onset POAG in an autosomal recessive mode of inheritance,[76,77] when present in heterozygous state. Mutations in this gene have also been found in Peters anomaly[78] and Axenfield Reiger syndrome.[79] The CYP1B1 gene spans about >12 kb genomic region containing 3 exons. Exon 1 represents untranslated regions and the exon 2; exon 3 encodes a 543 amino acid protein.[80]

The protein encoded by this gene was expressed in all studied tissues including the fetal retina[81] and TM.[75]

Reports suggests the involvement of cytochrome P450 enzymes in regulating oxygenated molecules that can act on signal transduction pathway receptors. These receptors regulate the differentiation and growth of tissues and hence, CYP1B1 may be involved in early ocular differentiation.[75] Therefore, mutations of CYP1B1 gene may interfere with the normal physiology of CYP1B1 and disturb normal anterior chamber growth and development. But the exact role of this gene in ocular development is still lacking.

CYP1B1 mutations have been observed more frequently in the cases which have positive family history, or parental consanguinity. More than 65 mutations and few polymorphisms were reported to be associated with 80 percent of the PCG cases in different ethnic groups. It has been reported that Gln48His (MYOC) mutation in combination with Pro437Leu (CYP1B1) and Arg368His (CYP1B1) mutation results in POAG and PCG phenotypes.[82] Mutations in CYP1B1 gene have been described in childhood glaucomas and in adult onset glaucoma as well. The role of genetic mutations in pathophysiology of glaucoma have been better understood of late by study of mouse models. In a mouse model with CYP1B1 mutation, anterior chamber angle development defects including trabecular meshwork abnormalities and an absence or small Schlemm's canal have been described. Study of mutations in albino mice have revealed that tyrosinase (present in pigmented and not albino mice) appears to have a protective effect, preventing severe anterior chamber anomalies otherwise seen in albinotic mice. In humans, congenital glaucoma has been reported in albinism.

FOXC1 (FKHL7) is another gene whose mutations have been reported to be associated with PCG–like features.

Most commonly the mutations in this gene are associated with anterior segment dysgenesis conditions.[83]

ADDITIONAL GENES ASSOCIATED WITH POAG

Along with the candidate genes, there are many other genes (Table 2)[14] that have been reported to be associated with POAG in various single population groups by different investigators. As there are some contradictory reports, further screening of these genes has to be carried with large sample size from different cohorts.

GENETIC LOCI ASSOCIATED WITH PRIMARY ANGLE-CLOSURE GLAUCOMA

Primary angle-closure glaucoma (PACG) is less common than POAG. The obstruction of the trabecular meshwork by iris tissue, prevents the aqueous humor outflow, which leads to elevation of intraocular pressure (IOP) and often damages the optic nerve. Based on the signs and symptoms of the disease at the time of diagnosis, PACG has been divided into acute, subacute and chronic cases.[112] The prevalence rate in Asian population is 0.8 percent.

PACG has been reported to have MYOC mutations in only isolated patients, including two with combined-mechanism glaucoma. Association of C677T polymorphism of MTHFR gene which is important for remodeling of the extracellular matrix, has been reported with a significance p value (p<0.01) in a Pakistani population.[113] No novel or previously reported sequence mutations were identified in MYOC, OPTN, WDR36, CYP1B1, OPA1 or OPA3 genes of Middle Eastern patients. In the same study, mtDNA nucleotide changes were identified with minimal rate, suggesting that anatomic factors might serve as more important determinants for PACG than the genetic and mitochondrial factors evaluated in the study.[114]

Table 2 Genes reported to be associated with POAG

Gene symbol	Gene name	Chromosomal location	Reference
AGTR2	Angiotensin II receptor, type 2	Xq22–q23	(Hashizume et al. 2005)[84]
APOE	Apolipoprotein E	19q13.2	(Copin et al. 2002)[85]
IL1A	Interluekin 1 alpha	2q14	(Wang et al. 2006)[86]
EDNRA	Endothelin receptor, type A	4q31.2	(Ishikawa et al. 2005)[87]
GSTM1	Glutathione S-transferase, mu-1	1p13.3	(Juronen et al. 2000)[88]
IGF2	Insulin-like growth factor II	11p15.5	(Tsai et al. 2003)[89]
IL1B	Interluekin 1 beta	2q14	(Lin et al. 2003a)[90]
MTHFR	5,10-methylenetetra-hydrofolate reductase	1p36.3	(Junemann et al. 2005)[91]
NOS3	Nitric oxide synthase 3	7q36	(Tunny et al. 1998)[92]
NPPA	Natriuretic peptide precursor A 108780		(Tunny et al. 1996)[93]
OCLM	Oculomedin	1q31.1	(Fujiwara et al. 2003)[94]
OLFM2	Olfactomedin 2	19p13.2	(Funayama et al. 2006)[95]
OPA1	Optic atrophy 1	3q28–q29	(Aung et al. 2002)[96]
TAP1	Transporter, ATP-binding cassette, major histocompatibility complex	6p21.3	(Lin et al. 2004)[97]
TNF	Tumor necrosis factor	6p21.3	(Lin et al. 2003b)[98]
TP53	Tumor protein p53	17p13.1	(Lin et al. 2002)[99]
OPTC	Opticin	1q32.1	(Acharya et al. 2007)[100]
CYP2D6	Cytochrome P450, Subfamily IID, Polypeptide 6	22q13.1	(Yang et al. 2009)[101]
PON1	Paraoxonase 1	7q21.3	(Inagaki et al. 2006a)[102]
CDH-1	Cadherin 1	16q22.1	(Lin et al. 2006)[103]
LMX1B	Lim Homeobox Transcription Factor 1	9q34.1	(Park et al. 2009)[104]
ANP	Atrial natriuretic polypeptide	1p36.2	(Tunny et al. 1996)[105]
P21	P21	6p21.2	(Tsai et al. 2004)[106]
HSPA1A	Heat shock 70 kDa protein 1A	6p21.3	(Tosaka et al. 2007)[107]
TLR4	Toll-like receptor 4	9q32–q33	(Shibuya et al. 2008)[108]
CYP46A1	Cytochrome P450, Family 46, Subfamily A, Polypeptide 1	14q32.1	(Fourgeux et al. 2009)[109]
PAI-1	Plasminogen activator inhibitor-1	7q21.3–q22	(Mossbock et al. 2008)[110]
ADRB1	beta-adrenergic receptors 1	10q24–q26	(Inagaki et al. 2006)[111]
ADRB2	beta-adrenergic receptors 2	5q32–q34	(Inagaki et al. 2006b)[111]

GENETIC LOCI ASSOCIATED WITH EXFOLIATION GLAUCOMA

Pseudoexfoliation (also termed exfoliation) glaucoma is a common form of secondary open-angle glaucoma resulting in deposition of fibrillar material throughout the anterior segment of the eye. This disease is characterized by increased intraocular pressure and optic nerve degeneration. The frequency of this syndrome varies from one ethinic group to the other.

Recently, a genome-wide association study has identified a locus on15q24 that is strongly associated with exfoliation patients in Icelandic and Swedish cohorts.[115] The gene has been identified

as the lysyl oxidase-like 1 (LOXL1) gene and spans 25kb genomic region containing seven exons. The investigators identified disease associated polymorphisms, two SNPs located within exon 1: rs1048661 (R141L), rs3825942 (G153D) and one located in intron 1: rs2165241.

The polymorphism rs3825942 showed consistent association where as no consistent association was found for rs2165241 or rs1048661, with XFS/XFG in different ethnic populations.[116]

The enzyme encoded by LOXL1 gene is part of a family of lysyloxidase genes (LOX) that are involved in the cross-linking of collagen and elastin polymers. LOXL1 oxidatively

deaminates the lysine residues of tropoelastin to allow it to form covalently cross-linked elastin fibers.[117] The expression of this protein has been shown in the cornea, iris, ciliary body, lens capsule, and optic nerve.[118] Future studies are required to understand the effect of LOXL1 mutations on the development of glaucoma in these patients.

GENETIC LOCI ASSOCIATED WITH ANTERIOR SEGMENT DYSGENESIS SYNDROMES

Anterior segment dysgenesis syndromes are developmental abnormalities of the anterior segment due to abnormal migration and differentiation of neural crest derived endothelial cells. These cells migrate as a continuous endothelium till the seventh or eighth gestational month and form connective tissues from the corneal endothelium to the lens and simultaneously differentiate with other structures of the drainage angle to form the outflow structures of the eye.[119,120] Alterations in the migration and/or differentiation of these cells can yield a "spectrum" of overlapping anterior segment abnormalities.[121]

Many loci have been identified to be linked to the anterior segment dysgenesis syndromes. *PITX2 (REIG1* locus) maps on chromosome 4q25-26[122,123] and *FOXC1 (FKHL7)* maps on chromosome 6q25[83,124] are the two transcription factor genes identified as the candidate genes for this syndrome. PAX6 gene maps on chromosome *11p13*,[125,126] *FOXE3* gene maps on chromosome 1p32[127] and the *CYP1B1* gene[128] have been identified with mutations in few numbers of the patients.

ROLE OF MITOCHONDRIAL DNA IN PATHOGENESIS OF GLAUCOMA

Mitochondria are morphologically dynamic organelles exhibiting a precise balance of ongoing fission and fusion during development and aging, which can be modified by disease. Glaucoma is a complex age related disorder characterized by elevated IOP as a significant risk factor. Based on the experiments carried out in animal models, it is not clear whether elevated IOP leads to mitochondrial alterations. In another point of view, primary mitochondrial abnormalities may disturb IOP regulatory mechanisms, there by leading to the elevation of IOP and initiation of neurodegenerative injury.[129]

Based on these observations mitochondrial genes seem to play crucial role in causing glaucoma. There is limited information available for involvement of mitochondrial genome in glaucoma. Studies suggest that mitochondrial abnormalities in patients with POAG, implicating oxidative stress and implying that mitochondria dysfunction may be a risk factor for POAG.[54] The same group attempted to elucidate, the role of mitochondrial DNA in PACG[114] and pseudoexfoliation glaucoma.[130] In both the cases, they have not identified any significant association.

SUMMARY

Attempts have been made by different research groups to identify the role of genetic variations in glaucoma causing genes. Three methods viz candidate genes approach, positional cloning and linkage analysis were followed to identify the candidate genes. By linkage analysis MYOC gene has been identified as the candidate gene. Several mutations have been reported in the MYOC gene of which many of them lie on the exon-3, which encodes olfactomedin domain of myocilin protein.

Various other genes viz OPTN, WDR36 have been reported to have mutations that are associated with POAG. Other forms of glaucoma like PCG, PXG and NTG have been studied using similar methodologies to unravel the role of mutations in the disease causing genes.

FUTURE ASPECTS
Efforts are ongoing towards:
- Identifying the new candidate genes.
- Gene expression and protein expression studies on myocilin.
- Understanding the structure-function relations of Myocilin.
- Collaboration between clinicians and the research groups to elucidate the phenotype-genotype correlation.

REFERENCES

1. Quigley HA. Number of people with glaucoma worldwide. Br J Ophthamol 1996;80:389-93.
2. Shields M, Ritch R, Krupin T. Classification of the glaucomas. Mosby, St Louis, USA, 1996.
3. Leske MC, Heijl A, Hyman L, Bengtsson B. The early manifest glaucoma trail group: Early manifest glaucoma trail. Design and baseline data. Ophthalmology 1999;106: 2144-53.
4. Wolfs RC, et al. Genetic risk of primary open-angle glaucoma. Population-based familial aggregation study. Arch Ophthalmol 1998;116(12):16405.
5. Goldwyn R, Waltman SR, Becker B. Primary open-angle glaucoma in adolescents and young adults. Arch Ophthalmol 1970;84:579-82.
6. Johnson AT, Drack AV, Kwitek AE, et al. Clinical features and linkage analysis of a family with autosomal dominant juvenile glaucoma. Ophthalmology 1993;100:524-9.
7. Thylefors B, Negrel AD. The global impact of glaucoma. Bull World Health Organ 1994;72:323-6.
8. Quigley HA. Proportion of those with open-angle glaucoma who become blind. Ophthalmology. 1999; 106:2039-41.
9. Challa P, Glaucoma Genetics. International Ophthalmology Clinics 2008;48(4):73-94.
10. Sheffield VC, Stone EM, Alward WL, Drack AV, Johnson AT, Streb LM, et al. Genetic linkage of familial open angle glaucoma to chromosome 1q21-31. Nat Genet 1993;4:47-50.
11. Meyer A, Valtot F, Bechetoille A, et al. Linkage between juvenile glaucoma and chromosome 1q in 2 French families. CR Acad Sci III 1994;317:565-70.
12. Richards JE, Lichter PR, Boehnke M, et al. Mapping of a gene for autosomal dominant juvenile-onset

open-angle glaucoma to chromosome Iq. Am J Hum Genet 1994; 54:62-70.

13. Wiggs JL, Haines JL, Paglinauan C, et al. Genetic linkage of autosomal dominant juvenile glaucoma to 1q21-31 in three affected pedigrees. Genomics 1994;21:299-303.

14. Ray K, Mookherjee S. Molecular complexity of primary open angle glaucoma: current concepts. J Genet 2009;88:451-67.

15. Stone EM, Fingert JH, Alward WL, Nguyen TD, Polansky JR, Sunden SL, et al. Identification of a gene that causes primary open angle glaucoma. Science 1997;275:668-70.

16. Rezaie T, Child A, Hitchings R, Brice G, Miller L, Coca-Prados M, et al. Adult-onset primary open-angle glaucoma caused by mutations in Optineurin. Science 2002;295:1077-9.

17. Monemi S, Spaeth G, DaSilva A, Popinchalk S, Ilitchev E, Liebmann J, et al. Identification of a novel adult-onset primary open-angle glaucoma (POAG) gene on 5q22.1. Hum Mol Genet 2005;14:725-33.

18. Stoilova D, Child A, Trifan OC, Crick RP, Coakes RL, Sarfarazi M. Localization of a locus (GLC1B) for adult onset primary open angle glaucoma to the 2cen-q13 region. Genomics 1996;36:142-50.

19. Wirtz MK, Samples JR, Kramer PL, Rust K, Topinka JR, Yount J, et al. Mapping a gene for adult-onset primary open-angle glaucoma to chromosome 3q. Am J Hum Genet 1997;60:296-304.

20. Trifan OC, Traboulsi EI, Stoilova D, Alozie I, Nguyen R, Raja S, et al. A third locus (GLC1D) for adult-onset primary open-angle glaucoma maps to the 8q23 region. Am J Ophthalmol 1998;126:17-28.

21. Sarfarazi M, Child A, Stoilova D, Brice G, Desai T, Trifan OC, et al. Localization of the fourth locus (GLC1E) for adultonset primary open-angle glaucoma to the 10p15-14 region. Am J Hum Genet 1998;62:641-52.

22. Wirtz MK, Samples JR, Rust K, Lie J, Nordling L, Schilling K, et al. GLC1F, a new primary open-angle glaucoma locus, maps to 7q35-6. Arch Ophthalmol 1999;117:237-41.

23. Monemi S, Spaeth G, DaSilva A, Popinchalk S, Ilitchev E, Liebmann J, et al. Identification of a novel adult-onset primary open-angle glaucoma (POAG) gene on 5q22.1. Hum Mol Genet 2005;14:725-33.

24. Suriyapperuma SP, Child A, Desai T, Brice G, Kerr A, Crick RP, et al. A new locus (GLC1H) for adult-onset primary open-angle glaucoma maps to the 2p15-6 region. Arch Ophthalmol 2007;125:86-92.

25. Allingham RR, Wiggs JL, Hauser ER, Larocque-Abramson KR, Santiago-Turla C, Broomer B, et al. Early adult-onset POAG linked to 15q11-13 using ordered subset analysis. Invest Ophthalmol Vis Sci 2005;46:2002-5.

26. Wiggs JL, Lynch S, Ynagi G, Maselli M, Auguste J, Del Bono EA, et al. A genomewide scan identifies novel early-onset primary open-angle glaucoma loci on 9q22 and 20p12. Am J Hum Genet 2004;74:1314-20.

27. Baird PN, Foote SJ, Mackey DA, Craig J, Speed TP, Bureau A. Evidence for a novel glaucoma locus at chromosome 3p21-2. Hum Genet 2005;117:249-57.

28. Pang CP, Fan BJ, Canlas O, Wang DY, Dubois S, Tam PO, et al. A genome-wide scan maps a novel juvenile-onset primary open angle glaucoma locus to chromosome 5q. Mol Vis 2006;12:85-92.

29. Wang DY, Fan BJ, Chua JK, Tam PO, Leung CK, Lam DS, et al. A genome-wide scan maps a novel juvenile-onset primary open-angle glaucoma locus to 15q. Invest Ophthalmol Vis Sci 2006;47:5315-21.

30. Wiggs JL, Allingham RR, Hossain A, Kern J, Auguste J, Del-Bono EA, et al. Genome-wide scan for adult onset primary open angle glaucoma. Hum Mol Genet 2000;9:1109-17.

31. Nemesure B, Jiao X, He Q, Leske M, Wu S, Hennis A, et al. A genome-wide scan for primary open-angle glaucoma (POAG): the Barbados Family Study of Open-Angle Glaucoma. Hum Genet 2003;112:600-9.

32. Lin Y, Liu T, Li J, Yang J, Du Q, Wang J, et al. A genome-wide scan maps a novel autosomal dominant juvenile-onset open-angle glaucoma locus to 2p15-6. Mol Vis 2008;14:739-44.

33. Charlesworth JC, Dyer TD, Stankovich JM, Blangero J, Mackey DA, Craig JE, et al. Linkage to 10q22 for maximum intraocular pressure and 1p32 for maximum cup-to-disc ratio in an extended primary open-angle glaucoma pedigree. Invest Ophthalmol Vis Sci 2005;46:3723-9.

34. Sunden SL, Alward WL, Nichols BE, et al. Fine mapping of the autosomal dominant juvenile open angle glaucoma (GLC1A) region and evaluation of candidate genes. Genome Res 1996;6:862-9.

35. Lange K, Boehnke M, Cox DR, Lunetta KL. Statistical methods for polyploid radiation hybrid mapping. Genome Res 1995;5:136-50.

36. Polansky JR, Fauss DJ, Chen P, Chen H, Lutjen-Drecoll E, Johnson D, et al. Cellular pharmacology and molecular biology of the trabecular meshwork inducible glucocorticoid response gene product. Ophthalmologica 1997;211:126-39.

37. Nguyen TD, Chen P, Huang WD, et al. Gene structure and properties of TIGR, an olfactomedin-related glycoprotein cloned from glucocorticoid-induced trabecular meshwork cells. J Biol Chem 1998;273:6341-50.

38. Polansky JR, Fauss DJ, Zimmerman CC. Regulation of TIGR/MYOC gene expression in human trabecular meshwork cells. Eye 2000;14:503-14.

39. Ortego J, Escribano J, Coca-Prados M. Cloning and characterization of subtracted cDNAs from a human ciliary body library encoding TIGR, a protein involved in juvenile open angle glaucoma with homology to myosin and olfactomedin. FEBS Lett 1997;413:349-53.

40. Kubota R, Noda S, Wang Y, Minoshima S, Asakawa S, Kudoh J, et al. A novel myosin-like protein (myocilin) expressed in the connecting cilium of the photoreceptor: molecular cloning, tissue expression and chromosomal mapping. Genomics 1997;41:360-9.

41. Kanagavalli J, Pandaranayaka E, Krishnadas SR, Krishnaswamy S, Sundaresan P. A review of genetic and structural understanding of the role of myocilin in primary open angle glaucoma. Indian J Ophthalmol 2004;52:271-80.

42. Aroca-Aguilar JD, Sanchez-Sanchez F, Ghosh S, Coca-Prados M, Escribano J. Myocilin mutations causing glaucoma inhibit the intracellular endoproteolytic cleavage of myocilin between amino acids Arg226 and Ile227. J Biol Chem 2005;280:21043-51.

43. Fingert JH, Ying L, Swiderski RE, Nystuen AM, Arbour NC, Alward WL, Sheffield VC, Stone EM. Characterization and comaprision of the human and mouse GLC1A glaucoma genes. Genome Res 1998;8:377-84.

44. Tomarev SI, Tamm ER, Chang B. Characterization of the mouse MYOC-MYOC. Biochem Biophys Res Commun 1998;245:087-93.

45. Ezequiel Campos-Mollo, Francisco Sánchez-Sánchez, María Pilar López-Garrido, Enrique López-Sánchez, Francisco López-Martínez, Julio Escribano. MYOC gene mutations in Spanish patients with autosomal dominant primary open-angle glaucoma: a founder effect in southeast Spain. Molecular Vision 2007;13:1666-73.

46. Ortego J, Escribano J, Coca-Prados M. Cloning and characterization of subtracted cDNAs from a human ciliary body library encoding TIGR, a protein involved in juvenile open angle glaucoma with homology to myosin and olfactomedin. FEBS Lett 1997;413:349-53.

47. Fautsch MP, Bahler CK, Jewison DJ, et al. Recombinant TIGR/MYOC increases outflow resistance in the human anterior segment. Invest Ophthalmol Vis Sci 2000;41:4163-8.

48. Borras T, Rowlette LL, Erzurum SC, et al. Adenoviral reporter gene transfer to the human trabecular meshwork does not alter aqueous humor outflow. Relevance for potential gene therapy of glaucoma. Gene Ther 1999;6:515-24.

49. Kim BS, Savinova OV, Reedy MV, et al. Targeted disruption of the myocilin gene (Myoc) suggests that human glaucoma-causing mutations are gain of function. Mol Cell Biol 2001;21:7707-13.

50. Gould DB, Reedy M, Wilson LA, et al. Mutant myocilin nonsecretion *in vivo* is not sufficient to cause glaucoma. Mol Cell Biol 2006;26:8427-36.

51. Senatorov V, Malyukova I, Fariss R, et al. Expression of mutated mouse myocilin induces open-angle glaucoma in transgenic mice. J Neurosci 2006;26:11903-14.

52. Sakai H, Shen V, Koga T, Park BC, Noskina Y, Tibudan M, et al. Mitochondrial association of myocilin, product of a glaucoma gene, in human trabecular meshwork cells. J Cell Physiol 2007;13:775-84.

53. He Y, Leung KW, Zhuo YH, Ge J. Pro370Leu mutant myocilin impairs mitochondrial functions in human trabecular meshwork cells. Mol Vis 2009;15:815-25.

54. Khaled K, Abu-Amero, Jose Morales, Thomas M, Bosley. Mitochondrial Abnormalities in Patients with Primary Open-Angle Glaucoma. Investigative Ophthalmology and Visual Science 2006; 47(6):2533-41.

55. Yuan He, Kar Wah Leung, Ye-Hong Zhuo, Jian Ge. Pro370Leu mutant myocilin impairs mitochondrial functions in human trabecular meshwork cells. Molecular Vision 2009;15:815-25.

56. Alex W Hewitt, David A, Mackey, Jamie E, Craig J. Myocilin Allele-Specific Glaucoma Phenotype Database Human Mutation 2008; 29(2):207-11.

57. Kanagavalli J, Krishnadas SR, Pandaranayaka E, Krishnaswamy S, Sundaresan P. Evaluation and understanding of myocilin mutations in Indian primary open angle glaucoma patients. Mol Vis 2003;9:606-14.

58. Kanagavalli J, Pandaranayaka PJ, Krishnadas SR, Krishnaswamy S, Sundaresan P. *In vitro* and *in vivo* study on the secretion of the Gly367Arg mutant myocilin protein. Mol Vis 2007;13:1161-8.

59. Zhou Z, Vollrath D. A cellular assay distinguishes normal and mutant TIGR/myocilin protein. Hum Mol Genet 1999;8:2221-8.

60. Jacobson N, Andrews M, Shepard AR, Nishimura D, Searby C, Fingert JH, et al. Nonsecretion of mutant proteins of the glaucoma gene myocilin in cultured trabecular meshwork cells and in aqueous humor. Hum Mol Genet 2001;10:117-25.

61. Joe MK, Sohn S, Hur W, Moon Y, Choi YR, Kee C. Accumulation of mutant myocilins in ER leads to ER stress, potential cytotoxicity in human trabecular meshwork cells. Biochem Biophys Res Commun 2003;312:592-600.

62. Liu Y, Vollrath D. Reversal of mutant myocilin nonsecretion and cell killing: implications for glaucoma. Hum Mol Genet 2004;13:1193-204.

63. Jia LY, Gong B, Pang CP, Huang Y, Lam DS, Wang N, et al. Correction of the disease phenotype of myocilin-causing glaucoma by a natural osmolyte. Invest Ophthalmol 2009;50:3743-9.

64. Li Y, Kang J, Horwitz MS. Interaction of an adenovirus E3 14.7-kilodalton protein with a novel tumor necrosis factor alpha-inducible cellular protein containing leucine zipper domains. Mol Cell Biol 1998;18:1601-10.

65. De Marco N, Buono M, Troise F, Diez-Roux G. Optineurin increases cell survival and translocates to the nucleus in a Rab8-dependent manner upon an apoptotic stimulus. J. Biol Chem 2006;281:16147-56.

66. Mao M, Biery MC, Kobayashi SV, et al. T lymphocyte activation gene identification by coregulated expression on DNA microarrays. Genomics 2004;83:989-99.

67. Skarie JM, Link BA. The primary open-angle glaucoma gene WDR36 functions in ribosomal –RNA processing and interacts with the p53 stress-response pathway. Hum Mol Genet 2008;17:2474-85.

68. Footz TK, Johnson JL, Dubois S, Bovini N, Raymond V, Walter MA. Glaucoma–associated WDR36 variants encode functional defects in a yeast model system. Hum MolGenet 2009;18:1276-87.

69. Pasutto F, Mardin CY, Michels-Rautenstrauss K, et al. Profiling of WDR36 missense variations in German patients with glaucoma. Invest Opthalmol Vis Sci 2008; 49:270-4.

70. Miyazawa A, Fuse N, Mengkegale M, et al. Association between primary open-angle glaucoma and WDR36 DNA sequence variations in Japanese. Mol Vis 2007;13:1912-9.

71. Fingert JH, Alward WL, Kwon YH, et al. No association between variations in the WDR36 gene and primary open-angle glaucoma. Arch Opthalmol 2007;125:434-6.

72. Hewitt AW, Dimasi DP, Mackey DA, et al. A glaucoma case-control study of the WDR36 gene D658G sequence variant. Am J Opthalmol 2006;142:324-5.

73. Hauser MA, Allingham RR, Linkroum K, et al. Distribution of WDR36 DNA sequence variants in patients with primary open-angle glaucoma. Invest Opthalmol Vis Sci 2006;47:2542-6.

74. Sarfarazi M, Akarsu AN, Hossain A, Turacli ME, Aktan SG, Barsoum-Homsy M, et al. Assignment of a locus (GLC3A) for primary open angle glaucoma (Buphthalmos) to 2p21 and evidence for genetic heterogeneity. Genomics 1995;30:171-7.

75. Stoilov I, Akarsu AN, Sarfarazi M. Identification of three different truncating mutations in cytochrome P4501B1 (CYP1B1) as the principal cause of primary congenital glaucoma (Buphthalmos) in families linked to the GLC3A locus on chromose 2p21. Hum Mol Genet 1997;6:641-7.

76. Acharya M, Mookherjee S, Bhattacharjee A, Bandyopadhyay AK, Daulat Thakur SK, Bhaduri G, et al. Primary role of CYP1B1 in Indian juvenile-onset POAG patients. Mol Vis 2006;12:399-404.

77. Bayat B, Yazdani S, Alavi A, Chiani M, Chitsazian F, Tusi BK, et al. Contributions of MYOC and CYP1B1 mutations to JOAG. Mol Vis 2008;14:508-17.

78. Vincent A, Billingsley G, Priston M, Williams-Lyn D, Sutherland J, Glaser T, et al. Phenotypic heterogeneity of CYP1B1: mutations in a patient with Peter's anomaly. J Med Genet 2001;38:324-6.

79. Chavarria-Soley G, Michels-Rautenstrauss K, Pasutto F, Flikier D, Flikier P, Cirak S, et al. Primary cogenital glaucoma and Rieger's anomaly: extended haplotypes reveal founder effects for eight distinct CYP1B1 mutations. Mol Vis 2006;12:523-31.

80. Murray GI, Melvin WT, Greenlee WF, et al. Regulation, function and tissue-specific expression of cytochrome P 450 CYP1B1. Annu Rev Pharmacol Toxicol 2001;41: 297-316.

81. Hakkola J, Pasanen M, Pelkonen O, et al. Expression of CYP1B1 in human adult and fetal tissues and differential inducibility of CYP1B1 and CYP1A1 by Ah receptor ligands in human placenta and cultured cells. Carcinogenesis 1997;18:391-7.

82. Chakrabarti S, Kaur K, Komatireddy S, Acharya M, Devi KR, Mukopadhyay A, Mandal AK, Hasnain SE, Chandrasekhar G, Thomas R, Ray K. Gln48His is the prevalent myocilin mutation in primary open angle and primary congenital glaucoma phenotypes in India. Mol Vis 2005;11:111-3.

83. Nishimura DY, Swiderski RE, Alward WL, et al. The forkhead transcription factor gene FKHL7 is responsible for glaucoma phenotypes which map to 6p25. Nat Genet 1998;19:140-7.

84. Hashizume K, Mashima Y, Fumayama T, Ohtake Y, Kimura I, Yoshida K, et al. Genetic polymorphisms in the angiotensin II receptor gene and their association with open-angle glaucomain a Japanese population. Invest Ophthalmol Vis Sci 2005;46:1993-2001.

85. Copin B, Brezin AP, Valtot F, Dascotte JC, Bechetoille A, Garchon HJ. Apolipoprotein E-promoter singlenu–cleotide polymorphisms affect the phenotype of primary open angle glaucoma and demonstrate interaction with the myocilin gene. Am J Hum Genet 2002;70:1575-81.

86. Wang CY, Shen YC, Lo FY, Su CH, Lee SH, Lin KH, et al. Polymorphism in the IL-1alpha (−889) locus associated with elevated risk of primary open angle glaucoma. Mol Vis 2006;12:1380-5.

87. Ishikawa K, Funayama T, Ohtake Y, Kimura I, Ideta H, Nakamoto K, et al. Association between glaucoma and gene polymorphism of endothelin type A receptor. Mol Vis 2005;11:431-7.

88. Juronen E, Tasa G, Veromann S, Parts L, Tiidla A, Pulges R, et al. Polymorphic glutathione S-transferase M1 is a risk factor of primary open-angle glaucoma among Estonians. Exp Eye Res 2000;71:447-52.

89. Tsai FJ, Lin HJ, Chen WC, Chen HY, Fan SS. Insulin-like growth factor-II gene polymorphism is associated with primary open angle glaucoma. J Clin Lab Anal 2003;17:259-63.

90. Lin HJ, Tsai SC, Tsai FJ, Chen WC, Tsai JJ, Hsu CD. Association of interleukin 1beta and receptor antagonist gene polymorphisms with primary open-angle glaucoma. Ophthalmologica 2003a;217:358-64.

91. Junemann AG, von Ahsen N, Reulbach U, Roedl J, Bonsch D, Kornhuber J, et al. C677T variant in the methylentetrahydrofolate reductase gene is a genetic risk factor for primary open-angle glaucoma. Am J Ophthalmol 2005;139:721-3.

92. Tunny TJ, Richardson KA, Clark CV. Association study of the 5' flanking regions of endothelial-nitric oxide synthase and endothelin-1 genes in familial primary open-angle glaucoma. Clin Exp Pharmacol Physiol 1998;25:26-9.

93. Tunny TJ, Richardson KA, Clark CV, Gordon RD. The atrial natriuretic peptide gene in patients with familial primary open-angle glaucoma. Biochem Biophys Res Commun 1996;223:221-5.

94. Fujiwara N, Matsuo T and Ohtsuki H. Protein expression, genomic structure and polymorphisms of oculomedin. Ophthalmic Genet 2003;24:141-51.

95. Funayama T, Mashima Y, Ohtake Y, Ishikawa K, Fuse N, Yasuda N, et al. SNPs and interaction analyzes of noelin 2, myocilin and optineurin genes in Japanese patients with open angle glaucoma. Invest Ophthalmol. Vis Sci 2006;47:5368-75.

96. Aung T, Ocaka L, Ebenezer ND, Morris AG, Krawczak M, Thiselton DL, et al. A major marker for normal tension glaucoma: association with polymorphisms in the OPA1 gene. Hum Genet 2002;110:52-6.

97. Lin HJ, Tsai CH, Tsai FJ, Chen WC, Chen HY, Fan SS. Transporter associated with antigen processing gene 1 codon 333 and codon 637 polymorphisms are associated with primary open-angle glaucoma. Mol Diagn 2004;8:245-52.

98. Lin HJ, Tsai FJ, Chen WC, Shi YR, Hsu Y, Tsai SW. Association of tumour necrosis factor alpha–308 gene polymorphism with primary open-angle glaucoma in Chinese. Eye 2003b;17:31-4.

99. Lin HJ, Chen WC, Tsai FJ, Tsai SW. Distributions of p53 codon 72 polymorphism in primary open angle glaucoma. Br J Ophthalmol 2002;86:767-70.

100. Acharya M, Mookherjee S, Bhattacharjee A, Thakur SK, Bandyopadhyay AK, Sen A, et al. Evaluation of the OPTC gene in primary open angle glaucoma: functional significance of a silent change. BMC Mol. Biol 2007;8:21.

101. Yang Y, Wu K, Yuan H, Yu M. Cytochrome oxidase 2D6 gene polymorphism in primary open-angle glaucoma with various effects to ophthalmic timolol. J Ocul Pharmacol Ther 2009;25:163-71.

102. Inagaki Y, Mashima Y, Funayama T, Ohtake Y, Fuse N, Yasuda N, et al. Paraoxonase 1 gene polymorphisms influence clinical features of open-angle glaucoma. Graefes Arch Clin Exp Ophthalmol 2006a;244:984-90.

103. Lin HJ, Tsai FJ, Hung P, Chen WC, Chen HY, Fan SS, et al. Association of E-cadherin gene 3_-UTR C/T polymorphism with primary open angle glaucoma. Ophthalmic Res 2006;38:44-8.

104. Park S, Jamshidi Y, Vaideanu D, Bitner-Glindzicz M, Fraser S, Sowden JC. Genetic risk for primary open-angle glaucoma determined by LMX1B haplotypes. Invest. Ophthalmol Vis Sci 2009;50:1522-30.

105. Tunny TJ, Richardson KA, Clark CV, Gordon RD. The atrial natriuretic peptide gene in patients with familial primary open-angle glaucoma. Biochem Biophys Res Commun 1996;223:221-5.

106. Tsai FJ, Lin HJ, Chen WC, Tsai CH, Tsai SW. A codon 31ser-arg polymorphism of theWAF-1/CIP-1/p21/tumor suppressor gene in Chinese primary open-angle glaucoma. Acta Ophthalmol. Scand 2004;82:76-80.

107. Tosaka K, Mashima Y, Funayama T, Ohtake Y, Kimura I. Association between open-angle glaucoma and gene polymorphism for heat-shock protein 70-1. Jpn J Ophthalmol 2007;51:417-23.

108. Shibuya E, Meguro A, Ota M, Kashiwagi K, Mabuchi F, Iijima H, et al. Association of Toll-like receptor 4 gene polymorphisms with normal tension glaucoma. Invest Ophthalmol Vis Sci 2008;49:4453-7.

109. Fourgeux C, Martine L, Bjorkhem I, Diczfalusy U, Joffre C, Acar N, et al. Primary Open Angle Glaucoma: Association with Cholesterol 24S-Hydroxylase (CYP46A1) Gene Polymorphism and Plasma 24-Hydroxycholesterol Levels. Invest Ophthalmol Vis Sci 2009;50:5712-7.

110. Mossbock G, Weger M, Faschinger C, Schmut O, Renner W. Plasminogen activator inhibitor-1 4G/5G gene polymorphism and primary open-angle glaucoma. Mol Vis 2008;14:1240-4.

111. Inagaki Y, Mashima Y, Fuse N, Funayama T, Ohtake Y, Yasuda N,

et al. Polymorphism of beta-adrenergic receptors and susceptibility to open-angle glaucoma. Mol Vis 2006b;12:673-80.

112. Ritch R, Lowe RF. Angle-closure glaucoma: mechanisms and epidemiology. In: Ritch R, Shields MB, Krupin T (Eds). The Glaucomas, 2nd edn. St. Louis: Mosby; 1996.pp.801-19.

113. Shazia Michael, Raheel Qamar, Farah Akhtar, Wajid Ali Khan, Asifa Ahmed. C677T polymorphism in the methylenetetrahydrofolate reductase gene is associated with primary closed angle glaucoma. Molecular Vision 2008;14:661-5.

114. Khaled K Abu-Amero, Jose Morales, Mazen N Osman, Thomas M Bosley. Nuclear and Mitochondrial Analysis of Patients with Primary Angle-Closure Glaucoma. Invest Ophthalmol Vis Sci 2007;48:5591-6.

115. Thorleifsson G, Magnusson KP, Sulem P, Walters GB, Gudbjartsson DF, Stefansson H, Jonsson T, Jonasdottir A, Jonasdottir A, Stefansdottir G, Masson G, Hardarson GA, Petursson H, Arnarsson A, Motallebipour M, Wallerman O, Wadelius C, Gulcher JR, Thorsteinsdottir U, Kong A, Jonasson F, Stefansson K. Common sequence variants in the LOXL1 gene confer susceptibility to exfoliation glaucoma. Science 2007;317(5843):1397-400.

116. Haoyu Chen, Li Jia Chen, Mingzhi Zhang, Weifeng Gong, Pancy Oi Sin Tam, Dennis Shun Chiu Lam, Chi Pui Pang. Ethnicity-based subgroup meta-analysis of the association of LOXL1 polymorphisms with glaucoma.

117. Liu X, Zhao Y, Gao J, et al. Elastic fiber homeostasis requires lysyl oxidase-like 1protein. Nat Genet 2004;36:178-82.

118. Hewitt AW, Sharma S, Burdon KP, et al. Ancestral LOXL1 variants are associated with pseudoexfoliation in Caucasian Australians but with markedly lower penetrance than in Nordic people. Hum Mol Genet 2008;17:710-6.

119. Smelser GK, Ozanics V. The development of the trabecular meshwork in primate eyes. Am J Ophthalmol 1971;1(1 Part 2):366-85.

120. Johnston MC, Noden DM, Hazelton RD, et al. Origins of avian ocular and periocular tissues. Exp Eye Res 1979;29:27-43.

121. Chandler PA, Grant WM, Epstein DL, et al. Chandler and Grant's Glaucoma, 4th edn. Baltimore: Williams & Wilkins 1997:xvi,670.

122. Semina EV, Reiter R, Leysens NJ, et al. Cloning and characterization of a novel bicoid-related homeobox transcription factor gene, RIEG, involved in Rieger syndrome. Nat Genet 1996;14:392-9.

123. Murray JC, Bennett SR, Kwitek AE, et al. Linkage of Rieger syndrome to the region of the epidermal growth factor gene on chromosome 4. Nat Genet 1992;2:46-9.

124. Mears AJ, Jordan T, Mirzayans F, et al. Mutations of the forkhead/ winged-helix gene, FKHL7, in patients with Axenfeld-Rieger anomaly. Am J Hum Genet 1998;63:1316-28.

125. Riise R, Storhaug K, Brondum-Nielsen K. Rieger syndrome is associated with PAX6 deletion. Acta Ophthalmol Scand 2001;79:201-3.

126. Hanson IM, Fletcher JM, Jordan T, et al. Mutations at the PAX6 locus are found in heterogeneous anterior segment malformations including Peters' anomaly. Nat Genet 1994;6:168-73.

127. Semina EV, Brownell I, Mintz-Hittner HA, et al. Mutations in the human forkhead transcription factor FOXE3 associated with anterior segment ocular dysgenesis and cataracts. Hum Mol Genet 2001;10:231-6.

128. Vincent A, Billingsley G, Priston M, et al. Phenotypic heterogeneity of CYP1B1: mutations in a patient with Peters' anomaly. J Med Genet 2001;38:324-6.

129. Tezel G, et al. The role of Glia, Mitochondria and the Immune system in glaucoma. Invest Ophthalmol Vis Sci 2009;5(3):1001-12.

130. Khaled K, Abu-Amero, Thomas M, Bosley, Jose Morales. Analysis of nuclear and mitochondrial genes in patients with pseudoexfoliation glaucoma. Molecular Vision 2008;14:29-36.

5 | Pathogenesis of Optic Nerve Head Changes in Glaucoma

Joshua Priluck, Deepak P Edward

CHAPTER OUTLINE

INTRODUCTION

Glaucoma is a progressive optic neuropathy characterized by degeneration of the retinal ganglion cells (RGCs) resulting in typical changes in the retina, optic nerve and brain. This chapter focuses on the pathologic changes at the optic nerve head and the theories and factors that play a role in glaucomatous damage specifically at the optic nerve head.

The optic nerve head is also referred to as the optic disc or papilla. However, these terms imply a flat surface to the optic nerve head that is in fact three-dimensional. The optic nerve head is the anatomical condensation of the nonmyelinated axons of the retinal ganglion cells in one location where they are organized into fascicles (also called bundles) surrounded by glial support cells. As these axons travel posteriorly towards the brain they transition into myelinated axons behind the lamina cribrosa.

The optic nerve head undergoes unique changes in glaucoma, both in primary open angle glaucoma (POAG) and normal-pressure glaucoma compared to other optic neuropathies. These changes include loss of neuroretinal rim tissue, progressive excavation of the optic nerve head and peripapillary changes. This chapter will discuss the normal anatomy of the optic nerve head, theories of glaucoma as they relate to the optic nerve head, changes both anatomical and histological of the optic nerve head in glaucoma and additional factors that contribute to the pathogenesis of glaucoma at the optic nerve head.

NORMAL OPTIC NERVE HEAD ANATOMY AND HISTOLOGY

The optic nerve head is defined as the intraocular portion of the optic nerve. The borders of the optic nerve head include the vitreous anteriorly, retina and sclera peripherally; and the posterior borders include the surrounding pial, arachnoid and dural meninges with cerebral spinal fluid located between the arachnoid and dural meninges[1] **(Figure 1)**. Recent use of histomorphometric reconstruction compared to disc photography has suggested that Bruch's membrane correlates to the clinically observed disc margin.[2] The whitish rim that occasionally is observed at the edge of the optic disc by ophthalmoscopy is exposed sclera.

There is variation in the size of the optic nerve head between individuals and its measurement further varies depending on the instrument used to make the measurements and software used to analyze it. Ethnic background has been shown to affect optic disc size, although gender and age do not. The role of refractive error and axial length in relation to optic disc size is controversial.[4,5]

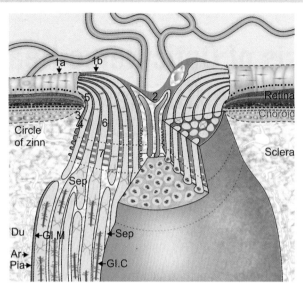

Fig. 1 Schematic drawing of optic nerve within and adjoining eyeball. Numbered regions: 1a, inner limiting membrane of retina; 1b, inner limiting membrane of Elschnig; 2, central meniscus of Kuhnt; 3, border tissue of Elschnig; 4, border tissue of Jacoby; 5, intermediary tissue of Kuhnt; 6, anterior portion of lamina cribrosa; and 7, posterior portion of lamina cribrosa. Du = Dura; Ar = Arachnoid; Sep = Septa. (*Courtesy*: Anderson DR. Ultrastructure of human and monkey lamina cribrosa and optic nerve head. Arch Ophthalmol 1969;82:800-14)

Accurate measurements of optic disc size are only available by histology or *in vivo* during vitrectomy. The range of reported average normal optic disc area by histology varies between studies[3] from 2.57 to 2.81 mm². Histologic studies report a normal average vertical disc diameter ranging from 1.86 to 1.88 mm and horizontal disc diameter ranging from 1.75 to 1.77 mm.[6]

Clinically, optic disc size can be measured in terms vertical and horizontal optic disc diameters. Reports of normal vertical and horizontal disc diameters based on clinical examination vary between an average horizontal length of 1.66 to 1.92 mm and vertical lengths of 1.57 to 1.76 mm.[6] The study of optic disc photographs or other imaging modalities allows quantification of optic disc area. Studies using optic disc photographs report the average disc area to range from 1.70 to 2.89 mm².[3] Racial differences in optic disc size have been demonstrated in black and white American patients using optic disc photographs with the mean disc area to be 2.63 mm² while black patients had a mean disc area of 2.94 mm².[4] A study in the south Indian population using optic disc photographs has been found consistent with the normal range without regard to race, with an average horizontal diameter of 1.77 mm and vertical disc diameter of 1.87 mm or a mean disc area of 2.58 mm².[7] Confocal scanning laser ophthalmoscopy studies report the average optic disc area to range from 1.74 to 2.47 mm² in white patients.[3] A study of the central Indian population using confocal scanning laser tomography found an average disc area of 2.25 mm² (+/- 0.51 mm²) and was felt to show a larger disc area in this study population compared to white patients.[8] Optical coherence tomography studies report the average optic disc area to range from 2.10 to 2.35 mm² in white patients.[3]

Histologically, the optic nerve head may be divided into four distinct regions.

These include (from anterior to posterior) the surface nerve fiber layer (NFL), prelaminar region, lamina cribrosa, and the retrolaminar region as defined by light microscopy, scanning electron microscopy and immunohistochemistry. **Figures 2A and B** demonstrates the optic nerve head in terms of its ocular location and distinct regions.

Nerve Fiber Layer

Overlying the surface NFL is the tissue of Elschnig, an internal limiting membrane between the vitreous and optic nerve head formed by astrocytes with a central area known as the central meniscus of Kuhnt.[9]

The surface nerve fiber layer (NFL) is composed mostly of nerve axons along with astrocytes. The RGC axons hold a retinotopic organization at the nerve head with areas of the retina such as arcuate nerve fibers being located at the superior and inferior poles of the nerve head (corresponding to Bjerrum area), the peripheral retinal fibers are more peripheral at the nerve head and the papillomacular fibers are more central at the nerve head.[10] The only connective tissue at this layer is in regions surrounding blood vessels.[9] The nonmyelinated axons of the retinal ganglion cells retain their retinotopic organization as they turn posterior and proceed through the prelaminar portion of the nerve.[1,11]

Prelaminar Region

The prelaminar portion of the optic nerve head is composed of type 1B astrocytes that segregate RGC axons into fascicles (also called bundles). The fascicles are contained within glial tubes of astrocytic processes for their continued course through the optic nerve head and optic nerve. Type 1B astrocytes also surround the blood vessels at this level.[1,11,12] Microglia are also located around the fascicles in the prelaminar region.[13]

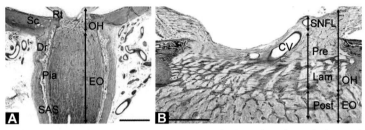

Figs 2A and B (A) Microphotograph showing a sagittal section through the optic nerve head and (B) A magnified view of the optic nerve head demonstrating the four distinct portions. The differences in the arrangement of connective tissue are apparent with this stain. Elastic fibers stained purple while collagen fibers are stained green. (aldehyde fuchsin-Masson Goldner stain) [Dr = Dura, Rt = Retina, SAS = Subarachnoidal space, Sc = Sclera, CV = Central retinal vein, OH = Optic nerve head, EO = Extraocular portion of the optic nerve, SNFL = Surface nerve fiber layer, Pre = Prelaminar, Lam = Laminar, Post = Postlaminar; scale bar in (A): 1 mm; scale bar in (B): 500 micrometer] (*Courtesy:* Oyama T, Abe H, et al. The connective tissue and glial framework in the optic nerve head of the normal human eye: light and scanning electron microscopic studies. Arch Histol Cytol 2006;69:341)

Laminar Region

The lamina cribrosa consists of approximately 10 horizontally parallel connective tissue sheets (cribriform plates) transmitting RGC axons. These fenestrated sheets are composed of collagen and elastin allowing the passage of the fascicles through the pores.[11,14] Located within the cribiform plates are the lamina cribrosa cells (detailed description of this cell is done further ahead in this chapter under the heading of glial support.) that extend thin processes into the core of the plates and connect with processes from the astrocytes.[12] Type IB astrocytes oriented perpendicular to the axons and line the horizontal cribriform plates. The astrocytes are separated from the collagen and elastic matrix of the plates by a basement membrane.[12] Microglia at this level are found in the glial columns and also in the extracellular matrix of the cribiform plates.[13]

The number of laminar pores reported in the literature is variable. One study reported that anteriorly at the level of the choroid, the lamina cribrosa has approximately 392 pores which increase in number posteriorly to 550 corresponding to increased branching of the fascicles as reported in one study.[15] However, another study reported an average of 227 pores measured at the middle of the lamina cribrosa and also that the size of the lamina cribrosa corresponded to the number of pores.[16] There does not appear to be any difference in laminar pore distribution between black and white patients.[17]

The normal course of RGC axons is not always directed posteriorly. One study estimates that 8 to 12 percent of axons have a course through the lamina cribrosa where they take a deviated path going parallel between cribrosal plates before turning and again proceeding posterior.[18] The significance of this unusual course is unclear.

The density of connective tissue and glial support cells in some human lamina cribrosa has been observed to vary by quadrant (superior, nasal, temporal and inferior). On dissection, a study of 25 human eyes found that 10 eyes had uniform tissue density, while nine had relatively greater tissue density in the nasal and temporal regions versus superior and inferior regions of the nerve. Five eyes had focal areas of decreased tissue density in the superior or inferior regions.[19] The lamina cribrosa has also been found to be thicker peripherally versus centrally signifying that the channels the axons pass through in the lamina cribrosa are longer for the peripheral axons.[20] The increased density of glial cells and smaller pore size in the nasal and temporal quadrants of the lamina cribrosa has been theorized to provide increased stiffness to the optic nerve head making these areas less susceptible to glaucomatous damage versus the superior and inferior quadrants.[21,22]

Retrolaminar Region

The retrolaminar portion of the optic nerve head is defined as the portion of the optic nerve posterior to the lamina and extends to the optic chiasm. In the retrolaminar portion of the nerve, the collagen sheaths separating the nerve fascicles become continuous with the pia mater.[9] The width of the nerve behind the nerve increases to 3 mm corresponding to the acquisition of myelination by oligodendrocytes and the surrounding meningial sheaths of pia, arachnoid and dura mater.[1,11] The optic nerve subarachnoid space is continuous with the rest of the central nervous system's subarachnoid space and contains cerebrospinal fluid. Cerebrospinal fluid (CSF) pressure is known to affect the optic nerve in conditions such as psuedotumor cerebri. Changes in the translaminar pressure (difference in pressure across the lamina cribrosa) have been suggested to play a role in optic nerve damage in glaucoma.[23] One study has found CSF opening-pressure to be significantly lower in patients with POAG versus controls by an average of 3.8 mm Hg.[24] The microglia in the retrolaminar region continue to be found in the glial columns around the optic nerve fascicles.[13]

Vasculature of the Optic Nerve Head

The vasculature of the optic nerve head varies in each of its four portions (superficial NFL, prelaminar, laminar, retrolaminar). All four portions receive the majority of their blood supply from the posterior ciliary arteries (PCAs) and the branches of the ophthalmic artery. There is an anatomical variation between individuals in the number posterior ciliary arteries. The most common number of PCAs is two, being found in 48 percent of individuals followed by three in 39 percent of individuals; it is also possible to have one, four, or five PCAs. The variation in number, size and location affects the PCAs distribution and may have consequences in optic nerve head disease. Fluorescein angiography demonstrates filling defects in watershed zones between zones of PCA distribution or along a single PCA distribution in cases of anterior ischemic optic neuropathy.[25]

The superficial NFL is supplied primarily from the arterioles in the adjacent retina. These vessels originate from capillaries of the peripapillary retinal arteries of the retinal circulation. There is no choroidal contribution to the blood supply of the superficial nerve fiber layer.

The prelaminar portion receives its blood supply via direct branches of the PCAs.[26] The prelaminar portion is believed to have a less effective blood-brain barrier allowing vasogenic elements easier access to the microstructural elements.[27,28]

The laminar portion is supplied like the prelaminar portion mostly by the short PCAs either directly or via the arterial circle of Zinn-Haller that arises from paraoptic branches of the short posterior ciliary arteries. The peripapillary choroidal vasculature may contribute small arterioles to the laminar portion.

The retrolaminar portion receives its blood supply from pial arteries that are branches of the ophthalmic artery and short posterior ciliary arterial system. The central retinal artery also

contributes occasional small branches within the retrolaminar optic nerve. The venous drainage of the optic nerve head is almost entirely via the central retinal vein. Occasionally small venous connections exist between the optic nerve head and peripapillary choroid at the prelaminar region.[26]

Glial Support

The optic nerve glial cells share a common embryologic and histologic heritage as the rest of the central nervous system. The optic nerve head glial cells create and regulate the microenvironment of the retinal ganglion cell axons. The glial cell types include oligodendrocytes, astrocytes, microglia and a unique lamina cribrosa cell.

Oligodendrocytes produce myelin, a protein that normally encompasses the neuronal axons and increases the speed of neuronal transmission. Oligodendrocytes are found normally only posterior to the lamina cribrosa. In less than 1% of the population myelination of the retinal nerve fiber layer occurs due to oligodendrocyte proliferation that is discontinuous with the myelination of the posterior optic nerve.[29]

Astrocytes are the primary glial cell of the optic nerve head and have many roles including, providing structural support to RGC axons and secreting extracellular matrix as well as acting as antigen presenting cells. The astrocytes of the human optic nerve head are divided into two subtypes: Type1A and Type 1B. Type 1A astrocytes are glial fibrillary acidic protein (GFAP) positive and neural cell adhesion molecule (NCAM) negative cells. Type 1B astrocytes are GFAP and NCAM positive cells that are the most common form of astrocyte.

Microglia are normally present quiescent macrophages and immune surveillance cells activated in response to neuronal injury and are located

throughout the optic nerve head.[13] They are identified as being HLA-DR positive cells which are located either perivascularly, around the small to medium sized blood vessels, or within the parenchyma in the optic nerve head.[30]

The lamina cribrosa cell: The lamina cribrosa also has a unique star-shaped glial cell known as the lamina cribrosa cell located inside cribiform plates. The cell is distinguished from astrocytes as it does not express the cell markers of astrocytes, microglia, or vascular specific markers. The origin of the lamina cribrosa cell remains undetermined.[12,31]

Extracellular Matrix

The optic nerve head at the prelaminar, laminar and retrolaminar regions is enclosed in an extracellular matrix that provides support and anchorage of the neural elements. The extracellular matrix contains collagen types I through VI, the noncollagenous glycoproteins laminin and fibronectin and proteoglycans.[32] The collagens of the extracellular matrix interconnect body tissue, direct differentiation, migration, and orientation of cells and form filtration membranes.[33]

Studies of the extracellular matrix of laminar cribrosa have shown that collagen types I, III and IV are produced actively throughout life. Astroglial cells in the lamina cribrosa as well as cells in the glial columns, vascular wall basement membrane and surrounding pial septa have been found to express collagen type IV using mRNA hybridization. In contrast, collagen type I was found to be expressed mainly in the cells of the cribriform plates.[34] Collagen types III production was localized mainly to endothelial cells of blood vessels in young subjects and present the lamina cribrosa in young and old subjects suggesting lifelong synthesis.[35] The collagen components of the optic nerve head are well demonstrated by the scanning electron micrograph in **Figure 3** showing a three-dimensional network in the optic nerve head laminar and retrolaminar optic nerve.

GLAUCOMATOUS NEURODEGENERATION AT THE OPTIC NERVE HEAD

The optic nerve undergoes a number of changes in glaucomatous optic neuropathy (GON). Some of these changes are visible at the macroscopic level to the clinician and other changes are microscopic and have been studied in histopathologic specimens in human and animal models. The changes seen are in the axons and the surrounding structures. Some of these changes are likely primary to the disease itself and others are secondary consequential reactive changes; differentiating a clear difference is not straightforward. This section will discuss currently recognized glaucomatous changes of the optic nerve head.

THEORIES OF THE PATHOGENESIS OF GLAUCOMA AT THE OPTIC NERVE HEAD

The optic nerve head is a site of interest in the pathogenesis of glaucoma because of evidence showing it to be the principal site of injury in glaucoma based on the pattern of visual field loss and anatomy of the optic nerve.[22,36] The arguments surrounding the pathogenesis of optic nerve head changes in glaucoma has for the last 150 years fallen between two camps: one favoring a biomechanical mechanism and the other favoring a vascular/ischemic mechanism. Experimental data and observational studies have revealed several mechanisms that have a role in producing GON. Both the mechanical (related to intraocular pressure) or vascular (ischemic) theories of glaucoma may work in concert creating GON.[37,38]

Biomechanical Model

In 1858, Müller first proposed a mechanical model of GON in which elevated IOP led to compression and subsequent neuronal death.[39] Elevated IOP is a known risk factor of glaucoma and evidence exists showing direct relationships. The mechanical model focuses on two aspects of the optic nerve head: mechanical factors affect the structural constituents of the optic nerve head and the geometric configuration of the optic nerve head. The structural constituent refers to the framework of supportive cells and changes that occur to them in response to elevated IOP. The geometric configuration refers to the previously mentioned distribution of glial tissue density in the optic nerve head. This refers to the superior and inferior quadrants having larger pores and less glial tissue corresponding to areas of common early glaucoma damage or the course of some RGC axons as they pass through the lamina cribrosa.[18,21,22]

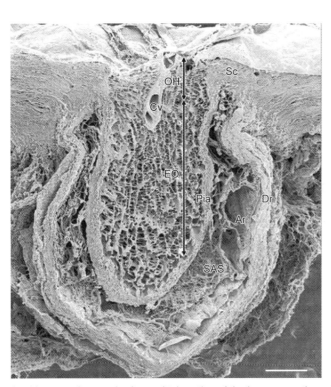

Fig. 3 Scanning electron micrograph of a sagittal section of the human eye through the optic nerve head and extraocular nerve. The collagen network of the retrolaminar optic nerve is continuous with the sclera and pia mater. Note the horizontal arrangement of the laminar fibers and vertically oriented collagenous meshwork of pial septa in the retrolaminar optic nerve. Also, note the fusion of the dura mater with sclera occurs within proximity to the subarachnoidal space and the lamina cribrosa. (AR = Arachnoidal membrane, CV = Central retinal vessels, DR = Dura mater, OH = Optic nerve head, EO = Extraocular portion of optic nerve, SAS = Subarachnoidal space, SC = Sclera; scale bar: 1 mm) (*Courtesy*: Oyama T, Abe H, et al. The connective tissue and glial framework in the optic nerve head of the normal human eye: light and scanning electron microscopic studies. Arch Histol Cytol 2006;69:341-56)

> **Biomechanical Model**
> ***Structural constituents***
> • Framework of supportive cells
> ***Geometrical constituents***
> • Distribution of glial tissue in ONH

The optic nerve head forms a discontinuity within the cornea-scleral shell allowing susceptibility to mechanical stress. These forces are described in engineering terms as stress and strain. Strain is a measure of local deformation while stress is the force acting on the tissue. Stress and strain are not directly proportional to each other because of soft tissue factors such as anisotrophy, nonlinearity and viscoelasticity. The lamina cribrosa deformation is difficult to observe directly. Evidence gathered from the optic nerve head surface has shown increases in optic cup when IOP is raised.[40] Presumably the deformation of the optic nerve head causes disturbances in axoplasmic flow or direct injury to the RGC axons.[37]

Vascular or Ischemic Model

In 1858, the same year that Müller proposed a mechanical model of GON, von Jaeger proposed a vascular cause of glaucoma pathogenesis.[41] The vascular model of GON focuses on ischemia related to the microvascular blood supply to the optic nerve head.

Proposed mechanisms of decreased blood supply leading to ischemic injury of the optic nerve head include compromised capillaries from elevated IOP, failure of autoregulation of blood flow, possible role of vasoactive substances that regulate vascular tone and systemic vascular influence effecting perfusion pressure (the difference between systolic and diastolic blood pressure).[37,42]

Alterations in blood flow at the optic nerve head have been demonstrated by laser Doppler flowmetry examining blood flow to each of the four quadrants of the optic nerve head. One study has compared patients with POAG with visual field deficits, POAG suspects without visual field deficits and controls. The study found a significant decrease in blood flow of 24 percent when POAG suspects were compared to controls. POAG patients with visual field defects had a 29 percent decrease in blood flow versus controls, not statistically significantly different from the POAG suspects. This study concluded that these observations suggested that

blood flow correlates with glaucoma early in the disease.[43]

One vasoactive substance of interest in GON is the vasoactive peptide endothelin-1 (ET-1). Patients with elevated serum ET-1 levels and POAG have been demonstrated to have glaucomatous progression despite adequate IOP control.[44,45] Elevated ET-1 levels have also been suggested to play a role in remodeling the extracellular matrix of the lamina cribrosa.[46] Ischemia of the optic nerve head and glaucomatous-like changes in structure induced by ET-1 administration has been demonstrated in rabbit and monkey models.[47-49] Ischemia of the optic nerve head would naturally lead to hypoxia and tissue injury. Presently, clinical tool to study tissue perfusion directly are not available. Therefore, direct evidence of ischemia playing a role in glaucomatous damage does not yet exist.[50] There is minimal histological evidence of ischemia playing a role, except for the presence of hypoxia-inducible factor 1-alpha which was identified in the optic nerve head of human donor eyes with glaucoma.[51]

CHANGES OF GLAUCOMATOUS OPTIC NEUROPATHY AT OPTIC NERVE HEAD AND THEIR PATHOGENESIS

The optic nerve demonstrates characteristic changes in glaucoma that have histological correlates. The first observation of optic nerve head cupping in glaucoma was by von Graefe in 1857. In 1854, during the era of early ophthalmoscopy, von Jaeger actually suggested the change was originally a "hilling" of the optic disc.[52] Specific changes discussed below occur in GON are seen at the various layers of the optic nerve head, glial cells and extracellular matrix.

Nerve Fiber Layer

Axonal loss in glaucoma is observed as a decreased density of the nerve fiber

layer observable by ophthalmoscopy or nerve fiber imaging such as scanning laser polarimetry, optical coherence tomography, or Heidelberg Retinal Tomograph.[53] Observable areas of nerve fiber defects correspond to axonal loss. It is of importance for clinicians to be aware that nerve fiber layer changes precede visual field changes detectable on static and kinetic perimetry.[54] In one study of 1344 eyes with elevated intraocular pressure, clinically observed nerve fiber layer loss occurred in 83 subject and of these 60 percent of eyes had nerve fiber layer loss found six years prior to a detectable visual field loss by Goldmann perimetry.[55] A histological study of patients with well documented glaucoma revealed that there needed to be at least a 25 to 35 percent loss of RGC to be associated with a significant visual field loss by automated Humphrey perimetry.[56]

Ophthalmoscopic examination of the optic nerve head may reveal notching, neural retinal rim loss, general cup enlargement and/or deepening, increased peripapillary atrophy and possible optic disc margin.[57] Glaucomatous optic disc changes are unique from other forms of optic atrophy in that the optic nerve head has an enlarging cup, but the color of the remaining neuroretinal rim remains normal.[21,22] The enlargement of the cup results from the loss of the axons and the neuroretinal rim at the optic nerve head and is accompanied by bowing of the lamina cribrosa posteriorly. In the advanced stages, the bowing results in the typical "bean pot" configuration of the optic nerve that has been associated with glaucoma as demonstrated in **Figures 4A and B**. It has been suggested that optic disc damage in glaucoma could be grouped into distinctive patterns. Four distinctive forms of glaucomatous cupping described include: focal glaucomatous with focal neuroretinal rim loss, myopic glaucomatous, senile sclerotic

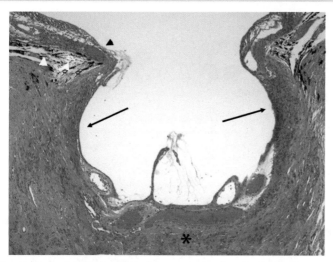

Fig. 4A Microphotograph showing optic nerve cupping in advanced glaucoma. Note the beanpot bowing of the lamina (black arrows) and laminar disorganization at the base (*). There is retinal nerve fiber layer atrophy (black arrowhead) and peripapillary atrophy also noted (white arrowhead). (Hematoxylin and eosin)

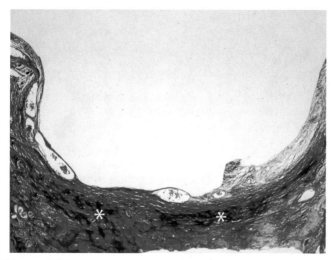

Fig. 4B Masson Trichrome staining highlighting the disorganization of the collagen in the laminar beams (*) (stains blue). (Original magnification x 4)

The peripapillary zone of nerve fiber layer undergoes characteristic chorioretinal atrophy in glaucoma known as peripapillary atrophy. Peripapillary atrophy has two distinct zones. The peripheral zone, or alpha zone, is distinguished by thinning of the chorioretinal tissue and irregular retinal pigmentation. The central zone, or beta zone, is an area of atrophy and thinning of the retinal pigment epithelium and underlying choriocapillaris allowing visibility of underlying sclera and choroidal vessels; occasionally even the circle of Zinn-Haller is visualized. Peripapillary atrophy is not pathognomic for glaucoma. It occurs in the normal population with a frequency of alpha zone presence estimated at 15 to 20 percent. The peripapillary atrophy of glaucoma is notable in the sense that the beta zone generally increases in size with disease severity, compared to normal and nonglaucomatous optic neuropathies. In addition, it is correlated with being greatest in the same quadrant corresponding to neuroretinal rim loss.[60,61]

Laminar Changes

Histopathological changes of the laminar portion of the optic nerve head show backward and lateral movement of the lamina include cribrosa (also known as bowing), remodeling of the extracellular matrix of the lamina cribrosa, and Schnabel cavernous degeneration in the prelaminar and postlaminar regions in which the space formerly occupied by the nerve fascicles is replaced by mucopolysaccharide.[21,22,62,63] In addition, the lamina cribrosa becomes less compliant (or stiffer) in glaucomatous eyes.[64] Recent advances in ocular imaging utilizing noninvasive three-dimensional high-speed optical coherence tomography have demonstrated the structure of the lamina cribrosa sheets and their bowing in patients with glaucoma and ocular hypertension.[65] On histopathologic examination, the optic

and generalized enlargement of the optic disc.[57]

Retinal hemorrhages at the optic disc margin are a feature that can be seen in most forms of glaucoma but more commonly in normal tension glaucoma and are a distinct risk factor for progression of visual field loss.[58] These hemorrhages are linear or flame-shaped and are typically seen at the optic disc margin. The hemorrhages follow the surface nerve fiber layer pattern arising from the prelaminar region of the optic nerve head.[59] The exact etiology of these hemorrhages remains undetermined. However, many theories have been proposed, most related to the mechanical effect of IOP on the capillaries, in addition to the possible role of loss of support cells leading to stretch and tear of optic nerve head capillaries, turbulence of blood flow at the optic nerve head and recently a weakness of the blood-brain barrier at the prelaminar region.[21,22,28,38,59] nerve head of patients with normal-pressure glaucoma demonstrated Schnabel's cavernous degeneration.[63]

Glial Changes

The role of glial cell changes in the pathogenesis of glaucoma has been extensively studied. For example, studies of gene expression using cDNA microarray of Type 1B astrocytes found a fivefold increase in the expression of 150 genes in glaucomatous eyes when compared to normal eyes. Isolating these genes and learning the role of their products will continue to enhance the understanding of how glial cells function.[66]

Astrocyte Changes

The type 1B astrocytes of the optic nerve head become "reactive" in glaucoma. These astrocytes undergo hypertrophy, hyperplasia and demonstrate increased expression of GFAP. The cells redistribute themselves within the fascicles of axons they normally surround.[67,68] Reactive astrocytes in the laminar and retrolaminar portions have been found to express increased matrix metalloproteinases (MMP's), tumor necrosis factor-alpha (TNF-alpha) and TNF-alpha-1 receptor.[69] Immunoperoxidase staining demonstrating increased presence of TNF-alpha is demonstrated in **Figures 5A to C.** The ability of optic nerve head astrocytes to migrate *in vitro* increases four to six fold under hydrostatic pressure along with enhanced expression of proteolytic enzymes.[66,70]

The MMP's are enzymes that digest extracellular matrix including collagen, proteoglycan, elastin and other glycoproteins in normal and pathologic conditions.[71] In glaucoma, MMP-2 and MMP-9 are upregulated in the astrocytes of the optic nerve head.[72] MMP-9 is also believed to be involved in the breakdown of the blood-brain barrier at the optic nerve head contributing to splinter hemorrhages.[28]

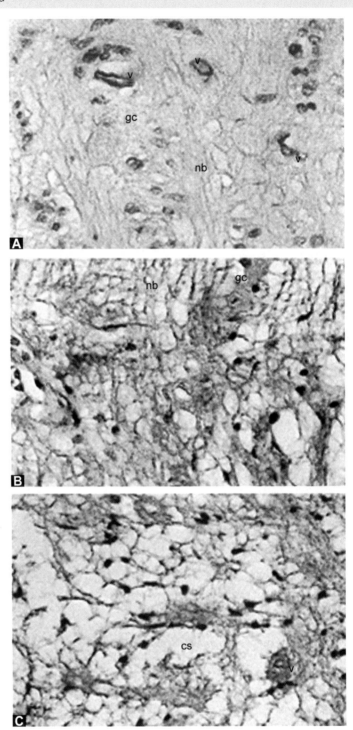

Figs 5A to C (A) Immunoperoxidase staining for TNF-alpha in the human optic nerve head shows faint immunostaining in control optic nerve head that is increased in the optic nerve with; (B) Primary-open angle glaucoma and (C) Normal-pressure glaucoma which also demonstrates cavernous spaces. TNF-alpha is among several molecules known to be expressed at increased levels in the optic nerve heads of patients with glaucoma. (GC = Glial column; NB = Nerve bundles; and CS = Cavernous spaces). (Chromagen, diaminobenzidine tetrahydrochloride, nuclear counterstain with Mayer hematoxylin, original magnification x 100) (*Courtesy*: Yan X, Tezel G, et al. Matrix metalloproteinases and tumor necrosis factor alpha in glaucomatous optic nerve head. Arch Ophthalmol 2000;118:666-73)

Microglia

Microglia are macrophage like cells of blood lineage that act to protect neural tissue and are believed to play a role in several diseases including multiple sclerosis, Alzheimer's disease, Parkinson's disease and acquired immunodeficiency syndrome dementia. In glaucoma, microglia cells activate and proliferate like astrocytes and also phagocytose, present antigens, produce neurodestructive molecules, eicosanoids and cytokines. Microglia in glaucomatous optic nerves produce increased levels of several molecules tumor growth factor-beta-2 (TGF-beta-2), TNF-alpha and proliferating cell nuclear antigens (PCNA). TGF-beta-2 is in a family of molecules that downregulates inflammation and increases remodeling of neural tissue after brain injury. TNF-alpha, in contrast to TGF-beta-2, injures the neurons by activating its receptor leading to neuronal apoptosis as well as by being directly toxic to neurons. Furthermore, molecules such as TNF-alpha can activate matrix metalloproteinases and cause weakening of the supportive matrix in neuronal tissue such as the optic nerve. The molecular expression of elevated levels of molecules such as TNF-alpha, TGF-beta-2, MMP-1, MMP-2, MMP-3, TIMP-1, PCNA, HSP27 and other molecules by microglia in glaucoma suggest that these cells play a role in the pathogenesis of glaucoma at the optic nerve head in concert with other glia cells and RGCs, but the exact relationship remains open-ended.[30]

Changes in the Extracellular Matrix

Astrocytes significantly contribute to remodeling of the extracellular matrix in glaucoma. Type 1B astrocytes from the lamina cribrosa may respond to an injurious insult such as shear and stress and may release cytokines, growth factors, cause activation of ion channels and degradation of the extracellular matrix.[62,73] The major element of the laminar extracellular matrix is elastin. Degeneration of elastin results in elastotic fibers in the lamina cribrosa found in patients with primary open angle glaucoma as well as patients with glaucoma associated with exfoliation syndrome.[74] The degeneration of the laminar extracellular matrix, particularly load-bearing connective tissue, can subsequently lead to laminar bowing, loss of axonal support and RGC axonal degeneration.[75]

Neurotrophic Support

There is growing evidence that neurotrophins play an important role for normal RGC function. Target-derived neurotrophins are transported in a retrograde fashion from the brain to the RGCs. Possibly an inhibition of retrograde transport by elevated IOP can result in neurotrophin deprivation and subsequent RGC damage. This has also been demonstrated to occur in ischemic conditions.[68] In glaucoma, it has been shown that blockade of retrograde transport of brain derived neurotrophic factor (BDNF) occurs at the optic nerve head in acute and chronic glaucoma.[76] BDNF binds the tyrosine kinase receptor B receptor (TrkB) which activates the mitogen-activated protein (MAP) kinase cascade which helps to maintain RGC's survival.[77] **Figures 6A and B** demonstrates the change in distribution of TrkB in the optic nerve head of monkeys with transected optic nerves and glaucoma. However, as in other possible contributing pathogenic mechanisms, abnormal neurotrophin axonal transport alone does not necessarily result in RGCs' death as evidenced by optic nerve recovery that can occur after prolonged papilledema.

Oxidative State

Oxidative stress has been implicated to serve a pathogenic role in many disease states such as cancer and aging. Molecular oxygen is highly stable, but reactive oxygen species (ROS) are unstable and cause cellular damage. ROS can be produced as by-products of normal metabolism or secondary messengers, or introduced by exogenous sources. The body has two forms of defensive mechanism against ROS; one is by enzymes such as glutathione peroxidase or superoxide dismutase and the other is by nonenzymatic molecules such as antioxidant vitamins or reduced

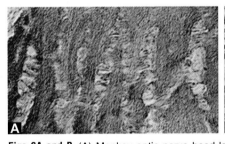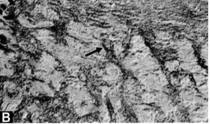

Figs 6A and B (A) Monkey optic nerve head labeled for TrkB the receptor for brain derived neuronal growth factor in normal subject shows uniform labeling of TrkB in nerve bundles and without labeling of optic nerve connective tissue; (B) After complete optic atrophy following nerve transection, the monkey optic nerve head shows increased connective tissue and zones formerly occupied by neural bundles are severely thinned; TrkB label is seen in areas known to be filled in by astrocytes (black arrow) after transection. Monkey optic nerve head with chronic, moderate glaucoma damage shows focal accumulations (black arrow) of TrkB in neural bundles compared to uniform staining of neuronal fascicle. (Magnification 240x) (*Courtesy*: Pease ME, Mckinnon SJ, et al. Obstructed Axonal Transport of BDNF and its Receptor TrkB in Experimental Glaucoma. Investigative Ophthalmology and Visual Science. 2000;41:764. *Copyright*: Association for Research in Vision and Ophthalmology)

glutathione.[51,78] There exists evidence from *in vitro* studies of the optic nerve head that astrocytes, retinal macroglia and retinal microglia have an immune response to ROS species demonstrated by increased amount MHC-II molecules.[79] In addition, decreased levels of plasma glutathione, a nonenzymatic antioxidant, have been found in patients with POAG.[78]

ADDITIONAL FACTORS IN THE PATHOGENESIS OF GLAUCOMA
Anomalous Immunity

Both humoral and cellular immunity may play a role in glaucoma. When autoantibodies against retinal, optic nerve and optic nerve head antigens were measured in high-pressure glaucoma, normal pressure glaucoma and patients without glaucoma, three distinct autoantibody patterns were identified. This signifies that there are common autoimmune phenomena in each of these patient populations.[80] There is keen interest regarding the role of the immune system in glaucoma because it is believed that if the immune system can be better regulated or even a vaccine developed to prevent or halt glaucomatous optic neuropathy.[81]

A set of autoantibodies has been found against small heat-shock proteins (HSP) (e.g. HSP-27, HSP-60 and alpha-crystallins) in patients with normal and high-tension glaucoma. These proteins are chaperone molecules that increase under conditions of ischemia and excitotoxicity. It is theorized that loss of these molecules predisposes a patient to RGC death by apoptosis.[82,83] The HSP-27 protein has been shown on immunostaining to be increased in postmortem eyes of patients with normal and high tension POAG. The majority of HSP-27 has been localized to the astrocytes of the laminar region.[84] In addition, Western blotting has demonstrated and immunohistochemistry confirmed the location of serum autoantibodies to be directed to glycosaminoglycans at the optic nerve head in normal-tension glaucoma.[85]

The first direct evidence of immune system alteration leading to GON has recently come from studies in a Lewis rat model. These rats were immunized against HSP-27 or HSP-60. These immunized rats demonstrated transient increases in T-cell levels (around day 14 and day 21 respectively) that were observed in the retinal parenchyma revealing the role of the immune system in retinal damage. These rats subsequently sustained RGC axon loss from apoptosis.[86]

Nitric Oxide

Nitric oxide (NO) is a potent mediator of cellular activity of some interest as playing a role in glaucoma as one study has identified isoforms of nitric oxide synthase in the astrocytes of the optic nerve head.[87]

Glutamate

Glutamate is a potent neurotoxin with excitotoxic effect causing over stimulation of the N-methyl-D-aspartate (NMDA) receptor. There have been several studies demonstrating elevated glutamate levels in the vitreous of humans and monkeys with glaucoma.[88-90] Studies done under similar condition have also found no difference in vitreous glutamate levels in experimental glaucomatous eyes making this an area of controversy.[91] In addition, memantine, a selective noncompetitive NMDA receptor antagonist used to treat Alzheimer's disease, was studied as a neuroprotective agent in the treatment of glaucoma in a clinical trial and the outcome was not successful.[92,93] Therefore, the role of neuroprotection though extensively studied in glaucoma, remains unclear.

SUMMARY

The accumulation of clinical, histopathologic and histochemical evidence supports the premise that the pathophysiology of glaucomatous optic neuropathy is multifactorial. The pathogenesis of glaucoma at the optic nerve head appears to involve both biomechanical and vascular components along with additional factors such as autoimmunity, oxidative stress and change in the expression of molecules in the optic nerve head microenvironment all possibly operating in concert in many glaucoma phenotypes. Future clinical and experimental research will continue to define causative mechanisms that will allow more efficacious directed therapeutic interventions of this potentially visually devastating disease.

REFERENCES

1. Agapova OA, Ricard CS, et al. Expression of matrix metalloproteinases and tissue inhibitors of metalloproteinases in human optic nerve head astrocytes. Glia 2001;33:205-16.
2. Anderson DR. Ultrastructure of human and monkey lamina cribrosa and optic nerve head. Arch Ophthalmol 1969;82:800-14.
3. Anderson DR. Ultrastructure of the optic nerve head. Arch Ophthalmol 1970;83:63-73.
4. Anderson DR, Hoyt HF. Ultrastructure of intraorbital portion of human and monkey optic nerve. Arch Ophthalmol 1969;82:506-30.
5. Berdahl JP, Allingham RR, et al. Cerebrospinal fluid pressure is decreased in primary open-angle glaucoma. Ophthalmology 2008;115:763-8.

6. Broadway DC, Nicolela M, et al. Optic disc appearances in primary open-angle glaucoma. Survey of ophthalmology 1999;43(Suppl 1):S223-43.

7. Burgoyne CF, Downs JC, et al. The optic nerve head as a biomechanical structure: a new paradigm for understanding the role of IOP-related stress and strain in the pathophysiology of glaucomatous optic nerve head damage. Prog Retin Eye Res 2005;24:39-73.

8. Cioffi G. Ischemic model of optic nerve injury. Transactions of the American Ophthalmological Society 2005;103:592-613.

9. Cioffi GA. Three common assumptions about ocular blood flow and glaucoma. Survey of ophthalmology 2001;45(Suppl 3):S325-31; discussion S332-4.

10. Dandona L, Quigley HA, et al. Quantitative regional structure of the normal human lamina cribrosa. A racial comparison. Arch Ophthalmol 1990;108:393-8.

11. Dichtl A, Jonas JB, et al. Course of the optic nerve fibers through the lamina cibrosa in human eyes. Graefes Arch Clin Exp Ophthalmol 1996;234:581-5.

12. Drance SM. Disc hemorrhages in the glaucomas. Survey of ophthalmology 1989;33:331-7.

13. Dreyer EB, Zurakowski D, et al. Elevated glutamate levels in the vitreous body of humans and monkeys with glaucoma. Arch Ophthalmol 1996;114:299-305.

14. Emre M, Orgül S, et al. Increased plasma endothelin-1 levels in patients with progressive open angle glaucoma. British Journal of Ophthalmology 2005;89:60-3.

15. Fechtner RD, Weinreb R. Mechanisms of optic nerve damage in primary open angle glaucoma. Survey of ophthalmology 1994;39:23-42.

16. Flammer J, Mozaffarieh M. What is the present pathogenetic concept of glaucomatous optic neuropathy? Survey of ophthalmology 2007;52(Suppl 2): S162-73.

17. Fledelius H. Optic disc size: are methodological factors taken into account? Acta Ophthalmologica 2008.pp.1-2.

18. Gherghel D. Systemic Reduction in Glutathione Levels Occurs in Patients with Primary Open-Angle Glaucoma. Investigative Ophthalmology and Visual Science 2005;46:877-83.

19. Goldbaum MH, Jeng SY, et al. The extracellular matrix of the human optic nerve. Arch Ophthalmol 1989; 107:1225-31.

20. Grieshaber MC, Flammer J. Does the blood-brain barrier play a role in Glaucoma? Survey of ophthalmology 2007;52(Suppl 2):S115-21.

21. Halpern DL, Grosskreutz CL. Glaucomatous optic neuropathy: mechanisms of disease. Ophthalmology clinics of North America 2002;15:61-8.

22. Hayreh SS. Inter-individual variation in blood supply of the optic nerve head. Its importance in various ischemic disorders of the optic nerve head and glaucoma, low-tension glaucoma and allied disorders. Documenta ophthalmologica Advances in ophthalmology 1985;59:217-46.

23. Hernandez M, Agapova O, et al. Differential gene expression in astrocytes from human normal and glaucomatous optic nerve head analyzed by cDNA microarray. Glia 2002;38: 45-64.

24. Hernandez MR. The optic nerve head in glaucoma: role of astrocytes in tissue remodeling. Prog Retin Eye Res 2000;19:297-321.

25. Hernandez MR, Igoe F, et al. Cell culture of the human lamina cribrosa. Investigative Ophthalmology & Visual Science 1988;29:78-89.

26. Hernandez MR, Pena JD. The optic nerve head in glaucomatous optic neuropathy. Arch Ophthalmol 1997; 115:389-95.

27. Hernandez MR, Wang N, et al. Localization of collagen types I and IV mRNAs in human optic nerve head by *in situ* hybridization. Investigative Ophthalmology and Visual Science 1991;32:2169-77.

28. Hoffmann EM, Zangwill LM, et al. Optic disc size and glaucoma. Survey of ophthalmology 2007;52:32-49.

29. Honkanen RA, Baruah S, et al. Vitreous amino acid concentrations in patients with glaucoma undergoing vitrectomy. Arch Ophthalmol 2003;121:183-8.

30. Inoue R, Hangai M, et al. Three-dimensional high-speed optical coherence tomography imaging of lamina cribrosa in glaucoma. Ophthalmology 2009;116:214-22.

31. Ishida K, Yamamoto T, et al. Disc hemorrhage is a significantly negative prognostic factor in normal-tension glaucoma. AJOPHT 2000;129:707-14.

32. Jaeger Ev. "Ueber Glaucom und seine Heilung durch Iridectomie." Z Ges der Aerzte zu Wien 1858;14(1858).

33. Jeffery G, Evans A, et al. The human optic nerve: fascicular organization and connective tissue types along the extra-fascicular matrix. Anat Embryol 1995;191:491-502.

34. Joachim S, Pfeiffer N, et al. Autoantibodies in patients with glaucoma: a comparison of IgG serum antibodies against retinal, optic nerve and optic nerve head antigens. Graefe's Arch Clin Exp Ophthalmol 2005;243:817-23.

35. Jonas JB. Clinical implications of peripapillary atrophy in glaucoma. Current opinion in ophthalmology 2005;16:84-8.

36. Jonas JB, Budde WM. Diagnosis and pathogenesis of glaucomatous optic neuropathy: morphological aspects. Prog Retin Eye Res 2000;19:1-40.

37. Jonas JB, Mardin CY, et al. Morphometry of the human lamina cribrosa surface. Investigative Ophthalmology and Visual Science 1991;32:401-5.

38. Jonas JB, Thomas R, et al. Optic disc morphology in south India: the

Vellore Eye Study. British Journal of Ophthalmology 2003;87:189-96.

39. Kerrigan-Baumrind LA, Quigley HA, et al. Number of ganglion cells in glaucoma eyes compared with threshold visual field tests in the same persons. Investigative Ophthalmology and Visual Science 2000;41:741-8.

40. Kim TW, Kang KB, et al. Elevated glutamate levels in the vitreous body of an *in vivo* model of optic nerve ischemia. Arch Ophthalmol 2000;118:533-6.

41. Levin LA. Pathophysiology of the progressive optic neuropathy of glaucoma. Ophthalmology clinics of North America 2005;18:355-64.

42. Levin LA, Peeples P. History of neuroprotection and rationale as a therapy for glaucoma. The American journal of managed care 2008; 14:S11-4.

43. Mackenzie P, Cioffi G. Vascular anatomy of the optic nerve head. Can J Ophthalmol 2008;43:308-12.

44. Minckler DS. The organization of nerve fiber bundles in the primate optic nerve head. Arch Ophthalmol 1980;98:1630-6.

45. Minckler DS. Histology of optic nerve damage in ocular hypertension and early glaucoma. Survey of ophthalmology 1989;33(Suppl):401-2; discussion 409-11.

46. Morgan JE, Jeffery G, et al. Axon deviation in the human lamina cribrosa. British Journal of Ophthalmology 1998;82:680-3.

47. Morgan WH, Yu DY, et al. The role of cerebrospinal fluid pressure in glaucoma pathophysiology: the dark side of the optic disc. J Glaucoma 2008;17:408-13.

48. Müler H. "Ueber Nervean-Veranderungen an der Eintrittsstelle des Schnerven." Archives of Ophthalmology 1858(4).

49. Nangia V, Matin A, et al. Optic disc size in a population-based study in central India: the Central India Eye and Medical Study (CIEMS). Acta Ophthalmologica 2008;86(1):103-4.

50. Neufeld AH. Microglia in the optic nerve head and the region of parapapillary chorioretinal atrophy in glaucoma. Arch Ophthalmol 1999;117:1050-6.

51. Neufeld AH, Hernandez MR, et al. Nitric oxide synthase in the human glaucomatous optic nerve head. Arch Ophthalmol 1997;115:497-503.

52. Noske W, Hensen J, et al. Endothelin-like immunoreactivity in aqueous humor of patients with primary open-angle glaucoma and cataract. Graefes Arch Clin Exp Ophthalmol 1997;235:551-2.

53. Oku H, Sugiyama T, et al. Experimental optic cup enlargement caused by endothelin-1-induced chronic optic nerve head ischemia. Survey of Ophthalmology 1999; 44(Suppl 1): S74-84.

54. Orgül S, Cioffi GA, et al. An endothelin-1-induced model of chronic optic nerve ischemia in rhesus monkeys. J Glaucoma 1996;5:135-8.

55. Orgül S, Cioffi GA, et al. An endothelin-1-induced model of optic nerve ischemia in the rabbit. Investigative Ophthalmology and Visual Science 1996;37:1860-9.

56. Osborne NN. Recent clinical findings with memantine should not mean that the idea of neuroprotection in glaucoma is abandoned. Acta Ophthalmologica 2009;87:450-4.

57. Oyama T, Abe H, et al. The connective tissue and glial framework in the optic nerve head of the normal human eye: light and scanning electron microscopic studies. Arch Histol Cytol 2006;69:341-56.

58. Pease ME, Mckinnon SJ, et al. Obstructed Axonal Transport of BDNF and Its Receptor TrkB in Experimental Glaucoma. Investigative Ophthalmology and Visual Science 2000;41:764.

59. Pena JD, Agapova O, et al. Increased elastin expression in astrocytes of the lamina cribrosa in response to elevated intraocular pressure. Investigative Ophthalmology and Visual Science 2001;42:2303-14.

60. Pena JD, Netland PA, et al. Elastosis of the lamina cribrosa in glaucomatous optic neuropathy. Experimental Eye Research 1998;67:517-24.

61. Pernet V, Hauswirth W, et al. Extracellular signal-regulated kinase 1/2 mediates survival, but not axon regeneration, of adult injured central nervous system neurons *in vivo*. J Neurochem 2005;93:72-83.

62. Piltz-Seymour JR, Grunwald JE, et al. Optic nerve blood flow is diminished in eyes of primary open-angle glaucoma suspects. AJOPHT 2001;132:63-9.

63. Quigley HA, Addicks EM. Regional differences in the structure of the lamina cribrosa and their relation to glaucomatous optic nerve damage. Arch Ophthalmol 1981;99:137-43.

64. Quigley HA, Addicks EM, et al. Optic nerve damage in human glaucoma. III. Quantitative correlation of nerve fiber loss and visual field defect in glaucoma, ischemic neuropathy, papilledema and toxic neuropathy. Arch Ophthalmol 1982;100:135-46.

65. Quigley HA, Addicks EM, et al. Optic nerve damage in human glaucoma. II. The site of injury and susceptibility to damage. Arch Ophthalmol 1981;99:635-49.

66. Quigley HA, Brown AE, et al. The size and shape of the optic disc in normal human eyes. Arch Ophthalmol 1990;108:51-7.

67. Radius RL, Gonzales M. Anatomy of the lamina cribrosa in human eyes. Arch Ophthalmol 1981;99: 2159-62.

68. Rao VR, Krishnamoorthy RR, et al. Endothelin-1-mediated regulation of extracellular matrix collagens in cells of human lamina

cribrosa. Experimental Eye Research 2008;86:886-94.

69. Reeves C, Taylor D. A history of the optic nerve and its diseases. Eye (London, England) 2004;18:1096-109.

70. Ridet JL, Malhotra SK, et al. Reactive astrocytes: cellular and molecular cues to biological function. Trends Neurosci 1997;20:570-7.

71. Schwartz M. Modulating the immune system: a vaccine for glaucoma? Can J Ophthalmol 2007;42:439-41.

72. Sigal IA, Ethier CR, Biomechanics of the optic nerve head. Experimental Eye Research 2009;88:799-807.

73. Sommer A, Katz J, et al. Clinically detectable nerve fiber atrophy precedes the onset of glaucomatous field loss. Arch Ophthalmol 1991;109:77-83.

74. Strouthidis NG, Yang H, et al. "Comparison of clinical and three-dimensional histomorphometric optic disc margin anatomy." Invest. Ophthalmol Vis Sci 2009; 50(5):2165-74.

75. Tarabishy AB, Alexandrou TJ, et al. Syndrome of myelinated retinal nerve fibers, myopia and amblyopia: a review. Survey of ophthalmology 2007;52:588-96.

76. Tezel G, Edward DP, et al. Serum autoantibodies to optic nerve head glycosaminoglycans in patients with glaucoma. Arch Ophthalmol 1999;117:917-24.

77. Tezel G, Hernandez MR, et al. *In vitro* evaluation of reactive astrocyte migration, a component of tissue remodeling in glaucomatous optic nerve head. Glia 2001;34:178-89.

78. Tezel G, Hernandez R, et al. Immunostaining of heat shock proteins in the retina and optic nerve head of normal and glaucomatous eyes. Arch Ophthalmol 2000;118: 511-8.

79. Tezel G, Seigel GM, et al. Autoantibodies to small heat shock proteins in glaucoma. Investigative Ophthalmology and Visual Science 1998;39:2277-87.

80. Tezel G, Wax MB. Hypoxia-inducible factor 1alpha in the glaucomatous retina and optic nerve head. Arch Ophthalmol 2004;122:1348-56.

81. Tezel G, Wax MB. Glaucoma. Chemical immunology and allergy 2007;92:221-7.

82. Tezel G, Yang X, et al. Mechanisms of Immune System Activation in Glaucoma: Oxidative Stress-Stimulated Antigen Presentation by the Retina and Optic Nerve Head Glia. Investigative Ophthalmology and Visual Science 2007;48:705-14.

83. Tso MO, Shih CY, et al. Is there a blood-brain barrier at the optic nerve head? Arch Ophthalmol 1975;93: 815-25.

84. Varma R, Tielsch JM, et al. Race-, age-, gender- and refractive error-related differences in the normal optic disc. Arch Ophthalmol 1994;112:1068-76.

85. Wamsley S, Gabelt BT, et al. Vitreous glutamate concentration and axon loss in monkeys with experimental glaucoma. Arch Ophthalmol 2005; 123:64-70.

86. Wax MB, Tezel G, et al. Clinical and ocular histopathological findings in a patient with normal-pressure glaucoma. Arch Ophthalmol 1998;116:993-1001.

87. Wax MB, Tezel G, et al. Induced auto-immunity to heat shock proteins elicits glaucomatous loss of retinal ganglion cell neurons via activated T-cell-derived fas-ligand. Journal of Neuroscience 2008;28:12085-96.

88. Woessner JF. Matrix metalloproteinases and their inhibitors in connective tissue remodeling. FASEB J 1991;5:2145-54.

89. Yan X, Tezel G, et al. Matrix metalloproteinases and tumor necrosis factor alpha in glaucomatous optic nerve head. Arch Ophthalmol 2000;118:666-73.

90. Ye H, Yang J, et al. Localization of collagen type III mRNA in normal human optic nerve heads. Experimental Eye Research 1994;58:53-63.

91. Yuan L, Neufeld AH, Activated microglia in the human glaucomatous optic nerve head. J Neurosci Res 2001;64:523-32.

92. Zangwill LM, Bowd C. Retinal nerve fiber layer analysis in the diagnosis of glaucoma. Current opinion in ophthalmology 2006;17:120-31.

93. Zeimer RC, Ogura Y. The relation between glaucomatous damage and optic nerve head mechanical compliance. Arch Ophthalmol 1989;107:1232-4.

6

Clinical Trials in Glaucoma

Valliammai Muthappan, Alan L Robin, A Jayaprakash Patil, Deepak P Edward

OVERVIEW OF MAJOR GLAUCOMA CLINICAL TRIALS

Valliammai Muthappan, Alan L Robin

Prior to the late 1980s, the practice of glaucoma suffered from a lack of clinical evidence backing up medical practice. To address this lack of evidence in daily therapeutic decisions, several large prospective clinical trials were organized. The careful design of these trials has limitations, but minimizes bias and the large sample sizes have adequate statistical power to answer pressing clinical questions relating to the treatment paradigms and the natural history of glaucoma. The regulations governing such trials ensured patient benefit and safety. The primary goals of these studies were to assess functional vision and visual field preservation, rather than IOP lowering alone. Clinical trials to date have addressed the spectrum of glaucomatous disease,

from ocular hypertension covered by the Ocular Hypertension Treatment Study (OHTS) to the Advanced Glaucoma Intervention Study (AGIS).[1] This chapter will discuss several of the seminal trials **(Table 1)**.

COLLABORATIVE INITIAL GLAUCOMA TREATMENT STUDY[2-15]

In 1993, the Collaborative Initial Glaucoma Treatment Study (CIGTS) was started to determine whether medical treatment or filtering surgery was more effective as the initial treatment in the patient with newly diagnosed open angle glaucoma. Smaller studies prior to this one had brought into question the practice of treating all newly diagnosed primary open angle glaucoma (POAG) with medical

therapy. Given the side effects of topical medications, quality of life with glaucoma therapy was studied as well.

Over 600 subjects were randomized to medication versus filtering surgery and followed for five years. If both eyes were eligible for the study, they were randomized to the same group. Recruited subjects ranged from age 25 to 75 with intraocular pressure (IOP) of 20 mm Hg or greater and evidence of optic nerve damage or visual field loss; patients with primary open-angle, pigmentary and pseudoexfoliation glaucoma but no other causes were eligible. The primary outcome was visual field changes and secondarily measured were quality of life by phone interviews, visual acuity, intraocular pressure and cataract development.

Table 1 Summary of studies (POAG = Primary open angle glaucoma; No. = Number)

Study	Disease	No. of subjects	Major findings
CIGTS	Newly diagnosed POAG	607	Filtering surgery and medical treatment equivalent at limiting progression at 5 years
EMGT	Newly diagnosed POAG	255	Early IOP lowering in newly diagnosed primary open glaucoma reduced risk of progression
OHTS	Ocular hypertension	1637	Treating ocular hypertensives prevented progression to glaucoma. Reduced central corneal thickness, advanced age, increased cup to disc ratio, IOP and pattern standard deviation are all risk factors for developing in an ocular hypertensive
AGIS	Advanced glaucoma	591 (789 eyes)	Treatment sequence starting with argon laser therapy was more beneficial for black patients while treatment starting with trabeculectomy was more beneficial for white patients. Mean IOPs below 14 mm Hg limited glaucoma progression
CNTGS	Normal tension glaucoma	230	IOP lowering therapy will reduce the rate of glaucomatous progression in normal tension glaucoma, though the presence of cataracts may obscure this effect

Patients in the medical treatment group were started on a single agent, generally a beta-blocker (as prostaglandin analogs had not yet entered clinical practice), with additional medications added for intraocular pressure control or evidence of progressive visual field loss. If maximum medical therapy failed to control progression, the subject underwent procedural interventions per conventional therapy, starting with laser trabeculoplasty and culminating with trabeculectomy as the final intervention. For the surgical treatment group, patients had immediate trabeculectomy. If the surgery failed, argon laser trabeculoplasty was tried and finally medical treatment was used.

The study found significant and sustained reduction in IOP in both arms, with few long-term disabling complications or major side effects from either surgery or medical therapy. Pressures in the medical treatment group were 17 to 18 mm Hg, showing a reduction of 38 percent; the surgical group had lower IOPs of 14 to 15 mm Hg, which was a reduction of 46 percent. Though in the first-three years, the surgical group had greater visual acuity loss as a result of lens opacification, over time results from both groups converged. At five years, visual field loss was 10.7 percent in the medical group and 13.5 percent in the surgical group. Of note, the rate of cataract removal was higher in the surgically treated group. The overall rate of progression was lower in this trial than in previous clinical studies, possibly as a result of more aggressive IOP goals and studying patients with earlier stage of disease.

From 43 symptoms surveyed in the quality of life aspect of this study, 12 visual function and local eye symptoms (blurred vision, problem with bright lights, problems with step as well as foreign body sensation, droopy lid) were significantly more in the surgical group and seven systemic symptoms (drowsiness, headache, wheezing, nausea, altered taste and smell, weight loss and dizziness) were significantly more in the medical group. Despite the symptomatic complaints, at 6 and 24 months, the surgical patients appeared happier. Approximately, half of patients initially were concerned they would go blind, but this feeling declined to only 25 percent of patients over time. This is still a marked number of patients, especially in a controlled study with many follow-up visits and much counseling from technicians, study coordinators and physicians.

Conclusion

Stringent IOP lowering minimizes visual field and disc progression. Both initial surgical and medical therapies can cause changes in the quality of life, but the changes are different for each initial therapy. Both filtering surgery and medical treatment strategies produced equivalent outcomes at five years of follow-up.

EARLY MANIFEST GLAUCOMA TRIAL[16-25]

The Early Manifest Glaucoma Trial started recruitment in 1993 to evaluate the effect of immediate IOP lowering as opposed to observation or delayed treatment in patients with newly diagnosed primary open-angle glaucoma (POAG). The study was supported by the United States National Eye Institute, but was performed primarily in two Swedish cities. The primary outcome was progression of glaucoma defined as worsening of the visual and/or increased optic disc cupping according to specified criteria. Secondarily studied were the extent of IOP reduction by medications, the characteristics that may influence glaucoma progression and the natural history of newly diagnosed POAG. This was the first trial to look at treatment of POAG as opposed to observation (unlike CIGTS, which compared medical treatment to surgery for POAG).

Over 250 patients between ages 50 and 80 were randomized to treatment or observation and followed for at least four years. The diagnosis of POAG was confirmed by two HVF tests and then randomization was performed to betaxolol with argon laser trabeculoplasty or no initial treatment. Patients with advanced visual loss, mean IOP greater than 30 or one IOP greater than 35 and visual acuity less than 20/40 were excluded.

HVF and IOP were obtained every three months while disc photographs were taken every six months. The visual fields and optic disc photos were evaluated by masked readers at designated centers. Additional follow-up visits were scheduled as necessary to confirm visual field progression and IOP elevation. If a patient in the treatment group had IOP > 25 mm Hg at two or more visits, latanoprost was prescribed. Similar treatment was given in the observation group for IOP >35 mm Hg at any visit. For continued elevation of IOP, individual treatment was prescribed.

In this study, 62 percent of observed or delayed treatment subjects progressed to glaucoma as compared to 45 percent of early treatment patients. Risk factors for progression included lack of treatment, older patients, higher IOP, pseudoexfoliation syndrome and bilateral disease as well as more severe visual field defects at baseline. Positive family history, refractive error, gender, blood pressure and remarkably, corneal thickness were not related to progression in this study. The relationship between IOP and progression was highlighted in the results of this study: per 1 mm Hg pressure reduction, there was a 10 percent decrease in progression; per each mm Hg elevation in IOP as measured at three months, there was

a 10 percent increase in progression. Consistently elevated IOPs caused a 13 percent increase in progression per mm Hg IOP elevation. Although not all eyes with optic disc hemorrhages progressed, their presence increased the risk of progression. As a side effect, nuclear sclerotic and cortical lens changes were seen more in the treated group.

Conclusion

IOP lowering in newly diagnosed primary open angle glaucoma significantly reduced risk of progression from 62 to 45 percent. However, the 45 percent rate of progression may be unacceptable in a large-scale population. Further work might be needed to better define the reasons that almost one-half of the treatment arm progressed during this relatively short period.

OCULAR HYPERTENSION TREATMENT STUDY[26-43]

Between 1994 and 1996, the ocular hypertension treatment study (OHTS) recruited over a thousand patients to evaluate the efficacy and safety of topical antihypertensive drops in preventing or delaying the onset of visual field loss and optic nerve damage in patients with elevated IOP. It should be noted that this study did not address the question of IOP lowering in delaying the onset, but whether medical therapy, given the problems of adherence and tolerability, could delay the onset. As a large prospective trial, OHTS was also designed to identify risk factors that predicted the development of POAG in ocular hypertensives, as well as characteristics of those patients who would benefit from early medical treatment.

The trial enrolled over 1600 subjects and intentionally enrolled nearly 25 percent African-Americans. African-Americans had been previously shown

to have a greater prevalence of open-angle glaucoma than white patients. The subjects in OHTS were followed for at least five years. The enrollees were between ages 40 and 80 with normal Humphrey visual fields (HVF) 30-2, normal optic discs and an untreated IOP of 25 to 32 mm Hg in the qualifying eye with an IOP of 21 to 32 mm Hg in the fellow eye. Excluded were patients with vision less than 20/40 in one or both eyes, previous ocular surgery, co-morbid diseases, secondary etiologies for elevated IOP including narrow angles and other ocular diseases that could cause progressive vision loss including diabetic retinopathy.

The patients were randomized to observation or any combination of topical medications. Biannual HVFs as well as annual dilated exam and optic disc photos were obtained. The treatment goal was to lower IOP by at least 20 percent, and the primary endpoint was reproducible visual field changes on three consecutive HVFs or progressive optic disc damage in either eye as determined by the masked photo readers. Secondary endpoints studied the utility of short wavelength automated perimetry (SWAP), as well as confocal scanning laser ophthalmoscopy (HRT), central corneal thickness and corneal endothelial cell counts.

This study unmasked several previously unknown findings. Hazard ratios showed increased risk with age (22%), IOP (10%), pattern standard deviation on HVF (27% for each 0.2 dB increase), horizontal cup to disc ratio (27% for each 0.1 increase), vertical cup to disc ratio (32% per 0.1 increase). A strong risk was associated with low central corneal thickness, with a hazard ratio of 81 percent per 40 microns decrease. Central corneal thickness was found to be 24 microns thinner on average in African-Americans (554 microns) than in all other groups combined

(578 microns). The only possible protective factor was found to be a history of diabetes mellitus with a hazard ratio of 37 percent. Many have postulated that this finding has been discounted due to the small number of subjects who had diabetes in the study and the study design, which excluded those with diabetic retinopathy and used self-reporting of diabetes rather than a documented medical diagnosis.

OHTS attained the goal for IOP lowering on treated subjects, with a 22.5 percent mean reduction; in the observation group, there was a 4.0 percent lowering. Correspondingly, only 4.4 percent of treated patients progressed to POAG compared to 9.5 percent of observed patients. Interestingly, patients with thicker corneas did not respond as well to beta-blockers. However, there was little evidence of increased systemic or ocular risk associated with the topical IOP lowering medications in either group.

The results also brought the interpretation and reproducibility of HVF testing. Of the over 21,000 regular follow-up visual fields performed, 745 were tests performed to confirm an abnormality on a reliable field. On retesting, the abnormality was not confirmed in 85.9 percent of the originally abnormal and reliable fields. Even from the initial visual field data, many abnormalities were not verified on retest. This uncovers a problem with the use of visual field testing as a marker of disease progression.

Conclusion

Treating ocular hypertensives prevented progression to glaucoma. The rate of conversion depended upon various factors, but surprisingly, one of the most important is central corneal thickness. Reduced central corneal thickness, advanced age, increased cup-to-disc ratio, IOP and pattern standard deviation on

HVF are all risk factors for conversion from ocular hypertensive to glaucoma.

ADVANCED GLAUCOMA INTERVENTION STUDY (AGIS)[44-55]

After the advent of laser trabeculoplasty, the question was raised of whether filtration surgery or a laser trabeculoplasty should be first line of non-medical intervention following trial with maximal tolerated medical therapy with inadequate IOP lowering. AGIS was designed to compare different procedural treatment sequences for patients with medically uncontrolled disease. The study began enrolling patients in 1988 and completed recruitment in 1992.

The trial included 789 eyes in 591 patients between ages 35 and 80 whose disease was not controlled by maximum medical therapy. The eyes were followed for at least five years. A successful IOP lowering was considered an IOP of 18 mm Hg or less. Each eye was randomized to one of two treatment sequences. In the first group, patients initially received argon laser trabeculoplasty. If this failed to control IOP, the subject's eye underwent trabeculectomy and if there was further failure trabeculectomy was repeated (ATT). The second group (TAT) started trabeculectomy and then graduated argon laser trabeculoplasty followed by repeat trabeculectomy in case of progressive treatment failures. Antifibrotic agents were used in eyes with previous invasive surgery. If a subject failed all three steps, further management was decided on an individual basis.

After the initial intervention, follow-up examinations were scheduled at one week, four weeks, three months and six months, and at six-month intervals thereafter. After subsequent interventions, patients were seen at one and four weeks. Additional visits were scheduled as necessary. The primary outcome was

not IOP lowering, but instead visual function decline, including either visual field loss or visual acuity loss attributable to no other cause than glaucoma. Also studied were sustained decrease in vision, failure rate of interventions, number of prescribed topical drops and IOP, reproducibility of perimetric loss. Additionally, supplementary study investigation of filtering bleb encapsulation was performed.

A multitude of findings and papers came out of AGIS and will be discussed by order of publication:

AGIS 1

In 1994, the first paper published the study design, methods and baseline characteristics required inclusion and exclusion of subjects.

AGIS 2

This paper presented the derivation of a visual field defect score that was based on the number and depth of adjacent depressed test points.

AGIS 3

The specific differences in baseline characteristics of white and black subjects were published, highlighting that while IOP and visual acuity were similar among whites and blacks, visual field defects were more severe in black subjects at baseline. There were significant differences in education level, marital status and family support systems between the two groups.

AGIS 4

In seven years of follow-up, mean IOP decreased more in the TAT group and failure was more likely after the first intervention in the ATT group. In black patients, the ATT sequence had less progression in visual field defects, less decrease in visual acuity and decrease in vision. In white patients, the TAT treatment sequence had more favorable results in the long-term, though initially the ATT sequence initially had better visual field defects and visual acuity outcomes. This was one of the first National Institute of Health studies finding a difference in treatments among racial groups.

AGIS 5

In eyes with previous ALT, the rate of encapsulated bleb formation was 18.5 percent, while the rate was 14.5 percent in eyes without previous ALT. However, this was not a statistically significant difference (p = 0.23). Additional findings showed a higher mean IOP in eyes without an encapsulated bleb at four weeks postoperation, but with re-initiation of topical therapy, the IOPs converged at one year.

AGIS 6

While visual fields and function improved after cataract removal, adjusting for this factor did not significantly change the conclusion that the ATT sequence is better for black patients while TAT had better outcomes for whites.

AGIS 7

Ad-hoc analyzes found eyes with mean IOPs greater than 17.5 mm Hg and averaged approximately 12 mm Hg had more worsening of the visual fields than eyes whose mean IOPs stayed below 14 mm Hg; this difference was seen in an analysis at two years and the worsening was even greater at seven years. Similarly, eyes whose pressures were always less than 18 mm Hg had nearly no mean change in visual defect scores while eyes with fewer than 50 percent of visits at 18 mm Hg had increasingly worse scores at two and seven years.

AGIS 8

Having a first trabeculectomy, regardless of prior ALT, increased the risk for cataract formation by 78 percent, though this was reduced to 47 percent

in patients who had no complications with the surgery while those with complications had a 104 percent risk. The increased risk of lens opacities and impairment was seen in CIGTS, the Collaborative Normal Tension Glaucoma study and the Early Manifest Glaucoma study also. A history of diabetes increased the risk of cataracts by 47 percent and each increased year of age at the time of study entry elevated the risk by seven percent.

AGIS 9

The risk of failure of first intervention was higher for whites than blacks in the ATT sequence, while the opposite was true in the TAT sequence, indicating that ALT may be preferred to trabeculectomy as the first procedural intervention in blacks who have failed medical therapy.

AGIS 10

Data from the study suggested the counterintuitive notion that partial notching of the optic disc rim was a lower risk for visual field loss than no notching of the disc. In a review of 26 disc photos, 11 photos had at least 93 percent agreement on degree of notching by the reviewing ophthalmologists. Subsequently, ten ophthalmologists re-graded the photographs with 80 percent agreement with previous classifications. The investigators recommended establishing a photographic classification of rim-notching to standardize findings.

AGIS 11

Factors associated with failure of ALT are younger age and higher IOP. Diabetes, postoperative complications, younger age and elevated IOP were implicated in trabeculectomy failure. Individual post-operative complications such as particularly high IOP post-procedure and marked inflammation were also associated with filtering surgery failure.

AGIS 12

Characteristics associated with visual field loss included less baseline visual field deficit (TAT and ATT sequences), male gender (ATT), worse baseline visual acuity (ATT) and diabetes (TAT). Characteristics associated with decreased visual acuity in both treatment sequences were better baseline visual acuity, older age and less formal education.

AGIS 13

Ten years results of the treatment sequences continued to support the ATT sequence for black patients and TAT sequence in white patients. Visual field loss was less in ATT for blacks though this was not statistically significant; the same finding was statistically significant in the TAT sequence for whites. Visual acuity loss was less in the ATT sequence for both groups, but IOP reductions were greater in the TAT sequence. For both black and white patients, first-intervention failure rates were substantially lower for trabeculectomy than for trabeculoplasty. Cumulative incidence of unilateral blindness in black subjects was 11.9 percent in the ATT group and 18.5 percent in the TAT group; in the white group, 9.9 percent of the ATT patients and 7.3 percent of the TAT patients were unilaterally blind.

AGIS 14

For an eye showing a visual field worsening of at least two decibels in mean deviation or two units of the visual field score, a single confirmatory test six months later had a 72 percent probability of predicting a sustained defect. If two confirmatory tests are used, the probability of a persistent defect increases to 84 percent.

Conclusion

Treatment sequence starting with argon laser therapy was more beneficial for black patients while treatment starting with trabeculectomy was more beneficial for white patients. Consistent mean IOPs below 14 mm Hg limited glaucoma progression.

COLLABORATIVE NORMAL TENSION GLAUCOMA STUDY[56,57]

The Collaborative Normal Tension Glaucoma Study was designed to assess the relationship between intraocular pressure and normal-tension glaucoma; particularly, the effect of aggressive IOP lowering on both optic nerve damage and visual field loss and the adverse events associated with such aggressive lowering were studied. The study was conducted over a several year period from 1989 to the early 1990s.

The trial recruited 230 patients between ages 20 and 90 and one eye of each patient was randomized to observation or to having IOP lowered by 30 percent from baseline. Patients with IOP < 24 mm Hg (mean of < 20 mm Hg) with typical visual field and optic nerve head changes were followed for five years. All subjects had either documented progression or central field loss to be included within the study.

Exclusion criteria included the use of systemic beta-blockers or clonidine, previous ocular procedures, eyes with non-glaucomatous field defects or with conditions that could cause such, narrow angles, best corrected visual acuity less than 20/30 or with visual fields with too many defects to detect progression reliably. Patients had a 4-week washout period if they were on prior topical therapy. They were then followed every three months for the first year and then every six months.

In the study of IOP lowering, 35 percent of the observed eyes and 12 percent of the treated eyes had evidence of glaucomatous optic disc progression or visual field loss; the treated group took about 1000 days longer to have progression, confirming a role for elevated IOP in the pathogenesis of normal tension glaucoma. Even in eyes in which the IOP is not that elevated, lowering IOP decreased the rate of glaucomatous progression. The main side effect of treatment was that more than twice as many patients developed cataracts in the treated group, with

most incidence in those who had filtration surgery. However, lens opacification also occurred in medically treated groups, confirming the fact that any type of IOP lowering may increase the rate of cataractous progression, but that surgery is associated with cataract more than medical therapy. In a second publication, the effectiveness of pressure reduction was examined. After patients in the treatment group had achieved the 30 percent reduction in IOP, new baseline visual acuity, visual fields and disc photos were obtained. It was not easy to lower the IOP consistently by this amount. Compared to these stabilized baseline data, there was no difference in visual field progression between the treated and untreated groups. When the cataracts were removed, however, a difference was unmasked.

Conclusion

IOP lowering therapy will reduce the rate of glaucomatous progression in normal tension glaucoma, though the presence of cataracts may obscure this effect.

REFERENCES

1. American Academy of Ophthalmology. Glaucoma. Basic Science and Clinical Course, Section 10. San Francisco, CA, 2010.
2. Mills RP, Janz NK, Wren PA, Guire KE, CIGTS Study Group: Correlation of visual field with quality-of-life measures at diagnosis in the Collaborative Initial Glaucoma Treatment Study (CIGTS). Journal of Glaucoma 2001; 10:192-8.
3. Lichter PR, Musch DC, Gillespie BW, Guire KE, Janz NK, Wren PA, Mills RP, CIGTS Study Group: Interim Clinical Outcomes in the Collaborative Initial Glaucoma Treatment Study (CIGTS) Comparing Initial Treatment Randomized to Medications or Surgery. Ophthalmology 2001;108:1943-53.
4. Janz NK, Wren PA, Lichter PR, Musch DC, Gillespie BW, Guire KE. The CIGTS Group: Quality of life in diagnosed glaucoma patients. The Collaborative Initial Glaucoma Treatment Study. Ophthalmol 2001;108:887-98.
5. Janz NK, Wren PA, Lichter PR, Musch DC, Gillespie BW, Guire KE, Mills RP. CIGTS Study Group: The Collaborative Initial Glaucoma Treatment Study (CIGTS): Interim Quality of Life Findings Following Initial Medical or Surgical Treatment of Glaucoma. Ophthalmol 2001;108:1954-65.
6. DC, Lichter PR, Guire KE, Standardi CL, CIGTS Investigators: The Collaborative Initial Glaucoma Treatment Study (CIGTS): Study design, methods and baseline characteristics of enrolled patients. Ophthalmol 1999;106:653-62.
7. Musch DC, Lichter PR, Guire KE, Standardi CL. CIGTS Investigators: The Collaborative Initial Glaucoma Treatment Study (CIGTS): Study design, methods and baseline characteristics of enrolled patients. Ophthalmol 1999;106:653-62.
8. Janz N, Wren PA. CIGTS Study Group: Implementing quality of life in a clinical trial, in Anderson DR, Drance SM (eds). The Collaborative Initial Glaucoma Treatment Study. Encounters in Glaucoma Research 3: How to Ascertain Progression and Outcome; 1996.pp.45-62.
9. Lichter PR, Mills RP. CIGTS Study Group: Quality of life study

determination of progression, in Anderson DR, Drance SM (eds). Encounters in Glaucoma Research 3: How to Ascertain Progression and Outcome, Amsterdam, Kugler Publications; 1996.pp.149-63.

10. Musch DC, Gillespie BW, Niziol LM, Cashwell LF, Lichter PR. CIGTS Study Group: Factors Associated with Intraocular Pressure before and during 9 years of Treatment in the CIGTS. Ophthalmol 2008;115:927-33.

11. Jampel HD, Frick KD, Janz NK, Wren PA, Musch DC, Rimal R, Lichter PR. CIGTS Study Group: Depression and Mood Indicators in Newly Diagnosed Glaucoma. Am J Ophthalmol 2007;144:238-44.

12. Parrish RK, Feuer WJ, Schiffman JC, Lichter PR, Musch DC. CIGTS Optic Disc Study Group. Five-year Follow-up Optic Disc Findings of the Collaborative Initial Glaucoma Treatment Study. Am J Ophthalmol 2009;147:717-24.

13. Musch DC, Gillespie BW, Lichter PR, Niziol LM, Janz NK. CIGTS Study Investigators: Visual Field progression in the Collaborative Initial Glaucoma Treatment Study: The Impact of Treatment and Other Baseline Factors. Ophthalmol 2009;116:200-7.

14. Janz NK, Wren PA, Guire KE, Musch DC, Gillespie BW, Lichter PR. The CIGTS Investigators. Fear of blindness in the Collaborative Initial Glaucoma Treatment Study: patterns and correlates over time. Ophthalmol 2007;114:2213-30.

15. Gillespie BW, Musch DC, Guire KE, Mills RP, Lichter PR, Janz NK, Wren PA. The CIGTS Study Group. The Collaborative Initial Glaucoma Treatment Study: baseline visual field and test-retest variability. Invest Ophthalmol Vis Sci 2003;44:2613-20.

16. Hyman L, Heijl A, Leske MC, Bengtsson B, Yang Z. The Early Manifest Glaucoma Trial Group. Natural History of Intraocular Pressure in the Early Manifest Glaucoma Trial: A 6-year follow-up. Arch Ophthalmol 2010;128:601-7.

17. Heijl A, Leske MC, Hyman L, Yang Z, Bengtsson B. For the EMGT group. Intraocular pressure reduction with a fixed treatment protocol in the Early Manifest Glaucoma Trial. Acta Ophthalmol E-publication March, 2010.

18. Heijl A, Bengtsson B, Chauhan BC, Lieberman MF, Cunliffe I, Hyman L, Leske MC. A comparison of visual field progression criteria of 3 major glaucoma trials in early manifest glaucoma trial patients. Ophthalmol 2008;115(9):1157-65.

19. Leske MC, Heijl A, Hyman L, Bengtsson B, Dong L, Yang Z. EMGT Group. Predictors of Long-Term Progression in the Early Manifest Glaucoma Trial. Ophthalmol 2007;114:1965-72.

20. Hyman LG, Komaroff E, Heijl A, Bengtsson B, Leske MC. Early Manifest Glaucoma Trial Group. Ophthalmology 2005;112(9):1505-13.

21. Leskea MC, Heijl A, Hyman L, Bengtsson B, Komaroff E. Factors for progression and glaucoma treatment: The Early Manifest Glaucoma Trial. Curr Opin Ophthalmol 2004;15:102-6.

22. Heijl A, Leske MC, Bengtsson B, Hussein M. Early Manifest Glaucoma Trial Group. Measuring Visual Field Progression in the Early Manifest Glaucoma Trial. Acta Ophthalmol Scand 2003;81:286-93.

23. Leske MC, Heijl A, Hussein M, Bengtsson B, Hyman L, Komaroff E. Early Manifest Glaucoma Trial Group. Factors for glaucoma progression and the effect of treatment: the early manifest glaucoma trial. Arch Ophthalmol 2003;121:48-56.

24. Heijl A, Leske MC, Bengtsson B, Hyman L, Hussein M. The Early Manifest Glaucoma Trial Group. Reduction of intraocular pressure and glaucoma progression: results from the Early Manifest Glaucoma Trial. Arch Ophthalmol 2002;120:1268-79.

25. Leske MC, Heijl A, Hyman L, Bengtsson B. Early Manifest Glaucoma Trial: design and baseline data. Ophthalmol 1999;106:2144-53.

26. Kass MA, Heuer DK, Higginbotham EJ, Johnson CA, Keltner JL, Miler JP, Parrish II RK, Wilson MR, Gordon MO. The Ocular Hypertension Treatment Study Group: The Ocular-Hypertension Treatment Study: A Randomized Trial Determines that Topical Ocular Hypotensive Medication Delays or Prevents the Onset of Primary Open-Angle Glaucoma. Arch Ophthalmol 2002;120:701-13.

27. Gordon MO, Beiser JA, Brandt JD, Heuer DK, Higginbotham EJ, Johnson CA, Keltner JL, Miller JP, Parrish II RK, Wilson MR, Kass MA. For the Ocular Hypertension Treatment Study Group: The Ocular Hypertension Treatment Study: Baseline Factors that Predict the Onset of Primary Open-Angle Glaucoma. Arch Ophthalmol 2002;120:714-20.

28. Brandt JD, Beiser JA, Gordon MO, Kass MA. The Ocular Hypertension Study Group. Central corneal thickness and measured IOP response to topical ocular hypotensive medication in the Ocular Hypertension Treatment Study. Am J Ophthalmol 2004;138:717-22.

29. Johnson CA, Keltner JL, Cello KE, Edwards M, Kass MA, Gordon MO, Budenz DL, Gaasterland DE, Werner E. The Ocular Hypertension Study Group. Baseline Visual Field Characteristics in the Ocular Hypertension Treatment Study Ophthalmol 2002;109:432-7.

30. Zangwill LM, Weinreb RN, Beiser JA, Berry CC, Cioffi GA, Coleman AL, Trick G, Liebmann JM, Brandt JD, Piltz-Seymour JR, Dirkes KA, Vega S, Kass MA, Gordon MO. Baseline Topographic Optic Disc Measurements are Associated with the Development

of Primary Open-Angle Glaucoma: The Confocal Scanning Laser Ophthalmoscopy Ancillary Study to the Ocular Hypertension-Treatment-Study-Group. Arch Ophthalmol 2005;123:1188-97.

31. Gordon MO, Kass MA. For the Ocular Hypertension Treatment Study Group. The Ocular Hypertension Treatment Study: Design and Baseline Description of the Participants. Arch Ophthalmol 1999;117:573-83.

32. Mansberger SL, Hugher BA, Gordon MO, Spaner SD, Beiser JA, Cioffi GA, Kass MA. For the Ocular Hypertension Treatment Study Group. Comparison of the Initial Intraocular Pressure Response with Topical Beta-Adrenergic Antagonists and Prostaglandin Analogues in African American and White Individuals in the Ocular Hypertension Treatment Study. Arch Ophthalmol 2007;125:454-9.

33. Brandt JD, Gordon MO, Beiser JA, Lin SC, Alexander MY, Kass MD. Ocular Hypertension Treatment Study Group. Changes in Central Corneal Thickness over Time. Ophthalmol 2008;115:1150-556.

34. Keltner JL, Johnson CA, Cello KE, Edwards MA, Bandermann SE, Kass MA, Gordon MO. For the Ocular Hypertension Treatment Study Group. Classification of Visual Field Abnormalities in the Ocular Hypertension Treatment Study. Arch Ophthalmol 2003;121:643-50.

35. Keltner JL, Johnson CA, Quigg JM, Cello KE, Kass MA, Gordon MO. For the Ocular Hypertension Treatment Study. Confirmation of Visual Field Abnormalities in the Ocular Hypertension Treatment Study. Arch Ophthalmol 2000;118:1187-94.

36. Mederios FA, Weireib RN, Sample PA, Gomi CF, Bowd C, Crowston JG, Zangwill LM. Validation of a Predicative Model to Estimate the Risk of Conversion From Ocular Hypertension to Glaucoma. Arch Ophthalmol 2005; 123:1351-60.

37. Keltner JL, Johnson CA, Levine RA, Fan J, Cello KE, Kass MA, Gordon MO. For the Ocular Hypertension Treatment Study Group. Normal Visual Field Test Results Following Glaucomatous Visual Field End Points in the Ocular Hypertension Treatment Study. Arch Ophthalmol 2005;123:1201-6.

38. Kass MA, Gordon MO, Gao F, Heuer DK, Higginbotham EJ, Johnson CA, Keltner JK, Miller P, Parrish RK, Wilson MR. For the Ocular Hypertension Treatment Study. Arch Ophthalmol 2010;128:276-87.

39. Kass MA, Heuer DK, Higginbotham EJ, Johnson CA, Keltner JL, Miller JP, Parrish RK, Wilson MR, Gordon MO. For the Ocular Hypertension Study Group. The Ocular Hypertension Treatment Study: A Randomized Trial Determines that Topical Ocular Hypotensive Medication Delays or Prevents the Onset of Primary Open Angle Glaucoma. Arch Ophthalmol 2002;120:701-13.

40. Higginbotham EJ, Gordon MO, Beiser JA, Drake MV, Bennet GR, Wilson MR, Kass MA. For the Ocular Hypertension Treatment Study Group. The Ocular Hypertension Treatment Study Group: Topical Medication Delays or Prevents Primary Open-Angle Glaucoma in African-American Individuals. Arch Ophthalmol 2004;122:813-20.

41. Zangwill LM, Weinreb RN, Berry CC, Smith AR, Dirkes KA, Coleman AL, Piltz-Seymour JR, Leibman JM, Cioffi GA, Trick G, Brandt JD, Gordon MO, Kass MA. For the Confocal Scanner Laser Ophthalmoscopy Ancillary Study to the Ocular Hypertension Treatment Study. Racial Differences in Optic Disc Topography: Baseline Results from the Confocal Scanning Laser Ophthalmoscopy Ancillary Study to the Ocular Hypertension Treatment Study. Racial Differences in Optic Disc Topography: Baseline Results from the Confocal Scanning Laser Ophthalmoscopy Ancillary Study to the Ocular Hypertension Treatment Study. Arch Ophthalmol 2004;122:22-8.

42. Keltner JL, Johnson CA, Levine RA, Fan J, Cello KE, Kass MA, Gordon MO. For the Ocular Hypertension Treatment Study Group. Normal Visual Field Test Results Following Glaucomatous Visual Field End Points in the Ocular Hypertension Treatment Study. Arch Ophthalmol 2005;123:1201-6.

43. Zangwill LM, Weinreb RN, Beiser JA, Berry CC, Cioffi GA, Coleman AL, Trick G, Leibmann JM, Brandt JD, Piltz-Seymour JR, Dirkes KA, Vega S, Kass MA, Gordon MO. For the Confocal Scanning Laser Ophthalmoscopy Ancillary Study to the Ocular Hypertension Treatment Study. Baseline Topographic Optic Disc Measurements are Associated with the Development of Primary Open-Angle Glaucoma. Arch Ophthalmol 2005;122:1188-97.

44. The Advanced Glaucoma Intervention Study Investigators: The Advanced Glaucoma Intervention Study (AGIS) 8: Risk of cataract formation after trabeculectomy. Arch Ophthalmol 2001;119:1771-80.

45. Gaasterland DE, Blackwell B, Dally LG, Caprioli J, Katz LJ, Ederer F. The AGIS Investigators: The Advanced Glaucoma Intervention Study (AGIS): 10. Variability among academic glaucoma subspecialists in assessing optic disc notching. Trans Am Ophthalmol Soc 2001; 99:177-85.

46. The AGIS Investigators: The Advanced Glaucoma Intervention Study (AGIS): 9. Comparison of glaucoma outcomes in black and white patients within treatment groups. Am J Ophthalmol 2001;132:311-20.

47. The AGIS Investigators: The Advanced Glaucoma Intervention Study (AGIS):

6. Effect of cataract on visual field and visual acuity. Arch Ophthalmol 2000;118:1639-52.

48. The AGIS Investigators: The Advanced Glaucoma Intervention Study (AGIS): 7. The relationship between control of intraocular pressure and visual field deterioration. Am J Ophthalmol 2000;130:429-40.

49. Schwartz AL, Van Veldhuisen PC, Gaasterland DE, Ederer F, Sullivan EK, Cyrlin MN. The AGIS Investigators: The Advanced Glaucoma Intervention Study (AGIS): 5. Encapsulated bleb after initial trabeculectomy. Am J Ophthalmol 1999;127: 8-19.

50. AGIS Investigators: Advanced Glaucoma Intervention Study (AGIS): 3. Baseline characteristics of black and white patients. Ophthalmol 1998; 105:1137-45.

51. AGIS Investigators: Advanced Glaucoma Intervention Study (AGIS): 4. Comparison of treatment outcomes within race: 7 years results. Ophthalmol 1998;105:1146-64.

52. The Advanced Glaucoma Intervention Study (AGIS) Data Management Handbook. Springfield, Virginia. National Technical Information Service, Document, No. PB96-137120, 1996.

53. The Advanced Glaucoma Intervention Study Investigators: The Advanced Glaucoma Intervention Study (AGIS): 1. Study design and methods and baseline characteristics of study patients. Controlled Clinical Trials 1994;15(4): 299-325.

54. The Advanced Glaucoma Intervention Study Investigators: The Advanced Glaucoma Intervention Study. 2. Visual field test scoring and reliability. Ophthalmol 1994;101:1445-55.

55. Kim J, Dally LG, Ederer F, Gassterland DE, VanVelhuisen PC, Blackwell B, Sullivan EK, Prum B, Shafranov G, Beck A, Spaeth GL. The AGIS Investigator: The Advanced Glaucoma Intervention Study (AGIS): 14. Distinguishing progression of glaucoma from visual field fluctuations. Ophthalmol 2004;111:2109-16.

56. The Collaborative Normal-Tension Glaucoma Study Group. Comparison of glaucomatous progression between untreated patients with normal-tension glaucoma and patients with therapeutically reduced intraocular pressures. Am J Ophthalmol 1998;126:487-97.

57. The Collaborative Normal-Tension Glaucoma Study Group. The effectiveness of intraocular pressure in the treatment of normal-tension glaucoma. Am J Ophthalmol 1998;126:498-505.

WHAT HAVE WE LEARNT FROM THE CLINICAL TRIALS IN GLAUCOMA?

A Jayaprakash Patil, Deepak P Edward

INTRODUCTION

Glaucoma is a leading cause of blindness in India and other developing countries. In India, glaucoma (of all types) ranks as the second major cause of blindness and accounts for 25.4 percent of all causes of visual impairment.[1-3]

Glaucoma is a major public health problem[4,5] since the disability caused by the disease is irreversible. The World Health Organization recommended that its member countries combat this public health problem through a programmed approach. To plan such strategies, it is important to better understand the natural history and progression of the disease[6] as well as clearly understand treatment outcomes. The current treatment protocols and evidence-based medicine in glaucoma are the result of several multicentric randomized clinical trials. In this chapter, we summarize some of these landmark studies that have revolutionized the management of glaucoma.

The practice of lowering intraocular pressure (IOP) in glaucoma management was questioned by Eddy and Billings.[7] Their arguments were based on a deficiency of clinical and experimental evidence to support the strategy of lowering IOP in patients with glaucoma and glaucoma suspects. These questions related to the optimal standardized management for glaucoma resulted in many of the clinical trials conducted over the last 20 years and have assisted in addressing several challenging dogmas and often-difficult clinical issues.[8]

EVIDENCE BASED MEDICINE

Historically, James Lind conducted the first comparative clinical trial in health care in 1747, in the treatment of scurvy. Evidence based medicine relies on the results of the well controlled clinical trials that has had rational experimental design and had fulfilled certain stringent norms of randomization, monitoring and meeting the end points. In this regards, the ongoing clinical trials in glaucoma are considered to be of high standard and potentially alter practice patterns and philosophy.

A methodologically sound trial forms the basis for formal treatment guidelines that can help the clinician choose the best treatment for their patients. In general, a clinical trial is formulated around a working hypothesis. The primary and secondary end points are picked up based on the existing evidence and the hypothesized concepts. There can be single end point (such as IOP lowering) or several endpoints (such as IOP lowering, visual field (VF) changes, nerve fiber layer changes) to a study. The trial should be well controlled, i.e. must compare the intervention with a standard or placebo treatment. A randomization process is used to ensure that the groups are comparable. The patients are monitored and the results analyzed in double-blind manner. The required number of patients is determined (sample size based on power calculations) based on the working hypothesis and the spontaneous variability of the primary endpoint. The experimental design (cross-over or parallel groups) is chosen according to the primary outcome measure and the disease characteristics. Finally, the results are analyzed using relevant statistical tests that provide information that can be extrapolated to clinical practice.[9]

CLINICAL TRIALS IN GLAUCOMA

The clinical trials that have been performed in glaucoma span the entire spectrum of the stages of open angle glaucoma especially focusing on outcomes related to the benefit of medical or surgical treatment.

The landmark clinical trials summarized in **Table 1**.

OCULAR HYPERTENSION TREATMENT STUDY (OHTS)

Introduction

This clinical study resulted from an analysis of existing literature that suggested that there was no consensus that medical reduction of IOP prevents or delays the onset of VF and/or optic nerve damage in ocular hypertensive (OHT) subjects. Despite the lack of convincing evidence for the efficacy of medical treatment in ocular hypertension, approximately 1.5 million glaucoma suspects in the United States were being treated with costly ocular hypotensive medications with potentially serious and even life-threatening side effects. The need for a well-controlled clinical trial to determine whether medical reduction of IOP can prevent or delay the onset of glaucomatous damage in OHT subjects was addressed by OHTS.

Objectives

- To determine whether medical reduction of IOP prevents or delays the onset of glaucomatous VF loss and/or optic disc damage in OHT subjects judged to be at moderate risk for developing primary open angle glaucoma (POAG).

Table 1 A summary of the salient features of some glaucoma clinical trials

Clinical trial	Diagnosis	No. of patients	Randomization	Follow-up (years)	IOP reduction	Outcome
OHTS	OHT	1636	Medical treatment vs Observation	5 years	20% Avg	- Treatment delays/prevents onset of POAG - Thinner CCT significant risk factor for progression POAG
EMGT	POAG	255	Treatment (ALT+Betaxolol) vs Observation	4–9 years	25% Avg	- Benefit in treating glaucoma was demonstrated - Every mm Hg lowering of IOP reduces the risk of glaucoma progression by 10%
AGIS	POAG	789	ALT vs Surgery	7 years	< 18 mm Hg at all visits	- In African-American patients with advanced glaucoma, laser surgery as initial treatment was more effective - IOP lowering halts glaucoma progression by at least 5–10 years.
CIGTS	POAG	607	Medical treatment vs Surgery	5 years	30% Avg	- Both treatments equally effective Early complication greater in surgical group
CNTGS	NTG	145	Medical treatment/ALT/ Surgery vs Observation	7 years	30% Avg	- With IOP lowering, visual field progression was minimal in both groups. Only a small percent of patients with NTG will eventually need surgery.

OHTS: Ocular hypertension treatment study; EMGT: Early manifest glaucoma trial; AGIS: Advanced glaucoma intervention study; CIGTS: Collaborative initial glaucoma treatment study; CNTGS: Collaborative normal tension glaucoma study; OHT: Ocular hypertension treatment; POAG: Primary open angle glaucoma; NTG: Normal tension glaucoma; ALT: Argon laser trabeculoplasty; IOP: Intraocular pressure; Avg: Average; CCT: Central corneal thickness

- To produce natural history data to assist in identifying patients at most risk for developing POAG and those most likely to benefit from early medical treatment.
- To quantify risk factors for developing POAG among OHT subjects.

Study Design

The OHTS was a long-term, randomized, controlled multicenter clinical trial. 1636 patients aged between 40 and 80 with IOP greater than or equal to 24 mm Hg but less than or equal to 32 mm Hg in at least one eye and IOP greater than or equal to 21 but less than or equal to 32 mm Hg in the fellow eye and with normal VFs and optic discs were included for the study. In the 1991 Baltimore Eye Survey, African-Americans were shown to have a prevalence of POAG four to five times higher than whites. Due to this high prevalence of glaucoma in the African-American population, it was decided to recruit approximately 25 percent of African Americans in the study.[10]

Patients presenting with best-corrected visual acuity worse than 20/40 in either eye, previous intraocular surgery, a life-threatening or debilitating disease, secondary causes of elevated IOP, angle-closure glaucoma or anatomically narrow angles, other diseases that can cause VF loss, background diabetic retinopathy, optic disc abnormalities that can produce VF loss or obscure the interpretation of the optic disc, or unwillingness to undergo random assignment were excluded from the trial. OHT subjects judged to be at moderate risk of developing POAG were randomly assigned to either close observation only or a stepped medical regimen. Medical treatment consisted of all commercially available topical antiglaucoma agents. After completion of baseline measures (IOP, VFs, disc photos) and randomization, the subjects were followed for a minimum of five years with automated threshold central static perimetry (Humphrey program 30-2) twice yearly and stereoscopic optic disc photographs once yearly.[11] Study endpoints were reproducible VF loss and/or progressive optic disc damage in either eye of a patient.

Results

In univariate and multivariate analyzes, baseline factors that predicted the development of POAG included older age, race (African-American), sex (male), larger vertical cup-disc ratio, larger horizontal cup-disc ratio, higher IOP, greater Humphrey VF pattern standard deviation, heart disease and thinner central corneal measurement.

During the course of the study, the mean ±SD reduction in IOP in the medication group was 22.5 ± 9.9 percent. The IOP declined by 4.0 ± 11.6 percent in the observation group. At 60 months, the cumulative probability of developing POAG was 4.4 percent in the medication group and 9.5 percent in the observation group. There was little evidence of increased systemic or ocular risk associated with OHT.[12]

Among African-American participants, 17 (8.4%) of 203 in the medication group developed POAG during the study (median follow-up, 78 months) compared with 33 (16.1%) of 205 participants in the observation group.

Recommendations

Topical ocular hypotensive medication was effective in delaying or preventing onset of POAG in individuals with elevated IOP.[13] Although this does not imply that all patients with borderline or elevated IOP should receive medication, clinicians should consider initiating treatment for individuals with OHT who are at moderate or high risk for developing POAG.

Kymes and his colleagues analyzed the cost-effectiveness of treating glaucoma based on the data from OHTS. This is particularly important in developing countries, where the pharmacoeconomics plays a significant role in the management of glaucoma. In this study, "Treat everyone" category, where all participants received treatment was found to cost more and was less effective than other options. Although the treatment of individual patients largely depends on their attitude toward the risk of disease progression and visual impairment, the treatment of those patients with IOP of greater than or equal to 24 mm Hg and a greater than or equal to 2 percent annual risk of the development of glaucoma was found to be cost-effective.[14] Whether these same models apply to developing countries is yet to be determined.

Complications

A borderline higher incidence of posterior subcapsular opacification in the medication group was noted on LOCS III (Lens Opacities Classification System) readings. In addition, an increased rate of cataract extraction and cataract/filtration surgery was noted in the medication group. However, there is no evidence to prove the role of topical hypotensive medication on the development of lens opacification.[15]

OHTS Follow-up Studies

Several follow-up studies of OHTS determined various other glaucoma diagnostic risk factors and follow-up strategies. The salient outcomes of some of these studies are summarized below:

1. OHTS was the first study to document that thinner central corneal thickness (CCT) was a strong predictive factor in the development of POAG. Participants with a corneal thickness of 555 µm or less had a 3-fold greater risk of developing POAG compared with participants who had a CCT of more than 588 µm. This inverse relationship was found across the ranges of baseline IOP and baseline vertical cup-disc ratios. CCT also influences the IOP measurement. Eyes with thicker corneas may have a true IOP that is lower than the measured IOP. Conversely, eyes with thin corneas have a true IOP that is greater than the measured IOP.[12] Cross-sectional studies have documented that CCT is greater in individuals with measured OHT compared with normotensive individuals or those with glaucoma.[16,17]

2. CCT was also found to correlate with measured IOP response to topical IOP lowering medication in the OHTS. CCT was inversely related to the IOP response after the initial one-eye therapeutic trial and during 12 to 60 months of follow-up (P < .05). However, mean CCT was not correlated with the number of different medications prescribed during follow-up, the total medication-months, or the percentage of visits at which IOP target was met. Individuals with thicker corneas had smaller measured IOP responses to ocular hypotensive medication than those with normal or thin corneas.[18]

3. Several segmental and global optic disc parameters showed significant changes in the converter group before confirmed VF changes could be seen. Changes in the confocal laser tomography (CSLO) parameters obtained with Heidelberg Retina Tomograph (HRT) were compared with changes of static VF measurements. HRT parameters such as cup area (CA), cup volume (CV), cup shape measure (CSM), rim volume (RV), retinal nerve fiber thickness (RNFLT) and contour height variation (CHV) were studied. A glaucomatous VF defect and therewith the conversion from OHT to POAG was defined as reproducible defect-cluster >20 dB of two or three single points at the same location. The linear model for the progression of the optic disc parameters detected only a small amount of the converters to glaucoma. It was suggested that a hit rate could be increased with the sectoral-based analysis. Cup shape measure showed the highest rate. The HRT could therefore be of some value in the sequential follow-up of those suspected of having glaucoma by identi-

fying eyes at risk of developing glaucoma.[19]

4. Due to the availability of a large database, it was also possible to determine the frequency with which VF abnormalities observed on follow-up VFs for patients in the OHTS were confirmed on retest. Of the 21,603 regular follow-up VFs, 1006 were follow-up retests performed because of an abnormality (n = 748) or unreliability (n = 258). 703 (94%) of the 748 VFs were abnormal and reliable and 45 (6%) were abnormal and unreliable. On retesting, abnormalities were not confirmed for 604 (85.9%) of the 703 originally abnormal and reliable VFs. Most VF abnormalities in patients in the OHTS were not verified on retest.[11] Thus, the OHTS study reaffirmed the concept that confirmation of VF abnormalities is essential for distinguishing reproducible VF loss from long-term variability.[20,21]

5. In both univariate and multivariate models, a history of diabetes mellitus appeared to be significantly protective against developing POAG. Of 191 participants who reported a history of diabetes mellitus at baseline, 6 (3.1%) developed POAG compared with 119 (8.3%) of 1427 participants who did not report a history of diabetes mellitus.[12]

THE EUROPEAN GLAUCOMA PREVENTION STUDY (EGPS)
Introduction
The EGPS was designed to determine whether medical lowering of IOP could prevent or delay the onset of glaucoma in patients with OHT.[22] The study design was similar to that of the OHTS with some differences in the treatment modalities used and baseline criteria.

Objectives
The randomized, double-masked, controlled trial was focused to study the efficacy of reduction of IOP by dorzolamide in preventing or delaying POAG in patients affected by OHT.

Study Design
1081 patients aged 30 years or more were enrolled in 18 different European centres. The patients had a baseline IOP of 22 to 29 mm Hg with a mean of 23.6 mm Hg. In OHTS, the baseline IOP was higher (24–32 mm Hg with a mean of 24.9 mm Hg). Of greater interest than this, a small difference in mean baseline IOP accounted for the different distribution of IOP in the EGPS group. Approximately 65 percent of EGPS patients would have been ineligible for inclusion in OHTS because their IOP would have been too low.[23] However, all participants had two normal and reliable VFs and normal optic disc as determined by the Optic Disc Reading Center. They were randomized to treatment with dorzolamide or placebo (the vehicle of dorzolamide). Efficacy end points were VF, optic disc changes, or both.

The VF endpoint was described by worsening of VF when at least one of the following criteria was met: (1) three or more horizontally or vertically adjacent points that differ 5 dB or more from baseline, (2) two or more horizontally or vertically adjacent points that differ 10 dB or more from baseline, (3) a difference of 10 dB or more across the nasal horizontal meridian at two or more adjacent points. A VF change during follow-up was confirmed by two further positive tests.

Worsening of the optic disc was defined as a visually recognizable (on stereophotographs) narrowing of the neuroretinal rim area (localized or diffuse) not attributable to photographic artifacts. This was detected by comparing follow-up stereoscopic optic disc slides with baseline stereoscopic optic disc slides.[24]

The safety end point was an IOP of more than 35 mm Hg on two consecutive examinations.

Results
During the course of the study, the mean percent reduction in IOP in the dorzolamide group was 15 percent after six months and 22 percent after five years. Mean IOP declined by 9 percent after 6 months and by 19 percent after five years in the placebo group. At 60 months, the cumulative probability of converting to an efficacy endpoint (conversion to glaucoma by either VF or disc changes) was 13.4 percent in the dorzolamide group and 14.1 percent in the placebo group. VF efficacy endpoint was defined as three or more horizontally or vertically adjacent points that differed by 5 dB or more from baseline or a difference of 10 dB or more across the nasal horizontal meridian at two or more adjacent points. A visually recognizable localized or diffuse (on stereophotographs) narrowing of the neuroretinal rim area was referred to as the optic disc efficacy end point. The cumulative probability of developing an efficacy or a safety end point was 13.7 percent in the dorzolamide group and 16.4 percent in the placebo group.[24]

Recommendations
The EGPS failed to detect a statistically significant difference between medical therapy and placebo in reducing the incidence of POAG. It is considered a good study of the natural history of OHT. The study did not detect differences between the two groups, unlike OHTS, possibly due to the large loss to follow-up of patients with higher IOPs and the placebo effect.[23]

Analysis of Combined Data of OHTS and EGPS[23]

The results of the OHTS showed that it is possible to prevent or delay the development of POAG in OHT patients by achieving an 18 percent net IOP reduction from baseline maintained at least for five years.[13] The EGPS failed to confirm the results of the OHTS in the primary analysis, which included the efficacy endpoints and in the secondary analysis that included the safety endpoints (described earlier). The incidence of efficacy endpoints (both VF and optic disc progressive changes) was higher in the EGPS than in the OHTS (9.8% vs 7.6%).[12]

In EGPS, treated arm had a mean IOP reduction ranging between 15 and 22 percent throughout the five years of the trial; however, a sustained placebo effect of approximately 9 to 19 percent was also seen. This is the first time such a meaningful and consistent placebo effect has been observed with chronic treatment. In fact, the mean IOP difference between the two treatment groups at each time point of the trial ranged between 1.1 and 1.3 mm Hg. The small difference between the IOP lowering effects of dorzolamide and placebo explained the failure to detect a statistically significant protective effect of medical treatment in the EGPS. However, the EGPS was powered to detect a much larger relative difference (40%) in the number of efficacy end points between the two arms, based on a greater expected difference in IOP reduction between dorzolamide and placebo.[13] Although a difference of even greater magnitude (approximately 60%) in the number of endpoints between the two study arms was observed in the OHTS.

Another possible limitation of the EGPS results may be the high dropout rate, which was 30.1 percent through the course of the study. It was higher (35.6%) in the dorzolamide group than in the placebo group (24.7%), which may be explained by the higher number of ocular side effects in the dorzolamide group. An additional explanation for such a high dropout rate may be the use of the placebo, which may create greater anxiety in the patients.

In conclusion, the EGPS failed to detect a protective effect of medical therapy (by means of dorzolamide) as compared with placebo for the development of POAG in OHT patients at moderate risk over a follow-up of approximately five years. This result can be explained mainly by a clinically significant effect of the placebo on IOP. Therefore, these results strongly support the need to evaluate or re-evaluate the efficacy of long-term medical therapy of OHT, POAG, or both by means of placebo-controlled, double-masked, randomized clinical trials.[25]

EARLY MANIFEST GLAUCOMA TRIAL (EMGT)
Introduction
Glaucoma is a common disease in older adults. Current treatment regimens aim at IOP lowering, but indications for therapy are not well defined. Furthermore, it is unclear whether IOP influences the natural history of glaucoma. Early diagnosis and rapid detection of progression are of paramount importance in limiting irreversible damage. The effectiveness of IOP lowering requires evaluation by controlled treatment trials.

Objectives
The EMGT was the first large, adequately powered, randomized controlled clinical trial to evaluate the effects of IOP lowering on the progression of newly detected POAG. This study intended to compare glaucoma progression in initially treated versus untreated patients with newly detected POAG. This also allowed for quantification of the effects of immediate IOP-lowering treatment on progression during the follow-up period.

The primary objective of this trial was to compare the effects of therapy to lower the IOP versus late or no treatment on the progression of newly detected open-angle glaucoma, as measured by increasing VF loss and/or optic disc changes. The secondary purposes were to determine the extent of IOP reduction attained by treatment, to explore factors that may influence glaucoma progression and to describe the natural history of newly detected glaucoma.

Study Design
Newly detected and untreated patients with POAG, aged between 50 and 80 years with reproducible VF defects by Humphrey perimetry, were included for the study. A total of 255 patients were identified by an extensive, population-based screening of successive age cohorts as well as by clinical referral. Exclusion criteria included: advanced VF loss (MD $\leq$ 16 dB); mean IOP > 30 mm Hg or any IOP > 35 mm Hg in at least one eye; VA < 0.5 in either eye; or any conditions precluding reliable fields or photos, use of study treatment, or 4-year follow-up.

Eligible patients were randomized to treatment with betaxolol and ALT (related group) or to no initial treatment (control group) with close follow-up of both groups. Patients in the treated group received latanoprost eye drops when IOP exceeded 25 mm Hg at more than one visit; patients in the control group received latanoprost eye drops when IOP reached 35 mm Hg or higher during the trial. If IOP remained high, treatment was individualized.[25] The study outcome of glaucoma progression was based on specific criteria derived from Humphrey VFs and masked evaluations of optic disc photographs. The perimetric outcome was defined as statistically significant deterioration (p < 0.05) of the same three or more test points in Pattern Deviation Change Probability Maps in three consecutive 30-2 Humphrey fields. Optic disc progression was determined by the presence of definite change (detected by comparison of follow-up photographs with baseline) by flicker chronoscopy in two follow-up photographs from the same visit.

Patients were followed for a minimum of four years and maximum of nine years to assess the development and progression of glaucoma. They were seen every three months for VF and IOP. Disc photographs were taken every six months. Additional follow-up visits were held to confirm VF progression and IOP elevation (>25 mm Hg in treated group, >35 mm Hg in control group).

Results

A mean IOP reduction of 25 percent reduced progression from 62 percent in the control group to 45 percent in the treatment group. The treatment delayed the progression by approximately two years. The study reported that for every one mm Hg lowering of IOP, the risk of glaucoma progression reduced by ten percent.[26]

Recommendations

Its intent-to-treat analysis showed considerable beneficial effects of immediate medical treatment that significantly delayed progression of POAG. Whereas progression varied across patient categories, treatment effects were present in both older and younger patients, high and normal pressure glaucoma and eyes with less and greater VF loss.

Complications

The treatment group had an increased incidence of nuclear lens opacities.

GLAUCOMA LASER TRIAL (GLT) AND GLAUCOMA LASER TRIAL FOLLOW-UP STUDY (GLTFS)[27-31]

Introduction

During the last decade, argon laser trabeculoplasty (ALT) has often been used instead of surgery as the treatment of choice in cases of POAG that could not be controlled by drugs. Sometimes it has been found to be effective in controlling glaucoma, although many eyes still require some medical treatment.

Objectives

The Glaucoma Laser Trial (GLT), a randomized, controlled clinical trial, was conducted to determine the safety and long-term efficacy of ALT with standard medical treatment for newly diagnosed POAG.

The GLTFS was a follow-up study of 203 of the 271 patients who enrolled in the GLT. By the close of the GLTFS, the median duration of follow-up since diagnosis of POAG was seven years with a maximum of nine years.

Study Design

A total of 271 patients aged 35 years and above and with IOP of 22 mm Hg or greater in each eye and evidence of optic nerve damage in at least one eye were included. Each of the 271 patients in the trial received ALT in one eye and standard topical medication in the other eye. The eye to be treated medically and the eye to be lasered were randomly selected.

The ALT was completed in two sessions, one month apart, with one-half of the trabecular meshwork treated with 45 to 55 laser burns in each session. Patients were followed up at every three months for at least two years. At each visit, IOP and visual acuity were examined. VF examinations were performed 3, 6 and 12

months after randomization and annually thereafter. Disc stereo photographs were taken 6 and 12 months after randomization and annually thereafter.[29] The results of these examinations determined whether treatment should be changed. If the IOP in either eye was still elevated, medication was changed or medication was instituted in the lasered eye according to a standardized procedure. If IOP was still not successfully reduced, surgery or further laser treatment was advised.

Results

Over the course of the GLT and GLTFS, the eyes treated initially with ALT had lower IOP and better VF and optic disc status than their fellow eyes treated initially with topical medication.[30] When compared with eyes initially treated with medication, eyes initially treated with ALT had a 1.2 mm Hg greater lowering in IOP (p < 0.001) and 0.6 dB greater improvements in the VF (p < 0.001) from entry into the GLT. The overall difference between eyes with regard to change in ratio of optic cup area to optic disc area from entry into the GLT was -0.01 (p = 0.005), which indicated slightly more deterioration for eyes initially treated with medication. After two years, ALT was as effective as medication, but more than half of the eyes initially treated with ALT required medications to control IOP.[28]

Recommendations

Initial treatment with ALT was at least as efficacious as initial treatment with topical medication.

Complications

ALT was associated with a transient rise in IOP in approximately 20 percent of patients;[27] however, no prophylaxis was used against an increase in IOP perioperatively in this trial.

ADVANCED GLAUCOMA INTERVENTION STUDY (AGIS)[32-34]

In advanced glaucoma, adequate IOP lowering with medication alone is difficult. Before 1980, filtration surgery, such as trabeculectomy, was the commonly practiced mode of intervention. With the advent of ALT to control IOP, it has become a popular alternative, although the outcome has been variable, in some cases lasting only a few weeks or months to years in others. So, it is more often used as a procedure, in a patient waiting for surgical intervention. Little was known about which sequence of intervention gives the best long-range outcome.

Objectives

To assess the long-term outcomes of sequences of interventions involving trabeculectomy and ALT in patients with failed initial medical treatment for glaucoma, visual function status was used in the study to compare two intervention sequences in managing the disease. The primary outcome variable was the average percent of eyes with substantial decrease of visual acuity or field that is due to glaucoma. Secondary outcome variables included sustained decrease of vision, failure of surgical or laser interventions, number of prescribed glaucoma medications, and level of IOP.

Study Design

A total of 789 eyes of 591 patients with advanced POAG, not optimally controlled by medication were enrolled. Eligible eyes were randomly assigned to one of two intervention sequences: (1) trabeculectomy (Trab), followed by ALT should trab fail, followed by a second trab should ALT fail (Trab → ALT → 2nd Trab) or (2) ALT, followed by trab should ALT fail, followed by another trab should the first trab fail (ALT → Trab → 2nd Trab). In eyes with previous surgery, antimitotic agents were used as an adjunct to

trabeculectomy. Eyes failing to respond to either of the intervention sequences were managed at the discretion of the physician. Laser or surgical interventions were supplemented with medical treatment as needed.[32,35]

Patients were followed under a standardized protocol for a minimum of five years to determine degree of visual function loss, failure rates of interventions, rates of complications and need for supplemental therapy. After the initial intervention, follow-up examinations were scheduled at one week, four weeks, three months, six months and every six months thereafter. After second and third interventions, follow-up examinations were scheduled at one and four weeks. Additional visits were scheduled as needed for the disease management.[36]

Results

After seven years of follow-up, results revealed that African-Americans and Caucasian-Americans differed in the way they benefited from the two treatment algorithms. The vision in eyes of African-American patients with advanced glaucoma tends to be better preserved in the program that started with the ALT. From initial treatment through seven years of follow-up, the average percent of eyes in African-American patients with decrease of vision was 28 percent in the program in which ALT was initially used, as compared with 37 percent in the program starting with a trabeculectomy.[35]

Through the first four years, the vision in eyes of Caucasian-American patients (as in the African-American population) with advanced glaucoma was better preserved in the program starting with ALT. Thereafter, the reverse was true; with seven years follow-up after the initial treatment, the average percent of eyes in Caucasian-American patients with decrease of vision was 31 percent in the program starting with a trabeculectomy, as

compared with 35 percent in the program starting with ALT.[37,38] Trabeculectomy without antimitotic agent stabilized perimetric sensitivities in 75 percent of African-Americans and 85 percent of Caucasian-Americans. Additional follow-up reports from AGIS suggested that ALT failure was associated with younger age and higher pre-intervention IOP. Also, trabeculectomy failure was associated with younger age, higher pre-intervention IOP, diabetes and one or more postoperative complications, particularly elevated IOP and marked inflammation.[39]

An important post hoc analysis of AGIS data looked at the relationship between IOP and preservation of the VF. Eyes with mean IOP of greater than 17.5 mm Hg had worsening of VF on subsequent follow-up. Associative analysis, in this study suggested that in eyes with IOP less than 18 mm Hg on 100 percent of visits over six years there was no VF change from baseline during follow-up, whereas eyes with less IOP less than 18 mm Hg at 50 percent of visits showed VF progression. This degree of worsening was greater at seven years than at two years. In both analyzes, low IOP was associated with reduced progression of VF, supporting evidence from earlier studies of a protective role of low IOP in VF deterioration.[37]

In another AGIS follow-up study, the role of IOP fluctuation to VF progression was investigated. 301 eyes of 301 patients enrolled in the AGIS were studied. VF progression was detected in 78 eyes (26%). There were statistically significant differences, between progressing and non-progressing eyes, for mean IOP ($P = 0.006$), IOP fluctuation ($P < 0.001$), mean length of follow-up ($P = 0.013$), mean number of VFs ($P = 0.005$) and mean number of medications ($P = 0.006$). Three variables that were associated with a higher probability of VF progression were greater IOP fluctuation ($P = 0.009$),

ALT (P = 0.004) and older age (P = 0.05). It was concluded that long-term IOP fluctuation is associated with VF progression in patients with low mean IOP but not in patients with high mean IOP. Long-term IOP fluctuation was defined as the standard deviation of IOP (mm Hg) at all visits after initial intervention until the time of VF worsening or end of follow-up, whichever came first.[40]

Recommendations

Based on the study results, it is recommended that African-American patients with advanced glaucoma begin a treatment program starting with laser surgery, which is consistent with current medical practice. In contrast, Caucasian-American patients with advanced glaucoma should begin a treatment program that starts with trabeculectomy. This recommendation is inconsistent with current medical practice. Since glaucoma is a chronic disease, long-term information is important. In addition, the importance of low IOP in preventing VF loss was demonstrated. Also further analysis of the data suggested long-term IOP fluctuation is associated with VF progression in patients with low mean IOP but not in patients with high mean IOP.

Complications

45 percent of operated eyes developed cataract over seven years. Rate of cataractogenesis was 47 percent more in uncomplicated trabeculectomy than in ALT group. This risk doubled if the surgery was complicated.[41,42]

FLUOROURACIL FILTRATION SURGERY STUDY (FFSS) [43-46]
Introduction

Filtration surgery adequately lowers IOP in most glaucoma patients; however, the prognosis is less favorable for aphakic patients with glaucoma or glaucoma in phakic eyes following unsuccessful filtration surgery. Failure of filtration surgery is due to the proliferation of fibroblasts at the filtering site. The use of 5-fluorouracil (5-FU), an antifibrotic agent has shown to inhibit the proliferation of fibroblasts in tissue culture and in preliminary studies it has increased the success of filtration surgery in a nonhuman primate model.

Objectives

The FFSS was a randomized, controlled clinical trial comparing the success rate of standard glaucoma filtration surgery to the success rate of filtration surgery with adjunctive 5-FU treatment. Another element of this study was to evaluate the frequency and severity of possible adverse effects related to 5-FU injections.

Study Design

A total of 213 patients with uncontrolled IOP greater than 21 mm Hg in one or both eyes despite maximal tolerated therapy were included in the study. Of 213 patients recruited into the study, 162 had previous cataract extraction and 51 had previous filtration surgery. After the investigators performed the filtration surgery and determined that the new outlet channel was functioning, patients were randomized to receive either 5-FU injections or standard postsurgical care without 5-FU. The patients treated with 5-FU received subconjunctival injections of 5 mg of 5-FU twice daily on postoperative days 1 through 7 and once daily on postoperative days 8 through 14. All patients were examined at 1 month, 3 months, 6 months, 1 year, 18 months and 2 years postoperatively and at yearly intervals thereafter until 5 years postoperatively. Possible concomitant risks of 5-FU treatment, such as toxic effects to the cornea, lens or retina were monitored.

Results

The data demonstrated improved surgical control of glaucoma using 5-FU in patients at high risk for trabeculectomy failure. At one year, the cumulative success rates as calculated by survival analysis were 80 percent for the 5-FU group and 60 percent for the standard surgery group; at three years the success rates were 56 percent for the 5-FU group and 28 percent for the standard group; and at 5 years the success rates were 48 percent in the 5-FU group and 21 percent in the standard. Success was defined as no repeat surgery for IOP control and no IOP over 21 mm Hg, at or after, the one-year visit.

Visual acuity in the 5-FU group was worse than results in the standard therapy group at one month; however, the visual acuity change from the qualifying visit was better in the 5-FU group at one, two, and three years. The difference was not statistically significant at four or five years. This study showed that, regardless of treatment group, patients with controlled IOP had less visual acuity loss than patients in whom IOPs were not controlled. No difference in VF sensitivity was noticed between treatment groups. Patients who underwent repeat surgery showed more VF loss than those who did not. The results also suggest that VF loss is associated with high IOPs. Both treatment groups lost visual acuity and VF throughout the five years of the study.

Other risk factors, other than treatment affecting the surgical outcome, included preoperative IOP, the number of previous ocular procedures with a conjunctival incision and the time interval between the last ocular surgery and the study filtration surgery. The risk of a suprachoroidal hemorrhage was not related to 5-FU; however, suprachoroidal hemorrhage was strongly associated with the preoperative IOP.[44] The development of a late-onset leak in the filtration bleb was more likely to occur in the 5-FU group (9%) than in the standard therapy group (2%). No other long-term adverse effects were significantly different between the two groups. Two cases of endophthalmitis developed in the 5-FU group versus one case in the standard group.

Recommendations

The FFSS group recommended the use of subconjunctival 5-FU after trabeculectomy in eyes that have undergone previous cataract surgery or unsuccessful filtration surgery. However, because of a higher risk of late-onset wound leaks, which may increase the risk of endophthalmitis, the study group cautions against the routine use of 5-FU in patients with good prognoses. The association between high preoperative IOP and acute postoperative hypotony was not suspected as a risk factor for the development of suprachoroidal hemorrhage prior to this study. This observation has contributed to a change in ophthalmic surgical practice. Patients with very high preoperative IOPs now undergo trabeculectomies with multiple tightly tied sutures or with releasable sutures in the scleral flap placed to minimize postoperative hypotony. Postoperative argon laser suture lysis or removal of releasable sutures may reduce the likelihood of large postoperative IOP fall and subsequent hypotony.

COLLABORATIVE INITIAL GLAUCOMA TREATMENT STUDY (CIGTS)
Introduction

In view of potentially inefficient IOP lowering by the conventional first-line medical treatment in some newly diagnosed patients with POAG, recent studies have suggested an effective IOP control by immediate filtration surgery. In addition, increased attention to the quality of life (QOL) has added another dimension in deciding upon appropriate treatment of such patients.

Objectives

CIGTS was conducted to compare the long-term effects of treating newly diagnosed POAG patients with conventional topical pharmacologic agents versus immediate filtration surgery.

Study Design

607 patients with newly diagnosed POAG were recruited for the study. Patients aged between 25 and 75 years with an IOP of 20 mm Hg or greater and evidence of optic nerve damage and/or VF loss in one or both eyes were included in the study. Eyes with other forms of glaucoma such as pigmentary glaucoma, or pseudoexfoliation were excluded. Patients were randomized to receive either a medical or surgical line of treatment to control their IOP. Patients, rather than eyes, were randomized to the two treatment arms; if both eyes were eligible for treatment, the treatment course for both eyes was same that was determined during randomization.[47] Patients randomized to the medication treatment arm received a stepwise regimen of topical medications, beginning with monotherapy (typically a beta blocker). Additional medications were added upon evidence of inadequate IOP control or progressive VF loss. If medications failed to control the patient's IOP, the treatment was furthered with ALT concluding in trabeculectomy in some. In the surgical treatment arm, patients underwent immediate trabeculectomy. With evidence of surgical failure, ALT was done, alongside the medications.

Patients had a standardized follow-up examination at three and six months after treatment and every six months thereafter; in addition, patients randomized to the surgical arm received a postsurgical follow-up at one day, one week, and one month. At every visit, evaluation of visual acuity, VF and IOP was done. Patients were interviewed over the telephone to assess their health-related QOL. A questionnaire including the sickness impact profile, visual activities questionnaire and other components were used.

Results

Interim results including 5-year follow-up visits were reported in 2001. Both treatment groups had substantial and sustained IOP lowering with the surgical group running IOPs about 2 to 3 mm Hg lower than the medical group; however, the surgical group had more VF and visual acuity loss in the first-three years of the study, but these differences largely disappeared over four and five years follow-up.[48]

In patients with early glaucoma, at least a 30 percent reduction in the IOP, maintaining a target IOP in upper teens was found adequate to prevent progression in the initial reports. QOL parameters indicated that both groups were satisfied with their line of treatment.[49-51]

Recommendations

Based on these interim follow-up data, the investigators do not recommend changes to current approaches to managing newly diagnosed POAG patients.

Complications

The medical group reported a variety of systemic symptoms, while the surgical group reported more local eye symptoms including foreign body sensation, ptosis, early visual fluctuation and cataract development. The surgical group warranted a greater need of cataract extractions than the medical group. However, other symptoms diminished with time.

COLLABORATIVE NORMAL TENSION GLAUCOMA STUDY (CNTGS)[53,54]
Introduction
Normal tension glaucoma (NTG), also known as normal pressure or low tension glaucoma is unique among the glaucomas in that damage to the optic nerve can happen without a rise in IOP above the statistically normal range. For many years, ophthalmologists have been uncertain about how to best treat NTG, as there was no solid evidence to show that lowering eye pressure prevents continued VF loss. This study was designed to attempt answering some of these difficult questions.

Objectives
The main focus of the study was to understand the disease itself, that is, to determine whether IOP was or was not a modifiable risk factor in the disease. The approach of the study was to compare the course of untreated disease with others who had successful lowering of the IOP.

Study Design
In this randomized clinical trial, 230 patients were enrolled from 24 collaborating centers. The eligible patients had unilateral or bilateral NTG evidenced by glaucomatous cupping of the disc and severity of field loss with a median IOP of 20 mm Hg or less in 10 baseline measurements. One eye of patients with NTG was randomized:

- To be followed without treatment until there was evidence of slight deterioration. The other eye was treated at the discretion of the treating physician, except that systemic carbonic anhydrase inhibitors were not used.
- To be placed on treatment with medication, ALT, filtration surgery, or any combination, as required to lower the IOP by 30 percent.

In both arms, neither eye received beta-blockers or adrenergic agonists, as they might have systemic cardiovascular effects that could conceivably alter the course of the treated or untreated disease, confounding the analysis of data. Some patients were randomized immediately, if the VF defect threatened the point of fixation or there was previously documented progression of the disease.[55] Other patients were randomized later if there was VF progression, progression of optic nerve head cupping, or a new disc hemorrhage.

By the end of the study, 145 eyes were randomized: 66 received treatment and 79 eyes served as untreated controls. Of the 66 assigned to treatment, five withdrew before achieving the IOP-lowering goal.

Results
A 30 percent lowering of IOP was achieved in patients with NTG with medical therapy and ALT about half the time.[56,57] In view of the fact that cataracts developed in some of the treated patients, predominantly those that had glaucoma surgery, it is fortunate that lowering of IOP has become easier with medications not permitted

in the CNTGS protocol and with drugs that have more recently become available. The fact that 30 percent lowering of IOP could be achieved so often in this group without surgery was unexpected and the study suggested that probably a smaller percentage of patients will require surgery to receive an effective degree of IOP lowering.[58] VF progression occurred at indistinguishable rates in the pressure-lowered (22/66) and the untreated control (31/79) arms of the study (P = .21). In an analysis with data censored when cataract affected visual acuity, VF progression was significantly more common in the untreated group (21/79) compared with the treated group (8/66).[57]

The study also pointed out that women, those with a history of migraine and history of disc hemorrhages, had a faster rate of progression. Also the rate of progression without treatment was highly variable, but often slow enough that half of the patients have no progression in five years.

Recommendations
The CNTGS showed lowering IOP prevents VF progression in majority of patients and that only a small percentage of patients would need surgical intervention to lower their IOP. It is also not yet known whether some patients may respond adequately with less IOP lowering, while others require more IOP lowering.

Complications
There was a higher incidence of cataract in the group undergoing filtration surgery and this masked the favorable effects of IOP lowering in the initial analysis.

REFERENCES

1. Dandona L, et al. Is current eye-care-policy focus almost exclusively on cataract adequate to deal with blindness in India? Lancet 1998;351: 1312-6.

2. Jain MR, Modi R. Survey of chronic simple glaucoma in the rural population of India (Udaipur) above the age group of 30 years. Indian J Ophthalmol 1983;31:656-7.

3. Murthy GV, et al. Current estimates of blindness in India. Br J Ophthalmol 2005;89:257-60.

4. Hitchings RA, Glaucoma screening. Br J Ophthalmol 1993;77:326.

5. Goldberg I, Graham SL, Healey PR. Primary open-angle glacoma. Med J Aust 2002;177:535-6.

6. Khandekar R, Mohammed AJ, Raisi AA. Prevalence and causes of blindness and low vision; before and five years after 'VISION 2020' initiatives in Oman: a review. Ophthalmic Epidemiol 2007;14:9-15.

7. Eddy DM, Billings J. The quality of medical evidence: implications for quality of care. Health Aff (Millwood) 1988;7:19-32.

8. Wilson MR, Gaasterland D. Translating research into practice: controlled clinical trials and their influence on glaucoma management. J Glaucoma 1996;5:139-46.

9. Jaillon P. [Controlled randomized clinical trials]. Bull Acad Natl Med 2007;191:739-56; discussion 756-8.

10. Higginbotham EJ, et al. The Ocular Hypertension Treatment Study: topical medication delays or prevents primary open-angle glaucoma in African-American individuals. Arch Ophthalmol 2004;122:813-20.

11. Keltner JL, et al. Confirmation of visual field abnormalities in the Ocular Hypertension Treatment Study. Ocular Hypertension Treatment Study Group. Arch Ophthalmol 2000; 118:1187-94.

12. Gordon MO, et al. The Ocular Hypertension Treatment Study: baseline factors that predict the onset of primary open-angle glaucoma. Arch Ophthalmol 2002;120:714-20.

13. Kass MA, et al. The Ocular Hypertension Treatment Study: a randomized trial determines that topical ocular hypotensive medication delays or prevents the onset of primary open-angle glaucoma. Arch Ophthalmol 2002;120:701-13.

14. Kymes SM, et al. Management of ocular hypertension: a cost-effectiveness approach from the Ocular Hypertension Treatment Study. Am J Ophthalmol 2006;141:997-1008.

15. Herman DC, et al. Topical ocular hypotensive medication and lens opacification: evidence from the ocular hypertension treatment study. Am J Ophthalmol 2006;142:800-10.

16. Argus WA. Ocular hypertension and central corneal thickness. Ophthalmol 1995;102:1810-2.

17. Wolfs RC, et al. Distribution of central corneal thickness and its association with intraocular pressure: The Rotterdam Study. Am J Ophthalmol 1997;123:767-72.

18. Brandt JD, et al. Central corneal thickness and measured IOP response to topical ocular hypotensive medication in the Ocular Hypertension Treatment Study. Am J Ophthalmol 2004;138:717-22.

19. Philippin H, et al. Ten-year results: detection of long-term progressive optic disc changes with confocal laser tomography. Graefes Arch Clin Exp Ophthalmol 2006;244:460-4.

20. Keltner JL, et al. Visual field quality control in the Ocular Hypertension Treatment Study (OHTS). J Glaucoma 2007;16:665-9.

21. Keltner JL, et al. Classification of visual field abnormalities in the ocular hypertension treatment study. Arch Ophthalmol 2003;121:643-50.

22. Quigley HA. European Glaucoma Prevention Study. Ophthalmol 2005; 112:1642-3: author reply 1643-5.

23. Parrish RK 2nd. The European Glaucoma Prevention Study and the Ocular Hypertension Treatment Study: why do two studies have different results? Curr Opin Ophthalmol 2006;17:138-41.

24. Miglior S, et al. Results of the European Glaucoma Prevention Study. Ophthalmol 2005;112:366-75.

25. Leske MC, et al. Early Manifest Glaucoma Trial: design and baseline data. Ophthalmol 1999;106:2144-53.

26. Heijl A, et al. Reduction of intraocular pressure and glaucoma progression: results from the Early Manifest Glaucoma Trial. Arch Ophthalmol 2002;120:1268-79.

27. The Glaucoma Laser Trial (GLT): I. Acute effects of argon laser trabeculoplasty on intraocular pressure. Glaucoma Laser Trial Research Group. Arch Ophthalmol 1989;107: 1135-42.

28. The Glaucoma Laser Trial (GLT): 2. Results of argon laser trabeculoplasty versus topical medicines. The Glaucoma Laser Trial Research Group. Ophthalmol 1990;97:1403-13.

29. The Glaucoma Laser Trial (GLT): 3. Design and methods. Glaucoma Laser Trial Research Group. Control Clin Trials 1991;12:504-24.

30. The Glaucoma Laser Trial (GLT): 6. Treatment group differences in visual field changes. Glaucoma Laser Trial Research Group. Am J Ophthalmol 1995;120:10-22.

31. The Glaucoma Laser Trial (GLT) and glaucoma laser trial follow-up study: 7. Results. Glaucoma Laser Trial Research Group. Am J Ophthalmol 1995;120:718-31.

32. The Advanced Glaucoma Intervention Study (AGIS): 1. Study design and methods and baseline characteristics of study patients. Control Clin Trials 1994;15:299-325.

33. Advanced Glaucoma Intervention Study. 2. Visual field test scoring and reliability. Ophthalmol 1994;101:1445-55.

34. The Advanced Glaucoma Intervention Study, 6: effect of cataract on visual field and visual acuity. The AGIS Investigators. Arch Ophthalmol 2000;118:1639-52.

35. The Advanced Glaucoma Intervention Study (AGIS): 4. Comparison of treatment outcomes within race. Seven-year results. Ophthalmol 1998;105:1146-64.

36. Gaasterland DE, et al. The Advanced Glaucoma Intervention Study (AGIS): 10. Variability among academic glaucoma subspecialists in assessing optic disc notching. Trans Am Ophthalmol Soc 2001;99:177-84;184-5.

37. The Advanced Glaucoma Intervention Study (AGIS): 7. The relationship between control of intraocular pressure and visual field deterioration. The AGIS Investigators. Am J Ophthalmol 2000;130:429-40.

38. The Advanced Glaucoma Intervention Study (AGIS): 9. Comparison of glaucoma outcomes in black and white patients within treatment groups. Am J Ophthalmol 2001;13:311-20.

39. The Advanced Glaucoma Intervention Study (AGIS): 11. Risk factors for failure of trabeculectomy and argon laser trabeculoplasty. Am J Ophthalmol 2002;134:481-98.

40. Caprioli J, Coleman AL. Intra-ocular pressure fluctuation a risk factor for visual field progression at low intraocular pressures in the advanced glaucoma intervention study. Ophthalmol 2008;115:1123-9.

41. The Advanced Glaucoma Intervention Study: 8. Risk of cataract formation after trabeculectomy. Arch Ophthalmol 2001;119:1771-9.

42. Schwartz AL, et al. The Advanced Glaucoma Intervention Study (AGIS): 5. Encapsulated bleb after initial trabeculectomy. Am J Ophthalmol 1999;127:8-19.

43. Fluorouracil Filtering Surgery Study one year follow-up. The Fluorouracil Filtering Surgery Study Group. Am J Ophthalmol 1989;108:625-35.

44. Risk factors for suprachoroidal hemorrhage after filtering surgery. The Fluorouracil Filtering Surgery Study Group. Am J Ophthalmol 1992;113:501-7.

45. Three-year follow-up of the Fluorouracil Filtering Surgery Study. Am J Ophthalmol 1993;115:82-92.

46. Five-year follow-up of the Fluorouracil Filtering Surgery Study. The Fluoro-uracil Filtering Surgery Study Group. Am J Ophthalmol 1996;121:349-66.

47. Musch DC, et al. The Collaborative Initial Glaucoma Treatment Study: study design, methods and baseline characteristics of enrolled patients. Ophthalmol 1999;106:653-62.

48. Lichter PR, et al. Interim clinical outcomes in the Collaborative Initial Glaucoma Treatment Study comparing initial treatment randomized to medications or surgery. Ophthalmol 2001;108:1943-53.

49. Janz NK, et al. Quality of life in newly diagnosed glaucoma patients: The Collaborative Initial Glaucoma Treatment Study. Ophthalmol 2001;108:887-98.

50. Mills RP, et al. Correlation of visual field with quality-of-life measures at diagnosis in the Collaborative Initial Glaucoma Treatment Study (CIGTS). J Glaucoma 2001;10:192-8.

51. Janz NK, et al. The Collaborative Initial Glaucoma Treatment Study: interim quality of life findings after initial medical or surgical treatment of glaucoma. Ophthalmol 2001;108:1954-65.

52. Comparison of glaucomatous progression between untreated patients with normal-tension glaucoma and patients with therapeutically reduced intraocular pressures. Collaborative Normal-Tension Glau-coma Study Group. Am J Ophthalmol 1998;126:487-97.

53. Anderson DR, Drance SM. "Not quite" natural history of NTG. Ophthalmol 2002;109:1041-2.

54. Schulzer M. Errors in the diagnosis of visual field progression in normal-tension glaucoma. Ophthalmol 1994;101:1589-95.

55. Drance S, Anderson DR, Schulzer M. Risk factors for progression of visual field abnormalities in normal-tension glaucoma. Am J Ophthalmol 2001;131:699-708.

56. Schulzer M. Intraocular pressure reduction in normal-tension glaucoma patients. The Normal Tension Glaucoma Study Group. Ophthalmol 1992;99:1468-70.

57. The effectiveness of intraocular pressure reduction in the treatment of normal-tension glaucoma. Collaborative Normal-Tension Glaucoma Study Group. Am J Ophthalmol 1998;126:498-505.

58. Anderson DR, Drance SM, Schulzer M. Natural history of normal-tension glaucoma. Ophthalmol 2001;108:247-53.

7 | Prevalence of Glaucoma in India and the World

SR Krishnadas

CHAPTER OUTLINE
- Regional Variations in the Prevalence of Glaucoma
- Prevalence of Glaucoma in India
- Glaucoma Blindness in India

INTRODUCTION

Glaucoma is the most common cause of irreversible blindness in the world. The World Health Organization estimates (2002) for the number of people blind from glaucoma were 4.4 million (12.3% of the blind worldwide). The majority of those with glaucoma remain undetected and one has to rely on the data from epidemiological studies to estimate the number of people afflicted by glaucoma and related blindness. With accumulation of a wealth of data from epidemiological surveys, it is understood that glaucoma affects all populations, though some regions and racial groups are more affected either due to higher prevalence and racial predilection or due to large populations in these regions resulting in the absolute number of persons with glaucoma being larger.[1]

REGIONAL VARIATIONS IN THE PREVALENCE OF GLAUCOMA

Europe and North America

Primary open angle glaucoma (POAG) is the predominant glaucoma in North America, Europe and European derived populations of Australia. The highest prevalence of glaucoma in these regions is observed in the African and Caribbean origin population in the USA and the Caribbean. Primary angle closure glaucoma (PACG) is relatively uncommon in Blacks and Caucasians living in these geographic areas.

Latin America

There are as yet no published data on the prevalence of glaucoma in populations of Central or South America, but the Los Angeles Latin American Study (LALES) demonstrated a relatively high prevalence of POAG (4.74%) amongst Latin Americans in USA. A study by Quigley et al[1] amongst Latin Americans revealed prevalence of glaucoma to be intermediate between those of Caucasians and Blacks.

Asia

Nearly half the population with glaucoma resides in Asia, owing to this region containing the two most populated nations in the world (India and China with 2.4 billion people account for a third of the global population). Prevalence surveys in Mongolia, Singapore, China and India have observed prevalence of primary angle closure glaucoma to be equal to that of POAG and the prevalence of POAG similar to that of Caucasians. A greater proportion of people in Asia are bilaterally blind from angle closure disease. 25 percent of those with PACG are blind as compared to 10 percent of those with POAG. Projection of these prevalence data to the predicted population growth in the Asian regions suggests that blindness from glaucoma is likely to be a major public health issue in the future.

Africa

The prevalence of combined glaucomas (primary and secondary) in the Tanzanian and South African studies was reported to be 5 percent. The predominant form of glaucoma was POAG, although exfoliation, aphakic and angle closure comprised the remainder. Glaucoma prevalence amongst the blacks in the USA is stated to be four times that of Caucasians. Since, the African-Americans and Caribbeans are of West African ancestry, the prevalence of glaucoma in West Africa is believed to be similar to that of the black population in North America and no cross-sectionals studies are currently available. In general, glaucoma affects a higher proportion of people of African ancestry, has a younger age of onset and results in greater visual morbidity as compared to most other populations.

A recent meta-analysis by Rudnicka et al[2] reviewed all surveys on POAG available in the literature and have estimated pooled prevalence by race. Similar prevalence figures have been applied to the projected worldwide population in the second decade of this century to estimate the absolute numbers of persons with glaucoma worldwide. It was expected that there will be about 45 million individuals with primary open angle glaucoma by 2010.

As far as primary angle closure glaucoma is concerned, data from Caucasian populations seems to suggest a relatively low prevalence of angle closure disease (0.04% in the Beaver Dam study and 0.6% in the Egna-Neumarkt studies). With a reported prevalence of about 0.5 percent in South Africa and Tanzania, the prevalence is also low in the African race. Surveys from Asia seem to suggest that angle closure glaucoma is more frequent in occurrence, although POAG is also equally common. Prevalence figures for angle closure glaucoma range from 0.8 to 0.85 percent in Mongolia and South India to 1 percent in Singapore and 1.5 percent in Guangzhou province in China. The estimates for number of persons with PACG in 2020 predict that China will account for 50 percent angle closure glaucoma and 85 percent of all individuals with angle closure glaucoma will reside in Asia. The increase in the predicted number of people with glaucoma is largely due to increased longevity.

PREVALENCE OF GLAUCOMA IN INDIA

Population based studies had estimated the prevalence of glaucoma in India to be about 11.9 million and 60.5 million in the World by the year 2010. Most data on prevalence of glaucoma has been from studies in South India and West Bengal, though one study is currently underway in Nagpur, Central India, and the data are yet to be made available. There is no data available from North India as of now. There have been four prevalence studies from South India: The Andhra Pradesh Eye Disease Study (APEDS), the Aravind Comprehensive Eye Survey (ACES),[3] the Chennai Glaucoma Study (CGS) and the Vellore Eye Study (VES). Though the methodology employed in each of these population based studies differ widely, all the studies based diagnosis of glaucoma on the appearance of optic disc and visual field defects on automated perimetry. No study relied on measurement of intraocular pressure for diagnosis of glaucoma except in situations where optic disc or visual fields were unavailable owing to lack of media clarity.

Primary Open Angle Glaucoma

Wide variation in the prevalence of glaucoma was reported between the different studies. The Vellore Eye Study (VES) reported the lowest prevalence rates, since, unlike other prevalence studies, this study included patients in the age group of 30 to 60 years. The prevalence of primary open angle glaucoma (POAG) increased with age in all the reported studies. There was also a low rate of performance of visual fields in the VES probably underestimating the prevalence of glaucoma in this population as both the optic disc and visual field defect criteria were required to detect glaucoma. The VES also had a high rate of non responders (51.5%) in a marked contrast to other prevalence studies, affecting case detection and possible underestimation of the prevalence.

The reported prevalence rates of glaucoma in an urban population were significantly higher as revealed in the Chennai glaucoma study (CGS)[4] and the Andhra Pradesh eye study (APEDS),[5] with the exception of VES.[6] Diabetes and cardiovascular diseases also have reported to have a higher prevalence in rural India. It is speculated that lifestyle changes and cardiovascular disease patterns in urban India may indirectly influence the prevalence of POAG. The proportion of persons with glaucoma who presented with a normal IOP (defined as within two standard deviation from the population mean) were relatively higher in all the studies: 65 percent of persons with POAG in APEDS, 45 percent in ACES (Aravind Comprehensive Eye Survey), 67 percent in CGS (rural) and 82 percent in CGS (urban) had normal IOP at the time of diagnosis **(Table 1)**. This emphasizes the unreliability of IOP measurement alone in screening

Table 1 Prevalence of POAG in India

	APEDS %	*ACES %*	*CGS (Rural) %*	*CGS (Urban) %*	*WBGS %*
40–49 years	1.27	0.34	0.63	2.26	–
50–59 years	2.31	1.57	1.62	3.57	2.55
60–69 years	4.89	1.83	2.58	4.08	2.69
>70 years	6.32	2.88	3.25	6.42	4.76
Reported prevalence %	2.56	1.7	1.62	3.51	2.99
(95% CI)	(1.22, 3.91)	(1.3, 2.1)	(1.42,1.82)	(3.04, 4.0)	

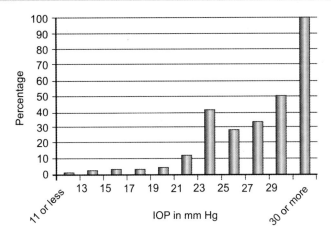

Fig. 1 Prevalence of POAG at each level of IOP—IOP is a significant risk factor for POAG. *(Vijaya et al. IOVS 2005)*

for glaucoma, and reinforces careful optic nerve head evaluation for accurate diagnosis of glaucoma. Increasing age and higher IOP was a consistent risk factor for glaucoma in all the prevalence studies. ACES reported male gender and myopia to be risk factors for POAG although no other studies observed gender or refractive errors to be associated with increased risk of POAG **(Figure 1)**.

Increased incidence of glaucoma with age is a cause for concern since India's population is aging and the prevalence is expected to increase exponentially in the decades to come. A significant proportion of individuals with glaucoma will reside in the Indian subcontinent by 2030. Quigley[1] had projected that number of persons with OAG older than 40 years would comprise 18.4 percent of the World's POAG population. In India, despite an inequitable distribution of eye care providers and ophthalmologists in urban areas, the prevalence of primary open angle glaucoma was reported to be twice in an urban population (3.47%) as compared to rural (1.62%).[7]

Primary Angle Closure Glaucoma
Owing to differing methodology and diagnostic criteria used in the definition of angle closure disease by the investigators, the prevalence of angle closure glaucoma reveals wide variation between the prevalence studies. Vellore Eye Study (VES) reported PACG to constitute a significant proportion of glaucoma in the population (4.32%). The stringent criteria used by VES investigators included both primary angle closure (PAC) and occludable angles (PACS) in the diagnosis of PACG thereby overestimating the prevalence of angle closure disease with glaucoma in the study population (urban, 30–60 years). 0.51 percent in the VES had angle closure disease with disc and field changes consistent with the dignosis of primary angle closure glaucoma.

This is similar to the prevalence of PACG reported in the other population studies. APEDS reported a lower prevalence of angle closure glaucoma, and the study especially highlighted a lower prevalence of PACS, partly accounted by a stricter criterion used to define occludability (nonvisibility of the pigmented trabecular meshwork for 270° or more of the filtering angle). The CGS used similar criteria as the VES to define occludable angles (180 of the filtering angle closed) and reported similar prevalence of angle closure

disease. The urban cohort of the CGS had a higher prevalence of angle closure disease than the rural population studied. A vast majority of persons with PACG had chronic, asymptomatic disease in the prevalence studies. Moreover, the CGS reported that in those diagnosed with glaucoma earlier, close to 40 percent were misclassified as POAG **(Table 2)**. Thus, Gonioscopy is an essential tool for appropriately classifying and treating glaucomas.

Blindness from angle closure disease is also reported to be higher than that from POAG. The Chennai glaucoma study reported 2 to 3 times increased unilateral and bilateral blindness from angle closure glaucoma as compared to POAG.[8] Interestingly, the prevalence of angle closure glaucoma and blindness from angle closure disease has been reported to be higher in urban than the rural cohort. One of the reasons speculated for this disparity is increased proportion of older population and later cataract extraction in the urban population.

Risk Factors for Angle Closure Disease and Glaucoma
Increasing age has been identified as a significant risk factor for PACG in all studies. CGS established female gender as a definite risk factor for PACG and PAC. The APEDS also reported more women with PACG though the association was not statistically significant. Both these studies also identified increased risk of PACG with hyperopia. Eyes with angle closure disease are reported to have shorter axial length, shallower anterior chambers and thicker crystalline lenses than normals in the population (CGS).

Exfoliation and Glaucoma
Exfoliation has been recognized to be the most common identifiable risk factor for ocular hypertension and glaucoma the world over. The prevalence of exfoliation

Table 2 Prevalence of angle closure disease in India

Age years	APEDS		CGS (Rural)			CGS (Urban)		
	PACG	PAC	PACG	PAC	PACS	PACG	PAC	PACS
40–49 years	0.00	0.76	0.44	0.38	4.29	0.07	1.27	4.86
50–59 years	1.54	3.08	1.02	0.81	7.31	0.63	3.30	7.77
60–69 years	2.17	3.80	1.01	1.01	7.96	2.21	4.19	9.27
>70 years	3.16	5.26	1.73	1.08	7.58	1.48	3.21	9.38
Reported Prevalence %	1.08	2.21	0.87	0.71	6.27	0.8	2.75	7.24
95% CI	(0.36, 1.80)	(1.15, 3.27)	(0.58, 1.16)	(0.45, 0.98)	(5.51, 7.03)	(0.6, 1.16)	(2.01, 3.49)	(6.58, 8.02)

VES reported prevalence of PACG 4.3 (2,3.01–5.63) (30–60 years)
ACES (40 years or more): 0.5% (0.3–0.7 and 95% CI)

glaucoma from hospital based data in India has been reported to be between 1.87 and 13.5 percent. Recently, population based data on exfoliation are available from the epidemiologic studies on glaucoma. The prevalence of exfoliation in South India has been estimated to be 3 to 6 percent in persons aged over 40. Amongst those with exfoliation, glaucoma has been reported to vary between 3 percent (APEDS), 7.5 percent (ACES) and 13 percent (CGS, rural cohort). Increasing age and occupation, outdoor as against indoor activity were identified to be significant risk factors. There was no gender predilection for glaucoma and an insignificant association of exfoliation and glaucoma were reported with lower socioeconomic status in the APEDS.

Secondary Glaucomas

The prevalence of secondary glaucomas in the population has been reported to be highly variable in the studies. The West Bengal Glaucoma Study (WBGS) reported 0.08 percent, the APEDS reported 0.21 percent in persons aged over 30 and ACES 0.3 percent in persons aged over 40 years. The Chennai Glaucoma Study, however, found a high prevalence of glaucoma (11.2%)[9] among persons with aphakia/pseudophakia. Such high prevalence of glaucoma following cataract extraction in this population prevailed

even after bilateral primary glaucomas were excluded from the study. The prevalence of glaucoma in aphakia and pseudophakia in this south Indian population is reported to be 0.82 percent which is higher than similar prevalence in African and Hispanic population. Aphakia, age, IOP and peripheral anterior synechiae exceeding 180° of the anterior chamber angle were significant risk factors. A history of prior cataract surgery remained a significant risk factor for glaucoma. Significantly, 22.2 percent of those with glaucoma following cataract surgery were blind in one or both eyes. 72 percent of those with glaucoma in aphakia and pseudophakia also had a normal IOP on presentation and most were undiagnosed until this population based study had detected them. Cataract surgery and intraocular lens implantation are the most common ophthalmic procedures performed and cataract continues to be the most common cause of preventable blindness in India. Such high rates of prevalence of glaucoma in eyes that have undergone cataract surgery calls for extreme caution in prevention of complications of cataract surgery and careful follow-up of individuals post cataract surgery.

GLAUCOMA BLINDNESS IN INDIA

Glaucoma has been declared to be the second common cause of blindness in

adult population in India. The proportion of persons bilaterally blind from POAG has been variably reported to be 11 percent (APEDS), 1.6 percent (ACES), 3.2 percent and 1.5 percent (CGS rural and urban population, respectively) and 5.2 percent (WBGS). In most of these studies, PACG was observed to cause one to four times the proportion of blindness as POAG: 16.6 percent (APEDS), 2.9 and 5.9 percent (CGS rural and urban). The high rate of blindness in the Indian population is due to high proportion of undiagnosed glaucoma in the community. Glaucoma was undetected in more than 90 percent of individuals identified in the population studies. The ACES also reported that 50 percent of persons detected with glaucoma had undergone an ophthalmic evaluation in the previous year and yet glaucoma was undetected in 80 percent of individuals identified by the study. Inadequate identification of glaucoma even in population undergoing ophthalmic evaluation continues to be a major determinant of preventable blindness due to glaucoma in India. Case detection needs to exponentially increase to address an important cause of preventable blindness in the country. Awareness of glaucoma, which is especially low in the rural community needs to be increased by public education and counseling and dissemination of relevant information on glaucoma through electronic and mass media.

REFERENCES

1. Quigley HA. Number of people with glaucoma worldwide. Br J Ophthalmol 1996;80:389.

2. Rudnicka AR, Mt-Isa S, Owen CG, et al. Variations in primary open angle glaucoma prevalence by age, gender and race: a Bayesian meta-analysis. Invest Ophthalmol Vis Sci 2006;47:4254.

3. Ramakrishnan R, Praveen NK, Krishnadas R. Glaucoma in a rural population in South India. The Aravind comprehensive eye survey. Ophthalmol 2003;110:1484.

4. Lingam V, George R, Paul P, et al. Prevalence of glaucoma in a rural population in South India. The Chennai glaucoma study. IOVS 2005; 46:4461.

5. Dandona L, Dandona R, Srinivas M, et al. Open angle glaucoma in an urban population in south India. Ophthalmol 2000;107:1702.

6. Jacob A, Thomas R, Koshy SP. Prevalence of primary open angle glaucoma in an urban population in South India. Indian Journal of Ophthalmology 1996;46:81.

7. Lingam V, George R, Bhaskaran M, et al. Prevalence of glaucoma in an urban population of South India. The Chennai glaucoma study. Ophthalmol 2008:115:648-54.

8. Lingam V, George R, Hemamalini A, et al. Prevalence of primary angle closure disease in an urban population and comparison with rural. Ophthalmol 2008;115:655-60.

9. Hemamalini A, George R, Raju P, et al. Glaucoma in aphakia and pseudophakia in the Chennai glaucoma study. Br J Ophthalmol 2005;89:699-703.

8

Vascular Factors in Glaucoma

Tanuj Dada, Shalini Mohan, Munish Dhawan

CHAPTER OUTLINE

INTRODUCTION

Primary open angle glaucoma (POAG) is a multifactorial optic neuropathy characterized by progressive retinal ganglion cell death and tissue remodeling of the optic nerve head (ONH). This is followed by visual field defects corresponding to the damage of the neuroretinal rim (NRR). Prevalence of glaucoma is 0.7 percent in the 5th decade and it increases to 7.7 percent in subjects over 80 years of age.[1]

Traditionally, diagnosis and treatment has been directed towards the control of increased intraocular pressure (IOP), which is the most important risk factor. However, all patients with glaucomatous ONH damage do not have elevated IOP, and glaucomatous neuropathy may progress even at IOP in the low teens, called as normal tension glaucoma (NTG). Some glaucoma patients continue to progress and subsequently develop irreversible loss of vision despite the medical lowering of IOP.

For instance, in the Early Manifest Glaucoma Trial (EMGT) the disease progression rate in the treatment group was 45 percent as compared to 62 percent in the control arm.[2]

In the Collaborative Initial Glaucoma Treatment Study (CIGTS) visual field progression occurred in $\geq$20 percent of participants during 8 years of follow-up.[3]

> Glaucoma actually represents a spectrum where mechanical damage predominates at high IOP and vascular factors increasingly contribute to damage at lower IOP levels. Both IOP and vascular factors are interrelated.

Specifically, increased incidence of visual field deterioration occurred with older age (increased risk of VF loss by 40% every 10 years), race (nonwhites had a 50% increased risk relative to whites) and diabetes (59% increased risk relative to non-diabetic patients).[3]

Likewise, 20 percent of normal tension glaucoma (NTG) patients show continued visual field loss even after 5 years of IOP reduction treatment.[4]

It is evident from these studies that the pathophysiological concept of glaucoma based only on IOP related damage is not complete. Glaucoma actually represents a spectrum where mechanical damage predominates at high IOP and vascular factors increasingly contribute to damage at lower IOP

levels. However, both factors are interrelated as an increase in IOP decreases the blood flow to the optic nerve head and *vice versa*. Compromised ocular blood flow and deranged vascular autoregulation in the ONH is emerging as an important causative and contributing to glaucomatous optic neuropathy.[5-9]

BLOOD SUPPLY OF THE OPTIC NERVE HEAD

The optic nerve head (ONH) consists of four distinct regions with a unique blood supply.[5,9-13] These regions from anterior to posterior aspect are as follows:

Surface Nerve Fiber Layer

This is the anterior most layer of the ONH. It contains the compact optic nerve fibers as they congregate from all over the retina and bend to run back. This part is essentially supplied by the retinal arterioles from the central retinal artery. However, in few cases the temporal part may be supplied by the posterior ciliary artery circulation from the underlying prelaminar region. When a cilioretinal artery is present, it supplies the corresponding part of the surface nerve fiber layer.

The Prelaminar Region

This part consists of optic nerve fibers arranged in bundles, surrounded by glial tissue septa, which contain capillaries. This region is supplied mainly by centripetal branches from the peripapillary choroid in a sectoral manner. The peripapillary choriocapillaris and central retinal artery play no role in its blood supply.

Lamina Cribrosa Region

This forms a band of dense, compact connective tissue extending transversely across the entire width of the ONH. It is laminar in nature, with collagen bundles alternating with glial tissue. The lamina cribrosa region is supplied by centripetal branches arising directly from the short posterior ciliary arteries or from the intrascleral circle of Zinn and Haller, when that is present. In the lamina cribrosa, the blood vessels, 10 to 20 microns in diameter, lie in the fibrous septa and form a dense capillary plexus which makes this part of the ONH a highly vascular structure.

Retrolaminar Region

This part of the optic nerve lies immediately behind the lamina cribrosa. It is enclosed by dura, arachnoid and pia. This region has centripetal and centrifugal vascular systems.

a. *The centripetal system* is the main and consistent vascular system, formed primarily by the recurrent pial branches from the peripapillary choroid and the circle of Zinn and Haller (or the short posterior ciliary arteries), with additional pial branches from the central retinal artery.

b. *A centrifugal system* may be seen in some nerves and consists of a few inconstant branches from the central retinal artery.

In summary, the primary source of blood supply to the ONH is the posterior ciliary artery circulation via the peripapillary choroid and short posterior ciliary arteries (or the circle of Zinn and Haller, when present).

FACTORS INFLUENCING BLOOD FLOW IN ONH

To understand the role of vascular insufficiency of the (ONH) in the pathogenesis of glaucoma, it is fundamental to understand the blood flow in the ONH in health and disease and the various factors that influence it. The blood flow depends upon three parameters:

1. Vascular resistance
2. Blood pressure
3. IOP.[6-13]

To calculate the ONH blood flow, the following formula is used:

$$\text{Blood flow} = \frac{\text{Perfusion pressure}}{\text{Vascular resistance}}$$

Perfusion Pressure

The perfusion pressure is essentially the difference between the mean arterial blood pressure (MABP) and the intraocular pressure (IOP).

Perfusion pressure = MABP – IOP
MABP = Diastolic BP + 1/3 (Systolic BP – Diastolic BP).

Based on the above equation it is clear that a decrease in BP or an increase in IOP reduces perfusion pressure.

Vascular Resistance

The resistance of the vasculature depends upon the state and caliber of the vessels feeding the ONH circulation and rheological properties of the blood which is influenced by a large variety of hematologic disorders, particularly those causing increase in blood viscosity.

The state and caliber of the vessels feeding the ONH may be altered by many factors, including the following:

1. *Autoregulation of blood flow* is to maintain a relatively constant blood flow, capillary pressure and nutrient supply in spite of changes in perfusion pressure. Evidences show that blood flow in both the retina and ONH is autoregulated by neural, endothelial and myogenic mechanisms.[14] The mediators of these mechanisms include oxygen, carbon dioxide, angiotensin-II, nitric oxide and endothelin-1. But various systemic and local factors can cause breakdown of this autoregulatory mechanism which are aging, arterial hypertension, diabetes mellitus, marked arterial hypotension from any cause, arteriosclerosis, atherosclerosis, hypercholesterolemia, vasospasm and probably regional vascular endothelial disorders.[15-18]

2. *Vascular endothelial vasoactive agents* play an important role in modulating the local vascular tone. The vascular endothelial cells release various known endothelial vasoactive agents, which include prostanoids, nitric oxide, endothelins, angiotensins, oxygen free radicals, smooth muscle cell hyperpolarization, thromboxane A2 and other agents.[19-21] Endothelial cells regulate vasomotor function not only by the vasoactive agents but can also function as mechanosensors. Pathophysiological changes in the vascular endothelial cell structure and/or function occur in most of the major cardiovascular diseases, including atherosclerosis, diabetes mellitus, hypertension and ischemia.

3. Vascular changes in the arteries feeding the ONH circulation may be produced by vasospasm, arteriosclerosis, vasculitis, drug-induced vasoconstriction or dilatation, and a host of other systemic and cardiovascular factors.

Arterial Blood Pressure

It is clear from the above equation that arterial blood pressure is a major factor which can affect the perfusion pressure in the ONH. Nocturnal arterial hypotension is an important risk factor for the development of ONH ischemic disorders. Therefore, it is important to record the night time BP as the daytime recording gives no information about the BP during sleep. Noctural fall in BP coupled with an increase in IOP may be deleterious for the optic nerve. Over-treatment of systemic hypertension in a glaucoma patient can lead to low blood pressure and progression of optic neuropathy despite an adequately controlled IOP.

Intraocular Pressure

There is an inverse relationship between IOP and perfusion pressure in the ONH. Studies have shown that subjects with a diastolic ocular perfusion pressure lower than 50 mm Hg may have a four times greater risk of OAG than those with a perfusion pressure of 80 mm Hg.[22] Lower systolic perfusion pressure more than doubled the relative risk (RR) and lower diastolic perfusion pressure (DPP) (<55 mm Hg) more than tripled the RR of OAG.[23]

In persons with normal BP and autoregulation, a much greater rise in IOP would be required before the ONH blood flow is compromised. By contrast, in persons with arterial hypotension, defective autoregulation or other vascular risk factors, even "normal" IOP may interfere with the ONH blood flow (e.g. in normal tension glaucoma). This mechanism is important in the pathogenesis of glaucomatous optic neuropathy, particularly in normal tension glaucoma.

> "Normal IOP" with may interfere with ONH blood flow in presence of nocturnal arterial hypotension, vascular risk factors or defective autoregulation.

Therefore, a rise in IOP during sleep and concurrent development of nocturnal arterial hypotension may together constitute an important risk factor for ONH ischemia in vulnerable subjects and lead to progression of glaucoma.

EVALUATION OF THE ONH CIRCULATION

The measurement of ocular perfusion is must as low perfusion pressure has been implicated as an important risk factor in the various studies.[24-26] The measurement of the ocular circulation is done by various imaging techniques such as color Doppler ultrasound imaging (CDI), transcranial Doppler, laser Doppler flowmetry, scanning laser Doppler flowmetry, magnetic resonance imaging, pulsatile ocular blood flow method, fluorescein fundus angiography, confocal scanning laser fluorescein angiography and retinal photography oximetry. These imaging techniques have there own limitations and none of them is currently accepted as a gold standard for measuring optic nerve head flow.[8] Another important aspect is that one time measurements are not sufficient and should be done throughout 24 hours so as to assess their variability and effect on perfusion in relation to the blood pressure.[18]

> **Limitations of Imaging Techniques**
> - Focus on the retinal circulation only
> - Only measure the blood flow velocity
> - No information about size of lumen
> - One time measurement
> - No information regarding variability.

Most of the recently advocated methods employ laser technology. All of them suffer from the fundamental flaw that the laser beam in all of them is focused on the surface of the optic disc to measure the amount of blood flow in the ONH. The surface layer of

the optic disc is supplied by the retinal circulation, whereas glaucomatous optic neuropathy is due vascular insufficiency in the deeper ONH circulation, supplied by the posterior ciliary artery circulation.[27] Experimental study in monkeys have confirmed that laser Doppler flowmetry predominantly measures the blood flow in the superficial layers of the ONH supplied by the retinal circulation.[28]

The same applies to Heidelberg retinal flowmetry (HRF) and to the laser speckle method. The other common error in blood flow measurements has been to equate blood velocity with the amount of blood flow in the ONH; the blood velocity does not provide information about the quantity of blood flow unless we know the size of the lumen of the vessels (e.g. use of color Doppler imaging). Therefore, none of the methods used so far provide scientifically valid information about the ONH blood flow and circulation.

Ocular Blood Flow and Visual Field Defects in Normal Tension Glaucoma

Recently, Logan et al. measured tissue blood flow in a 10×10 pixel box 200 µm from the disc margin in each quadrant, using the Heidelberg retina flowmeter (HRF, Heidelberg Engineering, Heidelberg, Germany).[29] They reported that glaucomatous subjects had lower retinal hemodynamic values than control subjects in these areas. The retinal nerve fiber layer in the inferior sector of the retina and the tissue in the inferior sector of the ONH have been reported to have lower blood flow/ unit nerve tissue volume than does the superior sector.[30] This would mean that the retinal ganglion cells and their axons in the inferior retina are more vulnerable to circulatory alterations than those in the superior retina. This corresponds with clinical findings that glaucomatous visual field defects are more commonly found in the superior visual field than in the inferior field.[31]

In addition, Yamazaki and Drance, using color Doppler imaging, reported that eyes with NTG and progressive visual field defects have significantly lower blood flow velocities and higher resistive indices in the short posterior ciliary and retinal arteries than eyes with relatively stable visual fields.[32] These studies suggest that alterations in the circulation in glaucomatous eyes are associated with the glaucomatous visual field changes. However, only limited information is available on whether the retinal hemodynamics is altered in eyes with glaucomatous visual field changes.[33,34]

Enrique Adan Sato et al.[35] determined the relationship between the blood flow parameters of the optic disc rim and the glaucomatous visual field changes. They measured tissue blood flow in the neuroretinal rim within the optic disc with the Heidelberg retina flowmeter (HRF) in 54 eyes of 54 patients with normal-tension glaucoma (NTG). Patients whose visual field defects were confined to either the superior or inferior hemifield were selected. Blood flow measurements were made in a $10 \times 2.5°$ area of the superior and inferior neuroretinal rim within the optic disc. The mean blood flow (MBF) was calculated by the automatic full-field perfusion image analyzer program and the ratio of the MBF in the superior to the inferior rim areas (the S/I ratio) was calculated from the same HRF image in order to minimize the variation in measurement conditions. They found out that the inferior rim blood flow was less than superior rim blood flow in patients with superior hemifield defect and superior rim blood flow was reduced compared to inferior in patients with inferior hemifield defect. The mean S/I ratios of the MBF in the patients with superior hemifield defect

was significantly higher than that in the patients with inferior hemifield defect and they concluded that the blood flow in the neuroretinal rim was found to correspond to the regional visual field defect in eyes with NTG. Reductions in flow were associated with reductions in function.

ROLE OF OCULAR BLOOD FLOW IN PATIENTS HAVING OBSTRUCTIVE SLEEP APNEA SYNDROME AND GLAUCOMA

Obstructive sleep apnea syndrome (OSAS) is characterized by snoring, excessive daytime sleepiness and insomnia. Epidemiological studies revealed prevalence between 2 and 20 percent. Among the risk factors, obesity, male gender, upper respiratory tract abnormality, consumption of alcohol, snoring and thick neck are worth mentioning.

In previous studies, retinal vascular tortuosity and congestion, floppy eyelid syndrome, keratoconus, papilledema and optic neuropathy have been described in patients with OSAS. It has been stressed that OSAS may be a predisposing condition for anterior optic neuropathy. Karakucuk S et al[36] studied the ocular blood flow in patients with OSAS since pathological ocular blood flow has been suggested as a major mechanism in the etiology of glaucoma and also to detect the glaucoma prevalence in the study group. They have concluded that in a group of patients with OSAS, a high prevalence was found (12.9%=4 glaucoma patients of 31 OSAS patients) and it is interesting to note that all four of the glaucoma patients were in the severe OSAS group. The positive correlation detected between OARI and MD, and also between CRARI and MD as well as LV, suggests that visual field defects may be due to optic nerve perfusion defects and that these field defects also increase as the RI increases. The presence and progression of glaucoma

should be investigated particularly in patients with severe OSAS in the long-term follow-up, and changes in retinal nerve fiber layer thickness and ocular Doppler ultrasonographic findings should also be monitored in such patients.

CLINICAL SIGNIFICANCE OF OCULAR PERFUSION PRESSURE IN THE DIAGNOSIS AND MANAGEMENT OF GLAUCOMA

It has been reported that ocular perfusion pressure may affect an individual patient's risk of developing and/or progression of glaucoma but currently there are multiple challenges to and limitations of accepting this concept.

> **PEARLS**
> Patient of NTG or POAG with progression despite good IOP control
> - Look out for nocturnal BP dips
> - Coexisting microvascular disease
> - History suggestive of OSAS.

Facts Favoring the Measurement of Ocular Perfusion Pressure in Glaucoma

1. Dysfunction of systemic vascular endothelium influences progression of Open Angle Glaucoma (OAG).[37]
2. Glaucoma, especially normal-tension glaucoma, is significantly associated with the occurrence of episodic asymptomatic myocardial ischemias.[38]
3. Importance of oxidative stress factors and mitochondrial function in OAG.[39,40]
4. Increasing ocular circulation improves oxidative stress in retinal tissues.[39,40]
5. OAG patients have abnormal autoregulatory response to changes in perfusion pressure.[39,40]
6. Documented role of OPP in progression of glaucoma in population based studies.[41,42]

7. Patients with NTG show increased variability of night-time blood pressure measurements.[43]

Facts Against the Measurement of Ocular Perfusion Pressure in Glaucoma

1. Conflicting results of Beijing eye study which did not demonstrate the association of OAG with SBP, DBP or ocular perfusion pressure.[44]
2. Brachial blood pressure unlikely to reflect true perfusion pressure at the optic nerve head.
3. Diurnal variation in IOP and BP.

4. Lack of universally accepted position (sitting or standing) to measure BP.
5. Influence of other variables on ocular perfusion pressure.[45]

CONCLUSION

To conclude, recent population based studies have described the potential effects of low ocular perfusion pressure in the development and progression of OAG. Despite conflicting reports (Beijing eye study) and the definite limitations on reliably measuring ocular perfusion pressure in patients with glaucoma, more work needs to be done in patients having documented low perfusion pressure and definite progression of glaucoma. The ophthalmologists need to evaluate the blood pressure in all glaucoma patients, especially in normal pressure glaucoma, POAG patients with documented progression and those with co-existing systemic microvascular diseases.

Patients on systemic antihypertensives with a low diastolic pressure or DPP < 50 mm Hg should be referred to the cardiologist for improving the perfusion of the optic nerve head.

REFERENCES

1. National Eye Institute. Statistics and Data. Prevalence of Blindness Data. Data Tables. http://www.nei.nih.gov/eyedata/pbd_tables.asp. Accessed on September 18, 2007.
2. Heijl A, Leske MC, Bengtsson B, et al. Early Manifest Glaucoma Trial Group. Reduction of intraocular pressure and glaucoma progression: results from the Early Manifest Glaucoma Trial. Arch Ophthalmol 2002;120:1268-79.
3. Lichter PR, Musch DC, Gillespie BW, et al. Interin clinical outcome in the collaborative initial glaucoma treatment study comparing initial treatment randomized to medications or surgery. Ophthalmol 2001;108:1943-53.
4. Collaborative Normal-Tension Glaucoma Study Group. The effectiveness of intraocular pressure reduction in the treatment of normal-tension glaucoma. Am J Ophthalmol 1998;126:498-505.
5. Hayreh S. Blood supply of the optic nerve head and its role in optic atrophy, glaucoma and oedema of the optic disc. Br J Ophthalmol 1969;53:721-48.
6. Hayreh SS. Factors influencing blood flow in the optic nerve head. J Glaucoma 1997;6:412-25,1998;7:71.

7. Hayreh SS. Blood flow in the optic nerve head and factors that may influence it. Prog Retin Eye Res 2001;20:595-24.
8. Hayreh SS. Evaluation of optic nerve head circulation: Review of the methods used. J Glaucoma 1997;6:319-30.
9. Hayreh SS. Pathophysiology of Glaucomatous optic neuropathy: Role of optic nerve head vascular insufficiency. J Curr Glaucoma Practice 2008;2:6-17.
10. Hayreh SS. The optic nerve head circulation in health and disease. Exp Eye Res 1995;61:259-72.
11. Hayreh SS. The blood supply of the optic nerve head and the evaluation of it—Myth and reality. Prog Retin Eye Res 2001;20:563-93.
12. Hayreh SS. Optic disc changes in glaucoma. Br J Ophthalmol 1972;56:175-85.
13. Hayreh SS. Structure and blood supply of the optic nerve. In: Heilmann K, Richardson KT (Eds). Glaucoma: Conceptions of a Disease. Stuttgart: Thieme 1978.pp.78-96.
14. Flammer J, Mozaffarieh M. Autoregulation, a balancing act between supply and demand. Can J Ophthalmol 2008;43:317-21.

15. Hayreh SS, Servais GE, Virdi PS. Fundus lesions in malignant Hypertension. V Hypertensive optic neuropathy. Ophthalmol 1986;93:74-87.
16. Hayreh SS, Bill A, Sperber GO. Metabolic effects of high intraocular pressure in old arteriosclerotic monkeys. Invest Ophthalmol Vis Sci 1991;32:810.
17. Hayreh SS, Bill A, Sperber GO. Effects of high intraocular pressure on the glucose metabolism in the retina and optic nerve in old atherosclerotic monkeys. Graefes Arch Clin Exp Ophthalmol 1994;232:745-52.
18. Haefliger IO, Meyer P, Flammer J, Lüscher TF. The vascular endothelium as a regulator of the ocular circulation: A new concept in ophthalmology? Surv Ophthalmol 1994;39:123-32.
19. Weinreb RN. Ocular blood flow in glaucoma. Can J Ophthalmol 2008;43:281.
20. Davies MG, Hagen PO. The vascular endothelium. A new horizon. Ann Surg 1993;218:593-609.
21. Rubanyi GM. Cardiovascular significance of endothelium-derived vasoactive factors (1st edn). Mount Kisco, NY: Futura; 1991.

22. Ryan US, Rubanyi GM. Endothelial regulation of vascular tone (1st edn). New York: Marcel Dekker; 1992.

23. Quigley HA, West SK, Rodriguez J, Munoz B, Klein R, Snyder R. The prevalence of glaucoma in a population-based study of Hispanic subjects: Proyecto VER. Arch Ophthalmol 2001; 119(12):1819-26.

24. Leske MC, Wu SY, Nemesure B, Hennis A. Incident open-angle glaucoma and blood pressure. Arch Ophthalmol 2002;120:954-9.

25. Leske MC, Heijl A, Hyman L, Bengtsson B, Dong L, Yang Z; EMGT Group. Predictors of long-term progression in the early manifest glaucoma trial. Ophthalmol 2007;114:1965-722.

26. Leske MC, Wu SY, Hennis A, Honkanen R, Nemesure B; BESs Study Group. Risk factors for incident open-angle glaucoma: the Barbados Eye Studies. Ophthalmol 2008;115:85-93.

27. Petrig BL, Riva CE, Hayreh SS. Laser Doppler flowmetry and optic nerve head blood flow. Am J Ophthalmol 1999;127:413-25.

28. Wang L, Cull G, Cioffi GA. Depth of penetration of scanning laser Doppler flowmetry in the primate optic nerve. Arch Ophthalmol 2001;119:1810-4.

29. Logan JF, Rankin SJ, Jackson AJ. Retinal blood flow measurements and neuroretinal rim damage in glaucoma. Br J Ophthalmol 2004;88:1049:54.

30. Harris A, Ishii Y, Chung HS, Jonescu-Cuypers CP, McCranor LJ, Kagemann L, Garzozi HJ. Blood flow per unit retinal nerve fiber tissue volume is lower in the human inferior retina. Br J Ophthalmol 2003;87:184-8.

31. Hart WM Jr, Becker B. The onset and evolution of glaucomatous visual field defects. Ophthalmol 1982;89:268-79.

32. Yamazaki Y, Drance SM. The relationship between progression of visual field defects and retrobulbar circulation in patients with glaucoma. Am J Ophthalmol 1997;124:28-95.

33. Grunwald JE, Piltz J, Hariprasad SM, DuPont J. Optic nerve and choroidal circulation in glaucoma. Invest Ophthalmol Vis Sci 1998;39(12): 2329-36.

34. Hayreh SS. The blood supply of the optic nerve head and the evaluation of it—myth and reality. Prog Retin Eye Res 2001;20:563-93.

35. Sato AE, Ohtake Y, Shinoda K. Decreased blood flow at optic nerve head corresponds with visual field defects in NTG. Graefe's Arch Clin Exp Ophthalmol 2006;244:795-801.

36. Karakucuk S, Goktas S, Aksu M, Erdogan N, Demirci S, Oner A, Arda H, Gumus K. Ocular blood flow in patients with obstructive sleep apnea syndrome (OSAS). Graefes Arch Clin Exp Ophthalmol 2008;246:129-34.

37. Buckley C, Hadoke PW, Henry E. Systemic vascular endothelial cell dysfunction in normal pressure glaucoma. Br J Ophthalmol 2002;86:227-32.

38. Waldmann E, Grasser P, Dubler B. Silent myocardial ischemia in glaucoma and cataract patients. Graefes Arch Clin Exp Ophthalmol 1996; 234:595-8.

39. Grieshaber MC, Flammer J. Blood flow in glaucoma. Curr Opin Ophthalmol 2005;16:79-83.

40. Tsai JC. Influencing ocular blood flow in glaucoma patients: the cardiovascular system and healthy lifestyle choices. Can J Ophthalmol 2008;43:347-50.

41. Tielsch JM, Katz J, Sommer A. Hypertension, perfusion pressure and primary open angle glaucoma. A population based assessment. Arch Ophthalmol 1995;113:216-21.

42. Leska MC, Wu S-Y, Hennis, et al. BESs studt group. Risk factors for open angle glaucoma. The Barbados Eye Studies. Ophthalmol 2008;115: 85-93.

43. Plange N, Kaup M, Daneljan L, Predel HG, Remky A, Arend O. 24-h blood pressure monitoring in normal tension glaucoma: night-time blood pressure variability. J Hum Hypertens 2006;20:137-42.

44. Xu L, Wang YX, Jonas JB. Ocular perfusion pressure and glaucoma: the Beijing eye study. Eye 2008;23:734-6.

45. Berdahl, JP, Fautsh MP, Sandra S. Intracranial pressure in primary open angle glaucoma, normal tension glaucoma and ocular hypertension. Invest Ophthalmol Vis Sci 2008;49:5412-8.

9 | Aqueous Humor Dynamics

Shalmali Ranaut, Mona Khurana, R Ramakrishnan

CHAPTER OUTLINE

- Functions of Aqueous Humor
- Aqueous Humor Dynamics
- Pathway of Circulation
- Aqueous Humor Production
- Composition of Aqueous Humor Aqueous Humor of BAB
- Aqueous Humor Formation and Secretion
- Steps of Aqueous Humor Formation
- Factors Affecting Aqueous Humor Production
- Aqueous Humor Drainage
- Measurement of Aqueous Humor Formation and Flow
- Measurement of Aqueous Humor Outflow and Facility of Outflow
- Measurement of Uveoscleral Outflow
- Factors Affecting Aqueous Humor Outflow

INTRODUCTION

Many prospective randomized controlled trials have shown that intraocular pressure (IOP) is the most important and currently the only modifiable risk factor in the management of glaucoma. Abnormalities in IOP are a result of altered aqueous humor dynamics (AHD), predominantly a deranged outflow. Thus, a knowledge of the normal aqueous humor dynamics and the factors regulating it is essential. The importance of understanding aqueous flow lies in both understanding of the pathogenesis of glaucoma and more importantly developing methods for lowering IOP. The ciliary body where the aqueous is produced and the trabecular meshwork, the principle site of outflow are closely related. This chapter will deal with the anatomy of the inflow and outflow system, the paths, dynamics and factors influencing AHD.

Aqueous humor is a fluid derived from the filtrate of plasma and secreted by the epithelium of the processes of the ciliary body into the posterior chamber.

FUNCTIONS OF AQUEOUS HUMOR

A stable production and drainage of aqueous humor is essential for the physiology of the eye and maintenance of normal visual function.

Optical

One of the major functions of aqueous humor is to maintain the intraocular pressure and structural integrity of the eyeball, and stabilizing its optical properties. Diurnal variations in IOP do not appear to alter the quality of the image formed on the retina. It provides an optically clear medium for the transmission of light along the visual pathway.

Nutrition

The aqueous humor delivers oxygen and nutrients like glucose, amino acids to the avascular ocular structures such as:
- Posterior part of cornea
- Trabecular meshwork
- Lens
- Anterior vitreous.

It removes metabolic wastes and potentially toxic substances like carbon dioxide, lactic acid. Thus, the aqueous humor provides an appropriate chemical environment for the proper function of these avascular structures. It delivers antioxidants like ascorbate to scavenge free radicals to protect against the effect of ultraviolet and other radiations.

Local Immunity

The aqueous humor participates in the immune responses of the eye and in paracrine signalling.

IOP

The IOP is maintained by a balance between aqueous production and outflow. The delicate balance between the aqueous humor production, resistance to its outflow and the episcleral venous pressure is important for maintaining the intraocular pressure. A normal IOP is essential for maintaining the structural integrity of the eye.

AQUEOUS HUMOR DYNAMICS

AHD is the study of the parameters that contribute to the creation, maintenance and variation of intraocular pressure. The factors and the relation between them is clearly summarized in the Goldmann equation **(Table 1)**.

AQUEOUS HUMOR: PATHWAY OF CIRCULATION

Modified from plasma within capillaries of ciliary processes, the aqueous humor is secreted into the posterior chamber. It then flows around lens, through pupil to anterior chamber. The temperature gradient is cooler towards the cornea causing a convection pattern. The aqueous humor then exits the eye by passing through the trabecular meshwork and then the Schlemm's canal and finally drains into the venous system through a system of collector channels. Part of it also leaves the eye through the uveoscleral pathway, that is through the root of the iris and the ciliary muscle to the suprachoroidal space and through the sclera. The anatomical and physiological details will be discussed in subsequent sections.

AQUEOUS HUMOR PRODUCTION
Ciliary Body

Ciliary body is a specialized part of the uveal tract and is associated with both aqueous humor production and outflow. It extends from the ora serrata posteriorly to the scleral spur anteriorly, forming a ring along the inner wall of the eyeball. It attaches to the scleral spur leaving a potential space called supraciliary space/suprachoroidal space between sclera and itself. Its anterior posterior length is 4.6 to 5.2 mm nasally to 5.6 to 6.3 mm

Table 1 Goldmann equation[1]

$P_0 = (F/C) + P_v$
• P_0 is the IOP in millimeters of mercury (mm Hg)
• F is the rate of aqueous formation in microliters per minute (µl/min)
• C is the facility of outflow (µl/min/mm Hg)
• P_v is the episcleral venous pressure in millimeters of mercury
• Resistance of outflow® is the inverse of facility (C).

temporally. It resembles a right angled triangle on sagittal section with its shortest side or the base facing anteriorly. One of its sides lies along the sclera, separated by a potential space continuous with the suprachoroidal space. The inner surface of the ciliary body (or the other side of the triangle) is divided into two parts: the anterior part being pars plicata and pars plana posteriorly.

Pars Plicata

Pars plicata (2-2.5 mm) is also called as the corona ciliaris. It is the anterior one-third of the ciliary body and has about 70 to 80 radiating ciliary processes of varying sizes. Ciliary processes are present on the inner, anterior part of pars plicata.

Pars Plana

The pars plana is the smooth posterior two-third part of the ciliary body. It is 5 mm wide temporally and 3 mm wide nasally.

The ciliary body consists of the following layers:
- Ciliary muscle
- Vessels and ciliary processes
- Basal lamina
- Ciliary epithelium
- ILM.

Ciliary Muscle

In the ciliary body, flat unstriated muscle cells are organized into bundles which are further organized into three groups of muscle fibers:
1. Outermost is the longitudinal muscle: It is attached to scleral spur (SS) with extensions into the trabecular meshwork (TM)
2. Middle: radial muscle
3. Innermost: circular muscle.

The radial and circular muscles form the base of the triangle. They can be seen as the ciliary body band (CBB) gonioscopically. The meridional one is attached to the scleral spur and is involved in aqueous outflow regulation.

Iris inserts into ciliary body. On gonioscopy, the ciliary body is visible between the root of the iris and scleral spur as the ciliary body band. The crystalline lens is suspended by zonules and separates the vitreous and the aqueous. The iris separates the anterior chamber and the posterior chamber. The angle of the anterior chamber is formed by the iris and cornea.

Each ciliary process consists of:
• Fibrovascular core
• Double layer of epithelium continuous with pars plana
• Microvasculature
• Blood aqueous barrier

Ciliary Processes[2-4]

Internal to the ciliary muscles are major (around 70) and minor radial ciliary processes (CP) which extend into the posterior chamber forming pars plicata. Collectively they are called the corona ciliaris. They arise just posterior to the iris root forming the ciliary sulcus. The major process are 2 mm long, 1 mm high with an irregular convoluted surface.

The pars plana overlies the ciliary muscle and extends from ciliary process to ora serrata. The lens zonules arise from between the nonpigmented epithelium (NPE) and are channeled between ciliary process to insert onto the anterior and posterior lens capsule.

The aqueous humor is formed by ciliary processes which provide a large surface area for aqueous production. Each ciliary process is composed of a double layer of epithelium, outer pigmented (PE) and inner nonpigmented (NPE) with apical surfaces facing each other. The core stroma is richly supplied by fenestrated capillaries, thus increasing surface area of proximity between the epithelium and capillaries. The capillaries are derived from the branches of the major arterial circle which is formed by the long posterior ciliary arteries.[2-4] This maximizes access of the secretions into the small space of the posterior chamber.

Capillaries occupy the center of the ciliary process and have a thin endothelium lining with false porous areas. They have fenestrations or "pores" which allow passage of macromolecules into ciliary process stroma. This is in contrast to the capillaries of the ciliary muscle which have an endothelial lining which is continuous and impermeable.

- The apical plasma membrane of PE and NPE appose each other establishing cell-to-cell communication through gap junctions.
- **NPE** – establish BAB by tight junctions proximal to apical–membrane.
- **PE** in contrast have a leaky epithelium allows movement of solutes through inter cellular spaces between PE.
- Active secretion allows precise control of composition of the fluid bathing essential structures.

Ciliary Epithelium[5-7]

It consists of two epithelial layers joined apex-to-apex, with the basal lamina of the pigmentary layer adjacent to stroma and that of NPE lining the posterior chamber. The ciliary NPE is continuous with the iris pigment epithelium (IPE) anteriorly and neurosensory retina posteriorly. The basolateral surface of the nonpigmented layer faces directly into the posterior aqueous chamber. The PE corresponds anteriorly to anterior myoepithelium and posteriorly to retinal pigmented epithelium (RPE). Gap junctions are present between the lateral interdigitations of the pigmented cells. Desmosomes also occur between the lateral interdigitations of the pigmented and nonpigmented epithelia and between their apical membranes.

- The ciliary epithelium is the responsible for aqueous humor secretion
- It is the site of blood aqueous barrier (BAB).

Pigmented Epithelium (PE)

These low cuboidal epithelial cells contain melanosomes, mitochondria, endoplasmic reticulum and Golgi apparatus. There are numerous melanin granules in the cytoplasm, hence the name. These cells are separated from stroma by an atypical basement membrane. The basal and the lateral surfaces of these cells show infoldings which increase the surface area facing the capillaries.

Nonpigmented Epithelium (NPE)

NPE consists of columnar cells separated from aqueous humor by a basement membrane. These are *metabolically active cells* having more mitochondria and endoplasmic reticulum (indicating protein synthesis) as compared to the PE and numerous microvilli protruding into the anterior chamber.[7] These epithelial cells lack melanosomes. There are more cells in the anterior part of the ciliary process. Tight junctions are present in the lateral interdigitations between the nonpigmented cells forming a barrier for the passage of larger molecules between the cells. Aquaporin-1 channels are present.

Blood Aqueous Barrier

The difference between the composition of the aqueous humor and plasma needs to be maintained in order to ensure the proper functioning of the avascular structures of the anterior segment. The blood aqueous barrier is responsible for this. It is both vascular and epithelial.

Vascular Part

The vascular part of this barrier are the tight junctions between the endothelial cells of the iris capillaries. These are in contrast to the fenestrated capillaries of the ciliary processes.

Epithelial Part: The Tight Junctions

They are present at the apex of intercellular clefts and are essential for formation and maintenance of osmotic gradient. The ciliary epithelium poses as a barrier preventing diffusion of fluids and solutes into the posterior chamber. The blood aqueous barrier is formed by zonula occludentes and zonula adherens located between inner nonpigment epithelium of ciliary body. The fluid and solutes from the ciliary stroma move easily into the spaces between the pigmented ciliary epithelium. On reaching the interface between the apical processes of PE and NPE, they are able to permeate the intercellular clefts. However, as they move forward between the adjacent NPEs, their progress is blocked by the apicolateral junctional complexes consisting of zonula occludens and zonula adherens and desmosomes. These are essential for the formation of aqueous humor and ensure a solute gradient across the epithelial bilayer. Thus, tight junctions between the apicolateral surfaces of the nonpigmented epithelium of the ciliary body and between the endothelial cells of the iris vasculature, prevent the passage of plasma proteins into the aqueous humor. However, this barrier is not absolute allowing a slow penetration of water-soluble substances of medium molecular weight such as urea, creatinine, certain sugars and highly lipid soluble substances.

COMPOSITION OF AQUEOUS HUMOR

The aqueous humor bathes the structures essential for normal vision. Thus, its composition is critical for their proper functioning. Moreover, metabolic interchanges occur constantly between the aqueous and the ocular tissues it bathes. Thus, the composition of aqueous humor is a dynamic equilibrium determined by its rate of inflow and outflow and its interaction with the surrounding tissues. It is devoid of blood cells and of more than 99 percent of the plasma proteins and is characterized by a marked excess of ascorbate and a marked deficit of protein. The difference in proteins is both in terms of quantity and composition. The fluid and the electrolyte composition of aqueous humor is similar to that of the plasma with a slight excess of chloride and slight deficit of bicarbonate. It is slightly hypertonic as compared to the plasma and has a pH of 7.2 in the anterior chamber. The various constituents of AH are discussed in **Tables 2 and 3**.

> **Note** There is a difference in the composition of aqueous humor across the anterior and posterior chamber. This alteration occurs as the aqueous flows across the hyaloid face, surface of the lens, iris blood vessels and corneal endothelium due to:
> - Active processes[8]
> - Passive dilutional transport[9]

The aqueous humor consists of:[8-10]
- Inorganic ions
- Organic ions
- Carbohydrates
- Proteins
- Glutathione and urea
- Growth modulatory factors
- Oxygen and carbon dioxide

Inorganic Ions
- Sodium, potassium, magnesium are present in similar concentration in aqueous humor and plasma
- *Calcium*—Concentration is half that of plasma
- Iron, copper, zinc—similar concentration in aqueous humor and plasma (1 mg/ml)
- *Anions:* Chloride and bicarbonate are the major ions in the aqueous humor. The aqueous humor has an excess of chloride ions and deficit of bicarbonate *as compared to the plasma*. Aqueous humor is slightly acidic as compared to plasma due to decreased bicarbonate

- *Phosphate:* It is present in a low concentration in aqueous humor and hence does not have any significant buffering capacity
- *Hydrogen ions (H+):* Excess.

Organic Anions
Lactate
It is present abundantly in a higher concentration than plasma. It results from glycolytic degradation of glucose by both the ciliary body and the retina. It diffuses into the posterior chamber where it is present at a marginally higher concentration than in the plasma at this site. However, it accumulates in the anterior chamber at considerably higher concentration than in the plasma.

Ascorbic Acid
It is an important antioxidant forming a unique component of the aqueous humor. The ascorbate concentration is 30 folds as compared to the plasma. Its levels are higher in diurnal mammals as compared to nocturnal. It is actively secreted by the ciliary epithelium from the stroma into the posterior chamber by Na^+-dependent L⁻ ascorbic acid transporter. Thus, its concentration is higher in the posterior chamber.

Hyaluronic acid is absent in plasma. Its source is the vitreous (during normal process of GAG removal).
Hydrogen peroxide is the key oxi-dant present in the aqueous humor.

Proteins
The protein composition of aqueous humor is essentialy different from plasma having 1/200 to 1/500 (0.02 gm/100 ml) of proteins found in the plasma, the ratio being 0.02/7 gm/dl. (Less than one percent of protein found in plasma). This difference in protein content due to the BAB and also reflects its integrity. Some proteins may diffuse into the aqueous through the root and anterior surface of the iris. The low

Table 2 Physical characteristics of aqueous humor
- Osmotic pressure: higher than blood
- Specific gravity slightly more than water
- pH: 7.2
- Refractive index:1.36
- Anterior chamber aqueous: 0.25 ml
- Posterior chamber aqueous: 0.5 ml
- Rate of formation: 2.3 µl/min (about 1% of AC vol/min)

Table 3 Aqueous humor composition in comparison to plasma
- Marked excess of ascorbate
- Marked deficit of protein
- Slight excess of:
  - Chloride
  - Lactic acid
- Slight deficit of:
  - Sodium
  - Bicarbonate
  - CO_2
  - Glucose
- Other components:
  - Amino acids
  - Sodium hyaluronate
  - Norepinephrine
  - Coagulation proteins
  - TPA

protein content maintains the optical clarity of the aqueous humor. The ratio of the levels of the lower molecular weight plasma proteins (such as albumin and the γ-globulins) to the higher molecular weight proteins (such as the α-lipoproteins and the heavy immunoglobulins) is much higher in aqueous in the normal healthy eye than in plasma. Albumin and *transferrin* (an iron scavenging protein) constitutes about half of the total protein in the aqueous humor. The A:G Ratio of aqueous humor is higher.

Other components include enzymes, amino acids (higher concentration than plasma) and immunoglobulins. IgG is present at a concentration of approximately 3 mg per 100 ml, while IgM, IgD, and IgA are absent, presumably because of their larger molecular structure.[10] Trace concentrations of active complement C2, C6, and C7 globulins are also present.

Crystallines (α and γ lens crystallins) may be increased in eyes with cataract. Trace quantities of several components of the fibrinolytic and coagulation system are present in the aqueous. Plasminogen and plasminogen proactivator are present at more significant concentration. Presence of trace quantities of the inhibitors of plasminogen activation are present in the aqueous, thereby ensuring that the aqueous outflow pathways remain free of fibrin.

Some proteins may be synthesized locally in the ciliary epithelium and secreted into the aqueous by the NPE cells. These include:

- **Plasma proteins:** Complement component C4, α_2-macroglobulin, selenoprotein P an antioxidant, apolipoprotein D which binds to hydrophobic substances, plasma glutathione peroxidases, angiotensinogen.

    Locally (intraocularly) produced polypeptides are also present:
    Immunoglobulin: Its source is local production via (iris) lymphocytes plasma cells.
- Growth factors like TGF-β are also present.

> **Note** The plasma derived proteins may be added to the aqueous just prior to entry into the outflow path bypassing the posterior chamber. They may contribute to the normal outflow resistance.

Neurotrophic and Neuroendocrine Proteins

The ciliary epithelia are derived from the neuroectoderm and are functionally similar to neuroendocrine glands.

As a result they have effect on both IOP regulation and neuroendocrine properties which may influence the composition of aqueous humor. These may determine the composition of aqueous humor. They may be responsible for circadian IOP rhythms. Neuropeptide processing enzymes are synthesized as large precursors and are cleaved to bioactive peptide and secreted by the ciliary epithelium into the aqueous. These include:

- Neuropeptide-processing enzymes (e.g. carboxypeptidase E, peptidyl-glycine-α-amidating monoxygenase)
- Neuroendocrine peptides (e.g. Secretogranin II, neurotensin, Galanin)
- Bioactive peptides and hormones (e.g. atrial natriuretic peptide, brain natriuretic peptide).
    Their exact function is not clear.

Growth Modulating Factors

Aqueous humor plays a substantial role in modulating the proliferation, differentiation, functional viability and wound healing of ocular tissues. These properties are influenced by a number of growth promoting and differentiation factors that are present in aqueous humor. They include:

- Transforming growth factor β 1 and 2 (TGF-β_1 and β_2)
- Acidic and basic fibroblast growth factor (α-FGF and β-FGF)
- Insulin—like growth factor 1 (IGF –I)
- Insulin—like growth factor binding proteins (IGFBPs)
- Vascular endothelial growth factor (VEGF)
- Transferrin.

Complex interaction between these growth factors may be responsible for the significant lack of mitosis of corneal and trabecular meshwork endothelium. The vascular endothelial growth factors and placental growth factors (PIGF) are present in the aqueous humor. Aqueous levels of VEGF-A are increased in response to anterior segment ischemia.

Glutathione and Urea

Glutathione is an important tripeptide, the source of which is diffusion from blood by an active transport system in ciliary epithelium. It stabilizes redox state of aqueous by converting ascorbate to its functional form after oxidation. It also removes excess hydrogen peroxide and plays a role in the detoxification of electrophilic compounds.

Glutathione S transferase is important in protecting tissue from oxidative damage and stress. This is highly expressed in the ciliary epithelium.

Urea: Concentration of urea in aqueous humor is 80 to 90 percent as compared to plasma. It is a small molecule and readily crosses the epithelial barrier and diffuses passively.

Proteinases

Proteinases like cathepsin D and cathepsin O are synthesized and secreted into the aqueous humor by the ciliary epithelial cells. Cathepsin D is involved in the degradation of neuropeptides and peptide hormones. Cathepsin O may be involved in normal cellular protein degradation and turnover.

Proteinase Inhibitors

Alpha 2 macroglobulin and alpha 1 antitrypsin are also present in the aqueous humor. Any imbalance between the proteinases and proteinase inhibitors may lead to an alteration in aqueous humor composition resulting in disease.

Enzymes

Activators, proenzymes and fibrinolytic enzymes are present in the aqueous and these enzymes could play a role in the regulation of outflow resistance. Some enzymes are increased in certain pathological condition due to their release after cellular damage. For example, in retinoblastoma. Most of the enzymes have no significant catalytic role in the normal aqueous. Exceptions are three enzymes:

1. *Hyaluronidase:* It is involved in the regulation of resistance to outflow of aqueous humor through the trabecular meshwork.
2. *Carbonic anhydrase:* It is present in trace amount and is significant in the catalysis of equilibrium between bicarbonate and CO_2 plus water even in low concentration.
3. *Lysozyme:* It provides significant antibacterial protection. The intraocular levels may be raised in case of ocular inflammation.

Glucose

The concentration of glucose in aqueous humor is 70 percent of that in plasma. It has a high rate of entry into the posterior chamber owing to facilitated diffusion. Aqueous humor glucose levels are increased in diabetics. Inositol, important for phospholipids synthesis occurs at a concentration of ten times that in plasma.

Oxygen

Source of O_2 and CO_2 is the blood supplied to ciliary body and iris. Corneal endothelium is critically dependent upon aqueous O_2 supply for active fluid transport that maintains corneal transparency. Lens and endothelial lining of trabecular meshwork also derive their oxygen supply from the aqueous humor. The partial pressure of oxygen in aqueous humor is about 55 mm Hg (one-third of its concentration in the atmosphere). It is derived from ciliary body and iris blood vessels. It is helpful in maintaining corneal transparency as the corneal endothelium is critically dependent on the aqueous oxygen.

Carbon Dioxide

The carbon dioxide content of the aqueous humor is 40 to 60 mm Hg. It contributes three percent of total aqueous bicarbonate. It is continuously lost to atmosphere, tear film by diffusion.

AQUEOUS HUMOR COMPOSITION FOLLOWING BREAKDOWN OF BAB

The blood aqueous barrier may be disturbed because of many factors. These include: intraocular infection, uveal inflammation, intraocular surgery, and certain drugs (topical and systemic) and cyclodestructive and laser procedures. The following changes are seen in the aqueous humor composition during the breakdown of the blood aqueous barrier:

- Increased protein—10 to 100 times especially high molecular weight
- Increased inflammatory mediators
- Imbalance of growth factors
- Hyperplastic response from lens epithelium, ciliary epithelium, trabecular epithelium.

AQUEOUS HUMOR FORMATION AND SECRETION

Three mechanism are involved in the production of aqueous humor. These include:

1. *Ultrafiltration:* It is a process by which a fluid and its solutes cross a semipermeable membrane under pressure. It is the bulk flow of blood plasma across the fenestrated ciliary capillary endothelia, into the ciliary stroma, which is increased by a hydrostatic force.
2. *Active secretion[8]* Active transport is an energy dependant process which selectively moves a substance against its electrochemical gradient. Most of the process of aqueous humor formation depends on the active secretion of ions into the intercellular

clefts between the nonpigmented epithelial cells. The precise details of the active transport mechanism have not been fully evaluated. Most of the process of aqueous humor formation depends on the active secretion of ions into the intercellular clefts between the nonpigmented epithelial cells. These clefts are small spaces between the NPE present beyond the tight junctions. Tight junctions between NPE ensure that the accumulation of ions in the intercellular clefts create an osmotic gradient along which water (H_2O) flows into the posterior chamber. Several secretory process are responsible for active solute transport across the ciliary epithelium and involve many channels (e.g. Na^+, K^+-$2Cl^-$ symport, Cl^- - HCO_3^- and Na^+, H^+ antiports, cation channels, water channels, Na^+ K^+ - ATPase, K^+ channels, Cl^- channels, H^+-ATPase).

3. *Diffusion[9]* Substances transported passively across a semipermeable membrane along their concentration gradient. Most capillary walls are permeable to water, dissolved gases, and many small molecules and ions. Substances of higher concentration on one side of a semipermeable membrane show a net movement to the side of lower concentration until the concentrations are equal on both sides. When equilibrium is reached, movement across the membrane still occurs, but the number of particles going in one direction equals the number going the other way, thus yielding no net movement. The solvent also participates with a net movement in the opposite direction of the solute. It should be noted that conditions for diffusion are markedly altered in a dynamic system

such as the ciliary processes, in which blood is flowing rapidly, aqueous humor is constantly being formed and circulated.

> **Note** Out of these three processes active secretion of ions across the ciliary epithelium is the primary mechanism for aqueous formation.

STEPS OF AQUEOUS HUMOR FORMATION

- Accumulation of plasma reservoir
- Uptake of plasma derived ions and water from the ciliary stroma by the PE cells at the stromal surface
- Movement of solutes and water from PE to NPE cells through gap junctions
- Transfer of solute and water by NPE cells into the posterior chamber.

Step 1: Accumulation of Plasma Reservoir

It is an important first step in aqueous humor formation by which plasma constituents gain entry into the ciliary process stroma. This occurs mainly by ultrafiltration and partly by diffusion. About 150 ml of blood flows into the ciliary processes every minute. As the blood passes through the capillaries of the ciliary processes, four percent of the plasma filters via the fenestrations into the stroma. The fluid movement is favored by the hydrostatic pressure difference between the capillary pressure and the interstitial fluid pressure. It is augmented by oncotic pressure of leaked proteins in the stroma and the high concentrations of colloids in the stroma of the ciliary processes favors the movement of water from the plasma to the ciliary stroma. At the same time, it also retards the movement of water from the stroma to the posterior chamber. This hydrostatic pressure is dependant on neuroregulatory and hormonal influences. It is

unlikely that ultrafiltration contributes to a large amount of aqueous formation but helps to move the fluid out of the capillaries and into the stroma. Many substances pass from the ciliary process capillaries, through the stroma of the ciliary processes and between the pigment epithelial cells finally accumulating behind the NPE tight junctions.

Step 2: Uptake of Solute and Water at the Stromal Surface by PE Cells

From the stroma of the ciliary processes, the solutes are taken up by the PE cells. This involves active exchangers, co-transporters and ion channels. Thus, the solutes move from the stroma of the ciliary processes into the pigment epithelium.

The uptake of sodium and chloride ions is mediated by the following:

- **$Na^+K^+2Cl^-$ symport:** Na and Cl is taken up by this symport into the PE cells. The K^+ is then recirculated back into the stroma. The driving force is provided by the intracellular chloride ion concentration.
- Paired Na^+/H^+ and Cl^-/HCO_3^- antiports actively transport Na and Cl from the stroma to the cells:
  - ❖ *Na^+H^+ antiport:* Na is taken up by the cells in exchange of H^+
  - ❖ *$Cl^- HCO_3^-$ antiport:* Chloride is taken up in exchange of bicarbonate.

> **Note** The cytoplasmic carbonic anhydrase II enhances the turnover at the antiports by providing H^+ and bicarbonate. Inhibition by carbonic anhydrase inhibitors reduces IOP by decreasing aqueous humor formation by influencing these antiports.

The driving force for solute uptake is dependent upon extracellular Cl^-.

Step 3: Movement of Solutes and Water from PE to NPE Cells through Gap Junctions

Gap Junctions

The solutes after uptake from the stromal fluids are transported to PE as described above. From here they move into the NPE cells via gap junctions present between NPE and PE. These gap junctions allow movement of solutes between the two layers of epithelial cells providing access for passive transport along the osmotic gradient via specific ion channels. They provide a low resistance pathway for transport between these cells.

Step 4: Transfer of Solute and Water by NPE Cells into the Posterior Chamber

Active Transport and Aqueous Humor Formation by NPE

The solutes are actively transported across the NPE and deposited in the clefts between the cells. Here they create a hyperosmotic environment and subsequent diffusion of water occurs into these spaces. At the apical end, these spaces are closed by tight junctions and open into the posterior chamber at the basal end. These tight junctions between the NPE cells ensure that the accumulation of ions creates an osmotic gradient which directs the flow of fluid into the posterior chamber. This is the standing gradient osmotic flow mechanism coupling water and solute transport.

The various secretory processes responsible include:

- Na^+—Active transport of the sodium ion is the key process in aqueous humor formation. Na^+ is transported into clefts using the NaK ATPase (Higher concentration in the lateral inter digitations of NPE). The electrochemical imbalance created is balanced by negatively charged ions which follow Na$^+$. The NPE cells extrude Na$^+$ via the Na$^+$K$^+$ATPase present in their basolateral cell membrane. It uses ATP to transport Na in exchange for extracellular K. This also establishes a transmembrane gradient required to drive the solute through the symports, antiports and uniports.

- Other Na$^+$ transporters include the Na$^+$K$^+$2Cl$^-$ symport, nonselective cation channels, parallel Na$^+$H$^+$ antiports and the sodium dependent vitamin C transporter 2. About 70 percent of sodium ions are actively transported in to the posterior chamber. The rest enters by diffusion and ultrafiltration. It is also the principle mechanism for H$_2$O movement. Na$^+$ is transported into clefts using the NaK ATPase.
- The NPE cells release chloride via the Cl$^-$ channels into the posterior chamber. The chloride channels at the basolateral surface of NPE are the rate limiting step in AHF and may play a role in its diurnal variation.
- Bicarbonate (HCO$_3^-$) is produced by the enzyme carbonic anhydrase (CA) in the NPE. This also maintains pH for proper function of NaK ATPase. It is released through the Cl$^-$ HCO$_3^-$ antiport and the chloride channels.
- Potassium ions are transported by active secretion and diffusion.
- Chloride ion is the major anion transported across the epithelium through Cl$^-$ channels. The classical view has been that chloride passively follows sodium ion secretion. However, there is also evidence that chloride ion is actively secreted into the posterior chamber. Na$^+$-K$^+$-2Cl$^-$ co-transporter as well as parallel Cl$^-$-HCO$_3^-$ and Na$^+$-H$^+$ exchanger/antiports are functioning in the pigmented and nonpigmented epithelial syncytium to bring sodium and chloride across into the posterior chamber in an electrically neutral way. Both the Na$^+$-K$^+$-2Cl$^-$ co-transpoter and the exchanger/antiport pair are commonly seen in secretory cells and have been located in the ciliary body in both pigmented and nonpigmented epithelial cells. These co-transporters and exchangers are responsible for maintaining intraocular pH and ion stability and, therefore, are very likely involved in secretory activity as well. The role of the co-transporters in Na$^+$ and Cl$^-$ transport has been amply documented with some questioning the role of the double exchangers at least as far as chloride transport is concerned.
- Ascorbic acid is also actively transported across the ciliary epithelium into the aqueous humor, at least in rabbit and cow and is linked to Na$^+$ transport.
- Chloride secretion is affected by pH and sodium ion concentration.

In addition, the natriuretic peptide precursor B (NPPB)-sensitive Cl channels at the basolateral surface in nonpigmented epithelial cells also play a crucial role in regulating the Cl movement across the functional syncytium.

Transport of Water
The mechanisms for the transport of water are less clear. Aquaporin water channels in the NPE cells facilitate the movement of water into the posterior chamber. Aquaporins are a family of proteins located in the cell membranes and are involved in active water transport. These channels are not present in the PE. Parallel PE and NPE couplets may transfer solute and water from the stroma to the posterior chamber.

Diffusion of O$_2$ and Glucose
Both oxygen and glucose are essential for health of cornea and lens. They pass the BAB by simple or facilitated diffusion. Their consumption from aqueous in the anterior chamber by the avascular structures establishes a gradient which is a driving force for the diffusion of these substances. Therefore, they do not depend on the rate of aqueous formation. A constant flow of aqueous is required to flush out waste products. Marked decreased in aqueous humor formation rate may increase concentration of potentially harmful substances.

Changes in Composition of AH in the Anterior Chamber
More nutrients are added by diffusion as the fluid moves through the anterior chamber. At the same time, some solutes are also removed from the aqueous humor by the ciliary epithelium.

Resorption of Aqueous Humor Across Ciliary Epithelium
There is a mechanism for transporting solute and water from the posterior chamber back into the stroma. In this unidirectional reabsorption another set of transporters may be involved in extruding Na$^+$, K$^+$ and Cl$^-$ back into the stroma. The excess stromal accumulation of water may lead to swelling of PE cells. This leads to ATP release and cAMP formation. The Cl channels are stimulated and excess chloride goes back into the stroma. This anion may be accompanied by Na and K. In the NPE, several transporters could be involved in the re absorption process. The exact significance of this process is unclear.

RATE OF AQUEOUS HUMOR FORMATION

Normal flow of aqueous humor is approximately 2.0 to 2.5 µl/min. The aqueous volume is turned over at a rate of 1 percent per minute.

It is measured by fluorophotometry. The most common method used to measure the rate of aqueous formation is fluorophotometry. Fluorescein is administered systemically or topically and the subsequent decline in its anterior chamber concentration is measured optically and used to calculate aqueous flow.

FACTORS AFFECTING AQUEOUS HUMOR PRODUCTION

Aqueous humor formation can be decreased by age, diurnal variation and exercise. Systemic factors like hypotension, decreased ciliary body blood flow, hypothermia and acidosis also reduce aqueous production. Uveitis, RD, choroidal detachment are also associated with decrease secretion of aqueous. Apart from these many pharmacological agents, trauma, laser (e.g. cyclophotocoagulation) and surgical procedures (e.g. cyclodialysis) reduce aqueous secretion. Some of these are discussed below.

- Sleep
- Age (as age increases aqueous production also decreases)
- Integrity of BAB
- Blood flow to ciliary body
- Neurohormonal regulation of vascular tissue and ciliary epithelium.

Circardian Rhythm and Sleep Suppression

Being a biological process, aqueous humor formation is subject to circardian rhythms. The rate of inflow of AH from 8 am to 12 pm in a normal young human reaches 3 microliter/min but falls by 60 percent (1.3 microliter/min) from 12 to 6 am. Interestingly, this magnitude of decline is greater than that achieved by drugs. This physiological regulation of AH flow seems insensitive to IOP as inflow does not change in glaucoma patients.

The mechanism that controls the aqueous humor suppression during sleep is incompletely understood. The endogenous catecholamines may stimulate aqueous humor formation and flow in daytime and their absence in sleep may be lower. Epinephrine and norepinephrine are the only hormones that can increase aqueous humor formation but in patients without adrenal glands normal rhythm of aqueous humor formation is maintained. This suggest additional mechanisms.

Decreased aqueous humor production is also seen in:

- Trauma
- Inflammation
- Carotid occlusive disease
- Drugs, e.g.
  - General anesthetics
  - Systemic hypotensive agents.

AQUEOUS HUMOR DRAINAGE

More than 90 percent of the aqueous humor exits via the conventional trabecular meshwork and the Schlemm's canal system. The Schlemm's canal communicates with the aqueous veins which are a part of the venous system via a series of collector channels. The two main pathways of aqueous humor drainage are:

1. **Conventional** or canalicular (Schlemm's canal). The flow of aqueous occurs down a hydrostatic pressure gradient between IOP and episcleral venous pressure.
2. **Unconventional** or uveoscleral and uveovortex pathway.

Trabecular Pathway[11-16]
Trabecular Meshwork

Most of the AH exits the eye via the trabecular meshwork-Schlemm's canal venous system. The trabecular meshwork (TM) is a wedge shaped band of tissue encircling the anterior chamber angle. The apex of this wedge is attached to peripheral edge of the cornea, the Schwalbe's line. Posteriorly it is attached to the scleral spur,[11] the stroma of ciliary body and the peripheral iris. The scleral spur projects into the base of this wedge. The trabecular meshwork consists of multiple layers of collagenous beams covered by endothelial cells about 200,000-300,000 in number. The cells have phagocytic activity. They may contain a large number of pigment granules in their cytoplasm.

The TM is divided into three parts:

1. **Uveal meshwork:** It is the innermost part of the trabecular meshwork and is adjacent to the anterior chamber. It extends from the iris root, ciliary body to the peripheral cornea. It consists of flat sheets with wide irregular perforations (25–75 µ diameter),[14] in multiple planes.

2. **Corneoscleral meshwork:** It consists of sheets which extend from the scleral spur to the lateral wall of the scleral sulcus. There are 8 to 15 perforated sheets 5 to 12 µm[15] in thickness with openings which are elliptical in shape and not aligned. The openings become progressively similar as they progress towards the canal of Schlemm's (diameter ranges between 5 and 50 microns).

    The components of the trabecular meshwork are:
    - Collagen types I, III, IV, V, VI, VIII
    - Laminin, fibronectin, heparin

    The trabecular sheets have four concentric layers:
    - Innermost core composed of collagen
    - Spiral fibers of collagen which provides flexibility

- ❖ A 'glass membrane' between the spiralling collagen and trabecular endothelial cells
- ❖ The outermost layer consists of the basement membrane of the trabecular endothelial cells. The trabecular endothelial cells have desmosomes and gap junctions, allowing a free passage of aqueous humor.

3. *Juxtacanalicular trabecular meshwork (JCT):* The major site of outflow resistance is adjacent to the Schlemm's canal and also forms its lateral wall. It is composed of three layers. The innermost is the trabecular endothelial layer which is a continuation of the trabecular meshwork. Outer to it is a connective tissue layer composed of collagen III. The outermost layer is the inner wall of the Schlemm's canal. It is lined by endothelial cells significantly different from the trabecular endothelium.

Schlemm's Canal

The Schlemm's canal is a single slit-like tube which runs circumferentially, resembling a lymphatic channel. It is 190 to 370 μm in width and is traversed by tubules.[15] Occasionally, it may branch in to a plexus like system. It is completely lined with endothelial layers that does not rest on a continuous basement membrane. The endothelial cells are irregular and spindle shaped. Its inner wall contains giant vacuoles which have direct communication with intertrabecular spaces. The inner wall endothelium has a high hydraulic conductivity due to the presence of 'pores' which may be intra- or intercellular. These pores are associated with giant vacuoles (out-pouchings of inner wall cells extending into the lumen of Schlemm's canal) which are seen to increase parallel to an increase in IOP. There may be 1000-2000 pores /mm sq. The outer wall does not contain pores.

Intrascleral Channels

These constitute a complex system of vessels connecting the Schlemm's canal to episcleral veins. The aqueous veins of Ascher[16] have been defined as originating at the outer wall of Schlemm's canal and terminating in episcleral and conjunctival veins in a laminations of aqueous humor and blood, referred to as the laminated vein of Goldmann. They are also called outflow channels or collector channels.

Two systems of channels have been identified:

1. A direct system of large caliber vessels, which run a short intrascleral course and drain directly in to the episcleral venous system
2. An indirect system of more numerous, finer channels, which form an intrascleral plexus before eventually draining into the episcleral venous system.

Episcleral Veins and Conjunctival Veins[17]

Most of the aqueous vessels drain into the episcleral veins and some into the conjunctival veins. The episcleral veins further drain into the anterior ciliary and superior ophthalmic vein which drain into the cavernous sinus. Conjunctival veins drain into superior ophthalmic and facial veins via the palpebral and angular veins. The pressure in the episcleral venous system is relatively stable. In humans, this pressure is measured by applying pressure to an area of the sclera occupied by these veins until they collapse. The end point is subjective.

Role of Ciliary Muscle Tension

The longitudinal ciliary muscle inserts onto the scleral spur and additionally sends extensions to the trabecular meshwork and the juxtacanalicular tissue. Cholinergic drugs lead to widening of the spaces in TM and JCT by increasing mechanical tension transmitted by the extensions of ciliary muscle to the TM.

Transcanalicular Flow

It occurs from uveal meshwork into corneoscleral meshwork, which further flows into juxtacanalicular meshwork. From there it enters the endothelial lining of Schlemm's canal. From it 20 to 30 collector channel connect to the intrascleral venous plexus, the episcleral venous plexus, the anterior ciliary plexus into the aqueous vein.

Characteristics of the transcanalicular flow system are that it is:

- Sponge like
- One way valve
- Prevents entry of toxic substance
- Phagocytosis (like RPE system)
- Absence of clotting factors
- Fibrinolytic activity
- Self cleaning filter.

Mechanism of Aqueous Transport Across Inner Wall of Schlemm's Canal

Various mechanisms have been proposed. These include:

- Vacuolation theory
- Leaky pores in endothelial cells
- Contractile microfilaments
- Sonderman's channels
- Aqueous outflow pump.

Sonderman's channels: They are of historical interest. Although originally described as endothelial lined channels, communicating between Schlemm's canal and intertrabecular spaces have subsequently been interpreted as tortuous communications wandering irregularly and obliquely through the meshwork or as deep grooves on cross-section, slit like spaces between cells or artifacts. It is unlikely that the structures, if they exist, have a significant role in aqueous humor outflow **(Figure 1)**.

Vacuolation Theory[18]

As vesicles and larger vacuoles are seen in endothelium, Tripathi et al. have suggested that these vacuoles open

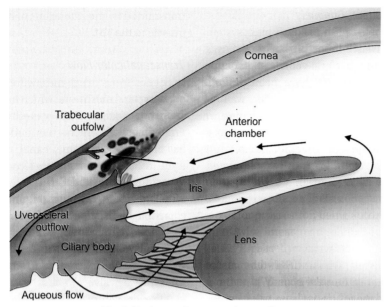

Fig. 1 Pathway of aqueous humor flow

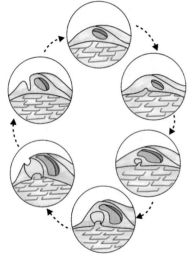

Fig. 2 Diagram illustrating the vacuolation theory

and close intermittently to transport aqueous from juxtacanalicular tissue to Schlemm's canal (**Figure 2**).

Aqueous Outflow Pump[19]

In this model, the trabecular pump controls flow and pressure. Flexible trabecular tissue movement pumps aqueous from the anterior chamber to Schlemm's canal through a series of valves. Trabecular tissue movement

then pumps aqueous from Schlemm's canal to the aqueous veins. The aqueous outflow pump receives its power from transient IOP increase during systole of the cardiac cycle, respiration, blinking and eye movement. These IOP transients cause deformation of the elastic structural elements of the trabecular tissues. During systole, the pressure increase moves the trabecular tissues outward, toward SC and eventually into it. Outward movement of the Schlemm's canal endothelium narrows SC, forcing aqueous from SC into collector channel ostia and then into the aqueous veins. Concurrently, the transient IOP increase forces aqueous from the trabecular meshwork interstices into one-way collector vessels or valves spanning Schlemm's canal. Decay of the pressure spike causes the elastic trabecular elements to respond by recoiling to their diastolic configuration. Trabecular tissue recoil causes a pressure reduction in Schlemm's canal that induces aqueous to flow from the aqueous collector vessels or valves into Schlemm's canal. Trabecular endothelial cells regulate trabecular tissue properties and act as

sensors constantly monitoring information related to pressure and flow.

Reduced outflow in glaucoma is explained by a failure of pump function which decreases trabecular tissue movement. Reduced trabecular tissue movement in turn results from two related abnormalities. This may be due to:

- Intrinsic trabecular tissue stiffening
- Abnormal persistence of trabecular tissue apposition to the external wall of Schlemm's canal due to excess intrinsic distention and extrinsic factors altering the position of trabecular tissue attachments to the scleral spur, Schwalbe's line and ciliary body.

Segmental Nature of Outflow

In adult eyes, there is a considerable resistance to the circumferential flow of aqueous in the Schlemm's canal. The Schlemm's canal in contrast to a freely communicating channel may behave as having separate segmental outflow pathways.

Uveoscleral Outflow (Nonconventional Outflow)

This constitutes 10 percent of the total aqueous outflow in contrast to primates where it is higher. Recent evidence questions the exact ratio. The aqueous seeps through the face of the ciliary body, passes through the ciliary muscle to reach the supraciliary and the suprachoroidal space. The aqueous humor reaching the ciliary muscle can exit via many routes. From here, it can pass through the sclera or along the nerves and vessels penetrating the sclera, the choroidal vessels. It can pass in and around vortex veins and into the ciliary processes. Ciliary muscle is the 'common' initial site of outflow whereas not all routes may include 'sclera'.

Traditionally, this pathway has been described as a 'pressure independent pathway'. As a result, it is not measurable by tonography. It is pressure independent or minimally pressure dependent at a normal or high range of IOP. However at low IOP, e.g. 4 mm Hg it is pressure dependent and reduced. The uveoscleral outflow decreases with age.

Clinical Significance
- Contraction of the ciliary muscle by cholinergic agents decreases outflow via this pathway.
- Cyclodialysis, i.e. detachment of the ciliary body may be associated with an enhanced uveoscleral outflow with the aqueous flowing into the suprachoroidal space.
- *Uveitis*: The increased uveoscleral outflow due to prostaglandin production may be one of the mechanisms of hypotony.

Factors Affecting Uveoscleral Outflow
Factors increasing uveoscleral outflow:
- Cycloplegia
- Adrenergic agents
- Prostaglandin analogs
- Cyclodialysis.

Factors decreasing uveoscleral outflow:
- Miotics
- Increasing age

Uveovortex Outflow
Movement of fluid from the aqueous humor to the iris vessels and vortex veins has been described. It is probably not clinically significant and its contributions is not clearly understood.

Trabecular outflow depends on the resistance in the trabecular meshwork and the pressure in the aqueous veins and episcleral vessels. Various methods have been developed to study these parameters.

EPISCLERAL VENOUS PRESSURE
It is one of the factors that contribute to the intraocular pressure. IOP generally increases with the increase in intraocular pressure. The normal range is 8 to 11 mm Hg.

MEASUREMENT OF AQUEOUS HUMOR FORMATION AND FLOW
Aqueous flow is defined as the rate of movement of aqueous from the posterior chamber into the anterior chamber through the pupil. Since, it does not include the small amounts of aqueous flow by other routes, it does not exactly equal aqueous production. Since, clinical assessment of aqueous humor production is not possible, the aqueous flow is used to estimate it.

The normal rate of aqueous flow is 2-3 µl/min. It slows at a rate of 2.4 percent per decade.

Fluorophotometry
Fluorescein can be injected into the bloodstream and maintain a high concentration there. Over a period of several hours, a small but measurable amount diffuses into the aqueous humor and reaches an equilibrated concentration. The level of the fluorescein in the blood declines rapidly due to renal clearance. The concentration in the aqueous, however, remains relatively constant over a short period of time, after which it starts to decrease, as fresh aqueous is formed not incorporating any fluorescein, because of low plasma levels. The rate of fresh aqueous formation can be calculated by measuring the declining concentration of fluorescein optically. This technique has been modified by using topically and is the current gold standard. Multiple drops of fluorescein are applied topically to establish a corneal depot or a reservoir which slowly releases fluorescein into the anterior chamber. This mixes with the aqueous humor by normal thermoconvective currents and almost 95 percent drains via the anterior chamber. Using a fluorophotometer, fluorescein concentrations in the corneal stroma and anterior chamber are measured periodically (every 45–60 minutes) for several hours. The fluorophotometer focuses an excitation beam of blue light on a defined region of the eye and collects the emitted fluorescence signal from the same site. The signals are then converted to ng/ml by reference to a standard curve. The mass of fluorescein is calculated by the product of their concentrations in the cornea and anterior chamber with their respective volumes. The flow rate is calculated by the mass of fluorescein lost from the cornea and the anterior chamber over time divided by the average concentration in the anterior chamber during the time interval.

The aqueous flow rate is a function of anterior chamber volume, slope of fluorescein decay curves and the ratio of mass of fluorescein in the corneal stroma to that in the anterior chamber.

Assumptions
- Fluorescein is evenly distributed in the anterior chamber. For this, measurements must start after at least four hours of topical administration.
- It is assumed that there is minimal diffusional loss of fluorescein into the limbal or iris vessels or the vitreous cavity.
- No optical obstructions like corneal scars which may scatter light.

Note This method cannot be used in eyes where fluorescein can exit the eye by routes other than the angle of the anterior chamber. It cannot be used in aphakic or pseudophakic eyes.

MEASUREMENT OF AQUEOUS HUMOR OUTFLOW AND FACILITY OF OUTFLOW
The facility of outflow is the rate at which the fluid can be expressed from the eye by pressure. It is the ease with which the aqueous leaves the eye and is hence the inverse of outflow resistance. The maximum resistance is

provided by the JCT. It varies widely is normal individuals ranging from 0.22 to 0.30 µl/min/mm Hg and decreases with age.

Outflow resistance is generally determined by measuring the inverse of outflow facility.

Factors affecting outflow facility
- Surgery
- Trauma
- Medications
- Endocrine factors

Various methods employed to estimate the outflow facility are listed below and two of these: *Tonography* and *fluorophotometry* are described ahead in the chapter. Invasive methods are used in an experimental setting. Clinically noninvasive methods are used.

Pressure Dependent Methods
- Tonography
- Suction cup
- Perfusion.

Tracer Methods
- Photogrammetry
- Radiolabeled isotopes.

Invasive Methods
Invasive methods to calculate the outflow facility (C) require cannulation of the anterior chamber and connection to a mock AH chamber from which AH is infused at two different rates. However, it does not avoid pseudofacility and ocular rigidity.

Uveoscleral Outflow
Currently, it cannot be measured directly. The Goldmann equation has been modified with respect to the pressure independent pathways.

$$F = (P0 - Pe)C + U$$

Where F = aqueous formation in microliters/minute, P0 = IOP in undisturbed eye in mm Hg, Pe is the sum of external pressure including episcleral venous pressure, U is the sum of pressure independent outflow including the uveoscleral outflow.[21]

Outflow Mechanics
Poiseuille Hagen Formula[20]
It states that resistance to flow of blood in a vessel is inversely proportional to 4th power of radius, hence flow in that vessel is directly proportional to the 4th power of radius.

Ohm's Law (V=IR)
The flow of aqueous through the trabecular meshwork (I) will depend on the pressure difference between the intraocular pressure and the EVP (V) divided by the resistance of the trabecular meshwork (R).

Conductance is inverse of resistance $\propto$ (I = VC) and TM conductance seems to decrease with increase IOP. Goldmann[21] proposed the rate of aqueous outflow (F) is proportional to the IOP(P_0)—Episcleral venous pressure.

Tonography
Estimation of Factor "C" (microliter/min/mm Hg)
Tonography was once a routine clinical practice in the diagnosis and management of glaucoma. Currently, it is used mainly for research purposes.[21] It provides a rapid assessment of the C value but is prone to errors. These include ocular rigidity and pseudofacility. Fluorophotometry avoids these errors but is time consuming and less practical in the clinical scenario and is currently of significance for

research especially to understand the mechanism of action of drugs. Tonography estimates C value by raising the IOP with the weight of an indentation tonometer and observing the decay curve in IOP. The weight causes raised IOP, leading to increased outflow and change in aqueous volume which is inferred from Friedenwald table relating volume change to Schiotz change.[20]

The normal value of "C" is 0.28 microliter/min/mm Hg.

Procedure
- A weighted tonometer is placed on the anesthetized cornea of a supine patient for four minutes. Measure IOP for four minutes and calculate the change in IOP. The standard weight increases the IOP and the drainage through the TM. As the fluid passes out, the IOP decreases. The change in IOP provides the volume of fluid which has exited the eye (by using Friedenwald tables). Assuming that this volume is the only factor responsible for the decrease in IOP, the rate of fluid outflow from the eye can be calculated as $\propto$ V/t. The outflow facility can be calculated.

  Rate of volume decrease = rate of outflow.
- Then C value is obtained from Grants equation:

$$F = C(P_0 - Pv) = V/T$$
$$C = V/T (P_0 - Pv)$$

P_0 is the IOP before the application of the weight when the IOP was stable and there was a balance between inflow and outflow.

P_v is the IOP at the end of the test time *t* when the outflow was greater than inflow.

Certain assumptions are made during this procedure. These include:

- Weight placed on the cornea does not affect AH inflow/production
- Change in pressure is entirely due to change in volume of AH moving out through the TM and not any other pathway
- Normal corneal curvature
- Normal ocular rigidity.

An assumption in tonography is that the rate of aqueous humors inflow into the anterior chamber during the measurement remains unchanged by the applied pressure. If pseudofacility and/or uveoscleral outflow facility are disturbed during the measurement, a change in tonographic outflow facility may not indicate a change in true trabecular outflow facility.

Pseudofacility: It is the facility of the flow of aqueous humor from the posterior chamber into the anterior chamber resulting from the probe induced increase in IOP. It is the artificial increase in the measured facility due to egress of the fluid via a nontrabecular route or decreased as production due to changes in ocular blood volume or extracellular fluid volume.

Sources of Error
- Variations in corneal curvature and rigidity. It makes no compensation for individual variations in ocular rigidity and assumes that it remains constant throughout the procedure. Thus, it is a confounding factor.
- Moses effect
- Consensual pressure drop
- Variations in line voltage
- Eye movement
- Patient relaxation effect
- Operator error
- Pseudofacility.

Note The outflow facility measured by tonography is the sum of trabecular outflow + pseudofacility + uveoscleral outflow.

Ocular Parameters Affecting Tonography
- Aqueous production
- Resistance to aqueous outflow
- Episcleral venous pressure
- Ocular rigidity
- Expulsion of uveal blood.

Fluorescein Fluorophotometry
It measures the change in flow across the trabecular meshwork. The procedure takes around six hours. It avoids the problem of pseudofacility and measures the change in ocular fluid flow directly. It does not require conversion tables or IOP measurements.

Procedure
Tonometry is used to measure IOP. Aqueous flow is determined by measuring the disappearance rate of a tracer from the anterior chamber. Next, an aqueous flow suppressant such as a acetazolamide, dorzolamide or timolol is given to reduce the IOP and aqueous flow. Brimonidine and apraclonidine are not appropriate for this purpose, because these drugs affect outflow as well as aqueous flow. The fluorescein decay curves are seen. After the drug has taken effect, IOP and aqueous flow are remeasured and the equation (given below) is used to calculate the outflow facility. The drug-induced change in IOP (IOP2–IOP1 is measured by tonometry, and the change in aqueous flow (F_2–F_1) is measured by fluorophotometry.

Outflow facility is calculated using the following equation:
$$C = (F_2 - F_1)/(IOP2 - IOP1).$$
C by fluorophotometry usually is labeled Cfl.

Assumptions
- Change in aqueous flow is caused by equal decrease in trabecular outflow (beta-blockers or oral CAIs)
- Assumes that uveoscleral flow is small and varies little with change in IOP.

Advantages
- Not affected by pseudofacility
- Not affected by scleral rigidity
- Detect changes missed by tonography.

Disadvantages
- Time—the procedure takes about six hours and cannot be used in daily clinical practice.
- This method does not work well in normotensive eyes in which aqueous flow suppressants cannot change the IOP effectively.

MEASUREMENT OF UVEOSCLERAL OUTFLOW
Currently, the only noninvasive means by which to assess uveoscleral outflow (Fu) is via mathematical calculation using equation.

Fu = F – C (IOP-P$_v$)
Aqueous humor flow (F) and Outflow facility are measured by any of the above mentioned methods. Episcleral venous pressure P_v is measured by venomanometry (Value of 9–10 mm Hg is often used as it may be difficult to obtain).

One limitation of the calculation method for uveoscleral outflow is the large standard deviations generated because of the inherent variability in each parameter in the equation. Large number of subjects are required to detect clinically relevant differences. Moreover, the calculated uveoscleral outflow can vary tremendously depending on which value of episcleral venous pressure is used in the equation.

Despite limitations it provides reasonable explanation for differences in IOP with respect to aging, pharmacological drugs, clinical syndromes, and surgical procedures. This may be helpful in treating the cause of IOP rise instead of the IOP itself.

Invasive methods for uveoscleral outflow measurement

Invasive methods involves infusing a radioactive or fluorescent tracer into the anterior chamber at a set pressure and for a specific period of time.

Intracameral tracer method

The total amount of tracer found in the uvea and sclera during the specified time interval is assumed due to the uveoscleral outflow.

Indirect isotope methods

These involve infusing a radioactive tracer in the anterior chamber and monitoring the rate of the tracer's appearance in the blood and the rate of the tracer's disappearance from the anterior chamber. Uveoscleral outflow is the difference between aqueous flow and trabecular outflow.

FACTORS AFFECTING AQUEOUS HUMOR OUTFLOW

- **Age:** A modest decline with age seen.
- **Hormones:** Corticosteroids decrease outflow facility
- Genetic factors
- Myopia
- Diabetes mellitus

- **Ciliary muscle:** Increased outflow facility
  - ❖ Accommodation
  - ❖ Electrical stimulation of IIIrd nerve
  - ❖ Posterior depression of lens
- Drugs.

Mechanisms of Drug Action (Table 4)

- Pilocarpine and cholinergic drugs increase outflow
- Epinephrine/dipivefrin/β-adrenergic agonist: increase conventional/unconventional flow
- Beta blockers, carbonic anhydrase inhibitors and alpha agonists: decrease aqueous humor production
- Prostaglandin analogues increase uveoscleral flow
- α-agonists increase uveoscleral flow.

Table 4 Mechanisms of drug action

Drug	Aqueous production	Trabecular outflow	Uveoscleral outflow
β-blockers	↓		
Pilocarpine		↑	
Adrenaline, Dipevefrine	↓?	↑	↑
Brimonidine	↓		↑
Prostaglandins		↑?	↑
Carbonic anhydrase (-)	↓		

REFERENCES

1. Goldmann H. Augendruck and Gluacom. Die Kammerwasservenen und das poiseuille'sche Gesetz. Ophthalmologica 1949:118:496.
2. Hogan MJ, Alvarado JA, Weddell JE: Histology of the Human Eye. An Atlas and Textbook. Philadelphia: WB Saunders Co., 1971:136-153,260-319.
3. Interchange 2n 3Funk R, Rohen JW. Scanning electron microscopy on the vasculature of the human anterior eye segment, especially with respect to ciliary processes. Exp Eye Res 1990;51(6):651.
4. Smelsker GK. Electron microscopy of a typical epithelial cell and of the human ciliary processes.Trans Am Acad Opth Otol 70:738,1966.
5. Wolosin JM, Schutte W. Gap junctions and interlayer communication in the heterocellular epithelium of the ciliary body. In: Civan MM, ed. The eye's aqueous humor from secretion to glaucoma, San Diego:Academic Press, 1998:135.
6. Raviola G, Raviola E. Intercellular junctions in the ciliary epithelium. Invest Ophthalmol Vis Sci 1978;17(10):958.
7. Hara K, Lutjen-Drscoll E, Prestel H, et al. Structural differences between the regions of the Ciliary body in Primates. Invest Ophthalmol Vis Sci 1977;16(10):912.
8. Gabelt BT, Kaufman PL. Aqueous humor hydrodynamics. In Kaufmann PL, Alm A eds. Adlers physiology of the eye C V Mosby and co, St Louis 2003:237.

9. Kinsey VE. Comparitive chemistry of aqueous humor in anterior and posterior segments of rabbits eye, its physiologic significance AMA Arch Ophthal 1953:50(4):401.

10. Sen DS, Sarin GS, Saha K. Immunoglobulins in human aqueous humor. Br J Ophthalmol 1977;61(3):216.

11. Spencer WH, Alvarado J, Hayes TL. Scanning electron microscopy of human ocular tissues: trabecular meshwork Invest OPhthal 1968;7(6):651.

12. R Rand Allingham, Sayoko E Moroi. Shield's textbook of Glaucoma. 6th edition. Lippincott Williams and Wilkins. Philedelphia.

13. Flocks M. The anatomy of the trabecular meshwork as seen in tangential section. AMA Arch Ophthal 1956; 56(5):708.

14. Rohen JW, Futa R, Lütjen-Drecoll E. The fine structure of the cribriform meshwork in normal and glaucomatous eyes as seen in tangential sections. Invest Ophthalmol Vis Sci 1981;21:574.

15. Rohen JW, Rentsch FJ. Morphology of Schlemm's Canal and related vessels in the human eye. Albrecht Von Grafe's Arch Klin Exp Ophthalmol 1968;176(4):309.

16. Ascher K. The aqueous veins: biomicroscopic study of Aqueous humor elimination. In: Monograph in the Banner-Stone division of American lectures in Ophthalmology, American Lecture Series, pub#403 Springfield,1961.

17. Tripathi RC. Mechanism of aqueous outflow across the trabecular wall of schlemm's canal. Exp eye res 1971; 11:116.

18. Frank NH.Introduction to mechanics and heat, 2nd ed New York: McGraw-Hill, 1939:246.

19. Johnstone MA. A new model describes an Aqueous outflow pump and explores causes of pump failure in glaucoma. Essentials in Ophthalmology (Glaucoma). Ed: Grehn F Stamper. Springer-Verlag Berlin Heidelberg 2006;3-32.

20. Friedenwald JS. Some problems in the calibration of tonometers. Am J Ophthal 1948;31:935.

21. Brubbacker RF. Goldmann's equation and clinical measures of aqueous humor dynamics. Exper Eye Res 2004; 78:633.

10 | When and How does Glaucoma Produce Visual Disability?

Pradeep Ramulu

INTRODUCTION

As glaucoma only affects visual acuity at very late stages of the disease, it has often been viewed as not having an impact on the patient until late in the disease process. However, in the late 1990s, several papers described lower quality of life scores amongst individuals with glaucoma.[1,2] Since, this time more focus has been placed on analyzing when and how glaucoma affects quality of life and produces measurable disability. Since these reports, the effect of glaucoma and/or visual field (VF) loss has been analyzed as part of several population-based studies[3-5] and multicenter clinical trials.[6] Many groups have also begun to directly observe how people with glaucoma perform tasks in order to characterize and quantify disability. This work has challenged the hypothesis that glaucoma affects the individual only at the latest stages of disease, and has demonstrated that the degree of VF loss necessary to affect functionality and produce noticeable visual symptoms may be less than previously believed.

IMPORTANCE OF RELATING GLAUCOMATOUS DAMAGE TO DISABILITY

Glaucoma affects approximately 2 percent of adults over the age of 40, and many more are suspects for the disease.[7] Glaucoma prevalence is several fold higher in older age groups,[8,9] which combined with the aging trends worldwide is expected to produce substantially more individuals with glaucoma.[7,8] While all these individuals suffer from the same pathophysiologic process, the functional consequences of their disease process and the visual symptoms associated with disease vary drastically across the spectrum of glaucoma severity.

Understanding which individuals with glaucoma are affected by disease, i.e. which have disability from disease, is important for several reasons. First, the goal of glaucoma treatment should be to apply the minimal amount of treatment and subject individuals to the least amount of risk en route to preventing visual disability over the course of a lifetime. Of course, accomplishing this requires an understanding of when glaucoma-related disability is likely to occur. Thus, understanding the relationship between glaucomatous VF loss and disability will help physicians make decisions regarding when treatment should begin and how aggressive treatment should be for various stages of disease. Understanding the symptoms consistent with various stages of disease will also help us understand whether any individual patient has been affected by their disease, and perhaps ought to be treated more aggressively. On a societal level, it will help us determine the stage at which it is important to diagnose glaucoma. Understanding the types of impairments caused by glaucoma will also allow us to identify and direct rehabilitative efforts towards individuals disabled from glaucoma, and also to set thresholds for activities such as driving which will improve the safety of both patients and society.

ASKING THE RIGHT QUESTIONS IN GLAUCOMA AND DISABILITY

While understanding the relationship between glaucoma and disability is clearly important, it is just as important to ask the question properly. In this chapter, we will attempt to describe "when glaucoma results in disability". To do so, we must define glaucoma, address the question of "when", and also determine what a disability is.

In restricting our analysis to glaucoma, we are still dealing with a disease process which affects visual acuity late, and may have no measurable visual defect early. Most subjects will have preserved central acuity with loss of peripheral vision in one or both eyes. However, individuals with VF damage do not necessarily have glaucoma. Thus, caution is indicated when analyzing studies which generically associate VF loss with disability. In most of these studies, VF loss occurs as a result of numerous eye conditions, including glaucoma, cataracts, and neuro-ophthalmic disease. While other eye conditions also produce visual field loss, they also produce different effects on visual acuity, contrast sensitivity and other parameters that cannot easily be accounted for. Additionally, 15 percent of subjects with VF loss in one study had no observable ocular problem,[10] and in subjects without glaucoma, lower VF mean deviation (MD) is strongly associated with cognitive function as measured by the Minimental state exam (SEE, unpublished).

Thus, the analysis of when glaucoma results in disability is best done by comparing subjects with and without glaucoma. When possible, inferences on VF loss from other conditions should not be used to answer the question of whether how glaucomatous VF loss produces disability.

GLAUCOMA AND DISABILITY— A QUESTION OF "WHEN" NOT "IF"?

As glaucoma is capable of completely eliminating sight in both eyes, the question of *if* it is capable of producing disability is obvious. The more important question, which bears relevance to clinical practice and decision-making, is *when* in the course of disease disability begins. Understanding when disability begins in the course of disease is important for all eye diseases, but is particularly relevant for glaucoma. First, most eye diseases produce a decrement in visual acuity, which has been strongly linked to difficulties in nearly every functional domain.[11] Glaucoma, on the other hand, usually only affects central vision late in the disease process, and more frequently results only in peripheral field loss, where the association with disability is less clear. Additionally, unlike diseases such as cataract, when treatment can be applied to individuals when they describe the onset of disability (i.e. describe symptoms), the onset of symptoms cannot be reversed in glaucoma, and treatment must be initiated to prevent disease progression to the stage where the likelihood of disability is increased as a result of disease.

Legal definitions for blindness and impairment as a result of VF loss suggest that significant disability from glaucoma does not happen until late in disease, until visual acuity is affected, or less than 10° of vision remains in the better-seeing eye. Indeed, evidence exists to support the idea that disability is mild until later stages of disease. For example, in the Collaborative Initial Glaucoma Study (CIGTS), where subjects had unilateral or early bilateral disease,[12] only weak correlations between difficulties with visual activities and better-eye VF loss were noted,

though correlations were statistically significant.[6] Additionally, less than ¼ of subjects with glaucoma are willing to trade off any years of life for perfect vision,[13,14] suggesting that 75 percent of glaucoma patients do not view their glaucoma as a major impediment.

On the other hand, data from the Los Angeles Latino Eye Study (LALES) has suggested that even mild (2 to 6 dB) unilateral VF loss is associated with lower quality of life scores.[3] Furthermore, perceived and measured VF deterioration are correlated, suggesting that subjects can tell the difference between different degrees of VF loss.[15] Finally, subjects with glaucoma in the Proyecto Ver eye project had lower vision-related quality of life than groups with cataract and diabetic retinopathy.[16] Moreover, the average magnitude of effect seen with glaucoma exceeded that seen for 2 lines of visual acuity loss within nearly every functional domain studied, suggesting a substantial impact even with routine levels of VF damage.[17]

The best analysis, however, should be done by analyzing disability within each functional domain separately, examining the stage of disease necessary to produce functional impairment in that domain, and looking at different types of evidence supporting the notion that glaucoma results in disability. Thus, in order to determine the association between glaucoma and disability, we must first discuss staging of glaucoma with regards to disability, which functional domains ought to be tested, and how the relationship between glaucoma and disability should be studied within a given functional domain.

> - ***The best analysis:*** Done by analyzing disability within each functional domain separately
> - ***Examine:*** The stage of disease necessary to produce functional impairment in that domain.

STAGING GLAUCOMA FOR PURPOSE OF DISABILITY

The ideal staging system for glaucoma would be constructed such that the stage of disease strongly correlated with the level of disability experienced. However, the manifestation of glaucoma are highly variable, in that disease can be unilateral or bilateral, may or may not affect vision, and may produce different degrees of visual field loss in different locations. Thus, constructing a simple staging system that explains the significant variability in disease is not simple.

Given the lack of a validated staging system for glaucoma-related disability, most studies relating VF loss to disability have simply related disability to the MD corresponding to the eye with more (worse-eye) or less (better-eye) VF loss. Others have also simply analyzed disability by the amount of VF loss present in the better or worse-seeing eye using scores from various clinical studies[18,19] or multicenter clinical trials,[20,21] some of which incorporate depth and/or location of a VF defect into the severity score.[18]

A few studies have gone further to either combine corresponding points in space from the right and left eye VFs to produce a simulated binocular field,[22,23] or to directly test the binocular VF using tests such as the Esterman VF.[24] True binocular VFs such as the Esterman method, however, are limited in that they are suprathreshold tests which may miss mild defects and cannot differentiate moderate defects from severe or total VF loss. Indeed, some studies, showed that combined monocular VF results more accurately predicted self-reported quality of life[25] as well as fitness to drive[23] than Esterman VFs. However, this entire approach is speculative, as overlapping VF loss has not been shown to produce more disability than non-overlapping VF loss. While it makes intuitive sense that overlapping VF loss would be particularly problematic, it remains possible that nonoverlapping VF loss results in loss of stereoacuity in portions of the visual field loss, producing a comparable level of disability. However, given the findings from multiple papers across multiple diseases that little or no impairment is present with unilateral VF loss[4,26] or visual acuity loss[27,28] or that binocular VF loss has a much more significant effect that unilateral VF loss,[3] it will be important to validate methods for measuring binocular VF loss or combining results from unilateral VFs and relate these binocular measures to disability.

Practically, systems which allow the clinician to estimate the level of severity without the use of any assisting software or computation offer the greatest benefit, as inferences about disability resulting from various degrees of glaucomatous damage can be directly translated towards meaningful clinical decisions. Therefore, until binocular fields become easier to directly measure or to generate using the standard visual field machinery, and also are more clearly established as the critical metric for disability, metrics easily generated from the individual monocular fields, i.e. metrics such as mean deviation of the better or worse eye, should be favored.

> • ***The Greatest Benefit:*** Methods which estimate the level of severity without the use of any assisting software or computation
> • Until binocular fields become easier to measure or generate metrics from monocular fields are a good option.

GLAUCOMA AND DISABILITY: WHICH TASKS AND FUNCTIONS ARE AFFECTED?

Studying disability in glaucoma also requires that one looks for disability in tasks that are likely to be affected by the disease. At the same time, it is important that vision-related tasks which are important to patients are examined.

If differences in quality of life scores amongst subjects with and without, glaucoma is the sole criteria for disability, then several papers suggest that nearly all types of tasks are affected by glaucoma, including items rarely associated with glaucoma such as color vision, mental health, and near vision.[6,16,21,29] While more specific effects were noted with questionnaires specifically designed to assess vision-related quality of life, similar effects were noted in some studies with generic health questionnaires,[30,31] though other studies using generic health questionnaires did not find an association of self-reported scores with disease severity.[2]

Other studies attempted to identify the most common problems associated with glaucoma, i.e. through focus groups[32,34] or standardized questioning of subjects entering a clinical trial.[35] Several of these studies identified tasks performed under specific lighting conditions as being the most common complaint of subjects with glaucoma, with members of Nelson's focus group most frequently complaining of glare (70%) and difficulty adapting to different levels of light (54%),[33] Lee's focus group most frequently describing trouble seeing in the dark (82% of glaucoma subjects vs 32% of controls),[34] and CIGTS patients most frequently describing difficulty with bright light (40%) and moving from light to dark (40%).[35] Outside of light-dependent complains, members of Nelson's focus group most commonly cited difficulties with mobility (49% walking steps, 42% shopping, and 36% crossing a road), reading (43% reading a newspaper), and face recognition (32%), with subjects not asked about driving.[33] The NEI-VFQ glaucoma focus group studied by Mangione most frequently described difficulty with mobility (including driving), reading, and social relations. In focus groups convened for other eye diseases in development of the NEI-VFQ, the most common complaints centered reading (#1) and driving (#2).[32] Viswanathan asked a series of questions to glaucoma patients regarding their most common complaints, and found that mobility tasks (i.e. stairs and bumping into things), and object finding (i.e. searching for something that has been dropped) were the most frequent complaints, though subjects were not asked about driving.[15]

> **Note** All studies have focused on developed Western nations where driving is a primary means of transportation, and may not reflect the tasks performed in India or other regions of the world.

Recent work has also focused on getting information on what vision-related tasks are viewed as most important by subjects with glaucoma **(Table 1)**. Burr, using a discrete choice experimental approach, noted that in the 286 glaucoma subjects studied, maximum importance was given to tasks of central and near vision, with the next highest importance given to mobility and other activities of daily living (driving was not included as an area of possible complaint).[36] Similar work from Bhargava suggested that the ability to continue to drive is a major priority for individuals with glaucoma, though domains such as walking, reading, and social interaction were

not evaluated.[37] A similar approach was taken by Aspinall and colleagues, who found that the most important visual tasks as rated by subjects with a range of glaucoma severity were reading (#1), followed by outdoor mobility (getting around outside the home). Less significant were glare, object bumping, and performance of household chores.[13] Altangerel and Spaeth directly tested the ability of glaucoma subjects to perform a variety of tasks, finding that the tasks most likely to be affected by glaucoma were reading small print in the dark, placing a stick into holes of different size, and finding objects.[38]

Combining these results together suggests that areas for study, based on importance of the task to patients as well as the likelihood that such tasks would be affected by glaucoma, include reading, mobility (i.e. walking and balance), and driving, and that the effect of low and very bright lighting on the performance of these tasks is particularly relevant.

UNDERSTANDING WHEN DISABILITY IS PRESENT

Perhaps the biggest challenge in relating glaucoma stage to disability is our ability to understand when disability is present in a given individual **(Figure 1)**. In determining when disability is present, the ideal comparison, i.e. the same individual without their level of glaucomatous field loss, is not available for comparison. Moreover, many potential confounders occur when comparing

subjects. For example, depression has been noted to have a high correlation with self-reported quality of life.[39-41] Additionally, numerous factors such as age, race, cognitive ability, education, and the presence of comorbid illnesses have been noted to both differ between subject with and without glaucoma, and to be highly predictive of tasks such as reading, mobility or driving.[42-44] Not adjusting for these important co-variates can result in drastically different results, as demon-strated by the analysis of reading ability, which showed substantial differences in reading speed between most bilateral glaucoma subjects and non-glaucoma subjects in univariate analyses, but no association (except in those with the most advanced glaucoma) after adjusting for age, race, education, and cognitive ability.[44]

> **Areas for assessment**
> * Reading
> * Mobility
> * Driving
> * Effect of lighting

The most common method for assessing when and whether disability occurs in glaucoma has been self-report. Numerous questionnaires have been constructed to have subjects self-report their general health,[45] difficulty with eye-related tasks,[32,46-48] or difficulty with tasks believed to be affected by glaucoma (previously reviewed by Altangerel et al.[49]). In addition to self-reporting difficulty with tasks, numerous studies have had individuals with glaucoma self-report outcomes, i.e. falls, or motor vehicle accidents. Self-report as a method for understanding disability is a necessary component of defining disability. Self-report methods incorporate people's perception of disease, and may be the only method for capturing rare events that would be hard to directly observe. These

Table 1 Clinically meaningful functional domains in glaucoma

Most common complaints*	Highest valued functions**
Vision in lighting extremes	Reading and seeing details
Mobility outside the home	Mobility outside the home
Reading and seeing details	Social Interactions
Social interactions	Self-care activities

* Mangione CM, 1998; Nelson P, 1999; Viswanathan AC, 1999; Janz NK, 2001
** Burr JM, 2007; Aspinall PA, 2008

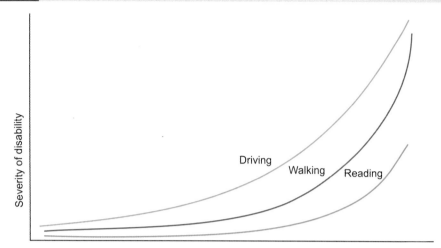

Fig. 1 Glaucoma and disability in different functional domains

techniques are subject to considerable reporting and recall bias.

Questionnaires: Self-reported methods
- Adjust for covariates like age, cognitive ability, education, comorbid illness
- Be aware of reporting and recall bias
- Yield numerical scores
- An important technique despite shortcomings

Direct observation of tasks: a critical adjunct
- Minimizes bias
- Yields quantitatively meaningful result

Self-report as a metric for disability also poses the potential for significant bias. Very few self-report studies have been performed on subjects who were unaware of their diagnosis, and awareness of diagnosis may lead to erroneous associations. For example, between 1/3 and 1/2 of subjects in CIGTS reported symptoms such as burning, irritation, eye pain and redness, even though they were newly diagnosed with glaucoma and had yet to receive treatment.[50] Despite the fact that these symptoms were almost certainly not a result of their glaucoma, over 70 percent of those experiencing the symptoms attributed the symptoms to their glaucoma.[50] Reporting bias may also occur when subjects are asked to report events that may have happened

in the past. For example, only moderate agreement was noted between self-reported and state reported accidents, leading to different conclusions about whether or not glaucoma led to more accidents.[51] On the other hand, subjects may not report disability in a functional domain if the domain is not relevant to them, i.e. a subject who feels unsafe walking may not report trouble with mobility tasks. In the SEE cohort, for example, only 1/4 of those who read slower than 80 words per minute, below which sustained reading is felt to not be possible, reported moderate or extreme difficulty reading.[52] Nonetheless, this disability may have a significant impact with regards to the patient's frailty, general health,

and also on the patient's family or caretakers, who require more effort to care for the individual. Many individuals are able to compensate for task difficulties by changing the frequency with which they perform the tasks or using assistive devices. However, these compensatory mechanisms have a limited lifespan, and research from SEE has shown that such compensations are the strongest predictor of incident self-reported disability.[53] Finally, self-report studies which measure self-reported difficulty with tasks (i.e. trouble reading fine print) as opposed to tangible outcomes (i.e. how many times in the last year did you fall), yield numerical scores of ability whose clinical significance is not clear. Despite these shortcomings, self-report is an important technique to identify the types of disability that occurs, to determine whether disability is likely to occur in a given functional domain, and to determine whether rare outcomes (i.e. falls) which could not be directly observed are more likely in glaucoma.

A critical adjunct to self-report in measuring disability is the direct observation of task performance **(Figure 2)**, and many studies in this line have been published over the last 5 years. Altangerel and Spaeth set-up a validated 5-item test to differentiate various levels of impairment in subjects with glaucoma.[38] Additionally,

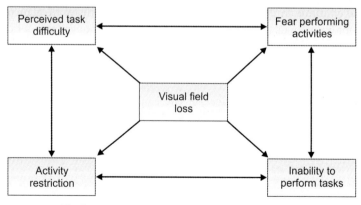

Fig. 2 Types of disability due to loss of visual field

the Salisbury Eye Evaluation was constructed to evaluate both self-reported and directly measured difficulty with task performance in a population-based sample from Salisbury Maryland.[54,55] In the fourth and final round of this longitudinal study, glaucoma status was determined,[9] allowing for a comparison of both self-reported[4,24] and direct measures[43,44] of task performance between 150 subjects with glaucoma and 1050 subjects without glaucoma. As direct measures of task performance are typically done in the clinical setting, it is critical that tests be set up to recapitulate how the task is normally performed at home. As part of SEE, for example, task performance at home and in the clinic was compared, with high correlations noted for most tested activities, and the highest correlation achieved for reading speed.[56] However, it is extremely difficult to set up tests of mobility or driving to recapitulate the variety of situations that an individual might encounter in their daily. Furthermore, direct testing may pick up disabilities that individuals have adapted to either with compensatory mechanisms (i.e. a cane for walking or magnifiers for reading), or by limiting or eliminating the activity from their routine. Identification of such disability can be viewed in one of two ways. First, one might suggest that picking up disabilities which subjects do not complain about is not particularly relevant. On the other hand, disabilities in functional domains such as walking and driving may have substantial impact on both the patient and their family, even if they have accepted it and do not find it something to complain about. Finally, direct observation minimizes reporting bias and yields quantitatively meaningful results.

The third important component of associating glaucomatous vision loss with disability is the suggestion of a plausible mechanism by which glaucoma might contribute to disability. For example, the idea that macular degeneration may affect reading is supported by the fact that vision is disturbed right at the point where subjects attempt to fixate on their reading targets. Below, we present studies which examine self-reported difficulty with tasks, studies which directly examined task performance, and studies which suggest a plausible mechanism for disability, focusing on the domains most likely to be affected by glaucoma as suggested above.

Walking and Balance

Walking and balance are important to healthy living in old age. Subjects with difficulty walking are more likely to enter into long-term care,[57] and more physical activity has been associated with better subjective well-being.[58] Nelson found that, aside from light-specific complaints, difficulty with walking were the most common category of complaint amongst subjects with glaucoma, with 49 percent describing difficulties with steps, 42 percent describing difficulty going shopping, and 36 percent describing difficulty crossing the road.[33] Similarly, Viswanathan noted reported difficulty with stairs and bumping into objects to be amongst the three strongest correlates with binocular VF loss.[15] Fear of falling can also lead to substantial restriction of activity,[59] and decreased physical activity has been associated with a wide array of negative consequences including decreased quality of life,[60] and higher morbidity[61-63] and increased mortality.[64-70]

Both glaucoma and VF loss from other causes have been clearly associated with more difficulty walking. All-cause VF loss in SEE was associated with slower walking speed and more bumping into objects, with particular trouble noted for VF loss in the central 20° most important in predicting trouble with walking speed and bumps.[71] Similar findings have been noted in subjects with low vision, where VF loss was more predictive of decreased walking speed, orientation errors, and bumping into objects than was loss of visual acuity.[72] Subjects with glaucoma have been noted to walk more slowly than similarly-aged controls,[73] with walking speed strongly correlated with the extent of worse-eye VF MD.[73] Walking may also require more concentration in glaucoma, as response time to a secondary task slowed in glaucoma subjects as VF damage worsened.[74] A population-based comparison of walking in subjects with and without glaucoma demonstrated that after adjusting for multiple covariates, subjects with bilateral, but not unilateral glaucoma, walked 2.4 meters/minute slower, and bumped into objects 1.65 times as frequently.[43] No difference in performance was observed going up and down a short staircase.[43] Simulation of VF loss in 20 normally sighted individuals demonstrated that when field of view was restricted to less than 11°, walking slowed, and more object bumping was observed, though less severe restrictions of the field of view could create difficulties at lower levels of contrast.[75]

Several studies have also examined balance in glaucoma. In SEE, subjects with bilateral, but not unilateral, glaucoma had more difficulty maintaining balance while performing tasks such as semi-tandem and tandem stands (where the heel of one foot is placed next to or in front of the big toe of the second food).[43] Other studies have demonstrated that individuals with glaucoma sway more when standing than normal individuals,[76] and that greater sway is noted with worsening better-eye VF MD.[77] No differences were observed between subjects with and without glaucoma, or with different levels of VF loss when testing was performed with eyes closed, strongly suggesting that the effect was due to loss of visual input, and not because of confounding variables.[76,77]

These difficulties with bumps and balance are corroborated by studies which report more frequent falling in glaucoma and with other VF loss. In the SEE, risk of falling increased with the degree of all-cause VF loss on suprathreshold VF testing, but did not increase with worsening acuity, contrast sensitivity or stereoacuity,[78] while Coleman described 1/3 of falls occurring as a result of severe binocular VF loss occurring from cataract, glaucoma or macular degeneration.[10] In participants of the Beaver Dam Eye Study, loss of VF not only doubled the risk of falls, but also doubled the risk of hip fractures.[79] Similar findings were noted in an analysis of Medicare recipients, where glaucoma subjects coded as visually impaired were more likely to have had a fall or accident (OR=1.6) as well as to have had a femur fracture (OR=1.6) than a glaucoma patient not coded to have visual loss.[80] Several studies provide data more specific to glaucoma. In the Blue Mountains Eye Study, falls were twice as likely when subjects were using a glaucoma medicine.[81] In the Singapore Malay Eye Study, glaucoma subjects had four times higher odds of falling than nonglaucoma subjects after adjusting for visual acuity, though conclusions were limited by the small number of glaucoma subjects.[82] A four-fold increased odds of self-reported falls was also noted in the clinic-based study of Haymes, though non-glaucoma controls may have represented an unusually healthy set of individuals (more frequently employed, fewer medical conditions, better acuity).[83] Colón-Emeric examined risk factors for entry into a skilled nursing facility with a hip fracture, and noted (using

Medicare data) that glaucoma was a risk factor in men, but not women.[84]

Reading

Reading is frequently associated with loss of visual acuity, and indeed loss of visual acuity is strongly associated with reading speed,[11] and loss of reading ability is the most frequent complaint amongst subjects with eye diseases which typically affect vision through degradation of acuity.[32] Possibly as a result, less focus has been placed on if or when glaucoma affects reading. Nonetheless, tasks of central and near vision, i.e. reading,[36] are listed as the most important visual function amongst subjects with glaucoma, and complaints regarding reading difficulty have been noted in over 40 percent of glaucoma subjects,[33] suggesting the importance of study in this domain.

In the Salisbury Eye Evaluation, subjects with bilateral glaucoma had nearly 5-fold higher odds of reporting severe difficulty with near activities than subjects without glaucoma,[4] confirming several clinic based studies which demonstrated lower scores amongst glaucoma subjects, or with worsening VF loss, with near activities such as reading.[21,16,29,30] Other work, however, has demonstrated significant discordance between reading speed and self-reported reading difficulty, particular amongst subjects who read poorly, highlighting the importance for direct testing of reading ability.[52]

Glaucoma subjects with worse Esterman scores also describe more difficulty following a line of print or finding the next line when reading,[15] providing a plausible mechanism by which loss in the visual field could make reading more difficult. Altangerel identified reading small print as one of the most visually demanding tasks in glaucoma subjects, and task performance in this domain was moderately

correlated with the extent of binocular VF loss measured with Esterman VFs.[38] The most extensive study of reading in glaucoma found slower reading speeds only in those with the most advanced bilateral glaucoma, at which point loss of visual acuity more likely accounted for slowed reading than loss of the visual field.[44] The reading test employed in SEE only tested reading for short durations, however, and may have missed difficulty with sustained reading, or word-finding tasks generally incorporated into the reading domain.

Driving

Driving is a critical function for the elderly, with cessation of driving leading to a nearly 5-fold increase risk of entry into long-term care,[85] in addition to higher rates of depression[86] and lower quality of life.[87] While some of those unsafe to drive may indeed stop or restrict their driving, large numbers of subjects with very advanced field loss continue to drive,[42] and some studies have suggested that even those who have experienced crashes are not more likely to stop driving.[88] Moreover, both patients and doctors are poor at reporting their decreased vision to the appropriate oversight agencies (where they exist, i.e. England).[89] Unsafe driving poses the risk of increase motor vehicle accidents, which poses a danger not only to elderly drivers, but also society at large. Accidents are particularly risky to elderly, whose risk of fatality associated with a motor vehicle accident is three times higher than for the average 20-year-old.[90] Additionally, the ability to move outside the home is cited as the one of the two most important visual functions amongst subject with glaucoma.[36,13] These issues are particular important as countries such as the United States age, resulting in higher number of older drivers in their eight and ninth decades,[91] approximately 10 percent of whom will have glaucoma in one or both eyes.[9,78] Additionally, driving difficulties can affect people other than the drivers, either as a result of collisions, or because subjects with no other drivers in the home are also more likely to enter into long-term care.[85]

Prior work has provided mixed information regarding whether or not subjects with glaucoma are more likely to crash. McGwin noted a 3-fold increase in the odds of crashes with glaucoma in cohort of elderly drivers when state records, but not self-report, was used to identify crashes.[51] A later case-control study of 406 subjects with various degrees of glaucoma confirmed these findings, with subjects with the most severe worse-eye mean deviation demonstrating showing roughly four-fold higher odds of a state-reported crash, though no effect was seen with worsening better-eye mean deviation.[92] As all subjects had glaucoma in this cohort, this suggests that the group with at least one severely effected eye had more accidents than those with minimal or no glaucoma damage in both eyes. As it is rare to have a single severely affected eye in glaucoma, it is likely that most of these subjects had bilateral glaucoma. Even greater odds of crashing were observed as a result of glaucoma by Haymes, who noted a 6.6 fold higher odds of a state-reported collisions in subjects with glaucoma.[83] However, controls in this study had cutoffs for visual acuity not applied to the glaucoma subjects, were recruited from workers (healthy-worker effect), and had extraordinarily good mean deviations, suggesting they may have been supranormal in their vision.[83] These results are contradicted by work from Hu, who found that state-recorded accidents were only slightly (OR=1.7) more common in males over the age of 65, but no more common in elderly women, McGwin,[93] who noted that subjects with glaucoma were less likely to crash than subjects without glaucoma (OR=0.67), and from Owsley, who noted in a prospective cohort study that VF defects from all causes had no effect on accident rates.[94] Early work by Johnson, who examined accident rates in 10,000 volunteers screened at a Department of Motor Vehicles visit, demonstrated a 2-fold increase in the age and sex-adjusted crash rate with binocular VF loss, though VF loss resulted from a mixture of cataract glaucoma, and retinal disease, and no effect was observed with unilateral VF loss.[26]

Recent work has also suggested that individuals with glaucoma are more likely to limit their driving or stop altogether. Recent work from SEE has demonstrated that subjects with bilateral, but not unilateral, glaucoma had nearly 3 times the odds of driving cessation after adjusting for a broad range of covariates.[42] This work corroborated previous work from the Blue Mountains Eye Study, which also identified glaucoma as a risk factor after adjusting only for age and sex, though the effect was not further investigated at different levels of glaucomatous damage.[95] The work is also supported by other work from SEE, which found more frequent driving cessation amongst subjects with all-cause baseline peripheral field loss, or incidence lower peripheral VF loss.[96] While it is unclear whether the decision to stop driving was that of the patient, or the local licensing agency, these findings run in parallel to work from the United Kingdom, where 20 percent of subjects had VFs worsen to the point where they were no longer qualified to hold a license over a 7 years period,[97] and 45 percent had vision insufficient for holding a license at the time of death (though nearly half of this could at least partially be attributed to diseases other than glaucoma).[98]

Many other studies have demonstrated that individuals with glaucoma may not stop driving, but instead restrict their driving. McGwin noted that subjects with glaucoma had two-fold higher odds of driving avoidance at night, in fog, in the rain, during rush hour, on the highway, and in high density, even after adjusting for multiple covariates, potentially explaining the lower crashes in glaucoma found as part of this study.[93] Adler found that glaucoma subjects were more likely to limit their driving at night (67% vs 43% of controls) and driving in unfamiliar areas (50% vs 30% of controls), but not to restrict driving on highways, bad weather, or during rush hour.[99] Freeman described that all-cause overlapping VF loss in the central 20° predicted cessation of night driving, while no effect was observed for changes in contrast sensitivity or visual acuity.[100] We described similar rates of night driving cessation, driving frequency, and cessation of driving in unfamiliar areas in a very elderly group of subjects with glaucoma, though subjects with glaucoma were more likely to report driving limitation (less frequent driving or cessation of night driving or driving in unfamiliar areas) attributable to difficulty with their vision.[42]

Finally, experiments which have examined driving patterns of subjects with and without visual field loss in driving simulators or on-road driving tests have demonstrated mixed results. Haymes compared on-road driving performance in subjects with and without glaucoma, and found that glaucoma subjects had more difficulty seeing pedestrians on the side of the road, or more frequently required a critical intervention from the driving evaluator.[101] Szlyk compared driving performance of subjects with and without glaucoma in a driving simulator, and found that simulated accidents correlated with the degree of constriction in the horizontal VF.[102] In a study of subjects with VF loss from a variety of conditions, more advanced horizontal and vertical VF loss was associated with difficulty maintaining lane position, keeping in the path of a curve, and poor anticipatory skills.[103] When VF loss was simulated in a group of normal subjects, monocular VF loss produced no difficulty driving, but binocular VF restriction produced slowed speeds when driving in reverse and lower reaction times to peripheral objects on a closed circuit course.[104] On the other hand, no significant difficulties with driving were noted amongst subjects with VF constriction from AMD, RP and glaucoma in a driving simulator.[105] Likewise, a group of 1,350 subjects with VF loss mainly as a result of stroke showed no overall worsening in an on-road driving performance evaluation.[106] Likewise, Szlyk found that glaucoma subjects did not differ from controls in any of 8 driving measures performed in a driving simulator, though less than 30 subjects were in each group.[102]

Subjects with glaucoma generally described more difficulty driving. SEE subjects with bilateral, but not unilateral glaucoma, had lower self-reported scores with regards to driving at night.[4] Several other studies have demonstrated lower driving scores in subjects with glaucoma,[21,107] with most such studies also demonstrating the strongest association between the degree of VF loss and self-reported difficulty noted in the driving domain.[1,107]

While these data suggest that glaucoma may be an important predictor of unsafe driving, the utility of specific cutoffs for maintaining a license, while reasonable, remains unsubstantiated. Moreover, other measures of visual impairment, such as the useful field of view, have been demonstrated to predict accidents much better than the presence of glaucoma.[27,51,94,108]

DISABILITY—IMPORTANCE OF LIGHTING CONDITIONS

The lighting conditions under which tasks are performed may be as important or even more important than the task itself. Nelson found the most common complaint amongst glaucoma subjects to be complaints of glare with bright lights (70%) and adapting to different levels of lighting (54%).[33] Similar findings were noted by Lee, who noted that 82 percent of glaucoma subjects described trouble seeing in the dark as compared to only 32 percent of controls.[34] Both Burr and Nelson noted that the greatest change in self-reported ability with extent of VF damage occurred in the domain of lighting and glare.[36,33] Questionnaires designed to assess vision problems under low luminance have been developed for macular degeneration, but have not be validate for or applied to subjects with glaucoma.[109]

However, relatively little testing has been done to elucidate how lighting affects the performance of various tasks. Altangerel tested reading with small print and under reduced illumination, and noted better Rasch analytic variables with reading small print. Kuyk examined mobility in 87 veterans with visual impairment from a broad range of conditions, noting that mobility under scotopic conditions resulted in lower walking speeds and more bumps, particularly in those with worse VF loss.[110] Similarly, Hassan noted broader fields of view for efficient navigation as contrast levels decreased.[75] These findings suggest that the lighting conditions under which tasks are performed may be more relevant to disability than the tasks itself. Future work should focus on assessing light-dependent task difficulty, as has been done for macular degeneration, and for directly observing task performance in glaucoma under varying light conditions.

GLAUCOMA—OTHER EFFECTS

Numerous other effects have been shown or suggested in glaucoma, though either the importance or significance of these tasks can be questioned. Finding objects has been noted to be particularly difficult in glaucoma, with Viswanathan noting a strong correlation between self-reported difficulty in this domain with binocular Esterman VF score.[15] Similarly, Altangerel noted the strongest correlation between VF loss and task difficulty in this domain.[38] However, the impact of difficulty in this domain is questionable, except as it relates to other tasks such as reading or driving. Evidence also exists that glaucoma may affect face recognition,[33] and focus groups have identified this as an important functional domain amongst subjects with glaucoma. No publications have studied the association of glaucoma and face recognition.

Little effect[4,111] and little importance[36,13] has been associated with household tasks and activities of daily living, suggesting that this is not a critical domain for study. While glaucoma patients have been noted to frequently complain of eye discomfort,[34,50] that these symptoms would frequently be attributed to glaucoma even prior to treatment suggests that those aware of disease are simply more likely to voice these complaints and attribute them to their known condition.[50]

Medicare data has suggested that subjects severely impaired from glaucoma are more likely to develop depression (OR = 1.6), though other studies have noted no association of depressive symptoms and glaucoma.[31,112]

However, a diagnosis of glaucoma may by itself increase anxiety, with 80 percent of patients describing negative emotions upon receiving the diagnosis of glaucoma, including 47 percent who described anxiety.[113] In CIGTS, nearly 50 percent worried about possible blindness as a result of their diagnosis.[50]

CONCLUSION

When we combine evidence from self-report studies and studies directly observing task performance, we find that glaucoma with bilateral visual field loss results in tangible symptoms and adverse outcomes, particular in important domains such as driving and mobility. No clear evidence supports the idea that unilateral VF loss results in significant disability. More work is required to determine if glaucoma affects other important domains such as reading. Future work should also corroborate findings in the driving and mobility domains as performed in patients' daily activities.

REFERENCES

1. Gutierrez P, Wilson MR, Johnson C, et al. Influence of glaucomatous visual field loss on health-related quality of life. Arch Ophthalmol 1997;115: 777-84.

2. Parrish RK, 2nd, Gedde SJ, Scott IU, et al. Visual function and quality of life among patients with glaucoma. Arch Ophthalmol 1997;115:1447-55.

3. McKean-Cowdin R, Varma R, Wu J, et al. Severity of visual field loss and health-related quality of life. Am J Ophthalmol 2007;143:1013-23.

4. Freeman EE, Munoz B, West SK, et al. Glaucoma and quality of life: The salisbury eye evaluation. Ophthalmol 2008;115:233-8.

5. Ivers RQ, Mitchell P, Cumming RG. Visual function tests, eye disease and symptoms of visual disability: A population-based assessment. Clin Experiment Ophthalmol 2000;28:41-7.

6. Mills RP, Janz NK, Wren PA, et al. Correlation of visual field with quality-of-life measures at diagnosis in the collaborative initial glaucoma treatment study (CIGTS). J Glaucoma 2001;10(3):192-8.

7. Friedman DS, Wolfs RC, O'Colmain BJ, et al. Prevalence of open-angle glaucoma among adults in the United States. Arch Ophthalmol 2004;122:532-8.

8. Quigley HA, Broman AT. The number of people with glaucoma worldwide in 2010 and 2020. Br J Ophthalmol 2006;90:262-7.

9. Friedman DS, Jampel HD, Munoz B, et al. The prevalence of open-angle glaucoma among blacks and whites 73 years and older. The salisbury eye evaluation glaucoma study. Arch Ophthalmol 2006;124:1625-30.

10. Coleman AL. Sources of binocular suprathreshold visual field loss in a cohort of older women being followed for risk of falls (an American Ophthalmological Society thesis). Trans Am Ophthalmol Soc 2007;105:312-29.

11. West SK, Rubin GS, Broman AT, et al. How does visual impairment affect performance on tasks of everyday life? the SEE project. salisbury eye evaluation. Arch Ophthalmol 2002; 120:774-80.

12. Mills RP. Correlation of quality of life with clinical symptoms and signs at the time of glaucoma diagnosis. Trans Am Ophthalmol Soc 1998;96:753-812.

13. Aspinall PA, Johnson ZK, Azuara-Blanco A, et al. Evaluation of quality of life and priorities of patients with glaucoma. Invest Ophthalmol Vis Sci 2008;49:1907-15.

14. Jampel HD, Schwartz A, Pollack I, et al. Glaucoma patients' assessment of their visual function and quality of life. J Glaucoma 2002;11:154-63.

15. Viswanathan AC, McNaught AI, Poinoosawmy D, et al. Severity and stability of glaucoma: Patient perception compared with objective measurement. Arch Ophthalmol 1999;117:450-4.

16. Broman AT, Munoz B, Rodriguez J, et al. The impact of visual impairment and eye disease on vision-related quality of life in a mexican-American population: Proyecto VER. Invest Ophthalmol Vis Sci 2002;43:3393-8.

17. Broman AT, Quigley HA, West SK, et al. Estimating the rate of progressive visual field damage in those with open-angle glaucoma, from cross-sectional data. Invest Ophthalmol Vis Sci 2008;49:66-76.

18. Mills RP, Budenz DL, Lee PP, et al. Categorizing the stage of glaucoma from pre-diagnosis to end-stage disease. Am J Ophthalmol 2006;141: 24-30.

19. Hodapp E, Parrish RK, Anderson DR. Clinical Decisions in Glaucoma. St. Louis: Mosby; 1993.

20. Katz J. Scoring systems for measuring progression of visual field loss in clinical trials of glaucoma treatment. Ophthalmol 1999;106:391-5.

21. Musch DC, Lichter PR, Guire KE, et al. The collaborative initial glaucoma treatment study: Study design, methods, and baseline characteristics of enrolled patients. Ophthalmol 1999;106:653-62.

22. Nelson-Quigg JM, Cello K, Johnson CA. Predicting binocular visual field sensitivity from monocular visual field results. Invest Ophthalmol Vis Sci 2000;41(8):2212-21.

23. Crabb DP, Fitzke FW, Hitchings RA, et al. A practical approach to measuring the visual field component of fitness to drive. Br J Ophthalmol 2004;88:1191-6.

24. Esterman B. Functional scoring of the binocular field. Ophthalmol 1982;89:1226-34.

25. Jampel HD, Friedman DS, Quigley H, et al. Correlation of the binocular visual field with patient assessment of vision. Invest Ophthalmol Vis Sci 2002;43:1059-67.

26. Johnson CA, Keltner JL. Incidence of visual field loss in 20,000 eyes and its relationship to driving performance. Arch Ophthalmol 1983;10:1371-5.

27. Rubin GS, Ng ES, Bandeen-Roche K, et al. A prospective, population-based study of the role of visual impairment in motor vehicle crashes among older drivers: The SEE study. Invest Ophthalmol Vis Sci 2007;48:1483-91.

28. Knudtson MD, Klein BE, Klein R, et al. Age-related eye disease, quality of life, and functional activity. Arch Ophthalmol 2005;123:807-14.

29. Ringsdorf L, McGwin G, Owsley C. Visual field defects and vision-specific health-related quality of life in African Americans and whites with glaucoma. J Glaucoma 2006;15:414-8.

30. Sherwood MB, Garcia-Siekavizza A, Meltzer MI, et al. Glaucoma's impact on quality of life and its relation to clinical indicators. A pilot study. Ophthalmol 1998;105:561-6.

31. Wilson MR, Coleman AL, Yu F, et al. Functional status and well-being in patients with glaucoma as measured by the medical outcomes study short form-36 questionnaire. Ophthalmol 1998;105:2112-6.

32. Mangione CM, Berry S, Spritzer K, et al. Identifying the content area for the 51-item national eye institute visual function questionnaire: Results from focus groups with visually impaired persons. Arch Ophthalmol 1998;116:227-33.

33. Nelson P, Aspinall P, O'Brien C. Patients' perception of visual impairment in glaucoma: A pilot study. Br J Ophthalmol 1999;83:546-52.

34. Lee BL, Gutierrez P, Gordon M, et al. The glaucoma symptom scale. A brief index of glaucoma-specific symptoms. Arch Ophthalmol 1998;116:861-6.

35. Janz NK, Wren PA, Lichter PR, et al. The collaborative initial glaucoma treatment study: Interim quality of life findings after initial medical or surgical treatment of glaucoma. Ophthalmol 2001;108:1954-65.

36. Burr JM, Kilonzo M, Vale L, et al. Developing a preference-based glaucoma utility index using a discrete choice experiment. Optom Vis Sci 2007;84:797-808.

37. Bhargava JS, Patel B, Foss AJ, et al. Views of glaucoma patients on aspects of their treatment: An assessment of patient preference by conjoint analysis. Invest Ophthalmol Vis Sci 2006;47:2885-8.

38. Altangerel U, Spaeth GL, Steinmann WC. Assessment of function related to vision (AFREV). Ophthalmic Epidemiol 2006;13:67-80.

39. Jampel HD, Frick KD, Janz NK, et al. Depression and mood indicators in newly diagnosed glaucoma patients. Am J Ophthalmol 2007;144:238-44.

40. Owsley C, McGwin G. Depression and the 25-item national eye institute visual function questionnaire in older adults. Ophthalmol 2004;111:2259-64.

41. Paz SH, Globe DR, Wu J, et al. Relationship between self-reported depression and self-reported visual function in latinos. Arch Ophthalmol 2003;121:1021-7.

42. Ramulu PY, West SK, Munoz B, et al. Driving cessation and driving limitation in glaucoma: The salisbury eye evaluation project 2009;116(10):1846-53.

43. Friedman DS, Freeman E, Munoz B, et al. Glaucoma and mobility performance: The salisbury eye evaluation project. Ophthalmol 2007;114:2232-7.

44. Ramulu PY, West SK, Munoz B, et al. Glaucoma and reading speed: The salisbury eye evaluation project. Arch Ophthalmol 2009;127(1):82-7.

45. Ware JE, Snow K, Kosinski M. SF-36 Health Survey Manual and Interpretation Guide. Boston, Mass.: The Health Institute, New England Medical Center; 1993.

46. Mangione CM, Lee PP, Gutierrez PR, et al. Development of the 25-item national eye institute visual function questionnaire. Arch Ophthalmol 2001;119:1050-8.

47. Mangione CM, Lee PP, Pitts J, et al. Psychometric properties of the national eye institute visual function questionnaire (NEI-VFQ). NEI-VFQ field test investigators. Arch Ophthalmol 1998;116:1496-504.

48. Kamel HK, Guro-Razuman S, Shareeff M. The activities of daily vision scale: A useful tool to assess fall risk in older adults with vision impairment. J Am Geriatr Soc 2000;48:1474-7.

49. Altangerel U, Spaeth GL, Rhee DJ. Visual function, disability, and psychological impact of glaucoma. Curr Opin Ophthalmol 2003;14:100-5.

50. Janz NK, Wren PA, Lichter PR, et al. Quality of life in newly diagnosed glaucoma patients: The collaborative initial glaucoma treatment study. Ophthalmol 2001;108:887-97; discussion 898.

51. McGwin G. Owsley C, Ball K. Identifying crash involvement among older drivers: Agreement between self-report and state records. Accid Anal Prev 1998;30:781-91.

52. Friedman SM, Munoz B, Rubin GS, et al. Characteristics of discrepancies between self-reported visual function and measured reading speed. Salisbury eye evaluation project team. Invest Ophthalmol Vis Sci 1999;40:858-64.

53. West SK, Munoz B, Rubin GS, et al. Compensatory strategy use identifies risk of incident disability for the visually impaired. Arch Ophthalmol 2005;123:1242-7.

54. Rubin GS, West SK, Munoz B, et al. A comprehensive assessment of visual impairment in a population of older americans the SEE study salisbury eye evaluation project. Invest Ophthalmol Vis Sci 1997;38:557-68.

55. Munoz B, West S, Rubin GS, et al. Who participates in population based studies of visual impairment? The salisbury eye evaluation project experience. Ann Epidemiol 1999;9:53-9.

56. West SK, Rubin GS, Munoz B, et al. Assessing functional status: Correlation between performance on tasks conducted in a clinic setting and performance on the same task conducted at home. The salisbury eye evaluation project team. J Gerontol A Biol Sci Med Sci 1997;52:M209-17.

57. Yu MS, Chan CC, Tsim RK. Usefulness of the elderly mobility scale for classifying residential placements. Clin Rehabil 2007;21:1114-20.

58. Garatchea N, Molinero O, Martinez-Garcai R, et al. Feelings of well-being in elderly people: Relationship to physicial activity and physical function. Arch Gerontol Geriatr 2009;48(3):306-12.

59. Deshpande N, Metter EJ, Lauretani F, et al. Activity restriction induced by fear of falling and objective and subjective measures of physical function: A prospective cohort study. J Am Geriatr Soc 2008;56:615-20.

60. Lynch BM, Cerin E, Owen N, et al. Prospective relationships of physical activity with quality of life among colorectal cancer survivors. J Clin Oncol 2008;26:4480-7.

61. Leon AS, Connett J, Jacobs DR,Jr, et al. Leisure-time physical activity levels and risk of coronary heart disease and death. The multiple risk factor intervention trial. JAMA 1987;258:2388-95.

62. Helmrich SP, Ragland DR, Leung RW, et al. Physical activity and reduced occurrence of non-insulin-dependent diabetes mellitus. N Engl J Med 1991;325:147-52.

63. Cummings SR, Kelsey JL, Nevitt MC, et al. Epidemiology of osteoporosis and osteoporotic fractures. Epidemiol Rev 1985;7:178-208.

64. Paffenbarger RS, Hyde RT, Wing AL, et al. Physical activity, all-cause mortality, and longevity of college alumni. N Engl J Med 1986;314:605-13.

65. Kaplan GA, Seeman TE, Cohen RD, et al. Mortality among the elderly in the alameda county study: Behavioral and demographic risk factors. Am J Public Health 1987;77:307-12.

66. Grand A, Grosclaude P, Bocquet H, et al. Disability, psychosocial factors and mortality among the elderly in a rural french population. J Clin Epidemiol 1990;43:773-82.

67. Rakowski W, Mor V. The association of physical activity with mortality among older adults in the longitudinal study of aging (1984-1988). J Gerontol 1992;47:M122-9.

68. Simonsick EM, Lafferty ME, Phillips CL, et al. Risk due to inactivity in physically capable older adults. Am J Public Health 1993;83:1443-50.

69. Ruigomez A, Alonso J, Anto JM. Relationship of health behaviours to five-year mortality in an elderly cohort. Age Ageing 1995;24:113-9.

70. Bijnen FC, Caspersen CJ, Feskens EJ, et al. Physical activity and 10-year mortality from cardiovascular diseases and all causes: The zutphen elderly study. Arch Intern Med 1998;158:1499-505.

71. Turano KA, Broman AT, Bandeen-Roche K, et al. Association of visual field loss and mobility performance in older adults: Salisbury eye evaluation study. Optom Vis Sci 2004;81:298-307.

72. Kuyk T, Elliott JL, Fuhr PS. Visual correlates of obstacle avoidance in adults with low vision. Optom Vis Sci 1998;75:174-82.

73. Turano KA, Rubin GS, Quigley HA. Mobility performance in glaucoma. Invest Ophthalmol Vis Sci 1999;40:2803-9.

74. Geruschat DR, Turano KA. Estimating the amount of mental effort required for independent mobility: Persons with glaucoma. Invest Ophthalmol Vis Sci 2007;48:3988-94.

75. Hassan SE, Hicks JC, Lei H, et al. What is the minimum field of view required for efficient navigation? Vision Res 2007;47:2115-23.

76. Shabana N, Cornilleau-Peres V, Droulez J, et al. Postural stability in primary open angle glaucoma. Clin Experiment Ophthalmol 2005;33:264-73.

77. Black AA, Wood JM, Lovie-Kitchin JE, et al. Visual impairment and postural sway among older adults with glaucoma. Optom Vis Sci 2008;85:489-97.

78. Freeman EE, Munoz B, Rubin G, et al. Visual field loss increases the risk of falls in older adults: The salisbury eye evaluation. Invest Ophthalmol Vis Sci 2007;48:4445-50.

79. Klein BE, Klein R, Lee KE, et al. Performance-based and self-assessed measures of visual function as related to history of falls, hip fractures, and measured gait time. The beaver dam eye study. Ophthalmol 1998;105:160-4.

80. Bramley T, Peeples P, Walt JG, et al. Impact of vision loss on costs and outcomes in medicare beneficiaries with glaucoma. Arch Ophthalmol 2008;126:849-56.

81. Ivers RQ, Cumming RG, Mitchell P, et al. Visual impairment and falls in older adults: The Blue Mountains eye study. J Am Geriatr Soc 1998;46:58-64.

82. Lamoureux EL, Chong E, Wang JJ, et al. Visual impairment, causes of vision loss and falls: The Singapore Malay eye study. Invest Ophthalmol Vis Sci 2008;49:528-33.

83. Haymes SA, Leblanc RP, Nicolela MT, et al. Risk of falls and motor vehicle collisions in glaucoma. Invest Ophthalmol Vis Sci 2007;48:1149-55.

84. Colon-Emeric CS, Biggs DP, Schenck AP, et al. Risk factors for hip fracture in skilled nursing facilities: Who should be evaluated? Osteoporos Int 2003;14:484-9.

85. Freeman EE, Gange SJ, Munoz B, et al. Driving status and risk of entry into long-term care in older adults. Am J Public Health 2006;96:1254-9.

86. Marottoli RA, Mendes de Leon CF, Glass TA, et al. Driving cessation and increased depressive symptoms: Prospective evidence from the new haven EPESE. Established populations for epidemiologic studies of the elderly. J Am Geriatr Soc 1997;45:202-6.

87. Eberhard JW. Driving is transportation for most older adults. Geriatrics 1998;53:S53-5.

88. Dellinger AM, Sehgal M, Sleet DA, et al. Driving cessation: What older former drivers tell us. J Am Geriatr Soc 2001;49:431-5.

89. Puvanachandra N, Kang CY, Kirwan JF, et al. How good are we at advising appropriate patients with glaucoma to inform the DVLA? A closed audit loop. Ophthalmic Physiol Opt 2008;28:313-6.

90. Evans L. Risk of fatality from physical trauma versus sex and age. J Trauma 1988;28:368-78.

91. Foley DJ, Heimovitz HK, Guralnik JM, et al. Driving life expectancy of persons aged 70 years and older in the United States. Am J Public Health 2002;92:1284-9.

92. McGwin G, Xie A, Mays A, et al. Visual field defects and the risk of motor vehicle collisions among patients with glaucoma. Invest Ophthalmol Vis Sci 2005;46:4437-41.

93. McGwin G, Mays A, Joiner W, et al. Is glaucoma associated with motor vehicle collision involvement and driving avoidance? Invest Ophthalmol Vis Sci 2004;45:3934-9.

94. Owsley C, Ball K, McGwin G, et al. Visual processing impairment and risk of motor vehicle crash among older adults. JAMA 1998;279:1083-8.

95. Gilhotra JS, Mitchell P, Ivers R, et al. Impaired vision and other factors associated with driving cessation in the elderly: The blue mountains eye study. Clin Experiment Ophthalmol 2001;29:104-7.

96. Freeman EE, Munoz B, Turano KA, et al. Measures of visual function and time to driving cessation in older adults. Optom Vis Sci 2005;82:765-73.

97. Owen VM, Crabb DP, White ET, et al. Glaucoma and fitness to drive: Using binocular visual fields to predict a milestone to blindness. Invest Ophthalmol Vis Sci 2008;49:2449-55.

98. Ang GS, Eke T. Lifetime visual prognosis for patients with primary open-angle glaucoma. Eye 2007;21:604-8.

99. Adler G, Bauer MJ, Rottunda S, et al. Driving habits and patterns in older men with glaucoma. Soc Work Health Care 2005;40:75-87.

100. Freeman EE, Munoz B, Turano KA, et al. Measures of visual function and their association with driving modification in older adults. Invest Ophthalmol Vis Sci 2006;47:514-20.

101. Haymes SA, LeBlanc RP, Nicolela MT, et al. Glaucoma and on-road driving performance. Invest Ophthalmol Vis Sci 2008;49:3035-41.

102. Szlyk JP, Taglia DP, Paliga J, et al. Driving performance in patients with mild to moderate glaucomatous clinical vision changes. J Rehabil Res Dev 2002;39:467-82.

103. Bowers A, Peli E, Elgin J, et al. On-road driving with moderate visual field loss. Optom Vis Sci 2005;82:657-67.

104. Wood JM, Troutbeck R. Elderly drivers and simulated visual impairment. Optom Vis Sci 1995;72:115-24.

105. Coeckelbergh TR, Brouwer WH, Cornelissen FW, et al. The effect of visual field defects on driving performance: A driving simulator study. Arch Ophthalmol 2002;120:1509-16.

106. Racette L, Casson EJ. The impact of visual field loss on driving performance: Evidence from on-road driving assessments. Optom Vis Sci 2005;82:668-74.

107. Bechetoille A, Arnould B, Bron A, et al. Measurement of health-related quality of life with glaucoma: Validation of the glau-QoL(c) 36-item questionnaire. Acta Ophthalmol Scand 2008;86:71-80.

108. Ball K, Owsley C, Stalvey B, et al. Driving avoidance and functional impairment in older drivers. Accid Anal Prev 1998;30:313-22.

109. Owsley C, McGwin G,Jr, Scilley K, et al. Development of a questionnaire to assess vision problems under low luminance in age-related maculopathy. Invest Ophthalmol Vis Sci 2006;47:528-35.

110. Kuyk T, Elliott JL, Fuhr PS. Visual correlates of mobility in real world settings in older adults with low vision. Optom Vis Sci 1998;75:538-47.

111. Nelson P, Aspinall P, Papasouliotis O, et al. Quality of life in glaucoma and its relationship with visual function. J Glaucoma 2003;12:139-50.

112. Wilson MR, Coleman AL, Yu F, et al. Depression in patients with glaucoma as measured by self-report surveys. Ophthalmol 2002;109:1018-22.

113. Odberg T, Jakobsen JE, Hultgren SJ, et al. The impact of glaucoma on the quality of life of patients in Norway. I. Results from a self-administered questionnaire. Acta Ophthalmol Scand 2001;79:116-20.

PART 2

Glaucoma—Diagnostics

11

History-taking

Arijit Mitra, R Ramakrishnan

History-taking is a very important and integral part of examination of a patient with glaucoma. In fact it is the very first-step of the doctor-patient interaction and plays a very major role in eliciting the diagnosis, winning the confidence of the patient and establishing the trust in the doctor-patient relationship. A good history can help in making the following steps of examination and management much easier. Although this holds true for all ophthalmic diseases, it is particularly important for glaucoma. It emphasizes the symptoms of the disease, present and past ocular problems and ocular medications. The history is intended to elicit any information that might be useful in evaluating and managing the patient.

GOALS OF HISTORY

The history should allow for the recording of a variety of important information that could affect the patients diagnosis and treatment.

The major goals of history-taking can be broadly classified as:
1. Identifying the patient
2. Obtaining a diagnosis
3. Identifying the previous treatment history
4. Selecting a management plan
5. Socioeconomic and other considerations.

IDENTIFYING THE PATIENT

All the demographic information pertaining to the patient should be recorded as: for example, name, date of birth, address, race, gender, profession and medical record number if any. Each point has its significance.

Age

The age of the patient is of great importance as certain glaucomatous conditions are common in certain age groups. Congenital glaucoma, developmental glaucoma, juvenile glaucoma as their names suggest are more prevalent in the younger population groups.

Pigmentary glaucoma is common in the younger age group especially males. Primary open angle glaucoma and angle-closure glaucoma are more prevalent in the middle age groups. Exfoliation glaucoma is more common in the older population groups.

Race

It is also an important factor as certain glaucomatous conditions are prevalent in certain races. African Americans are four times as more likely than Caucasians to develop glaucoma. Open angle glaucoma also occurs earlier among people of African ancestry than among Caucasians, and develops more rapidly. African Americans and Caucasians with advanced glaucoma respond differently to laser and surgical treatment options. The incidence and prevalence of angle-closure glaucoma is much higher amongst the Eskimo (Inuit) population as well as amongst the South East Asians. The prevalence of exfoliation syndrome and exfoliation glaucoma has a wide variation.

Location

The address or location can help us to note the incidence and prevalence of certain disease conditions and the reverse also holds true. Thus, we can get an idea of certain disease conditions which are known to be prevalent in those regions.

OBTAINING A DIAGNOSIS

The likely diagnosis or at least a reasonable differential diagnosis can often be suspected merely on the basis of a good history and allows for the planning and tailoring of a more useful and efficient examination. A proper documentation of each complaint according to the severity and the duration should be recorded. Even though the lesser problems may not seem relevant they should be noted and followed up.

Some General Questions

The following general areas of enquiry are given as suggestions for developing a preliminary diagnostic information:

Time and Manner of Onset

Was it sudden or gradual?
In cases of angle closure the onset in usually sudden although it is not always the rule as a large number of cases may have subclinical attacks and subtle symptoms. The open angle cases are almost always innocuous and have a very gradual mode of progress.

The lens induced glaucomas like phacomorphic and phacolytic glaucoma also present dramatically with pain and redness in the involved eye. However there is a history of an initial gradual decrease of vision in that eye. This can be elicited if the right questions are asked.

A patient with pigment dispersion may present with a sudden onset of pain or blurring of vision following an episode of exercise due to the dispersed pigments blocking the trabecular meshwork and causing a pressure spike.

Severity

Has the problem improved, worsened or remained the same?
Glaucoma is a very slowly progressive disease condition. It usually takes years for the disease to manifest itself barring the childhood glaucomas which present early. Thus it is sometimes not possible for the patient to grade the severity of the disease and to quantify the progression if at all.

Influences

What might have precipitated the condition, made it better or worse?
Asking about prior therapeutic efforts is important. It is helpful to know when the patients refractive prescription was last changed. Episodes of pain, redness or discomfort on entering a dark room or a theater may point to the diagnosis of an angle closure patient and if the patient is diagnosed early, a simple peripheral iridotomy may be only treatment required. A similar episode precipitated after exercise may point to the diagnosis of pigmentary glaucoma.

Constancy and Temporal Variation

Has the problem been intermittent or does it worsen at a particular time of day? If so, were there any influences that seemed to precipitate exacerbations or remissions?

Laterality

Is the problem unilateral or bilateral?
Primary open angle glaucoma is usually a bilateral condition although the changes may be asymmetrical. Primary angle closure patients usually have the similar narrow angles in both eyes. In case of unilateral glaucoma one must suspect an underlying secondary cause.

Documents

Old records like disc photographs, baseline IOP records, medications used can be of immense value in planning the management. Their significance will be discussed ahead in the chapter.

> **Note** In glaucoma a proper documentation of the findings is very important, be it the history or the examination results. The initial mode of presentation and the patient's complaints at the first visit and at the subsequent visits may give an idea as to the status of the disease and the progression.

SYMPTOMS
Blurred Vision

POAG is an asymptomatic disease aptly called the silent thief of sight. The patients are usually unaware of their field defects until the disease is quite advanced. The open angle glaucoma patients will usually present with an innocuous history or they may complain of a slight blurring of vision which is usually painless and progressive. However, these patients may also complain of difficulty in near work and a frequent change of presbyopic glasses. In some forms of glaucoma there is a forward shift of the crystalline lens leading to symptoms of myopia. A hyperopic shift may be seen in cases of choroidal effusion due to elevation of the retina and choroid due to suprachoroidal fluid.

Blurred Vision with Colored Haloes

When IOP is suddenly elevated, fluid moves into the cornea exceeding the capacity of the corneal endothelial pumps to remove it. This results in corneal epithelial edema which produces symptoms of blurred vision and colored haloes. These haloes are more common in acute angle closure glaucoma but can also be appreciated by patients of open angle glaucoma with a rapid elevation of IOP. Other conditions in which the patients complain of seeing colored haloes along with blurred vision should be excluded.

Pain

A rapid elevation of IOP leads to pain. This may be accompanied by nausea and vomiting. The patients with angle-closure glaucoma, however, have a more dramatic mode of presentation. They may complain of acute intense pain radiating along the distribution of the fifth cranial nerve. They may, however, also complain of headache with nausea and vomiting and can be mistaken for a bilious attack. Thay may also present with marked dimness of vision, redness, lacrimation and photophobia.

Field of Vision

Most patients of POAG are unaware of their visual field defects which are mostly peripheral. Patients with normal tension glaucoma or Myopia may have field loss close to fixation and may be symptomatic. Patients with a sustained high IOP can develop loss of visual acuity accompanied by pallor of the optic nerve head.

PAST OCULAR HISTORY

Prior ocular problems can have a bearing on the patients current status. The existence of any such problems should be discovered so that their possible role in the present illness can be evaluated and so that they can be managed effectively. These include:

- Use of eyeglasses or contact lenses; the date of the most recent prescription may be recorded
- Use of ocular medication in the past
- Any previous ocular surgery or laser
- Ocular trauma: This may point to the fact that an angle recession might have occurred and the glaucoma which is present now is a manifestation of the damage to the trabecular meshwork sustained at the time of injury

- History of ambloypia or of ocular patching in the childhood
- In secondary glaucoma due to ocular conditions like CRVO, Uveitis, or lens induced, history regarding these conditions is valuable
- History of refractive surgery
- Pigmentary dispersion syndrome.

OCULAR MEDICATIONS

Knowledge of the patients use of ocular medications is essential for the following reasons:

- *Selecting a therapy:* It is necessary to know how the patient responded to prior therapy. It will reveal the varying levels of efficacy of the drugs and help in modifying treatment accordingly.
- *Allergy* or adverse reactions to certain drugs will come to light.
- Certain drugs like brimonidine are not well tolerated by the patients. The various prostaglandin analogues have also been reported to have numerous side effects on the ocular and periocular tissues. Thus the history of the use of such agents will immediately give an idea as to the cause of the redness, stinging, burning, periocular pigmentation or lash lengthening and the simple step of discontinuation of the drug will suffice in controlling the condition.
- Recent therapy can affect the patients present status, because toxic and allergic reactions to topical medications and preservatives sometimes resolves slowly.
- The duration of use of antiglaucoma medications can be a prognostic indicator as to the success of an operative intervention along with other factors such as age and race.
- *Assessing compliance:* Certain patients may appear to be non-compliant to the therapeutic advice right from the very onset. This helps in deciding management as it may

be futile to recommend multiple drug or combination drug regimens to these patients and surgery might be a better option in controlling the condition in these patients.

> **Note** All current and prior ocular medications used for the present illness should be recorded including dosages, frequency and duration of use. Practitioners who have treated the patient may be contacted for additional information. Regarding the previous medications used if the patient is unable to provide any information. Old records may also reveal the baseline parameters of the patients.

SYSTEMIC DISEASE

All medical and surgical problems should be recorded along with the approximate dates of onset, medical treatments or surgeries when possible.

A pertinent review of systems tailored to the patients complaints should be conducted including questions about diabetes mellitus, hypertension, dermatologic, cardiac, renal, hepatic, pulmonary, gastrointestinal, central nervous system and autoimmune collagen vascular diseases.

The patients present and past systemic history is important for the following reasons:

- Hypertension has been associated with POAG.
- Glaucomas that are associated with specific conditions. For example, Sturge Weber syndrome neovascular glaucomas secondary to diabetes.
- Many ocular diseases are manifestations of, or are associated with, systemic diseases.
- Systemic medications can cause ocular, preoperative, intraoperative and postoperative problems and can provide clues to systemic disorders the patient might have.
- Some systemic medication may mask glaucoma and also decrease response to medication.

- History of use of aspirin and other anticoagulant agents as they can cause intraoperative and postoperative bleeding.
- The general medical status must be known to perform a proper preoperative evaluation.
- History of any steroids use in the form of oral or topical should be taken as even topical or inhalational can lead to or aggravate increase in intraocular pressure.
- Many of the antiglaucoma medication have potential systemic side effects and also interact with other systemic medications.
- Forms of arthritis are also associated with uveitis and may lead to uveitic glaucoma.

ALLERGIES

The patient's history of allergies to medications is important for avoiding drugs to which the patient is allergic. This includes both topical and systemic medications. Patients with allergy to sulphonamides are also allergic to carbonic anhydrase inhibitors. It is important to differentiate between true allergic reactions from side effects or other nonallergic side effects of medications.

LIFESTYLE AND DAILY ACTIVITIES

History of any vigorous exercises, or any yoga practices should be taken.

Water drinking: Large amounts of water consumed rapidly cause a transient rise in IOP in many glaucomatous eyes. This is the basis for water drinking test.

Rarely high levels of caffeine intake in patients of POAG have been associated with some IOP elevation.

Playing wind instruments like the trumpet also increase the IOP briefly.

Driving habits: One must enquire as to the driving habits of the patient to guide them depending upon their field of vision.

SOCIOECONOMIC HISTORY

The socioeconomic condition also has to be kept in mind when recommending a particular drug. Thus recommending a prostaglandin analogue to a patient of lower socioeconomic strata might not be a good option as the patient may not adhere to the therapy simply because of the economic reasons. Also certain prostaglandin analogues require refrigeration and thus may not be a suitable drug for a number of patients.

The treatment regimen might be very confusing if a number of drugs are prescribed to a patient. This holds specially true if the drugs prescribed are different for the two eyes based on the glaucomatous damage. Thus the best therapeutic option requiring the minimal number of drops is to be selected and the treatment is to be tailor made on the basis of the patients needs, occupation and lifestyle.

The components of history are:
- Chief complaints
- Present Illness
- Past ocular history
- Ocular medications
- General medical and surgical history
- Systemic medications
- Allergies
- Social history
- Family history

FAMILY HISTORY

The role of family history in glaucoma is of paramount importance. A positive family history has consistently been shown to be major risk factors. It is generally recognized that genetic factors play an important role.

Glaucoma: Important points in history-taking:
- Steroid use—aggravate or cause increased IOP
- Ocular injury
- Family history
- Drug allergy especially sulphonamide
- Aspirin/Anticoagulant use
- Asthma/COPD
  - ❖ May worsen
  - ❖ Patient may be using steroids
- CCF—Worsen after carbonic anhydrase inhibitors or hyperosmotic
- Renal failure
- Vasospastic condition
- History of previous hemodynamic crisis (severe blood loss)
- Diabetic mellitus
- Sickle cell disease
- CVS disease
- Hypercholesterolemia
- Arthritis

12 | Tonometry

Mani Bhaskaran

TONOMETRY BASICS AND NEWER TECHNIQUES

INTRODUCTION

Tonometry in reference to the eye, is the measurement of intraocular pressure (IOP). A **tonometer** is an instrument that exploits the physical properties of the eye to permit measurement of intraocular pressure without the need to cannulate the eye.

The first practical tonometer was invented by Maklakov in 1885. Fick is credited with inventing a second applanation tonometer employing a fixed area produced by an adjustable force. This instrument was a forerunner of the **Goldmann Applanation Tonometer (1954)** which is today considered the most accurate clinical tonometer.

From a functional standpoint, a normal IOP is one that does not result in optic nerve damage. All eyes do not respond similarly to a particular IOP, so a normal pressure cannot be represented as a specific measurement. Various studies of IOP distribution have shown a mean IOP of 15.5 ± 2.6 mm Hg and the upper limit has been demonstrated to be two standard deviations above the mean IOP; that is 20.5 mm Hg.

TYPES OF TONOMETERS

The physical properties of the normal cornea determine the limits of accuracy of tonometry.

When the cornea is deformed by a tonometer, the resulting fluid displacement causes the remainder of the globe to distend. The tendency of the wall of the eye is to resist stretching; deformation of the cornea raises the IOP. Tonometers in which the IOP is negligibly raised during tonometry, for example less than five percent are termed *low-displacement tonometers*. The Goldmann tonometer displaces only 0.5 ml of aqueous humor and raises IOP by only three percent. Tonometers that displace a large volume of fluid and consequently raise IOP significantly are termed *high-displacement tonometers*. In a normal eye, IOP is more than double during Schiotz tonometry. High-displacement tonometers are mostly less accurate than low-displacement tonometer.

CLASSIFICATION

Tonometry can be broadly classified into two types, **direct and indirect**.

Direct Method

A catheter is inserted into the anterior chamber of the eye and the other end is connected to a manometric device from which the pressure is calculated. Though this is the most accurate method available, it is not feasible because of its invasive nature.

Indirect Method

It is based on the eyes response to an applied force. The indirect methods can be broadly divided into **contact and noncontact methods**. Basic types of contact tonometers differ according to shape and magnitude of deformation.

Noncontact Tonometers

They measure the time required to deform the standard amount of corneal surface in response by jet of air.

Contact Tonometers

IOP measurement is performed by deforming the globe and correlating the force responsible for deformation to the pressure within the eye. Both indentation and applanation tonometers effect a deformation of globe but the magnitude varies.

Palpation Method

IOP is estimated by response of eye to pressure applied by finger pulp (indents easily/firm to touch).

INDENTATION TONOMETERS

They are used to measure the amount of deformation or indentation of the globe in response to a **standard weight** applied to the cornea or the area flattened by a **standard force**. The shape of corneal deformation is a truncated cone **(Figure 1A)**. It displaces large intraocular volume so conversion tables based on empirical data are used to estimate IOP. The prototype is Schiotz tonometer **(Figure 2)**.

APPLANATION TONOMETERS

They are used to measure force necessary to flatten a small, standard area of cornea. The shape of corneal

deformation is simple flattening **(Figure 1B)**. The shape is constant so IOP is derived from mathematical calculation. They are of two types on basis of the variable that is measured.

1. Variable Force
- Area of cornea on applanation is held constant, force varies.
- Prototype: Goldmann tonometer **(Figures 3A to C)**.

2. Variable Area
- Force applied to cornea is held constant, area varies
- Volume displacement is sufficiently large to require conversion table
- Prototype: Maklakov.

SCHIOTZ TONOMETER

Type: Indentation tonometer

Instrument: It consists of a metal plunger that slides through a hole in a concave metal plate. The plunger supports a hammer device connected to a needle that crosses a scale. The extent to which cornea is indented by the plunger is measured as the distance from the foot plate curve to the plunger base and a lever system moves a needle on calibrated scale. The indicated scale reading and the plunger weight are converted to an IOP measurement.

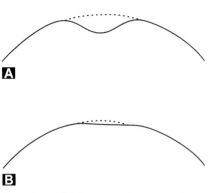

Figs 1A and B (A) Indentation: The shape of the corneal deformation is a truncated cone; (B) Applanation: A small standard area of the cornea is flattened

More the plunger indents the cornea, higher the scale reading and lower the IOP.

Standard Instrument (Figure 4A)
- ***Foot plate:*** Concavity of 15 mm radius of curvature, weight 11 gm
- ***Plunger:*** 3 mm diameter, weight 5.5 gm including the force of the lever resting on top of the plunger
- Additional weights are added to the plunger to increase it to 7.5, 10 or 15 gm
- The scale reading is zero when the plunger extends 0.05 mm beyond foot plate curve
- Each scale unit represents 0.05 mm protrusion of the plunger.

Basic Concept

The weight of tonometer on the eye **(Figure 4B)** increases the **actual IOP (Po)** to a higher level **(Pt)**. The change in pressure from Po to Pt is an expression of the resistance of the eye (scleral rigidity) to the displacement of fluid. Determination of Po from a scale reading Pt requires conversion which is done according to **Friedenwald conversion tables**.

Friedenwald generated an empirical formula for linear relationship between the log function of IOP and the ocular

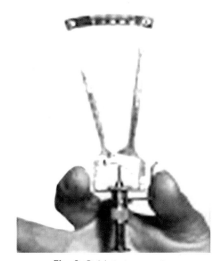

Fig. 2 Schiotz tonometer

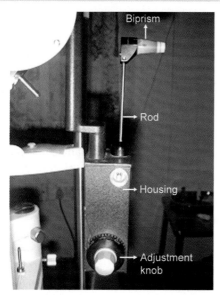

Fig. 3A Goldmann applanation tonometer

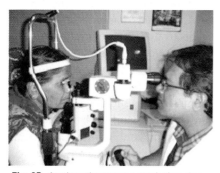

Fig. 3B Applanation tonometry being done

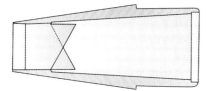

Fig. 3C Goldmann tonometer showing biprism inside

distension. This formula has 'C' a numerical constant, the coefficient of ocular rigidity which is an expression of dispensability of eye. Its average value is 0.025.

Technique

The patient should be in supine position, looking up at a fixation target while the examiner separates the lids and lowers the tonometer plate to rest on the anesthetized cornea so that plunger is free to move vertically (**Figure 4C**). A fine movement of needle on the scale

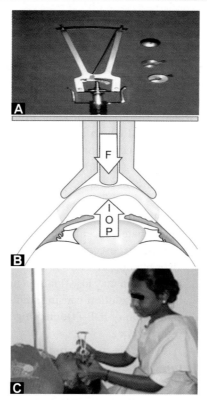

Figs 4A to C (A) Schiotz tonometer; (B) Principle of Schiotz tonometry; (C) Schiotz tonometry being performed

is seen in response to ocular pulsations. Scale reading is an average of the extremes of these excursions. The 5.5 gm weight is initially used. If scale reading is four or less, additional weight is added to plunger. Conversion table is used to derive IOP in mm Hg from scale reading and plunger weight. The instrument is **calibrated** before each use to check whether the scale reading is zero.

Sources of Error

- Accuracy is limited as ocular rigidity varies from eye to eye. As conversion tables are based on an average coefficient of ocular rigidity, an eye that varies significantly from this value give erroneous IOP.
  - ❖ *High-ocular rigidity* is seen in high hyperopia, extreme myopia, long standing glaucoma, ARMD and vasoconstrictor therapy. High rigidity gives a falsely high IOP.

- ❖ *Low-ocular rigidity* is seen in high myopia, increasing age, miotics, vasodilators, after RD surgery (vitrectomy, cryopexy, SB) and intravitreal injection of compressible gas. Low ocular rigidity gives a falsely low IOP reading.
- The variable expulsion of intraocular blood during Schiotz tonometry may influence IOP measurement.
- Repeated measurements lower the IOP.
- Either a steeper or thicker cornea cause greater displacement of fluid during tonometry giving a falsely high IOP measurement.

GOLDMANN APPLANATION TONOMETER

Type: Variable force applanation tonometer.

Basic Concept

Based on Imbert-Fick law: An external force (**W**) against a sphere equals the pressure in the sphere (**P**) times the area flattened (applanated) by external force (A)

$$W = P \times A$$

Cornea being aspherical, wet, slightly inflexible fails to follow the law. Moisture creates surface tension (**S**) or capillary attraction of tear film for tonometry head. Lack of flexibility requires force to bend the cornea (**B**) which is independent of internal pressure. As central thickness of cornea is $\cong 0.55$ mm, so outer area of corneal flattening differs from inner area of flattening (A1). It is this inner area which is of importance. Modified Imbert-Fick law

$$= W + S = PA1 + B$$

When A1 = 7.35 mm^2, S balances B and W = P. This internal area of applanation is achieved when the diameter of the external area of corneal applanation is around 3.06 mm. Using this diameter, the grams of force applied to flatten the cornea multiplied by ten is directly converted to mm Hg.

Instrument

The instrument is mounted on the end of a lever hinged on the slit-lamp **(Figures 3A to C)**. The examiner views through the center of a plastic biprism, which is used to applanate the cornea. Two beam splitting prisms within the applanating unit optically convert circular area of corneal contact in two semicircles **(Figures 5A to C)**. The edge of corneal contact is made apparent by instilling fluorescein while viewing in cobalt blue light. By manually rotating a dial calibrated in grams, the force is adjusted by changing the length of a spring within the device. The prisms are calibrated so that the inner margins of semicircles touch when 3.06 mm of the cornea is applanated. The biprism is attached by a rod to a housing which contains a coil spring and series of levers that are used to adjust the force of the biprism against the cornea.

Technique

Cornea is anesthetized and the tear film is stained with sodium fluorescein. The cornea and the biprism are illuminated by a cobalt blue light. Fluorescein facilitates visualization of tear meniscus at margin of contact. Fluorescent semicircles are viewed through the biprism.

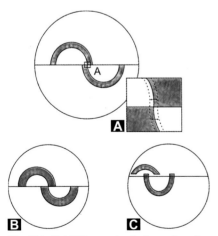

Figs 5A to C (A) The end-point in applanation tonometry; (B) Wide meniscus; (C) Incorrect end-point due to improper vertical alignment applanation tonometry

Force against the cornea is adjusted until the inner edges overlap. Ocular pulsations create excursions of semicircular tear meniscus and IOP is read as the median over which arc glides **(Figures 5A to C)**. This is the end point at which a reading can be taken from a graduated dial which indicates grams of force applied to tonometer and so this number is multiplied by 10 to obtain IOP in mm Hg.

Sources of Error

- Inadequate concentration of fluorescein in precorneal tear film gives hypofluorescence.
- Fluorescein may lose fluorescence in acidic solution causing underestimation of IOP—**Quenching of fluorescence**.
- Wider meniscus or improper vertical alignment gives higher IOP readings **(Figures 5A to C)**.
- Thin corneas underestimates and thick corneas overestimates the IOP.
- For every 3D increase in corneal curvature, IOP rises $\cong$ 1 mm Hg as more fluid is displaced under steeper corneas causing increase in ocular rigidity.
- > 3D astigmatism produces an elliptical area on applanation giving erroneous IOP.
- 4D of With the Rule (WTR)/Against the Rule (ATR) of astigmatism underestimates/overestimates the IOP. To minimize this, tonometer biprism should be rotated so that axis of least corneal curvature is opposite the red mark on the biprism. This results in a separation of 43 degrees and an applanation of an area of approximately 7.35 mm².
- The other method is to obtain measurements in both vertical and horizontal meridians and average these readings.
- Mires may be distorted on applanating irregular corneas.

Effect of Central Corneal Thickness (CCT)

Variations in corneal thickness change the resistance of the cornea to indentation so that this is no longer balanced entirely by the tear film surface tension thus affecting the accuracy of IOP measurement. A thinner cornea may require less force to applanate it, leading to underestimation of true IOP while a thicker cornea would need more force to applanate it, giving an artifactually higher IOP.

The Goldmann applanation tonometer (GAT) was designed to give accurate readings when the CCT was 520 μ. As shown by Ehlers et al., there can be under estimation or overestimation of IOP when the corneal thickness is lesser than 520 μ or greater respectively. He interpolated that deviation of CCT from 520 μ yields a change in applanation readings of 0.7 mm Hg per 10 μ. IOP measurements are also modified by both PRK and LASIK giving lower readings on applanation and thinning of central cornea is believed to be the cause.

Hand-Held Goldmann Type Tonometers
Perkin's

Type: Variable force applanation tonometer.

It uses same prisms as Goldmann but is counterbalanced so that tonometry is performed in any position **(Figures 6A and B)**. The prism is illuminated by battery powered bulbs. The force on the prisms is adjusted manually. Being portable, it is practical when measuring IOP in infants/children and for use in operating rooms.

Draeger

Type: Variable force applanation tonometer.

Similar to Perkin's but uses different set of prisms and operates with a motor adjusting the force on these prisms.

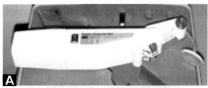

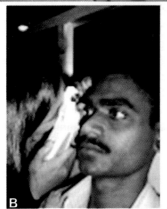

Figs 6A and B Perkin's tonometer

MACKAY MARG TONOMETER (MMT)

Type: Variable force applanation tonometer.

Basic Concept

Force required to keep the flat plate of a plunger flush with a surrounding sleeve against the pressure of corneal deformation.

It incorporates a 1.5 mm diameter plunger affixed to a rigid spring that extends 10 microns beyond the plane of surrounding rubber sleeve. Movement of the plunger is electronically monitored by a transducer and recorded on a moving paper strip. When the tonometer is placed against cornea, the tracing that represents the force applied to the plunger begins to rise.

At 1.5 mm of corneal area applanation, tracing reaches a peak and the force applied is equal to IOP + Force required to deform the cornea.

At 3 mm flattening, force required to deform cornea is transferred from plunger to surrounding sleeve, creating a dip in tracing corresponding to IOP.

More than 3 mm of area gives artificial elevation of IOP.

It is most accurate in eyes with scarred, edematous and irregular corneas.

Other Mackay Marg Type Tonometers

They have an internal logic program which automatically selects the acceptable measurement and three or more good IOP readings are averaged and displaced on screen, e.g. CAT 100 Applanation Tonometer, Biotronics Tonometer.

Tonopen

It is portable and battery operated **(Figures 7A and B)**. Principle is same as Mackay Marg Tonometer. The tip has a strain gauge that is activated when in contact with cornea. The built-in microprocessor logic circuit senses a trough force and records until an acceptable measurement is achieved. Four to ten such measurements are averaged to give a final IOP which is displayed.

The probe tip is applied perpendicularly to cornea until it is just indented. An audible click indicates that the measurement is acceptable. The process is repeated 2 to 10 times until a beep indicates a statically valid average reading.

Pneumotonometer

It is similar to MMT in that a core sensing mechanism measures IOP while force required to bend the cornea is transferred to surrounding structures. The sensor is air pressure unlike electronically controlled plunger in MMT. It can also be used for continuous IOP monitoring. It gives significantly higher IOP estimates.

MAKLAKOV APPLANATION TONOMETER

Type: Constant force applanation tonometer.

Basic Instrument

IOP is estimated by measuring the area of cornea flattened by a known weight. It has dumb-bell shaped metal cylinders with flat end plates of polished glass on either end with diameter of 10 mm. Identical instruments weighing 5, 7.5, 10, and 15 gm are used to measure the IOP. Cross-action wire handle to support instrument on the cornea is used. A thin layer of dye is spread onto the bottom of either end plate and the instrument is made in contact with anesthetized cornea in supine position for one second. A circular white imprint on the end plate corresponds to the area of corneal flattening. The area is measured and IOP is read from a conversion table in the column corresponding to the weight used.

NONCONTACT TONOMETER

It was introduced by Grolman. A puff of room air, creates a constant force that

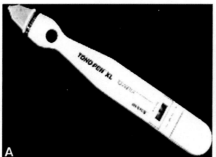
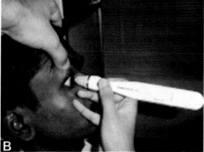

Figs 7A and B Tonopen

momentarily flattens the cornea. The time from an internal reference point to the moment of flattening is measured and converted to IOP.

The corneal apex is deformed by a jet of air. The force of air jet which is generated by a solenoid activated piston increases linearly over time. Original NCT has three subsystems.

1. **Alignment system:** Aligns patient's eye in three dimensions.
2. **Optoelectronic applanation monitoring system**
   ❖ Transmitter directs a collimated beam of light at corneal apex
   ❖ Receiver and detector accepts only parallel coaxial rays of light reflected from cornea
   ❖ Timer that measures from an internal reference to the point of peak light intensity
3. **Pneumatic system:** Generates a puff of room air directed against cornea.

When the reflected light is at peak intensity, the cornea is presumed to be flattened. The time elapsed is directly related to the force of jet necessary to flatten the cornea and correspondingly to IOP. NCT is accurate if IOP is nearly normal, accuracy decreases with increase in IOP and in eyes with abnormal cornea or poor fixation **(Figure 8)**.

New NCT, Pulsair is a portable hand held tonometer **(Figures 9A and B)**.

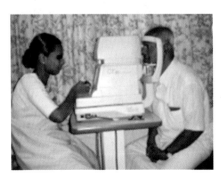

Fig. 8 Technique of noncontact tonometer

CONTINUOUS IOP MONITORING DEVICES

Devices under investigation include:
- Flush fitting silastic gel contact lens instrumented with strain gauges that measures changes in meridional angle of corneoscleral junction caused by variations in IOP.
- A similar device using a pressure transducer made in form of a cylindrical guard ring applanation tonometer.
- A scleral gauge embedded in an encircling scleral band to measure the distension of globe.

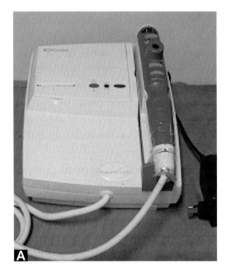

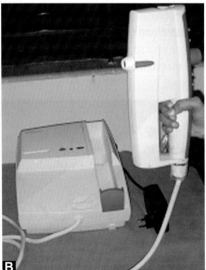

Figs 9A and B Portable noncontact tonometer

- An instrument using suction cups for B/L recording for IOP for up to one hour in supine subjects.

HOME TONOMETRY
- **Schiotz tonometry**
- **Self-tonometer**—applanation principle
- **Impact tonometer**—measures time of contact of a spring driven hammer with the eye.
- **Vibra tonometer**—measures the frequency of vibrating probe in contact with the cornea (Other methods of home tonometry are discussed further ahead in the chapter).

COMPARISON, CALIBRATION AND STERILIZATION OF DIFFERENT TONOMETERS
Comparison of Tonometers
Comparison of GAT in Eyes with Regular Cornea

In eyes with regular corneas, GAT is generally accepted as the standard against which other tonometers must be compared. Even with GAT, inherent variability must be taken in account.

Schiotz Tonometer

Studies indicate that Schiotz reads lower than GAT even when the postural influence on IOP is eliminated by performing both measurements in supine position. The magnitude of difference between the two tonometers and the influence of ocular rigidity are such that Schiotz indicates only that the IOP is within a certain range and is of limited value even for screening purposes.

Perkin's Applanation Tonometer

It compares favorably against GAT. In one study, difference between readings with the two instruments was 1.4 mm Hg. It is subject to the same influence of corneal thickness as the GAT. It is useful in infants and children and is accurate in horizontal as well as vertical position.

Draeger Applanation Tonometer

Comparative studies with GAT have given inconsistent results because of its more complex design. It is more difficult to use than the Perkin's and patient's acceptance tends to be worse.

Mackay Marg Tonometer

Highly significant correlation between IOP readings Mackay Marg Tonometer (MMT) and GAT with MMT values systematically higher and GAT systemically lower than their mean results.

Mackay Marg Type Tonometers

Tonopen has compared favorably against manometric readings in human autopsy eyes although it may cause a significant increase in IOP during measurements. It has good correlation with GAT readings within normal IOP ranges. But most studies indicate that it **under estimates GAT IOP in higher ranges and over estimates in the lower range.**

Pneumatic Tonometer

Correlates well with GAT readings. However, it gives significantly higher IOP estimates.

Noncontact Tonometer

Reliable within the normal IOP range, although reliability is reduced in higher IOP ranges and is limited by abnormal corneas or poor fixation. Corneal thickness has greater influence on NCT than on GAT. The hand held pulsair NCT has compared favorably with Goldmann readings in normal and glaucomatous eyes. It tends to read lower IOPs above the normal range.

Tonometry on Irregular Corneas

- Accuracy of GAT and Maklakov type AT and NCT is limited in eyes with irregular corneas.
- MMT considered to be the most accurate in scarred or edematous corneas. As MMT applanates a small surface area, the effects of corneal resistance to deformation and surface tension of tears are less than that with GAT.
- Pneumotonometer has also been shown to be useful in eyes with diseased corneas
- Tonopen compares favorably with MMT on irregular corneas.

Tonometry Over Soft Contact Lens

MMT, pneumotonometer and tonopen can measure the IOP through bandage contact lens (CL) with reasonable accuracy although soft CL of different powers created a bias with tonopen.

Applanation tonometers are affected by the power of CL with high water content and correction tables are developed to compensate this.

The power of soft CL influenced the difference in IOP between the paired readings by NCT.

Tonometry Over Gas Filled Eyes

- Intraocular gas significantly influences scleral rigidity rendering indentation tonometry unsatisfactory.
- Pneumotonometer underestimates GAT readings in gas filled eyes while Tonopen compared favorably with GAT readings.

CALIBRATION OF GAT

It is essential that GAT be calibrated periodically, at least monthly (Figures 10A and B). It is done in a stepwise manner.

Steps

1. ***Check at measuring drum setting 0***
   Check position –0.05: Turn the zero calibration on the measuring drum downwards by the width of one calibration marking, against the index marker. When the feeler arm is in the free movement zone, it should then move itself against the stop piece in the direction of the examiner.

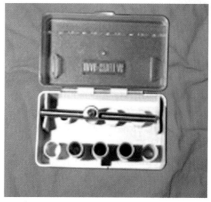

Fig. 10A Calibration rod for Goldmann applanation tonometer

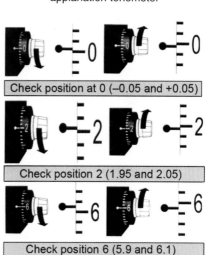

Check position at 0 (–0.05 and +0.05)

Check position 2 (1.95 and 2.05)

Check position 6 (5.9 and 6.1)

Fig. 10B Calibration of Goldmann applanation tonometer

Check position +0.05: Turn the zero calibration on the measuring drum upwards by the width of one calibration marking, against the index marker. When the feeler arm is in the free movement zone, it should then move itself against the stop piece in the direction of the patient.

2. ***Check position at drum setting 2:*** For, this the check weight or calibration rod provided with the instrument is used. Five circles are engraved on the weight bar. The middle one corresponds to drum position 0, the two immediately to the left and right to position 2 and the outer ones to position 6.

   One of the marks on the weight corresponding to drum

position 2 is set precisely on the index mark of the weight holder.

Holder and weight are then fitted over the axis of the tonometer so that the longer part of the weight points towards the examiner.

Check position 1.95: The feeler arm should move towards the examiner.

Check position 2.05: The feeler arm should move in the direction of the patient.

3. ***Check at measuring drum setting 6:*** Turn the weight bar to scale calibration 6, the longer part shows in the direction of the examiner.

Check position 5.9: The feeler arm should move towards the examiner.

Check position 6.1: The feeler arm should move in the direction of the patient.

STERILIZATION
Schiotz Tonometer

Dissemble between each use and the barrel is cleaned with two pipe cleaners, the first soaked in alcohol and the second dry. The footplate is cleaned with alcohol swab. All surfaces must be dried before reassembling.

GAT

Variety of techniques are described for disinfecting tonometer tips:

- Soaking applanation tip for 5 to 15 minutes in diluted sodium hypochlorite, 3% H_2O_2 or 70% isopropyl alcohol or by wiping with alcohol, H_2O_2, povidone iodine or 1: 1000 merthiolate
- Ten minutes of rinsing in running tap water
- Soap and water wash
- Disposable film covers for tips
- Exposure to UV light.

Tonopen

Tip is protected by disposable latex cover.

Pneumotonometer

Tip should be cleaned with an alcohol sponge, taking care to dry the surface before use. An alternative is the use of disposable latex cover over the tips.

BIBLIOGRAPHY

1. Armaly MF. On the distribution of applanation pressure. I. Statistical features and the effect of age, sex, and family history of glaucoma. Arch Ophthalmol 1965;73:11.
2. Bengtsson B. Comparison of Schiotz and Goldmann tonometry and tonography in a population. Acta Ophthalmol (Copenh) 1972;50:455.
3. Craven ER, et al. Applanation tonometer tip sterilization for adenovirus type 8. Ophthalmology 1887;94:1538.
4. Drance SM. The coefficient of scleral rigidity in normal and glaucomatous eyes. Arch Ophthalmol 1960;63:668.
5. Dunn JS, Brubaker RF. Perkins applanation tonometer, clinical and laboratory evaluation. Arch Ophthalmol 1973;89:149.
6. Durhan DG, Bigliano RP, Masino JA. Pneumatic applanation tonometer. Trans Am Acad Ophthalmol Otolaryngol 1965;69:1029.
7. Finlay RD. Experience with the Draeger applanation tonometer. Trans Ophthalmol Soc 1970;90:887.
8. Forbes M, Pico GJ, Goldmann B. A noncontact applanation tonometer description and clinical evaluation. Arch Ophthalmol 1974;91:134.
9. Friedenwald JS. Standardization of tonometers decennial report. Trans Am Acad Ophthalmol Otolaryngol 1954;58:1954.
10. Friedenwald JS. Contribution to the theory and practice of tonometry. Am J Ophthalmol 1937;20:985.
11. Friedman E, et al. Increased scleral rigidity and age related macular degeneration. Ophthalmology 1989;96:104.
12. Glouster J, Perkins ES. The validity of the Imbert-Fick law as applied to applanation tonometry. Exp Eye Res 1963;2:274.
13. Grolman B. Noncontact applanation tonometry. Optician 1973;166:4.
14. Hollows FC, Graham PA. Intraocular pressure, glaucoma, and glaucoma suspects in a defined population. Br J Ophthalmol 1966;50:570.
15. Imbert A. Theories ophthalmotonometers. Arch Ophthalmol 1885;5:358.
16. Kaufman HE, Wind CA, Waltman SR. Validity of Mackay-Marg electronic applanation tonometer in patients with scarred irregular corneas. Am J Ophthalmol 1970;69:1003.
17. Khan JA, et al. Comparison of Oculab Tonopen readings obtained from various corneal and scleral locations. Arch Ophthalmol 1991;109:1444.
18. Krieglstein GK, Waller WK. Goldmann applanation versus hand-applanation and Schiotz indentation tonometry. Graefes Arch Clin Exp Ophthalmol 1975;194:11.
19. Kronfeld PC. Tonometer calibration empirical validation: the committee on standardization of tonometers. Trans Am Acad Ophthalmol Otolaryngol 1957;61:123.
20. Langham ME, McCarthy E. A rapid pneumatic applanation tonometer: comparative findings and evaluation. Arch Ophthalmol 1968;79:389.
21. Macri FJ, Brubakar RF. Methodology of eye pressure measurement Biorheology 1969;6:37-45.
22. Markiewitz HH. The so-called Imbert Fick law (corresp). Arch Ophthalmol 1960;64:159.
23. McMillan F, Forster RK. Comparison of Mackay-Marg, Goldmann and Perkins tonometers in abnormal corneas. Arch Ophthalmol 1975;93:420.
24. Moses RA. Fluorescein in applanation tonometry. Am J Ophthalmol 1960;49:1149.
25. Moses RA. The Goldmann applanation tonometer. Am J Ophthalmol 1958;46:865.

26. Pepose JS, et al. Disinfection of Goldmann tonometers against human immunodeficiency virus type I. Arch Ophthalmol 1989;107:983.

27. Perkins ES. Hand-held applanation tonometer. Br J Ophthalmol 1965;49:591.

28. Petersen WC, Schlegel WA. Mackay-Marg tonometry by technicians. Am J Ophthalmol 1973;76:933.

29. Posner A. Practical problems in the use of the Maklakov tonometer. EENT J 1963;42:82.

30. Posner A. An evaluation of the Maklakov applanation tonometer. EENT J 1962;41:377.

31. Rootman DS, et al. Accuracy and precision of the Tonopen in measuring intraocular pressure after keratoplasty and epikeratophakia in scarred corneas. Arch Ophthalmol 1988;106:1697.

32. Schmidt T. The clinical application of the Goldmann applanation tonometer. Am J Ophthalmol 1960;49:967.

33. Schwartz NJ, Mackay RS, Sackman JL. A theoretical and experimental study of the mechanical behavior of the cornea with application to the measurement of intraocular pressure. Bull Math Biol 1966;28:285.

34. Schields MB. The noncontact tonometer: Its value and limitations. Surv Ophthalmol 1980;24:211.

35. Starrels ME. The measurement of intraocular pressure. Int Ophthalmol Clin 1979;19:9.

36. Stepanik J. Tonometry results using a corneal applanation 3.53 mm in diameter. Klin Monatsbl Augenheilkd 1984;184:40.

37. Ventura LM, Dix RD. Viability of herpes simplex type I on the applanation tonometer. Am J Ophthalmol 1887;103:48.

RECENT ADVANCEMENTS IN TONOMETRY—MERITS AND DEMERITS

INTRODUCTION

Increased IOP is considered the main risk factor for the onset of glaucoma. The precise technique to measure IOP is direct cannulation of the anterior chamber, with a needle connected to a manometer. Obviously, such a procedure may only be performed in animals for experimental investigation. The measurement of IOP by a noninvasive device (a tonometer) is defined as tonometry. This conventionally involves applying a force against the cornea that produces a distortion of the globe. A number of tonometers based on this principle have been introduced into clinical practice. There are two techniques, according to the shape of the corneal distortion-indentation tonometry or applanation tonometry.

The latter may be performed with a variable force or with a constant force. However, the central corneal thickness and other variables involved in measurement in applanation tonometry have been a problem identified for quite sometime now. Various new tonometers have come into the market claiming better accuracy, however, are prone for problems in actual clinical scenario.[1]

This chapter deals with the principles, merits and demerits of:

a. The recent modifications or improvements made by manufacturers in existing tonometers
b. The recent tonometers which came into the practice for various reasons including the experimental models.

TONOMETERS WITH RELEVANT MODIFICATIONS

Some of the tonometers widely used and the relevant modifications are as follows:

Noncontact Tonometry or Air-puff Tonometry

Measuring the time it takes from the initial generation of the puff of air to where the cornea is exactly flattened (in milliseconds) to the point where the timing device stops gives an indirect measurement of IOP. Noncontact tonometer have generally been considered a fast and simple way to screen for high IOP. The TOPCON CT-80, one of the popular devices, takes its original measurement method using two sensors; one for light and one for pressure. When the air puff applanates the cornea a light sensor detects the applanation moment, while at the same time another sensor monitors the internal chamber to obtain the intraocular pressure. Measurement range is 0 to 60 mm Hg. Keeler pulsair tonometer is the portable version of noncontact tonometer to become popular in recent times. The pulsair tonometer emits air at half of the pressure exerted by previous air-impulse tonometers. The pulsair instrument enables the operator to obtain measurements with the patient in the standing, seated or supine positions. The operator achieves correct alignment by focusing on the image of two mires of red light projected onto the cornea. The instrument then evaluates the pressure needed to produce a corneal depression measuring 3.00 mm in diameter; this is then converted to a pressure value that can immediately be read from a digital display. According to the manufacturers, the pulsair is equipped with a device that is activated by pressing the "subflex" button, which enables the operator to perform tonometry even in cases in which the cornea presents abnormalities of form or transparency. In a study of 160 patients with IOP ranging from 10 to 44 mm Hg by GAT,

the mean difference between them was noted to be –0.48 mm Hg and the 95 percent CI of the limits of agreement was noted to be 1.75 to –2.72 mm Hg. However, the noncontact technique is bound to show larger variations with central corneal thickness and IOP variations, making it difficult to interchange the results with GAT.[2]

Tonopen
Tono-Pen XL

It is a portable electronic, digital pen-like instrument that determines IOP by making contact with the cornea, after use of topical anesthetic eyedrops. This is especially useful for very young children, patients unable to reach a slit-lamp due to disability, patients who are uncooperative during applanation tonometry, or patients with corneal disease where contact tonometer cannot be accurately performed. It is based on Mackay Marg principle. It is contained within a large tubular hand piece that has a small footplate at the end. Within the footplate is a protruding plunger connected to a sensitive electrical position transducer. As it is pushed against the cornea, both corneal rigidity and IOP resist indentation and plunger is forced back into the footplate. When cornea is flattened by footplate, corneal rigidity is largely negated and equilibrium exists between plunger's force and IOP. IOP is determined when tip of plunger is in same plane as footplate. It overestimates low IOP and underestimates high IOP in most studies.

The Reichert Tono-Pen AVIA

The Reichert Tono-Pen AVIA tonometer has a lightweight, ergonomic design and advanced electronic measurement technology that enables operators to take fast and accurate IOP measurements. This utilizes micro-strain gauge technology and a 1.0 mm transducer tip. The device displays the average of 10 independent readings along with a statistical confidence indicator. Its measurement range is 5 to 55 mm Hg.

Electronic Schiotz Tonometer

The electronic Schiotz tonometer has a continuous recording of IOP that is used for tonography. The scale is also magnified which makes it easier to detect small changes in IOP. This was mainly of interest in experiments where coefficient of rigidity was calculated, however, of academic interest in the present era.

Pneumotonometer

A pneumotonometer utilizes a pneumatic sensor (consisting of a piston floating on an air bearing). It is touched to the anesthetized cornea. A precisely regulated flow of filtered air (from an internal air pump) enters the piston. A small (5 mm diameter) fenestrated membrane at the end of the piston reacts to both the force of the air blowing through it and to the force represented by the pressure behind the cornea, against which it is being pressed. The balance between these two forces represents the precise intraocular pressure. In a study of 479 subjects, the mean difference between GAT and pneumotonometer was found to be 0.5 mm Hg and the 95 percent CI of the limits of agreement was 7 to –5.5 mm Hg and was affected by CCT.[3]

Perkin's Tonometer

It is a special type of portable applanation tonometer, which allows measurement of IOP in children, patients unable to cooperate for slit-lamp exam, and in anesthetized patients who may be in a supine position.

Self-tonometry
Ocuton S

The interest for self-tonometry has increased lately. The function of Ocuton S is based on Goldmann's principle of applanation. The instrument was introduced in 1999 and is equipped with a multifunctional microprocessor capable of calculating IOP instantaneously. After instillation of a drop of local anesthetic the Ocuton S tonometer is positioned at a fixed distance of 10 mm from the corneal apex of the eye to be measured. Once aligned with the center of the cornea with the aid of an internal luminous viewfinder, the measurement prism emerges automatically from the instrument until contact with the corneal surface for two seconds. The IOP is automatically estimated after the contact.

Recent Advancements in Tonometers
PASCAL Dynamic Contour Tonometer

It is a relatively new device introduced in 2002 that uses principle of contour matching to measure IOP instead of applanation to eliminate the systematic errors inherent in previous tonometers **(Figure 11)**. These factors include the influence of corneal thickness, rigidity, curvature and elastic properties. It is supposedly not influenced by mechanical changes, such as those seen in refractive surgery that would, otherwise, cause error in applanation tonometers. PASCAL uses a miniature pressure sensor embedded within a tonometer tip contour-matched to the shape of the cornea. The tonometer tip rests on the cornea with a constant appositional force of one gram. This is an important difference from all forms of applanation tonometry in which the probe force is variable. When the sensor is subjected to a change in pressure, the electrical

resistance is altered and the PASCAL's computer calculates a change in pressure in concordance with the change in resistance. The contour matched tip has a concave surface of radius 10.5 mm, which approximates the cornea's shape when the pressures on both sides of it are equal. This is the key to the PASCAL's ability to neutralize the effect of intraindividual variation in corneal properties. Once a portion of the central cornea has taken up the shape of the tip, the integrated piezoresistive pressure sensor begins to acquire data, measuring IOP 100 times per second. A complete measurement cycle requires about eight seconds of contact time. During the measurement cycle, audio feedback is generated, which helps the clinician to ensure proper contact with the cornea. The tip requires a disposable cap with a membrane housing.[1] Ku et al., in their study of 116 patients, demonstrated that DCT measures 2 ± 2.1 mm Hg higher than GAT and the 95 percent limits of agreement range from –6.2 to 2.3 mm Hg. The variability increased with higher corneal thickness. Even though DCT cannot be used in place of GAT, they suggested it showed least variability with CCT and so it may be used in extremes of corneal thickness.[4]

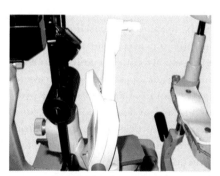

Fig. 11 The PASCAL dynamic contour tonometer—the concave tip houses the miniature pressure sensor

Merits

Unlike applanation tonometers, which are influenced by corneal thickness and other characteristics of the cornea and hence may produce misleading estimates of IOP, a contour tonometer provides IOP which is relatively independent of interindividual variations in corneal properties. IOP measurement may work correctly even on post-LASIK eyes. PASCAL detects and accurately measures the dynamic pulsatile fluctuations in IOP and thus permits a more detailed assessment of the pressure range to which the eye is subjected due to pulsatile ocular blood flow. No fluorescein staining is required for the measurement. It prints all the values shown on the LCD display and the actual IOP curve.

Demerits

The equipment and the disposable tip is more expensive than GAT and measures slower than GAT. There is a fair amount of training required for the measurement technique.[1]

Transpalpebral (Diaton) Tonometer

Diaton transpalpebral tonometry was introduced in 2006 and is a unique approach for measuring intraocular pressure through the eyelid. It is a pen-like, hand-held, portable device using a free falling thin rod on the stretched upper eyelid. The measuring principle of the tonometer is based on processing the rod acceleration time resulting from its free fall and interaction with the elastic surface of the eye to be measured. The device has a position sensor to determine the rod position in the process of its free fall from the constant height and the interaction with eye through the eyelid. The head is kept horizontally while lying down and the patient has to keep the eyeball at 45° to horizontal, while the rod is placed closer to the upper lid cilia so that it can freely fall on the sclera below through

the lid near the limbus. The digital display shows the IOP value calculated from the rod acceleration-deceleration time through the in-built processor of the device. In a group of 200 normal, glaucoma and ocular surface disorders subjects, the mean difference between GAT and Diaton tonometry was –1.8 mm Hg and the 95 percent CI of limits of agreement was 7.6 to –11.2 mm Hg suggesting wide variations and a systematic bias **(Figure 12)**.

Merits

Transpalpebral tonometry requires no contact with the cornea, therefore, sterilization of the device and anesthetic drops are not required and there is very little risk of infection. Transpalpebral tonometry is used in those for whom Goldmann tonometry is not indicated, such as in children, those with corneal pathology, or those who have had corneal surgery. Diaton tonometer is suggested for a wide range of applications: at the patient's bedside, in geriatrics homes, in children hospitals, for the military and for home use.

Demerits

This tonometer is prone for measurement errors due to large systematic bias especially if wrong technique is used. The contraindications of the tonometer's

usage are as follows: Upper lid pathology (inflammatory diseases, scars, eyelid deformation), Scleral exposure and/or conjunctiva pathology in the measuring area. Errors in measurements can be due to incorrect patient position, incorrect instrument position or incorrect eyelid positions.

Ocular Response Analyzer

Reichert's ocular response analyzer measures corneal hysteresis. Corneal hysteresis is determined through inducing the cornea to move (effect) following an air pulse (cause). First, a short 20 ms air impulse causes the cornea to move inward, through applanation and into a slight concavity.

Then, only milliseconds after the induced applanation, the air pump shuts off and the cornea moves through a second applanation while returning from concavity back to its baseline convexity. An electro-optical collimation detector, designed to monitor the corneal curvature of the central cornea throughout the movement, establishes two applanation event times. The difference in pressure values at the "inward" and "outward" applanation event times is defined as corneal hysteresis and their average provides a corrected IOP measurement for more accurate IOP monitoring. Corneal hysteresis is

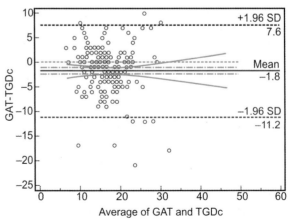

Fig. 12 Bland Altman test for agreement between two methods—shows wide limits of agreement between GAT and Diaton tonometry

a measure of viscous damping during the inward and outward applanation events and hence turns out to be an important indicator of the biomechanical properties of the cornea. A lower corneal hysteresis value, but not CCT, was recently found to be associated with progressive visual field loss in patients with primary open angle glaucoma. In addition, lower than average hysteresis values have been observed in patients with normal tension glaucoma (NTG). In a study of 165 subjects, the mean difference between normalized ORA IOP and GAT was 0.1 mm Hg and the 95 percent limits of agreement was –6.6 to 6.8 mm Hg.[5]

Merits
The ability of the ORA to measure these properties enables the calculation of an IOP measurement called IOPcc (Corneal Compensated IOP). This is an IOP measurement that is supposedly less influenced by corneal properties such as resistance or thickness. Since IOPcc compensates for corneal influence, it facilitates post-LASIK pressure measurements that are not artificially lower than pre-LASIK values.

Demerits
The IOP value is a calculated value and not the true IOP; is prone for errors similar to the noncontact tonometers.

Icare or Rebound Tonometer
The Icare or rebound tonometer (RBT) **(Figure 13)** was introduced in 1997 and consists of a pair of coils coaxial with the probe shaft, a solenoid coil and a sensing coil. A lightweight probe is propelled towards the cornea by the solenoid and the sensing coil monitors the movement. The probe consists of a steel wire shaft with a round plastic tip of 1.7 mm diameter. The speed immediately before impact, the deceleration during impact and the ratio of these parameters, are correlated to the

IOP. The method does not need any anesthetics. The main advantage of the RBT is that the IOP measurements can be taken without the need for topical anesthesia even in pediatric population. Also, the RBT has disposable tips. This could be an advantage in situations involving a high-risk of cross-barrier infection. In addition, although it was suggested for home monitoring, one must take into account that there is a high degree of variability in individual patients. In a study of 23 glaucoma patients, mean difference between GAT and rebound tonometer readings was 1.9 mm Hg and 95 percent limits of agreement was 7.9 to –4.2 mm Hg **(Figure 14)**.

Merits
It is portable and has disposable tips to be used in specific situations of high-risk of infection. It can be used in children without anesthetic agents.

Demerits
The accuracy of the instrument was questioned in some studies and it tends to overestimate IOP compared to GAT.

Smartlens
The hand-held dynamic observing tonometer, SmartLens® was introduced in 1999. It has a contact lens that incorporates an electronic pressure sensor, which is able to measure IOP and ocular pulse amplitude continuously by applanation of the central cornea. It weighs approximately 25 gm. In the center of the contact lens surface there is a Mylar-membrane covered bore hole that provides a 2.5 diameter applanation zone. The cavity behind the membrane is filled with silicon oil and is connected with a piezo-electric pressure transducer that is offset in the housing of the lens. The measure of IOP is achieved by the transmission of pressure through the oil to the transducer when the applanation membrane is

displaced during its contact with the cornea. Pressure recordings at the lens are sampled at a frequency of 100 Hz and are transmitted telemetrically to a base unit where the data is stored. This lens formed the precursor for the PASCAL dynamic contour tonometer later. This instrument is used mainly in experimental studies.

Proview®—pressure Phosphene Tonometer
The pressure phosphene tonometer (PPT) is made available as a patient self-monitoring device for IOP **(Figure 15)**. The PPT was introduced by Fresco, utilizes a psychophysical technique based on entopic phenomenon of pressure phosphenes. It is a spring compression device consisting of a spring loaded plunger encased within a plastic sleeve and marked with a graded scale. Pressure applied to plunger moves an indicator across the scale. The threshold pressure for creating a phosphene spot may provide an indication of IOP. The action of the PPT is based on a calibrated spring attached to a flat circular probe, with a diameter equal to the Goldmann type applanation tonometer. The scale on the PPT is divided into 2 mm Hg units and runs from 10 to 40. The PPT indicator remains at the position

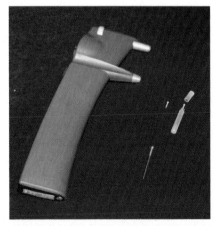

Fig. 13 Icare or rebound tonometer (the lightweight probe is propelled on cornea upon activation of the instrument)

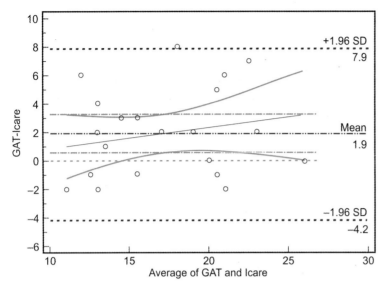

Fig. 14 Bland Altman test for agreement between two methods—shows wide limits of agreement between GAT and rebound tonometry

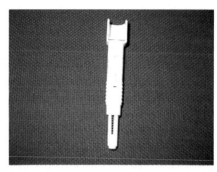

Fig. 15 Proview® (Pressure Phosphene tonometer) shows the spring compression console and the mobile tip

Applanation Resonance Tonometer

The development of the new applanation resonance tonometer probe was based on continuous and simultaneous sampling of both contact area and contact force. The area-measuring device consisted of a piezoelectric element made of Lead Zirconate Titanate (PZT) with a pick-up part. A feedback circuit processed the signal from the pick-up and powered the PZT element in order to sustain the oscillations at resonance frequency. A convex contact piece was glued onto one end of the PZT element. The resonance frequency depends on the geometry, the material properties of the PZT element and contact piece, the suspension of the element and the frequency characteristics of the feedback circuit. Thus, a force transducer was attached to the PZT element and they were mounted into a sensor module.

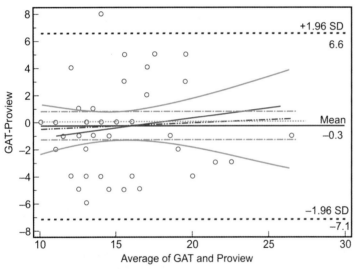

Fig. 16 Bland Altman test for agreement between two methods—shows wide limits of agreement between GAT and pressure phosphene tonometer

of the highest value measured. In a study consisting of 45 subjects including normals and glaucoma patients, Bland Altman test showed a mean difference of –0.3 mm Hg between GAT and PPT and 95 percent confidence interval of limits of agreement was +6.6 to –7.1 mm Hg (**Figure 16**).[6] However, other studies give wide scatter of difference even up to 12 to 16 mm Hg between GAT and PPT.[7]

Merits

This appeals as a simple, inexpensive home monitoring device in very well trained subjects.

Demerits

The merit is overshadowed by its inconsistency and the variable results in many studies. Many individuals may not appreciate the phosphene.

When the sensor is brought in contact with the cornea, the acoustic impedance of the cornea will mechanically load the sensor and a new oscillating system is formed with a new resonance frequency. Since the degree of load on the resonance system depends on the contact area, the resonance frequency of the system is related to the contact area between the sensor and the cornea. Resonance sensor technology gives multipoint method for measuring IOP. It reduces errors in the clinical measurement of IOP, especially after corneal surgery. However, it is position dependent and measures are being taken to rectify this issue. This tonometer is still in the experimental stage only.[8]

IMPLANTABLE IOP SENSORS (UNDER DEVELOPMENT)

There are several implantable sensors that are being developed for use in and out of the eye for continuous recording of IOP. Most of these devices aim to use wireless technology to receive data from the instruments, which will be received by a telemetric device. The sensors will be used in contact lens, implanted in the choroidal space or encapsulated and attached to IOL, etc.

IOP-IOL Probe

a. A sensor for continuous monitoring of IOP, incorporated in the haptics of an IOL was proposed. The sensor consists of a capacitative spiral circuit, needing no energy, correlating its resonance frequency to the actual IOP. An external device located in a spectacle frame remotely and non-invasively detects this resonance frequency and calculates the IOP.

b. A completely encapsulated intra-ocular pressure (IOP) sensor equipped with telemetric signal and energy transfer integrated into a silicone disc for implantation into the eye is also proposed.[9]

Contact Lens Sensor

The method chosen for measuring the evolution of the IOP in the sensing contact lens is indirect and correlates the spherical deformation of the eyeball with the changes in IOP. It has been proven by previous studies that a change of IOP of 1 mm Hg causes the radius of curvature of the central cornea of the human eye to change by approximately 3 μm over a typical radius of 7.8 mm. To measure this change, a soft contact lens was designed in which microfabricated strain gauges were inserted in a Weatstone bridge configuration. This allows high-precision measurements to be made and compensates for thermal drift. The sensor is made from two active strain gauges, which are placed circumferentially and two passive strain gauges for thermal compensation, which are placed radially. The sensor is stimulated by a DC current and gives an output voltage that is proportional to the strain and consequently to the IOP variation. A telemetry microchip when added inside the

contact lens, as well as an antenna, the whole console becomes wireless.[10]

Choroid-IOP Sensor

Small changes in IOP can be measured by a sensor in contact with the surface of the choroids. The sensors have been tested in two modes:

Fixed: Using the sensor in contact with choroid at 0 to 2 mm depth of scleral surface.

Sutured: Sensor sutured to the surface of sclera with the probe touching the choroidal surface.[11]

CONCLUSION

All the above devices may have varying roles in the patient's management and some of these devices may be proven redundant in due course. The clinician should carefully evaluate these characteristics before getting any of these instruments to utilize in their day-today practice. As of now, the GAT remains the gold standard and seems to remain with our practice for a long-time.

The dynamic contour tonometry may be useful in specific circumstances such as in postrefractive surgery and extremes of corneal thickness along with GAT. The implantable sensors may gain popularity once proven by clinical studies and may unravel the pathophysiology of glaucoma in a better manner in future.

REFERENCES

1. Herndon LW. Measuring intraocular pressure—adjustments for corneal thickness and new technologies. Curr Opin Ophthalmol 2006;17:115-9.

2. Parker VA, Herrtage J, Sarkies NJ. Clinical comparison of the Keeler Pulsair 3000 with Goldmann applanation tonometry. Br J Ophthalmol 2001; 85(11):1303-4.

3. Gunvant P, Baskaran M, Vijaya L, Joseph IS, Watkins RJ, Nallapothula M, Broadway DC, O'Leary DJ. Effect of corneal parameters on measurements

using the pulsatile ocular blood flow tonograph and Goldmann applanation tonometer. Br J Ophthalmol 2004; 88(4):518-22.

4. Ku JF, Danesh Meyer HV, Craig JP, et al. Comparison of intraocular pressure measured by Pascal dynamic contour tonometry and Goldmann applanation tonometry. Eye 2006;20:191-8.

5. Kotecha A, Elsheikh A, Roberts CR, Zhu H, Garway-Heath DF. Corneal thickness and age-related biomechanical properties of the cornea

measured with the ocular response analyzer. Invest Ophthalmol Vis Sci 2006;47(12):5337-47.

6. Baskaran M, Ramani KK, Ramesh SVe, et al. Comparison of Proview Phosphene Tonometer with the Goldmann Applanation Tonometer in Myopic and Nonmyopic Eyes. Asian J Ophthalmol 2006;8:57-61.

7. Chew GS, Sanderson GF, Molteno AC. The pressure phosphene tonometer - a clinical evaluation. Eye 2005;19(6): 683-5.

8. Eklund A, Hallberg P, Lindén C, Lindahl OA. An applanation resonator sensor for measuring intraocular pressure using combined continuous force and area measurement. Invest Ophthalmol Vis Sci 2003; 44(7):3017-24.

9. Walter P, Schnakenberg U, vom Bögel G, Ruokonen P, Krüger C, Dinslage S, Lüdtke Handjery HC, Richter H, Mokwa W, Diestelhorst M, Krieglstein GK. Development of a completely encapsulated intraocular pressure sensor. Ophthalmic Res 2000;32(6): 278-84.

10. Leonardi M, Leuenberger P, Bertrand D, Bertsch A, Renaud P. First steps toward noninvasive intraocular pressure monitoring with a sensing contact lens. Invest Ophthalmol Vis Sci 2004;45(9):3113-7.

11. Rizq RN, Choi WH, Eilers D, Wright MM, Ziaie B. Intraocular pressure measurement at the choroid surface: a feasibility study with implications for implantable microsystems. Br J Ophthalmol 2001; 85(7):868-71.

Gonioscopy

Gus Gazzard, Arun Rajan, Paul Foster, Keith Barton

DEFINITION

Gonioscopy is the biomicroscopic examination of the anterior chamber angle of the eye. It enables the glaucomas to be classified into two main groups, angle-closure glaucoma and open-angle glaucoma. Gonioscopy is helpful diagnostically, prognostically, and therapeutically in glaucoma.[1-4]

HISTORY OF GONIOSCOPY[5]

In 1907, Trantas visualized the angle in an eye with keratoglobus by indenting the limbus. He later coined the term gonioscopy, meaning *observation of the angle*. Salzmann, realizing that the angle was not visible due to total internal reflection, introduced the goniolens in 1914. Koeppe improved it 5 years later by designing a steeper lens and using it in combination with the Zeiss slit-lamp. Otto Barkan established the use of gonioscopy in the management of glaucoma. He used a slit-lamp suspended from a celling, a hand held illuminator and a Koeppe lens to view the angle and classified glaucoma into "deep chamber" and "shallow chamber". He also performed goniotomy using these lenses. Troncoso also contributed to gonioscopy by

developing a self-illuminating monocular gonioscope for magnification and illumination of the angle. In 1938, Goldmann introduced indirect gonioscopy using the Goldmann mirrored contact lens. The Allen lens which had a totally refractive prism instead of mirror was developed and later modified in to the Allen Thorpe gonioprism. Gradle and Sugar (1940) were the first to grade the angle and Schie subsequently (1957) developed system of grading based on visible angle structure. The popular Shaffer technique was developed in 1960 and further modified by Spaeth in 1971.

OPTICAL PRINCIPLES

Normally, the angle of the anterior chamber cannot be viewed during slit lamp examination as the light rays emanating from the angle strike the cornea at an angle steeper than the critical angle (46°) and are refracted back into the eye due to total internal refection **(Figure 1)**. The solution to this problem is to eliminate the cornea (optically). This can be done by using gonioscopy lenses which are designed to overcome the total internal refection and exceed the critical angle by altering

the cornea-air-fluid interface. These include:

Direct Goniolenses

In direct gonioscopy, the anterior curve of the contact lens (goniolens) is such that the critical angle is not reached, and the light rays are refracted at the contact lens-air interface **(Figure 2)**.

The Koeppe lens is the prototype diagnostic goniolens and is available in different diameters and radii of posterior curvature. A gonioscope, or hand biomicroscope, provides 15Å to 20Å magnification. It may be handheld or suspended from the ceiling with a counterbalance or on an elastic belt.[6] The light source is usually a separate handheld unit, such as the Barkan focal illuminator, although it may be attached to the gonioscope.

Direct gonioscopy is performed with the patient in a supine position, preferably on a movable diagnostic table or chair. After applying a topical anesthetic, the goniolens is positioned on the cornea, using a bridge of balanced salt solution, a viscous preparation such as methylcellulose, or the patient's own tears. The examiner usually holds the gonioscope in

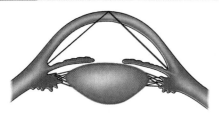

Fig. 1 Light coming from the angle of anterior chamber undergoes total internal reflection at the tear-air interface. Thus the angle can not be visualized directly

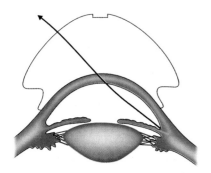

Fig. 2 Direct gonioscopy: Performed with a step concave lens which permits light from the angle to exit the eye closer to the perpendicular at lens air interface

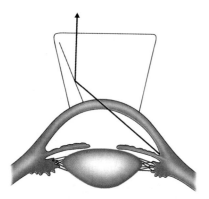

Fig. 3 Uses mirrors or prisms to overcome the problem of total internal reflection

one hand and a light source in the other. Occasionally, an assistant may be needed to move the goniolens to the desired position. Alternatively, a gonioscope with mounted light source may be used, which allows the examiner to control the goniolens with the other hand. In either case, the examiner scans the anterior chamber angle by shifting his or her position until all 360 degrees have been studied.

Indirect Goniolens

In indirect gonioscopy, the light rays are reflected by a mirror in the goniolens and leave the lens at nearly a right angle to the contact lens-air interface (**Figure 3**). These are more popular because they can be used to understandard examination circumstances, with the patient sitting at the slit-lamp. They can further be of two types (**Table 1**):

1. Those whose surface is slightly larger than the cornea and that require a gonioscopic coupling gel (e.g. Goldmann lens); (**Figures 4A and B**).
2. Those whose surface is smaller than the cornea and that use the patient's tear film as a coupling agent (e.g. Zeiss or Sussman four-mirror lens) (**Figures 4C to E**).

The Goldmann single-mirror lens is the prototype. The mirror in this lens has a height of 12 mm and a tilt of 62 degrees from the plano front surface. The central well has a diameter of 12 mm and a posterior radius of curvature of 7.38 mm.

A Goldmann three-mirror lens has two mirrors for examination of the fundus and one for the anterior chamber angle, which is tilted at 59 degrees. The posterior radius of curvature of both standard Goldmann diagnostic gonioprisms is such that a viscous material must be used to fill the space between cornea and lens. However, a modified Goldmann-type lens has been developed with an 8.4 mm radius of curvature, which eliminates the need for a viscous bridge.[7] Goldmann-type lenses have also been modified

with antireflection coating for use with laser trabeculoplasty.

In the Zeiss four-mirror lens all four mirrors are tilted at 64 degrees for evaluation of the angle, thereby eliminating the need to rotate the lens. The original four-mirror lens is mounted on a holding fork (Unger holder), while newer models have a permanently attached holding rod (Posner lens) or are held directly (Sussman lens). An adjustable slit-lamp mount has also been developed for the Zeiss four-mirror gonioprism. The posterior curvature of each of these four-mirror lenses is similar to that of the cornea, which allows the patient's own tears to be used as the fluid bridge.

The mirrored arrangement of both of these types of lenses causes the observed image of the angle to be reversed but not crossed. In other words, that which is seen in the mirror is 180 degrees away, but its detail is not altered with respect to right and left. The other important adjustment the novice gonioscopist need master is to apply the absolute minimum amount of pressure of the contact lens on the cornea, especially while maneuvering the slit-lamp beam and the lens to maximize visualization.

CLEANING OF DIAGNOSTIC CONTACT LENSES

Any instrument that contacts the eye creates the potential hazard of transmitting bacterial and viral infection. Human immunodeficiency virus and other infectious agents have been isolated in the epithelium of the eye

Table 1 Indirect gonioscopic lenses

Goldmann single mirror	Mirror inclined at 62°
Goldmann three mirror	Mirror for gonioscopy is at 59°
Zeiss four mirror	Mirrors inclined at 64°, requires a holder (Unger)
Posner four mirror	Modified Zeiss with attached handle
Sussmann four mirror	Finger (Hand) held Zeiss type
Thorpe four mirror	4 mirrors inclined at 62° requires fluid bridge
Ritch trabeculoplasty lens	2 mirrors at 59° and 2 at 62° with convex lens over two.

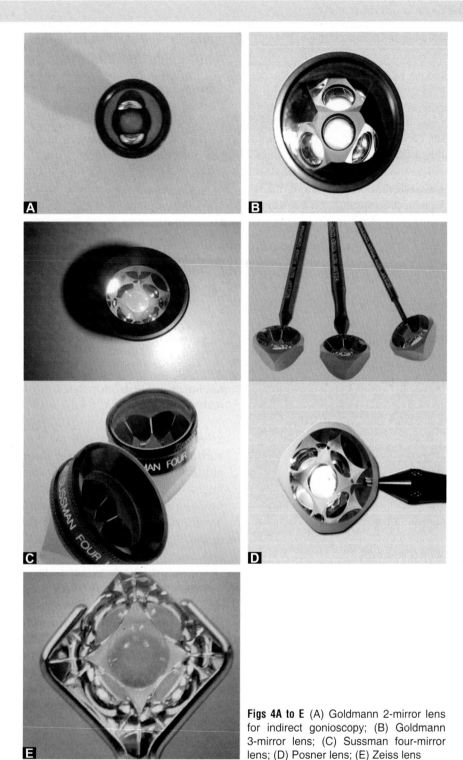

Figs 4A to E (A) Goldmann 2-mirror lens for indirect gonioscopy; (B) Goldmann 3-mirror lens; (C) Sussman four-mirror lens; (D) Posner lens; (E) Zeiss lens

phenol. Unfortunately, many gonioscopic lenses are quite fragile and may be damaged by some of the recommended techniques for disinfection.

In 1988 the American Academy of Ophthalmology, the National Society to Prevent Blindness, and the Contact Lens Association of Ophthalmologists jointly issued guidelines for disinfection. They suggested inverting the contact lens and wiping the surface with an alcohol sponge. For added protection the lens can be inverted and the concave contact area filled with a solution of 1:10 household bleach, which is left for 5 minutes and then rinsed off with water (American Academy of Ophthalmology, 1989). Some manufacturers recommend soaking lenses in 2 percent glutaraldehyde or dilute (1:10) household bleach (Ocular Instruments, Bellevue, Washington) **(Table 2)**. Most lenses can be gas-sterilized and some glass lenses can be autoclaved. With all lenses the manufacturer's instructions for disinfection should be followed to prevent damage to the lens.

TECHNIQUE OF GONIOSCOPIC EXAMINATION

Clinical Application of Gonioscopy

Gonioscopy is a fundamental clinical test that should be performed on all patients with glaucoma, suspected glaucoma and a family history of glaucoma, whereas some assessment of the width of the angle should be routinely performed on all patients on presentation to any eye-care practitioner **(Table 3)**. Gonioscopy is part of a comprehensive eye examination. The examination should specifically aim to identify anatomical characteristics and pathological phenomena that are associated with an increased risk of glaucoma, for example, iridotrabecular contact (angle-closure), pigment deposition (pigment dispersion and exfoliation syndromes, trauma, angle-closure,

and in tears. Although transmission of human immunodeficiency virus has not been documented in ophthalmic examinations, it is important to disinfect lenses after each use. The human immunodeficiency virus is sensitive to heat and to a variety of commonly used disinfectants such as alcohol, glutaraldehyde, sodium hypochlorite, (household bleach), formalin and

Table 2 Guidelines by American Academy of Ophthalmology

- Invert the contact lens
- Wipe the lens with alcohol sponge
- Fill concave area with 1:10 solution of household bleach
- Leave for 5 minutes
- Rinse with water
- Some manufactures also recommend 2% glutaraldehyde
- Most lenses can be gas sterilized and some glass lenses can be autoclaved

Table 3 Uses of gonioscopy*

Diagnostic	Therapeutic
Visualization of anterior chamber angle	Argon laser trabeculoplasty
In eyes with narrow peripheral anterior chamber depth	Laser goniopuncture after NPGS
In eyes with clinical/historical evidence of angle closure	Reopening of trabecular ostium
For classification of glaucoma	
Family history of glaucoma	
Glaucoma suspects	
To note the presence and extent of neovascularization	
To asses angle recession	
Evidence of inflammation	
Extent of tumors	
Degenerative or developmental anomaly	
Planning management	

* Gonioscopy is a part of a comprehensive eye examination

uveitis), neovascularization, angle recession, and other pathologies such as iris and ciliary body tumors, or foreign bodies.

> **Note** It is important to emphasize the *dynamic* nature of angle anatomy, and particularly that lighting, posture, autonomic function and systemic medication can all affect angle configuration. For accurate assessment of the risk of angle-closure, all examinations must be carried out in the dark as even small amounts of extraneous illumination can influence angle width.

It is important to remember that an eye's gonioscopic status is not static and determined in perpetuity by a single baseline examination. Long-term dynamic factors such as lens changes, medication effects, aging, and disease processes make periodic gonioscopy an important feature of appropriate glaucoma management.

Why Gonioscopy?

Gonioscopy is an essential component of ocular examination because primary open angle glaucoma is ultimately a diagnosis of exclusion: one must demonstrate that angle closure is not occurring in order to make the diagnosis.

Iridotrabecular contact, or sign of previous contact, is the defining characteristic of primary angle closure. Similarly, the diagnosis of secondary glaucomas associated with pigment dispersion, pseudoexfoliation and uveitis can be supported by gonioscopic signs. Gonioscopy is also an important prelude to treatment—not only of angle closure (with peripheral iridotomy or iridoplasty) but also laser trabeculoplasty for open angle glaucomas.

Examination Prior to Gonioscopy
Central anterior chamber depth estimation

Before examining the anterior chamber angle itself, it is useful to consider other aspects of the patient. It helps to know about the age of first reading spectacle use, current refraction, or a history of amblyopia.

It is important to assess the anterior chamber depth, and in particular to compare the eyes. A shallow central anterior chamber is associated with angle closure and more pupil block, whereas marked asymmetry can be a sign of posterior segment mechanisms of angle-closure.

Limbal chamber depth estimation—a modified van Herick

The limbal chamber depth (LCD) is assessed at a slit-lamp with the illumination column offset from the axis of the microscope by 60 degrees. The brightest, narrowest possible vertical beam of light is directed at the temporal limbus, with the beam of light perpendicular to the ocular surface, and viewed from the nasal aspect.

The beam is positioned at the most peripheral point that gives a clear view of both anterior chamber and peripheral iris and then viewed at maximum magnification. The limbal chamber depth may be graded according to classic grading schemes, e.g. 1 to 4 **(Table 4)** but more recently has been graded as a percentage of the adjacent corneal thickness, and recorded as a percent such as 0, 50 or 100 percent. It gives an idea of the likelihood of angle-closure on gonioscopy as well as an impression of the iris profile. Concave iris profiles will be seen to sweep posteriorly in the periphery, down to the lens equatorial sulcus, before rising anteriorly across the anterior surface

Table 4 Van Herick estimate of angle width from anterior chamber depth at the periphery

Grade 4	Anterior chamber depth = Corneal thickness
Grade 3	Anterior chamber depth = 1/4 to 1/2 corneal thickness
Grade 2	Anterior chamber depth = 1/4 corneal thickness
Grade 1	Anterior chamber depth = Less than 1/4 corneal thickness
Slit angle	Anterior chamber depth = Slit-like (extremely shallow)
Closed angle	Absent peripheral anterior chamber

Table 5 SEAGIG (South-East Asia Glaucoma Interest Group) guidelines for gonioscopy

- Use a magnification of 10-25x
- Use a fairly short and narrow beam (2-3 mm)
- Use a dark room
- Pupillary constriction makes a narrow angle appear more open. The slit beam should not cross the pupillary margin

of lens and zonules. Conversely, steep iris profiles will in some cases be seen to rise almost in parallel to the corneal endothelium. It is very uncommon to be able to identify a plateau configuration using this technique.

The limbal chamber depth is also helpful in identifying cases where gonioscopy artefact has altered the *in vivo* anatomy of the angle. If limbal chamber assessment identifies peripheral iridocorneal contact, but an open angle is seen on gonioscopy, it strongly suggests that gonioscopy is causing artifactual opening of the angle. Using more categories (from 0 to >100%) has been shown to give better screening performance for angle-closure than the traditional "van Herick" method in high-risk populations. Standard photos

are available in the report on this technique have been published.[2]

Which Lens to Use?

The best choice of gonioscope is the subject of much debate. Lenses that are steeper than the corneal curvature (Goldmann-style) require coupling fluid while those that are less curved do not. Many ophthalmologists feel the 4-mirror lenses have the advantage of rapidity in identifying normal, open angles, avoid the need for contact media, and allow more effective compression examination.

In contrast the Goldmann-style lenses offer a more stable, clearer view. A very popular lens is for the ocular instruments Magnaview (a magnifying Goldmann-style lens). Carbomer 90 or Hydroxypropyl-methylcellulose 0.5 percent are suitable coupling agents.

Dynamic examinations are to some extent possible with the Goldmann type lenses. The possibility of artefact occurring from the use of one or the other is again a matter of debate. The examiner should use the lens that (s)he is comfortable with, and gives the best view in the circumstances. Glaucoma specialists should certainly have access to both.

Direct view lenses, such as the Koeppe lens, are generally only used in the operating theater but are able to give a wide field direct view of the angle.

The Procedures
Adequate anesthesia, patient positioning and explanation

Before even touching the patient it is important to obtain full topical anesthesia: that sufficient for applanation tonometry is often inadequate for successful pain-free gonioscopy. It is vital to have the patient, slit-lamp and doctor carefully positioned for what might be a lengthy, detailed assessment: a rest for the ophthalmologist's elbow will prove invaluable. It is also important to give the patient a clear explanation of what to expect—they may well never have had any ocular examination before and can feel very threatened by a gonioscope in a darkened room!

Illumination

It is absolutely essential to have the lowest possible background room illumination for error-free angle examination: the lights must be off, the blinds closed, curtains drawn and even the Snellen chart dimmed. Just a small amount of light-induced pupillary miosis can pull a closed angle open—many a case of angle closure has been missed because the room lights were on **Table 5**.

For the same reasons, the slit-lamp beam that is used should be the dimmest that permits landmark structures to be seen. With a standard

Comparison between Goldmann and Zeiss gonioscopic lenses

Type of lens	Goldmann single	Goldmann three	Goldmann-Zeiss 4-mirror
Diameter of corneal contact	12 mm	12 mm	9 mm
Overall diameter	15 mm	18 mm	9 mm
Size of rim	1.5 mm	3 mm	none
Mirror angulation (degrees)	62 d	59 d	64 d
Mirror height	17 mm	12 mm	12 mm
Distance from central cornea	3 mm	7 mm	5 mm
Radius of curvature	7.4 mm	7.4 mm	7.85 mm
Coupling fluid	Required	Required	Not required
Dynamic gonioscopy	Manipulation	Manipulation	Indentation

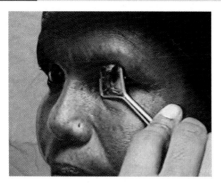

Fig. 5 Gonioscopy being performed with a Zeiss 4-mirror lens

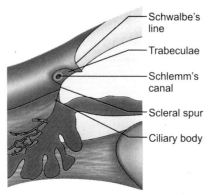

Schwalbe's line

Trabeculae

Schlemm's canal

Scleral spur

Ciliary body

Fig. 6 Gonioscopic anatomy of the angle of the anterior chamber

Haag-Streit it is usual to perform the initial examination with the filter in and a thin 1 mm beam. The beam should not cross the pupillary margin. It may be necessary to brighten the beam temporarily in order to identify reliably the corneal wedge, but then dim it again to look for iridotrabecular contact.

Lens Insertion

The larger Goldmann style lenses, such as the high magnification Magnaview, can be awkward to insert in some patients. Inserting a goniolens is made easier by asking the patient to look upwards. Then gently insert the lens with its leading upper edge holding the upper lid margin to prevent any reflex blink—being very careful not to place any pressure on the cornea. The patient should then look directly ahead, or at

the examiner's contralateral ear with the other eye.

In very sensitive patients with a lot of reflex blepharospasm it may be necessary to stop, check there is adequate anesthesia, and repeat the process with fresh coupling fluid, if used **(Figure 5)**.

GONIOSCOPIC ANATOMY

The anterior chamber angle is the recess between the iris on one side and the corneal endothelium, Schwalbe's line, trabecular meshwork, scleral spur and ciliary body face on the other.

The root of the iris usually inserts into the ciliary body face but the exact level is variable. The iris itself is highly mobile and can vary in profile a great deal with the degree of pupil block or position of more posterior structures such as ciliary processes or lens. Starting at the root of the iris and progressing anteriorly toward the cornea, the following structures can be identified by gonioscopy in a normal angle in an adult **(Figure 6)**.

Ciliary Body Band

This structure is the portion of ciliary body that is visible in the anterior chamber as a result of the iris insertion into the ciliary body. The width of the band depends on the level of iris insertion, and tends to be wider in myopia and narrower in hyperopia. The color of the band is usually gray or dark brown.

Scleral Spur

This is the posterior lip of the scleral sulcus, which is attached to the ciliary body posteriorly and the corneoscleral meshwork anteriorly. It is usually seen as a prominent white line between the ciliary body band and functional trabecular meshwork, unless it is obscured by dense uveal meshwork or excessive pigment dispersion. Variable numbers of fine, pigmented strands may frequently be seen crossing

the scleral spur from the iris root to the functional meshwork. These are referred to as iris processes, and represent thickenings of the posterior uveal meshwork.

Functional Trabecular Meshwork

This is seen as a pigmented band just anterior to the scleral spur. Although the trabecular meshwork actually extends from the iris root to Schwalbe's line, it may be considered in two portions:

a. The anterior part, between Schwalbe's line and the anterior edge of Schlemm's canal, which is involved to a lesser degree in aqueous outflow.

b. The posterior (or functional) part, which is the remainder of the meshwork and is the primary site of aqueous outflow (especially that portion immediately adjacent to Schlemm's canal).

The posterior, more functional part of the trabecular meshwork is usually pigmented, though variably so. In poorly pigmented eyes it can be hard to distinguish the TM on color alone and it is essential to be able to identify the corneoscleral junction.

The appearance of the functional meshwork varies considerably depending on the amount and distribution of pigment deposition. It has no pigment at birth, but color develops with age from faint tan to dark brown, depending on the degree of pigment dispersion in the anterior chamber. The distribution of pigment may be homogeneous for 360 degrees in some eyes and irregular in others. In the functional portion of the meshwork, especially when lightly pigmented, blood reflux in Schlemm's canal may sometimes be seen as a red band.

Schwalbe's Line

This is the junction between the anterior chamber angle structures and the cornea. It is a glistening white line just anterior to the meshwork which represents the posterior most termination of Descemet's membrane. There is also a transition from the scleral curvature to the steeper corneal curvature at this line which can cause settling of pigment in this area, especially inferiorly.

Normal Blood Vessels

Blood vessels are normally not seen in the angle, although loops from the major arterial circle may appear in front of the ciliary body band and less commonly over the scleral spur and trabecular meshwork. These vessels typically take a circumferential route in the angle.

In addition, an anterior ciliary artery may occasionally be seen as a more radially oriented vessel in the ciliary body band of lightly pigmented eyes. Circumferential and radial vessels may also occasionally be seen in the peripheral iris of lightly colored eyes. Radial vessels are more common in the peripheral iris, whereas the circumferential type are more common on the ciliary body.

Iris processes are fine physiological extensions of peripheral iris to the trabecular meshwork that are highly variable from individual to individual. The important distinction is between normal iris processes and peripheral anterior synechiae (PAS). PAS are usually broader and cause an irregularity in the contour of the surface of the iris.

GONIOSCOPIC LANDMARKS
The Corneal Wedge

The most important step in gonioscopy to identify is the corneal wedge (**Figure 7**). To find this the illumination beam must be slanted off axis to be able to view simultaneously the corneal epithelial and endothelial reflections. For superior and inferior angles the illumination column should be horizontally offset from the axis of

the microscope and the beam vertical. For the nasal and temporal angles the beam should be horizontal and offset vertically, by tilting the illumination column.

The corneal wedge is that point at which the two lines converge. Its apex marks the termination of Descemet's membrane—the site of Schwalbe's line. This is formed by the junction of the beam on the endothelium/trabecular meshwork surface and the beam falling across the corneoscleral junction. The trabecular meshwork starts immediately posterior to this structure. Its location helps confidently identify the where meshwork starts even in densely pigmented angles, or those with extensive iris processes. With experience, it can be seen that the corneal wedge may be acute or obtuse in its approach. Once this is realized, it can be seen in almost all cases without difficulty—provided the angle is open.

If the apex of the corneal wedge is not visible then iris is obscuring the trabecular meshwork. If neither epithelial nor endothelial line is visible then there may be obscuring corneal pannus or scarring. The next step is to identify whether there is iridotrabecular contact and assess the angular width between the peripheral iris and the trabecular meshwork/peripheral cornea.

Level of Iris Contact—Looking 'Over the Hill'

In some eyes a convex iris profile can obscure a narrow gap between iris and trabecular meshwork when viewed in the primary position. That is the angle will appear closed when it is not.

There is always debate regarding how much an eye can be moved from the primary position in the assessment of an angle. A very gentle rotation of the lens may be all that is needed to 'look over the hill' and confirm that there is no iridotrabecular contact (**Figure 8**). However, if too great an 'off axis' view

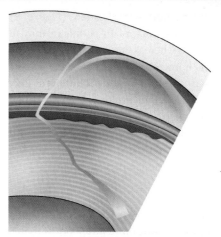

Fig. 7 The corneal wedge

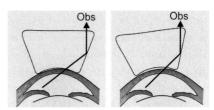

Fig. 8 Principle of *Over the Hill* view

is attempted in order to 'look over the hill' then accidental indentation may occur with the edge of the lens and an artefactually wider angle be seen. (This is what is done deliberately when indenting with a Goldmann-style lens). It is difficult to ask the patient to make small changes in direction of gaze to facilitate this. Movement of the lens is the best approach.

Estimate Width, Iris Profile and Structures Seen

Assessment of angular width is done by mentally constructing tangents to the trabecular meshwork and the peripheral iris and then estimating the geometric angle between these two lines. It may be helpful to envisage a 90 degree angle cut in half and remember that forms 45 degrees. The average—or range if it varies a lot—for each quadrant is usually recorded. It is usually possible to assign values of 0 (closed), 10, 20, 30 and 40 degrees (or greater in an aphakic eye for example).

Spaeths' classification **(Figure 9)** uses the average of the peripheral third of the iris whereas Foster suggests using the iris immediately adjacent to the trabecular meshwork and Schwalbe's line. The overall iris profile is then described (as steep, regular, flat, concave or in a plateau configuration) and a record made of the deepest angular structure visible without indentation.

Indentation

The first gentle examination in the primary position is intended to determine the level of iris contact with the eye-wall and the angular width of the anterior chamber angle. In the absence of iridotrabecular contact, the level of iris insertion is determined. If iridotrabecular contact is present then it is important to determine whether this is purely "appositional", i.e. it can be easily reversed, or synechial, i.e. a permanent adhesion. Indentation (or 'manipulative') gonioscopy achieves this by applying pressure to the central cornea, and so increasing the anterior chamber pressure and forcing aqueous fluid into the angle. This pushes the iris posteriorly and away from the meshwork in those areas in which it can separate—thus revealing the true point of iris insertion or the level to which abnormal adhesions have formed **(Figures 10A and B)**. Additional signs of abnormal iris curvature over posterior structures (the 'double-hump' or 'volcano' signs) also rely on indentation to be revealed.

Indentation is best performed with 4-mirror lenses which have a smaller contact area. Traditionally, it was considered impossible to perform indentation gonioscopy with Goldmann-style goniolenses. However, it may be possible to indent and open many closed angles with a Goldmann-style lens using three specific maneuvers:

1. Increase the illumination to a bright, wide beam falling onto the pupil.

2. The patient refixates and looks towards the mirror of the gonioscope.

3. The rim of the gonioscope over the mirror is rotated towards the patient to indent the central cornea.

> **Note** In cases where all angle structures still cannot be visualized clearly, a four-mirror lens should be used with gentle forward pressure, to produce greater direct central pressure. However, too great a pressure will distort the cornea and cause folds that obscure the view and the lower magnification can make subtle signs harder to see.

Standardize the Examination Routine

As with any clinical examination it helps to develop a routine, as you are less likely to omit something. For example, examine the superior and inferior then nasal and temporal angles in turn and of course, begin with identifying the corneal wedge, assess angle width and then and only then indent.

You must then remember the common mistakes and avoid them!

Recording and Classification— Grading Schemes

There remains much confusion about different grading schemes. The choice is between one of the three "s" schemes and Foster's recent modifications thereof.

They are often confused:

- *Scheie:* Describes the structures seen[5] **(Table 6)**
- *Shaffer:* Estimates geometric angle between iris and cornea[6] **(Table 7, Figure 11)**
- *Spaeth:* Describes features identified by Scheie and Shaffer schemes, as well as the iris profile and level of true and apparent iris insertion[7] **(Table 8, Figure 9)**
- *Foster's modified Spaeth:* Spaeths' classification uses the average of the peripheral third of the iris whereas Foster suggests using the iris immediately adjacent to the trabecular meshwork and Schwalbe's line. This is because the most peripheral iris may be almost in contact but then very quickly diverge from the endothelium—the average value can therefore be misleading. To the original three grades of iris profile (steep, regular and concave), a fourth grade of plateau was added.

The detail required varies with the clinical setting. The most detailed information is needed for careful longitudinal follow-up of borderline angle-closure cases. PAS are increasingly more common in eyes with a narrower geometric angle width. Angular width thus, seems the most appropriate angle measure. A full assessment will include the angular width, the structures seen, the level of iris insertion, the iris profile,

Table 6 Scheie system of grading

Grade 0	CBB seen	No angle closure
Grade I	CBB narrow	No angle closure
Grade II	CBB not seen, SS seen	Rarely closure possible
Grade III	PTM not seen	Closure likely
Grade IV	Schwalbe's line not seen	Gonioscopically closed

Table 7 Shaffer and modified Shaffer grading of angle width

	Grade 0	Grade I	Grade II	Grade III	Grade IV
Shaffer	Closed	10°	20°	30°	40°
Modified Shaffer	Schwalbe's line not visible	Schwalbe's line visible	Anterior TM visible	Scleral spur visible	Ciliary band visible

Table 8 Spaeth system of grading of angle

Peripheral iris configuration

- b = 'bows 1 to 4 plus' (usually indicative of optically-appearing closure, altering with indentation)
- p = 'plateau' (comparable to older 's' designation)
- f = 'flat approach': the commonest iris appearance (comparable to the older 'r' designation)
- c = 'concave' as in posteriorly bowed iris (comparable to the older 'q' designation)

Angular width of angle recess

- 10°, 20°, 30°, 40°

Level of iris insertion

- A (anterior to schwalbe's line)
- B (just behind schwalbe's line)
- C (at the scleral spur)
- D (deep angle CBB seen)
- E (extremely deep angle)

Iris processes

- U along angle recess
- V up to trabecular meshwork
- W up to Schwalbe's line

Pigmentation of posterior trabecular meshwork

- 0 — no visible pigmentation
- 1+ — just perceptible pigmentation
- 2+ — definite but mild
- 3+ — moderately dense
- 4+ — dense black pigmentation

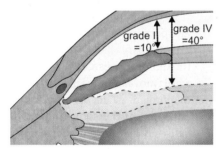

Fig. 9 Spaeth system of grading

the presence, height and distribution of peripheral anterior synechiae and the types and pattern of pigment seen.

FOSTERS' QUESTIONS FOR GONIOSCOPY

There are four cardinal questions that need to be answered in angle-closure gonioscopy, and the answers described as clearly as possible:

1. Does the iris touch the trabecular meshwork?

2. If there is no touch, is there evidence that it has been in contact previously?

3. If there is touch, is the contact reversible?

4. If the touch is not reversible, what is the extent of synechial contact (height, pattern and circumference)?

Pigment

Patterns of pigment deposition can vary a great deal but also give useful clues to pathology. A wide range of mild-to-moderate intratrabecular pigment can be normal while localized geographical blotches of moderate/dense "milk chocolate" pigment on the TM of eyes with brown irises is often a sign that intermittent angle-closure is occurring.

A dusting of "dark chocolate" granular pigment on the TM/iris/cornea/

zonular insertions is frequently seen with pigment dispersion and pseudo-exfoliation syndromes.

It is homegeneous in pigment dispersion and patchy in pseudoexfoliation syndrome.

Common Pitfalls and Misdiagnoses in Gonioscopy of Angle-Closure

There are a number of common mistakes made in gonioscopy that can mislead the unwary. Careful identification of the corneal wedge and a high magnification view of the signs can help the observer avoid most pitfalls.

Open or Closed?

One common error is to mistake a fully closed angle for one that is open with a featureless, pale trabecular meshwork. In this situation the corneal wedge would of course not be visible and an abnormally high point of iris contact should be detected.

Pigment: Normal or Abnormal?

Another is to misinterpret pigment smudging due to intermittent iridotrabecular contact—and therefore pathological—as normal trabecular pigmentation. Different races may show different degrees of pigment deposits in the angle, but pathological 'smudging' is identified by it's paler color (more similar to the anterior iris surface) and irregular geographical or blotchy appearance. Pigment in the superior, nasal or temporal angles is of greater significance than that in the inferior angle in which gravity may play a part.

Peripheral Anterior Synechiae

- A further subtle sign of angle-closure that is easy to miss are low peripheral anterior synechiae (PAS) that do not extend to the trabecular meshwork. These may only be detectable as localized variations in the apparent insertion of the iris on indentation of a

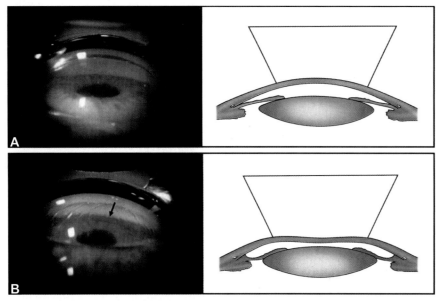

Figs 10A and B (A) Indentation gonioscopy. No angle structures are seen in Figure A; (B) On indentation, all the angle structures can be visualized (Arrow). Note the corneal folds on indentation

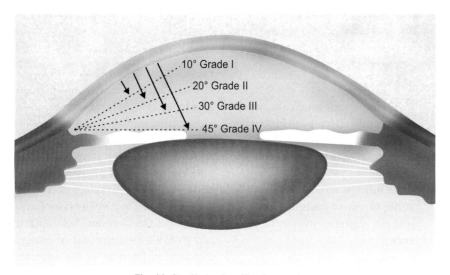

Fig. 11 Shaffer's classification system

Table 9 Gonioscopic difference between iris processes and peripheral anterior synechiae (PAS)

Features	Iris processes	PAS
Shape	Fine, lacy	Broad, Irregular
Extension	Up to inferior portion of TM	Up to Schwalbe's line
Special feature	Follow concavity of recess	Bridge underlying structures
During indentation gonioscopy	Do not inhibit movement of iris	Drag iris vessels with them
Interference with	Absent	Present

narrow angle. They may be distinguished from physiological iris insertion variation by their greater variability in height and more localized nature. These subtle signs are revealed by careful comparison of the angles of each eye—which can also reveal subtle degrees of angle recession that might in isolation be passed off as normal.

- Peripheral anterior synechiae (PAS) or iris processes (**Table 9**) (**Figures 12 and 13**).

Mechanism of Angle-Closure

- Once angle-closure has been detected and described it is important to diagnose the mechanism and assess the contribution of pupil block and nonpupil block mechanisms. Pupillary block alone will lead to a convex iris curvature or 'bombe'. Pronounced iris bombe can obscure other mechanisms such as "crowded" angles, a prominent last iris roll and various plateau iris configurations.

- It also is important to differentiate pupillary block and anterior nonpupillary block mechanisms (including plateau iris) from forward movement of the iris-lens diaphragm—such as occurs in aqueous misdirection and other causes posterior to the lens equator. These cases are often unilateral and there will be a pronounced asymmetry of the central anterior chamber depths.

  Difference between Neovascularization of angle (NVA) and normal iris vessels is discussed in **Table 10**.

OTHER USES OF GONIOSCOPY

The examination discussed, so far has been focussed on the detection and assessment of angle-closure. Obviously there is a wide range of other angle

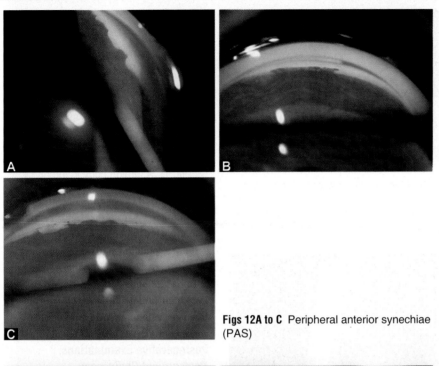

Figs 12A to C Peripheral anterior synechiae (PAS)

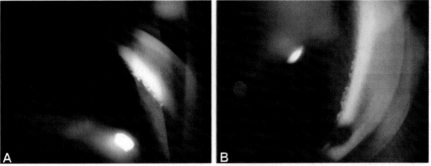

Figs 13A and B Gonioscopic view of prominent iris processes

Table 10 Angle blood vessels

Normal vessels	Neovascularization
• Radially oriented (peripheral iris)	• Fine
• Circumferentially oriented (ciliary body)	• Branching
• Thick	• Usually cross the scleral spur
• Nonbranching	
• Do not cross the scleral spur	

pathology that is of importance to the glaucoma specialist such as pigment dispersion, uveitic synechiae and pigment damage, silicone oil droplets and neovascularization. Experience, a good atlas of gonioscopic pathology and careful gonioscopy should identify these.

A few examples of nonangle closure pathology that illustrate the range of signs seen.

• Pigment dispersion causes uniform pigment throughout the angle that may be dense, obscuring the trabecular meshwork, or more subtle **(Figures 14A and B)**.

• In pseudoexfoliation syndrome there may be pigment shedding and patchy deposits together with deposits of pseudoexfoliative material **(Figures 15A and B)**.

• Silicone oil glaucomas often have multiple emulsified oil droplets throughout the superior angle (not to be confused with heavy liquid deposits in the inferior angle).

• Iris neovascularization has to be distinguished from simply dilated iris vessels and variants of normal angle vasculature. The abnormal vessels are fine, branching vessels that cross the angle rather than running along the length of it, which are associated with peripheral synechiae.

• In angle recession, there is an irregular widening of the ciliary body band. In severe cases, this may only be detectable with careful comparison of both eyes **(Figures 16A and B)**.

• Peripheral anterior synechiae from iridocorneal endothelial syndrome can be dramatic.

• Lastly cyclodialysis clefts in hypotonous eyes can be notoriously difficult to identify. The low IOP leads to easy compression and distortion of the cornea with loss of clarity and small clefts are often obscured by iridotrabecular contact of even frank peripheral anterior synechiae. It is sometimes necessary to inject viscoelastic into the anterior chamber to give sufficient chamber stability for a successful examination.

Easily overlooked causes of secondary glaucoma can be revealed by careful inspection at the time of gonioscopy: finding a foreign body in an angle **(Figure 17)**; seeing holes in the peripheral iris caused by the passage of an intraocular foreign body; observing a traumatic angle recession; appreciating precipitates on the trabecular surface; or recognizing blood in Schlemm's canal,

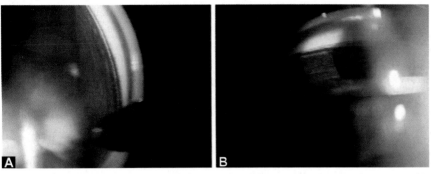

Figs 14A and B (A) Gonioscopic view of the angle of the anterior chamber in an eye with pigmentary glaucoma. Note the dense, homogeneous (grade 4) pigmentation of the trabecular meshwork; (B) Gonioscopic view in pigmentary glaucoma. Note the concave iris configuration

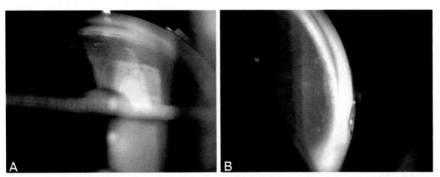

Figs 15A and B The dandruff like exfoliation material can be seen in the angle in eyes with exfoliation. The trabecular meshwork shows patchy pigmentation with pigment deposition anterior to the Schwalbe's line, especially in the inferior angle (Sampaolesi's line)

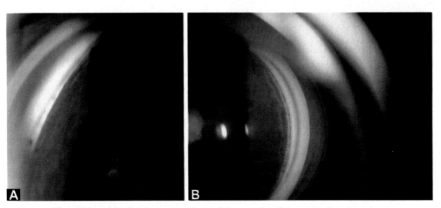

Figs 16A and B Gonioscopic view of the angle of the anterior chamber showing angle recession

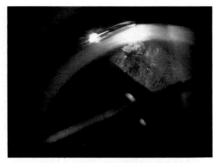

Fig. 17 A foreign body in the angle along with PAS

should be re-evaluated after therapy has begun. Occasionally, miotics narrow the angle further as a result of forward lens shift and enhanced pupillary block. Therefore, in narrow-angled eyes, any change in therapy should be monitored by periodic and frequent gonioscopy.

Postoperative Examinations
Postsurgical Gonioscopy
While it is possible to gonioscope an eye soon after cataract surgery it is rarely necessary in the immediate postoperative period due to the risk of inadvertent compression, reopening of the wound and possibility of infection. A sutured wound will of course be much safer than an unsutured section but both have risks if compressed.

If it is essential to perform gonioscopy then very gentle placement of a 4-mirror lens, which requires less manipulation to insert and minimal rotation, can be safely used: for example, in post-trabeculectomy patients in whom the patency of a sclerostomy must be assessed **(Figures 18A and B)**.

The success of iridotomy in opening an angle and can be evaluated promptly by gonioscopy. After filtering procedures, the surgical ostium can be seen gonioscopically. If filtration is impaired, the appreciation of a patent ostium will direct attempts to restore the bleb by addressing the episcleral surface—suture lysis, bleb needling, or resections of scar tissue beneath the

suggestive of increased venous pressure or inflammation. If no obstruction at the trabecular meshwork can be seen, the block to outflow must be beyond the trabecular surface—and by default the diagnosis is open-angle disease.

Use of mydriatics might cause the angle to close completely in eyes with narrow angles, precipitating an acute rise of IOP. If miotics become necessary for the management of glaucoma in an eye with a narrow angle, the angle

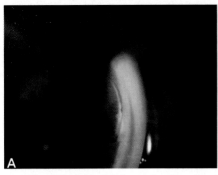 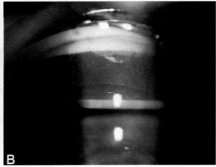

Figs 18A and B Gonioscopic view showing the haptic of the PCIOL in the angle

conjunctiva. If the ostium is occluded by the iris or adhesions, it may be reopened using laser.

Conditions Other Than Glaucoma

The diagnosis of peripheral tumors or cysts often can be made by gonioscopy. Their extent can be determined by an accurate view of the extent to which the iris and ciliary body are involved, supplemented by anterior segment imaging with UBM. Foreign bodies in the angle and holes in the peripheral iris from penetrating foreign bodies may be discovered. Inflammatory and traumatic conditions, such as keratic precipitates covering the meshwork and iridodialysis, can be visually evaluated. When a portion of the cornea is hazy, it may be possible by gonioscopy to look through a clear portion of cornea to see the reason for the haze. Tears in Descemet's membrane, epithelial downgrowth, and areas of

vitreous adhesions can be diagnosed in this way.

CYCLOSCOPY

This technique allows direct visualization of ciliary processes under special circumstances, such as the presence of an iridectomy, wide iris retraction, aniridia, and some cases of aphakia. Although special contact prisms with scleral indentors have been developed for cycloscopy, the procedure is still limited by the small percentage of eyes in which circumstances are favorable for good visualization of the ciliary processes. The main value of the technique thus, far has been in research studies of the ciliary processes, and in conjunction with laser therapy to the ciliary processes (transpupillary cyclophotocoagulation).

Imaging—UBM/OCT

Gonioscopy is limited by poor interobserver reproducibility and the need to

use visible light. Objective, quantifiable and reproducible measures of the angle can now be achieved by ultrasound biomicroscopy (UBM) and anterior-segment OCT. These can be performed in true dark-room conditions and the resulting cross-sectional angle images are very amenable to automated analysis and quantitative comparisons.

UBM and AS-OCT complement rather than replace gonioscopy however, which remains essential to assess PAS, angle pigmentation, vessels and other subtle angle characteristic.

CONCLUSION

The diagnostic basis of any glaucoma should be in correlation to the gonioscopic findings whenever, possible. The management and prognosis of the disease depends on a complete diagnosis that includes a routine gonioscopic evaluation. Gonioscopy widens our scientific understanding of the disease process and guides us to manage the disease more effectively.

The approach to gonioscopy that we have outlined here describes a clear, rational and evidence-based technique to elicit the signs of angle pathology. There is no substitute for carefully gathered experience and thoughtful reflection upon every patient examined—only with practice do we become proficient and only with practice do we improve.

REFERENCES

1. van Herick W, Shaffer RN, Schwartz A. Estimation of the width of the angle of anterior chambers: incidence and significance of the narrow angle. Am J Ophthalmol 1969;68: 626-9.
2. Foster PJ, Devereux JG, Alsbirk PH, Lee PS, Uranchimeg D, Machin D, et al. Detection of gonioscopically occludable angles and primary angle-closure glaucoma by estimation of limbal chamber depth in Asians: modified grading scheme. Br J Ophthalmol 2000;84: 186-92.
3. Alsbirk PH. Optical pachymetry of the anterior chamber. A methodological study of errors of measurement using Haag-Streit 900 instruments. Acta Ophthalmol 1974;52:747-58.
4. Foster PJ, Alsbirk PH, Baasanhu J, Munkhbayar D, Uranchimeg D, Johnson GJ. Anterior chamber depth in Mongolians. Variation with age, sex and method of measurement. Am J Ophthalmol 1997;124:53-60.
5. Scheie HG. Width and pigmentation of the angle of the anterior chamber. A system of grading by gonioscopy. Arch Ophthalmol 1957;58:510-2.
6. Becker B, Shaffer RN. Diagnosis and therapy of the glaucomas. St Louis: CV Mosby 1965l.pp.42-53.
7. Spaeth GL. The normal development of the human anterior chamber angle: a new system of descriptive grading. Transactions of the Ophthalmological Societies of the United Kingdom 1971; 91:709-39.

14 | Central Corneal Thickness and Its Relevance in Glaucoma Diagnosis and Management

Manish Shah

CHAPTER OUTLINE

❖ Estimation of True IOP from Goldmann Applanation Tonometer Readings

❖ Is CCT an Independent Risk Factor to Predict Glaucoma Progression?

Discussions on the role of central corneal thickness in glaucoma diagnosis and management came to occupy center stage in various meetings and journals after the publication of the Ocular Hypertension Treatment Study results where CCT was looked upon as a risk factor for progression in a prospective follow up of ocular hypertensive patients. More studies such as the European Glaucoma Prevention Study and the Early Manifest Glaucoma Management Trial looked at these factors as well.

The central points of relevance on the subject are:

1. How to estimate the true intraocular pressure in a patient from the reading of the Goldmann Applanation Tonometer (GAT).
2. The role of CCT as a risk factor for glaucoma progression independent of the confounding role it plays in GAT recording.

ESTIMATION OF TRUE IOP FROM GOLDMANN APPLANATION TONOMETER READINGS

Currently the most reliable technique available for IOP recording is the GAT which is based on the Imbert Fick Law.

The law states that the force required to applanate the anterior corneal surface is equal to the true IOP X area of the applanated on the posterior corneal surface. Practically speaking the anterior corneal curvature is not equal to the posterior corneal curvature as the cornea is not evenly thick. This unevenness is exaggerated after ablative corneal refractive surgery. Thus applanation of the anterior corneal surface does not mean applanation of the posterior corneal surface. In addition the cornea is not sufficiently soft, it has an average thickness of 520 and resists the applanation force. In addition the modulus of elasticity of the cornea may vary among individuals and affect the IOP recordings. For example the cornea of elderly, male and non myopic is likely to be more rigid as compared to young, female, myopic and keratokonic patients. Corneas of eyes which have had refractive surgery and corneal edema are likely to be less rigid. The differences in amount and characteristics of tear film among individuals may also affect the surface tension and the intermolecular force of the tear film and thereby affect the IOP recordings.

Goldmann and Schmidt expected an empirical balance between the surface tension and the force required to deform the cornea. The surface tension may be fairly constant among subjects but the force required to deform the cornea varies with the corneal thickness and the modulus of elasticity of the cornea, thus resulting in a cornea dependent error in IOP reading.

Goldmann and Schmidt reported that IOP recordings by the GAT can be affected by corneal thickness, curvature, modulus of elasticity (a term indicating rigidity, which is a preferred term over "ocular rigidity") and tear film. Investigation of the relationship between CCT and GAT readings started with pioneering works of Hansen and Ehlers and associates. There have been many reports on a positive correlation between CCT and measured IOP recordings.

Several investigators have attempted to calculate the Error (ΔP = IOPT-IOPG, IOPT is true IOP and IOPG is the IOP recorded by the GAT) by empirical clinical studies and others by theoretical means. There is a gross agreement that underestimation of IOP decreases

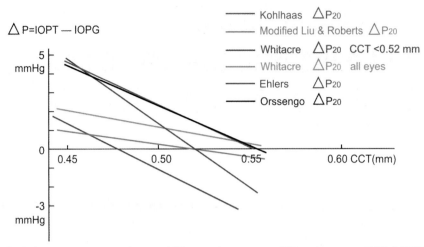

Fig. 1 Correlation between the error (difference between true IOP and measured IOP at IOPT of 20 mm Hg) and central corneal thickness (CCT). Underestimation of the IOP decreases with an increase of CCT in both the clinical study and theoretical estimation by Orssengo

with an increase of CCT in both clinical study and theoretical estimation by Orssengo **(Figure 1)**. But at this stage there is no formula or reference table from which a clinician can get true IOP from his clinical recording on the GAT.

IS CCT AN INDEPENDENT RISK FACTOR TO PREDICT GLAUCOMA PROGRESSION?

This is a question that researchers on the subject continue to ask themselves. An attempt to reanalyze the OHTS figures after correcting the intraocular pressure measured by Goldmann Applanation with the central corneal thickness failed to eliminate CCT as a risk factor. This lead to two possibilities, one that the correction algorithms were not good and that seems to be so from the discussion given above. The second that CCT is indeed an independent risk factor. The EMGT provides another opportunity to test this hypothesis. With 11 years progression data available now there is indication that CCT appears to be a predictive risk factor for progression in patients with higher IOP at baseline but not in patients with lower IOP at baseline. Nether of the studies prove that CCT is a risk factor for progression but this is a hypothesis that requires further independent testing.

SUMMARY

At this stage of knowledge, knowing a patients central corneal thickness seems to be of importance in ocular hypertension as there is irrefutable evidence that this may be used in deciding whether to treat that patient or not. In normal tension glaucoma the evidence is not that strong but definitely it may be considered whether a patient having a very thin cornea has erroneous readings on the GAT leading to misclassification as normal tension glaucoma. In established open angle glaucoma whether we may rely on CCT as a tool to identity patients who are at higher risk of progression hence require more aggressive treatment seems to be indicative but still further investigation is needed before we accept it whole heartedly.

15

Back to Basics: Structural Changes in Glaucoma and Clinical Evaluation of the Optic Nerve Head

R Ramakrishnan, Mona Khurana

CHAPTER OUTLINE

- ❖ Optic Nerve Head Evaluation Techniques
- ❖ Morphology of the Normal Optic Nerve Head
- ❖ Glaucomatous Optic Nerve Head

- ❖ Summary of Some Commonly Used Disc Evaluation Terms
- ❖ Differentiating Glaucomatous and Nonglaucomatous Optic Discs

- ❖ How to Document the Appearance of the Disc?
- ❖ Disc Damage Likelihood Scale

INTRODUCTION

The diagnosis of glaucoma can be fairly straightforward at times and at many a times be elusive. *Is glaucoma always present in the presence of raised intraocular pressure? Can glaucoma be present in the absence of any visual field defect or raised IOP?* These are the questions one often encounters in clinical practice. Both intraocular pressure (IOP) and visual field examination have their limitations. Elevated intraocular pressure is a risk factor for glaucomatous damage to the optic nerve.[1] However, it is not always associated with glaucomatous damage. On the other hand, some patients with a statistically normal IOP may develop glaucoma.

Visual field loss on standard achromatic perimetry may occur only after 25-35 percent of retinal ganglion cells in a local area have been lost. A number of histological and clinical studies have convincingly shown that optic nerve damage in patients with glaucoma occurs and can be detected before

conventional achromatic computerized perimetry uncovers early visual field defects.[2-11] Glaucoma itself is defined on the basis of structural appearance of the optic nerve head.[12,13] It is a progressive optic neuropathy characterized by degeneration of the retinal ganglion cells (RGCs) resulting in typical changes in the retina, optic nerve, and brain. While intraocular pressure reduction remains the mainstay of therapy, assessment for progressive disease depends solely on periodic assessment of the structure and function of the optic nerve. Careful, accurate clinical assessment and documentation of the appearance of the optic nerve head can yield a number of clues and is indispensable for early detection of the disease and monitoring its progression. In the present era of fast emerging technology, it is easy to rely on the various newer technologies to make a diagnosis of glaucoma and its progression. However, these only complement and do not replace a thorough clinical

evaluation which can detect subtle glaucomatous changes in the optic nerve head which has a wide range of biological variability in its normal appearance. This chapter aims to take the reader *back to the basics* and refocuses attention on a thorough clinical evaluation of the optic nerve head.

OPTIC NERVE HEAD EVALUATION TECHNIQUES

The overlap seen between normal and those with glaucoma is great. A thorough clinical examination of the optic nerve head despite the availability of sophisticated technology to quantify the structure of the optic nerve and surrounding retina is essential to distinguish between the two.

Before discussing the techniques of optic nerve head (ONH) evaluation one should be clear as to its goal. The purpose of ONH evaluation is:
- To assess the health of ganglion cell axons and to distinguish between the healthy and the diseased ONH

- Grouping the patients into categories such as healthy, mild, moderate, and advanced glaucoma
- Monitoring change/progression
- Quantifying the rate of any change that has occurred.

There are several ways to clinically examine the optic nerve head. Ideally the examination should be under magnification and a stereoscopic view. This is easily possible with slit-lamp biomicroscopy **(Figure 1A)**. Other techniques include indirect ophthalmoscopy and direct ophthalmoscopy. Monocular techniques rely mainly on color changes between neuroretinal rim (NRR) and optic cup to estimate the cup to disc ratio (CDR) and one needs to look for clues whereas stereoscopic methods allow examination of the topographic contour of optic cup and careful assessment of NRR. Although the examination of the ONH can be performed through an undilated pupil, a stereoscopic view may be possible only if the pupil is dilated.

Slit-lamp Biomicroscopy

Slit-lamp biomicroscopy is the *preferred method* of examination. The advantage is the quality of stereopsis and magnification. It is performed using a slit-lamp along with a variety of lenses. Indirect condensing lenses, such as a 60, 66, 78 or 90 diopter lens can be used **(Figure 1B)**. These are quite convenient to use and provide an inverted image and a reasonable view through a small pupil and relatively opaque media. Patients tolerate the procedure well. The lens is held 1 to 2 cm from the patient's eye. The disadvantage is that the image is reversed and inverted.

- **+78D, +66D lens:** Provide a wide enough field for a view of the entire posterior pole.
- **+60D lens:** It gives more magnification and a smaller field of view.

- **+90D lens:** Wider field of view, less magnification. Especially useful when pupillary dilatation is poor.

> **Note** Tinted lenses may be comfortable for the patient but the presence of a color artifact limits their usefulness. They can make the disc look healthier than it is and a proper examination of RNFL is not possible, so **a clear lens is preferable**.

- **The Hruby lens:** (–55D) It is a planoconvex lens that provides a direct and upright image which is not laterally reversed. The main disadvantage is the small field of view which is smaller than all other lenses. Small movements of the lens or patient have a negative effect on the quality of the image. It requires good fixation making patient cooperation extremely important. It is less convenient to use and the quality of the image is easily degraded by media opacities. It does not give a very good view in the presence of a small pupil.
- **Contact lenses:** A contact lens such as a Goldmann 3 mirror or the center of a gonioscope can be used but the coupling agent usually makes the examination more cumbersome. The image is a true and direct image **(Figures 1B(a to d))**.

Direct Ophthalmoscope

The direct ophthalmoscope provides a two-dimensional view. It provides a view that is too magnified, nonstereoscopic and leads to an underestimation of cupping. However, the use of parallax and attention to the bending of vessels after they cross the disc margin provides a reasonably fair idea about the contour of the rim. In the present times the use of direct ophthalmoscope has decreased significantly. However,

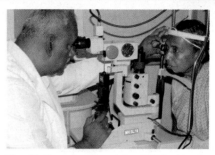

Fig. 1A Examination of the ONH with slit-lamp biomicroscopy and +90D lens

it may be one of the few tools that can be used to screen for glaucomatous discs in outreach screening camps.

Indirect Ophthalmoscope

The indirect ophthalmoscope provides a stereoscopic view but the image is too small, inverted and is difficult to identify the changes is in the contour of the ONH.

> The ONH cupping and contour can look different with different tools. Examination of the ONH should be performed with a similar method each time, preferably slit-lamp biomicroscopy in a dilated pupil using +78 or 90 D lenses.

NORMAL OPTIC NERVE HEAD

The optic nerve is composed of about 1.2 million axons (700,000 to 2 million)[14,15] which originate from cell bodies of the ganglion cells of the retina and ultimately synapse in the lateral geniculate body (LGB). The **optic nerve** head is the distal part of the optic nerve. It extends from the retinal surface to the myelinated part of the optic nerve just behind the sclera and lamina cribrosa. The optic nerve head is called so because of its three-dimensional structure. The term 'optic disc' gives the false impression of a two-dimensional, flat structure.

Composition

The ONH is composed of nerve fibers that arise from the ganglion cell

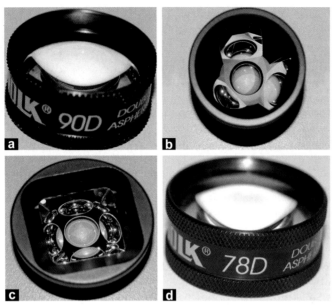

Figs 1B(a to d) Slit-lamp biomicroscopy can be done using a variety of lenses: (a) +90 diopter lens; (b) Goldmann 3 mirror lens; (c) Centre of a 4 mirror gonioscopy lens; (d) +78 diopter lens

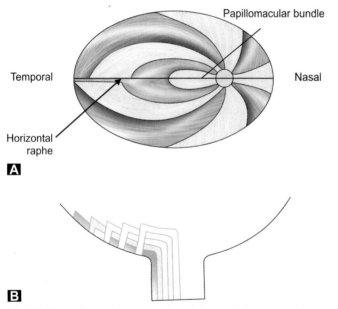

Figs 2A and B (A) Fibers from the temporal periphery originate on either side of the horizontal raphe and arch over the or below the fovea as arcuate fibers. The papillomacular and nasal fibers follow a direct course to the optic nerve. Arrangement of axons in the normal nerve fiber layer; (B) Axons from the periphery are located deep in the RNFL and have peripheral location in the optic nerve

angles and cascading over the rim, while axons from the central regions occupy a more superficial position and cascade over the top of the deeper fibers to occupy a more central position in the optic nerve **(Figures 2A and B)**. The area they form is the neuroretinal rim (NRR).

Other constituents of the neuroretinal rim are capillaries, glial cells and astrocytes. The capillaries provide nutrition as well as a reddish orange hue to the neuroretinal rim. Connective tissue support is provided by the glial cells and astrocytes. The axons at the superior and inferior poles have less structural support and are more prone to glaucomatous damage. The axons exit the globe through a fenestrated scleral canal, the *lamina cribrosa*. The scleral canal varies in size with diameters ranging from 1000 to 3000 microns in a normal healthy population. The area may also vary in normal eyes. Its size determines the size of the optic nerve head which in turn is determined genetically.[16] The diameter of the optic nerve expands to about 3 mm once the axons become myelinated in the retrolaminar part.

Since, the number of axons in the retina is relatively constant they will occupy a similar area in the optic nerve head no matter what the size of the scleral canal is. The area that they form is termed as the **neuroretinal rim** and the remaining empty space in the center of the ONH is termed as the **optic cup**. The optic cup is pale due to the visibility of the lamina cribrosa and presence of connective tissue. The lamina cribrosa has fenestrations which appear as dots. These may be more pronounced in case of glaucomatous damage. **The size of the cup varies with the size of the disc**. The normal optic disc is vertically oval while the cup is horizontally oval and slightly displaced superiorly. Thus, the inferior rim is the thickest. This is because the fovea is below the

layer and converge upon the ONH. Ninety percent of the neuroretinal rim is made of these ganglion cell axons. They travel in the superficial retinal nerve fiber layer in an organized pattern. At the ONH they make a 90 degrees turn and remain at the outer edge of the ONH. As these bundles of axons approach the scleral canal they are organized such that the axons from the most peripheral sites are the deepest within the retina turning at right horizontal center of the optic disc and the papillomacular bundle arising from it adds bulk to the inferior rim. It is next thickest superiorly followed by nasal, temporal being the thinnest.

> **Note** The vertical cup to disc ratio is measured by judging the vertical height of the cup against the vertical height of the disc. It is usually symmetrical between the fellow eyes with a similar disc size.

The optic nerve head is also the site of entry and exit of the retinal blood vessels. The retinal blood vessels show a great variation as they emerge. Usually they arise nasally in the cup. Cilioretinal arteries are present in 25 percent of the normal population and arise from the temporal side.[17]

Divisions of ONH (Figure 3)
Surface Nerve Fiber Layer
It is the innermost part of the ONH and composed predominantly of axonal nerve fibers of the ganglion cells along with interaxonal glial tissue.

Prelaminar Region
This is composed of axons, astrocytes and astroglial tissue. The glial tissue is more than that present in the surface nerve fiber layer. The transition from prelaminar to laminar region is gradual.

Lamina Cribrosa
This specialized extracellular matrix consists of fenestrated sheets of collagen through which fascicles of axons exit the globe. Astrocytes line the fenestrae and separate the sheets. Each trabeculum has a central capillary. It is described in detail further in the chapter.

Retrolaminar Region
The axons become myelinated in the retrolaminar region. The posterior extent of the retrolaminar region is not clear. It is covered by dura, arachnoid and pia. The connective tissue septa are

in contact with the pia on the outside, tissue surrounding the central vessels in the center and lamina cribrosa in front. The septa are covered by an astroglial layer which separates the nerve fiber from the connective tissue.

Vascular Supply of the Optic Nerve Head[17-24]
Arterial supply: The posterior ciliary artery is the main source of blood supply to the ONH with the exception of the surface nerve fiber layer which is supplied by the retinal circulation. The ONH has a sectoral distribution of blood supply.

The vascular supply to the various parts of the optic nerve head is as follows:

Surface Nerve Fiber Layer
It has a rich capillary network supplied mostly by the retinal arteries, intraocular branches of central retinal artery. These anastomose with the vessels of the prelaminar region (posterior

ciliary circulation). In some cases branches from the cilioretinal artery when present supply the corresponding sector.

The Prelaminar Region
This region receives blood supply from the centripetal branches of the peripapillary choroidal vessels. Branches from the circle of Zinn Haller (when present) penetrate the optic nerve to supply this region. When the circle of Zinn Haller is absent direct branches from the short posterior ciliary artery supply this region.

Lamina Cribrosa Region
It receives its blood supply from centripetal branches of the short posterior ciliary arteries and some from the recurrent pial branches from the peripapillary choroid. These branches may arise from the circle of Zinn Haller (when present) formed by the anastomosis between temporal and medial

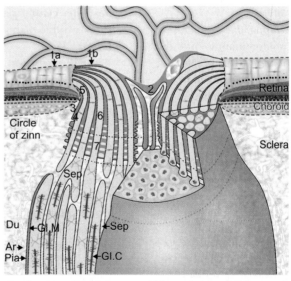

Fig. 3 Schematic drawing of optic nerve within and the adjoining eyeball. Numbered regions: 1a, inner limiting membrane of retina; 1b, inner limiting membrane of Elschnig; 2, central meniscus of Kuhnt; 3, border tissue of Elschnig; 4, border tissue of Jacoby; 5, intermediary tissue of Kuhnt; 6, anterior portion of lamina cribrosa; and 7, posterior portion of lamina cribrosa. Du = Dura; Ar = Arachnoid; Sep = Septa. (*Courtesy:* Anderson, DR (1969). Ultrastructure of human and monkey lamina cribrosa and optic nerve head. Arch Ophthalmol)

posterior ciliary arteries. The blood vessels lie in the fibrous septa and form a dense capillary plexus which makes it a highly vascular structure.

The Retrolaminar Region

This area has two circulatory systems. The main supply is from the branches of posterior ciliary artery:

- The axial centrifugal circulatory system consists of small branches from the central retinal artery
- A peripheral centripetal circulatory system consisting of retrograde vessels from:
  - Recurrent pial branches present all around the retrolaminar part arising from the peripapillary choroids or circle of Zinn Haller
  - Pial branches of central retinal artery arising during its intraorbital course
  - Pial branches from collaterals of the ophthalmic artery or its intraorbital branches.

Venous Drainage

The ONH including the retrolaminar part drains predominantly into the central retinal vein. The prelaminar part also drains into the choroidal veins. Communications between the two systems may occasionally enlarge: Retinociliary veins (when blood flows from retinal to choroidal circulation) or cilio-optic veins (choroidal to retinal circulation). The vortex veins receive blood from the choroid, iris and ciliary processes.

> **Note** Although derived from both retinal and ciliary circulation, the capillaries resemble more closely the features of retinal capillaries with tight junctions, abundant pericytes, nonfenestrated endothelium (no leak of fluorescein).

Astroglial Tissue, Connective Tissues and Nerve Sheaths

Astrocytes: Provide a continuous layer between the nerve fibers and blood vessels in the ONH. They also cover parts of the ONH. The space which they occupy increases from the RNFL to the laminar region and then again decreases in the retrolaminar part. **Two subtypes: Type 1A and Type 2B** astrocytes are present.[25] They play a major role in the remodeling of the extracellular matrix, synthesis of growth factors and other mediators. Their processes envelope the nerve fibers and provide structural and functional support.

Müller cells processes group axons into different bundles.

The astroglial tissue provides covering for various parts of the ONH:[26-30]

- *Connective tissue of Elschnig:* It separates the ONH from the vitreous and is continuous with internal limiting membrane (ILM) of the retina. It is a condensation of ILM just anterior to the optic nerve head. Its central part is referred to as central meniscus of Kuhnt **(Figure 3)**.
- *Central meniscus of Kuhnt:* It is traditionally described as the central thickened part of the ILM that overlies the optic disc.
- *Intermediate tissue of Kuhnt:* It separates the nerve from the retina and consists of mainly Muller cells.
- *Border tissue of Jacoby:* Separates the nerve from the choroid and is mainly a thin layer of astroglia.
- *Border tissue of Elschnig:* This rim of connective tissue extends between the choroid and optic nerve tissue especially temporally. It lies between the nerve fibers and the sclera.

- *Nerve sheaths:* Posterior to the globe, the optic nerve is surrounded by meningeal sheaths (pia, arachnoid and dura).

Lamina Cribrosa

The lamina cribrosa consists of a series of collagen plates arranged over one another with hundreds of (about 500–600) perforations or *'pores'* through which axons of the RGC pass to the retrolaminar part. These are not completely aligned. It is a three-dimensional meshwork of astrocyte covered, capillary containing connective tissue beams. A specialized glial cell, the lamina cribrosa cell is also present in the cribriform plates. The pores are nearly round in physiological discs whereas eyes with glaucoma have compressed pores.[31] The superior and inferior poles have larger pore area (single pore as well as total) with thinner connective and glial tissue as compared to nasal and temporal sectors.[32-35]

The axonal nutrition here depends upon the movement of oxygen and nutrients from the laminar capillaries through the laminar extracellular matrix (ECM) into the laminar astrocyte process within the beam finally reaching the central axon of each bundle. The connective tissue beams are anchored to a circumferential ring of collagen and elastin within the parapapillary sclera and bear the IOP related stress and strain. It is exposed to circumferential as well as anteroposterior forces. It is not as strong as the sclera which is about 1.5 mm thick whereas the lamina cribrosa is only 300 to 400 microns thick and full of holes containing axons, with a pressure differential across it (inside and out). *It is a place where million axons bend and pass out of the globe without getting damaged!*

This specialized ECM has components that are different from those in the sclera or pial septa.[37,38] It is composed of collagen I-VI, laminin, and fibronectin. The cribriform plates are composed of a core of elastin fibers with a patchy distribution of collagen III coated with collagen IV and laminin. Proteoglycans and cell adhesive proteins are also present. In excavated discs the laminar plates usually become compressed.[36-38]

NORMAL ONH MORPHOLOGY

The normal optic nerve head demonstrates biological variability in relation to its shape, size and other parameters. A thorough knowledge of the clinical appearance of the normal optic nerve head **(Figure 4)** is thus essential to detect any early change in morphology which is one of the early and reliable signs of glaucomatous damage.

Size

Normal Population

The optic disc size can be measured in terms of vertical and horizontal diameter and disc area. The optic nerve head shows a marked inter individual variability **(Figures 5A to C)** of about 0.80 to almost 6.00 mm² (disc area) or about 1:7 in a normal population (Caucasian).[39-45] It is independent of age beyond the age of 3 to 10 years. In the Baltimore Eye Survey, the optic disc area ranged from 1.15 to 4.94 mm² in white adults and from 0.90 to 6.28 mm² in black adults.[45] Studies in the Indian population also show a similar inter-individual variability with a *mean disc area* ranging from 2.25 to 3.37 mm².[46-51] The size may be larger in men according to some studies.[39,40,42,43,45] Within a range of –5D to +5D the size is independent of refractive error.[40,42,45]

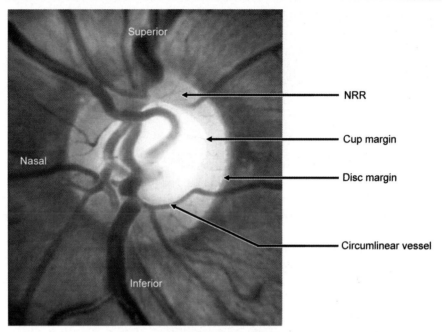

Fig. 4 The normal ONH

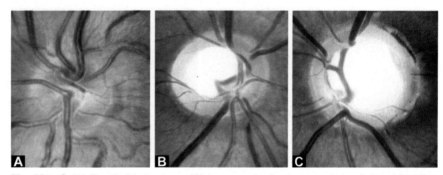

Figs 5A to C (A) Small; (B) Average; (C) Large optic disc in normal population. Note that the size of the cup varies according to the disc size. The large optic disc has a larger cup

Significance

Disc size affects the disc morphology. It correlates positively with the cup to disc ratio. The disc size is significantly larger in high myopia and significantly smaller in marked hypermetropia (more than +5D). Large optic discs in healthy individuals tend to have large cups, which can lead to an erroneous diagnosis of glaucoma. On the other hand, small cups can be glaucomatous in small optic discs and are likely to be underdiagnosed **(Figures 6A to C)**. Moreover larger optic discs have a larger neuroretinal rim area as compared to smaller optic discs, with less crowding of nerve fibers and a larger area of lamina cribrosa pores.

Disc size depends on the ethnic background. Caucasians have relatively small optic discs followed by Mexicans, Asians and Africans in increasing order (*Mean disc area* 2.14 to 3.75 mm² in African Americans compared with

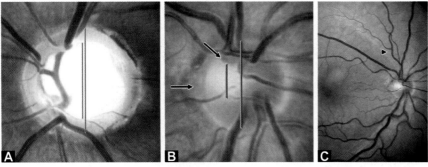

Figs 6A to C (A) A Large disc with physiological cupping (CDR0.77); (B and C) A Small disc with glaucomatous cupping (CDR0.4). Note the presence of an early notch, PPA (arrows in B) and RNFLD (arrowhead in C)

Table 1 Morphological anomalies associated with optic disc size

Small optic discs	Large optic discs
• Optic nerve head drusen	• High myopia
• Nonarteritic AION	• Optic disc pits
• Pseudopapilledema	• Morning glory syndrome
	• Coloboma of the optic disc

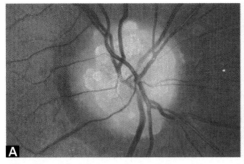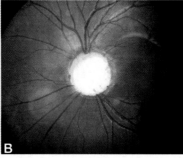

Figs 7A and B (A) A small sized disc with an optic nerve head drusen; (B) A large sized disc with a coloboma

1.73 to 2.63 mm² in Caucasians). As mentioned earlier, studies in different parts of India have found *mean disc area* ranging from 2.25 to 3.37 mm².[46-51] Some of these studies have found the disc area to be larger than Caucasians whereas others have reported similar results. The measurement depends on the technique used. Ramakrishnan[49] et al compared optic disc size measurements using OCT to measurements with planimetry and found a mean disc area of 2.37 mm² (OCT) and 2.83 mm² (planimetry). The optic disc size is also related to certain morphological anomalies as shown in **Table 1** and **Figures 7A and B**.

Based on a Gaussian distribution of optic disc area, very small and very large discs can be defined morphometrically. A **macrodisc**[42,52] is one that is larger than 2 standard deviations of the normal population whereas a **microdisc** is one which is smaller than 2SD of the normal population.

Primary Macrodiscs

Their size is independent of age after the first few years of life. They are independent or only slightly dependant on the refractive error. They may be further divided into 'asymptomatic' and 'symptomatic' with morphological and functional defects such as pit or morning glory syndrome.

Secondary Acquired Macrodiscs

These eyes increase in size after birth (as the refractive error continues to increase with age in these highly myopic eyes). Below –8 diopters, the optic disc size increases, probably owing to myopic stretching. The high myopia can be 'primary' which is caused by unknown reasons or 'secondary' due to congenital glaucoma.[52a]

> The optic disc size may also vary according to the method used for measurement in that particular study.

Clinical Methods for Evaluating Disc Size

Clinically there are various methods to measure optic disc size:

Direct ophthalmoscope: The optic disc size can be subjectively assessed by using a direct ophthalmoscope.[53] The 5° spot of light from the Welch-Allyn ophthalmoscope projects a circle of light with a diameter of 1.5 mm and an area of 1.77 mm square (slightly smaller than an average sized optic disc) on the retina when the ophthalmoscope is held in the usual range used for ophthalmoscopy. The spot may be aligned either over or adjacent to the optic disc and the size of the optic disc is compared to the size of the spot of light. If the optic nerve head is smaller than the spot of light, the disc can be estimated as small. If the optic nerve head is more than the size of the light spot, the optic disc size is large. This way, the disc can be classified as small, average or large in size.

Slit-lamp biomicroscopy: Another method consists of using a slit-lamp and hand held high power convex lenses (e.g. Volk 66D, 78D or 90D). It is easy rapid and relatively inexpensive. It shows an acceptable intra- and interobserver variability coefficient.[54,55] A vertical slit is placed over the optic disc and the beam is adjusted until it approximates the vertical disc diameter. The measurement is then read off the calibrated knob on the slit-lamp. Correction factors are needed depending upon the power of the lens being used (×1.0 for +60D lens, ×1.1 for 78D lens and ×1.3 for 90D lens).[56-58] These measurements are influenced by axial length, but not by the distance of the lens to the cornea or by changes in refractive errors up to eight diopters of ametropia. The presence of clinical situations such as tilted optic discs may limit the ability to evaluate optic disc size due to the imprecise definition of the scleral ring and optic disc margins.[59]

Note Examination of the optic disc without pupillary dilation can lead to significantly poorer interobserver agreement compared to dilated pupils.[60] The values measured from the slit-lamp do not represent the actual size, but they approximate the relative size. Appropriate correction factors need to be applied. These methods also help in the clinical comparison of optic nerve head size between fellow eyes.

Shape
Normal Population

The optic nerve head is slightly vertically oval **(Figures 8A to C)** with the vertical diameter being 7 to 10 percent larger than the horizontal one.[42] The optic nerve head shape does not correlate with height, weight, gender. An abnormal optic nerve head shape is significantly correlated with increased corneal astigmatism and amblyopia.[42,,61,62] The orientation of the longest disc diameter can indicate the axis of astigmatism.

The Tilted Myopic Disc

The clinical assessment of the optic nerve head and retinal nerve fiber layer (RNFL) is an important method to diagnose and monitor the progress of glaucomatous optic neuropathy but is often difficult in eyes with tilted

discs which are a common feature in myopia. Clinically, there are 2 orientations of tilting of the optic nerve head: temporal and inferior. In these eyes, the optic nerve fibers exit the sclera at an acute angle and at a turn of more than 90 degrees nasally. This is associated with a slightly recessed temporal perineural border of retinal pigment epithelium (RPE) producing a 'temporal crescent'. There is an ectasia of the inferonasal fundus. This accounts for the relative depression of the superotemporal isopters, not respecting the vertical meridian in the visual field of such patients (refractive scotoma). The stimuli fall short of their retinal focal plane retarding their recognition. Alternatively, visual field defects may result due to a partially hypoplastic optic nerve which may be associated with a tilted disc.

Myopic astigmatism less than −8D: In individuals with myopic astigmatism of less than −8D, the nerve head shape in normal and glaucomatous eyes does not differ significantly. In such glaucomatous eyes, the optic nerve head shape is not correlated with the mean NRR area or the mean perimetric defect suggesting that the glaucoma susceptibility is largely independent of disc shape.[61]

Myopic astigmatism more than −8D: The abnormal shape is more pronounced in refractive errors of more than −8D **(Figure 8C)**. It becomes more

elongated and oblique. Marked and asymmetric traction on these discs may be responsible for a high susceptibility to glaucoma.[52,63]

Note Considering the relation between the distance of central retinal vessel trunk and exit on lamina cribrosa and location of neuroretinal rim loss, the evaluation of disc shape becomes important as the disc shape influences this distance.

Tips for Clinical ONH Examination

Accurate recognition of the disc margin is necessary for the assessment of the disc parameters **(Figure 9)**.

- The disc margin is the internal edge of the scleral ring and is easily identifiable in most cases. However, it can be difficult in small crowded discs, highly myopic and tilted discs.
- NRR is identified by its pink color and the change of contour from the cup.
- Sloped or saucerized cups are most often present in the sclerotic type. Precise determination of the types of the optic disc cup is difficult and requires a detailed stereoscopic examination.
- Follow the trajectory of the vessels to identify the contour of the NRR.
- Pay attention to rim contour rather than cup, disc size, corroborating findings between rim and RNFL.

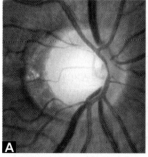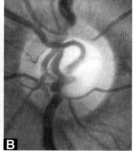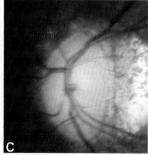

Figs 8A to C (A and B) Color fundus photographs showing the physiological variations in optic disc shape in the normal population; (C) Shows the appearance of the optic disc in high myopia

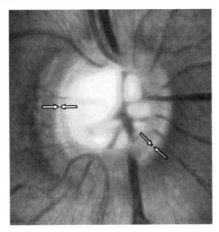

Fig. 9 Identifying the disc margins. The inner margins of a thin rim of sclera appearing as a white rim marks the disc margins (white arrows)

> **Note** The peripapillary scleral ring itself does not belong to the optic disc. This is of utmost importance for all optic disc measurements, because the inclusion of the outer margin of the peripapillary scleral ring into the optic disc area markedly enlarges the area of the neuroretinal rim and decreases the cup/disc ratios.[64] The inner margin of the scleral ring must be used for all measurements.

The Optic Cup

In normal eyes, the shape of the optic cup is horizontally oval and the horizontal diameter is about 8 percent longer than the vertical diameter. The combination of the horizontally oval shape of the optic cup and the vertically oval shape of the optic disc explains the configuration of the normal neuroretinal rim, which has its broadest parts in the inferior and superior disc regions and its smallest parts in the temporal and nasal region of the optic disc.[42]

In normal eyes, the optic cup depth depends on the cup area and, indirectly, on the disc size: the larger the optic cup, the deeper it is.[61] The ratio of cup diameter to disc diameter, i.e. the cup/disc ratio is dependent on the size of the optic disc and cup. The high interindividual variability of the optic disc and cup diameters

(**Figure 5**) explain why the cup/disc ratios range in a normal population from 0.0 to almost 0.9.[42] Because of this correlation between disc area and cup area[39,40,42,43,49,65-67] cup to disc ratios are low in small optic nerve heads and are high in large optic discs. An unusually high cup to disc ratio, therefore, can be physiologic in eyes with large optic nerve heads whereas an average cup to disc ratio is uncommon in normal eyes with small optic discs (**Figures 6A to C**).

> **Note** In the diagnosis of glaucomatous optic nerve damage, this interindividual variability of cup to disc ratios and their dependence on the optic disc size has to be accounted for. Eyes with physiologically high cup/disc ratios in macrodiscs should not be overdiagnosed and considered glaucomatous. On the other hand eyes with increased IOP, small optic nerve heads, and average or low cup to disc ratios should not be underdiagnosed as being "ocular hypertensive".

Four types of normal cupping have been described in literature:[42]

- No cupping
- Well demarcated cups with steep sides
- Cups with partially sloping temporal rim
- Cups with entire temporal rim sloping (including superotemporal, horizontal temporal, and inferotemporal rim).

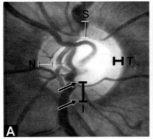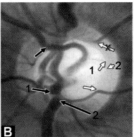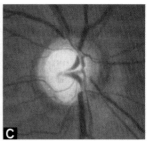

Figs 10A to C (A) The normal neuroretinal rim follows the ISNT rule. The NRR is broadest in the inferior region followed by superior, nasal and temporal being thinnest; (B) Marking the correct margins of the NRR and optic cup based on contour changes; (C) A glaucomatous optic nerve head (for comparison). Note that the ISNT rule is not followed as the inferior rim is the thinnest

Neuroretinal Rim (NRR)

Due to the wide range of the optic disc cupping in the normal population, changes in neuroretinal rim contour may provide more useful information in the diagnosis of glaucoma. Identification of the neuroretinal rim width in all sectors of the optic disc is of fundamental importance for detection of diffuse and localized rim loss due to this disease. The rim width is the distance between the border of the optic disc delimited by the inner margin of the scleral ring and the border of the contour cup indicated by the position of blood vessel bending (**Figures 10A to C**).

Normal Population

The neuroretinal rim exhibits a characteristic configuration in normal eyes based on a vertically oval shape of the optic disc and the horizontally oval shape of the optic disc cup. In a majority of eyes the rim shape follows the **ISNT rule,** (a mnemonic) that is, it is usually broadest in the inferior disc region, followed by the superior disc region, the nasal disc area and finally the temporal disc region where the rim is the thinnest.[42,68] If the optic disc itself has a normal shape, the tendency of the normal neuroretinal rim to obey the ISNT rule appears to be largely independent of disc size, cup size, cup–disc ratio or neuroretinal rim area. In the normal population, the rim size demonstrates the same interindividual variability as the optic disc size. In glaucoma, neuroretinal rim is lost in all sectors of the optic disc with regional preferences, depending on the stage of the disease.

Looking at the Neuroretinal Rim: ISNT Rule

Two factors need to be evaluated during clinical examination of the ONH:
- The relative thickness of the inferior with respect to the superior rim (glaucomatous damage most commonly manifests as thinning of the inferior rim).
- To check whether the temporal rim is the thinnest. A thinner superior/inferior than temporal rim is considered highly suspicious of glaucomatous damage.

Exceptions to the Rule

This rule should be carefully evaluated because the inferior sector of the optic disc may not be the thickest rim in 37.8 percent of normal eyes.[69]

Studies in Indian populations have also noted violations in the ISNT rule. In a Heidelberg retina tomograph (HRT) study in normal North Indian eyes, Sihota et al. reported the inferior rim area to be more than the superior rim area followed by the temporal rim area in 71 percent of normal eyes and violation in 29 percent eyes.[70] Arvind H et al., reported that the temporal rim was not the thinnest in 12 percent of eyes in a study in normal population in the southern part of India.[51]

Factors Influencing Assessment of the Shape of the NRR

Disc shape: A shorter vertical-to-horizontal disc diameter (i.e. a more horizontally oval disc) increases the relative availability of space for arrangement of nerve fibers at the superior and inferior poles, and decreases the space available nasally and temporally,

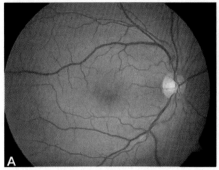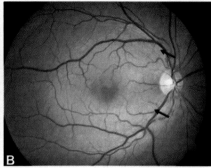

Figs 11A and B Color fundus and red free photographs showing the normal pattern of RNFL. Note the bright striations (arrows) where the RNFL is thickest, that is the superior temporal and the inferior temporal region

necessitating that the nerve fibers be bunched thicker at the latter positions. *Sloping optic disc cups:* Oblique arrangement of fibers in the horizontal temporal region in discs with sloping cups may contribute to measurement of wider rim widths temporally. Nasal or temporal torsion of the disc would change the relative rim positions measured at the 12 (for superior) and 6 (inferior) o'clock positions and contribute to relatively thinner rim measurement inferiorly than for a nontorted disc. So these torted discs which are otherwise non glaucomatous may not have a thicker inferior than superior rim. In the absence of other glaucomatous features, an inferior rim with width at least 90 percent of the superior rim may be normal, especially if the disc is torted.[69]

> Disc shape, astigmatism, and any oblique arrangement of nerve fibers must be taken into consideration while assessing the NRR.

Retinal Nerve Fiber Layer

Qualitatively this can be examined with slit-lamp biomicroscopy and a condensing lens using a red free light. In normal eyes, bright striations are visible and the retina glistens in the regions where the retinal nerve fiber layer (RNFL) is thickest: superior temporal and inferior temporal from the disc, followed by superior nasal

and inferior nasal regions. The peripapillary vessels are buried within the nerve fiber layer and may look blurred in healthy eyes **(Figures 11A and B)**. The visibility of RNFL decreases with age. It is discussed in detail ahead in the chapter.

Parapapillary Area

The junctional zone between the retina, with the underlying choroid and sclera and the optic nerve is often poorly defined. A thin rim of sclera, appearing as an even thin white rim (the Elschnig ring) marks the disc margin. This is the extension of the sclera between the choroid and the ONH. Peripheral to this, may be present areas concentric to the disc where the retina and the choroid do not appear to extend to the margin but stop short. The normal optic nerve head may be surrounded by zones that vary in width, circumference and pigmentation. These include the alpha zone, the beta zone and the temporal scleral crescent **(Figures 12A and B)**.

Zone alpha is the parapapillary zone of increased pigmentation and may represent the embryonic fold with a double layer or irregularity of RPE.

Zone beta represents the retraction of RPE from the disc margin and is often associated with thinning/atrophy of RPE, choriocapillaris and or absence of choroid adjacent to the disc.

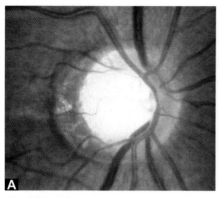
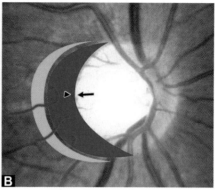

Figs 12A and B PPA is divided into two zones: alpha (light blue) and beta zone PPA (dark blue). Note that alpha zone PPA is characterized by irregular hypo- and hyperpigmentation of the retinal pigment epithelium and thinning of the chorioretinal tissue layer. The beta zone is adjacent to the optic disc and is characterized by atrophy of the retinal pigment epithelium and choriocapillaris, thinning of chorioretinal tissues, and visible sclera and choroidal vessels

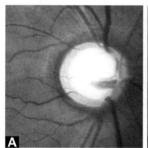
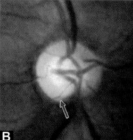
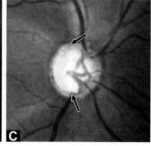

Figs 13A to C (A) Concentric enlargement of cup due to diffuse loss of neuronal tissue; (B) Unipolar cupping (blue arrow); (C) Bipolar cupping with corresponding RNFLD

GLAUCOMATOUS OPTIC NERVE HEAD

In glaucoma, there is a progressive loss of retinal ganglion cells. This manifests as characteristic structural changes in the optic nerve head, retinal nerve fiber layer and parapapillary area. The various mechanisms for pathogenesis of these characteristic changes are discussed in a separate chapter.

ONH Size and Shape

The first step in the correct interpretation of glaucomatous optic nerve head is the estimation of its size. The size determines the apparent estimation of the neuroretinal rim and the cup disc ratio. Structural characteristics associated with large discs include a larger number of nerve fibers, more and larger lamina cribrosa pores, a larger

neuroretinal rim area, and a higher cup to disc ratio. Although few studies have directly addressed this issue, there is no conclusive evidence that disc size is an independent risk factor for glaucoma. Along with the disc size, it is also important to document the shape of the optic disc.

ONH Cupping

Increased cupping of the optic nerve head has been recognized as an important characteristic of glaucomatous change.

Cup to disc ratio (CDR): Quantification of the optic disc cup and its relation to the disc size is termed as the cup disc ratio. The estimation of the vertical cup to disc ratio is one of the most frequently performed clinical

methods for a simple assessment of the optic disc in glaucoma diagnosis and follow-up. It can range from 0.0 to 0.9 in the healthy population and there is considerable overlap between normal and glaucomatous eyes.[42] The vertical cup to disc ratio is positively associated with optic disc size in normal and glaucomatous eyes.[71] Vertical elongation of the cup is a characteristic feature of glaucomatous optic neuropathy. This is due to the preferential loss of NRR in the superior and inferior poles. In some cases a concentric enlargement may occur where the vertical cup disc ratio may not be larger than the horizontal. A value of vertical CDR of more than 0.7 is commonly used as a cut off to separate healthy from glaucomatous eyes as it is found only in 2.5 percent of the healthy population. However, it has limitations when used as the sole measure for the diagnosis of glaucoma due the wide variation in the normal population. This variation is attributable to the variations in optic disc size. Thus, assessment of vertical cup disc ratio taking into account the optic disc size improves accuracy. In fact, in a study by Jonas[72] the vertical cup to disc ratio adjusted for optic disc size showed the highest accuracy in the discrimination of preperimetric glaucoma eyes from normal eyes. However, it had a low sensitivity of 31.5 percent with 95 percent specificity and cannot be solely relied upon. When patients with glaucomatous field loss were compared with healthy individuals, NRR area was a better parameter followed by vertical cup disc ratio (adjusted for disc size) with a sensitivity of 77 percent.

Pattern of Cupping

The optic disc cupping can occur in a variety of patterns (**Figures 13A to C**):
- Concentric enlargement of cup (**Figure 13A**)
- Unipolar enlargement of the optic cup (**Figure 13B**)

Bipolar enlargement of the optic cup (**Figure 13C**).

- *Nasal cupping:* Rarely, in some patients the NRR loss may not follow this pattern and there may be marked rim loss in the nasal region. In this case the nasal vessels which normally lie on the nasal neuroretinal rim are separated from the rim by an extension of the cup. This is highly suggestive of glaucoma.

- *Pattern of cupping in inverse discs:* Here the principle vessels may leave the disc on the temporal side rather than nasal. Thus, the first cupping in such discs may be nasal and the field defect temporal.

To Re-emphasize

- A physiological optic cup is horizontally oval. A vertically larger cup is uncommon in healthy eyes.
- Margins of the optic cup should be assessed using the contour not the color. In glaucoma the cup is larger than the area of pallor.
- The cup-disc ratio should always be interpreted in context with the disc size.
- In small optic discs glaucomatous changes can go unnoticed unless a high degree of suspicion is maintained as cup to disc ratios remain small until the late course of the disease (**Figures 6A to C**).

Asymmetry of ONH Cup Size

Healthy individuals have similar sized optic disc cups and therefore cup disc ratios in both the eyes, unless there is an asymmetry in disc size. However, the presence of an asymmetry in the optic cup size in discs of similar size is suggestive of glaucomatous damage. This is because glaucoma tends to asymmetric between the fellow eyes of the same individual. Armaly[73] using a direct ophthalmoscope found less than 1 percent of healthy individuals to have an asymmetry of more than 0.2 in the

Table 2 Causes of inter eye cup-disc ratio asymmetry

- Asymmetric disc size
- Asymmetrical POAG
- Anisometropia (**Figures 14A and B**)
- Unilateral glaucoma (including secondary glaucoma)
- Disc hypoplasia
- Morning glory syndrome
- Coloboma of the ONH
- Congenital pit of the ONH

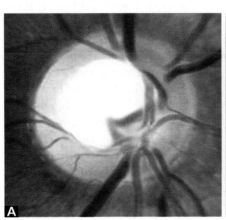 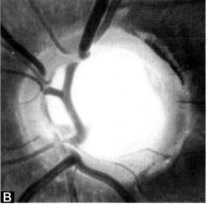

Figs 14A and B Asymmetric cup to disc ratio between the fellow eyes of a patient due to difference in disc size. The disc size and vertical CDR of the left eye is larger than the right eye

vertical cup-disc ratio. Jonas[42] using morphometric analysis found an asymmetry of more than 0.2 in the vertical cup to disc in 4 percent of healthy population and more than 0.3 in less than 1 percent of the healthy population. However, this parameter at a 0.2 cut off has a low sensitivity and if used as a sole criterion for diagnosis majority of glaucoma can go undiagnosed.

> **Note** Asymmetry in the vertical cup disc ratio more than 0.2 between fellow eyes (with similar disc size) more common in glaucoma but may also occur in healthy eyes.[45,74,75] Nevertheless, it should raise the suspicion of glaucoma especially when not associated with any asymmetry in disc size. At the same time it should be correlated with other disc characteristics (Table 2).

Deepening of Cup

It may sometimes be the predominant pattern in glaucomatous disc damage. In the initial stages lamina cribrosa is

not exposed. An overpass vessel may be seen which later collapses into the cup. Later, the underlying lamina cribrosa may become exposed and its fenestrations are seen (**laminar dot sign**). In the initial stages they are dot like but in advanced cases become striate.

Neuroretinal Rim

The neuroretinal rim is identified by its pink color and characteristic contour changes. It represents the axons of the ganglion cells and changes in the neuroretinal rim (NRR) reflect the nerve fiber damage occurring in glaucoma. Loss of neuroretinal rim in glaucoma can be in a diffuse or localized pattern (**Figures 15A to C**).

Diffuse loss results in neural tissue loss from the entire sectors and generates a concentric enlargement of the cup (**Figure 13A**). This may be difficult to differentiate from a large physiological disc. However, it has been seen that even in concentric enlargements preferential regional loss is frequent and ISNT rule is violated. The normal horizontally oval shape is lost indicating a preferential superior and inferior damage. The temporal rim may be affected first **(temporal unfolding)**. In early glaucomatous damage, loss predominantly occurs in the temporal superior and temporal inferior sector leading to a vertical elongation of the cup.

Localized rim loss can sometimes take the form of a notching of the rim **(Figures 15A to C)**. *A notch* is a localized defect in the neuroretinal rim on the cup side, the rim/disc ratio being smaller in that area than the surrounding and the extent being less than 2 clock hours.[76] There is some disagreement in literature regarding the definition of a notch. A notch represents an extension of localized loss which eventually results in complete absence of NRR in that area. It starts at the inner surface of neuroretinal rim and extends peripherally and posteriorly. The loss of neural tissue exposes the pores of the lamina cribrosa. The deeper the cup, better the visibility of the notch which may go unnoticed in shallow cups. It is most commonly present in the inferotemporal sector followed by superior.

Advanced NRR loss with advanced glaucomatous damage, the temporal rim is also lost and ultimately only the nasal rim may remain.

Why are the Poles Affected?

- This may be due to regional differences in the character of the lamina cribrosa. The laminar pores are larger in the superior and inferior part with thinner connective tissue making these areas more susceptible to deformation which could be associated with increased axonal damage.

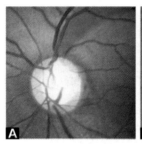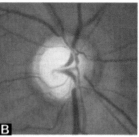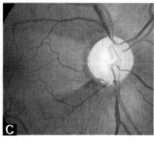

Figs 15A to C Color fundus photograph showing patterns of neuroretinal rim loss: (A) Superior notch with RNFLD; (B) Inferior notch; (C) Bipolar notch with RNFLD

- The poles are occupied by larger axons which may be preferentially damaged in glaucoma.
- The larger the distance of the central vessel trunk exit from the rim, the more pronounced the rim loss. Since the vessels mostly exit from the superonasal part, the inferotemporal and superotemporal sectors are most susceptible. The vessel trunk could act as a stabilizing element in the lamina cribrosa making a mechanical deformation in that area more difficult.[77] In eyes with anomalous position of exit of the central vessel trunk, the rim loss may not follow the usual pattern.

Neuroretinal Rim Color

The color of the neuroretinal rim is important. Pallor of the rim increases the likelihood that a nonglaucomatous optic neuropathy is present, especially when pallor is greater than cup size. Nonglaucomatous optic neuropathy may sometimes show optic disc cupping. Studies have found pallor of the neuroretinal rim to be 94 percent specific for nonglaucomatous atrophy and cupping, whereas focal or diffuse obliteration of the neuroretinal rim with preservation of color of any remaining rim tissue to be 87 percent specific for glaucoma.[78]

However, one must keep in mind that a localized rim pallor may be seen after an acute rise in pressure in glaucomas associated with very high pressures.

Retinal Nerve Fiber Layer

Hoyt drew attention to the importance of the retinal nerve fiber layer (RNFL) in diagnosing glaucoma.[79,80]

Defects in the RNFL were found to have an increased prevalence in glaucoma. Subsequently, RNFL defects were often found to precede the visual field defects and often were the first detectable sign of glaucomatous damage.

The RNFL is composed of axons of ganglion cells, astrocytes and components of Muller cells. It follows a specific arrangement. Axons from the periphery are located deep in the RNFL and have peripheral location in the optic nerve head. Ganglion cells in the peripapillary retina send axons to the superficial part of RNFL and occupy a more central part in the ONH. The arcuate nerve fibers (arching over the papillomacular bundle) are located at the superior and inferior poles of the nerve head (corresponding to Bjerrum area), the peripheral retinal fibers are more peripheral at the nerve head, and the papillomacular fibers are more central at the nerve head. The papillomacular and nasal fibers follow a more direct course to the optic nerve. The RNFL is thickest in the peripapillary area with the superior and inferior poles being thicker leading to the characteristic double hump pattern seen during imaging. This corresponds with the physiological pattern of the neuroretinal rim.

Retinal nerve fiber layer can be assessed qualitatively during the clinical examination.[81,82] This can be done with slit-lamp biomicroscopy using a red free light. The RNFL reflects a substantial amount of light owing to the presence of microtubules in the axons of the ganglion cells. The remaining light is absorbed by the RPE and choroid due to the presence of melanin. The brightness is produced by light reflected from the RNFL. The reflectance absorbance property of light depends on the wavelength of the light. Red light (long wavelength) penetrates deeply and is not reflected whereas blue light (short wavelength) is almost totally reflected by the RNFL. However, direct observation of blue light is difficult. In clinical practice a *red free light* is preferred as it is well reflected by the RNFL and the remaining light absorbed by the RPE and choroid provides a dark background to contrast with the bright reflections from RNFL.

The brightness, texture and pattern of the RNFL as it emerges from the optic nerve head and the visibility of blood vessels is noted. In normal eyes, bright striations are visible and the retina glistens in the regions where the RNFL is thickest: superior temporal and inferior temporal from the disc, followed by superior nasal and inferior nasal regions. The peripapillary vessels are buried within the nerve fiber layer and margins appear indistinct in healthy eyes. The glial tissue reflects less light appearing as dark lines. In glaucoma, the loss on RNFL affects their brightness, texture and visibility of blood vessels. There is loss of brightness and attenuation of texture and increased visibility of blood vessels. As the RNFL

is lost, the borders of blood vessels become clearer and their appearance dark.

The pattern of loss can be slit like, localized, diffuse, or mixed **(Figure 16)**.
- *Localized loss:* Localized RNFL loss occurs in about 20 percent or more of all glaucomatous eyes[83] **(Figures 16A to C)**.
- *Wedge shaped:* The RNFL defect appears as wedge-shaped dark areas emanating from the optic disc. These defects follow an arcuate pattern as would be expected from the normal RNFL anatomy.[84-86] They should be distinguished from the physiological slitlike defects.
- *Slit defects:* These are splits or cleavages in the RNFL **(Figures 16E and F)**. Normally, dark glial bands formed by the processes of the Müller cells which have different optical properties separate the nerve bundles. They can sometimes be quite wide and be mistaken for RNFL defects. However, these are always narrower than the large caliber peripapillary blood vessels, not wedge shaped and rarely extend up to the optic nerve head border. They can mimic a true defect especially in high myopia.[87]
- *Diffuse loss (Figure 16D):* In diffuse RNFL loss there is a diffuse reduction of brightness. The normal pattern of coarse striations in the superior and inferior arcuate area is lost and the striations become finer and more defined as the nerve fiber loss increases and the striations finally disappear in advanced loss. There is better visualization of the edges of the parapapillary blood vessels. This pattern is more difficult to detect as compared to localized.

- *Mixed pattern:* Both diffuse and localized RNFL defects may coexist.
- *Advanced Diffuse Loss (Reversal of Pattern):* This is seen in advanced diffuse RNFL loss when the papillomacular bundle appears bright as compared to the superior and inferior RNFL. The reverse is seen in normal eyes where the opposite is true due to a greater thickness of the RNFL at the superior and inferior poles **(Figures 16G and H)**.

Limitations in the Examination of RNFL

The ability to assess RNFL loss depends upon the pigmentation of the fundus, media clarity, pupillary dilation and the pattern of RNFL loss. In some cases 50 percent of nerve fibers can be lost without any clinical evidence of nerve fiber defects.[86] This is because loss of axons located in the deeper layers produces no visible effect in the superficial aspect of the RNFL. Another limitation is the directional reflectance of the nerve fibers as a result of their cylindrical configuration. The brightness observed during examination depends upon the angle of observation. The nerve fibers which are visible when illuminated from one direction may disappear when illuminated from another.

It should also be remembered that localized RNFL defects are not pathognomonic for glaucoma since they may occur in eyes with optic nerve atrophy due to other reasons[88,89] **(Table 3)**.

Changes in Lamina Cribrosa
Visualization of lamina cribrosa in discs with glaucomatous damage is more common as compared to normal. The loss of the neural tissue exposes the

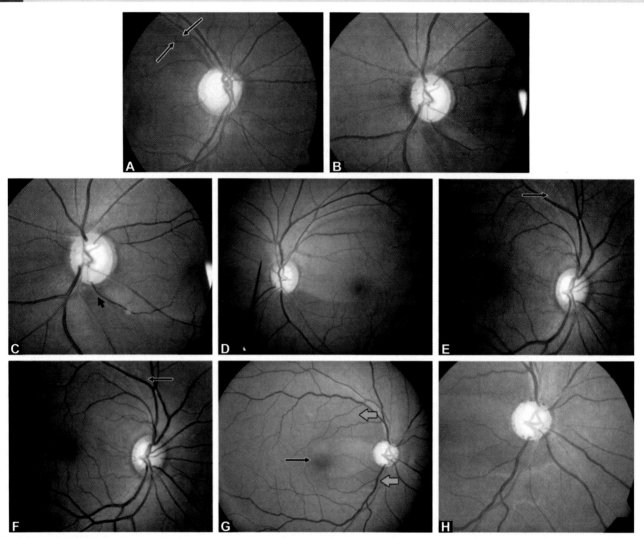

Figs 16A to H (A) Color fundus photograph showing localized early RNFLD in the superotemporal sector (arrows) along with a corresponding early notch of the NRR; (B and C) Color and red free fundus photograph showing localized, wedge shaped RNFLD in the inferotemporal part along with a corresponding notch of the NRR. Note the lack of striations and the dark appearance of vessels in the area of the defect; (D) Red free fundus photograph of a diffuse RNFL defect. The striations are absent and the blood vessels are not covered by the bright reflex in the area of the RNFL defect; (E and F) Slit RNFL defects indicated by the arrows (color and red free fundus photographs); (G and H) Pattern reversal following advanced diffuse loss of RNFL. The black arrow indicates the papillomacular bundle and the blue arrows indicate areas of RNFL loss. The papillomacular bundle appears brighter due to the loss of the normal brighter striations in the superior and inferior poles due to advanced RNFL loss. Compare with the normal RNFL pattern in Figure 11

Table 3 Nonglaucomatous causes of RNFL defects

- Optic disc drusen
- Optic disc pit
- Optic disc coloboma
- Toxoplasma retinochoroidal scars
- Ischemic retinopathies (e.g. BRVO)
- Optic neuritis
- Diabetic retinopathy

laminar pores. This is known as the laminar dot sign **(Figures 17A and B)**. These pores can also be seen in healthy discs with large physiological cups. Thus, it is not specific for glaucoma. Their presence in small discs does however suggest a glaucomatous damage as small discs do not have visible pores.

The shape of the pores also changes as the glaucomatous process progresses. It changes from round in early glaucoma to oval in moderate and striated or elongated in cases with advanced visual field loss. This is because the pores become elongated as the disease progresses due to changes in the connective tissue, backward and lateral bowing of the lamina cribrosa, strain and compression.[90-95]

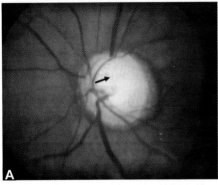 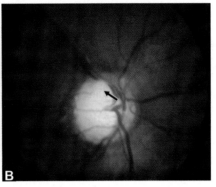

Figs 17A and B The laminar dot sign. Note the prominent pores of the lamina cribrosa with striations (arrow)

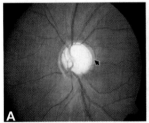 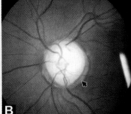 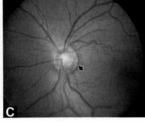

Figs 18A to C (A and B) The fundus photograph (color and red free) showing parapapillary atrophy encircling the ONH 3600: the 'glaucomatous halo'; (C) More localized PPA in a small glaucomatous disc. Note that the area of PPA corresponds to the area of rim loss

Pearls

- Examine the base of the optic cup.
- Look for the visibility of the Laminar Dots and their shape.
- Scrutinize for APONs (acquired pit of optic nerves).

Advanced Cupping

In the advanced stage, all neural tissue is lost resulting in total cupping. The ONH clinically appears white and the vessels appear to bend at the margin. There is an undermining of the disc margin with extreme posterior bowing of the lamina cribrosa (Bean potting).

Parapapillary Changes

Association between parapapillary atrophy (PPA) and glaucoma was first described by Elschnig and Bucklers.[96-98] It was called "glaucomatous halo" **(Figures 18A to C)** encircling 360 degrees of the optic

nerve head in advanced glaucoma. Primrose[99] showed that the presence of PPA was twice as common in eyes with glaucoma as compared to healthy eyes. Parapapillary region is the area located just outside the optic disc. Parapapillary atrophy (PPA) refers to the thinning and degeneration of the chorioretinal tissue just outside of the optic disc. Ophthalmoscopicaly, it can be divided into a central beta zone and a peripheral alpha zone.

Zone alpha is characterized by a region of irregular hypopigmentation and hyperpigmentation of the retinal pigment epithelium (RPE) and thinning of the chorioretinal tissue layer. It is characterized mainly by irregularities in RPE. It corresponds to a relative scotoma on visual field examination.

Zone beta is associated with marked atrophy of the RPE, reduction in photoreceptors and choriocapillaris leading to good visibility of

the large choroidal vessels and sclera. Thus, it corresponds to an absolute scotoma. Zone beta is more common and extensive in eyes with glaucoma than in healthy eyes. It becomes more important when associated with other findings suggestive of glaucomatous damage. The area of PPA is spatially correlated with the area of neuroretinal rim loss, with the atrophy being largest in the corresponding area of thinner neuroretinal rim.

The alpha and beta zones should be differentiated from the myopic scleral crescent in eyes with high myopia and from the inferior scleral crescent present in eyes with tilted optic discs. A larger beta zone has been reported in myopic eyes.[74,100,101]

Scleral crescent: Here there is a misalignment of tissues due to the differential growth of the eyeball. Only the ILM and RNFL cover the sclera whereas in beta zone the Bruch's membrane and choroid is present between the sclera and remaining retina.

In highly myopic eyes, three zones are seen:

1. Internal surface of the scleral canal covered by only RNFL and appears white. All other layers are missing.
2. **Beta zone:** RNFL and Bruch's membrane present, photoreceptor and RPE atrophy.
3. **Alpha zone:** RPE changes.

Alpha and beta zone may be present in normal eyes with the beta zone in 15 to 20 percent.[102] In normal eyes, both alpha zone and beta zone are largest and most frequently located in the temporal horizontal sector, followed by the inferior temporal area and the superior temporal region. They are smallest and most rarely found in the nasal parapapillary area. Jonas found a significantly higher prevalence of PPA in glaucomatous eyes. In a population based study[47] the optic disc morphology including parapapillary atrophy was found not to be markedly different between European and Indian (in the southern part of India) subjects.

The beta-zone PPA is associated with glaucomatous visual field loss which has been demonstrated by standard automated perimetry and short-wavelength automated perimetry.[103] Patients with eventual progression of glaucomatous visual field defects (VFDs) have a significantly larger beta-zone PPA than patients with a stable visual field.[104] Its presence and size in ocular hypertensive patients is related to the development of visual field damage.[105,106]

In the region of parapapillary atrophy, fundus autofluorescence is increased as a sign of increased lipofuscin accumulation. Fundus autofluorescence in the parapapillary region can be significantly larger in ocular hypertensive eyes than in normal eyes, and can be larger in eyes with glaucomatous visual field defects than in ocular hypertensive eyes.[107]

PPA in Various Types of Glaucoma
Myopic and senile sclerotic discs have larger areas of PPA whereas focal ischemic glaucoma have more localized areas of PPA. The findings in focal normal pressure glaucoma however are contradictory.[72,103,108-110]

PPA and Progression
Both presence and size of beta zone PPA is a risk factor for progression.[111-115] It has been suggested that once beta-zone PPA has developed, the ensuing, continued insult to the regional optic nerve complex (optic disc, RNFL, and parapapillary region) results in a greater susceptibility to progression that is relatively more important than its actual size.[116] The enlargement of the area of PPA is associated with progressive ONH damage and visual field defects. The assessment of any increase in size of PPA can be especially useful in detecting progression in highly myopic discs and to establish the presence of glaucoma in case of small discs where cup to disc ratios may be small inspite of NRR loss. The presence and extension of PPA in patients with ocular hypertension is known to be associated with an increased risk of development of glaucomatous change and the development of field defects. In a retrospective study, Teng et al. evaluated the presence of beta zone as a risk factor for progression using automated point wise linear regression. The beta zone PPA based on stereophotography, measured by HRT-II, and an adequate number of Visual Fields after the HRT image were evaluated for progression. They found that glaucomatous eyes with beta zone PPA progressed faster than eyes without beta zone PPA, and the presence of any amount of beta zone PPA increased the risk of progression.[116]

PPA and Disc Hemorrhages
Parapapillary atrophy is closely associated with a disc hemorrhage in glaucoma patients. It is also one of the optic disc characteristics that antedate disc hemorrhage.[117,118] A higher frequency of beta zone and a significantly larger beta zone has been noted in glaucomatous eyes with disc hemorrhages as compared to contralateral eyes with no hemorrhages.[117] Beta zone parapapillary atrophy area is an independent significant factor associated with disc hemorrhage.

Pathogenesis of PPA: It is not yet clear whether it predisposes to glaucomatous change or merely accompanies it. It could be indicative of an area of greater glaucomatous susceptibility. On the other hand it could be an entry door to various circulating vasoconstricting substances due to an altered blood retinal barrier making the optic nerve more susceptible to ischemic damage. The role of microglia for the development of PPA has also been proposed.[119-125]

Significance
- PPA is more common in glaucomatous eyes. It correlates with the NRR area, optic cup size, RNFL loss and visual field defect. The area of PPA is larger near notches and areas of NRR thinning.
- Alone it is not sufficient to permit differentiation between glaucomatous and nonglaucomatous changes. Observation of the area of PPA has a greater value when assessed along with other disc variables increasing or decreasing the suspicion that a glaucomatous change is present.
- Disc hemorrhages occur more often in eyes with PPA and, if PPA is present, more commonly in the region of its greatest extent.[117,126] The presence of PPA should suggest a more careful examination of the corresponding NRR.
- In eyes with small optic discs, glaucomatous optic nerve damage may be indicated more sensitively by parapapillary changes than by cup-to-disc ratios.
- It is also helpful in differentiating discs with large physiological cups which are less likely to have PPA from discs with glaucomatous cupping.
- In contrast to glaucomatous optic neuropathy, nonglaucomatous optic nerve damage does not usually lead to an enlargement of PPA.

Note Parapapillary chorioretinal atrophy is one among several morphologic variables to detect glaucomatous abnormalities in the optic nerve head. In a ranking list of optic disc variables for the detection of glaucomatous optic nerve damage, it is a variable of second order[72] and is useful for the differentiation of the various types of the primary and secondary open-angle glaucomas.

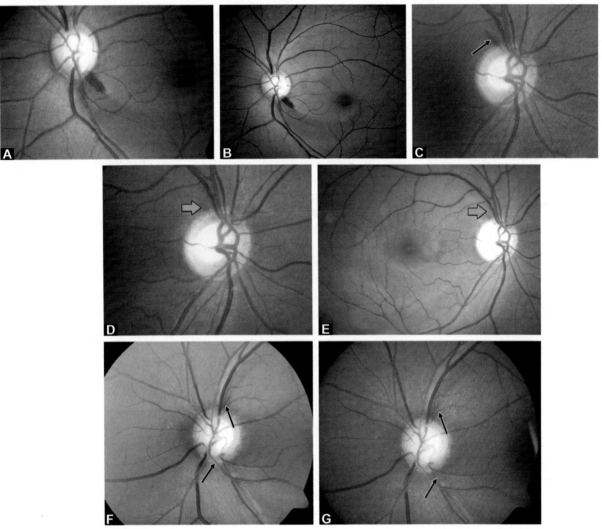

Figs 19A to G (A to C) Color fundus photographs showing the various ways in which a disc hemorrhage may present. They occur most commonly in the inferior temporal and superior temporal sectors in the region of pre-existing RNFLD and notching; (D and E) Color fundus and red free photograph showing a resolving disc hemorrhage with an evolving RNFLD after a few weeks (blue arrows); (F and G) Multiple disc hemorrhages may be present at a given time (black arrows)

Since eyes with nonglaucomatous optic nerve atrophy, including eyes postarteritic anterior ischemic optic neuropathy, do not show an enlargement of parapapillary atrophy, evaluation of the parapapillary atrophy can be helpful in the differential diagnosis of glaucomatous versus nonglaucomatous optic nerve damage.[127-129]

Vascular Signs in Glaucoma
Disc Hemorrhages

The association between optic disc hemorrhage and glaucoma was first described by Bjerrem in 1889.[130] Splinter-shaped or flame-shaped hemorrhages at the border of the optic disc are a hallmark of glaucomatous optic nerve atrophy **(Figures 19A to G)**. Drance and Berg reported the association between disc hemorrhage and development of VFD in glaucoma.[131] These hemorrhages are present in the nerve fiber layer and are thus feathery in shape. They may be located on the retina or cross the disc margin and retina or just at the disc margin. The ones located deep in the lamina cribrosa assume a circular shape. Sometimes the bleeding is minimal and occurs near blood vessels making them difficult to detect. They are transient and usually visible for a few weeks to months and but may recur.[132]

They are usually located in the inferotemporal or temporal superior sectors, although they can occur in any sector on the disc. They tend to occur in association with notching of the neuroretinal rim, retinal nerve fiber layer defects and localized parapapillary atrophy. Their frequency increases from

Table 4 Nonglaucomatous causes of disc hemorrhages

- Posterior vitreous detachment
- Diabetic retinopathy
- Hypertension
- Peripapillary neovascular membranes
- Ischemic optic neuropathy
- Blood dyscrasias
- Vascular occlusive diseases
- Optic disc drusens
- COPD
- Patients on anticoagulants

an early stage of glaucoma to a medium advanced stage and decreases again towards a far advanced stage.[133] While more common in normal tension glaucoma, they can be present in all types. Frequency of detected disc 'bleedings' is lower in patients with juvenile-onset glaucoma, age related atrophic POAG, and highly myopic POAG. Rarely or very rarely found in normal eyes, disc hemorrhages are detected in about 4 to 7 percent of eyes with glaucoma.[133,134]

About 2 months after the initial bleeding, a localized defect of the RNFL or a broadening of a localized RNFL defect can often be detected correlating with the visual field defect.[132-144]

The diagnostic importance of disc hemorrhages is based on their high specificity. In two epidemiologic studies, frequency of disc hemorrhages in nonglaucomatous eyes was about 1 percent.[145,146]

Recurrent optic disc hemorrhage in cases of glaucoma may reflect more rapid optic nerve head damage and progression than a single disc hemorrhage. They have been reported as one of the main risk factors for progression.[147,148]

Glaucoma, however, is not the only optic nerve disease in which optic nerve disc hemorrhages can be found (**Table 4**).

Pathogenesis of Disc Hemorrhages

Disc hemorrhages can be found in all types of the chronic open-angle glaucomas, suggesting that the pathogenic mechanism associated with disc hemorrhages may be present in all these types.

Theories for Pathogenesis

The exact mechanism remains unknown. It has been postulated that the rapid movements of the lamina cribrosa tear the superficial blood vessels of the optic disc, resulting in a break and subsequent circumscribed bleeding. A mechanical effect of IOP may damage the capillary network at the lamina cribrosa. There may also be a weakness in the barrier at capillaries in the prelaminar region. The commonly held belief that disc hemorrhages indicate an ischemic event may be contradicted by the fact that they are never associated with a cotton-wool spot, which is the typical sign for an ischemic infarct in the RNFL.

> **Note** The presence of an optic disc hemorrhage indicates that the process of glaucoma is still active which will be reflected in the subsequent appearance or progression of a structural or functional defect. Such patients should be considered for additional treatment of lowering for IOP and require close monitoring.

Position of the Exit of the Central Retinal Vessel Trunk on the Lamina Cribrosa Surface

The local susceptibility for glaucomatous neuroretinal rim loss partially depends on the distance to the exit of the central retinal vessel trunk on the lamina cribrosa surface. The longer the distance to the central retinal vessel trunk exit, the more marked the glaucomatous loss of neuroretinal rim and the loss of visual field in the corresponding visual field quadrant. The location of the central retinal vessel trunk exit can, therefore, be one of several factors influencing local glaucoma susceptibility. This relationship is also valid for parapapillary atrophy.[149-151] This is in agreement with the spatial relationship between glaucomatous neuroretinal rim loss inside of the optic disc and enlargement of parapapillary atrophy outside of the optic disc border. As mentioned earlier, it can be hypothesized that the retinal vessel trunk could act as a stabilizing element against glaucomatous changes in the lamina cribrosa. Alternatively, the vascular supply to the adjacent tissue is better in close vicinity of the retinal vessel trunk than in the periphery.

Vascular Changes seen on the Optic Disc

As the cup enlarges, the normal course of vessels on the disc may be altered.

Nasalization of Vessels[76,152-155]

Normally, the retinal vessels enter the eye along the nasal border of the optic nerve head. In a large cup, which may be physiological or glaucomatous, the vessels appear nasally displaced as a result of the normal anatomic configuration. Jonas found that in both glaucomatous and normal discs the central retinal artery was located nasal to the vein and both were displaced nasally and superiorly with respect to the vertical and horizontal meridian respectively. The magnitude of the nasal and superior displacement showed a positive correlation with the disc size. It is of little value in differentiating large physiological cups from glaucomatous.

> **Note** Progressive nasalization may occur as a result of progressive NRR loss.[154,155] The change in position of the blood vessels over time may indicate progression of glaucomatous damage.

Bayoneting of Vessels

In areas where the neuroretinal rim is thin or absent, a retinal vessel may pass under the overhanging edge of the cup and make a sharp bend as this crosses the cup margin. This is known as **bayoneting**. It is due to the neural tissue loss extending below the edge and is named so because of its resemblance to the sharp angle of a rifle bayonet. The bayonet must not be mistaken for a blood vessel that perforates the neuroretinal rim which is a normal sign.

> **Note** Bayoneting is rarely seen in normal discs even in the presence of a large physiological cup.

Overpass Vessels

Normally, the retinal vessels crossing the disc margin pass on or through the surface of the neuroretinal rim. If the underlying rim is lost, the vessel may appear to "hang in the air" without any contact with the underlying tissue. This is known as "overpass vessel".[156]

Narrowing of Retinal Arterioles

Diffuse and focal[157] arteriolar narrowing occurs frequently in glaucoma but also in nonglaucomatous optic atrophy. Eyes with advanced glaucoma show a greater degree of narrowing. In normal eyes arterioles become progressively narrower as they branch towards the periphery. Focal arteriolar narrowing implies that the diameter of an arteriole is narrower at the immediate region around the optic disc compared to its diameter in a more peripheral region of the retina.

Studies have noted that the vessel diameter reduces with decreasing area of the neuroretinal rim, diminishing visibility of the RNFL and increasing visual field defects.[158] When compared to age matched controls with patients with NTG a significantly greater narrowing has been seen. It is more localized to the area of greater rim loss and increases with significantly increasing NRR loss. The mechanism responsible for this lumen stenosis could be an autoregulatory response secondary to a decreased metabolic demand or secondary to vasoactive substances.

> **Note** The importance of focal arteriolar narrowing in glaucoma has not been well established. It is typical of optic nerve damage but not characteristic of glaucoma as the reduction of the vessel caliber is also found in eyes with nonglaucomatous optic nerve damage, such as descending optic nerve atrophy[129,159] and nonarteritic anterior ischemic optic neuropathy.

Baring of Circumlinear Vessel

Baring of circumlinear vessel (BCLV) is a clinical sign first described by Herschler and Osher.[160,161] A circumlinear vessel is a small branch of the central retinal vein or artery following a curved path along the optic cup margin. When the cup enlarges, the margin recedes from the vessel leaving a space between the margin and the vessel **(Figure 20A)**. It is often present in glaucomatous discs. However, the presence of BCLV is not specific for glaucoma. It may also be seen in large physiological cups and other diseases of the optic nerve. Sutton et al. reported the presence of BCLV in 14 percent of normal eyes.[162]

> Practically, the presence of a BCLV should prompt an examiner to look for other signs of glaucoma. In conjunction with other signs it is highly suggestive of glaucomatous damage to the ONH.

Collaterals[163,164]

Collaterals on the optic disc occur in 3 percent of patients with glaucoma or ocular hypertension **(Figure 20B)**. They occur as a result of chronic obstruction of venous efflux. Pre-existing blood vessels become patent to allow redirection of blood flow from an obstructed site and represent a communication between central retinal vein and parapapillary choroidal vessels or between two retinal veins. The mechanism of collateral formation in glaucoma is not clear. Some factors responsible could be increased IOP, arteriosclerosis and structural changes associated with optic disc cupping. Mechanical stretching of the blood vessels and a loss of supporting tissue could make the blood vessels more sensitive to the raised IOP leading to venous obstruction and development of collaterals. Although associated with glaucoma they are not specific. They can also occur as a congenital anomaly or in any condition associated with optic nerve and central retinal venous obstruction like meningiomas of the optic nerve sheath, orbital lesions and chronic papilledema.

Acquired Pit of the Optic Nerve

Acquired pit of the optic nerve (APON)[165] represents a deep localized excavation in the neuroretinal rim with a sharply localized depression and

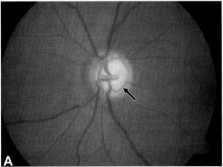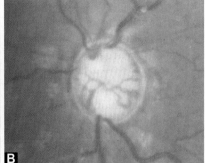

Figs 20A and B (A) Disc photograph showing baring of the circumlinear vessel (arrow) along with an inferior notching of the NRR; (B) Disc photograph showing collaterals in an advanced case of glaucoma

loss of normalized architecture of the lamina cribrosa. The affected area is pale with little or no remaining NRR. It is more localized, well defined and pronounced than a notch. Its presence is pathognomic of glaucoma. The most common location is in the inferotemporal part of the disc in 70 to 80 percent cases, followed by the superior. The low density of pores in the lamina cribrosa in these regions makes them more susceptible to structural changes. APONs are seen more commonly in normal tension glaucoma and are associated with VFD close to or involving fixation.

The difference between a notch and an acquired pit is that an APON is a localized loss of optic nerve tissue extending deep into the lamina and disc margin. The notch does not extend deep into the lamina and there is no focal laminar insufficiency. They also differ from congenital pits of the optic nerve which are usually in the temporal margin of the optic nerve head and may be associated with serous macular detachment.

Patterns of Glaucomatous Damage to Optic Nerve Head

Various patterns of optic disc alterations have been recognized in patients with glaucoma. Many classification schemes have been proposed to clinically distinguish subtypes of glaucoma based on optic disc appearance. Nicolela and colleagues classified the optic disc appearances into four types: the focal ischemic (FI) disc type; myopic (MY) disc type; senile sclerotic (SS) disc type; and generalized enlargement (GE) disc type.[166] They found that patients with SS were less likely to have a progression of the optic disc morphology and visual field defects than patients with the other types of discs with similar IOPs.[167] One must keep in mind that there is a considerable overlap of clinical features in daily practice. The patterns from various studies are summarized below:

Focal Ischemic Optic Nerve Head

The optic nerve head is usually normal in shape and size. The cupping is characteristic with a steep and distinct edge to the cup, with the deep cup remaining visible as it progresses to manifest rim notches, disc hemorrhages, focal wedge shaped RNFL defects.[168] The remainder of the rim remains intact **(Figure 21A)**. Parapapillary atrophy may not be very prominent.[133] The associated clinical signs are a higher frequency in females, scotomas near fixation and a positive history of migraine.[169] Circulatory abnormalities in the orbital circulation have been demonstrated. The inclusion of the term ischemic is probably based on the clinical impression of frequent disc hemorrhages in these eyes which rarely demonstrate high IOP.[170]

Age Related Atrophic Type (Senile Sclerotic)

The size and shape of the optic nerve head is normal. It is usually associated with diffuse changes in the fundus such as choroidal sclerosis/tessellation. The parapapillary atrophy is prominent, so it is important to distinguish the optic disc margin.[140] The cup is shallow saucerized and often gives a moth eaten appearance. The cupping progresses in a concentric manner and focal changes are uncommon **(Figure 21B)**. Looking for a color contour discrepancy is thus important. Overlooking it often leads to underdiagnosis of the extent of glaucomatous damage. A comparison with the other eye also helps. The visual field defects appear more advanced as compared to the disc changes. Clinical associations are a tessellated fundus, lower IOP, associated hypertension and ischemic heart disease.[166] Disturbances of orbital blood flow velocities have also been noted.[170] The visual field progression is less as compared to other patterns.[167]

Juvenile Open Angle Glaucoma Type (JOAG Type)

The disc is normal in size and shape. The cup is deep and steep edged. Laminar pores are exposed. The enlargement of the cup is concentric with focal changes occurring infrequently **(Figure 21C)**. The disc findings in young patients with glaucoma have been found to be similar to discs subjected to high pressure from a secondary cause (secondary open angle glaucoma).[141]

POAG (Generalized Enlargement)

This pattern is commonly seen in eyes with POAG and high IOP. The ONH is normal in size and shape. There is diffuse and concentric enlargement of the cup due to a more or less homogeneous neuroretinal rim loss. Even though the enlargement is diffuse, a bias towards temporal rim known as "temporal unfolding" may be seen. It should be compared with the other eye and any asymmetry should be noted. Diffuse and focal retinal nerve fiber layer defects are present **(Figure 21D)**. Such a pattern of glaucomatous damage is also commonly seen in pigmentary glaucoma and exfoliation syndrome.[171]

High Myopia Disc Patterns

Myopic discs present a dilemma in the detection and management of glaucoma. Considering that glaucoma is more common in myopes adds to the problem.[63] The problem is further compounded by a low scleral rigidity and a thinner cornea in some myopic eyes. Highly myopic eyes with open angle glaucoma have an abnormally shaped optic disc. The cupping is shallow as compared to normal

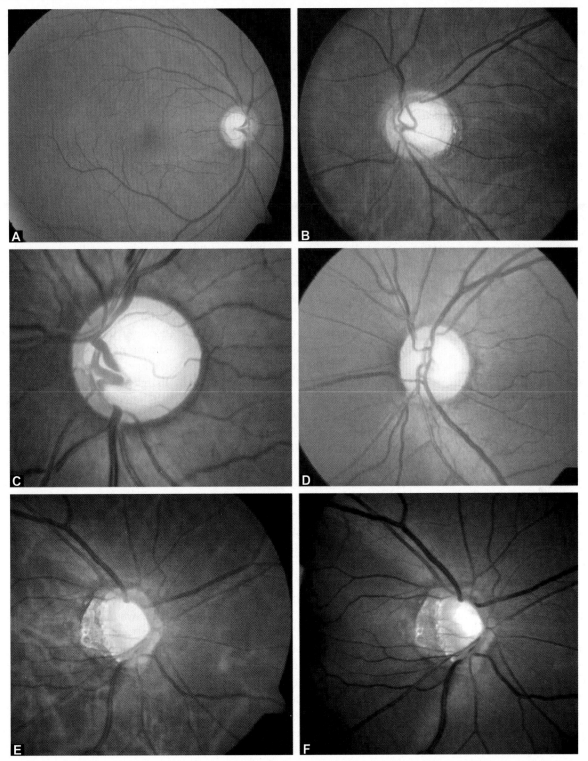

Figs 21A to F Color and red free fundus photographs of various patterns of disc cupping: (A) Focal ischemic type; (B) Senile sclerotic type; (C) JOAG type; (D) POAG or generalized enlargement type; (E and F) Color and red free fundus photographs of high myopic type. Note that the bending of vessels, RNFLD and presence of large beta zone provide valuable clues for the correct assessment of glaucomatous changes in these myopic discs or hyperopic eyes due to a smaller distance between the level of lamina cribrosa and retina.[172] Thus, a cupped myopic disc will have a shallow excavation which may be difficult to appreciate clinically. Furthermore, the cupped myopic disc may be masked by the conus, tilting of the disc and parapapillary atrophy. Clinically, the enlargement of the blindspot may be incorrectly attributed to these factors or vice versa. *In the cupped myopic disc, the key factors aiding in diagnosis are to look for sloping, loss of rim volume and kinking of vessels* (**Figures 21E and F**).

> **Note** It should be emphasized that in a large number of patients optic discs cannot be classified into a single pattern and may show characteristics of more than one group.[173]

Progressive Glaucomatous Damage to the ONH

Identification and monitoring of progressive glaucomatous damage to the optic nerve head is an important part of management of glaucoma. It is central to the management of a patient with established glaucoma as well as one who is perceived to be at a high risk of developing glaucoma, e.g. ocular hypertensives. This helps in assessing the immediate and long-term risk of functional visual loss and the efficacy of treatment. Change means an alteration in the optic nerve head appearance in comparison to its previous appearance. Clinical examination and drawings are subjective and not very accurate. Stereo-disc photographs especially simultaneous are a better option. However, with these too the examination is subjective, depending upon the quality of the photographs, magnification and the skill of the examiner. While evaluating disc photographs for progression one should observe and compare changes in contour with clues given by bending of vessels and any BCLV. One should compare each

sector of the neuroretinal rim including the nasal one. Any changes in RNFL, enlargement of PPA and presence of disc hemorrhage should be noted (**Table 5**).

SUMMARY OF SOME COMMONLY USED DISC EVALUATION TERMS[174]

Disc margin: The inner edge of the peripapillary scleral ring of Elschnig.

Cup margin: When the cup is steep and punched out and the demarcation of the cup margin is clear. Bending of vessels provides valuable clues.[174, 175]

Neural rim: The area between disc margin and cup margin.

Contour cup versus pallor cup: The glaucomatous process causes a progressive backward bowing of the ONH tissue which may result in changes in contour. It may lead to a fairly deep extension of the cup in one direction or a gentler sloping. With the loss of substance there is a loss of color also. However, the key parameter is the change in contour or the ***contour cup*** rather than ***the pallor cup***.

Sloping rims refers to more horizontally or obliquely arranged nerve fibers at the optic nerve head.

Steep rims represent a more compact arrangement of nerve fibers which bend posteriorly at an almost 90° angle at the optic disc.[42]

Saucerization (as in a saucer plate): Refers to a mild change in depth of the rim. The term has evolved to indicate a subtle change in the rim contour, in the early course of the disease. There is a mild change in depth and is a pattern of early glaucomatous change in which diffuse shallow cupping extends to the disc margin with retention of the central pale cup.

Chandler and Grant[174] used the term to indicate an uncommon, more generalized backward bowing in the periphery of a part of the disc or the whole disc like a saucer plate in contrast to excavation where it may

Table 5 Signs of progressive ONH damage

- Changes in NRR contour
- Development/enlargement of a notch
- Shift in position of blood vessels
- Disc hemorrhage especially recurrent
- Progressive changes in RNFL
- Enlargement of PPA (beta zone)
- Development of focal NRR pallor

resemble the contour of a teacup. It usually involves more than one quadrant, sometimes the entire disc. The nasal quadrant may also be involved. It is rare and indicates an early change. A visual field defect may not be present (**Figures 22A and B**).

Focal saucerization refers to a more localized shallow sloping cup usually in the inferotemporal quadrant. The normal neural rim color may be retained initially *(tinted hollow)* but as the glaucomatous damage progresses it is replaced by a grey area *(shadow sign)* and an increased visibility of laminar pores *(laminar dot sign)*.

Shelving: Intermediate change in depth of the rim (**Figure 22C**).

Excavation: Indicates a precipitous appearance of the wall of the cup (**Figures 22D and E**).

Torsion: The optic disc is considered torted when the vertical axis of the optic disc is rotated more than 15° from the vertical meridian.[100]

Tilting: The optic disc is considered tilted when there was (three-dimensional) angulation of the (anteroposterior) optic cup axis.[100]

Sometimes in an enlarged cup is difficult to evaluate particularly if it is sloped or saucerized. In a saucerized optic nerve head, the area of cupping is larger than the area of pallor and a pink neuroretinal rim slopes to the disc margin. Using a stereoscopic view to determine whether saucerization is present is important. It is also helpful to follow the small vessels as they approach the rim of the ONH. Normally, these

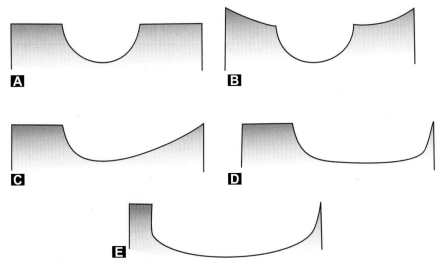

Figs 22A to E (A) A diagram illustrating a cross-sectional view of the physiological cup; (B) Cross-sectional view of a disc with saucerization. Note that there is a backward bowing of the entire rim without any enlargement of the physiological cup; (C) A cross-sectional view showing shelving; (D) Unipolar excavation; (E) Bipolar excavation

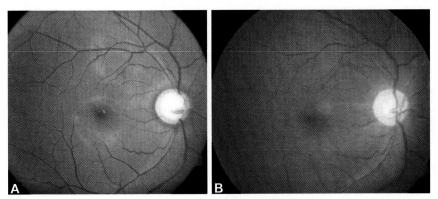

Figs 23A and B Color and red free fundus photographs showing reversal of optic disc cupping after successful surgical lowering of IOP in a young boy with JOAG: (A) Before surgery; (B) After 1 year of surgery. Note the change in the position of the blood vessels

vessels usually travel straight across the neuroretinal rim at the plane of the retina until they reach the cup. If they turn at the edge of the ONII, it suggests that the cup slopes all the way to the edge of the ONH.

Reversal of Cupping

Since axonal loss is irreversible, reversal of cupping is rarely seen in glaucoma. Some conditions where a partial reversal has been observed are children especially in the first year of life following successful control of IOP. However,

it has been reported in adults[176] also after a marked reduction of IOP. In all situations, the reversal is only mechanical and not due to an increase in the neuronal tissue **(Figures 23A and B)**.

GLAUCOMATOUS OR NONGLAUCOMATOUS

Is all Cupping Glaucomatous?

Optic disc cupping is a consequence of a myriad of disorders. Cupping can be seen in neurological disorders which may be life-threatening or treatable. The clinician must be

vigilant to detect such uncommon but potentially threatening causes of optic disc cupping and not mistake them for glaucoma. One must also keep in mind that both conditions can also coexist with known cases of glaucoma developing concomitant neurological disease. On the other hand cupping can be physiological or due to congenital anomalies. The primary distinction between physiologic cupping and pathologic cupping, and *the accurate subclassification* of eyes with pathologic cupping is vitally important.

Certain points are helpful in differentiation. In contrast to glaucomatous optic neuropathy, nonglaucomatous optic nerve damage is not always associated with neuroretinal rim loss and consequently, the shape of the neuroretinal rim is not markedly altered. Also the optic cup does not *markedly* enlarge in eyes with nonglaucomatous optic nerve damage. In addition to parapapillary atrophy, disc pallor, and depth of the optic cup, the increase in cup area is, thus, an important marker to differentiate between glaucomatous and nonglaucomatous optic nerve damage. The other features which may alert the examiner as to a nonglaucomatous cause are listed in **Table 6**.

Some conditions where optic disc cupping is seen in the absence of elevated intraocular pressure (IOP) are as follows **(Figures 24A to C)** (Some important conditions have been explained in detail):

These excavated optic disc anomalies include (apart from glaucoma):

- Congenital or physiological cupping
- Megalopapilla
- Congenital optic-disc anomalies [e.g. coloboma, pits, hypoplasia, tilted discs, ONH drusen, morning glory syndrome, septo-optic dysplasia (DeMorsier)]
- Arteritic anterior ischemic optic neuropathy (AAION) and much

Table 6 Red flags for nonglaucomatous causes of optic disc cupping

- Neuroretinal rim pallor: a greater depth of pallor is seen
- Pallor out of proportion to the degree of cupping (Pallor > Cupping)
- Marked asymmetry between fellow eyes (nonglaucomatous cupping is mostly unilateral or highly asymmetrical)
- Visual-field defects out of proportion and not correlating to the degree of cupping
- Visual field defects not typical of glaucoma
  - ❖ Defects respecting the vertical midline
  - ❖ Temporal > nasal defects
  - ❖ Central scotoma
- Decreased visual acuity out of proportion to the amount of cupping or visual field loss
- Decreased central visual acuity in the early course of disease
- Unilateral or asymmetrical dyschromatopsia
- Relative afferent pupillary defect (RAPD) especially in the presence of CDR asymmetry < 0.3
- Younger age
- Unilateral progression (structural or functional) despite equal IOP in both eyes
- Progression despite well controlled IOP in a glaucomatous eye (after ruling out causes like diurnal variation, adherence)*
- Associated history and clinical findings that are not typical of glaucoma
- A high index of suspicion is required

* Both conditions (glaucoma and nonglaucomatous causes of cupping) can coexist adding to the diagnostic dilemma

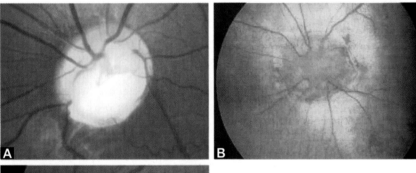

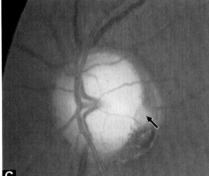

Figs 24A to C (A) Optic disc coloboma; (B) Morning glory disc; (C) Optic disc pit (arrow)

more rarely in posterior ischemic optic neuropathy

- Compression from fusiform aneurysms of the intracranial carotid arteries or tumors compressing the anterior visual pathway
- 'Shock' optic neuropathy
- Traumatic optic neuropathy
- Hereditary (Leber's and autosomal dominant optic neuropathies)
- Radiation optic neuropathy
- Methanol poisoning
- Excavated optic disc anomalies have been associated with periventricular leukomalacia and papillorenal syndrome.

Megalopapilla

It is a common variant in which an abnormally large optic disc (greater than 2.1 mm in diameter) retains an otherwise normal configuration.[177,178] This form of megalopapilla is usually bilateral and is often associated with a large cup-to-disc ratio, which almost invariably raises the suspicion of normal tension glaucoma. However, the optic cup is usually round or horizontally oval with no vertical notching or encroachment, so that the horizontal to vertical cup-to-disc ratio remains normal.

Anterior ischemic optic neuropathy

Among the anterior ischemic optic neuropathy (AION) it is giant cell arteritis (GCA) induced AION which is more commonly associa-ted with NRR thinning and cupping closely resembling glaucomatous cupping.[128,179] Disruption of the pial vessels induces ischemia and axonal necrosis ultimately resulting in axonal loss and cupping. Similar to patients with glaucoma, patients with arteritic anterior ischemic optic neuropathy develop glaucoma-like cupping of the optic disc with loss of neuroretinal rim and deepening of the optic cup especially in end stage. Several features distinguish the cupping produced by arteritic AION from the classic cupping of glaucoma. **The location of pallor** seems to be the most useful feature. In glaucoma, pallor usually does not extend beyond the area of the cup. The intensity of the pallor is usually greater in AION and there is no focal loss of the ONH rim in arteritic AION as observed in discs with glaucoma with similar cups. In contrast to glaucoma, arteritic anterior ischemic optic neuropathy does not lead to an enlargement of parapapillary atrophy.

> **Note** Clinical differentiation between glaucomatous and nonglaucomatous changes can at times be challenging. The presence of NRR pallor larger than cupping strongly suggests the presence of nonglaucomatous atrophy. However, in glaucoma associated with high pressure and in end stage cupping in advanced glaucoma. NRR can be found to be pale. A notch of the rim is present in glaucoma but has also been noted in AION. However, in AION even if a notch is present, diffuse pallor of the intact rim differentiates it from glaucoma. An associated diffuse area of pallor is present in AION whereas in glaucoma the intact rim is healthy. Moreover the clinical profile is also characteristic with a history of sudden vision loss in AION.

Compressive lesions

Compressive lesions developing cupping have been described in several case studies.[180-184] Suprasellar lesions, tumors, intracranial aneurysm compressing the optic nerve, are associated with cupping of the optic disc. Kupersmith and Krohn[183] presented the first significant series of 16 patients with lesions compressing the anterior visual pathway that developed glaucoma-like cupping. Later studies by Bianchi-Marzoli et al.[182] found that the cup-to-disc ratio in patients with compressive lesions was greater compared with controls and to the fellow eye. Rarely, retrobulbar compressive lesions may be associated with optic nerve head cupping. They can manifest as asymmetric cupping with visual field defects similar to glaucoma. These discs usually show pallor, temporal cup saucerization and asymmetric cup to disc ratios.

The presence of pallor more than cupping, visual field defects respecting the vertical meridian, age less than 50 years and a best corrected visual acuity of less than 20/40 warrants a neuroimaging. Defective color vision and an RAPD are the other red flags.

Optic disc coloboma

Optic disc coloboma is an inherited dominant trait with variable expressivity and penetrance. It is characterized by a sharply delimited, glistening white, bowl-shaped excavation that occupies an enlarged optic disc **(Figure 24A)**. The excavation is decentered inferiorly, reflecting the position of the embryonic fissure relative to the primitive epithelial papilla. The inferior neuroretinal rim is thin or absent, while the superior neuroretinal rim is relatively spared. Rarely, the entire disc appears excavated; however, the colobomatous nature of the defect can still be appreciated because the excavation is deeper inferiorly.[185] The defect may extend further inferiorly to include the adjacent choroid and retina. Progressive cupping and neuroretinal rim decrease in patients with autosomal dominant optic-nerve coloboma have also been observed.[186]

Morning glory disc anomaly

It is a congenital, funnel-shaped excavation of the posterior fundus that incorporates the optic disc and is named so because of its resemblance to the morning glory flower. Ophthalmoscopically, the disc is markedly enlarged, orange or pink in color, and may appear to be recessed or elevated centrally within the confines of a funnel-shaped peripapillary excavation **(Figure 24B)**. A wide annulus of chorioretinal pigmentary disturbance surrounds the disc within the excavation. The retinal vessels appear increased in number, appear to emerge from the disc periphery, and have an abnormally straight radial configuration. It is unilateral in most cases.

Peripapillary staphyloma

Peripapillary staphyloma is an extremely rare, usually unilateral anomaly, in which a deep fundus excavation surrounds the optic disc. In this condition, the disc is seen at the bottom of the excavated defect and may appear normal or show temporal pallor. The walls and margin of the defect may show atrophic changes in the retinal pigment epithelium and choroid.

Optic disc pit

An optic disc pit is a round or oval, gray, white, or yellowish depression in the optic disc **(Figure 24C)**. Optic pits commonly affect the temporal portion of the optic disc but may be situated in any sector. They are often accompanied by adjacent peripapillary pigment epithelial changes. One or two cilioretinal arteries emerge from the bottom or the margin of the pit in more than 50 percent of cases. Although optic pits are typically unilateral, bilateral pits are seen in 15 percent of cases.[177] In unilateral cases, the affected disc is slightly larger than the normal disc. They should be differentiated from the acquired pits of the optic nerve seen in glaucoma.

Papillorenal syndrome

The papillorenal syndrome, also previously known as renal-coloboma syndrome, was first described by Rieger in 1977.[187] In this syndrome, the centrally excavated optic disc is normal in size, and may be surrounded by variable pigmentary disturbance. Peripheral visual field defects corresponding to areas of retinal hypoplasia are often present. The central optic disc excavation and peripheral field defects can simulate a coloboma as well as normal tension glaucoma. Patients with PAX2 mutations have similar ophthalmologic features and a wider spectrum of renal abnormalities, which may include hypoplasia, variable proteinuria, vesiculoureteral reflux, recurrent pyelonephritis, microhematuria, echogenicity on ultrasound, or high resistance to blood flow on Doppler ultrasound.

Congenital-tilted disc syndrome

The tilted disc syndrome is a non-hereditary, usually bilateral condition in which the superotemporal optic disc is elevated and the inferonasal disc is posteriorly displaced, resulting in an oval-appearing optic disc, with its long axis obliquely oriented. This configuration is accompanied by situs inversus of the retinal vessels, congenital inferonasal conus, thinning of the inferonasal RPE and choroid, and bitemporal hemianopia (refractive scotoma) that does not respect the vertical midline. Histopathologically, the optic nerve enters the eye at an extremely oblique angle, the superior or superotemporal portion of the disc is elevated, and there is posterior

ectasia of the inferior or inferonasal fundus and optic disc. **Tilted optic discs** may or may not have excavation of the ONH. With the displacement of the optic disc peri-pherally with oblique insertions of the vessels it can be difficult to assess the cup-to-disc ratio.

> **Note** The bitemporal hemianopia in patients with tilted discs is typically incomplete and does not respect the vertical meridian, being confined primarily to the superior quadrants. It is, in fact, a refractive scotoma, secondary to regional myopia localized to the inferonasal retina.[188,189]

Methanol toxicity

Following ingestion of methanol, patients experience intoxication followed by a latent period of 24 hours, after which the systemic toxicity begins. This is marked by metabolic acidosis, depressed level of consciousness, stupor, coma, and death. Edema of the disc and peripapillary retina are the first findings followed by optic atrophy and excavation in the severely affected. Rim pallor is seen along with cupping.[190]

Radiotherapy

Optic neuropathy with optic disc cupping is a rare but important complication of **radiotherapy** used in the treatment of cancers of the head and neck.

Optic disc dysplasia

Optic disc dysplasia is a term that connotes a markedly deformed optic disc that fails to conform to any recognizable diagnostic category.

Hereditary optic neuropathies also

produce optic disc cupping. *Dominant optic atrophy (DOA)*, the most common hereditary optic neuropathy, may be associated with optic disc cupping.[191]

Genetic linkage studies have localized the DOA gene *(OPA1)* to a region on chromosome 3. It is diagnosed on the basis of several criteria, often including autosomal dominant inheritance with variable penetrance and expression, insidious onset in the first-two decades of life, and mild-to-moderate symmetrical central or cecocentral vision loss. It is associated with dyschromatopsia, temporal disc pallor, and wedge-shaped temporal excavation of the optic disc.[192]

Optic disc cupping in *Kjer type DOA* can lead to confusion with glaucoma. A triangular cupping with temporal pallor has been described as a characteristic finding. A cup disc ratio of more than 0.5 has been noted in more than 90 percent of the eyes. The patients are younger and the condition bilateral. The patients manifest with characteristic tritanopic color vision defects. The disc pallor is associated with decreased visibility of the papillomacular bundle in red free light on slit-lamp biomicroscopy. The visual field defects are central or cecocentral with sparing of the peripheral visual fields.

Leber's hereditary optic neuropathy

Several cases of nonglaucomatous cupping with leber's hereditary optic neuropathy (LHON) have been reported in the literature. It is a maternally inherited disease (maternal mitochondrial DNA mutation) affecting males between the ages of 10 to 30 years. It is characterized by a slow central visual loss secondary to bilateral optic degeneration. LHON presents with elevation of the disc and peripapillary thickening (in early stages), peripapillary telangiectasias, and tortuous arterioles before visual loss transpires. There is a preferable loss of unmyelinated axons (these have more mitochondria) making the RNFL a more vulnerable site for damage. Cupping may be seen in the atrophic stage. Usually the other associated features of LHON help in differentiating it from glaucoma.[193]

How to Distinguish Nonglaucomatous from Glaucomatous Cupping?

Acquired excavation of the ONH is most frequently associated with glaucoma. Cupping as a result of optic neuropathies other than glaucoma occurs infrequently and inconsistently. Even in the optic neuropathies that produce disc excavation, only very small fractions are considered to have an appearance that may be mistaken for glaucoma. Distinguishing glaucomatous from nonglaucomatous optic disc cupping on clinical examination is difficult. In a study Trobe[194] et al. demonstrated that clinicians can misdiagnose glaucomatous cupping in stereophotographs in a significant number of eyes. Interestingly, 13 out of 29 (44%) eyes with nonglaucomatous optic neuropathy were classified as glaucomatous by at least one out of the three masked observers. However, the case selection was biased towards cases with a difficult differential diagnosed. The characteristic optic disc pallor helpful in differentiating may be absent especially in early cases or masked because of the lenticular changes. A variation in the degree of flash illumination during fundus photography is also an issue.

Common Features

In addition to glaucoma, an enlargement of the optic cup and a loss of neuroretinal rim may be found in patients after arteritic anterior ischemic optic neuropathy and in a few patients with intrasellar or suprasellar tumors. Glaucomatous and nonglaucomatous optic neuropathy have in common both a decreased diameter of the retinal arterioles, including the occurrence of focal arteriole narrowing, and a reduced visibility of the RNFL. Localized RNFL defects can be found in glaucoma and in

many types of nonglaucomatous optic nerve damage, such as in optic disc drusen and long-standing papilledema.

Differentiating Features

Compared with nonglaucomatous optic nerve atrophy, the optic cup enlarges and deepens in glaucomatous optic neuropathy, and, in a complementary manner, the neuroretinal rim decreases. Parapapillary atrophy does not usually occur in eyes with nonglaucomatous optic nerve damage and is helpful for the differentiation of glaucomatous versus nonglaucomatous optic neuropathy. Greenfield[78] found several risk factors that predicted nonglaucomatous causes of optic disc cupping. Age younger than 50 years was 93 percent specific for nonglaucomatous optic atrophy. Optic disc pallor greater than cupping, visual-field defects that obey the vertical meridian, and visual acuity of less than 20/40 were 90 percent, 81 percent, and 77 percent specific for nonglaucomatous cupping, respectively. Visual field defects not correlating with disc changes are suggestive of nonglaucomatous causes of cupping. Glaucomatous patients have larger cup-to-disc ratios, greater vertical elongation of the cup, horizontal visual-field defects, a family history of glaucoma, and more frequent parapapillary atrophy and disc hemorrhages. Glaucomatous nerve fiber loss is usually symmetrical; and asymmetrical colour vision deficits are rare. Other factors are listed in **Table 6**.

Note Neuroimaging is warranted in patients with cupping, normal IOP, visual-field loss, and nonglaucomatous optic atrophy with associated risk factors including age younger than 50 years, visual acuity of less than 20/40, vertically aligned visual-field defects, pallor of the residual neuroretinal rim, field defects approaching the vertical meridian, symmetrical loss of color vision, an afferent pupillary defect, cranial pain, and symptoms of hypothalamic–pituitary dysfunction.

HOW TO DOCUMENT THE APPEARANCE OF THE DISC?
Documentation Techniques
Documentation of the appearance of the optic disc is critical to longitudinal patient care. There are various techniques ranging from simple drawings of the disc to the newer automated technology.

Disc Drawings

Drawings of the optic disc are far more superior to just documentation of the cup disc ratio. They provide more detail about the rim and the cup **(Figure 25)**.

Disc Photographs

Optic nerve head photography is the longest established and most widely used imaging technique. In simple terms it is color picture of the optic disc. In fact, it is the only full color image technology available. Serving as a permanent record of the patients optic nerve in the era of ever changing technology it has the additional benefit of recording features like disc hemorrhages, parapapillary atrophy and rim pallor which are not readily detected by newer automated technology. Traditionally taken by a fundus camera on a 35 mm film, it is now mostly replaced by digital photographs taken on a charged coupled device (CCD). The resolution of the image is determined by the number and size of pixels in the CCD chip. They provide instant good

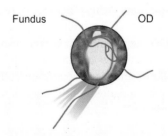

Fig. 25 Disc drawings can be used for documentation of the disc changes in clinical practice

quality images which can be viewed on a computer screen. The added advantage is the easy storage and transfer of mass data which can be used for teaching, telemedicine and research. The photographs may be monoscopic or stereoscopic; the latter preferred due to a better interobserver agreement. But even monoscopic pictures are better than disc drawing. Stereoscopic images may be acquired simultaneously or sequentially. Simultaneous stereophotographs are preferred as they give a more reliable estimation of cup depth and rim changes. These can be viewed on a computer screen with the help of a stereoscope. *Software for newer technologies for disc imaging keeps changing with time. In such a fast changing scenario, disc photos taken 20 years back can easily be compared to a photo taken at any time point making detection of any change simple.*

Serial disc photography can be done to assess progression. In trained hands its sensitivity is fair to good and has been used in clinical trials. It is limited by its reliance on the judgment of expert graders/observers especially for detecting progression. The greatest barrier to the routine clinical use of stereoscopic disc photographs is the lack of viewing systems.

Disc Planimetry

Planimetry provides quantitative optic disc measurements by plotting disc stereophotographs on paper and measuring them manually or with the help of computerized techniques. There is good inter- and intraobserver agreement for experienced observers using planimetry. It is a time consuming technique, and also depends upon the subjective judgment of the edge of the optic disc.

Systems of Staging Disc Damage

Grouping patients into categories, monitoring change, and quantitating the rate of change all require some type of quantitative staging of the amount of damage. In a critical review Spaeth et al. identified eight systems, including the cup/disc ratio system of Armaly.[195] Most of the earlier systems suffer from a failure to take into account the importance of the size of the optic disc. Disc Damage Likelihood Scale (DDLS),[196-198] which appears to offer substantial advantages over the other systems is discussed in detail.

Disc Damage Likelihood Scale (DDLS)

It is a clinical grading scale deviced by Spaeth, based on rim width/disc ratio and incorporates the effect of disc size and focal rim width. It is highly reproducible and correlates with the degree of field loss.

First step-disc classification: The disc is categorized into small (< 1.5 mm), medium (1.5 – 2 mm) or large (>2 mm) (measured on slit-lamp biomicroscopy with condensing lens). Appropriate correction factors for disc size are applied.

Second step-NRR assessment: The width of the thinnest part of the rim is measured. If no rim is present (value = 0), the circumferential extent of absence of the neuroretinal rim is measured in degrees. Caution must be taken to differentiate the actual absence of rim from sloping of the rim as, for example, can occur temporally in some patients with myopia.

There are **10 DDLS stages, (Figure 26)** extending from 1 to 10. Considering average-sized optic discs (1.5 to 2.0 mm of diameter), a DDLS stage 1 would represent a disc with a rim/disc ratio of 0.4 or more at its narrowest position.

Similarly, stage 2 would comprise 0.3 to 0.39 of the narrowest rim/disc ratio, stage 3 from 0.2 to 0.29, stage 4 from 0.1 to 0.19, and stage 5 less than 0.1 (but more than 0).

Rim/disc ratios reach 0 (no rim present at any location) from DDLS stages 6 to 10. These stages are separated by the circumferential extent of rim absence. The circumferential extent of rim absence (0 rim/disc ratio) is measured in degrees. In stage 6 it is less than 45°; in stage 7, between 46° and 90°; in stage 8, between 91° and 180°; in stage 9, between 181° and 270°; in stage 10, more than 270°.

For small discs (diameter less than 1.5 mm) the DDLS stage is increased by 1; for large discs (diameter O 2.0 mm) it is decreased by 1.

Limitations

The DDLS has limitations. The location of rim narrowing is not considered, and non-contiguous areas of less extensive narrowing are not taken into account. There is no room for unclassifiable discs, discs with congenital anomalies or other atypical discs which do not fit well into any staging scale and are best described individually. The rim width characterizations are also subjective. At first sight the DDLS may appear to be complex.

Advantages

The DDLS has been found to be highly reproducible, with higher interobserver and intraobserver reproducibility than Armaly's cup/disc ratio system. The DDLS is useful for four aspects of optic disc examination:
1. Diagnosis
2. Grouping into categories of severity
3. Monitoring change
4. Determining the rate of change.

DDLS Stage	Narrowest width of rim (rim/disc ratio)			DDLS Stage	Examples		
	For Small Disc <1.50 mm	For Average Size Disc 1.50-2.00 mm	For Large Disc >2.00 mm		1.25 mm optic nerve	1.75 mm optic nerve	2.25 mm optic nerve
1	.5 or more	.4 or more	.3 or more	0a			
2	.4 to .49	.3 to .39	.2 to .29	0b			
3	.3 to .39	.2 to .29	.1 to .19	1			
4	.2 to .29	.1 to .19	less than .1	2			
5	.1 to .19	less than .1	0 for less than 45°	3			
6	less than .1	0 for less than 45°	0 for 46° to 90°	4			
7	0 for less than 45°	0 for 46° to 90°	0 for 91° to 180°	5			
8	0 for 46° to 90°	0 for 91° to 180°	0 for 181° to 270°	6			
9	0 for 91° to 180°	0 for 181° to 270°	0 for more than 270°	7a			
10	0 for more than 180°	0 for more than 270°		7b			

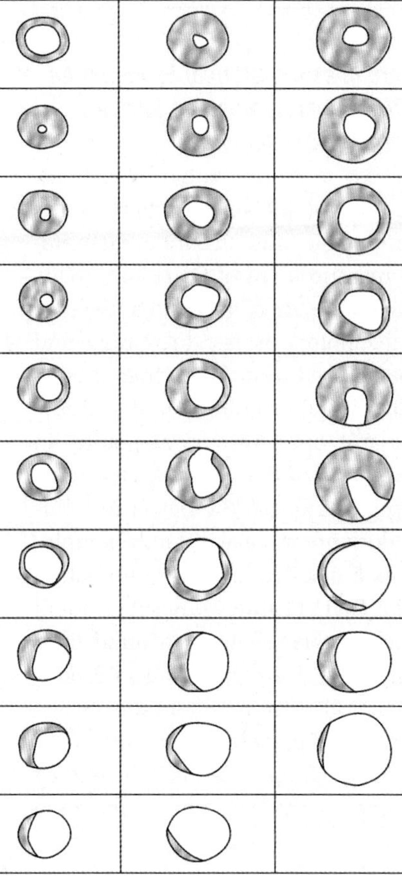

Fig. 26 The Disc Damage Likelihood Scale: Spaeth GL, Henderer J, Liu C, et al. The disc damage likelihood scale. Reproducibility of a new method of estimating the amount of optic nerve damage caused by glaucoma. Trans Am Ophthalmol Soc 2002;100:181-5

The DDLS forces the examiner to determine the disc size and alerts the observer as to which disc is large or small. It also formalizes the evaluation of the NRR. The use of 10 stages of damage makes it possible to grade the amount of deterioration in steps that are far enough apart to allow clinically meaningful separation and yet close enough to permit high sensitivity. Since each grade is assigned a numerical value, it can be used to determine severity or progression.

Newer Technology

Automated devices present an attractive option. They have the potential to quantify parameters and a high inter-individual repeatability. Three devices employing different technologies are commonly used to assess the ONH and RNFL (Optical Coherence tomography: OCT, confocal scanning laser ophthalmoscope: HRT and slit-lamp polarimetry or GDx). The details of these are beyond the scope of this chapter and are discussed separate chapters. Each technique has its advantages and limitations which should be kept in mind while interpreting them. They should be used to compliment and never replace a detailed clinical examination.

- Documentation by disc drawings is not alone adequate to monitor progression
- Baseline stereophotographs are a better option' after photographs
- Newer technology to complement clinical examination.

Where does the Clinical Examination of ONH Stand Against the Various Emerging Technologies?

It is easy to be fascinated by technology. It is fast and simple, offers a fairly reproducible and accurate quantitative measurement of ONH and RNFL. In fact there are concerns that reliance on technology is fast increasing and is being used more often than a thorough clinical examination, disc drawings and optic disc photographs in some parts of the world.[199] One must keep in mind that the newer technology does not replace but only complements a detailed clinical examination of the ONH **(Table 7)**. Results should be interpreted keeping in mind their limitations. A detailed clinical examination is also important for the clinical diagnosis of glaucoma in a busy practice in which these recently developed imaging techniques such as scanning laser tomography or retinal nerve fiber layer polarimetry are not yet available. A thorough clinical examination may additionally show the value of certain optic nerve head variables, such as parapapillary atrophy, torsion, pallor that cannot reliably be measured by confocal scanning laser tomography or polarimetry **(Figure 27)**.

CONCLUSION

Ideally, we should be able to identify glaucoma in its earliest stages. By the time patients experience visual field loss on standard achromatic perimetry, they have already progressed from early to moderate disease. Studies, including histologic evaluations, have shown that optic nerve abnormalities, retinal ganglion cell death and defects in the retinal nerve fiber layer (RNFL) precede visual field defects by as much as 6 years. As glaucoma progresses from optic nerve damage to visual field loss, we can observe a distinct correlation between optic nerve structure and function. Quadrants with fewer axons correlate with regions of greatest field loss.[2] Clinical measurements of the disc rim and RNFL thickness correlate quantitatively with visual function in glaucoma.[5,6] Thus, it is important that we monitor and document early optic nerve changes. Unfortunately, a high degree of variability in optic nerve morphology among healthy people can make it difficult to detect early glaucomatous changes. For this reason, we must be especially vigilant when evaluating high-risk patients. A detailed examination of the ONH, RNFL and the parapapillary area along with disc drawings and stereodisc photography can be done to document degenerative changes in the optic nerve. Although stereodisc photography is still the *gold standard*, new user-friendly computerized imaging techniques are providing a unique perspective on assessing and tracking disease progression. These complement the clinical examination and documentation but do not replace it. Focusing our diagnostic acumen on the optic nerve head can help us detect glaucoma earlier, giving us a chance to prevent progressive visual field loss. It is worthwhile to start with the basics and perform a thorough clinical evaluation of the ONH and document it.

Table 7 Steps in clinical examination of ONH

1.	Determine disc size
2.	Check for unusual disc shape
3.	Determine the vertical cup to disc ratio
4.	Determine cup and rim size in relation to disc size
5.	Evaluate rim shape (which is the narrowest rim) and apply the ISNT rule
6.	Check RNFL (red free illumination)
7.	Look for disc hemorrhages
8.	Look for vascular changes: Bending of vessels, BCLV, collaterals anteriolar constriction
9.	Parapapillary atrophy (Beta zone)
10.	High myopia: Rule out glaucoma
11.	Rule out nonglaucomatous causes of cupping
12.	Correlate visual fields with optic disc changes

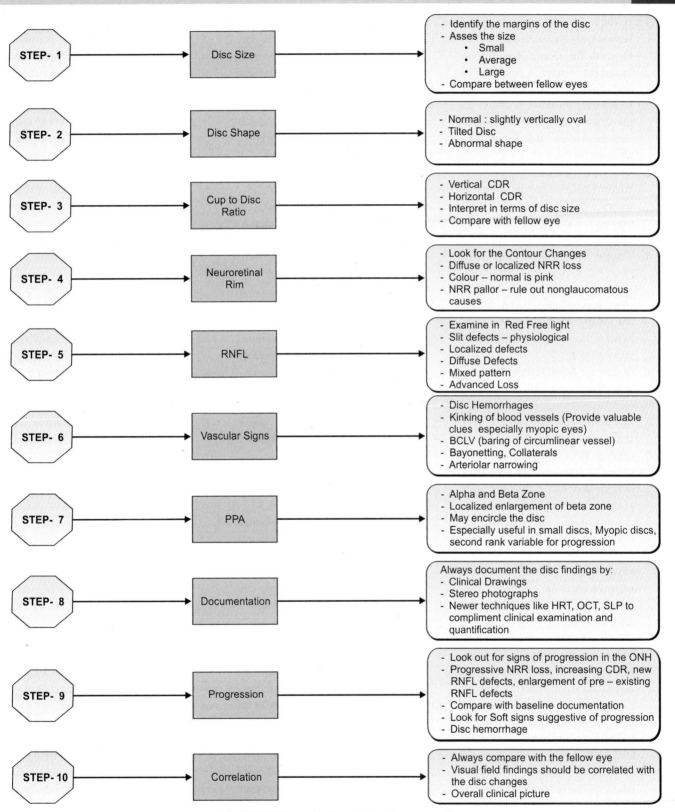

STEP- 1 → Disc Size →
- Identify the margins of the disc
- Asses the size
  - Small
  - Average
  - Large
- Compare between fellow eyes

STEP- 2 → Disc Shape →
- Normal : slightly vertically oval
- Tilted Disc
- Abnormal shape

STEP- 3 → Cup to Disc Ratio →
- Vertical CDR
- Horizontal CDR
- Interpret in terms of disc size
- Compare with fellow eye

STEP- 4 → Neuroretinal Rim →
- Look for the Contour Changes
- Diffuse or localized NRR loss
- Colour – normal is pink
- NRR pallor – rule out nonglaucomatous causes

STEP- 5 → RNFL →
- Examine in Red Free light
- Slit defects – physiological
- Localized defects
- Diffuse Defects
- Mixed pattern
- Advanced Loss

STEP- 6 → Vascular Signs →
- Disc Hemorrhages
- Kinking of blood vessels (Provide valuable clues especially myopic eyes)
- BCLV (baring of circumlinear vessel)
- Bayonetting, Collaterals
- Arteriolar narrowing

STEP- 7 → PPA →
- Alpha and Beta Zone
- Localized enlargement of beta zone
- May encircle the disc
- Especially useful in small discs, Myopic discs, second rank variable for progression

STEP- 8 → Documentation →
Always document the disc findings by:
- Clinical Drawings
- Stereo photographs
- Newer techniques like HRT, OCT, SLP to compliment clinical examination and quantification

STEP- 9 → Progression →
- Look out for signs of progression in the ONH
- Progressive NRR loss, increasing CDR, new RNFL defects, enlargement of pre – existing RNFL defects
- Compare with baseline documentation
- Look for Soft signs suggestive of progression
- Disc hemorrhage

STEP- 10 → Correlation →
- Always compare with the fellow eye
- Visual field findings should be correlated with the disc changes
- Overall clinical picture

Fig. 27 ONH examination: A stepwise approach

REFERENCES

1. Kass MA, Heuer DK, Higginbotham EJ, et al. The Ocular Hypertension Treatment Study: a randomized trial determines that topical ocular hypotensive medication delays or prevents the onset of primary open-angle glaucoma. Arch Ophthalmol 2002;120:701-13.

2. Harwerth RS, Carter-Dawson L, Smith EL 3rd, et al. Neural losses correlated with visual losses in clinical perimetry. Invest Ophthalmol Vis Sci 2004;45:3152-60.

3. Kerrigan-Baumrind LA, Quigley HA, Pease ME, Kerrigan DF, Mitchell RS. Number of ganglion cells in glaucoma eyes compared with threshold visual field tests in the same persons. Invest Ophthalmol Vis Sci 2000;41:741-8.

4. Quigley HA, Dunkelberger GR, Green WR. Retinal ganglion cell atrophy correlated with automated perimetry in human eyes with glaucoma. Am J Ophthalmol 1989;107:453-64.

5. Quigley HA, Katz J, Derick RJ, Gilbert D, Sommer A. An evaluation of optic disc and nerve fiber layer examinations in monitoring progression of early glaucoma damage. Ophthalmol 1992;99:19-28.

6. Sommer A, Katz J, Quigley HA, et al. Clinically detectable nerve fiber atrophy precedes the onset of glaucomatous field loss. Arch Ophthalmol 1991;109:77-83.

7. Quigley HA, Addicks EM, Green WR, Maumenee AE. Optic nerve damage in human glaucoma, III: quantitative correlation of nerve fiber loss and visual field defect in glaucoma, ischemic optic neuropathy, papilledema and toxic neuropathy. Arch Ophthalmol 1982;100:135-46.

8. Sommer A, Pollack I, Maumenee AE. Optic disc parameters and onset of glaucomatous visual field loss, I. methods and progressive changes in disc morphology. Arch Ophthalmol 1979;97:1444-8.

9. Pederson JE, Anderson DR. The mode of progressive disc cupping in ocular hypertension and glaucoma. Arch Ophthalmol 1980;98:490-5.

10. Balazsi AG, Drance SM, Schulzer M, Douglas GR. Neuroretinal rim area in suspected glaucoma and early open-angle glaucoma. Correlations with parameters of visual function. Arch Ophthalmol 1984;102:1011-4.

11. Caprioli J, Miller JM, Sears M. Quantitative evaluation of the optic nerve head in patients with unilateral visual field loss from primary open-angle glaucoma. Ophthalmol 1987; 94:1484-7.

12. American Academy of Ophthalmology: Primary open angle glaucoma preferred practice patterns, San Francisco, American Academy of Ophthalmology; 2005.

13. Foster PJ, Buhrmann R, Quigley HA, Johnson GJ. The definition and classification of glaucoma in prevalence surveys. Br J Ophthalmol 2002;86:238-42.

14. Curcio CA, Allen KA. Topography of ganglion cells in human retina. Int J Neurosci 1972;4:77.

15. Radius RL, Anderson DR. The course of axons through the retina and optic nerve head. Arch Ophthalmol 1979;1154.

16. Aramaly MF. Genetic determinants of cup/disc ratio of the optic nerve. Arch Ophthalmol 1967;78:25.

17. Hayreh SS. The blood supply of the optic nerve head and the evaluation of it-myth and reality. Prog Retin Eye Res 2001;20:563.

18. Onda E, Cioffi GA, Bacon DR, et al. Microvasculature of the human optic nerve. Am J Ophthalmol 1995;120:92.

19. Lieberman MF, Maumenee AE, Green WR. Histologic studies of the vasculature of the anterior optic nerve. Am J Ophthalmol 1976;82:405.

20. Anderson DR, Braverman S. Re-evaluation of the optic disk vasculature. Am J Ophthalmol 1976;82:165.

21. Ko MK, Kim DS, Ahn YK. Morphological variation of the peripapillary circle of Zinn-Haller by flat section. Br J Ophthalmol 1999;83:862.

22. Goder G. The capillaries of the optic nerve. Am J Ophthalmol 1974;77:684.

23. Zaret CR, Choromokos EA, Meisler DM. Cilio-optic vein associated with phakomatosis. Ophthalmol 1980;87: 330.

24. Hayreh SS. Structure and blood supply of the optic nerve. In: Heilmann K, Richardson KT (Eds). Glaucoma: Conceptions of a Disease. Stuttgart: Thieme; 1978.pp.78-96.

25. Trivino A, Ramirez JM. Salazar JJ, et al. Immunohistochemical study of human optic nerve head astroglia. Vision Res 1996;36:2015.

26. Anderson DR, Hoyt WF, Hogan MJ. The fine structure of the astroglia in the human optic nerve and optic nerve head. Trans Am Ophthalmol Soc 1967;65:275.

27. Anderson DR. Ultrastructure of the optic nerve head. Arch Ophthalmol 1970;83:63.

28. Anderson DR, Hoyt WF. Ultrastructure of intraorbital portion of human and monkey optic nerve. Arch Ophthalmol 1969;82:506.

29. Heegaard, Jensen OA, Prause JU. Structure of the vitreous face of the monkey optic disc (Macaca Mulatta). SEM on frozen resin-cracked optic nerve heads supplemented by TEM and immunohistochemistry. Graefes Arch Clin Exp Ophthalmol 1988;226:377.

30. Hernandez MR. The optic nerve head in glaucoma. Role of astrocytes in tissue remodeling. Prog Retin eye Res 2000;19:297.

31. Maeda H, Nakamura M, Yamamoto M. Morphometric features of laminar cribrosa observed by scanning laser ophthalmoscopy. Jpn J Ophthalmol 1999;43:415.

32. Quigley HA, Addicks EM. Regional differences in the structure of the lamina cribrosa and their relation to

glaucomatous optic nerve damage. Arch Ophthalmol 1981;99:137.

33. Radius RL, Gonzales M. Anatomy of the lamina cribrosa in human eyes. Arch Ophthalmol 1981;99:2159.

34. Radius RL. Regional specificity in anatomy at the lamina cribrosa. Arch Ophthalmol 1981;99:478.

35. Jonas JB, Mardin CY, Schlotzer-Schrehardt U, et al. Morphometry of the human lamina cribrosa surface. Invest Ophthalmol Vis Sci 1991; 32:401.

36. Hernandez MR, Luo XX, Igoe F, et al. Extracellular martix of the human lamina cribrosa. Am J Ophthalmol 1987;104:567.

37. Rehnberg M, Ammitzboll T, Tengroth B. Collagen distribution in the lamina cribrosa and the trabecular meshwork of the human eye. Br J Ophthalmol 1987;71:886.

38. Goldbaum MH, Jeng SY, Logemann R, et al. The extracellular matrix of the human optic nerve. Arch Ophthalmol 1989;107:1225.

39. Bengtsson B. The variation and covariation of cup and disk diameters. Acta Ophthalmol 1976;54:804-18.

40. Betz P, Camps F, Collignon-Brach J, et al. Biometric study of the disk cup in open-angle glaucoma. Graefes Arch Clin Exp Ophthalmol 1982;218: 70-4.

41. Franceschetti A, Bock RH. Megalopapilla. A new congenital anomaly. Am J Ophthalmol 1950;33: 227-35.

42. Jonas JB, Gusek GC, Naumann GOH. Optic disk, cup and neuroretinal rim size, configuration, and correlations in normal eyes. Invest Ophthalmol Vis Sci 1988;29:1151-8.

43. Ramrattan RS, Rolfs RCW, Hoffman A, de Jong PTVM. Are gender differences in disk and rim area due to differences in refractive error or height? The Rotterdam Study . Invest Ophthalmol Vis Sci 1997;38:S824.

44. Tomita G, Takamoto T, Schwartz B. Glaucoma like disks without increased intraocular pressure or visual field loss. Am J Ophthalmol 1989; 108:496-505.

45. Varma R, Tielsch JM, Quigley HA, et al. Race-, age-, gender and refractive error- related differences in the normal optic disk. Arch Ophthalmol 1994;112:1068-76.

46. Sekhar GC, Prasad K, Dandona R, John RK, Dandona L. Planimetric optic disc parameters in normal eyes: a population-based study in South India. Indian J Ophthalmol 2001;49: 19-23.

47. Jonas JB, Thomas R, George R, et al. Optic disc morphology in south India. The Vellore Eye Study. Br J Ophthalmol 2003;87:189-96.

48. Agarwal HC, Gulati V, Sihota R. The normal optic nerve head on heidelberg retina tomograph II. Indian J Ophthalmol 2003;51:25-33.

49. Ramakrishnan R, Kader MA, Budde WM. Optic disc morphometry with optical coherence tomography. Comparison with planimetry of fundus photographs and influence of parapapillary atrophy and pigmentary conus. Indian J Ophthalmol 2005;53:187-91.

50. Nangia V, Matin A, Bhojwani K, et al. Optic disc size in a population based study in central India. The Central India Eye and Medical Study (CIEMS). Acta Ophthalmol 2008:86: 103-4.

51. Arvind H, George R, Raju P, et al. Neural rim characteristics of healthy South Indians. The Chennai Glaucoma Study. Invest Ophthalmol Vis Sci 2008;49:3457-64.

52. Jonas JB, Gusek GC, Naumann GOH. Optic disk morphometry in high myopia. Graefes Arch Clin Exp Ophthalmol 1988;226:587-90.

52a. Jonas JB. Optic disc size correlated with refractive error. Am J Ophthalmol 2005;139:346-8.

53. Gross P, Drance S. Comparison of simple ophthalmoscopic and planimetric measurement of glaucomatous neuroretinal rim areas. J Glaucoma 1995;4:314-6.

54. Haslett RS, Batterbury M, Cuypers M, Cooper RL. Interobserver agreement in clinical optic disc measurement using a modified 60 d lens. Eye 1997;11:692-7.

55. Spencer AF, Vernon SA. Optic disc measurement. A comparison of indirect ophthalmoscopic methods. Br J Ophthalmol 1995;79:910-5.

56. Garway-Heath DF, Rudnicka AR, Lowe T, et al. Measurement of optic disc size: Equivalence of methods to correct for ocular magnification. Br J Ophthalmol 1998; 82: 643-9.

57. Jonas JB, Papastathopoulos K. Ophthalmoscopic measurement of the optic disc. Ophthalmol 1995;102: 1102-6.

58. Ansari-Shahrezaei S, Maar N, Biowski R, Stur M. Biomicroscopic measurement of the optic disc with a high-power positive lens. Invest Ophthalmol Vis Sci 2001;42: 153-7.

59. Sussana Jr R, Vessani RM. New findings in the evaluation of the optic disc in glaucoma diagnosis. Curr Opin Ophthalmol 2007;18:122-8.

60. Kirwan JF, Gouws P, Linnell AE, et al. Pharmacological mydriasis and optic disc examination. Br J Ophthalmol 2000;84:894-8.

61. Jonas JB, Papastathopoulos KI. Optic disk shape in glaucoma. Graefes Arch Clin Exp Ophthalmol 1996;234: S167-73.

62. Jonas JB, Kling F, Gründler AE. Optic disk shape, corneal astigmatism and amblyopia. Ophthalmol 1997; 104:1934-7.

63. Perkins ES, Phelps CD. Open-angle glaucoma, ocular hypertension, low-tension glaucoma, and refraction. Arch Ophthalmol 1982;100: 1464-7.

64. Jonas JB, Budde WM, Joonas SP. Ophthalmoscopic Evaluation of the Optic Nerve Head. Surv Ophthalmol 1999;43:293–320.

65. Betz P, Camps F, Collignon-Brach D, Weekers R. Photographic stéréoscopique et photogrammétrie de l'excavation physiologique de la papille. J Fr Ophthalmol 1981;4:193-203.

66. Caprioli J, Miller JM. Optic disk rim area is related to disk size in normal subjects. Arch Ophthalmol 1987;105:1683-5.

67. Varma R, Steinmann WC, Spaeth GL, Wilson RP. Variability in digital analysis of optic disk topography. Graefes Arch Clin Exp Ophthalmol 1988;226:435-42.

68. Jonas JB, Gusek GC, Naumann GOH. Optic disk morphometry in chronic primary open-angle glaucoma. I. Morphometric intrapapillary characteristics. Graefes Arch Clin Exp Ophthalmol 1988;226:522-30.

69. Budde WM, Jonas JB, Martus P, Grundler AE. Influence of optic disc size on neuroretinal rim shape in healthy eyes. J Glaucoma 2000;9:357-62.

70. Sihota R, Srinivasan G, Dada T, et al. Is the ISNT rule violated in early primary open-angle glaucoma: a scanning laser tomography study? Eye 2008;22:819-24.

71. Crowston JG, Hopley CR, Healey PR, et al. The effect of optic disc diameter on vertical cup to disc ratio percentiles in a population based cohort: The Blue Mountain Eye study. Br J Ophthalmol 2004;88:766-70.

72. Jonas JB, Bergua A, Schmitz-Valckenberg P, et al. Ranking of optic disc variables for detection of glaucoma damage. Invest Ophthalmol Vis Sci 2000;41:1764-73.

73. Armaly MF. Cup/disk ratio in early open-angle glaucoma. Doc Ophthalmol 1969;26:526-33.

74. Ramrattan RS, Wolfs RCW, Jonas JB, et al. Determinants of optic disc characteristics in a general population. The Rotterdam Study. Ophthalmol 1999;106:1588-96.

75. Ong L, Mitchell P, Healy PR, et al. Asymmetry in optic disc parameters. The Blue Mountain Eye Study. Invest Ophthalmol Vis Sci 1999;40:849-57.

76. Spaeth GL, Lopez JM, Junk AK, et al. Systems for staging the amount of optic nerve damage in glaucoma. A critical review and new material. Surv Opthalmol 2006;51:293-315.

77. Jonas JB, Fernández MC. Shape of the neuroretinal rim and position of the central retinal vessels in glaucoma. Br J Ophthalmol 1994;78:99-102.

78. Greenfield DS, Siatkowski RM, Glaser JS, et al. The cupped disc. Who needs neuroimaging? Ophthalmol 1998;105:1866-74.

79. Hoyt WF, Newman NM. The earliest observable defect in glaucoma? Lancet 1972;1:692-3.

80. Hoyt WF, Schlicke B, Eckelhoff RJ. Fundoscopic appearance of a nerve fiber bundle defect. Br J Ophthalmol 1972;56:577-83.

81. Quigley HA, Sommer A. How to use nerve fiber layer examination in the management of glaucoma. Trans Am Ophthalmol Soc 1987;85:254-72.

82. Jonas JB, Dichtl A. Evaluation of the retinal nerve fiber layer. Surv Ophthalmol 1996;40:369-78.

83. Jonas JB, Schiro D. Localized wedge shaped defects of the retinal nerve fiber layer in glaucoma. Br J Ophthalmol 1994;78:285-90.

84. Airaksinen PJ, Heijl A. Visual field and RNFL in early glaucoma after optic disk haemorrhage. Acta Ophthalmol 1983;61:186-94.

85. Airaksinen PJ, Mustonen E, Alanku HI. Optic disk haemorrhages precede retinal nerve fibre layer defects in ocular hypertension. Acta Ophthalmol 1981;59:627-41.

86. Quigley HA, Addicks EM. Quantitative studies of retinal nerve fiber layer defects. Arch Ophthalmol 1982;100:807-14.

87. Chihara E, Chihara K. Apparent cleavage of the retinal nerve fiber layer in asymptomatic eyes with high myopia. Graefes Arch Clin Exp Ophthalmol 1992;230:416-20.

88. Chihara E, Matsuoka T, Ogura Y, Matsumara M. Retinal nerve fiber layer defect as an early manifestation of diabetic retinopathy. Ophthalmol 1993;100:1147-51.

89. Jonas JB, Schiro D. Localized retinal nerve fiber layer defects in nonglaucomatous optic nerve atrophy (letter). Graefes Arch Clin Exp Ophthalmol 1994;232:759.

90. Quigley HA, Addicks EM, Green WR, Maumenee AE. Optic nerve damage in human glaucoma: II. The site of injury and susceptibility to damage. Arch Ophthalmol 1981;99:635-49.

91. Sussana Jr. The lamina cribrosa and visual field defects in open angle glaucoma. Can J Ophthalmol 1983;18:124-6.

92. Miller KM, Quigley HA. The clinical appearance of lamina cribrosa as a function of the extent of glaucomatous nerve damage. Ophthalmol 1988;95:135-8.

93. Pena JD, Netland PA, Vidal I, et al. Elastosis of the lamina cribrosa in glaucomatous optic neuropathy. Exp Eye Res 1998;67:517-24.

94. Quigley HA. Neuronal death in glaucoma. Prog Retinal Eye Research 1999;18:39-57.

95. Fontana L, Bhandari A, Fitzke FW, et al. *In vivo* morphometry of the lamina cribrosa and its relation to visual field loss in glaucoma. Curr Eye Res 1998;17:363-9.

96. Elschnig A. Das Colobom am Sehneneintritte und der Conus nach unten. Archiv Ophthalmol 1900;51:391-430.

97. Elschnig A. Der Normale Sehneveneintritt Des Menschlichen Auges. Denkschriften Der Kaiserlichen Akademie Der Wissenschaften. Mathematisch-Naturwissenschaftliche Classe 1901;70:219-304.

98. Bücklers M. Anatomische Untersuchung über die Beziehungen zwischen der senilen und der myopischen circumpapillären Aderhautatrophie: Unter Beifügung eines Falles von

hochgradiger Anisometropie. Archiv Ophthalmol 1929;121:243-83.

99. Primrose J. The incidence of the peripapillary halo glaucomatosus. Trans Ophthalmol Soc UK 1971;89:585-8.

100. Vongphanit J, Mitchell P, Wang JJ. Population prevalence of tilted optic disks and the relationship of this sign to refractive error. Am J Ophthalmol 2002;133:679-85.

101. Dichtl A, Jonas JB, Naumann GOH. Histomorphometry of the optic disc in highly myopic eyes with glaucoma. Br J Ophthalmol 1998;82:286-9.

102. Jonas JB. Clinical implications of peripapillary atrophy in glaucoma. Curr Opin Ophthalmol 2005;16:84-8.

103. Kono Y, Zangwill L, Sample PA, et al. Relationship between parapapillary atrophy and visual field abnormality in primary open-angle glaucoma. Am J Ophthalmol 1999;127:674–80.

104. De Moraes CG, Juthani VJ, Liebmann JM, Teng CC, Tello C, Susanna R, Ritch R. Risk factors for visual field progression in treated glaucoma. Arch Ophthalmol 2011;129(5):562-8.

105. Tezel G, Kolker AE, Wax MB, et al. Parapapillary chorioretinal atrophy in patients with ocular hypertension. II. An evaluation of progressive changes. Arch Ophthalmol 1997;115:1509-14.

106. Tezel G, Dorr D, Kolker AE, et al. Concordance of parapapillary chorioretinal atrophy in ocular hypertension with visual field defects that accompany glaucoma development. Ophthalmol 2000;107:1194-9.

107. Viestenz A, Mardin CY, Langenbucher A, Naumann GO. *In vivo* measurement of autofluorescence in the parapapillary atrophic zone of optic discs with and without glaucomatous atrophy. Klin Monatsbl Augenheilkd 2003;220:545-50.

108. Tezel G, Kass MA, Kolker AE, Wax MB. Comparative optic disc analysis in normal pressure glaucoma, primary open angle glaucoma, and ocular hypertension. Ophthalmol 1996; 103:2105-13.

109. Jonas JB, Xu L. Parapapillary chorioretinal atrophy in normal pressure glaucoma. Am J Ophthalmol 1993;15;115:501-5.

110. Park KH, Park SJ, Lee YJ, et al. Ability of peripapillary atrophy parameters to differentiate normal-tension glaucoma from glaucoma-like disk. J Glaucoma 2001;10:95-101.

111. Quigley HA, Enger C, Katz J, et al. Risk factors for the development of glaucomatous visual field loss in ocular hypertension. Arch Ophthalmol 1994;112:644-9.

112. Uchida H, Ugurlu S, Caprioli J. Increasing peripapillary atrophy is associated with progressive glaucoma. Ophthalmol 1998;105:1541-5.

113. Araie M, Sekine M, Suzuki Y, Koseki N. Factors contributing to the progression of visual field damage in eyes with normal tension glaucoma. Ophthalmol 1994;101:1440-4.

114. Jonas JB, Budde WM. Diagnosis and pathogenesis of glaucomatous optic neuropathy. Morphological aspects. Prog Retin Eye Res 2000;19:1-40.

115. Kwon YH, Kim YI, Pereira ML, et al. Rate of optic disc cup progression in treated primary open-angle glaucoma. J Glaucoma 2003;12:409-16.

116. Teng CC, De Mores CGV, Prata TS, et al. Beta-zone parapapillary atrophy and the velocity of glaucoma progression. Ophthalmol 2010;117:909-15.

117. Ahn JK, Kang JH, Park KH. Correlation between a disc hemorrhage and peripapillary atrophy in glaucoma patients with a unilateral disc hemorrhage. J Glaucoma 2004;13:9-14.

118. Law SK, Choe R, Caprioli J. Optic disk characteristics before the occurrence of disk hemorrhage in glaucoma patients. Am J Ophthalmol 2001; 132:411-3.

119. Hayreh SS. *In vivo* choroidal circulation and its watershed zones. Eye 1990;4:273-89.

120. Cioffi GA, Van Buskirk EM. Micro-vasculature of the anterior optic nerve. Surv Ophthalmol 1994;38:S107-16.

121. Raitta C, Sarmela T, Fluorescein angiography of the optic disc and the peripapillary area in chronic glaucoma. Acta Ophthalmol 1970; 48:303-8.

122. Ulrich A, Ulrich C, Barth T, et al. Detection of disturbed autoregulation of the peripapillary choroid in primary open angle glaucoma. Ophthalmic Surg Lasers 1996;27:746-57.

123. O'Brart DPS, de Souza Lima M, Bartsch DU, et al. Indocyanine green angiography of the peripapillary region in glaucomatous eyes by confocal scanning laser ophthalmoscopy. Am J Ophthalmol 1997;123:657-66.

124. Neufeld AH. Microglia in the optic nerve and the region of parapapillary chorioretinal atrophy in glaucoma. Arch Ophthalmol 1998;117:1050-6.

125. Yan, Neufeld AH. Activated microglia in the human glaucomatous optic nerve head. J Neurosci Res 2001;64:523-32.

126. Radcliffe NM, Liebmann JM, Rozenbaum I, et al. Anatomic relationships between disc hemorrhage and parapapillary atrophy. Am J Ophthalmol 2008;146:735-40.

127. Rath EZ, Rehany U, Linn S, Rumelt S. Correlation between optic disc atrophy and aetiology. Anterior ischaemic optic neuropathy vs optic neuritis. Eye 2003;17:1019-24.

128. Hayreh SS, Jonas JB. Optic disc morphology after arteritic anterior ischemic optic neuropathy. Ophthalmol 2001;108:1586-94.

129. Jonas JB, Fernández MC, Naumann GOH. Parapapillary atrophy and retinal vessel caliber in nonglaucomatous optic nerve damage. Invest Ophthalmol Vis Sci 1991;32:2942-7.

130. Bjerrum J. Om en Tilfojeke til den Saedvanlige Synsfelfundersogelse samt om Synfeletved Glaukom. Nord Ophthalmol Tskr (Copenh) 1889;2:141-85.

131. Drance SM, Begg IS. Sector hemorrhage. A probable acute disk change in chronic simple glaucoma. Can J Ophthalmol 1970;5:137-41.

132. Heijl A. Frequent disk photography and computerized perimetry in eyes with optic disk haemorrhage. Acta Ophthalmol 1986;64:274-81.

133. Jonas JB, Xu L. Optic disk hemorrhages in glaucoma. Am J Ophthalmol 1994;118:1–8.

134. Jonas JB. What are the ophthalmoscopic signs of glaucomatous optic neuropathy. In: Susanna Jr R, Weinreb RN (Eds). Answers in Glaucoma. Rio de Janeiro. Cultura Me´dica; 2005.

135. Caprioli J. Correlation between disk appearance and type of glaucoma. In: Varma R, Spaeth GL (Eds). The Optic Nerve in Glaucoma. Philadelphia, Lippincott; 1993. pp. 91-8.

136. Drance SM. Disk hemorrhages in the glaucomas. Surv Ophthalmol 1989; 33:331-7.

137. Geijssen HC, Greve EL. The spectrum of primary open-angle glaucoma. I. Senile sclerotic glaucoma versus high tension glaucoma. Ophthalmic Surg 1987;18:207-13.

138. Jonas JB, Dichtl A. Optic disk morphology in myopic primary open-angle glaucoma. Graefes Arch Clin Exp Ophthalmol 1997;235:627-33.

139. Jonas JB, Gründler AE. Optic disk morphology in "age related atrophic glaucoma." Graefes Arch Clin Exp Ophthalmol 1996;234:744-9.

140. Jonas JB, Gründler AE. Optic disk morphology in juvenile primary open-angle glaucoma. Graefes Arch Clin Exp Ophthalmol 1996;234:750-4.

141. Kitazawa Y, Shirato S, Yamamoto T. Optic disk hemorrhage in low-tension glaucoma. Ophthalmol 1986; 93:853-7.

142. Spaeth GL, Katz LJ, Terebuh AK. Managing glaucoma on the basis of tissue damage. A therapeutic approach based largely on the appearance of the optic disk. In: Krieglstein GK (Ed). Glaucoma Update V. Heidelberg, Kaden-Verlag; 1995.pp.118-23.

143. Healey PR, Mitchell P, Smith W, Wang JJ. Optic disk hemorrhages in a population with and without signs of glaucoma. Ophthalmol 1998;105:216-23.

144. Klein BEK, Klein R, Sponsel WE, et al. Prevalence of glaucoma. The Beaver Dam Eye Study. Ophthalmol 1992; 99:1499-504.

145. Kim SH, Park KH. The relationship between recurrent optic disc hemorrhage and glaucoma progression. Ophthalmol 2006;113:598-602.

146. Drance S, Anderson DR, Schulzer M. Risk factors for progression of visual field abnormalities in normal-tension glaucoma. Am J Ophthalmol 2001;131:699-708.

147. Ishida K, Yamamoto T, Sugiyama K, Kitazawa Y. Disk hemorrhage is a significantly negative prognostic factor in normal tension glaucoma. Am J Ophthalmol 2000;129:707-14.

148. Prata TS, Teng CC, et al. Factors Affecting Rates of Visual Field Progression in Glaucoma with Optic Disc Hemorrhages. Ophthalmol 2010;117: 24-9.

149. Jonas JB, Budde WM, Németh J, Gründler AE. Exit of central retinal vessel trunk on the lamina cribrosa and location of parapapillary atrophy in glaucoma. Ophthalmol; 2001. pp.1059-64.

150. Jonas JB, Fernández MC, Naumann GOH. Glaucomatous parapapillary atrophy: Occurrence and correlations. Arch Ophthalmol 1992;110: 214-22.

151. Jonas JB, Naumann GOH. Parapapillary chorioretinal atrophy in normal and glaucoma eyes: II. Correlations. Invest Ophthalmol Vis Sci 1989;30:919-26.

152. Armaly MF. The Optic cup in the Normal Eye. Cup Width, Depth, Vessel Displacement, Ocular Tension and outflow Facility. Am J Ophthalmol 1969;68:401-7.

153. Jonas JB, Mardin CY, Schlotzer-Schrehardt U, GO Naumann GO.9. Morphometry of the human lamina cribrosa surface. Invest Ophthalmol Vis Sci 1991;32:401-5.

154. Varma R, George L, Spaeth GL, Hanu C, Steinmann WC, Feldman RM. Positional Changes in the Vasculature of the Optic Disk in Glaucoma. Am J Ophthalmol 1987;140:457-64.

155. Heuck M, Sonnsjoe B, Krakau CET. Measurement of progressive disc changes in glaucoma. Ophthal Surg Lasers 1992;23:672-9.

156. Kronfeld PC. The optic nerve. Symposium on Glaucoma, St. Louis: Mosby; 1967.p.62.

157. Radar J, Feuer J, Anderson DR. Peripapillary vasoconstriction in the glaucoma and anterior ischemic optic neuropathy. Am J Ophthalmol 1994;117:72-80.

158. Jonas JB, Nguyen XN, Naumann GOH. Parapapillary retinal vessel diameter in normal and glaucoma eyes: I. Morphometric data. Invest Ophthalmol Vis Sci 1989;30:1599-603.

159. Frisén L, Claesson M. Narrowing of the retinal arterioles in descending optic atrophy. A quantitative clinical study. Ophthalmol 1984;91: 1342-6.

160. Herschler J, Osher RH. Baring of the circumlinear vessel. An early sign of optic nerve damage. Arch Ophthalmol 1980;98:865-9.

161. Herschler J, Osher RH. Baring of the circumlinear vessel. A prospective study. Arch Ophthalmol 1981;99:817-8.

162. Sutton EG, Motolko MA, Phleps CD. Baring of the circumlinear vessel in glaucoma. Arch Ophthalmol 1983;101:739-44.

163. Varma R, Spaeth GL, Katz LJ, Robert M, Feldman RM. Collateral Vessel Formation in the Optic Disc in Glaucoma. Arch Ophthalmol 1987;105:1287.

164. Tuulonen A. Asymptomatic Miniocclusions of the Optic Disc Veins in Glaucoma. Arch Ophthalmol 1989; 107:1475-80.

165. Radius RL, Maumenee AE, Green WR. Pit-like changes of the optic nerve head in open-angle glaucoma. Br J Ophthalmol 1978;62:389-93.

166. Nicolela MT, Drance SM. Various glaucomatous optic nerve appearances: clinical correlations. Ophthalmol 1996;103:640-9.

167. Nicolela MT, McCormick TA, Drance SM, et al. Visual field and optic disc progression in patients with different types of optic disc damage: a longitudinal prospective study. Ophthalmol 2003;110:2178-84.

168. Spaeth GL. A new classification of glaucoma including focal glaucoma. Surv Ophthalmol 1994;S9:38.

169. Geijssen HC, Greve EL. Focal ischemic normal pressure glaucoma versus high pressure glaucoma. Doc Ophthalmol 1990;75:291.

170. Nicolela MT, et al. Various glaucomatous optic nerve appearances: a color Doppler imaging study of retrobulbar circulation. Ophthalmol 1996; 103:1670.

171. Jonas JB, Papastathopoulos KI. Optic disk appearance in pseudoexfoliation syndrome. Am J Ophthalmol 1997;123:174.

172. Goldmann H. Problems in present day-glaucoma research. In: Streiff EB, Babel F (Eds). Modern problems in ophthalmology, Basel, S Karger; 1957.

173. Nicolela MT, Drance SM, Broadway DC. Agreement among clinicians in the recognition of patterns of optic disc damage in glaucoma. Am J Ophthalmol 2001;132:836-44.

174. Epstein DL. Examination of the optic nerve. In: Epstein DL, Allingham RR, Schuman JS (Eds), Chandler and Grant's Glaucoma; 1997.p.85-93.

175. Feuer WJ, Parrish RK 2nd, Schiffman JC, et al. The Ocular Hypertension Treatment Study. Reproducibility of cup/disk ratio measurements over time at an optic disc reading center. Am J Ophthalmol 2002;133:19-28.

176. Pederson JE, Herschler J. Reversal of glaucomatous cupping in adults. Arch Ophthalmol 1982;100:246.

177. Brown G, Tasman W. Congenital Anomalies of the Optic Disc. New York, Grune and Stratton; 1983. pp.31-215.

178. Franceschetti A, Bock RH. Megalopapilla: A new congenital anomaly. Am J Ophthalmol 1950;33:227-35.

179. Danesh-Meyer H, Savino PJ, Sergott RC. The prevalence of cupping in endstage arteritic and nonarteritic anterior ischemic optic neuropathy. Ophthalmol 2001;108:593-8.

180. Dutton GN. Congenital disorders of the optic nerve. Excavations and hypoplasia. Eye 2004;18:1038-48.

181. Portney GL, Roth AM. Optic cupping caused by an intracranial aneurysm. Am J Ophthalmol 1982;84:98-103.

182. Bianchi-Marzoli S, Rizzo JF III, Brancato R, Lessell S. Quantitative analysis of optic disc cupping in compressive optic neuropathy. Ophthalmol 1995;102:4-40.

183. Kupersmith MJ, Krohn D. Cupping of the optic disc with compressive lesions of the anterior visual pathway. Ann Ophthalmol 1984;16:948-53.

184. Kalenak JW, Kosmorsky GS, Hassenbusch SJ. Compression of the intracranial optic nerve mimicking unilateral normal-pressure glaucoma. J Clin Neurophthalmol 1992;12:230-5.

185. Dattani M, Martinez-Barbera JP, Thomas PQ, et al. Mutations in the homeobox gene HESX1/HESX1 associated with septo-optic dysplasia in human and mouse. Nat Genet 1998;19:125-33.

186. Moore M, Salles D, Jampol LM. Progressive optic nerve cupping and neural rim decrease in a patient with bilateral autosomal dominant optic nerve colobomas. Am J Ophthalmol 2000;129:517-20.

187. Rieger G. Zum Krankheitsbild der Handmannschen Sehnerven-anomalie: "Windenbluten" -(Morning Glory) Syndrom? Klin Monatsbl Augenheilkd 1977;170:697-706.

188. Flueler UR, Guyton DL. Does a tilted retina cause astigmatism? The ocular imagery and the retinoscopic reflex resulting from a tilted retina. Surv Ophthalmol 1995;40:45-50.

189. Vuori ML, Mäntyjärvi M. Tilted disc syndrome may mimic false visual field deterioration. Acta Ophthalmol 2008;86:622-5.

190. Sharma M, Volpe NJ, Dreyer EB. Methanol-induced optic nerve cupping. Arch Ophthalmol 1999;117:286.

191. Buono LM, Foroozan R, Sergott RC. Unexplained visual loss. Surv Ophthalmol 2003;48:626-30.

192. Kline LB, Glaser JS. Dominant optic atrophy. Arch Ophthalmol 1979;97: 1680-6.

193. Piette SD, Sergott RC. Pathological optic-disc cupping. Curr Opin Ophthalmol 2006;17:1-6.

194. Trobe JD, Glaser JS, Cassady J, Herschler J, Anderson DR. Non-glaucomatous excavation of the optic disc. Arch Ophthalmol 1980;98: 1046-50.

195. Armaly MF. The optic cup in the normal eye. I. Cup width, depth, vessel displacement, ocular tension and outflow facility. Am J Ophthalmol 1969;68:401-7.

196. Spaeth GL, Henderer J, Liu C, et al. The disc damage likelihood scale. Reproducibility of a new method of estimating the amount of optic nerve damage caused by glaucoma. Trans Am Ophthalmol Soc 2002;100:181-5, discussion 185-6.

197. Spaeth GL, Henderer J, Steinmann W. The disc damage likelihood scale, its use in the diagnosis and management of glaucoma. Highlights Ophthalmol 2003;31:4-16.

198. Spaeth GL, Hwang S, Gomes M. Disc damage as a prognostic and therapeutic consideration in the management of patients with glaucoma. In: Grehn F (Ed). Pathogenesis and risk factors of glaucoma. Berlin, New York, Springer; 1999.pp.135-44.

199. Fremont AM, Lee PP, Mangione CM, et al. Patterns of Care for Open-angle Glaucoma in Managed Care. Arch Ophthalmol 2003;121:777-83.

Interpretation of a visual field printout should help to:
- Identify a field defect
- Decide whether the field defect is due to glaucoma
- Set a target IOP
- Decide whether a defect is progressive or not.

Definition of Visual Field

A visual field is defined as that part of the environment that is visible to the steadily fixing eye. The extension is superiorly 60 degrees, temporal 100 degrees, nasal 60 degrees and inferior 75 degrees **(Figures 1 and 2)**.

MEASUREMENTS OF VISUAL FIELDS

The visual field can be measured by kinetic perimetry **(Figure 3)** and static perimetry.

Kinetic Perimetry

When the island hill of vision is kinetically explored along the X-Y axis (i.e. a plane parallel to the surface of the sea), the locations of points with the same threshold are identified. These are isopters **(Figure 3)**.

Disadvantages

It is suprathreshold and is not always reproducible and highly dependent on skill of the technician.

Static Perimetry

When the island of the hill of vision is statically explored along the Z axis (i.e. a plane perpendicular to the surface of the sea), the varying points of sensitivity are identified. These are the thresholds displayed as a meridional cut **(Figure 4)**.

Static perimetry is done to find out the threshold of the retina at various fixed points. It is a technique where the patient looks at a small fixation point, located at the center of a white hemispherical bowl and the light stimuli are briefly presented at fixed stationary locations usually for about 200 milliseconds duration. The patient presses a response button when the stimulus is detected.

Factors affecting the stimulus visibility are stimulus size, background illumination and brightness of the stimulus. Typically, in static perimetry the size of the stimulus and background illumination remain constant, the light intensity is varied according to

staircase (bracketing) procedure which defines the minimum intensity necessary for the detection of stimulus.

Stimulus Size

The standard size for all perimeters is Goldmann size III **(Table 1)**. Size V does not have a normative data and is generally reserved for patients with macular disorders and advanced glaucoma.

Background Illumination

Background illumination for different field analyzer is:
- Octopus 101—4 asb (1.27 cd/m^2)
- Octopus 1-2-3—31.4 asb (10 cd/m^2)
- Humphrey 700—31.5 asb (~10 cd/m^2)
- Dicon—31.5 asb (~10 cd/m^2).

Stimulus intensity is varied by use of attenuation filters. Attenuation of light is expressed in logarithmic unit and is more commonly in tenths of log units which are known as decibel (dB). 1 decibel = 1/10 log unit of attenuation of maximum available stimulus (10,000 asb units for current Humphrey perimeters).

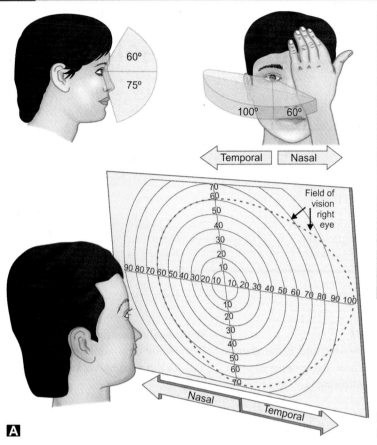

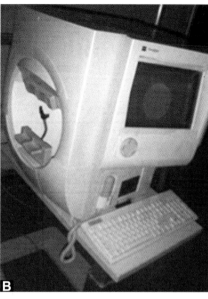

Figs 1A and B (A) Boundaries of the normal visual field; (B) The Humphrey visual field analyzer

Definition of Threshold

If a particular intensity of light is shown 100 times and if it is appreciated 50 times then that particular intensity of light is termed as threshold. Threshold for a given point is defined as that stimulus intensity which has a 50 percent probability of being seen. If the stimulus is seen >50 percent of times, it is termed suprathreshold and if it is seen <50 percent of times, it is termed as infrathreshold **(Figure 5)**.

Units for Light Intensity and Retinal Sensitivity

Apostilbs (asb units): They are the fundamental units for expressing light sensitivity. *Maximum intensity of light projected by the Humphrey* perimeter is 10,000 asb units, brightness being controlled by filters. This is *labeled as 0 decibel.* In Humphrey field analyzer '0' dB value = 10,000 asb units. Therefore, 0 dB is the brightest light that is projected by the perimeter.

Conversion of asb Units to Decibel Units

The attenuation of light is expressed in logarithmic units and is more commonly in tenths of log units called as decibel (dB). 1 dB = 1/10 log unit of attenuation of maximum available stimulus (10,000 asb units for the current Humphrey perimeters). The 10 dB stimulus is one log unit less intense that the maximum stimulus of 10,000 asb units, that is 1/10 of 10,000 asb units which is equal to 1000 asb units. The 20 dB stimulus is two log unit less intense than the maximum stimulus of 10,000 asb units, that is 1/100 of 10000 asb units which is equal to 100 asb units. 40 dB stimulus is 4 log units less intense than the maximum stimulus of 10000 asb units, that is 1/10000 of 10000 asb units which is equal to 1 asb unit. Apostilbs are absolute units of light intensity. In contrast the decibels are relative units. This means the decibel value depends on the maximum intensity projected by each perimeter. As the brightest light projected by each perimeter varies, the dB value also varies. The 10 dB stimulus on Goldmann perimeter which is equal to 100 asb units is not the same intensity as a 10 dB stimulus on Humphrey field analyzer, which is equal to 1000 asb units **(Figure 6)**.

> When we use dB to express light sensitivity, a high dB value indicates dim light and a low dB value indicates bright light.

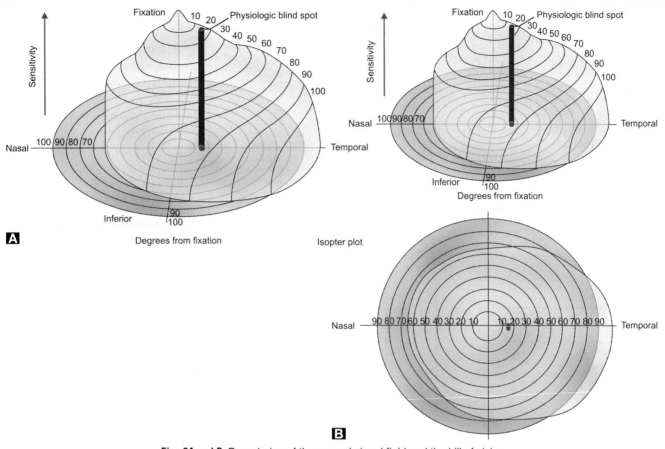

Figs 2A and B Boundaries of the normal visual field and the hill of vision

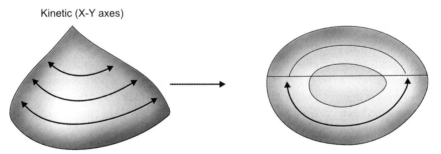

Fig. 3 Kinetic perimetry

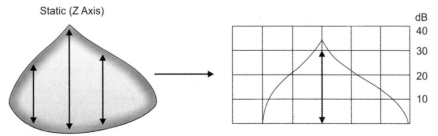

Fig. 4 Static perimetry

Table 1 Goldmann's stimulus sizes

Size	Angular subtended (degrees)	Stimulus area on 30 cm bowl (mm²)
0	0.05	1/16
I	0.11	1/4
II	0.22	1
III	0.43	4
IV	0.86	16
V	1.72	64

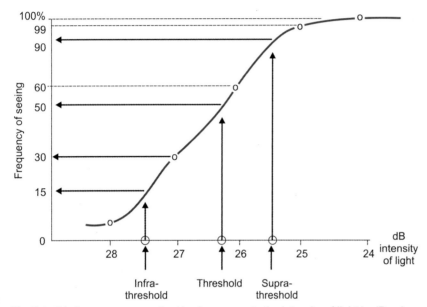

Fig. 5 In this frequency curve, the X axis represents the intensity of light in dB values and the Y axis represents the percentage of frequency of seeing

The main disadvantage of using asb units for expressing retinal sensitivity is that retinal sensitivity is inversely proportional to asb value because a high asb value indicates bright light and a low asb value indicates dim light.

The fall of retinal threshold from 40 dB, the resultant new threshold value and the stimulus intensity needed to get the response to the new retinal threshold values are shown in **Table 2**.

- Fall of retinal sensitivity by 3 dB indicates that the retina has lost its sensitivity by 2 times.
- Fall of retinal sensitivity by 5 dB indicates that the retina has lost its sensitivity by 3 times the original threshold stimulus.

The visual field tests of Humphrey field analyzer are broadly divided into two types depending on the testing strategies used during the test **(Flow chart 1)**.

Point Patterns of the Threshold Tests
Group 1
Point patterns used in suspected and established cases of glaucoma are as follows **(Table 3)**:

30-2 Point Pattern
- Extent of the field to be tested is a 30 degrees radius of a circle with the fixation point as a center.
- There are no points on both the horizontal and vertical axis.
- Distance between point to point is 6 degrees.
- 76 points are distributed in this entire area.

- In this point pattern the bare area around the fixation spot is a circle of 3 degrees radius because the distance between the point to the axis is 3 degrees.

24-2 Point Pattern: A Subset of 30-2 Program
- The extent of the field to be tested is a 24 degrees area of a circle from the fixation point.
- There are no points on both the horizontal and vertical axis.
- The distance between point to point is 6 degrees.
- 54 points are distributed in this entire area.

Note In this point pattern the bare area around the fixation spot is a circle of 3 degrees radius because the distance between the point to the axis is 3 degrees.

The bare area: An area of 3 degrees radius of a circle around fixation point is devoid of any test points in 30-2 and 24-2 point patterns and hence is not tested. This is called a bare area. In the 10-2 point pattern there is only an area of 1 degree radius of a circle around fixation spot that is devoid of test points. In 10-2 most of the central area around fixation point is being tested and hence is a test of choice in advanced cases of glaucoma to know the macular status.

Threshold Testing Strategies
The test strategy refers to the method of presenting stimuli to the patient to attain the desired information. There are 2 types of strategies:
1. Screening and suprathreshold testing strategies.
2. Threshold testing strategies.

In a suprathreshold test, each stimulus is intense enough to be seen by all normal individuals and it provides only general, qualitative information about the visual field and consumes

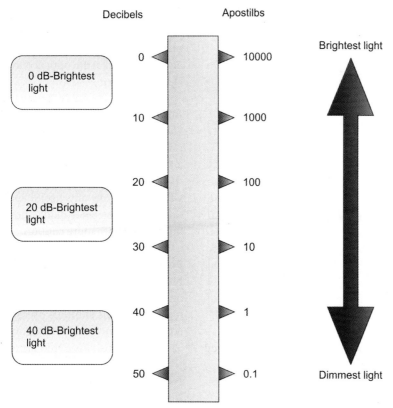

Fig. 6 The decibel—Apostilbs (asb) scale of Humphrey field analyzer

Table 2 Fall of retinal threshold from 40 dB

Fall of retinal threshold from 40 dB	Retinal threshold	Stimulus intensity
− 0 dB	40 dB	1 asb
− 1 dB	39 dB	1.3 asb
− 3 dB	37 dB	2 asb
− 4 dB	36 dB	2.5 asb
− 5 dB	35 dB	3.2 asb
− 10 dB	30 dB	10 asb
− 20 dB	20 dB	100 asb
− 30 dB	10 dB	1000 asb
− 35 dB	5 dB	3162 asb
− 36 dB	4 dB	3981 asb
− 37 dB	3 dB	5012 asb
− 38 dB	2 dB	6310 asb
− 39 dB	1 dB	7943 asb
− 40 dB	0 dB	10, 000 asb

less time. While threshold testing strategies consume more time, they provide detailed, quantitative information to find out the threshold at each selected point of retina (**Figures 7 and 8**). They are of the following types:

1. **Standard threshold strategies**
   ❖ Full threshold strategy
   ❖ Fast pac

2. **Newer threshold strategies**
   ❖ SITA standard
   ❖ SITA fast
   SITA stands for *Swedish Interactive Threshold Algorithm*

Selection of Point Patterns

In **suspicious** cases of glaucoma, in order to know whether there is a field defect or not we prefer the 24-2 point pattern. In *established* cases of glaucoma, one would like to know how much field is lost (**Flow chart 2**). Therefore, prefer 24-2. 24-2 point pattern is the test of choice even for glaucoma suspects because:

- The outer set of points in 30-2 are not considered while selecting the 7th best sensitivity point of TDNP.
- These points are not included in the 5 zones of glaucoma hemifield test (GHT).
- These points are not considered in Anderson's criteria to pick up early field defects.
- As they are tested last, the patient may get fatigued.
- Average normative data value of peripheral points has a wide range.

Advanced Cases of Glaucoma

In advanced cases, our main aim is to know how much central field is retained around the fixation spot. For this, we select the 10-2 point pattern. It can be done with standard size III stimulus or if the sensitivity is low, the test is done using a size V stimulus. It is used to determine a macular split. If there is a split with size III stimulus, the test should be repeated with size V stimulus, the absence of which in size V stimulus carries a better visual prognosis after glaucoma surgery (snuff-out syndrome). It is used only when 5 degrees central field is remaining.

UNDERSTANDING A SINGLE FIELD PRINTOUT

A single field printout can be divided into 10 zones (**Figure 9**):

- **Zone 1:** Patient data and test data
- **Zone 2:** Reliability indices and foveal threshold
- **Zone 3:** Raw data
- **Zone 4:** Gray scale
- **Zone 5:** Total deviation numerical plot
- **Zone 6:** Total deviation probability plot

Flow chart 1 Classification of Humphrey visual field tests

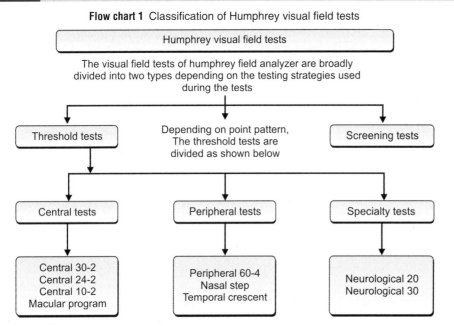

- **Zone 7:** Pattern deviation numerical plot
- **Zone 8:** Pattern deviation probability plot
- **Zone 9:** Global indices
- **Zone 10:** Glaucoma Hemifield test.

Zone 1: Patient Data and Test Data
Fixation Targets
Fixation targets are of four types **(Figure 10)**:

- **Central:** Yellow light in the center of the bowl
- **Small diamond:** It is located below central target and should be used if the patient cannot see the central fixation light, e.g. macular degeneration. The patient should look at the center of the diamond formed by the 4 lights.
- **Large diamond:** It is located below the central target and is used for patients with a central scotoma who cannot see either center fixation light or small diamond.
- **Bottom LED:** When testing with the superior 64 or superior 36 screening specialty tests, the bottom LED is the default fixation target.

Stimulus size—size III is used routinely.

Age of the Patient
The analysis of raw data by STATPAC is age-dependent. The accurate date of birth of the patient should be entered, otherwise the patient's raw data will be compared to mean normal threshold values of a wrong age group.

Size of the Pupil
The pupil size should be between 3 and 4 mm. A constricted pupil gives rise to diffuse visual field depression or edge scotomas.

Refractive Error
Proper correction of the patient's near vision should be done otherwise the field may show generalized depression or possibly a scotoma. Proper placement of glasses in the frame is also important to avoid artefacts.

Zone 2: Foveal Threshold and Reliability Indices
Foveal Threshold and Visual Acuity
It is useful to measure the foveal threshold at the very beginning of the test. If visual acuity is good and there is significant reduction in foveal threshold then the technician should become alert and check if the optical correction is correct or not.

Reliability Indices
These include fixation losses, false positive errors, false negative errors and short-term fluctuations. Even if they are low, it does not mean that it will not provide any useful information, only that such fields should be interpreted with more caution.

Fixation Losses
Five percent of stimuli will be presented on to the blind spot. The patient's response to this stimulus presentation is due to shift of fixation. Fixation losses >20 percent are considered unreliable.

False Positive Response
If the patient pushes the response button to the nonprojected stimulus it will be recorded as false positive response. If false positive rate exceeds 33 percent, the printout will indicate by showing 'XX' next to the rate. White scotomas appear on the gray scale printout.

False Negative Response
Failure to respond to the brightest stimulus in an area previously determined to have some sensitivity is a false negative response. It may indicate lack of attentiveness, fatigue or hypnosis. A value of twenty percent or greater in adults is considered significant, although by default the machine sets it at 33 percent. In patients with advanced glaucomatous optic nerve damage we may get more than 50 percent false response which can be attributed to small shifts in fixation **Table 4**.

It is important to locate the blind spot before starting the visual field examination **(Figure 11)**.

Table 3 Point patterns of the threshold tests

Test pattern	Point density (degrees)	No. of test points	Notes
10-2	2°	68	Test points straddle the horizontal and vertical meridians. The region tested is the same as the Amsler grid.
24-2	6°	54	Test points straddle the horizontal and vertical meridians and used for routine glaucoma monitoring.
30-2	6°	76	Test points straddle horizontal and vertical meridians. Used for first glaucoma field.
Macular program	2°	16	For testing extent of macular lesions or central scotoma.
Nasal step		14	50 degrees extension of the field. Screen for nasal step.
24-1	6°	56	Test points fall on horizontal and vertical meridians. Not used much.
30-1	6°	71	Test points fall on horizontal and vertical meridians. Not used much.

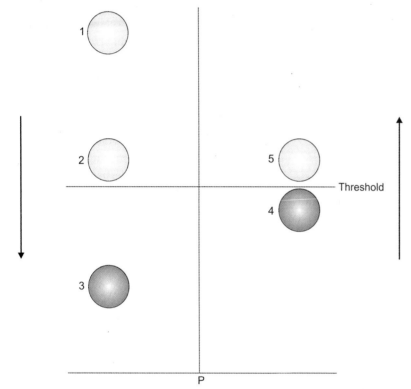

Fig. 7 Threshold determination at a visual field point P, blue circle indicates patient response to stimulus. Brown circle indicates no response to stimulus. Down arrow indicates stimuli decreasing in 4 dB steps. Up arrow indicates stimuli increasing in 2 dB steps. Numbers indicate order of stimulus presentation. This method is used in full threshold strategy

Note Raw data is strategy specific, different strategies will have different raw datas. Hence for comparison, same test strategy should be used in the same patient.

Zone 4: The Gray Scale

Retinal sensitivity values from the best retinal sensitivity value 50 dB to absolute scotoma 0 dB are divided into 10 groups. Each step of pattern corresponds to a change of 5 dB intensity, except the first column which is represented by 50 to 41 dB. In gray scale form, areas of high sensitivity are denoted by lighter shades and areas of low sensitivity are denoted by darker shades. One should not make any definitive diagnosis on basis of gray scale. It only gives an idea about the pattern and depth of field defect. High false positive areas will show white scotomas. High false negative will show a clover leaf appearance. It is more useful to explain the seriousness of the condition to the patient (**Figures 12 and 13**).

Zone 3: Raw Data

It is the exact retinal sensitivity in dB units of selected points calculated by field analyzer. Only numerical data is displayed and db units are omitted. '0' indicates absolute scotoma (no response to brightest light stimuli 10,000 asb units in Humphrey field analyzer). The number 40 indicates response to 1 asb unit. It is the highest sensitivity that can be recorded by HFA.

The raw data will be compared with the mean normal value stored in the computer and calculates the difference between measured retinal sensitivity and mean normal retinal sensitivity at all points and plots them as total deviation numerical plot. The retinal sensitivity at 5 degrees from fovea is always higher than the retinal sensitivity at 10 degrees from the fovea. So the normal slope of the hill of vision is smooth.

Zone 5: Total Deviation Numerical Plot (TDNP)

The measured retinal sensitivity of each point (raw data) is compared with the normative data of same age group and calculates the difference between the measured sensitivity and the normative data at each point and plots the deviation values from the normative data as TDNP. If the measured retinal sensitivity is equal to the mean normal values of the same age group, 0 will be displayed

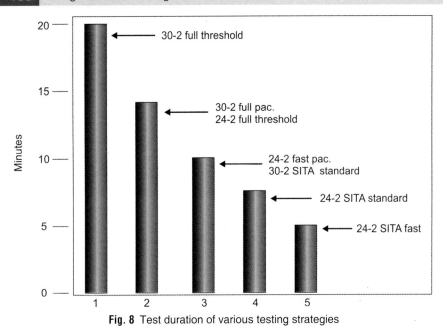

Fig. 8 Test duration of various testing strategies

Flow chart 2 Approach of interpretation of visual fields defects according to the stage of glaucoma

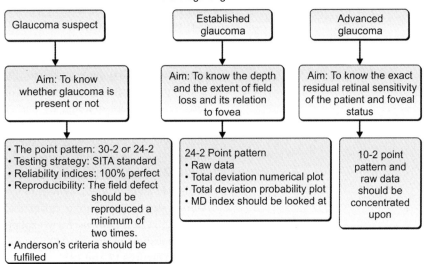

platform for calculation of global indices (MD and PSD) **(Figure 14)**.

Zone 6: Total Deviation Probability Plot (TDPP)

The loss of retinal sensitivity at each point is expressed in terms of its probability or P value and each P value is given a symbol. The probability plots are defined to know the extent and the pattern of the field defect. Probability statements are based on the distribution seen in the normal population. The darker the symbol the greater the probability of abnormality as indicated by P value **(Figures 15 and 16)**. Lesser the P value more statistically significant it becomes. Each numerical value in the total deviation numerical plot depending on its P value is assigned the corresponding symbol of P value. The main aim of creating the probability plots is to give the pattern and extent of the field defect in the form of symbolic representation of P value of loss of retinal sensitivity at each point. Once the field defect becomes generalized, the pattern of the field defect is not known in the TDPP.

> **Note** STATPAC calculates the P value for the points where there is loss of sensitivity. P value is not calculated for those points where sensitivity is better than normal.

Significance of P value and probability plots: Global indices which include MD and PSD are also expressed in terms of their P values. Glaucoma hemifield test is also P value dependent.

Zone 7: Pattern Deviation Numerical Plot (PDNP)

The pattern deviation plot is created to know the pattern and the extent of the deep scotomas masked by the generalized depression in the total deviation probability plot. The generalized field defect is removed from the

in the total deviation numerical plot. If the measured retinal sensitivity is better, no sign is given and if the measured retinal sensitivity is less than mean normal values of the same age group a negative sign (–) is allotted to the deviation value. The (–) dB value indicates the depth of the field defect. They are directly proportional to each other.

If there is a localized field defect it can be identified by localizing areas of high negative values. If there is irregular loss of sensitivity, TDNP contains dissimilar deviation values and the difference between highest negative dB value and lowest negative dB value will be very high. Reverse is true in cases of uniform field loss. TDNP is the

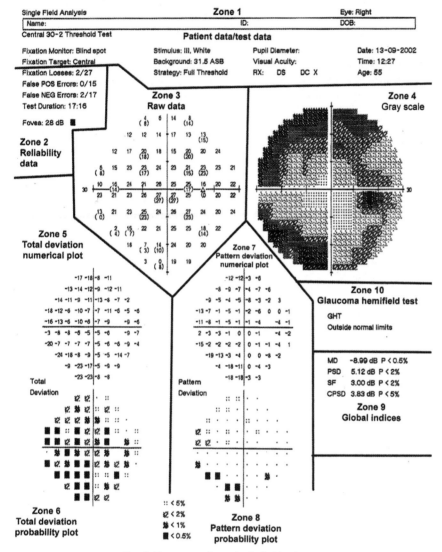

Fig. 9 Ten zones in a single field printout

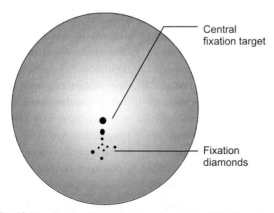

Fig. 10 The fixation lights in Humphrey visual field analyzer

total deviation plot by elevating each point's sensitivity by certain dB value to form the new numerical plot and corresponding probability plot will expose the pattern of the deep scotomas masked in the TDNP. The most important point is the selection of 7th best sensitivity point of the TDNP. **The dB value that converts the 7th best sensitivity point of the total deviation numerical plot to 0 deviation, is added to all points of TDNP to convert it to pattern deviation numerical plot.** Before selecting 7th best sensitivity point in TDNP the following points are to be noted **(Figures 17A to C)**.

- In the 30-2 point pattern only points of 24-2 point pattern is considered.
- In the 24-2 point pattern 3 points adjacent to the blind spot area are ignored.
- In 10-2 point pattern all points are considered since there is no blind spot in 10 degrees field.

Zone 8: Pattern Deviation Probability Plot (PDPP)

The pattern deviation probability plot tells whether the generalized field defect in the total deviation probability plot is of uniform generalized type or irregular generalized type **(Figures 17A to C)**. If it is an irregular generalized type, the pattern and the extent of the deep scotomas masked under generalized depression in the TDPP are highlighted in the PDPP. If it is of a uniform generalized type the PDPP will be normal and a uniform generalized field defect will be seen in conditions like cataract, media opacities, small pupil and improper refractive correction.

Note The pattern deviation plot is nothing but the total deviation plot minus a generalized field defect worth of the dB value that converts the 7th best sensitivity point of TDNP to 0 deviation.

Table 4 Sources of error

Technician faults	Patients lack of performance skill
Age of the patient not properly entered	High fixation losses < 33%
Refractive error not properly corrected for near vision	High false (+) ve error >33%
Pupil size <3 mm	High false (–) ve error >33%
Improper positioning of the patients head	Short-term fluctuation >2.5 dB

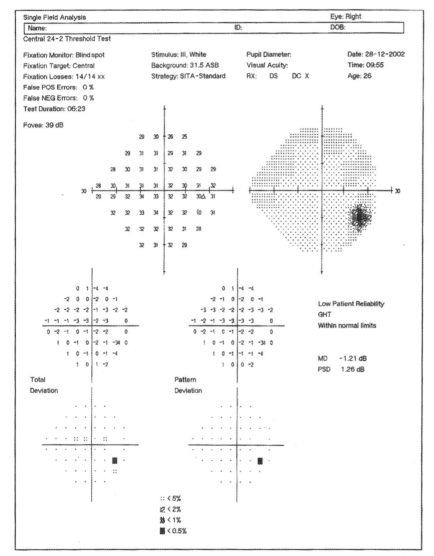

Fig. 11 Importance of locating blind spot before interpreting the visual field printout

dB value	41 to 50	36 to 40	31 to 35	26 to 30	21 to 25	16 to 20	11 to 15	6 to 10	1 to 5	0
Shade										

Fig. 12 The gray scale

Zone 9: The Global Indices
Mean Deviation Index (MD)

The MD signifies the average of overall severity of field loss. It is the average of all the numbers shown in the total deviation numerical plot except for the two points in the area of the blind spot. Points with low variance, i.e. those closer to fixation affect the MD value more as compared to the more eccentric points. The mean deviation is expressed in terms of dB units with P value. A positive value indicates that the patient's overall sensitivity is better than the normal observer whereas a negative value indicates that patient's overall sensitivity is worse than average normal individual.

Diagnosis of early glaucoma: This must be interpreted along with other clinical signs:

1. 2 dB difference of MD between 2 eyes.
2. An average difference of 1.5 dB MD must be maintained between 2 eyes on 2 consecutive tests.
3. An average difference of 1 dB must be maintained between the 2 eyes on 4 consecutive tests.

Note During Follow-Up tests, the most important index to assess field progression is MD index. The increase in MD > 0.08 dB per year should be considered abnormal.

Pattern Standard Deviation (PSD)

PSD is an index to express dissimilar deviation values in the total deviation numerical plot or in other words to express the contour of hill of vision whether it is smooth or rough. The roughness of the hill is usually due to loss of sensitivity or due to the measured sensitivity being better than normal values. PSD does not carry a + or – sign in front of it. It will be without a P value if the roughness of the hill is not significant.

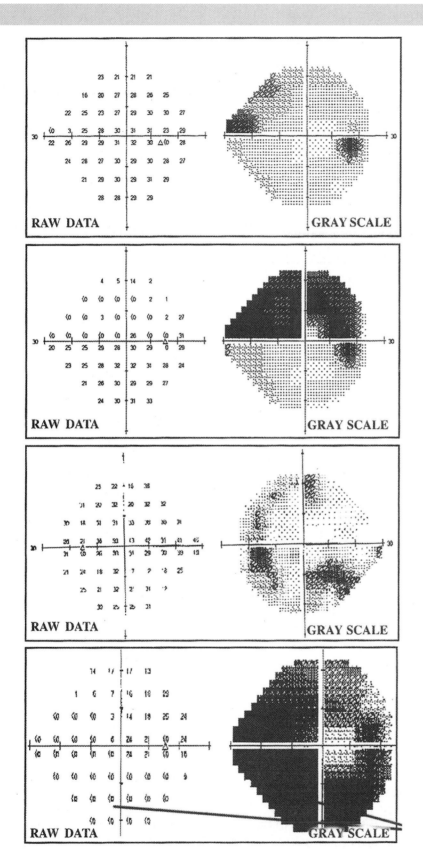

Fig. 13 Some of the uses of gray scale

Localized Field Defect (Figures 18A and B)

- TDNP will contain dissimilar deviation values
- The contour of the hill of vision will be irregular
- Hence PSD values will be high with significant P values.

Irregular Generalized Field Defect (Figures 19A and B)

- PSD will be high in irregular generalized field defect.
- Contour of hill of vision will be irregular in irregular generalized field defect.

Uniform Generalized Field Defect (Figures 20A and B)

- Loss of sensitivity at all points is almost same in uniform generalized field defect.
- The TDNP contains similar deviation values.
- As a result PSD will be low.
- The contour of hill of vision is smooth.

Role in Assessing Progression

- Increase in MD and change in PSD index indicate that there is progression of field defect and it may be localized to an area or to a localized area in generalized depression.
- Increase in MD index and no change in PSD indicate that there is progression of field defect and it is of uniform generalized type.

Short-term Fluctuations (SF)

SITA strategies do not calculate SF and hence corrected pattern standard deviation (CPSD) cannot be calculated. Only FAST PAC and full threshold strategies calculate them. SF is an index of intratest variation. The sensitivity is calculated twice at ten preselected points. The SF is almost always less than 3 dB and is usually between 1 and 2.5 dB.

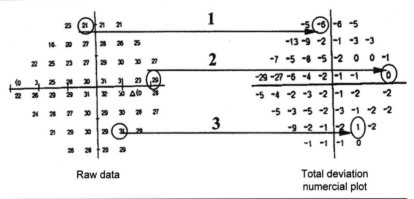

Raw data

Total deviation numercial plot

The raw data is expressed as deviation from normal values in the total deviation numeric plot

Fig. 14 Total deviation numeric plot (TDNP)

∷ < 5%   P < 5% indicates that this degree of loss sensitivity of that point is seen in < 5% of normal population. The P<5% is represented by- ∷ <5%

✗ < 2%   P < 2% indicates that this degree of loss sensitivity of that point is seen in < 2% of normal population. The P<2% is represented by- ✗ <2%

✗ <1%   P < 1% indicates that this degree of loss sensitivity of that point is seen in < 2% of normal population. The P<1% is represented by- ✗ <1%

■ <0.5%   P < 5% indicates that this degree of loss sensitivity of that point is seen in < 2% of normal population. The P<0.5% is represented by ■ <0.5%

Fig. 15 The P value

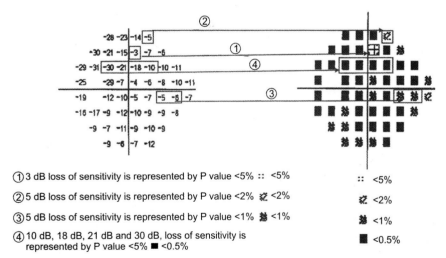

① 3 dB loss of sensitivity is represented by P value <5% ∷ <5%

② 5 dB loss of sensitivity is represented by P value <2% ✗ <2%

③ 5 dB loss of sensitivity is represented by P value <1% ✗ <1%

④ 10 dB, 18 dB, 21 dB and 30 dB, loss of sensitivity is represented by P value <5% ■ <0.5%

∷ <5%

✗ <2%

✗ <1%

■ <0.5%

Fig. 16 Example of conversion of total deviation plot to total deviation probability plot

Note If the 10 preselected points are pathological, it will show greater variability. If all these fixed tested points are normal, a high SF index would indicate low reliability.

Corrected Pattern Standard Deviation

SF when removed from PSD gives us CPSD. SF and corrected pattern standard deviation (CPSD) are not mentioned

in SITA programs, and thus not a part of Anderson's criteria.

Zone 10: Glaucoma Hemifield Test (GHT)

The glaucoma hemifield test was developed to pick up the dissimilarity among the sensitivities of the corresponding points on either side of horizontal axis to diagnose glaucoma at an early stage. GHT evaluates 5 zones in the upper field and compares these zones to their mirror image zones in the lower field **(Figure 21)**. The zones are constructed in approximate arrangement of retinal nerve fiber layers. A score assigned to each zone based on the location of the zones and their deviation values in the PDNP. A comparison of each upper zone is made with the corresponding lower zone and the difference in scores between the upper and lower zones is calculated. The difference is compared with significant limits taken from a database of normal subjects. Five possible results can appear.

1. ***Outside normal limits:*** Indicates that one of the two conditions has been met:
    A. When the score in the upper zones are compared with those of the lower zones, at least one sector pair's score difference must exceed that found in 99 percent of the normal population.
    B. The individual zone score in both members of any zone pair exceed that found in 99.5 percent of normal individuals.
2. ***Borderline:*** In comparing the upper and lower zones, at least one sector pair difference exceeds that found in 97 percent of normal individuals.
3. ***General reduction of sensitivity:*** This appears when neither of the conditions for the 'outside normal limits' is met, but general height calculation shows the best part

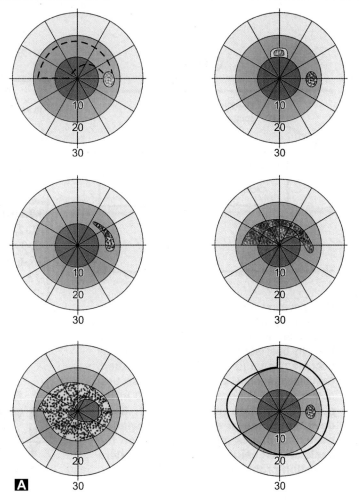

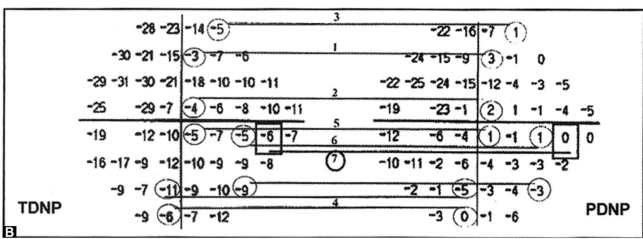

Figs 17A and B

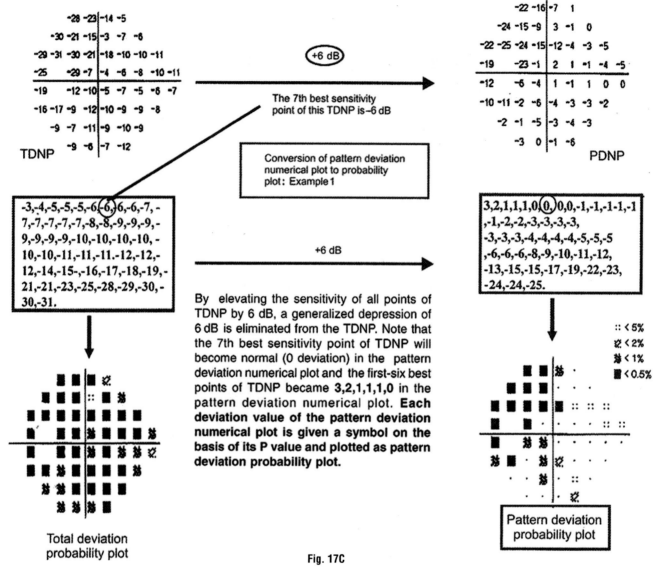

Fig. 17C

Figs 17A to C Zone 8: The pattern deviation probability plot

of the field to be depressed to a degree that occurs in fewer than 0.5 percent of normal population.

4. **Abnormally high sensitivity:** This indicates that the overall sensitivity in the best part of the field is higher than that found in others. In the phase of abnormally high sensitivity, the comparison of upper with lower zones is not made.

5. **Within normal limits:** This message appears if none of the above four conditions are met.

Note
- 'Borderline' and 'general reduction in sensitivity' are the only two that can appear together.
- The GHT is not designed to detect a temporal wedge defect.

SINGLE FIELD ANALYSIS PRINTOUT

Step 1: Verify whether the patient data and test data are properly entered.

Step 2: Decide whether the test is reliable or not.

Step 3: Measured foveal sensitivity should correlate with the visual acuity.

Indicates that refractive error correction for near is correct.

Step 4: Locate the blind spot correctly, whether it is in normal position.

Step 5: Analyze TDPP and PDPP.

Localized defect: TDPP and PDPP almost look similar (**Figure 22**).

- For example, glaucomatous damage, AION, optic nerve pathway defects, occipital lobe infarcts.

Irregular generalized field defect: A generalized defect in TDPP and a localized defect in PDPP (**Figure 23**).

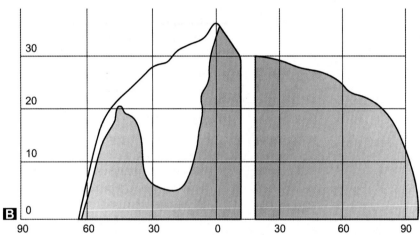

```
              0  1 | -1  0
         -3 -1 -1 |  2  2   0
          3  3  0 -3 | -1  0  -1  -5
         -1    -7 -3 | -3 -4 -10 -10 -18
         ─────────────────────────────
          1    -1 -3 | -5 34 -33 -29 -28
          2  1 -5 -6 | -4 -8  -6 -30
            -1 -2 -2 | -3 -6 -11
             1 -1 |  0 -5
```

A   TDNP

Figs 18A and B (A) Localized defect; (B) Rough contour of hill of vision PSD—high

- For example, pure advanced stage of glaucoma or cataract associated with glaucoma.

Uniform generalized field defect: A generalized defect in the TDPP and normal PDPP **(Figure 24)**.

- For example, media opacities cataract, small pupil, refractive error, advanced end stage of glaucoma and optic neuritis.

Step 6: GHT and PSD are two indices developed to pick up early cases of glaucoma. They should be outside normal limits (PSD <5 percent and GHT- borderline or outside normal limits) to pick up glaucoma at an early stage.

Step 7: Look at the TDNP and MD index (depth of field defect). In order to know the exact loss of sensitivity at each point, concentrate on the TDNP. MD index represents the average loss of sensitivity of all points of TDNP. In a case of localized field defect, the loss of sensitivity is confined to a particular area and there is no loss of sensitivity (0 deviation in TDNP) at the remaining points. MD index represents the average of normal and abnormal points.

Step 8: Look at the pattern deviation numerical plot in order to know the extent and depth of field defect and whether it is caused by glaucoma, cataract or both.

Step 9: The role of raw data. If the probability plot shows a black square, we cannot conclude a relative or an absolute scotoma. Only if raw data shows a 0 dB, we know it is an absolute scotoma.

> **Note** Never come to a conclusion of foveal split unless you see the 0 dB sensitivity at any four points on 1 degree circle around fixation point of 10-2 raw data.

Step 10: Always correlate clinically. Assess whether the pattern of visual field loss is consistent with the optic nerve head changes and other clinical findings.

Identification of artifacts:

- Size of pupil **(Figures 25A and B)**
- Refractive error correction **(Figures 26A and B)**
- Reliability indices **(Figures 27 to 29)**
- Rim artifacts **(Figures 30A and B)**.

ANDERSON'S CRITERIA

Minimal Criteria for Glaucomatous Damage (30-2)

- Glaucoma hemifield test—outside normal limits on at least 2 consecutive occasions.
- Cluster of 3 or more nonedge points in a location typical for glaucoma, all of which are depressed on PSD at a P < 5 percent level and one of which is depressed at P<1 percent, on two consecutive occasions.
- CPSD/PSD that occurs in less than 5 percent of normal individuals on 2 consecutive fields **(Figure 32)**.

Criteria to Label as Early Defect

- MD is better than –6 dB
- 25 percent of the points in total deviation plot should have P value 5 percent and less than 10 points have P value of 1 percent.
- No point in the central 5 degrees has sensitivity less than 15 dB.

A **moderate defect** exceeds 1 or more of the criteria required to keep it in the early defect category but does not meet the criteria to be severe.

A severe defect has any of the following:

- MD index worse than –12 dB
- More than 50 percent of the points in TDP should have P value of 5 percent.
- More than 20 points depressed at P value 1 percent.

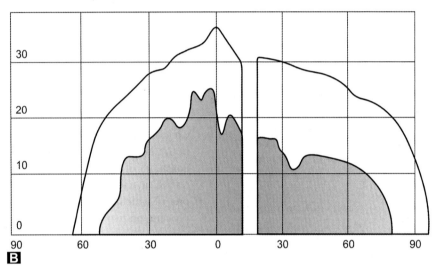

```
              -8 -10  | -9  -8
           -7 -7  -9  | -9  -7 -12
       -6 -9 -11  -7  |-15 -17 -14 -15
       -7     -6  -4  |-12 -17 -19 -18 -16
       ───────────────┼──────────────────
       -6     -7  -5  | -4  -9 -22 -18 -18
    -9 -7 -7  -6       | -8 -14 -15 -19
           -9 -6  -8  |-12  -7  -9
              -5  -9  |-13 -10
```

A   TDNP

Figs 19A and B (A) Irregular generalized field defect; (B) Rough contour of hill of vision PSD—high

A point in the central 5 degrees with the 0 dB sensitivity or points closer than 5 degrees fixation under 15 dB sensitivity in both the upper and lower hemifields. *Few examples:* Some examples have been shown in **Figures 33 to 43**.

Follow-up Visual Field Examination

Glaucoma is a progressive disease, hence the field defect gradually increases over time as the disease progresses **(Figures 31A to F)**. To know whether the disease is stable or progressing, we must have a baseline field and the follow-up fields. The most important point to be remembered is the follow-up tests should be conducted by the same testing strategy used in the baseline field test. During the interpretation of these follow-up tests, we should always keep in mind the effect of pupil size, refractive error correction and long-term fluctuation. There is nothing like a fixed time interval for follow-up visual field examination. The frequency of the visual field examination depends on clinical circumstances. The Humphrey field analyzed has the STATPAC to print the follow-up fields in four formals.

1. Overview printout
2. Change analysis printout
3. Glaucoma change probability analysis printout
4. Glaucoma progression analysis printout **(Flow chart 3)**.

OVERVIEW PRINTOUT

The main advantage of the overview printout is that all the single field analysis examinations up to 16 tests can be seen on a single page. They are printed in chronological order. Except visual acuity and refractive error everything that is present on a single field printout is present in overview printout. The printout must be analyzed on judgment alone as no statistical assistance is available. The following information is provided in an overview printout:

Patient Data
Name, date of birth, size of pupil.

Test Data
This includes point pattern and strategy. The point pattern should be same as the first test for all the follow-up test to analyze the change in MD index.

Testing Strategy
It is important to know that in an overview printout field tests with different testing strategies may be present simultaneously. For example, we can get an overview printout if we select a SITA fast test strategy for a follow-up test even if the previous test was done using SITA standard. This must be kept in mind during interpretation.

Reliability Data
Fixation losses, false negative errors, false positive errors of the previous tests and follow-up test should be kept in mind.

Foveal Sensitivity
One should know whether the refractive error correction given is correct or not for all the tests. This can be known by correlating visual acuity and foveal sensitivity. Always see the foveal sensitivity of the previous test and the follow-up test before analyzing the MD index.

Interpretation of Overview Printout for Glaucoma Progression
Step 1: Confirm that increase in MD index is not due to the improper refractive correction, pupil size, high FN, different point patterns and different testing strategies.

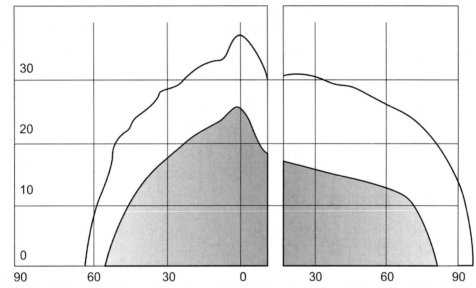

```
              -7 -7 | -9 -7
          -12 -8 -8 | -8 -6 -7
       -13 -9 -8 -9 | -8 -7 -6-7
        -7    -7 -7 | -9 -8 -8-6 -2
         ─────────────────────────
        -6    -5 -8 | -9 -8 -7-6 -3
       -9-10 -8 -9  | -9 -9 -7 -7
          -9 -9 -9  |-10 -8 -8
             -9 -8  | -8 -9
```

A TDNP

```
30
20
10
 0
   90    60    30     0    30    60    90
```

B

Figs 20A and B (A) Generalized depression; (B) Smooth contour of hill of vision PSD–low

If the increase in MD index is not due to any of the above factors then only can we analyze MD index, raw data and probability plots.

Step 2: No change in PSD (uniform loss of sensitivity) indicates cataract and other media opacities or glaucoma associated with cataract.

With change in PSD and irregular loss of sensitivity, we assume damage is due to glaucoma.

Step 3: Look at the:
• Probability plots (extent and depth in few occasions)
• Raw data (to assess change in measured retinal sensitivity)
• Gray scale (change in shade of gray scale during its progression).

CHANGE ANALYSIS PRINTOUT

Like the overview printout, the change analysis printout shows more than 10 tests on one sheet. The STATPAC produce analytical summary of changes in the patients visual field from the time of earliest test included in the summary to the time of the most recent test included. The changes analysis printout consists of three components: (i) A box plot with its relation to the dB scale, (ii) The summary of the global indices, and (iii) Linear regression analysis of mean deviation. The indices are the same four presented in the single field analysis. But this time, they are plotted over time to indicate the changes in the patient's visual field.

Changes analysis printout of full threshold strategy will contain normal box plot display on the left side of the dB scale. All the components of the global indices (mean deviation, PSD, SF, CPSD) are represented in graphic forms.

Change analysis printout of FASTPAC strategy will contain normal box plot display on the left side of the dB scale. All the components of the global indices (mean deviation, PSD, SF, CPSD) are represented in graphic forms.

Change analysis printout of SITA-standard strategy will not contain normal box plot display on the left side of the dB scale.

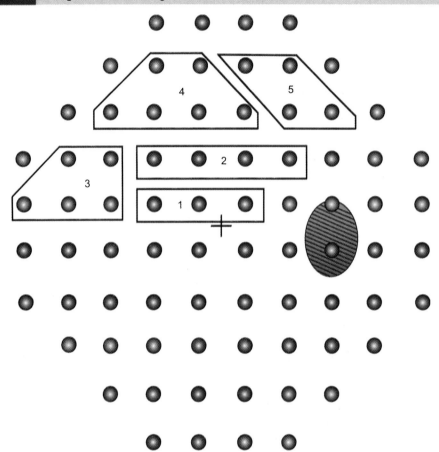

Fig. 21 The glaucoma Hemifield test

The values of mean deviation and PSD are represented in graphic forms.

Change analysis printouts of SITA strategies do not calculate SF and CPSD an hence they will not be represented in the graphic forms.

The box plots are helpful in making a quick determination about the nature and the extent of visual field analysis overtime. The box plot is a modified histogram that gives a five number summary of test results. To interpret box plot, one should have a very clear concept about how the box plot is being constructed.

Construction of the Box Plot

The basis for the construction of the box plot is the total deviation numerical plot (TDNP) of the single field analysis printout. The deviations displayed in TDNP are ranked according to the degree of deviation. The decibel deviations (from age-matched normal) are arranged according to their sensitivities in chronological order and they are divided into three groups. These three groups constitute the box plot.

The vertical rectangle (box) represents the range of deviations for 70 percent of the locations. The median deviation value (not to be confused with the mean deviation global index) is indicated by a flanked heavy bar in the box. The extremes of the deviations are shown with the extended vertical lines above and below the box, incorporating 15 percent of points in each direction. The ends of the vertical lines thus indicate the total range of deviations from normal values for all points included in the analysis.

For example, in the 30-2 field the test points are 76.

First group: Fifteen percent best points are represented by upper tail

The best sensitivity point (100th percentile) in the field analysis: Eleven points represent the upper tail (15% of 76 test points = 11 points) 11th best point (85th percentile).

Seventy percent next best points are represented by rectangular box.

Fifty-two points will be represented by the box (70% of 76 test points = 52 points).

The worst 15% points represented by lower tail.

63rd ranked point (15th percentile) 11 points represent the lower tail (15% of 76 test points = points).

76th least sensitivity point (0 percentile) field analysis.

Normal Position of the Box Plot in Relation to Decibel Scale

In normal visual field, it would not be expected that the threshold sensitivity estimated could be exactly equal to the average normal values at all locations. At a fewer locations, the estimate may be slightly better than the normal values; and at other points, the estimate may be slightly worse. Experience shows that the majority are close to mid-normal value as the deviations are typically near zero dB for a median (50th percentile) point in the normal field.

In 30-2 central field, 70 percent of the points range from approximately 3 dB above to 3 dB below the average normal value. All deviations including 30 percent of two tails are expected to fall within the 10 decibel range from 4 to – 6 dB.

For interpretation, the main points to be noted are:
- Overall shape of the box—how elongated or compact it is the location of the three dark lines inside the box that indicate the median

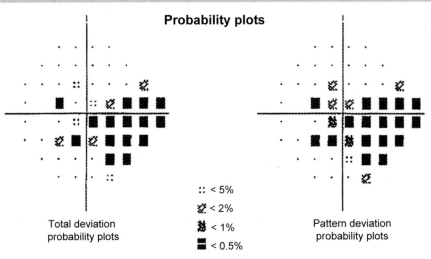

Probability plots

```
::  < 5%
🌀  < 2%
🐾  < 1%
■  < 0.5%
```

Total deviation
probability plots

Pattern deviation
probability plots

Fig. 22 Features of a localized field defect:
- TDPP and PDPP look identical
- PSD is high
- Mean deviation index depends on the size and on the depth of localized defect

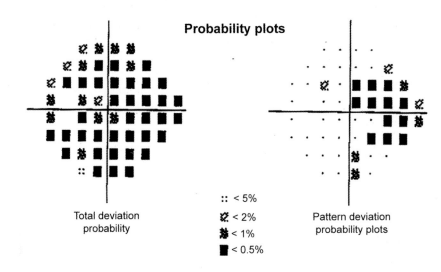

Probability plots

```
::  < 5%
🌀  < 2%
🐾  < 1%
■  < 0.5%
```

Total deviation
probability

Pattern deviation
probability plots

Fig. 23 Features of irregular generalized field defect:
- Generalized depression in the TDPP
- Localized field defect in the PDPP
- High PSD value
- High MD index

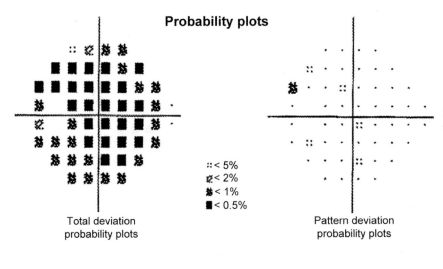

Probability plots

```
::  < 5%
🌀  < 2%
🐾  < 1%
■  < 0.5%
```

Total deviation
probability plots

Pattern deviation
probability plots

Fig. 24 Features of uniform generalized field defect:
- Generalized depression in the total deviation probability plot
- Almost normal pattern deviation probability plot
- The mean deviation index value is equal to deviation values of most points of TDNP
- Low PSD value

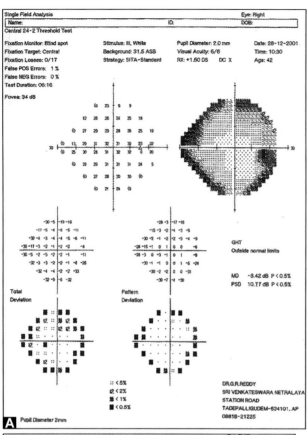

Single field analysis printout with 2 mm

Pupil size

Point pattern and testing strategy

24-2, SITA standard

Reliability indices-

FL - 0/17

FN- 1%

FP - 0%

PSD 10.77 dB P<0.5%

GHT Outside normal limits

MD - 8.42 dB P<0.5%

Foveal sensitivity 34dB

7th best sensitivity point of TDNP (-2dB)

Whenever tehere are the edge scotomost (The significant P value symbols on the outmost set oof points of any point pattern is called as edge scotomass) remember that these scotomas may be due to small pupil high false (-) ve errors or lens rim artifacts.

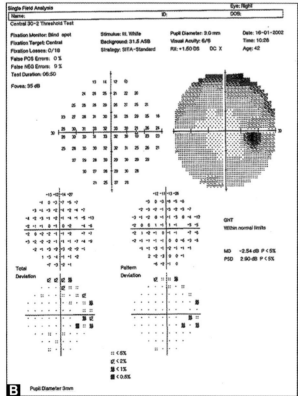

Single field analysis printout with 3 mm pupil size of

the same patient

Point pattern and testing strategy

30-2–SITA standard

Reliability indices–

FL - 0/18

FP - 0%

FN - 9%

PSD 2.90 dB P<5%

GHT - with in normal limits

MD - 2.54 dB P<5%

Foveal sensitivity 35 dB

7th best sensitivity point of TDNP (-1dB)

Figs 25A and B Edge scotomas

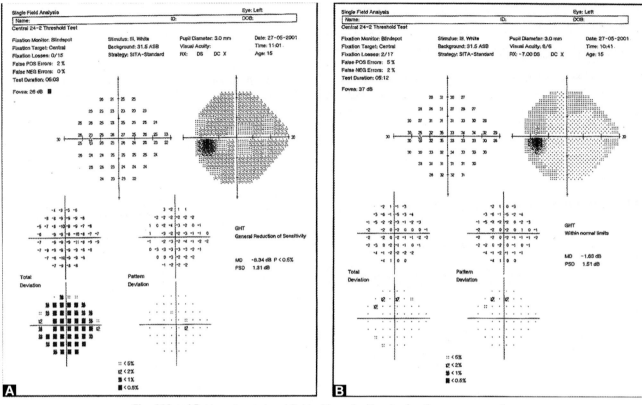

Figs 26A and B Humphrey visual field with and without refractive error correction

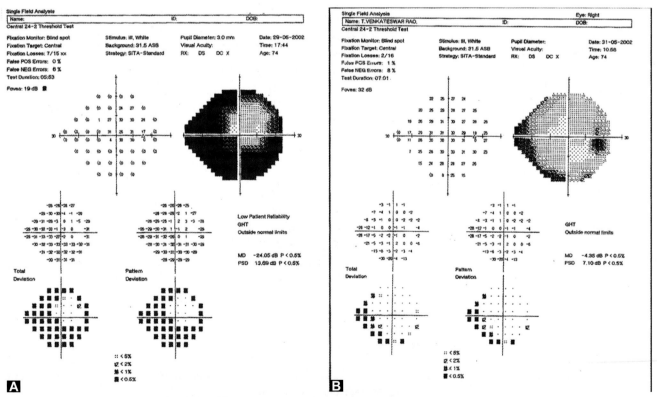

Figs 27A and B Humphrey visual field with and without fixation losses

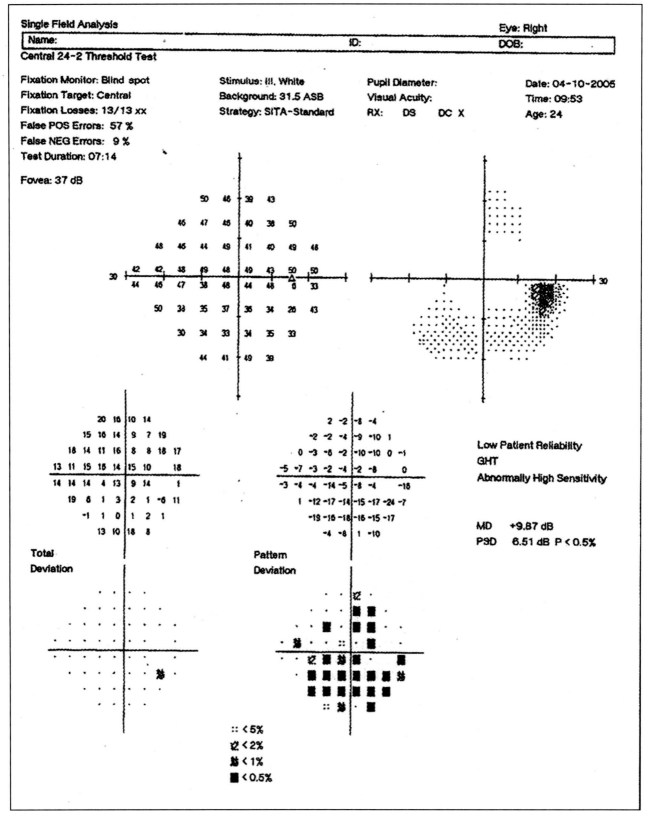

Fig. 28 High false positive errors

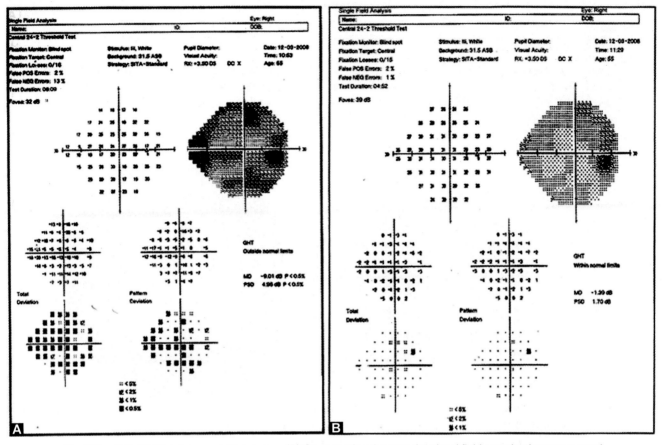

Figs 29A and B (A) High false negative errors; (B) On repeating the test, the visual field examination was normal

- The length of the upper and the lower tails
- Length of the box
- The top and the bottom end points of a line along which the box lies, the position of the box plot in relation to decibel scale.

The change analysis printouts of SITA strategies do not contain the normal box plot figure left to the dB scale unlike what we see the normal box plot left to the dB scale with full threshold and FASTPAC change analysis printout.

The change analysis printout is not a substitute for single field analysis printout. The change analysis printout should always be attached with single field analysis printout for its interpretation. In isolation, we cannot interpret the change analysis printout for the following reasons:

1. It does not contain details of the patient's data like visual acuity, pupil size, near vision correction.
2. Foveal threshold of the patient is not recorded.
3. Reliability indices are not recorded. Only the selection of the test and date of birth of the patient are recorded in the printout. So we do not know whether the change analysis printout is reliability or not. That is why, it should always be attached to the single field analysis printout. The other pitfalls of change analysis printout are that, all the points of the total deviation probability plot will be analyzed without eliminating the

edge scotoma of 30-2 central field. Sometimes the edge scotomas may give an impression as a localized a scotoma represented by the long lower tail of the box plot.

4. The change analysis printout does not show the location of the scotoma whether they are in the arcuate area, nearer to fixation or at fixation.

Field Defects: Box Plot Analysis

In localized depression, some points will have normal sensitivity value, so, the upper tail position of the box plot will always be normal. The length of the other components of the box plot depends on the size of the field defect. If only 15 percent of the points lose their retinal sensitivity, we see the

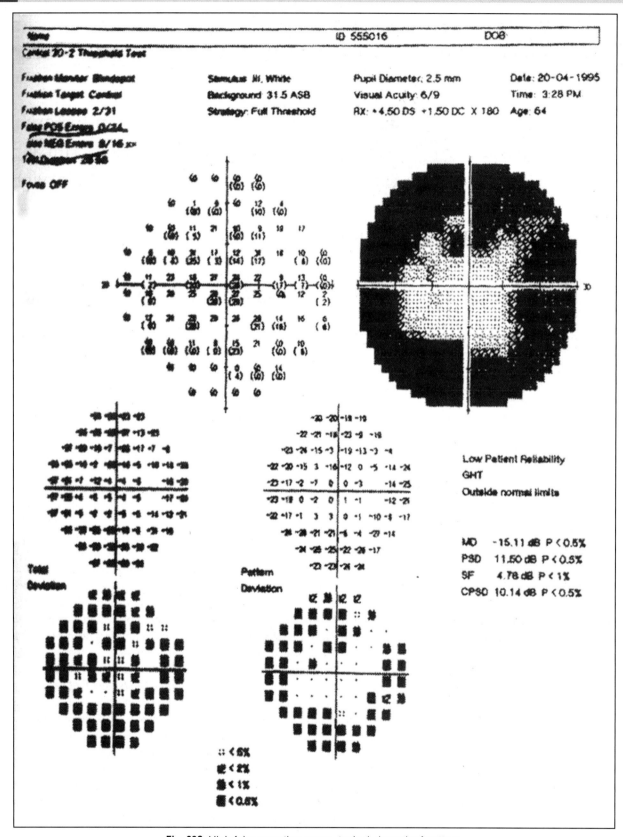

Fig. 29C High false negative errors, typical clover leaf pattern

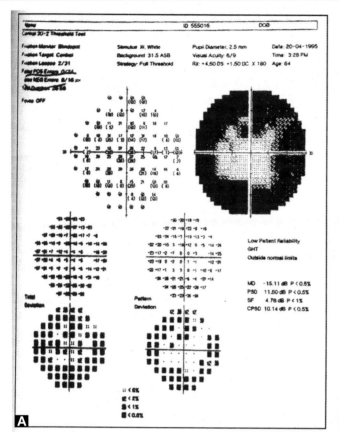 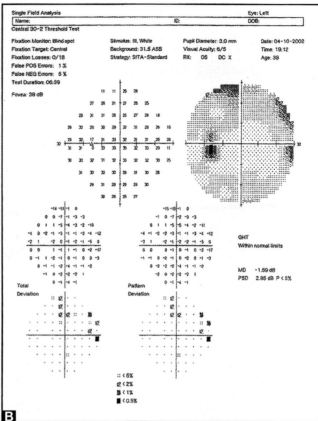

Figs 30A and B Rim artifacts (before and after)

lengthening of the lower tail of the box plot without any shift of the box plot from its normal position. If 50 percent of the points lose their retinal sensitivity, we see the lengthening of the lower tail and lower half of the box without any shift of the box plot from its normal position. Hence, the most important point to be noted in localized depression is the change in the length of the box plot without shift in the position of the upper tail.

Uniform Generalized Depression

The entire box plot is shifted downwards and the shift depends on the degree of field loss, but the length of the box plot is not changed, which means all the points lost their sensitivity equally. The most important point to be noted in uniform generalized depression is the length of the box plot is unaltered.

Irregular Generalized Depression

The entire box plot is shifted downwards along with change in the length of the box plot. Because the loss of retinal sensitivity of all points is not equal, the length of each component of box plot will be different. The most important point to be noted in irregular generalized depression is the length of the box plot is altered.

GLAUCOMA PROGRESSION ANALYSIS

To analyze glaucoma progression, Humphrey introduced a new software glaucoma progression analysis and Guided Progression Analysis 2. It has been introduced to overcome the drawback of glaucoma change probability analysis where that the comparisons are made between the raw data (TDNP) of the baseline and the follow-up tests. As the raw data (TDNP) is affected both transient and progressive generalized

changes (e.g. those caused by learning effects, long-term fluctuation or media changes), we do not know whether the changes are either due to disease progression or due to long-term fluctuation. The SITA strategies do not have glaucoma change probability analysis option. In order to avoid these drawbacks, the glaucoma progression analysis (GPA) has been introduced by Humphrey in GPA, the comparisons are made between the baseline pattern deviation numerical plot and the pattern deviation numerical plot of the follow-up test. The SITA strategies have the GPA option. GPA uses SITA and pattern deviation to identify glaucoma specific progression.

Step 1: Establishing the Baseline Data (Pattern Deviation Numerical Plot)

The first step in glaucoma progression analysis is the establishment of baseline

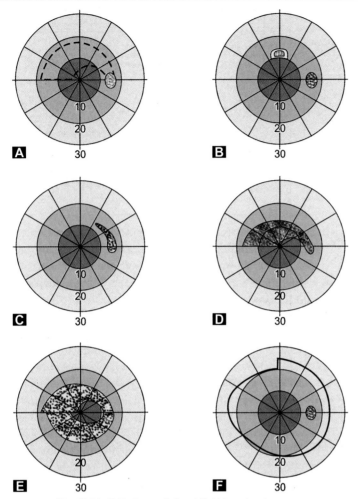

Figs 31A to F Pattern of visual field loss in glaucoma

data (pattern deviation numerical plot). If the patient undergoes the field test for three or more times, the field analyzer generates the baseline printout depending on the data of the first 2 tests.

Step 2: Establishing the Decibel Deviation Plot in Follow-up Test Printout

Now the follow-up test result (pattern deviation numerical plot) is compared to the baseline pattern deviation numerical plot and the difference as deviation from the baseline plot in the follow-up test printout is calculated.

Step 3: Establishing the Progression Analysis Probability Plot in Follow-up Test Printout

Now each deviation from the baseline is compared to intertest variability typical of stable glaucoma patients and then point locations in progression analysis plot which have changes significantly are depicted as symbols. The progression analysis consists of four symbols.

Symbols

▲ = Progression at 95 percent significance level

△ = Progression point repeated in 2 consecutive exams

▲ = Progression point repeated in three consecutive exams

X = Out of range

The criteria for identifying progression in visual fields:

• Minimum of three tests required: 2 baseline and 1 follow-up exam

• Each follow-up compared to average thresholds of 2 baseline exams

• Additional follow-up compared both to baseline and 2 most recent follow-ups.

GPA alert TM: Three-▲ in one exam denotes "possible progression" and three ▲ indicates likely progression.

Glaucoma Progression Analysis Baseline Printout

The GPA consists of two components: The data of the first 2 tests presented in baseline printout just an overview printout of the two tests.

The change in mean deviation is presented in the baseline printout just as linear regression analysis of mean deviation of change analysis printout.

So the baseline printout of GPA is nothing but the combination of the overview printout and linear regression analysis of mean deviation of change analysis printout.

The patients name, the eye tested, date of birth, the selection of the test will appear on the top of the GPA printout. The baseline printout of GPA presents the results of each test in four plots—gray scale, RAW data, total deviation probability plot and pattern deviation probability plot. The foveal threshold, the reliability parameters and global indices are also printed at the bottom of each test.

The linear regression analysis of mean deviation component of GPA consists of the mean of the value of mean deviation index of the baseline tests and the follow-up tests and the STATPAC calculates linear regression analysis of mean deviation.

Guided Progression Analysis

This new GPA presents baseline, VFI plot, progression analysis plot and GPA alert all on one page.

Visual Field Index

The visual field index (VFI) is calculated as a percentage of the of normal visual field after adjustment for age. VFI of 100 percent implies that the visual field is normal whereas a VFI

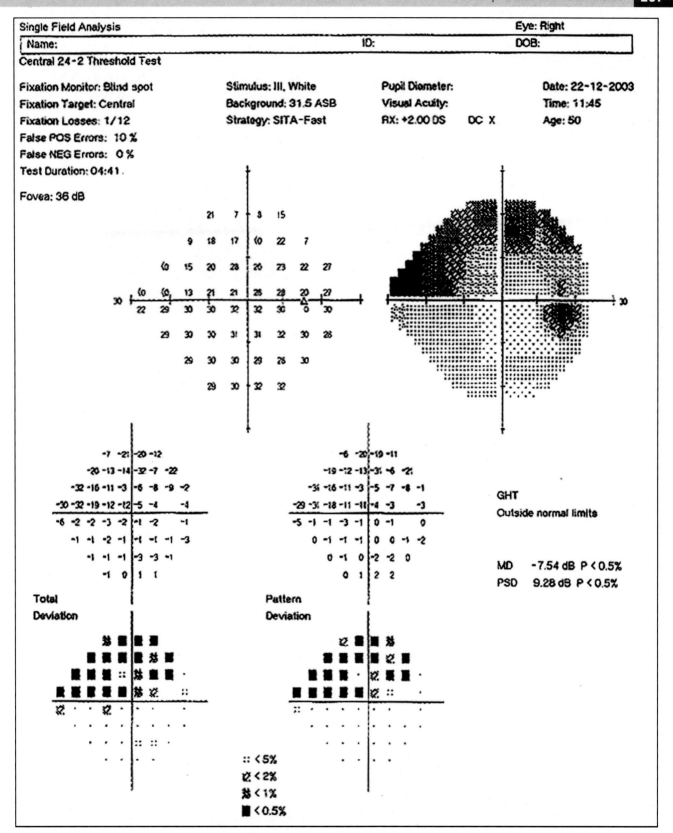

Fig. 32 Localized field defect is fulfilling the Anderson's criteria to say that the loss of retinal sensitivity is due to glaucoma

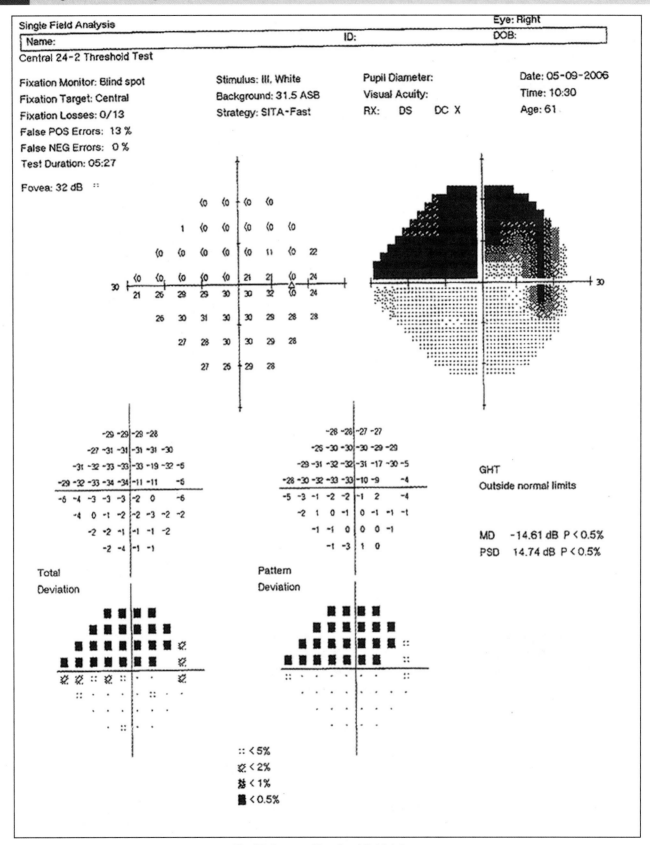

Fig. 33 A case of localized field defect

of 0 percent means that the patient is perimetrically blind. It is based on both total and pattern standard deviation probability maps and also weighs points according to their location in the visual field. The central points are given more weight as compared to the peripheral. The final VFI score is thus a mean of the weighted scores of all the points. It is plotted against age and as a trend analysis. It is less affected by media opacities as compared to MD and helps in estimation of progression in patients with cataract and glaucoma.

The VFI also provides an estimate of additional visual field loss that may occur in the next 5 years if the same rate of progression is maintained.

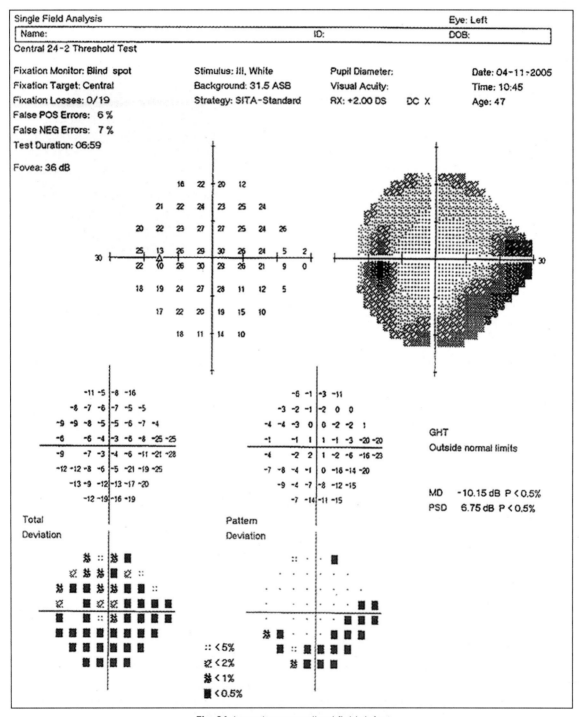

Fig. 34 Irregular generalized field defect

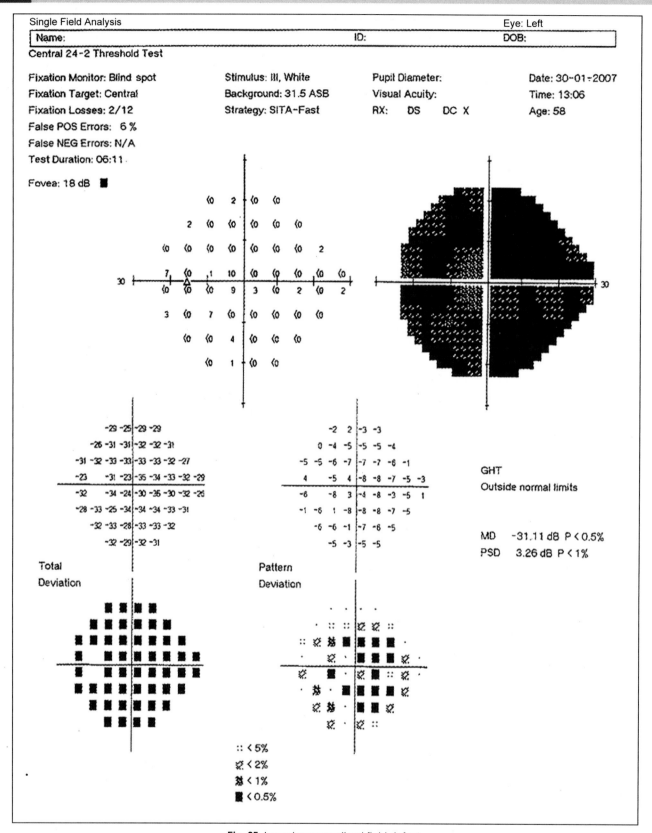

Single Field Analysis   Eye: Left

Name: ID: DOB:

Central 24-2 Threshold Test

Fixation Monitor: Blind spot   Stimulus: III, White   Pupil Diameter: Date: 30-01-2007
Fixation Target: Central   Background: 31.5 ASB   Visual Acuity: Time: 13:06
Fixation Losses: 2/12   Strategy: SITA-Fast   RX: DS   DC X   Age: 58
False POS Errors: 6 %
False NEG Errors: N/A
Test Duration: 06:11

Fovea: 18 dB

GHT
Outside normal limits

MD   -31.11 dB P < 0.5%
PSD   3.26 dB P < 1%

Total Deviation

Pattern Deviation

:: < 5%
✗ < 2%
✗ < 1%
■ < 0.5%

Fig. 35 Irregular generalized field defect

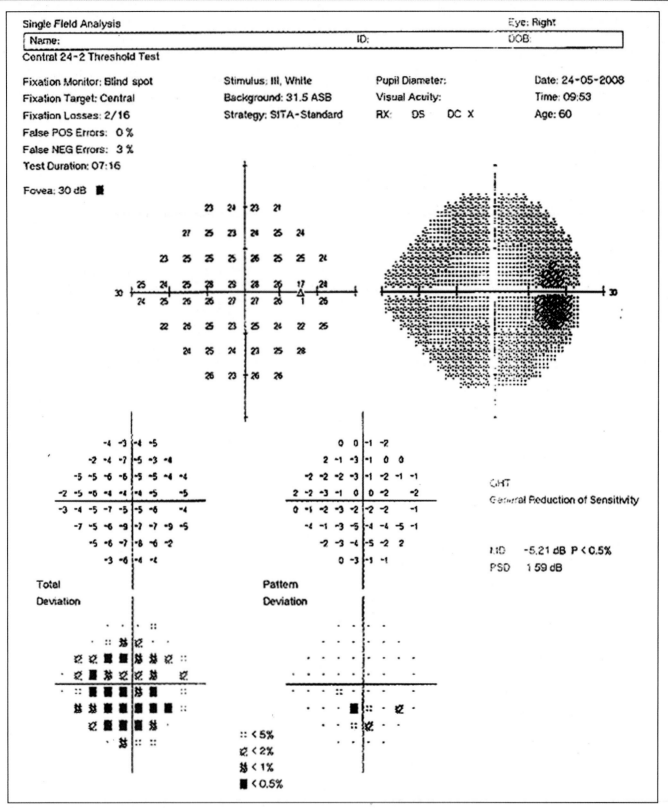

Single Field Analysis   Eye: Right

| Name: | ID: | DOB: |

Central 24-2 Threshold Test

Fixation Monitor: Blind spot   Stimulus: III, White   Pupil Diameter: Date: 24-05-2008
Fixation Target: Central   Background: 31.5 ASB   Visual Acuity: Time: 09:53
Fixation Losses: 2/16   Strategy: SITA-Standard   RX: DS   DC   X   Age: 60
False POS Errors: 0 %
False NEG Errors: 3 %
Test Duration: 07:16

Fovea: 30 dB

CHT
General Reduction of Sensitivity

MD   -5.21 dB P < 0.5%
PSD   1.59 dB

Total Deviation

Pattern Deviation

:: < 5%
⦂ < 2%
⅏ < 1%
■ < 0.5%

Fig. 36 The visual field is not suggestive of glaucoma

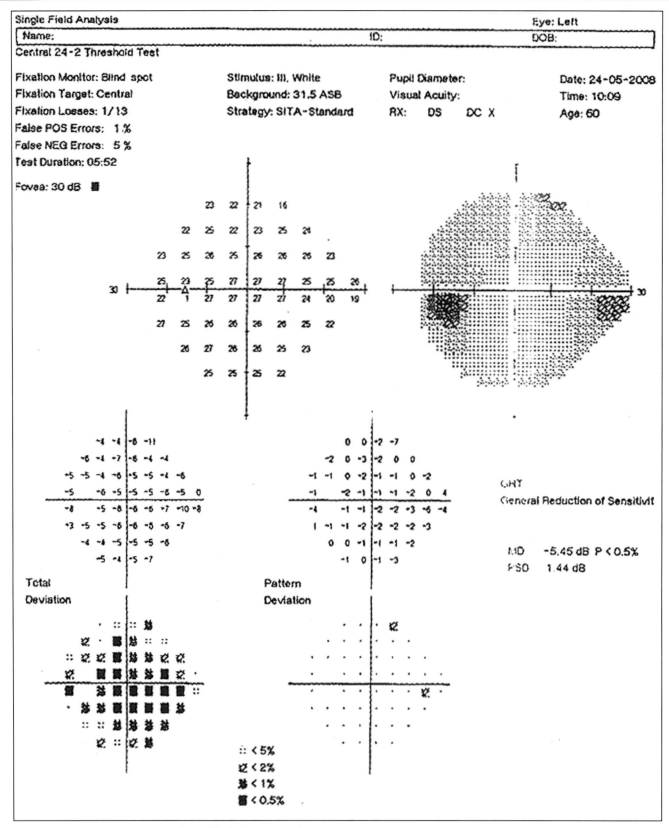

Fig. 37 The visual field is not suggestive of glaucoma

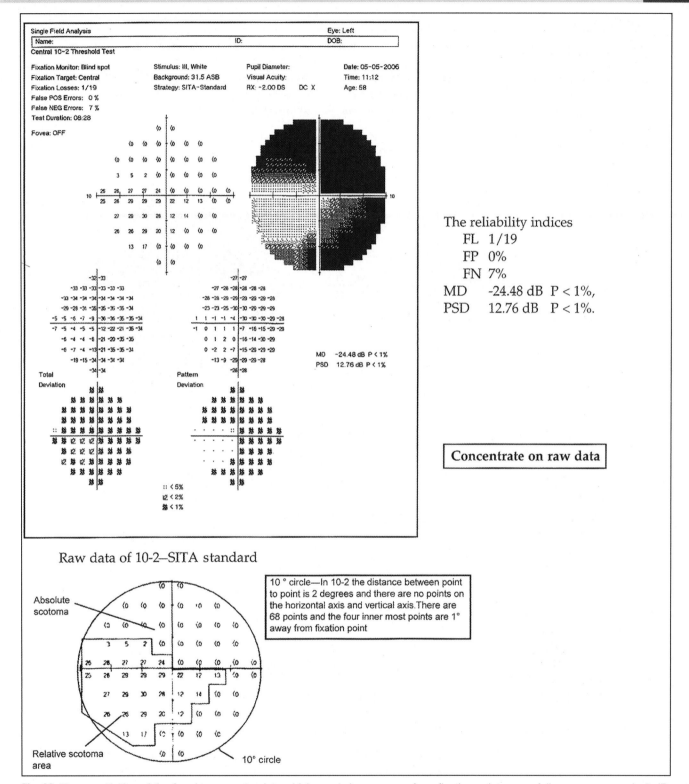

Fig. 38 The sensitivities of the four inner most points which are 1 degree away from fixation point are as follows: upper nasal <0 dB; lower nasal 22 dB; upper temporal 24 dB; lower temporal 29 dB. The upper nasal point is also showing 0 dB. So there is foveal involvement in the upper temporal quadrant. In the remaining quadrants there is good sensitivity

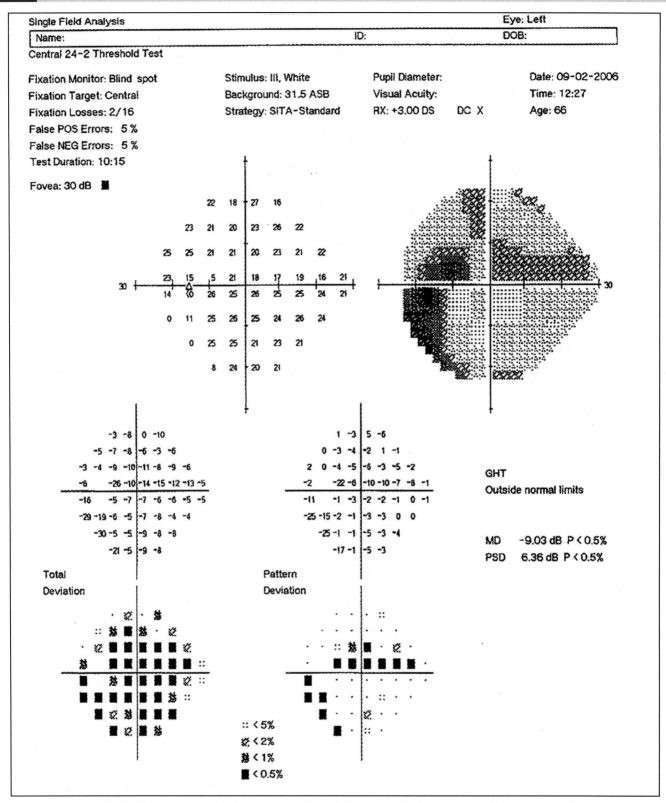

Single Field Analysis   Eye: Left

Name: ID: DOB:

Central 24-2 Threshold Test

Fixation Monitor: Blind spot   Stimulus: III, White   Pupil Diameter: Date: 09-02-2006
Fixation Target: Central   Background: 31.5 ASB   Visual Acuity: Time: 12:27
Fixation Losses: 2/16   Strategy: SITA-Standard   RX: +3.00 DS   DC X   Age: 66
False POS Errors: 5%
False NEG Errors: 5%
Test Duration: 10:15

Fovea: 30 dB

GHT
Outside normal limits

MD   -9.03 dB P < 0.5%
PSD   6.36 dB P < 0.5%

Total
Deviation

Pattern
Deviation

:: < 5%
< 2%
< 1%
< 0.5%

Fig. 39 Cataract producing uniform generalized field defect and when associated with glaucoma,
it will produce irregular generalized field defect

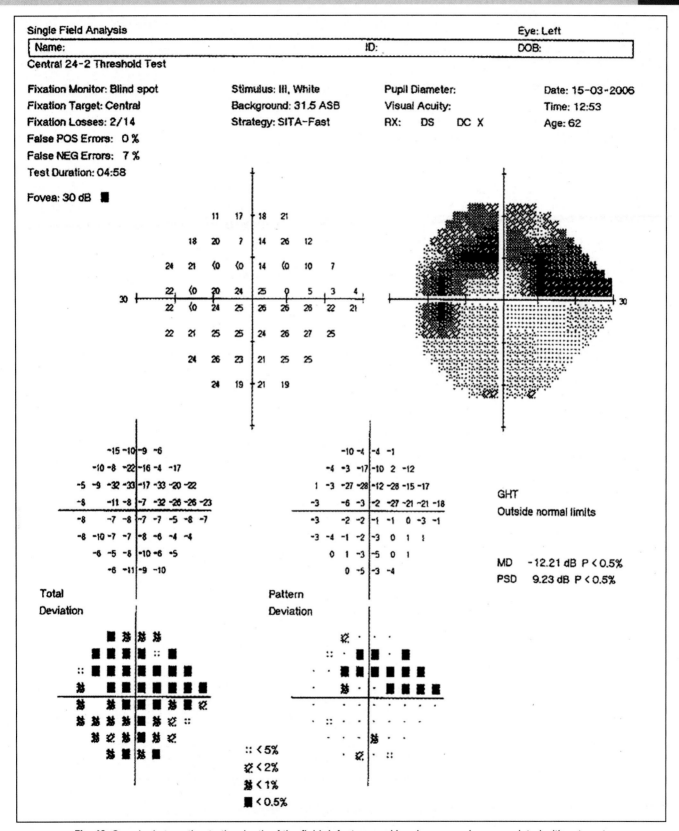

Fig. 40 Our aim is to estimate the depth of the field defect caused by glaucoma when associated with cataract. Follow-up visual field examination is required

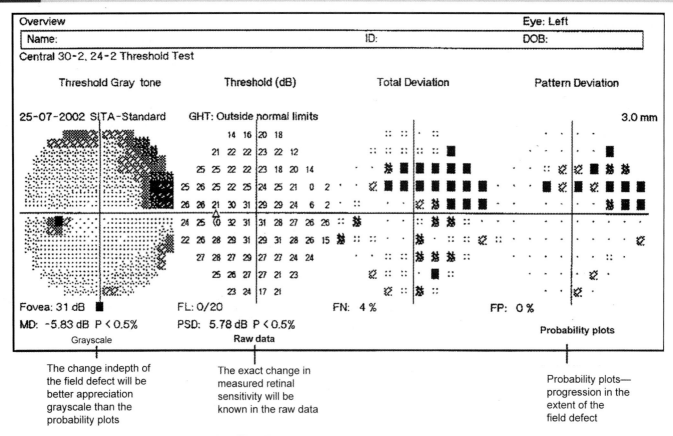

Fovea: 31 dB

FL: 0/20   FN: 4 %   FP: 0 %

MD: -5.83 dB P < 0.5%   PSD: 5.78 dB P < 0.5%

Grayscale   Raw data   Probability plots

The change indepth of the field defect will be better appreciation grayscale than the probability plots

The exact change in measured retinal sensitivity will be known in the raw data

Probability plots— progression in the extent of the field defect

Fig. 41 Increase in MD index and change in PSD indicate that there is progression of field defect and it may be confined to a localized area or to a localized area in generalized depression (irregular generalized loss). Increase in MD index and no change in PSD index indicate that there is progression of the field defect and it is uniform generalized type

Flow chart 3 Classification of follow-up visual field printouts

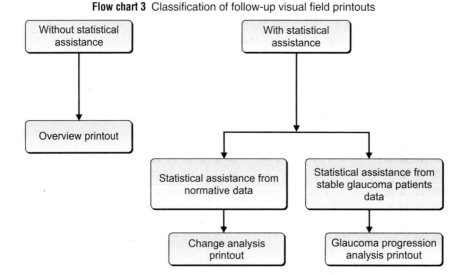

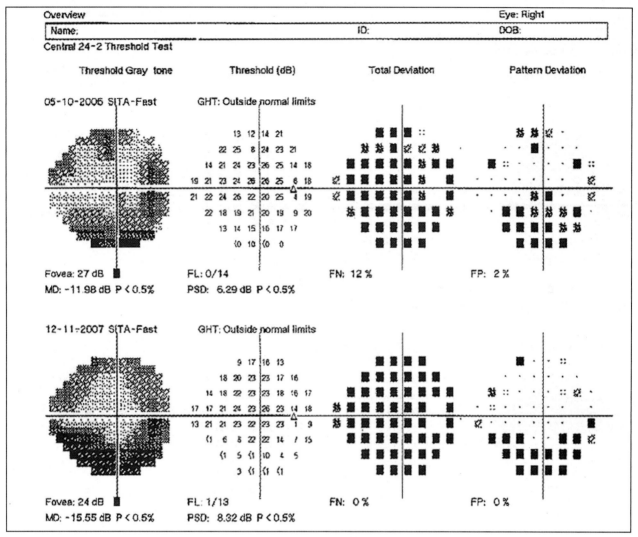

Fig. 42 MD index 1st test −11.98 dB P < 0.5% and 2nd test −15.55 dB P < 0.5%. Average loss of sensitivity in lower nasal quadrant is 3.67 dB in 1st test and in second test it is 7.49 dB. *Conclusion:* There is definite progression of the field defect

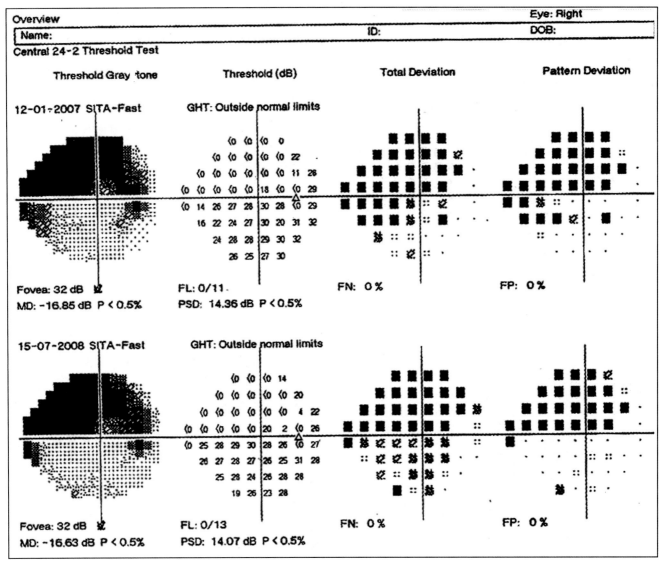

Fig. 43 MD index 1st test –16.58 dB P < 0.5% and 2nd test –16.63 dB P < 0.5%

- No significant change in MD index
- Both tests done on 24-2 program
- Reliability indices are 100% perfect in both tests
- Foveal sensitivity in both tests is 32 dB which indicates that the refractive correction for near vision is perfectly given during the tests

Conclusion: There is no progression of the field defect

17 | Octopus Perimetry: A Synopsis

NR Rangaraj, Murali Ariga

CHAPTER OUTLINE

- ❖ Visual Field Evaluation
- ❖ Basic Definitions
- ❖ Measurement Strategies
- ❖ Systematic Interpretation of Octopus Seven in One Single Field Report, 'The Ten Step Approach'
- ❖ Octopus Examination Programs
- ❖ Octopus Perimeter Reports

VISUAL FIELD EVALUATION

Perimetry is the evaluation of visual field. Many eye diseases like glaucoma alter the visual function in a characteristic pattern which makes computer assisted perimerty a valuable tool for diagnosis and follow-up **(Figure 1)**. Visual field testing compliments other parameters like intraocular pressure and structural changes in the optic nerve head in decision making as in glaucoma to chart progression of the disease. The central 30° visual field examination using automated perimetry is currently the gold standard in evaluation, management and follow-up of glaucoma. Non-glaucomatous causes of visual field changes may also be diagnosed and followed up.

Evolution of Octopus Perimeter

Visual field as a tool in diagnostics was known since 1668 when Mariotte first discovered blind spot. Goldmann in 1945 gave standardization to the mapping of visual fields with the introduction of a cupola. The Goldmann Perimeter **(Figure 2)** too was only as good as the operator behind it.

Introduction of automated perimetry as it is known today was from the school of Goldmann in Berne, Switzerland **(Figure 3)**. In 1972 Fankhauser et al, developed the first computer assisted static automated perimeter.[1] **(Figure 4)** Sphar investigated the basic concept of threshold determination.[2] Bebie **(Figure 5)**,

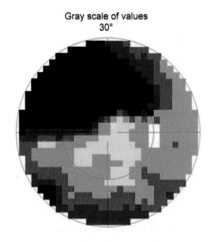

Gray scale of values
30°

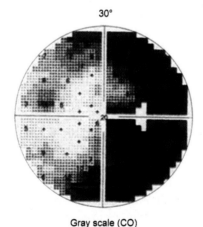

Gray scale (CO)

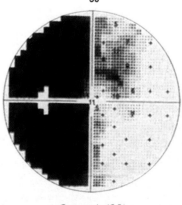

Gray scale (CO)

Fig. 1 Gray/color scale

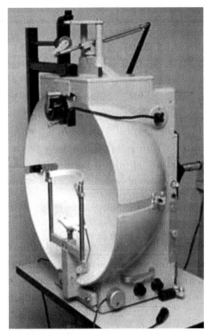

Fig. 2 Goldmann perimeter (Reprinted with permission of HAAG-STREITAG)

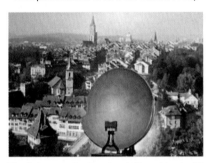

Fig. 3 Berne, Switzerland (Reprinted with permission of HAAG-STREITAG)

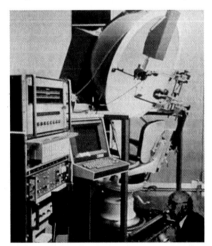

Fig. 4 Fankhauser with the original perimeter (Reprinted with permission of HAAG-STREITAG)

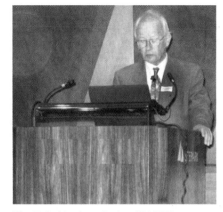

Fig. 5 Bebie, introducing 'RAMP' strategy

Fankhauser, Hirsbrunner contributed the concepts which formed the mathematical and statistical model into a workable software for the Automated static perimetry which included behavior pathology of the tested locations over time. 1985 saw the introduction of a new program called the G1 by Flammer that had a new set of locations based on the retinal nerve fiber topography and the fields could be summed up with visual field indices.[3] The **'Bebie Curve'** or the cumulative defect curve was added to the printout presentation for additional information.[4] Modifications to the normal strategy by staging and phases made the procedure of the automated visual field analysis shorter without much loss of information since the information gained in the first tested locations were more reliable than the locations tested latter in the test.

Recent progress in faster strategies to determine the differential light sensitivity[5] like the TOP and Dynamic on the Octopus perimeters gives good quality of visual field report in a much shorter time. Reliability of performance of the visual field test by the patient was found to have an inverse function with time with both physical and retinal fatigue contributing to errors.[6]

The TOP strategy was based on the algorithm of repetitive extrapolation of local visual field information at the tested location and in neighborhood groups of the tested locations. This strategy allowed 59 tested points as in G1 to be extrapolated with 294 adjustments to give the final results in the visual field results. The results of the visual field analysis from TOP are available in 2 to 3 minutes on an average.

The Dynamic strategy[7] steers the staircase test according to the steepness of the frequency of seeing curve. The steps being larger at test points where depth of local depression (differential light sensitivity) is deeper and smaller steps of differential sensitivity when the test point is within 4 dB of the age corrected estimated hill of vision. The Dynamic takes a little longer than TOP since it is a modification of the regular normal threshold program.[8] This gain in test time and improved patient compliance could contribute to loss of information that can be adequately made up when there is structure function correlation as in diseases such as glaucoma.

Newer perimetry methods like the Blue on Yellow were an attempt to detect early visual field loss. This visual field test is very demanding visually with the inability to visualize the blue stimulus in presence of even minimal opacities.[9] Octopus introduced the **Flicker perimetry** to overcome the disadvantage of opacities in the media. The **Critical Fusion Frequency (CCF)** is the point at which the eye no longer sees's the light as a flicker but as a continuous glow. The CCF has similar characteristics as blue on yellow perimetry with opaque media no longer a barrier to detection of early visual field loss, as in combined cataract and glaucoma management.[10]

The Octopus family of perimeters has two distinct models. The traditional 101 and the 900 series are the cupola type of perimeters and the 123 and 300 series are infinity projection system models from Octopus **(Figure 6)**. The

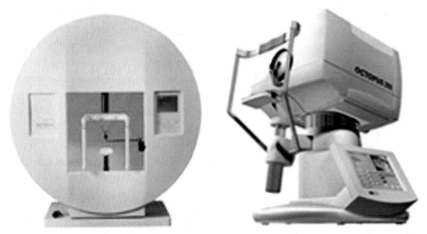

Fig. 6 Octopus perimeters models

101 and 900 series is also capable of semiautomated Kinetic perimetry with the software to perform the traditional Goldmann Kinetic perimetry. The Octopus perimeter has undergone six generations of design evolution since the first clinical model was introduced in the late 70s to the latest 900 series cupola perimeter and the infinity projection perimeter of the 300 series. The two on one or the left to right print-out presentation of the visual field results is unique to Octopus, which at one glance gives the estimation of the visual fields from both eyes. This is particularly useful in demonstrating congruence or noncongruence of loss of visual field in neuro-ophthalmic conditions or the nasal step in glaucomatous optic nerve damage. Version upgrades for the automated perimeters can be done over the internet from the Octopus website and new feature functions may be unlocked with only the appropriate number key. All computing is done on the external Personal Computer and the perimeters have flash memory cards to do all relevant computing functions on the machine. The advantage being new strategies and programs may be upgraded by switching to new memory cards in the older machine without having to replace the machine.

BASIC DEFINITIONS
Visual Field

It is the area seen by the steadily fixating eye. This area of visual field when measured for follow-up and comparison is done under standard conditions of color, background illumination that is fixed for a particular machine. Stimulus size may vary for normal estimations and for low vision conditions. The visual field tests the subject's ability to perceive the faintest light stimuli against the uniformly illuminated background, in effect measures the least difference between the stimuli and the background illumination.

The Patient's Threshold

It is defined as the stimulus luminance which is perceived for a given background illumination, with a probability of 50 percent chance of seeing or not seeing which is described by the frequency of seeing curve (FOSC) as function of stimulus luminance.

Threshold

It is expressed in decibel (dB) scale in clinical practice. In reality the threshold is not a fixed point, it fluctuates during the test when it is being conducted and over long periods of time at the same test points. The FOSC is very steep normally. This is due to the consistency

of response to the projected light stimulus during visual field examination. This ability to perceive the 50 percent threshold illumination is very sharp in normal individual at all test points in the visual field, about 4 bandwidth (**Figure 7A**). The test points which are abnormal due to disease show inconsistency of response and the bandwidth of response becomes more than 4dB which makes the FOSC flat (**Figure 7B**). Generalized depression of the field causes the FOSC shift to the right but remains steep.

The Octopus perimeter has standard test conditions so that, consistent data may be obtained from one visit to the next. This consistent data obtained during each visit helps in follow-up and comparison to be made with age related normals. The standard test conditions adopted in the Octopus 101 and 300 series along with the Humphrey 700 series perimeter test conditions as in **Table 1**.

Background illumination plays an important part in the shape of the hill of vision. Lower background illumination in static perimetry increases the dynamic range and highlights areas of depressed sensitivity better because of the flatter slope of the hill of vision (**Figure 8**). The draw back of lower background illumination is longer period of adaptation before the test is started. The Goldmann Kinetic perimetry uses a 31.4 asb as the background illumination. **The direct projection perimeters like the Octopus 123 and 300 use a background illumination of 31.5 asb hence can be used in normal clinic lighting conditions with a shortened adaptation time.**

The stimulus exposure time is 100 ms in the Octopus perimeter since this time is enough to reach temporal summation of the stimulus luminance. Any exposure longer than 200 ms will provoke fixation reflex and give erroneous results (**Figure 9**). Setting the stimulus interval

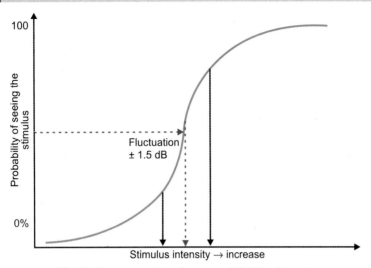

Fig. 7A Frequency of seeing curve (FOSC)—Normal

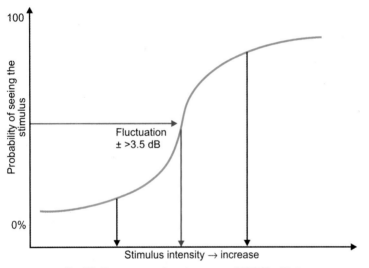

Fig. 7B Frequency of seeing curve (FOSC)—Flat

for an expected pattern of visual field loss expected in the particular disease process. New strategies like TOP and Dynamic give quantitative results in the same time. Hence, the two zone testing and screening strategies are of only academic value now.

Octopus perimeters offer

- The normal full threshold testing strategy
- The dynamic strategy (Weber)
- Tendency oriented perimetry (TOP).

It is important to understand the **Classical normal strategy** introduced by Flammer since it forms the basis of automated perimetry.

Normal Testing Strategy

The normal strategy tests all points in a random manner in steps of decreasing luminance such that a yes or no answer is obtained to the least amount of stimulus at all test points. The perimetry being computerized helps in correlating all the randomized stimulus intensities and answers in a printout. To make things easy for the patient and duration of test shorter, testing starts at one point in each of four visual field quadrants called **anchor points**. The anchor points test the general slope of the hill of vision to the age corrected normal values. The visual field determination starts at all test points from the expected age corrected minus 4 decibels. A 'no' answer drops the stimulus luminance by 6 dB if the first response to a minus 4 dB start is negative. A brighter light stimulus is projected which is 8 dB less to quickly approach the depressed sensitivity of the test point. Once the anchor points are determined further testing in a 4-2-1 dB step approach at each of the predetermined test points are determined from the data obtained from the estimated hill of vision rather than starting from normal hill of vision values which

takes into consideration the NO answer and the next stimulus. The adaptive stimulus presentation keeps track of the average time of response and proceeds with the completion of the test either faster or slower. The normal interval is set between 1.5 and 4 seconds.

MEASUREMENT STRATEGIES

It is important to understand that the **How** of testing is the strategy and the **Where** is the program or the set of test points being tested. The choice of test strategies is offered in the Octopus 300/900 series perimeter to meet the different clinical situations of diagnosis and follow-up. The two main testing procedures offered across all perimeters are the Screening tests (Qualitative) and the Quantitative tests as offered by the full threshold tests in the 4-2-1 dB steps.

Traditional screening strategies give qualitative results in a yes or no format to save time to get a general idea of the visual field to help in looking

Table 1 Standard test conditions

Parameter	Octopus 101	Octopus 300	HFA 700
Background luminance	4 asb	31.1 asb	31.5 asb
Stimulus			
• Size	Goldmann I-V	Goldmann III,V	Goldmann I-V
• Duration	100 ms	100 ms	200 ms
• Luminance for 0 dB	1,000 asb	4,800 asb	10,000 asb
Measuring range	0-40 dB	0-40 dB	0-40 dB
Test strategies	4-2-1 dB bracketing	4-2-1 dB bracketing	4-2-1 dB bracketing
	Dynamic strategy	Dynamic strategy	SITA standard
	TOP	TOP	SITA fast
Normal values	Age correction per year		

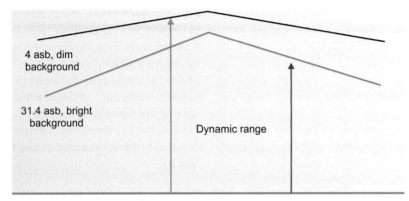

Fig. 8 Dynamic range with low and high background illumination

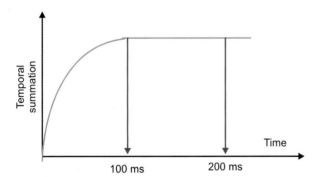

Fig. 9 Stimulus duration in ms and temporal summation

would make the testing tedious. This is approximately five questions per test point hence sensitive enough to detect shallow pathology. Normal strategy takes about 15 to 18 minutes per eye to complete a visual field examination **(Figure 10)**.

Octopus introduced new strategies to minimize the effects of physical and retinal fatigue, which are implemented in all models of the perimeters as below:

- Staging and phases
- Dynamic strategy
- Tendency oriented perimetry (TOP).

Octopus Staging and Phases
Staging of Visual Field
Visual field analysis testing was traditionally done in a single pass, i.e. the first to last test result is needed before a test result is printed out **(Figure 11)**. Normal strategy typically takes 18 to 20 minutes to complete for final results of the test. The single pass visual field test was modified by Octopus into staged modules to run in a sequence of diagnostically relevant stages and test points so that the first tested points give the best results without the influence of fatigue, physical or retinal. Each of the four stages behaving as independent test with result outcome accumulated thus far. The need to continuation into the next stage could be dependant on need for more diagnostic information. This visual field result can now be saved, printed or restarted from the last tested point. The results obtained in the first two stages account for almost 80 percent of the result **(Figure 12)**. The Octopus perimeters have an online 'defect level' indicator in the screen which statistically facilitates if the current visual field examination is 'normal', 'borderline' or 'depressed'. In cases of borderline, the test could be continued in the next two stages of the visual field test to get a complete analysis.

Test Phases in Octopus Perimeter
After one or two stages of visual field testing in the first phase, one of four options now exist in second phase of visual field testing.

1. The test may be saved, printed or stopped.
2. The test points may be retested to ascertain the short-term fluctuations.

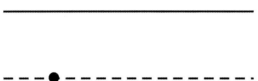

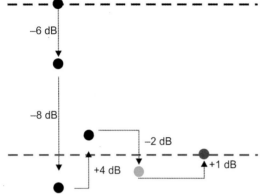

Fig. 10 Schematic of 4-2-1 bracketing strategy

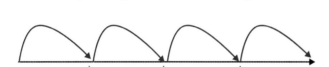

Fig. 11 Single Pass visual field testing

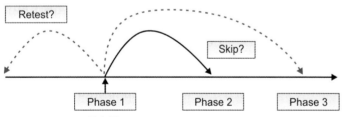

Fig. 12 Schematic of staging concept

Fig. 13 Test phases after 1st stage

3. Quantify relative defects.
4. When data already indicates deviation from normal then additional peripheral test points may be tested to confirm clinical findings. This concept of phasing allows standardized data to be obtained by selectively testing for a specific pathology at the expected test points with very little loss of information and economizing the time duration taken for the test **(Figure 13)**.

Dynamic Test Strategy

Weber introduced the Dynamic strategy of visual field testing. The stimulus luminance step size (bracketing) adapts to the slope of the FOSC. When the depth of the defect is deep, the step size increases from increments steps of 2 dB to 10 dB to achieve final calculated value from the last two tested values. The accuracy obtained with this test is comparable to the regular full threshold test with a 4-2-1 dB strategy. This strategy provides quantitative data, which may be represented as the gray scale, Bebie curve and global indices. Quantitative values are useful for follow-up and to track changes over time. The test duration is about 40 to 50 percent in severely depressed fields and 30 to 40 percent in marginally depressed fields when compared to normal threshold. Short-term fluctuation values may also be calculated by retesting all locations in the second phase if additional information is needed. Dynamic strategy provides data of the visual field comparable to the regular full threshold determination done in four stages **(Figures 14A and B)**.

Tendency Oriented Perimetry

Tendency oriented perimetry (TOP) strategy introduced by Prof González de la Rosa reduces the time taken to complete the visual field analysis by 80 percent to the time taken by normal threshold. TOP takes the neighboring test locations into account when the results are interpreted. TOP strategy can be applied to all test methods like blue on yellow and flicker or programs like macular-M2. The neighboring zones exhibit a topographical interdependence, which establishes a tendency between adjacent points under examination.

TOP evaluates every 'yes' and 'no' in two ways, the test location under test is evaluated for the differential sensitivity, which is called the vertical bracketing and the neighboring points are also adjusted by interpolation. A 'yes' answer at the test location will influence the neighboring point positively and a 'no' answer will influence the neighboring point negatively on the

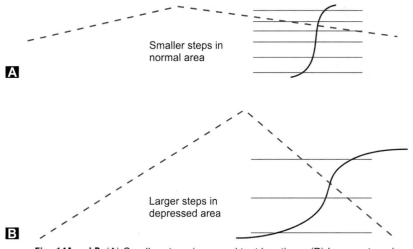

Figs 14A and B (A) Smaller steps in normal test locations; (B) Larger steps in depressed areas

decibel scale. In regular full threshold perimetry every test location is tested at least 4 to 6 times before arrival at the final value of differential sensitivity. A single answer in TOP is adjusted five times from the results of the neighboring test locations in the grid for final results.

TOP divides the test location in the visual field into evenly intermingling grids. The four grids are examined one after another and the locations of the other three matrices are adjusted to get new values by interpolation. The examination starts at half the value of the expected age corrected value, which in dB is 8/16 of the expected normal value. Then the testing begins with steps in relation to the patients age corrected value, i.e. 4/16, 3/16, 2/16 and finally a 1/16. These steps may be in either direction to determine the final threshold of dl sensitivity (**Figure 15**). Gray scales show a rounded effect in TOP compared to regular threshold gray scale values because of the adjustments of the neighboring points. Hence, the average sensitivity values obtained may be a little 'shallow' compared with regular threshold testing (**Figure 16**). This difference is not of any significance when the parameter in follow-up is only change over time,

since the pathology is already established and the patient compliance is improved for follow-up testing. Note the difference in MD values of only 0.1 between the two strategies (**Figure 16**). The gray/color scale shows some spread and shallowness of the color scale in the TOP strategy.

Qualitative 2 Level Testing
With the introduction of faster full threshold testing, these screening tests are almost obsolete. 2-level testing uses a maximum of two questions per location and provides a simple quantification of the tested location. The test starts with a stimulus –4 dB less than the age corrected value. A 'yes' answer sums up the test result of that location. A 'no' answer provides the same location the brightest stimuli and a 'yes' tags the test location as relative defect. A 'no' to the brightest stimulus is classified as an absolute defect. The Octopus perimeter allows these relatively tested points to be quantified in the second phase and thus convert a qualitative test result into a quantified test result.

OCTOPUS EXAMINATION PROGRAMS
A white on white visual field testing procedure needs two questions to be answered, 'which' locations need to be

tested—program and 'how' should it be tested—strategy. A third additional question could be—'what method' i.e. flicker, kinetic or blue on yellow Perimetry.

Table 2 illustrates the combinations of test programs, test strategy and perimetry method that may be chosen depending on the pathology to be tested on octopus perimeters 900, 101, 123 and 300 series. **A neurologic examination** may be done with program 32 using TOP, dynamic and rarely or never with normal strategy on a white/white perimetry method. The table sums up the various combinations that could be used (**Table 2**).

Test program, test strategy and perimetry method may be appropriately chosen for a given pathology under investigation. Octopus perimeter offers test locations or programs for specific pathology, e.g. glaucoma, macular degeneration or neurological examination.

The test programs that are offered on the Octopus perimeters, which are commonly used are as follows:

Program G1/G2[11]
The two programs are identical in the central 30° consisting of 59 test point locations and differ only in the peripheral 15 additional points tested between the 30° and 60° in G2. The G2 is a program optimized for Octopus 101/900 series perimeter. The G1 program test locations respect the topography of the nerve fiber layer and are weighted to detect the nasal step in glaucoma (**Figure 17A**). The foveal and paracentral areas have resolution of 2.8° in the G1/G2 programs compared to 4.2° resolution in a classical program 32 test location. The increased resolution in the foveal area gives a good follow-up when there is a fixation threat, with out the need of an additional visual field test for the fovea. Depressed areas have a high false

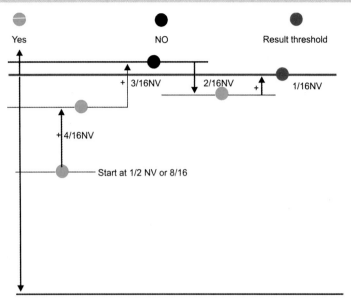

Fig. 15 Schematic representation of the bracketing in TOP

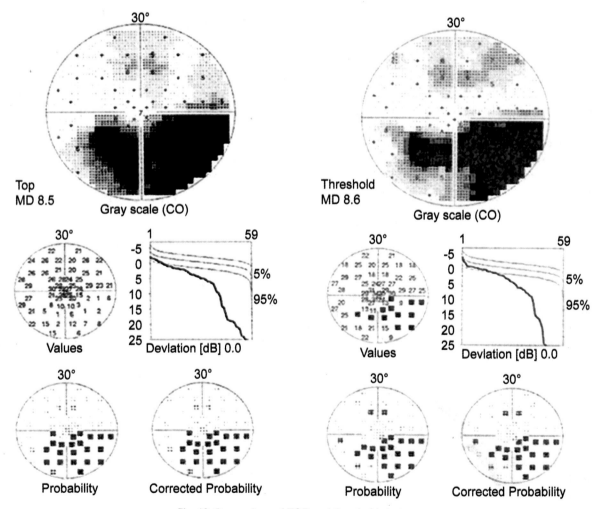

Fig. 16 Comparison of TOP and threshold strategy

Table 2 Combination of test program

Examination Procedure	Test Program +	Test Strategy +	Perimetry Method
	G1, G2	Normal Strategy	White /White
	Program 32	Dynamic Strategy	Flicker
	Program M2	TOP Strategy	Blue/Yellow

negative behavior because of a flatter FOSC and extend the test duration.

All strategies can run on the G1 and G2 program **(Figure 17B)**. The 300 Octopus perimeters allow the phase 2 retesting of all the test locations in the dynamic and normal strategy. The phase 3 (screening the periphery) and phase 4 (quantifying the periphery) runs in the 101 and 900 series. These perimeters are used in research and teaching settings. The 4 dB background illumination increases the dynamic range of the tested locations. Most clinical needs are satisfied with the 300 series Octopus perimeter. Having an additional test points between the 30° and 60° of testing does not give additional information but only confirms what is seen in the central 30° field.

Program 32

This is the classic 'off axis' program introduced by Octopus and later by other perimeters as the 30-2 program. There are 76 test locations in a grid pattern with a resolution of 6°. This program is not related to the topography of the nerve fiber layer or pathology with both eyes having identical pattern of test locations. The area where the blind spot appears marks the right and left eye. The program 32 is still an option if old follow-up was done with this program. It may also be used in neurological cases where this program defines the vertical and horizontal meridians well. Phase 2 testing may be done to asses the short-term fluctuation in normal and dynamic strategy **(Figure 18)**.

Program M2

The macular program was designed for detection and follow-up of central and paracentral visual field defects in patients with neurological diseases, macular or perimacular diseases.

The M2 program has 45 test locations which are tested in two stages consisting of the central 4° and the area between 4° and 9°. The 45 test locations in the central 4° gives a 0.7° resolution with a Goldmann Size III which is 0.43° in diameter **(Figure 19)**. The additional 36 test locations situated in the outer 4° to 9° gives this program the highest resolution in the central 10° of the visual field. Additional test locations may also be tested between 9.5° and 26° if need be.

The M2 program can be run using the TOP, dynamic or normal strategy to define the visual field pathology in question.

Other Octopus Programs

The N1 neurologic program is a multistep examination program which takes into account the possible displacement of blind spot due to extraocular muscle and avoids artifacts due to hemianopia or hemineglect.

Program STX/ST—Glaucoma (2-Level) screening test: The test locations are the same as G1 except that the only qualitative data is obtained in 3 to 4 minutes.

> **Note** New strategies of visual field evaluation have made screening tests obsolete with quantitative data of the visual field presented in a shorter time than the screening tests.

SYSTEMATIC INTERPRETATION OF OCTOPUS SEVEN IN ONE SINGLE FIELD REPORT, 'THE TEN STEP APPROACH'

The Octopus seven in one printout contains the raw results from the visual field examination and easy to read data interpreting the results of the test. The single field printout also presents the statistical calculations, images, graphs, plots and indices. The 'Ten Step Approach' to the single field printout makes the interpretation of visual fields in a clinic setting easy to read and correlate the clinical findings **(Figure 20)**.

The seven in one report is interpreted in the following order:

1. **Patient data:** Information about the patient.
2. **Examination data:** Details about the examination and reliability.
3. **Value table:** This table shows the measured values. All further statistical and graphical details are derived from this set of raw data.
4. **Comparison table:** Representing the local difference between the measured values and the normal values valid for the patient's age.
5. **Corrected comparison table:** Shows the defects discounting any uniform depression caused by a cataract or other diffuse loss, e.g. refractive errors.
6. **Gray scale (in color or in B/W):** An overview of the pattern of visual field defects for the doctor and can be used to explain the nature of the problem to the patient.
7. **Cumulative defect (Bebie) curve:** An arrangement of all test data from the highest value to least

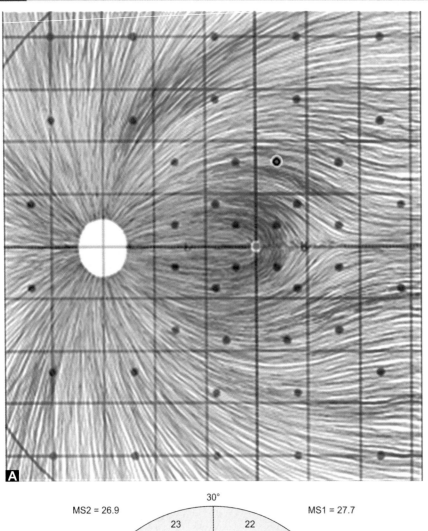

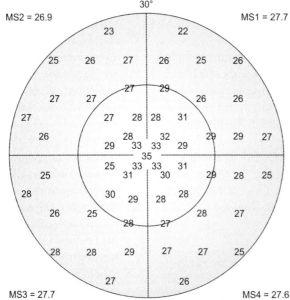

Figs 17A and B (A) G1 test points superimposed on the nerve fiber layer (Reprinted with permission of HAAG-STREITAG); (B) Typical G1 locations of test points

from left to right which is overlaid on a statistically age corrected normal for comparison.

8. ***Probability plots:*** Graphical representation of the probability or significance of a defect.
9. **Visual field indices**: Condenses the visual field results in a few numbers.
10. **Structure function correlation**.

Patient Data

The demographic data of the patient should be checked. The name, both first and last is to be entered in the same way so that the software understands the name as the 'same patient' and all the visual field tests are bunched together in the peritrend database. *The date of birth entry* in the machine is used for age corrected values and comparison. Hence, a young patient with a wrong date of birth (older) will show unusually high sensitivity expected for the age. *The notes field* is used for entry of the intraocular pressure and central corneal thickness values **(Figure 21)**.

Examination Data

This field highlights the *examined eye* and the *size of pupils* on the top. The Octopus measures the pupil's size automatically and is important for comparisons with previous fields and normal data. The *examination program and strategy* should be prefixed according to the pathology and user preference e.g., glaucoma G1/P32 program and TOP/Dynamic so that all future data are collected for follow up with the same selection. *Comparing data obtained with P32/Dynamic strategy and compared with G1/TOP will make follow-up unreliable.* The other data in this section includes the date, time, and test duration. The total number of questions and repetitions are also displayed. The repetitions occur due

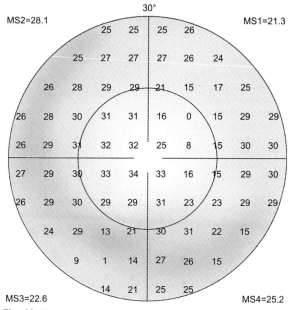

MS2=28.1   30°   MS1=21.3

MS3=22.6   MS4=25.2

Fig. 18 Test point locations in the P32 or the 30-2 program

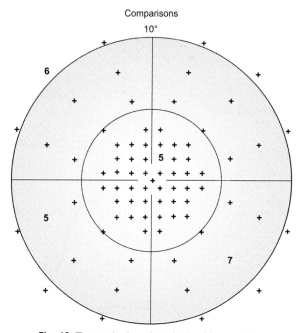

Comparisons
10°

Fig. 19 Test point locations in the M2 program

was responded to with less bright stimulus. Negative catch trials are increased in neighboring test locations of pathology in the visual fields because of a flat FOSC caused by wide variation in differential sensitivity of more than 5 dB. Unusually, high negative catch trials do not sometimes indicate unreliable fields when taken in the context of the pathology under investigation. The percentage of missed catch trails of both categories defines the "Reliability factor" (RF) together within the visual field indices. The percentage of wrong answers should not be higher than about 15 percent (Reliability factor = 15). If the patient has difficulty in performing the test and the value is higher than 20 percent this is noted so as to use this data in subsequent follow-up.

Value Table

The actual measured values of local sensitivities in decibels (dB) at each of the test locations are shown in the value table (VA) **(Figure 23)**. The other graphs, plots and images are derived from this 'raw' data by calculations based on normal data and statistical methods. *It is important to remember that a person's normal sensitivity value decreases with age with the hill of vision becoming steeper in the periphery.*

Comparison Table

The comparison (CO) table presents the age corrected values of the test locations from the measured actual values from the values table. The normal values are presented in '+' symbol and the numerical values are representation of the deviation from normal. This '+' symbol corresponds to the 4 dB bandwidth which is the age corrected normal bandwidth in the Bebie Curve. The '+' symbol simplifies the representation of normal value for every age correction without the need to remember age corrected numerical values for

to lost fixation and blink at the time of presentation of the stimulus. The increase in repetitions does not influence the quality of the test since only valid questions and answers are used to give the final results. Repetitions are common in anxious and fatigued patients **(Figure 22)**.

The catch trials are indicators for the reliability of the results of the actual examination. The positive catch trials indicate the number of times the patient has answered when stimulus was not presented. The negative catch trials are the number of times did not respond to a brighter stimulus which

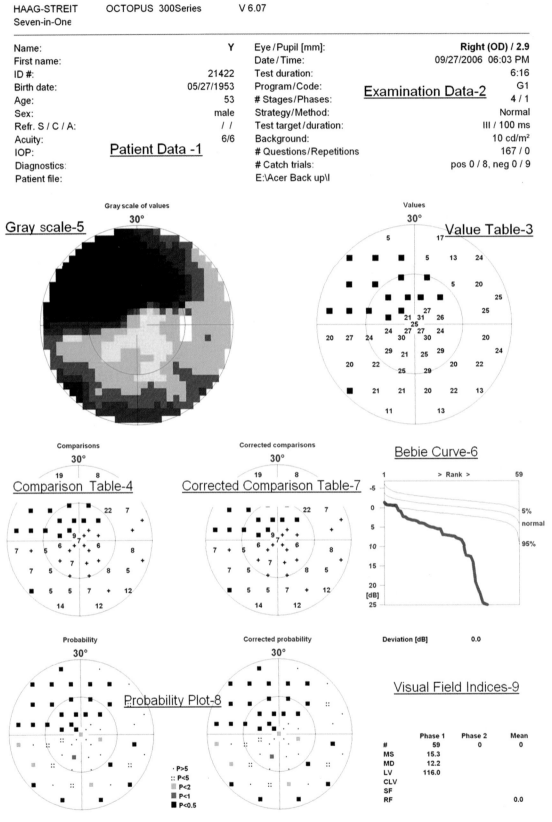

Fig. 20 Seven-in-one report

HAAG-STREIT	OCTOPUS 300 Series
Seven-in-One	
Name:	Y
First name:	:
ID #:	21422
Birth date:	05/27/1953
Age:	53
Sex:	male
Refr. S/C/A:	/ /
IOP:	6/6
Diagnostics:	
Patient file:	

Fig. 21 Patient data-1

Eye/Pupil (mm):	Right (OD)/2.9
Date/Time	09/27/2006 06:03 PM
Test duration:	6:16
Program/Code:	G1
# Stages/Phases:	4/1
Strategy/Method:	Dynamic/Normal
Test target/Duration:	III/100 ms
Background:	10 cd/m²
# Questions/Repetitions:	167/0
# Catch trials:	pos 0/8, neg 0/9
E:/Acer Back up/	

Fig. 22 Examination data-2

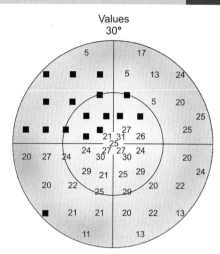

Fig. 23 Value table-3

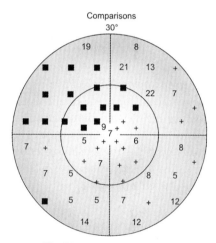

Fig. 24 Comparison table-4

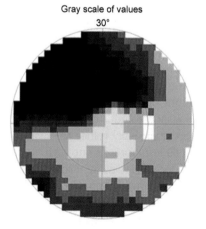

Fig. 25 Gray/color scale table-5

all ages. Significant deviation over 4 dB is represented by the actual numerical deviation from the age match normal **(Figure 24)**.

Gray Scale

The Gray scales are the first graphical presentation on the single field report. The single field print out depicts the gray scales in the actual measured sensitivity values and a graphical presentation of the value table. The gray scale is the presentation of the hill of vision in two dimensions, the center of the graph may be light in color due to higher sensitivity and the periphery darker because of lower sensitivity. The darker peripheral areas just represent 'normal' lower sensitivity. A graphic presentation of the normal comparison (CO) table would be white completely since it indicates normal values in the visual field and any dark area alerts abnormal areas. The medical utility of the gray scale is minimal other than to alert topographically the affected areas in the visual field, which can be correlated with defect on the Bebie curve. The pattern of loss of visual field also point to specific patterns of visual field loss **(Figure 25)**.

Cumulative Defect Curve

The cumulative defect curve (CD) graphically presents the measured sensitivity values sorted in order of increasing depth from left to right. The cumulative defect curve was introduced by Bebie and gives a quick assessment of the depth and characteristic of defect along with the pattern of diffuse loss of sensitivity as in cataract. The index, mean defect is the horizontal portion on the curve and loss variance (LV) is the slope on the left of the Bebie curve. *The most important highlight of the defect curve is the zone of age corrected normality with a bandwidth of +/– 2 dB (4 dB) representing the 90 percent confidence interval of the normal population which are represented by the two lines on the top of the curve.* The ranking numbers are the sorted sensitivity of the test points from rank 1 which is the highest to the lowest on the left. The Bebie curve gives details of the depth of defect without the topography or the location of the defect in the visual field defect. A typical G1 program has 59 test points which are presented in decreasing sensitivity from the left to right. *The diffuse loss calculated and represented at the bottom of the Bebie curve is the deviation in dB.* This deviation may be pathological when cataract is present **(Figure 26)**.

Corrected Comparison Table

The corrected comparison table is the result of the CO table minus the deviation measured in the Bebie curve. This table depicts the true sensitivity behind the diffuse loss, e.g. cataract associated with Glaucoma **(Figure 27)**.

Probability Plot

The 'Probability plot' is the graphic display in symbols of the comparison values in the CO table. The plot displays the statistical significance of the local defects in different shades, darker being most significant with P < 0.5 percent. When P < 0.5 percent at a test location it means that this value is normal in 0.5 percent of the normal population. This in normal understanding means that the test location has an abnormal response and is considered to be a defect. Probability values are such that with 60 test locations one such 'significant' location may by chance find its way in a perfectly normal field. Hence,

conclusions should be drawn with care and correlated with clinical findings. The lowest significant value is P > 5 percent indicating that these values are normal in 5 percent of the population **(Figure 28)**.

Corrected Probability Plot

The 'Corrected probability' is the graphic display of the corrected comparison values. Localized defects such as nerve fiber bundle defects are highlighted. The symbols represent the increasing significance with darker shades **(Figure 29)**.

Visual Field Indices

Visual field indices summarize the characteristics of the visual field into few key numbers. These numbers provide a global perspective of the visual field that are useful to understand diffuse loss and focal loss at a glance and are useful in comparing visual fields over time. Flammer introduced these indices in the Octopus perimeters in 1985. The visual field indices are more precise since the effect of scattering and inaccuracies of the test points are reduced by averaging the results over all tested test points. The fluctuations are also reduced by the square root of the number of test locations by a factor of 8 in a typical G1 program in the Octopus perimeter.

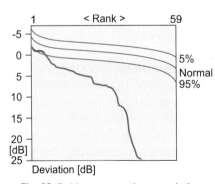

Fig. 26 Bebie curve or the cumulative defect curve-6

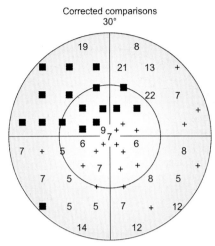

Fig. 27 Corrected comparisons table-7

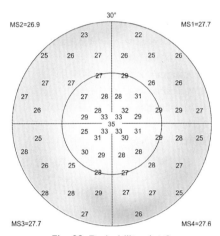

Fig. 28 Probability plot-8

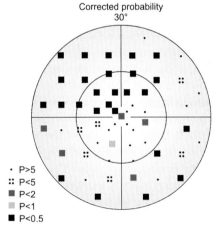

Fig. 29 Corrected probability plot-8

Deviations from known normal range then indicate pathology.

The visual field indices are mathematical expressions of the all test locations, though complex calculations are done this is often not of much clinical interest since these are clinically evaluated functions which can be used in day to day practice **(Figure 30)**.

Mean Sensitivity

Mean sensitivity (MS) is the first index to be displayed in the table. MS is the average of all test locations which is measured in dB. MS is an arithmetic mean of all test locations and is a raw value. MS cannot be compared since it is neither corrected for age or diffuse losses. MS gives a general picture of the sensitivity of the visual field test.

Mean Defect

Mean defect (MD) is age corrected mean sensitivity. This age correction makes MD independent of age. The normal value of MD is zero. Ninety percent of fields have a normal value between –2.0 and +2.0. Borderline MD values of more than 2.4 need a retest to confirm damage. The trend of MD over time is a good indicator of global damage.

Loss Variance

Loss variance (LV) is the square value of the standard deviation of the local defects in the CO tables. LV is a very sensitive index to early localized

	Phase 1	Phase 2	Mean
#	59	0	0
MS	15.3		
MD	12.3		
LV	116.0		
CLV			
SF			
RF			0.0

Fig. 30 Visual field indices-9

damage. LV increases exponentially to the damage until masked by the general depression caused to the MD values, this characteristic of LV highlights early defects. The square root of LV is called sLV or PSD (Pattern Standard Deviation). sLV is used as an index to follow change over time in trend analysis. sLV as a number being the square root is more smooth on a follow-up trend analysis graph. sLV as an index does not feature in a single field analysis visual field report.

Short-term Fluctuation

Short-term fluctuations (SF) are values obtained from retesting locations already tested in the same session a second time. This index value, which normally varies between 1.5 and 2.5 dB, is used to judge the reliability of the local test values and to determine the index CLV. Short-term fluctuations are measured in the second phase of visual field test, retesting the previously tested test locations. Most new strategies do not display this value, e.g. TOP and Dynamic in the first phase.

Corrected Loss Variance

The corrected loss variance (CLV) is an index, which measures localized loss that is independent of short-term fluctuations. CLV is below 2.5 for 90 percent of the population. The SF and CLV are no longer used in newer strategies for measurements of visual field loss. These results are flagged only when retest values are available.

Reliability Factor

The Reliability Factor (RF) is calculated from the positive and negative catch trial questions. RF is the sum of the false positive answers and false negative answers divided by the total number of catch trial questions. RF is an indicator of the patient's cooperation. RF value

of '0' is excellent and figures below 15 to 20 percent are an indicator of a fair visual field test.

Structure Function Correlation

The visual field printout report should be correlated with the clinical fundus findings and should be consistent **(Figures 31A to C)**. A fundus picture is a good additional tool for follow-up, though a good optic disc diagram should be enough 'in case of cost constraints'.

OCTOPUS PERIMETER REPORTS
Seven-in-One Report

The seven-in-one printout is the most popular format since it gives all the data collected from each of the test points along with global indices. The seven in one printout presents the 'raw' data and corrected data in values, graphs and indices. The ten-step approach to interpretation is based on the seven in one visual field printout report.

Combination Report

Reports may be printed out depending on the pathology investigated. Neuro-ophthalmological examinations may be better presented with a value and comparison table, gray scale values, cumulative defect curve of Bebie and visual field indices.

Large Graphics

The gray scale or value table may be printed as large graphics to help the patient understand the disease process on the visual field.

Two-on-One Report

The 'Two-on-one printout' on the Octopus 300 series is a excellent presentation of the left and right eye visual fields in a left eye to right eye format on the printout. Symmetrical or asymmetrical patterned loss of visual field

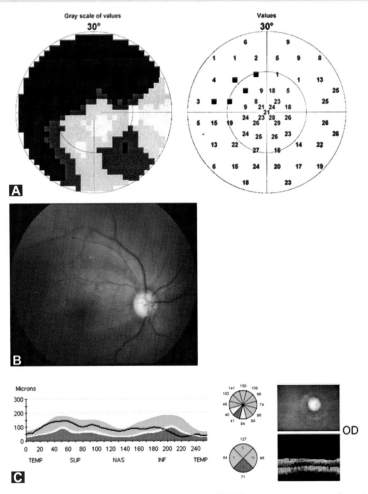

Figs 31A to C (A) Perimetry function/structure correlation-10; (B) Disc photo, structure/function correlation-10; (C) RFNL average thickness report on a status OCT-10

is immediately apparent with a single glance. The overview of fields from both eyes is always necessary to weed out neurological diseases while following up for glaucoma. A patterned loss of visual field in both eyes is a pointer and very well displayed on a 'Two on one' print out. This printout is currently available from the print command on selecting both left and right eye visual fields from the perimeter only **(Figure 32)**.

Peritrend PC Software

Peritrend software is used in conjunction with all models of Octopus perimeters. The software can be used to import, store, manage, display and print. The software can be used in a PC

network and all stations on the network may view the visual field test files. The MD and sLV are the two indices used to follow-up fields over time. The graphic display is made very easy by the color of the lines on the printout display **(Figure 33)**.

The significance of trend is highly dependant on the number of examinations and the reliability of the examinations for a small value of 'σ' (Sigma). The sigma value becomes less significant as more data points or examinations values becomes avaiable to follow progression over time **(Figure 34)**. Follow-up requires same strategy and program for proper follow-up. Peritrend software automatically

groups the tests from the same patient together classifed into right and left eye. A minimum of three follow-up fields are required for trend analysis.

Four questions need to be answered when evaluating fields, Is the visual field normal? Significant change in consecutive visual fields? Changes in visual field indices and finally how the local changes behave over time. Reliable examinations are a prerequisite for interpretation of fields over time, i.e. have a small sigma. Follow-up softwares in current development is the Octopus field analysis in the Beta version addresses the issue of trend analysis in a pointwise **(Figure 35)** and cluster analysis as well over time **(Figure 36)**.

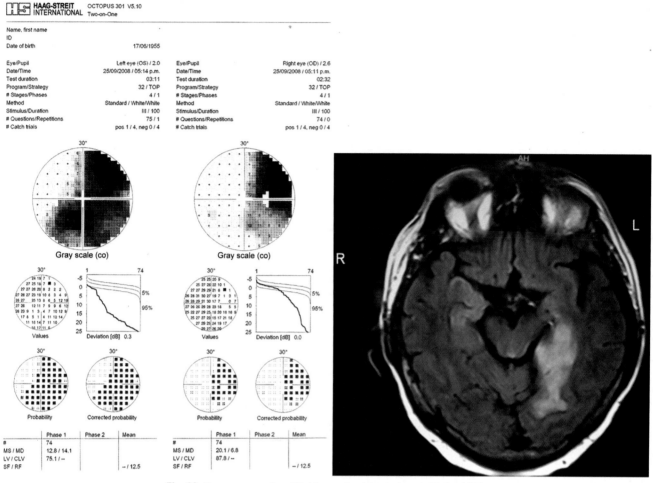

Fig. 32 Two-on-one visual field report printout along with the MRI

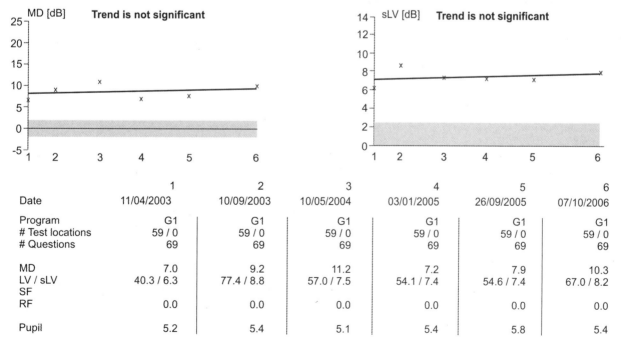

	1	2	3	4	5	6
Date	11/04/2003	10/09/2003	10/05/2004	03/01/2005	26/09/2005	07/10/2006
Program	G1	G1	G1	G1	G1	G1
# Test locations	59 / 0	59 / 0	59 / 0	59 / 0	59 / 0	59 / 0
# Questions	69	69	69	69	69	69
MD	7.0	9.2	11.2	7.2	7.9	10.3
LV / sLV	40.3 / 6.3	77.4 / 8.8	57.0 / 7.5	54.1 / 7.4	54.6 / 7.4	67.0 / 8.2
SF						
RF	0.0	0.0	0.0	0.0	0.0	0.0
Pupil	5.2	5.4	5.1	5.4	5.8	5.4

Fig. 33 Trend analysis MD, sLV

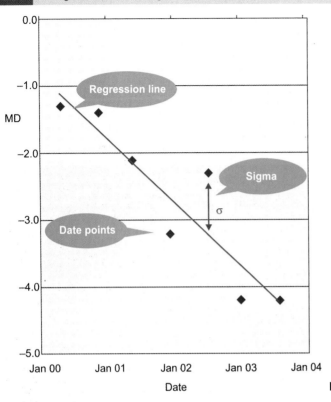

Fig. 34 Trend line of MD values over time

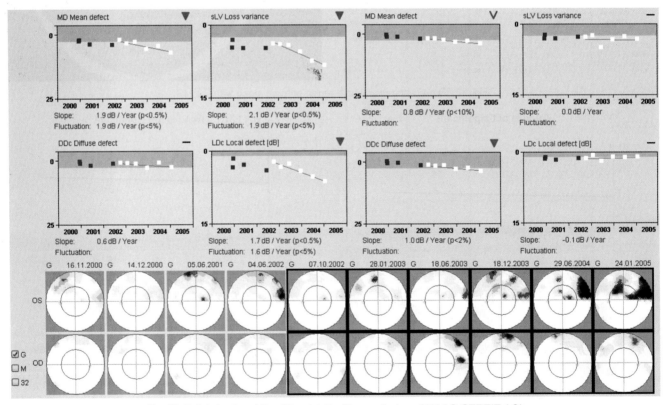

Fig. 35 Pointwise trend line (Reprinted with permission of HAAG-STREIT AG)

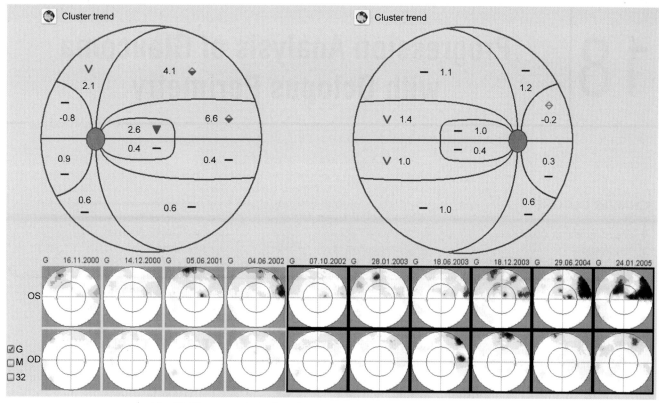

Fig. 36 Cluster analysis (Reprinted with permission of HAAG-STREIT AG)

REFERENCES

1. Fankhauser F, Koch P, Roulier A. On automation of perimetry. Graefe's Arch Clin Exp Ophthalmol; 1972.pp. 126-50.

2. Bebie H, Fankhauser F, Spahr J. Static perimetry: Strategies. Acta Ophthalmol 1976;54:325-32.

3. Flammer J, Jenni A, Bebie H. The OCTOPUS G1 Program. Glaucoma 1987;9:67-72.

4. Bebie H, Flammer J, Bebie T. The cumulative defect curve: Separation of local and diffuse components of visual field damage. Graefes Arch Clin Exp Ophthalmol 1989;227:9-12.

5. Flammer J, Drance SM, Fankhauser F, Augustini L. Differential light threshold in automated static perimetry. Arch Ophthalmol 1984;102:876-9.

6. Gonzàlez de la Rosa M, Pareja A. Influence of the fatigue effect and the mean deviation measurement in perimetry. Eur J Ophthalmol 1997;7:29-34.

7. Weber J, Klimaschka T. Test time and efficiency of the dynamic strategy in glaucoma perimetry. German J Ophthalmol 1995;4:24-31.

8. Morales J, Weitzmann M, Gonzàlez de la Rosa M. Comparison between tendency oriented perimetry (TOP) and Octopus threshold perimetry. Ophthalmology 2000;107:134-42.

9. Moss I. The influence of age-related cataract on blue-on-yellow perimetry. Invest Ophthalmol Vis Sci 1995;36:764-73.

10. Gallardo Sánchez LM. Findings using flicker perimetry and the top strategy in patients with ocular hypertension and normal subjects. 76th Meeting of the Sociedad Española de Oftalmología. October; 2000.

11. Dannheim F. First experiences with the new Octopus G1-program in chronic simple glaucoma. IPS Meeting; 1986.

18 | Progression Analysis of Glaucoma with Octopus Perimetry

NR Rangaraj

CHAPTER OUTLINE

INTRODUCTION

The open angle glaucomas are chronic, progressive optic neuropathies, that have in common characteristic morphological changes at the optic nerve head and retinal nerve fiber layer in the absence of other ocular disease or congenital anomalies. Progressive retinal ganglion cell death and visual field loss are associated with these changes.[1]

Visual function changes and progression are characteristic in glaucoma by definition. Major trials have also demonstrated progression as inevitable in well-managed and untreated glaucoma. In the light of this knowledge management and follow-up of glaucoma is based on tracking visual field progression which may be global or focal in nature. The rate of progression of the glaucoma in turn influences the therapeutic decision to alter treatment to suite the changing needs and quality of vision for the patient. When a diagnosis of glaucoma is made the quality of life has a direct bearing on the visual field damage.[2] When the damage to visual field is minimum quality of vision and life is not an issue, however, significant damage to the visual field in both eyes leads to deterioration of quality life itself. Hence, identification of patients who are at risk of visual impairment which affects the quality of vision becomes important. Identification of these high-risk individuals are difficult in clinical situations due to variations in the number of visual fields and frequency with which visual fields are done.[3]

Progression analysis of visual field in glaucoma takes into consideration the age of the patient and the amount of damage at diagnosis. This is well-illustrated in the **Figures 1A to C**. Visual fields of patients with minimal loss at diagnosis with progression of less than or equal to 0.1dB/year will be expected to last a life time. Advanced visual field loss with rapid progression impacts quality of life since the patient will be visually impaired in his life time.

The goal of progression analysis is to intervene and reduce the IOP to preserve visual function (green arrow), untreated glaucoma would progress to significant visual impairment during the patient's life time.

BARRIERS TO FOLLOW-UP

Common clinical problems with follow-up are when sufficient number of visual field tests are done, a large volume of data is generated which may be difficult to interpret by 'eyeball technique.' There is no clinical evidence based rational to monitor the progression which sets out the number and frequency of tests to be conducted on the patient at the time of diagnosis. This leads to making therapeutic decisions based on inadequate information due to insufficient number of fields done infrequently leading to severe visual disabilities while the patient is under care and supervision.[4-6]

Standard white on white automated static perimetry is the gold standard in measuring progression of visual fields. All major landmark trials in glaucoma have used visual fields done on automated static perimetry with white on white as the primary end point for progression. Monitoring progression is exclusively done with standard automated white on white perimetry and clinically this translates into better care for the patient under follow-up.

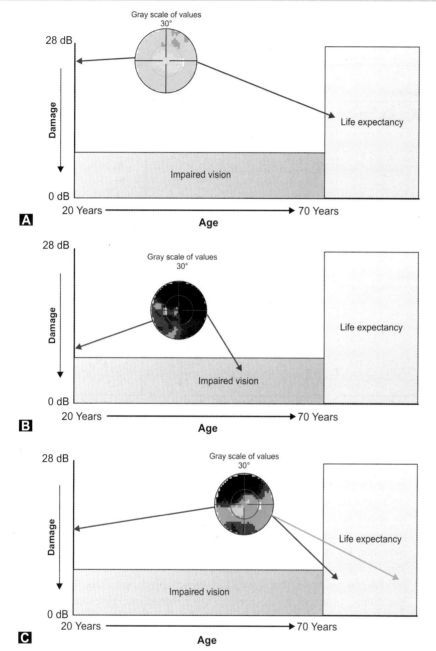

Figs 1A to C (A) Normal visual fields; (B) Severe visual fields loss; (C) Moderate visual field loss

up to 8 dB.[8] This makes progression analysis difficult to interpret. Grouping of test location or clusters is a means of reducing the magnitude of fluctuation and provides recognition of abnormality, making local changes easy to identify. Global indices like mean defect and loss variance give a summary of the whole field in a single number. These global indices are influenced by effects of cataract, refraction and reliability of fields. *Local defect* and *diffuse defect* are new indices introduced by Octopus to reduce this effect and present the true picture of the visual field.

Detecting Rate of Progression of Visual Field Loss

The rate of change of mean defect in most glaucoma patients is anywhere between 0 and 2.5 dB per year depending on the severity of the disease. Progression was greater than 2.8 dB in seven years only in the worst 2.5 percent study group in the AGIS study.[9] Recognition of these changes in the range of 0 to 2.0 dB needs a proper frequency and follow-up of visual field analysis depending on risk factors. Risk factors like inadequate control of IOP, pseudoexfoliation and advanced visual field loss influence the number of tests to be conducted per year. Practical recommendations are summarized below:[10]

- Perform six visual fields in the first two years, this will effectively rule out any rapid progression of more than 2.8 dB/year and establish a good base line data for progression follow-up.

- Analysis of progression can be done only when the same threshold algorithm and test pattern is used each time. Octopus recommends the G1 program with dynamic or TOP strategy, i.e. use only G1 with TOP or G1 with

MEASUREMENT OF VISUAL FIELD PROGRESSION

There are many approaches to measurement and detection of progression. Global indices along with sectors of visual field and clusters are analyzed to detect the rate of progression and change in visual fields. There is evidence that normal as well as pathological visual fields have test locations which are relative to one another.[7] A single test location can fluctuate normally

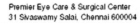

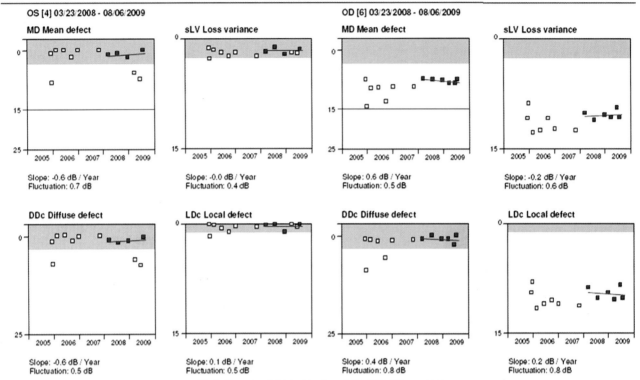

Fig 2 Trends of Global indices MS, MD, DD and LD

dynamic and not once with G1 TOP and another with G1 dynamic.

• Pay attention to quality of the test performed, since this becomes the basic data entry for charting progression. Reliance on reliability indices should be taken into consideration along with the optometrist notes during the performance of the test by the patient. When obvious artifacts like learning effects, poor centration, wrong refractive correction, high false positives errors and rim effects are present the test should be removed from the data set. Poor quality of visual field examination will lead to under or over estimation of progression and wrongly influence clinical decision.

• Measuring the rate of visual field progression, i.e. dB/year, is a basic guide for clinical and therapeutic decisions for estimating the risk of visual impairment during the patient's life time. Establishing a base line for visual field progression requires good follow-up for several years. Stable treated glaucoma progresses at about 0.1 dB/year.[8]

Method of Measurement of Visual Field Progression

Standard white on white static automated perimetry is used to measure visual field progression. Octopus has the traditional global indices MD (Mean defect) and LV (Loss variance) or sLV (Square root of loss variance). The graphical display of resulting values is better when sLV is used for analysis of data. Newer indices introduced by Octopus, the local defect

(LD) and diffuse defect (DD) are found to be more stable in presence of false positives and diffuse defect due to refraction and cataract. The indices summarize the global nature of the defect without information on the topography of the defect **(Figure 2)**.

Topographical results of the visual field analysis are quantified and represented by the cluster graphs and polar graphs. Statistical tools combined with customized software help in analysis of the rate of change and detection of change of visual field. The EyeSuite™ combines both trend analysis and event analysis to display progression in glaucoma. Trend analysis of the global indices gives the rate of change in decibels per year but does not display that change has occurred **(Figure 3)**. The event analysis in EyeSuite™ is displayed by the cluster and polar graphs

Y, Academic, 05/27/1953
ID 21422

Premier Eye Care & Surgical Center
31 Sivaswamy Salai, Chennai 600004

OS [4] / 03/23/2008 - 08/06/2009
Corrected cluster trend

OD [6] / 03/23/2008 - 08/06/2009
Cluster trend

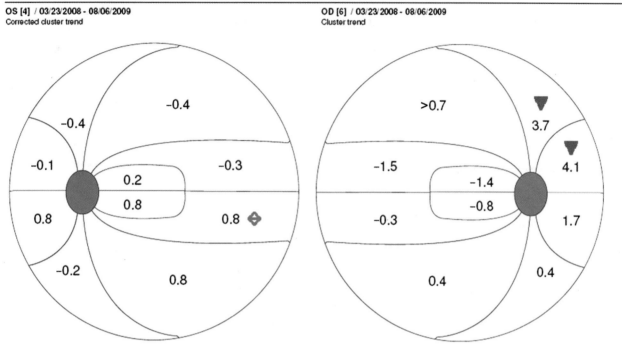

Fig. 3 Sectorwise analysis of the cluster trends

and shows that change indeed has occurred but does not display rate of change. Hence, both types of analysis are complimentary and help the clinician to analyze even the subtle changes in the visual fields.

EyeSuite™: Perimetry software introduced by Haag-Streit is a solution for storing, analyzing, printing and display of visual field examination data from the all models of Octopus perimeters (300 and 900 series) on the personal computer or network. The highlight of the software is the ability to combine structural with functional findings. The software also mathematically identifies and highlights relevant change occurring in the progressing visual field. This mathematical model based on population based statistics is more specific in judging truly progressing visual fields and in specific areas of the visual field.[11] The rate of progression of global indices is calculated in dB/year and is displayed in accordance with the EGS guidelines along with the fluctuations and the significance of the displayed values from the test result. The cluster trend displays the fast regional changes even though the global indices (average) do not flag the progression. The polar graph displays the correlation of the visual function to the structure, there by increasing diagnostic accuracy which may have been misinterpreted as measurement noise.

The EyeSuite™ Software

Clinicians need follow-up with results displayed in the form of global indices and regional trends with details of the rate of loss per year compared with stable glaucoma population to take therapeutic decisions for their patients.

EyeSuite™ displays these results in a very simple format:

1. The global indices are displayed as global trend graphs for each of the four global indices.
2. Topographical trend display as the cluster trends and cluster graph.
3. The polar trend and graph are oriented to the optic disc to facilitate structure function correlation.

EyeSuite™ has two new indices the diffuse defect (DD) and local defect (LD) based on the Bebie curve in addition to the mean defect (MD) and sLV (Square root of loss variance). Diffuse defect is not very representative by itself, but the local defect (LD) is derived from diffuse defect. **Figure 4** displays the diffuse defect, this value subtracted from the comparison derives the corrected comparisons. The single field analysis introduced in the EyeSuite™ software calculates the values as described.

Values of diffuse defect is displayed below the defect (Bebie) curve.

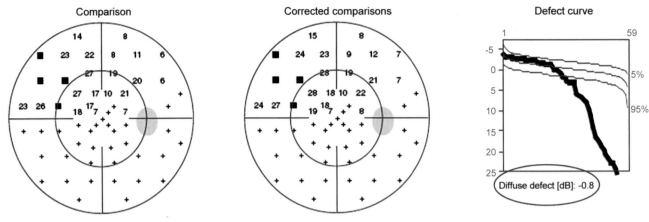

Fig. 4 Values of diffuse defect is displayed in the defect (Bebie) curve. This value subtracted from the comparison derives the corrected comparisons

Diffuse Defect and Local Defect (Figure 5)

The diffuse defect and local defect are the two new indices that are based on the Bebie curve introduced in the EyeSuite™ software. The Bebie curve has two distinct parts, the first is the general height of the Bebie curve which indicates the diffuse loss and the second, is the drop that indicates the focal or local loss. The one-third of the Bebie curve is spared from increased fluctuation in the initial phase of glaucoma progression.[12,13] To calculate the DD and LD, first the general height of the diffuse loss is estimated from the average of the rank values between 12th and 16th values. The reason for estimating this averaged value is that even when 20 percent of test locations are abnormal as in moderate glaucoma there is less influence of the global change on the value of the diffuse defect.[14] This averaged value also avoids the false positive peak on the left of the Bebie curve that may arise due to trigger happy behavior and influence the value of the general height. The rank values in the Bebie curve are not physical neighboring values but these test points share a common abnormal response behavior.

Diffuse Defect

Diffuse defect (DD) is the difference between this general height and the visual fields individual height indicated by the dark blue band in the **Figure 6**. Estimation of this value is important since it varies from the old peritrend which calculated the diffuse height from the 6th rank value. This estimation is important since it filters the effect of diffuse loss due to cataract and effect of fluctuations in the patient while on a long follow-up.

Local Defect

Local defect (LD) is the area between the patient's defect curve and the 50th percentile of the defect curve when shifted by DD. This index correlates highly with the sLV (or the PSD). Local defect is less influenced by false positive responses. Local defect is the area highlighted with dark blue in the **Figure 7**, is expressed in dB and normalized to be comparable between different program patterns.

Global Trend Graph (Figures 8 and 9)

The trend of the global indices is shown with the baseline on top and the 95 percent of normality is indicated in the gray range. To make interpretation visually simple to interpret, a descending trend line always means an increasing visual field defect. Calculations for the slope in decibels per year, the amount of fluctuation and their statistical significance are given highlighted

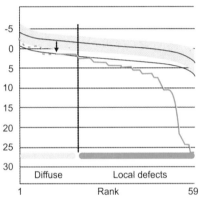

Fig. 5 Diffuse and local defects

at the bottom of the graph as in EGS guidelines. The icons on the top right corner when present, flag the significance of worsening of the trend line as below.

Statistical representation with icons is used universally in all the printouts of EyeSuite™. This makes reading the significance of worsening easy and hard to miss.

Worsening at ▼ 1 percent (Closed triangle) and ⋁ 5 percent significance (Open triangle).

Improvement at ▲ 1 percent (Closed triangle)/⋀ 5 percent significance (Open triangle).

Fluctuation at ◆ 1 percent (Closed diamond)/◇ 5 percent significance (Open diamond).

The progression rate (mathematical slope) is calculated in dB per year,

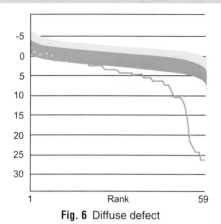

Fig. 6 Diffuse defect

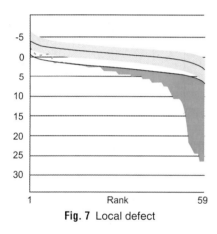

Fig. 7 Local defect

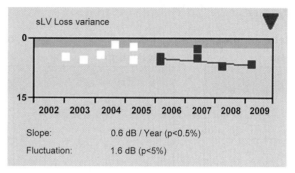

Fig. 8 Closed triangle showing significance at 1 percent

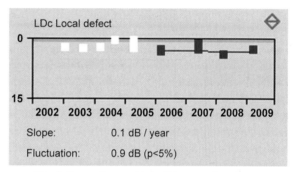

Fig. 9 Open diamond, significance at 5 percent

allowing therapeutic decisions to be made to suit the needs of every individual patient. This means that when significance is at the level of 1 percent, then this is hardly by accident. A value of 1.9 dB per year in a patient having a current defect of 7 dB will have a reserve of 15 dB if 22 dB is considered as blindness, then the visual loss may be expected in 7 to 8 years.

Display of Probability Values

The probability values are displayed as an Icon on the top right hand corner of the graph of the global trend. This icon displays the worsening by applying population based statistics to identify worsening visual fields. The global trend display is displayed for all indices, MD, sLV, DD and LD. All the global values need to be taken into

consideration when estimating the progression in a visual field since glaucoma has a diffuse component and a local component.

Traditional Global Indices

MD is the mean defect and is the average sensitivity difference compared to age corrected normal. It is pertinent to know that negative values indicate oversensitivity compared to normal. sLV is the square root of loss variance and an indicator for local variation and displays the existing defects if any.

DISPLAY OF DATA IN THE EYESUITE™ Global Trends (Figure 10)

The trends for all the global indices MD, sLV, DD and LD from both eyes are displayed together with the series overview of the visual fields to give a proper perspective of the visual field defect. The software by default selects the recent six tests along with the time slot of the tests under evaluation and

calculates the rate of change along with significance. The icons on the graphic display of the statistical significance and the values at the bottom of each graph give the slope calculated in dB/year along with fluctuation. The series printout of the color/gray scale gives the topography of the defect in the visual field since glaucoma has a very characteristic pattern of visual field loss. This display allows selection or deselecting of tests which have high variability and do not contribute to the follow-up. Using windows convention of Ctrl + Click will alter the selection of any visual field. The operator may also select all visual fields manually if the need be, though the last six tests are most appropriate. The selection button allows switching of representation from global to cluster trend and polar trend which is available in the pro version of the software. The global trend is available in the light version of the software.

Global Trend Printout

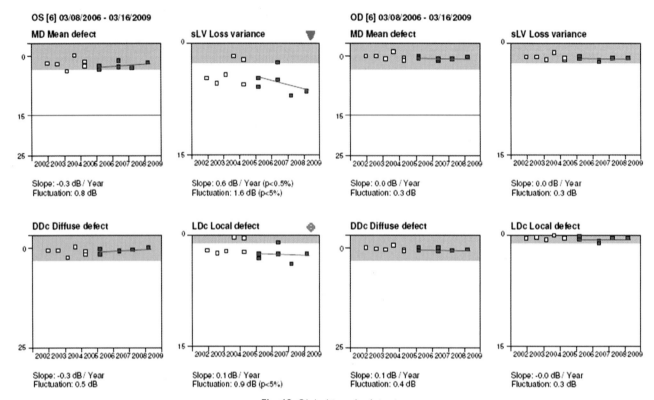

Fig. 10 Global trend printout

Cluster Graph

The test locations in the visual fields are grouped together into 10 clusters according to the nerve fiber distribution. The upper and lower halves of the clusters are not mirror images due to the asymmetry in the distribution of the nerve fibers. The clusters help to identify the differences between the clusters and to absolute measures at each individual test points. The 10 clusters are schematically represented as in the **Figure 11**. The cluster graph is a combination display of probability and deviation from normal. The '+' sign represents the normal, the normal font number displays cluster defect that deviates at 5 percent probability level and bold indicates significance at 1 percent probability level.

Cluster Trend (Figure 12)

The cluster trend represents regions of change, the rate of change and significance of the trend. Areas of interest or significant changes are highlighted with icons. Marked fluctuations may indicate early change in the cluster area. The number on the cluster area indicates the rate of change in dB per year from that representative area.

Polar Graph

The polar graph displays the depth of the defect and location with a red line with its length corresponding with depth of the defect and the location at the nerve fiber angle on the optic disc. **Figure 13** illustrates the test point and the corresponding nerve fiber angle on the polar graph. The orientation is vertically mirrored to the representation in the visual field to match morphologic representation of a fundus photo or HRT images. The orientation thus being superior, nasal, inferior and temporal with the gray

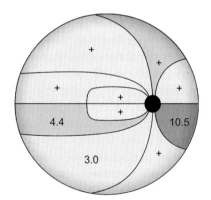

Fig. 11 Cluster graph

areas indicating the defect range of –4 dB to +4 dB with the blue rings indicating the 10/20/30 dB local defects. 30 dB being the maximum loss at a given test location.

Polar Trend (Figure 14)

The polar trend is a pointwise linear regression using the polar graph. The red and green lines indicate the

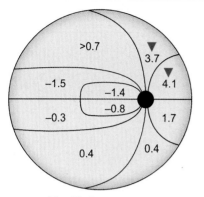

Fig. 12 Cluster trend

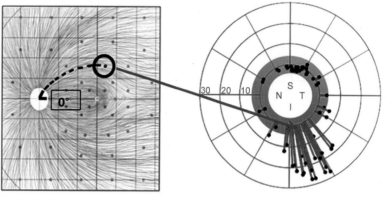

Fig. 13 Polar graph

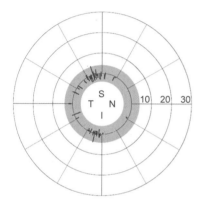

Fig. 14 Polar trend

pointwise linear regression analysis for each of the test location at the corresponding nerve fiber angle at the optic disc. Red indicates worsening and the outer end corresponds to the actual depth of defect which may be measured in relation to the blue rings at the 10/20/30 dB values indicated in the graph. The length of the line is the worsening in dB as calculated by the point wise linear regression. The mirror orientation helps in comparing the function to structure with the HRT printout. Small changes are highlighted which normally may have been missed. Correlating function with structure helps the clinician in making a better diagnosis.

EXAMPLES TO HIGHLIGHT CONCEPTS OF EYESUITE™ SOFTWARE
Time Series
EyeSuite™ software selects the last six tests as default to display the trend **(Figure 15)**. This time window selection is important to display the current global trend. Selection of all tests shows a worsening of 1 percent significance. The second figure displays same test series with the last six visual field test that displays a stable glaucoma. This may be due to good control of IOP achieved during follow-up. The selections of the number of visual fields may be increased in order to understand the trend in a particular patient. Tests which may show gross variation or artifacts may be excluded from the analysis.

Global versus Cluster Changes
EyeSuite™ software graphically displays the global changes highlighting the regions from where the changes occurred **(Figure 16)**. A 1.9 dB change per year in the global index may mask the average from the clusters. When the range of cluster values are noted to be from –0.8 dB to 6.7 dB per year, with the maximum value of 6.7 dB per year being from the area near the macula,

it highlights the extent of worsening in the quality of vision for the patient. This situation may require a more aggressive therapeutic intervention.

COMPONENTS OF THE EYESUITE™ PRINTOUT
The printout is a simplified display of the results of the visual field over a time line that is calculated by the EyeSuite™ software. The printouts are similar across all printouts, e.g. global trend or cluster trend.

The demographic details of the patient are displayed on the top left corner with the name and ID number. The next line displays the eye and the time window which has been selected for analysis. The four graphs to the left represent the left eye and the four graphs to the right represent the right eye. The individual global indices of interest are the mean defect, square root of loss variance and local defect. Diffuse defect is needed to derive local defect.

The mean defect is the first display graph. The graph is made easy-to-read with color coding. The horizontal axis indicates the time line of the test selections in all the graphs. The vertical line with 0, 15 and 25 indicates the values in decibels. The gray band indicates the

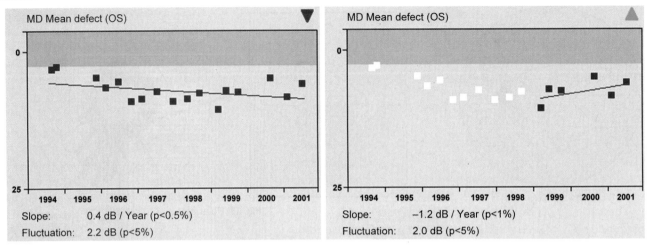

Fig. 15 Examples of the importance of test selection

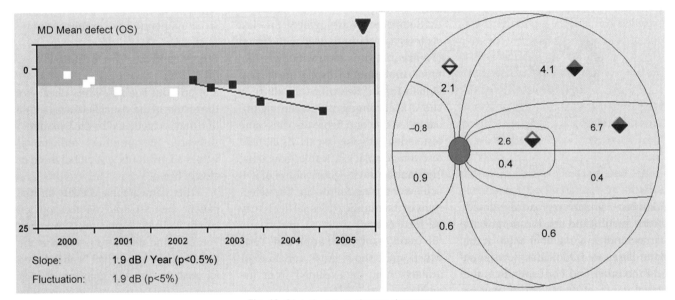

Fig. 16 Global versus cluster changes

normal bandwidth of 4 dB and values in this area are considered normal with the age matched population. The red line at 15 dB indicating any value being classified as significant worsening of visual field affecting the quality of vision. The tests which are selected or deselected are indicated by the color code since widely varying fields may be excluded from the follow-up. A summary of comments of the graph are at the bottom in plain language giving the values of the slope in dB/year and

the fluctuation in the values obtained in the selected tests.

The square root of loss variance is the next display, the difference is the values in the vertical line from 0 to 15 and the gray band of normality having a width of 2.5 dB to the age matched population. Values below the gray band indicate focal loss. Statistical icons flag when significant focal loss is present by means of open (at 5% significance) and closed (at 1% significance) triangles. Open diamond is significance at

5 percent and closed diamond being significance at 1 percent of the fluctuation of the selected values for follow-up. This display scheme is uniform across the cluster trends, cluster graphs, polar trend and graph.

GLOBAL TREND PRINTOUT

Typical global trend printout has details of the patient name, date of birth and identification number.

The above printout **(Figure 17)** shows visual field follow-up from the

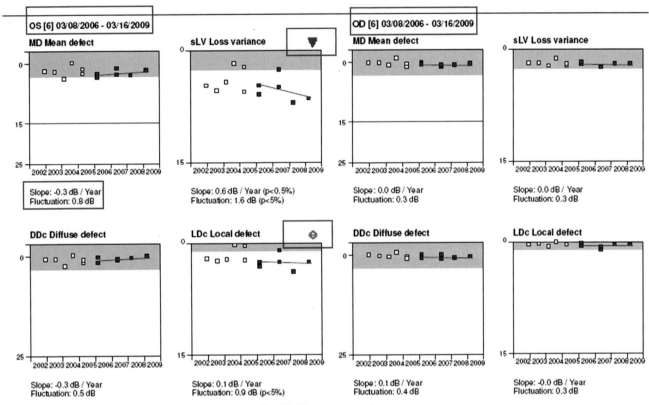

Fig. 17 Global trend printout

year 2002 to 2009 which is indicated in the time slot along with the eye under consideration. The last six tests are selected for this display, this happens by default in the software. Selected tests are blue in color and the color scales are highlighted with black squares. The global trend of the MD looks normal and is not flagged. sLV is flagged with a closed red triangle indicating a 1 percent significance of the value, that is only 1 percent of the population would have that value normally. The rate of progression of the slope is 0.6 dB/year with a fluctuation of 0.8 dB. The local defect also confirms this finding but with an open diamond flag indicating a significance of 5 percent, e.g. this is expected to be normal in only 5 percent of the population. The right eye visual field looks normal. No flags have appeared on the global indices, the slope of each global index is calculated at the bottom of each graph.

CLUSTER ANALYSIS

The cluster analysis also gives the demographic details in the uniform display. The cluster analysis displays the rate of progression in dB/year in sectorwise detail. This example in **Figure 18** shows the closed triangle indicating a 1 percent significance with a rate of 1.1 dB/year in the affected sector. This enables the clinician to take a therapeutic decision based on the regions from which the loss is greater which may not be reflected in the global index. The numerals on the graph are the rate of progression in dB/year. The same icons are used to flag areas of worsening and fluctuation. The demographic and eye details along with the time window selected are as in the global trend printout.

POLAR TREND

The polar trend printout (**Figure 19**) follows the same convention for

demographic details and time window which is selected for the progression analysis. The orientation of the graph is used to correlate with Optic disc image from fundus picture or HRT. The outer edge of the line denotes the depth of defect and the length of the line to the point wise linear regression analysis for each test location at the corresponding nerve fiber angle at the optic disc in dB.

SUMMARY OF THE PRINTOUTS

The sLV global trend shows rate of worsening at 0.6 dB per year with a red inverted triangle icon with 1 percent significance and a fluctuation of 1.6 dB. This effect of fluctuation ironed out in the global trend displayed in the LD, which shows a rate of worsening at 0.1 dB per year and an open diamond icon with 5 percent significance. The cluster trend shows sector wise details of worsening at 1 percent significance with a rate of 1.1 dB/year from that

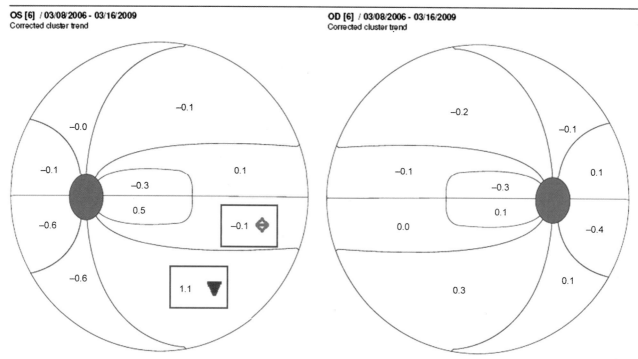

Fig. 18 Printout of cluster analysis

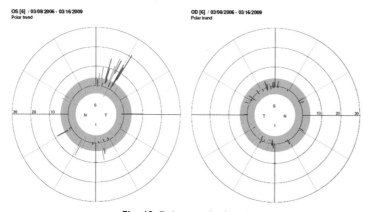

Fig. 19 Polar trend printout

sector. The polar trend displayed to help structure function correlation shows the point wise linear regression analysis of the test points that are represented at the nerve fiber angle. Hence, this field needs to be watched for any further rate of worsening in both global and cluster trends.

TYPICAL EXAMPLES OF EYESUITE™ PRINTOUT WITH INTERPRETATION

Example 1: 77-year-old female patient diagnosed to have POAG on Prostaglandin eye drops for the past 9 years with IOP of 10 mm Hg in both eyes.

The two on one left to right color scale printout shows deep defects in the left nasal area. The right eye visual field looks normal.

Global trends of typical global indices when seen on computer screen by the clinician. A systematic approach to interpretation makes understanding easy in a clinical situation when the results need to be conveyed to the patient for any modification in treatment plan.

Screen display global trend: The global indices MD, sLV, DD and LD are displayed for both the eyes in the left to right format. The selected visual fields are highlighted in blue (Last six visual fields as a default selection) and the corresponding color scales are highlighted in black outline in the onscreen view. Moving the cursor of the mouse on the icon on the screen displays the statistical significance and the date of exam when dragged on the date line.

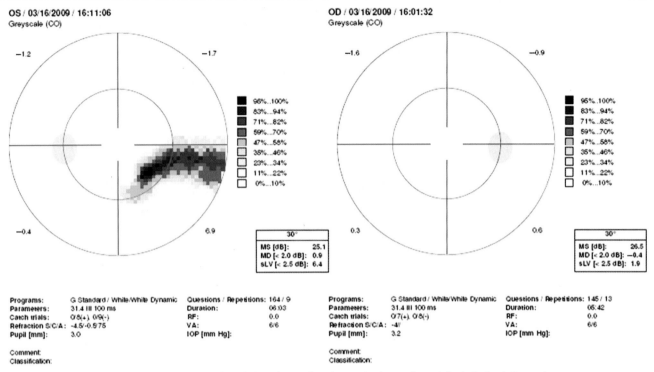

Example 1 The two on one left to right color scale printout: It shows deep defects in the left nasal area.
The right eye visual field looks normal

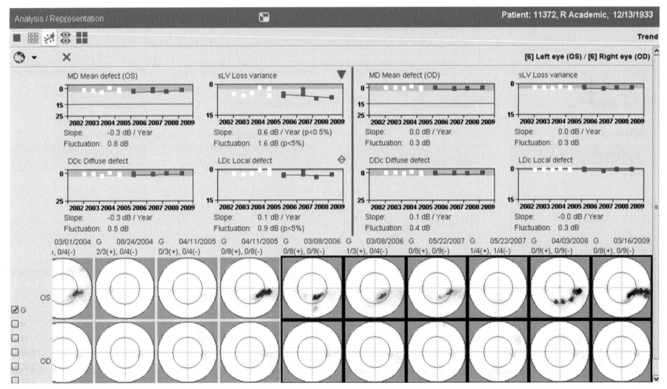

Example 1 Screen display of global trend

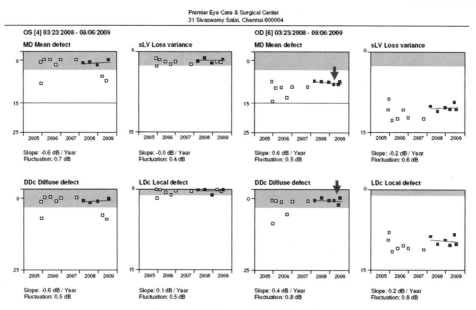

Example 2 Printout of global trend

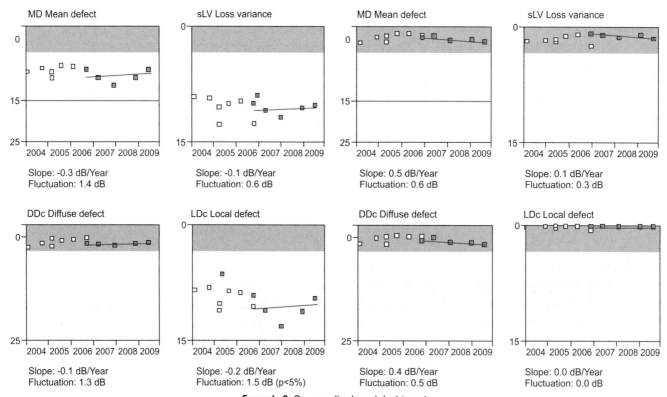

Example 2 Screen display global trend

Example 2: A male patient diagnosed to have POAG underwent cataract surgery in the right eye. His IOP remains at 12 mm Hg both eyes. Note the right eye MD and DD trend line showing a change before and after surgery (red arrow).

Summary: This display shows the effect of cataract on follow-up of patient with glaucoma and the recovery of MD values after cataract surgery. Interpretation of visual fields should always take the clinical findings, e.g. cataract in this case before therapeutic changes are made. The red arrow

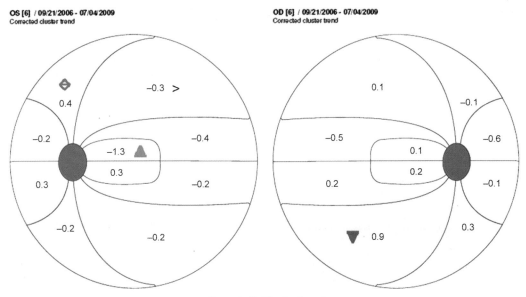

OS [6] / 09/21/2006 - 07/04/2009
Corrected cluster trend

OD [6] / 09/21/2006 - 07/04/2009
Corrected cluster trend

Example 3 Cluster trend

shows the effect of cataract. Right eye shows a MD slope of 0.6 dB/year with a fluctuation of 0.5 dB. DD shows a slope of 0.4 dB/year with fluctuation of 0.8 dB. The diffuse defect corrects for the loss of sensitivity due to cataract in this case and shows the corrected rate of loss per year. The icons for any statistically significant worsening are not displayed in this printout.

Example 3: A female patient diagnosed with POAG on follow-up with visual fields.

Global trend: The Demographic details of the patient are reconfirmed, all global indices MD, sLV, DD and LD are displayed with the plain language interpretation of the slope in dB/year with relevant statistical information. Note the slope. The MD is below the gray line which indicates the area of normality and the patient's MD is midway from 0 to 15 dB.

Cluster trend: Cluster trend displays the regional trends in dB/year. This gives an idea of the range from which the global indices are derived and

indicates areas where worsening is progressing faster.

The four-in-one printout displays the color scale, Bebie curve, cluster analysis and polar analysis. This four in one printout is customized to show a summary of changes that have taken place in the visual field in the affected eye along with a polar analysis which is mirrored to compare with optic disc image. Hence, even subtle changes are highlighted.

Summary: Global trend of MD showing moderate visual field loss with a loss of –0.1 dB/year correlated with sLV and LD trends showing stable values. The cluster trends showing areas of worsening at 1 percent significance and area of no response (Black symbol). The four-in-one printout shows the color scale in the area of worsening. The cluster analysis shows the numerical deviation from normal with the font being bold, showing a 1 percent significance of the estimate values of the sensitivity. The polar analysis is convenient for structure function correlation. The

four-in-one printout follows the same convention in display of the global indices and demographic details with a table giving the values of MS, MD and sLV.

CONCLUSION

EyeSuite™ perimetry software displays global changes along with regional changes which are responsible for the global values. When functional changes correlate with structural defects even subtle changes dismissed as 'noise' are correctly interpreted. The trend based analysis detects the rate of progression and the event based analysis detects if the change has indeed progressed. The EyeSuite™ perimetry software provides answers to both these questions with the global trends and cluster trends to detect the rate of progression globally and sector wise changes. The combination of global and cluster rate of change is sensitive to detect small changes in the affected areas before detection that actual change has indeed progressed.

U, Academic, 09/20/1951
ID 3785

OS / 07/04/2009 / 16:32:11
Four-in-One

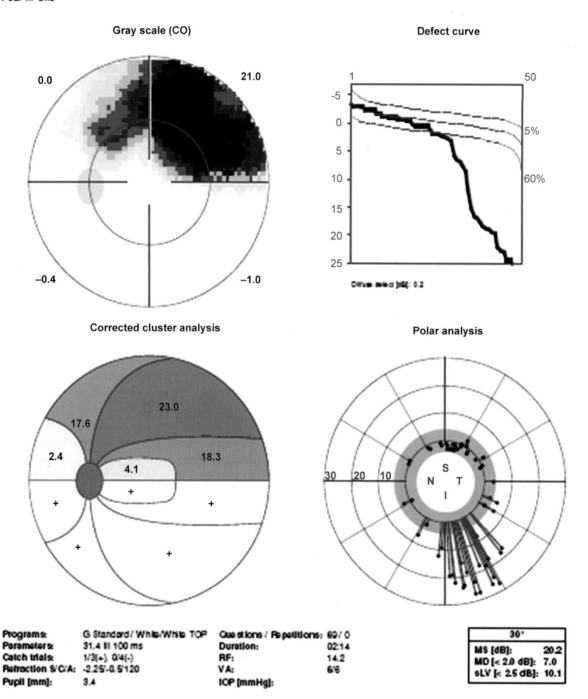

Example 3 Four in one printout showing the color scale, bebie curve, cluster analysis and polar analysis

REFERENCES

1. European Glaucoma Society Guidelines 3rd Edition.

2. Hyman LG, Komaroff E, Heijl A, Bengtsson B, Leske MC. Treatment and vision related quality of life in the early manifest glaucoma trial. Ophthalmology 2005;112:1505-13.

3. Hertzog LH, Albrecht KG, LaBree L, Lee PP. Glaucoma care and conformance with preferred practice patterns. Examination of the private, community-based ophthalmologist. Ophthalmology 1996;103:1009-13.

4. Oliver JE, Hattenhauer MG, Herman D, Hodge DO, Kennedy R, Fang-Yen M, et al. Blindness and glaucoma: a comparison of patients progressing to blindness from glaucoma with patients maintaining vision. Am J Ophthalmol 2002;133:764-72.

5. Chen PP. Blindness in patients with treated open-angle glaucoma. Ophthalmology 2003;110:726-33.

6. Forsman E, Kivela T, Vesti E. Life time visual disability in open-angle glaucoma and ocular hypertension. J Glaucoma 2007;16:313-9.

7. Heijl A, et al. Inter-point correlations of deviation of threshold values in normally and glaucomatous visual fields, Perimetry Updates, Amsterdam: Kugler publications; 1988–89.pp.177-83.

8. Flammer J, Drance SM, Zulauf M. Differential light threshold. Short and long-term fluctuation in patients with glaucoma, normally control, and patients with suspected glaucoma, Arch Ophthalmol, 1984;102:704-6.

9. AGIS7. Am J Ophthal 2000;130:429-420.

10. Practical Recommendations for Measuring Rates of Visual Field Change in Glaucoma. Balwantray C Chauhan, David F Garway-Heath, Francisco J Goñi, Luca Rossetti, Boel Bengtsson, Ananth Viswanathan and Anders Heijl.

11. Hans Bebie, Ernst Bürki, Receiver Operating Characteristics of a Novel Method of Visual Field Trend Analysis, ARVO 2008: program1154.

12. Funkhouser A, Flammer J, et al. A comparison of five methods for estimating general glaucomatous visual field depression, Graefes Arch Clin Exp Ophthalmol 1992;230:101-6.

13. Zulauf M, Becht C, Bernoulli D, False positive peak of the Bebie curve as a reliability parameter, Perimetry Updates, Amsterdam: Kugler Publications; 1996-97.pp.185-90.

14. Fankhauser F, et al. pp. Simulation in perimetry—program Perisim 2000, Ophthalmologica 2005;219:123-8.

19 Ultrasound Biomicroscopy in Glaucoma

Aditya Neog, L Vijaya

CHAPTER OUTLINE

- Technique of Examination
- Ultrasound Biomicroscopy in Normal Eye
- Ultrasound Biomicroscopy in Glaucoma
- Other Conditions in which Ultrasound Biomicroscopy may be Helpful
- Quantitative Measurements
- Future Trends

INTRODUCTION

Ultrasonography has been used as a diagnostic tool in ocular and orbital diseases since a long time. Ultrasound biomicroscopy or UBM is a method of high frequency ultrasound imaging, which has great use in the evaluation of selected anterior segment pathologies. It is possible to generate images approaching light microscopic resolution up to a depth of about 4 mm from the surface using the UBM. Anterior segment structures like the cornea, iris, ciliary body, zonules and anterior sclera can be imaged and their morphology assessed.

Pavlin, Sherar, and Foster[1] developed the UBM. The original technology of the UBM was developed by examining the eye with 50 to 100 MHz transducers.[1-3] Higher frequency transducers provide finer resolution of more superficial structures, whereas lower frequency transducers provide greater depth of penetration with less resolution.[10] The acoustic spectrum is spread over a wide range of frequencies and includes mechanical waves and vibrations. This extends from the audible range to the phonons, which comprise the vibrational states of matter. Clinical ultrasound frequencies range from 1–100 MHz and comprise routine diagnostic imaging, high frequency ultrasound and ultrasound biomicroscopy.

The UBM probe has a moving transducer without a protective membrane. The transducer oscillates during image acquisition. The principle of scanning is similar to conventional B-scan ultrasound (**Figure 1**). The images can be viewed real-time on the screen and also be stored for later analysis.

The commercial machines have transducers scanning in the range of 35 to 50 MHz. The commercially available instruments provide lateral and axial physical resolution of approximately 50 and 25 micrometers respectively.[10]

In some instruments, the UBM probe is suspended from a gantry arm to decrease artifacts. Some of the instruments have very light probes, which can be hand held. The plastic eyecup is inserted between the lids, to hold them open. The coupling solution, methylcellulose or normal saline is filled in the cup.

TECHNIQUE OF EXAMINATION

The technique used for examination is the immersion technique using a fluid stand off. The procedure is done under topical anesthesia. It is usually done with patient in supine position, but in UBM it has been described for both prone and sitting positions.[4] An eyecup is used to keep the lids open

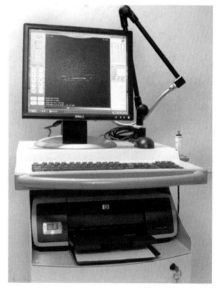

Fig. 1 Ultrasound biomicroscopy (UBM) machine

and a coupling medium in the used. The coupling medium can be methylcellulose or normal saline. The transducer is immersed in the solution and placed directly over the part to be scanned. The cornea and anterior segment can be easily studied, and the conjunctiva, sclera and peripheral retina up to the limits of rotation of the eye in various directions. The transducer should be properly oriented so that the scanning ultrasound beam strikes the target surface perpendicularly to ensure maximum detection of the reflected signal.

Scans are performed in radial and transverse meridians, as illustrated in **Figure 2**.[5] Patient cooperation is necessary, as the eyeball has to be moved to scan various quadrants and areas of interest. The moving transducer is very near the ocular surface and there is possibility of corneal injury. A bandage contact lens can be used to protect the cornea. [6]

After the procedure, the probe and the eyecup have to be cleaned as per the manufacturer's instructions.

ULTRASOUND BIOMICROSCOPY IN NORMAL EYE

During UBM imaging of the eye, the structures of the anterior segment—cornea, anterior chamber, iris, ciliary body, posterior chamber and the iris can be imaged well **(Figure 3)**. The zonular apparatus can also be imaged on routine scanning.

The scleral spur is the structure taken as the landmark to assess the angle status. The scleral spur is located where the trabecular meshwork meets the interface line between the sclera and the ciliary body.

> **Note** The anterior segment structures undergo morphological changes in different lighting conditions and on accommodation of the eye; therefore, these factors should be kept constant especially when quantitative information is gathered.[7]

ULTRASOUND BIOMICROSCOPY IN GLAUCOMA

Glaucoma may be broadly classified as open angle or closed angle based on the status of the anterior chamber angle. UBM can be used to assess the anterior chamber angle and ciliary body in detail **(Table 1)**. The UBM images can be very useful in explaining the rationale for any treatment to the patient.[8]

The most studied entities with UBM are angle-closure glaucoma and pigment dispersion glaucoma.[8]

> **Scleral spur:** It is taken as the landmark to assess the angle
> **Location:** Where the trabecular meshwork meets the interface line between the sclera and the ciliary body

Angle-Closure Glaucoma

Contact between the iris and trabecular meshwork causing obstruction in the outflow of aqueous humor is the diagnostic feature of this condition. This iris —trabecular meshwork apposition can be due to various factors. There can be four different anatomic locations where the block can occur:
- The iris (pupillary block)
- The ciliary body (plateau iris)
- The lens (phacomorphic glaucoma)
- Behind the iris by a combination of various forces (malignant glaucoma and other posterior pushing glaucoma types).[9]

Differentiating the affected sites is the key to provide effective treatment. UBM is extremely useful for achieving this goal.[10] Some eyes with primary angle closure glaucoma may have presence of uveal effusion.[11]

Pupillary Block

This is the most common type of angle-closure glaucoma. There is resistance to aqueous flow from the posterior to the anterior chamber at the area of iris-lens contact. The unequal pressure gradient between the two chambers pushes the iris forwards. This abnormal resistance causes anterior iris bowing, angle narrowing, and acute or chronic angle-closure glaucoma **(Figure 4)**.

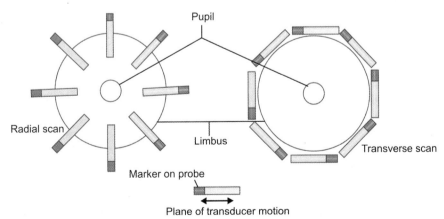

Fig. 2 Schematic diagram showing the orientation of the transducer in relation to the eye during UBM imaging. Scans are performed in radial and transverse meridians

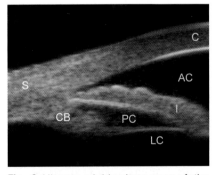

Fig. 3 Ultrasound biomicroscopy of the normal eye. The sclera (S), cornea (C), ciliary body (CB), iris (I), anterior chamber (AC), posterior chamber (PC), and lens capsule (LC) are marked

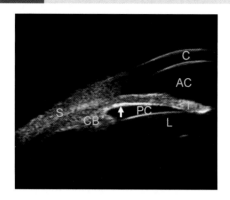

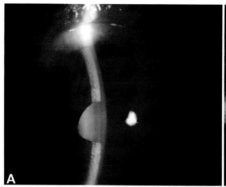

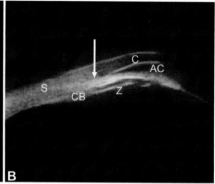

Fig. 4 Ultrasound biomicroscopy (UBM) of pupillary block. White arrow denotes forward bowing of iris causing angle closure

Figs 6A and B (A) Slit lamp clinical photograph showing shallow anterior chamber with forward displacement of lens in a patient with malignant glaucoma; (B) UBM in malignant glaucoma. White arrow denotes the closed angle. The ciliary processes, iris, zonules and lens are pushed forward causing angle closure and very shallow anterior chamber

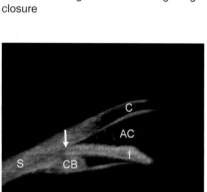

Fig. 5 Ultrasound biomicroscopy (UBM) of plateau iris. White arrow denotes the closed angle. The ciliary body is large and positioned anteriorly. It causes angle closure by pushing the iris root against the cornea

Laser peripheral iridotomy (LPI) equalizes the pressure gradient between the anterior and posterior chambers and flattens the iris. This results in a widened anterior chamber angle.

UBM clearly shows the changed iris configuration pre- and postlaser iridotomy.

Plateau Iris

In this condition, a large or anteriorly positioned ciliary body (pars plicata) pushes the iris root mechanically up against the trabecular meshwork. The iris root may be short and inserted anteriorly on the ciliary face (**Figure 5**). The

anterior chamber is usually of medium depth, and the iris surface is flat or slightly convex. On indentation gonioscopy, the "double hump" sign is observed. Even after laser iridotomy, the angle does not open well as the peripheral iris is prevented from falling back by the ciliary body.[12]

Indentation UBM is a special technique of examination that imposes mild pressure on the peripheral cornea with the skirt of a plastic eyecup so that one can simulate indentation gonioscopy.[13] Features of plateau iris can be confirmed by performing indentation UBM.[10]

Phacomorphic Glaucoma

An intumescent cataractous lens or an anterior subluxated lens may cause angle-closure glaucoma. This is because of the lens pushing the iris and ciliary body toward the trabecular meshwork. UBM imaging shows the presence of shallow anterior chamber. There is usually no pupillary block present.

Aqueous Misdirection (Malignant Glaucoma)

This condition is also known as ciliary block glaucoma or aqueous misdirection syndrome. Angle closure is due to anterior rotation of the ciliary body

around its attachment to the scleral spur (**Figure 6A**). This condition is very challenging to diagnose and treat.

UBM shows that the anterior segment structures are displaced forwards (**Figure 6B**).[10] UBM imaging sometimes shows shallow supraciliary effusion that is not detectable on routine B-scan ultrasonography.[8]

UBM has demonstrated the anterior rotation of ciliary processes to make the diagnosis of malignant glaucoma.[14] Leibmann et al[15] have classified malignant glaucoma into two groups on the basis of UBM — one with supraciliary effusion, which responds to medical management better, and another without effusion that usually requires surgical management. **UBM helps in deciding the course of management at an early stage.**

Other Causes of Angle Closure

Lesions in the region of the ciliary body pushing the iris forward can cause angle closure. UBM imaging can reveal the pathology, which may not be feasible on clinical examination.

Iridociliary cysts may cause a focal angle closure while multiple cysts may cause a "pseudoplateau" iris syndrome with angle closure. UBM is helpful in confirming the underlying mechanism and guiding therapy (**Figure 7**).[16]

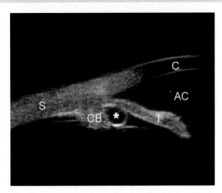

Fig. 7 Ultrasound biomicroscopy (UBM) showing a iridociliary cyst marked by white asterix (*)

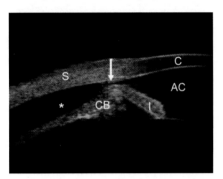

Fig. 8 Ultrasound biomicroscopy (UBM) in cyclodialysis. White arrow denotes point where ciliary body is detached from the sclera. White asterix (*) denotes the supraciliary space filled with fluid from AC

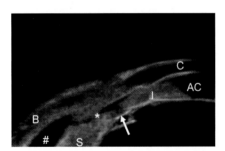

Fig. 9 Ultrasound biomicroscopy (UBM) in a patient with a large overfiltering bleb with a shallow AC. White arrow marks the peripheral iridectomy, white asterix marks the trabeculectomy ostium (#) shows the large bleb space. The bleb wall (B) is imaged. AC is shallow and there is iridocorneal touch in the periphery

Other entities such as iridociliary tumor, ciliary body enlargement due to tumor or inflammation can also cause angle closure.

Intraoperatively injected air, gas or silicone oil can precipitate angle closure.

Open Angle Glaucoma

Pigment dispersion syndrome shows some characteristic findings on UBM evaluation. In this disease, there is pigment release from the iris due to mechanical friction between the anterior zonules and the posterior iris surface. Typical UBM features are a widely opened angle, an iris with slight concavity (bowing posteriorly), and increased iridolenticular contact. There is a relative pressure gradient between the anterior and posterior chamber with the anterior chamber being at higher pressure. This condition is called "reverse pupillary block", in contrast to pupillary block where the posterior chamber is at a higher pressure.[17] Laser iridotomy helps to eliminates this pressure gradient, resulting in a flattened iris configuration.[18]

OTHER CONDITIONS IN WHICH ULTRASOUND BIOMICROSCOPY MAY BE HELPFUL

Post-traumatic cyclodialysis clefts can cause hypotony and may sometimes not be evident on clinical examination. UBM can be used to evaluate cyclodialysis **(Figure 8)**.[19,20]

Angle recession can be a cause for glaucoma after trauma. UBM can be used to evaluate for the same.[20]

Virtual gonioscopy can be done in cases of corneal opacity precluding view of the anterior chamber. This helps in the management of clinical entities like sclerocornea, Peter's anomaly.[8]

Assessment of the filtering bleb is of prime importance in patients undergoing glaucoma surgery.

Demonstration of the trabeculectomy stoma, its patency and the bleb can be demonstrated on UBM **(Figure 9)**. Yamamoto et al have described a bleb classification system.[21]

Suprachoroidal effusion due to reaction to drugs can cause secondary angle closure glaucoma, which may be of sudden onset. The management of these conditions depends on the arriving at the correct diagnosis. UBM can detect the presence of the supraciliary effusion and ciliary body edema.[22]

Assessment of the position of the implant after glaucoma seton surgery is important.

UBM imaging can be used in patients with media opacities to assess the position of the tube of a glaucoma drainage device in the anterior segment.[23]

QUANTITATIVE MEASUREMENTS

Quantitative assessment of the anterior segment using UBM is more difficult than the initial qualitative assessment.[8]

Quantitative measurements in UBM can be done using various measurement parameters **(Table 2)**. These were proposed by Pavlin et al.[2]

While calculating these measurements, the scleral spur is taken as the reference point as it is possible to identify the scleral spur with consistency during UBM imaging. Using these measurements, intraobserver reproducibility was reasonably good, but interobserver reproducibility was not, as reported by Tello et al.[7] Urbak et al had similar results.[24,25]

Pavlin described **Angle Opening Distance (AOD)** as the measure for assessing the anterior chamber angle **(Figures 10 and 11)**. While measuring AOD, the iris surface is taken as a straight line, but in real-life the iris contour may not be straight and there may be irregularities.

To account for any iris irregularity, Ishikawa et al[26] defined the **Angle Recess Area (ARA)**. This is defined as the triangular area bordered by the anterior iris surface, corneal endothelium, and a line perpendicular to the corneal endothelium drawn to the iris surface from a point 750 µm anterior to

Table 1 Salient UBM features in different types of glaucoma

Types of glaucoma	UBM findings	Clinical significance
Angle-closure glaucoma		
1. Pupillary block	Appositional closure due to anterior bowing of iris.	Reversal with LPI seen as a flattened iris and deep anterior chamber
2. Plateau iris	a. Large, anteriorly positioned ciliary body b. Peripheral iris roll c. Iris surface flat d. "Double hump" sign with indentation UBM	Responsible for failure of LPI
3. Malignant glaucoma	a. Anterior rotation of ciliary processes b. Supraciliary effusion	Presence of (b) indicates that medical management may be successful
4. Secondary angle glaucoma	a. Iris-ciliary body cysts b. Tumor of iris or ciliary body c. Intraocular gas bubble d. Ciliary body edema/supraciliary effusion due to inflammation	May be the cause for failure of conventional treatment of angle-closure
Open-angle glaucoma		
Pigment dispersion syndrome	a. Deep a/c with concave iris b. Increased iridolenticular contact c. Iridozonular contact	Demonstration of (c) is an indication for peripheral iridotomy

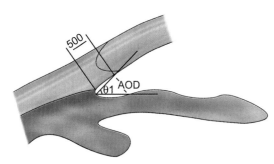

Fig. 10 Angle opening distance (AOD), as proposed by Pavlin. (Distance in µm, see Table 2)

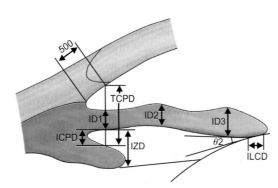

Fig. 11 Pavlin's measurement parameters. Distance in µm

Table 2 Parameters for quantitative measurements using UBM

Normal and abbreviation	Description
Angle opening distance (AOD)	Distance between the trabecular meshwork and the iris at 500 µm anterior to the scleral spur
Trabecular-iris angle (TIA θ1)	Angle of the angle recess
Trabecular-ciliary process distance (TCPD)	Distance between the trabecular meshwork and the ciliary process at 500 µm anterior to the scleral spur
Iris thickness (ID1)	Iris thickness at 500 µm anterior to the scleral spur
Iris thickness (ID2)	Iris thickness at 2 mm from the iris root
Iris thickness (ID3)	Maximum iris thickness near the pupillary edge
Iris-ciliary process distance (ICPD)	Distance between the iris and the ciliary process along the line of TCPD
Iris-zonule distance (IZD)	Distance between the iris and the zonule along the line of TCPD
Iris-lens contact distance (ILCD)	Contact distance between the iris and the lens
Iris-lens angle (ILAθ2)	Angle between the iris and the lens near the pupillary edge
Angle recess area (ARA)	The triangular area bordered by the anterior iris surface, corneal endothelium, and a line perpendicular to the corneal endothelium drawn to the iris surface from a point 750 µm anterior to the scleral spur

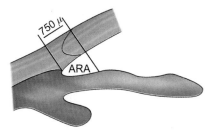

Fig. 12 Angle recess area (ARA). Distance in µm (also see Table 2)

the scleral spur **(Figure 12)**. UBM Pro 2000, a semiautomated software can be used to calculate ARA.[10]

Quantitative parameters have been used for various studies in relation to glaucoma. These studies have looked at various aspects of the anterior segment of the eye. Kobayashi et al[27] looked at the development of the angle in normal infants and children in relation to age.

UBM can be used for objective quantification of angles and AOD can

be a reliable and standard parameter to grade angle width.[28] Marchini et al found the anterior segment is more crowded in patients with primary angle closure glaucoma compared to normal subjects.[29]

Krishna Kumar et al studied and compared anterior chamber parameters between normal patients and primary angle closure suspects and found significant difference between the two groups.[30]

In a cross-sectional study, Esaki et al[31] reported that the anterior chamber angle opening in normal Japanese eyes narrowed with age.

UBM can also be used to evaluate the effect of drugs on anterior segment structures.[32,33]

FUTURE TRENDS

Research is going on newer aspects of UBM use.

High frequency doppler: Instrumentation is being developed to analyze ocular microcirculation.

Corneal arc imaging: Imaging the cornea in an arc along its curvature as opposed to a linear scan will help to map corneal changes after refractive surgery.

Three-dimensional scanning has been under development and may enable users to get three-dimensional sections of the eye in the future.

CONCLUSION

UBM has evolved as a diagnostic tool which plays an important role in glaucoma management, especially in patients posing a clinical challenge. The superior image quality and resolution highlights the pathology of the various clinical conditions.

REFERENCES

1. Pavlin CJ, Sherar MD, Foster FS. Subsurface ultrasound microscopic imaging of the intact eye. Ophthalmology 1990;97:244-50.
2. Pavlin CJ, Harasiewicz K, Foster FS. Ultrasound biomicroscopy of anterior segment structures in normal and glaucomatous eyes. Am J Ophthalmol 1992;113:381-9.
3. Pavlin CJ, Harasiewicz K, Sherar MD, et al. Clinical use of ultrasound biomicroscopy. Ophthalmology 1991; 98:287-95.
4. Esaki K, Ishikawa H, Liebmann JM, Ritch R. A technique for performing ultrasound biomicroscopy in the sitting and prone positions. Ophthalmic Surg Lasers 2000;31:166-9.
5. Pavlin CJ, Foster FS. Ultrasound Biomicroscopy of the eye. 1st edn. Spring-Verlag, New York Inc; 1995.
6. Tello C, Potash S, Liebmann J, Ritch R. Soft contact lens modification of the ocular cup for high-resolution ultrasound biomicroscopy. Ophthalmic Surg 1993;24: 563-4.

7. Tello C, Liebmann J, Potash SD, Cohen H, Ritch R. Measurement of ultrasound biomicroscopy images: intraobserver and interobserver reliability. Invest Ophthalmol Vis Sci 1994; 35:3549-52.

8. Liebmann JM, Ritch R, Esaki K. Ultrasound biomicroscopy. Ophthalmology Clinics of North America 1998;11:421-33.

9. Ritch R, Liebmann JM, Tello C. A construct for understanding angle-closure glaucoma: The role of ultrasound biomicroscopy. Ophthalmology Clinics of North America 1995;8:281-93.

10. Ishikawa H, Schuman JS. Anterior segment imaging: ultrasound biomicroscopy. Ophthalmology Clinics of North America 2004;17:7-20.

11. Sakai H, Morine-Shinjyo S, Shinzato M, Nakamura Y, Sakai M, Sawaguchi S. Uveal effusion in primary angle-closure glaucoma. Ophthalmology 2005;112:413-9.

12. Pavlin CJ, Ritch R, Foster FS. Ultrasound biomicroscopy in plateau iris syndrome. Am J Ophthalmol 1992; 113:390-5.

13. Ishikawa H, Inazumi K, Liebmann JM, Ritch R. Inadvertent corneal indentation can cause artifactitious widening of the iridocorneal angle on ultrasound biomicroscopy. Ophthalmic Surg Lasers 2000;31:342-5.

14. Trope GE, Pavlin CJ, Bau A, Baumal CR, Foster FS. Malignant glaucoma. Clinical and ultrasound biomicroscopic features. Ophthalmology 1994; 101:1030-5.

15. Liebmann JM, Weinreb RN, Ritch R. Angle-closure glaucoma associated with occult annular ciliary body detachment. Arch Ophthalmol 1998;116:731-5.

16. Shukla S, Damji KF, Harasymowycz P, Chialant D, Kent JS, Chevrier R, Buhrmann R, Marshall D, Pan Y, Hodge W. Clinical features distinguishing angle closure from pseudoplateau versus plateau iris. Br J Ophthalmol 2008;92:340-4. Epub 2008 Jan 22.

17. Potash SD, Tello C, Liebmann J, Ritch R. Ultrasound biomicroscopy in pigment dispersion syndrome. Ophthalmology 1994;101:332-9.

18. Breingan PJ, Esaki K, Ishikawa H, Liebmann JM, Greenfield DS, Ritch R. Iridolenticular contact decreases following laser iridotomy for pigment dispersion syndrome. Arch Ophthalmol 1999;117:325-8.

19. Gentile RC, Pavlin CJ, Liebmann JM, Easterbrook M, Tello C, Foster FS, Ritch R. Diagnosis of traumatic cyclodialysis by ultrasound biomicroscopy. Ophthalmic Surg Lasers 1996;27:97-105.

20. Ozdal MP, Mansour M, Deschênes J. Ultrasound biomicroscopic evaluation of the traumatized eyes. Eye 2003;17:467-72.

21. Yamamoto T, Sakuma T, Kitazawa Y. An ultrasound biomicroscopic study of filtering blebs after mitomycin C trabeculectomy. Ophthalmology 1995;102:1770-6.

22. Panday VA, Rhee DJ. Review of sulfonamide-induced acute myopia and acute bilateral angle-closure glaucoma. Compr Ophthalmol Update. 2007;8:271-6.

23. Carrillo MM, Trope GE, Pavlin C, Buys YM. Use of ultrasound biomicroscopy to diagnose Ahmed valve obstruction by iris. Can J Ophthalmol 2005;40:499-501.

24. Urbak SF. Ultrasound biomicroscopy. I. Precision of measurements. Acta Ophthalmol Scand 1998;76:447-55.

25. Urbak SF, Pedersen JK, Thorsen TT. Ultrasound biomicroscopy. II. Intraobserver and interobserver reproducibility of measurements. Acta Ophthalmol Scand 1998;76:546-9.

26. Ishikawa H, Esaki K, Liebmann JM, Uji Y, Ritch R. Ultrasound biomicroscopy dark room provocative testing: a quantitative method for estimating anterior chamber angle width. Jpn J Ophthalmol 1999;43: 526-34.

27. Kobayashi H, Ono H, Kiryu J, Kobayashi K, Kondo T. Ultrasound biomicroscopic measurement of development of anterior chamber angle. Br J Ophthalmol 1999;83: 559-62.

28. Arun N, Vijaya L, Shantha B, Baskaran M, Sathidevi AV, Baluswamy S. Anterior chamber angle assessment using gonioscopy and ultrasound biomicroscopy. Jpn J Ophthalmol 2004;48:44-9.

29. Marchini G, Pagliarusco A, Toscano A, Tosi R, Brunelli C, Bonomi L. Ultrasound biomicroscopic and conventional ultrasonographic study of ocular dimensions in primary angle-closure glaucoma. Ophthalmology 1998;105:2091-8.

30. Ramani KK, Mani B, Ronnie G, Joseph R, Lingam V. Gender Variation in Ocular Biometry and Ultrasound Biomicroscopy of Primary Angle Closure Suspects and Normal Eyes. J Glaucoma 2007;16:122-8.

31. Esaki K, Ishikawa H, Liebmann JM, Greenfield DS, Uji Y, Ritch R. Angle recess area decreases with age in normal Japanese. Jpn J Ophthalmol 2000;44:46-51.

32. Kobayashi H, Kobayashi K, Kiryu J, Kondo T. Pilocarpine induces an increase in the anterior chamber angular width in eyes with narrow angles. Br J Ophthalmol 1999;83: 553-8.

33. Marchini G, Babighian S, Tosi R, Perfertti S, Bonomi L. Comparative study of the effects of 2% ibopamine, 10% phenylephrine, and 1% tropicamide on the anterior segment. Invest Ophthalmol Vis Sci 2003;44:281-9.

20 | Confocal Laser Scanning Tomography: Principles and Clinical Utility

Vinay Nangia

INTRODUCTION

The optic disc is an important site of glaucomatous damage. In addition, this is accompanied by changes in the retinal nerve fiber layer and adjacent peripapillary tissues. Clinical examination of the optic nerve remains an important tool in the day to day diagnosis and management of subjects with optic neuropathy. Stereoscopic magnified evaluation of the optic nerve has become the norm of clinical optic disc examination. Clinical notes and drawings of the optic nerve has been followed for several decades. Optic nerve photography became adopted as a tool for documentation and comparison of disc photographs which complimented the clinical stereoscopic evaluation and the disc drawings. Stereodisc photography using cameras specially designed for it was also adopted though not universally. Subjective assessment both clinically and on photography is an important consideration. A shift in techniques and technology towards a more objective and accurate documentation system which allows for follow up over time was an important goal. This was the basis of the development

of several objective and accurate imaging tools amongst which is the confocal scanning laser ophthalmoscope (CSLO) also known as the Heidelberg retina tomograph (HRT).

CONFOCAL SCANNING LASER TOMOGRAPHY

Basis of Function

The Heidelberg retina tomograph is a scanning laser ophthalmoscope specially designed to acquire three dimensional images of the optic nerve head, retinal nerve fiber layer and posterior pole. A rapid scanning 670 nm diode laser is used to acquire images, without mydriasis. Images are obtained non invasively, at low illumination and rapidly. The HRT II and HRT III acquire reflectance images (16–64) to a depth of 4 mm. These are consecutive and equidistant two dimensional optical section images. Each successive scan plane is 0.0625 mm deeper. Thus, if scanning of 1 mm depth is needed, 16 imaging planes will be scanned. If it is 2 mm depth then there will be 32 imaging planes and so on to a maximum depth of 4 mm. These are joined together to provide a three dimensional contour

map of the optic disc surface. An area of 15 degree by 15 degree is imaged. The topographical image consists of more than 147000 independent local height measurements. The images obtained have high spatial resolution. A lateral resolution of 10 μ (microns) is achieved. Three scans are included for analysis and storage from the prescans. The software automatically aligns these scans and averages the values to create the mean topography scan for the individual.

Method of Imaging Optic Disc

The patient is asked to sit in front of the instrument and to look at the internal fixation target (Figure 1). The actual imaging may take place in 10 seconds and in practice the eye may be imaged in less than a minute. The corneal curvature has to be entered for the subject. A cylinder of more than 1 diopter refractive error is corrected by attaching cylindrical lenses to the HRT. Each scan gives a standard deviation value. A value of under 20 μm indicates an excellent image. 20 to 30 microns is a very good image and 30 to 40 microns an acceptable image.

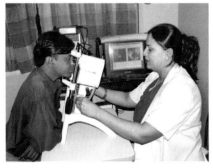

Fig. 1 The operator and subject using the Heidelberg retina tomograph

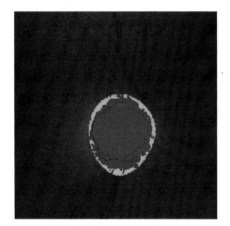

Fig. 2 Color coded optic disc

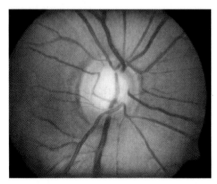

Fig. 3 Optic disc of the subject for whom the CLSO images are shown

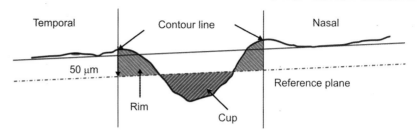

Fig. 4 Reference plane is located 50 μm below the mean height of the retinal surface along the contour line, between 350° and 356° (papillomacular bundle). Volume enclosed by the contour line and located above the reference plane is the rim. Below is the cup

The Contour Line

Once the image has been obtained the contour line should be drawn **(Figure 2)**. This identifies the margin of the optic disc. The reflectance image may be used for this. When in doubt about the exact border of the optic disc, one may look at the contour of the blood vessels, the peripapillary atrophy, and other visual cues. It is also helpful to visualize the color optic disc photograph **(Figure 3)** to delineate the margin with the help of the drawing tool provided. This is the most important manual part of the imaging. Once this is done the several parameters of the image will automatically be generated.

Reference Plane

Once the contour line is done, the software automatically creates a reference plane, **(Figure 4)** parallel to the peripapillary retinal surface and located 50 μm below the retinal surface as measured along the contour line in the papillomacular bundle (350°–356°). This reference line serves as the base with which the height of the retinal nerve fiber layer is measured along the retinal surface all around the disc along the contour line. In addition the reference plane serves to separate the disc into the rim and the cup **(Figure 4)**. The color coded optic disc image provides for identification of the rim (green), rim slope (blue) and cup (red) **(Figure 2)**.

Parameters

The morphometric parameters besides the optic disc area include cup area, cup disc area ratio, rim area, cup volume, cup depth, retinal nerve fiber layer thickness and cross sectional retinal nerve fiber layer area. These parameters are available for the entire optic disc (global) and for the different segments of the optic disc. The optic disc in the HRT imaging for purposes of measurements, analysis and follow-up be segmented in various ways. The most common is in six segments: superotemporal, temporal, inferotemporal, inferonasal, nasal and superonasal **(Figure 5)**. A selection of the measurements that are generated by the HRT are as follows **(Figure 2)**.

1. **Disc area (mm²):** This is the area bounded by the contour line, indicating the area of the optic disc.
2. **Cup area (mm²):** This is the area of the optic disc cupping and is seen as the area enclosed by the contour line, which is located beneath the reference plane. It appears as a red overlay on the topography image.
3. **Rim area (mm²):** This is the area of the neuroretinal rim and is seen as the area enclosed by the contour line, which is located above the reference plane. It appears as either blue or green on the topography image (Blue-sloping and green-stable neuroretinal rim).
4. **Cup volume:** The volume of optic disc cupping, defined as the volume enclosed by the contour line and located below the reference plane.
5. **Cup/disc area ratio:** Ratio of area of optic disc cupping to area of the optic disc.
6. **Linear cup/disc ratio:** The average cup disc diameter ratio calculated as the square root of the cup/disc area ratio.

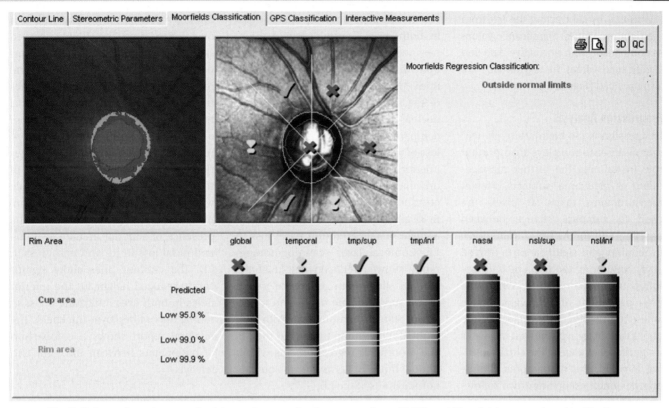

Fig. 5 Color coding of neuroretinal rim and cup, optic disc segments on CLSO and Moorfields regression classification

7. ***Mean retinal nerve fiber layer thickness:*** The mean thickness of the retinal nerve fiber layer measured along the contour line, and measured relative to the reference plane.

8. ***RNFL cross-section area (mm²):*** This is the total cross-sectional area of the retinal nerve fiber layer along the contour line, and measured relative to the reference plane.

PRINCIPLES AND CLINICAL UTILITY

In the printout, the parameters from the normative database of the particular ethnic group (Caucasians, African Americans and Indians) are given and compared with values obtained in the particular patient. When the parameters are different from the normative values, significance values are highlighted helping the clinicians in the interpretation.

Moorfields Regression

The Moorfields regression was derived at Moorfields Hospital on normal subjects. The regression has as its basis the log of the rim area plotted against the disc area. Thus if for a particular disc, the rim area/disc area ratio is less than expected in a normal population, then one may suspect that the patient has glaucoma. The Moorfields regression analysis may also be performed for the different segments of the optic disc. The upper limit of the disc size to be acceptable for the MRA was about 2.8 mm². However, the new databases may enable the MRA to be acceptable for disc sizes between 1 and 3.6 mm² (Caucasian database). It may not be utilized or only with caution in discs smaller or larger than mentioned. The Moorfields regression is represented in a bar form representing the rim as green and the red as the cup. There are three lines that cross the red- green bar.

The predicted line, which is the average or predicted relationship between log neuroretinal rim area and optic disc area. The lower three lines represent the lower 95 percent, 99.0 percent and 99.9 percent prediction intervals for the same relationship. Thus for the 95.0 percent prediction interval, 95.0 percent of normal eyes would be expected to have a neuro-retinal rim area above that interval line. The same principal would apply for the lines representing 99.0 percent and 99.9 percent prediction intervals **(Figure 5)**.

Bilateral Printout

An informational printout of both eyes is now available. It includes information about the patient and the disc area. It further includes the linear cup disc ratio, cup-shaped measure, rim area, rim volume, height variation contour and retinal nerve fiber layer thickness. Values are provided for each eye, including the asymmetry by subtracting the left from the right eye values. Significance values as comparison with normative data and significance values for asymmetry are also provided **(Figure 6)**.

Progression Analysis

Progression is the hallmark of glaucomatous disease and plays an important role in defining the further management of glaucoma subjects. Height measurements taken at pixels are used to compare change between baseline and follow-up examinations. Probability and significance is arrived at by comparing the baseline with the follow-up measurements. When the error probability of the height change is less than 5 percent for rejecting the equal variances hypothesis it indicates a significant change at the corresponding location. For topographic change analysis one baseline and two follow-up examinations are required. In the image for topographic change analysis, there is a change map, a probability map and a significance map. Areas in red are those which show a depression and areas in green are those which show elevation. The exact values in area and volume and the change can be obtained by pressing the mouse at the location of change **(Figure 7)**. A cluster change graph may also be obtained which shows the area along the Y axis on the left, the volume on the Y axis on the right and the time interval and examination date on the X axis. A change in the normalized values of stereometric parameters vs time may also be displayed in a graph for different segments.

CLINICAL CASES
Case 1

A 60-year-old gentleman **(Figures 8 to 11)** presented with visual acuity of RE 6/9 and LE 6/18. He was using Beta-blockers in both eyes. IOP RE was 18 mm Hg and LE was 34 mm

Hg. Gonioscopy showed open angles in both eyes. Central corneal thickness was RE 536 and LE 535 μm. The optic disc area was 2.29 mm² and 1.89 mm². Optic disc RE, showed sloping of the superior neuroretinal rim and decreased visibility of RNFL superiorly compared to inferiorly. The LE showed loss of neuroretinal rim superiorly and inferiorly with RNFL loss more superiorly than inferiorly. Automated perimetry showed early visual field changes in RE and superior paracentral, inferior arcuate, paracentral and nasal loss in LE. Confocal laser scanning tomography showed reduced height of the contour line from reference plane in the superior pole of RE and a flattened plateau contour line with loss of the double hump pattern in the LE. The Moorfields regression was within normal limits in RE and it was outside normal limits in the LE.

Values for Case 1

Table 1 shows the values for case 1.

Case 2

A sixty year elderly lady **(Figures 12 to 15)** presented with a visual acuity of 6/9 in RE and 6/9 in LE. She was using prostaglandins once a day in both eyes. IOP was BE 14 mm Hg. Gonioscopy showed open angles in both eyes. Central corneal thickness was RE 519 μm and LE 517 μm. The optic disc size was RE 1.72 mm² and LE 2.09 mm². Optic disc RE was obliquely oval with

inferior extension of the cup with loss of inferior rim. The RNFL showed significant loss inferiorly. There was narrowing of the inferior temporal retinal arteriole with increased inferior tesselation. Optic disc in LE was horizontally oval with inferior loss of neuroretinal rim and generalized retinal nerve fiber layer thinning inferiorly. LE also showed narrowing of the inferior temporal retinal arteriole with increased inferior tesselation. Automated perimetry showed the presence of superior arcuate scotoma and nasal loss in RE and nasal loss in LE. The contour lines show significantly reduced height for the inferior poles in both eyes indicating a loss of retinal nerve fiber layer thickness. The bilateral report shows a comparison of parameters between the right and left eye.

Values for Case 2

Table 2 shows the values for case 2.

CLINICAL IMPLICATIONS AND CONCLUSION

Qualitative evaluation of the optic disc remains a very important and reliable expertise in the diagnosis and management of glaucoma. However, it is important that subjective and qualitative clinical expertise is supported by objective measurements. This is the relevance of confocal scanning laser tomography or HRT. HRT measurements are reproducible and have small

Table 1 Values for case 1

Parameters (OD)	Global	Parameters (OS)	Global
Disc area (mm²)	2.28	Disc area (mm²)	1.88
Cup area (mm²)	0.49	Cup area (mm²)	1.13
Rim area (mm²)	1.79	Rim area (mm²)	0.75
Cup/disc area ratio	0.21	Cup/disc area ratio	0.6
Cup volume (mm²)	0.07	Cup volume (mm²)	0.37
Mean RNFL thickness (mm)	0.26	Mean RNFL thickness (mm)	0.11
RNFL cross-sectional area (mm²)	1.4	RNFL cross-sectional area (mm²)	0.55
Linear cup/disc ration	0.46	Linear cup/disc ration	0.77

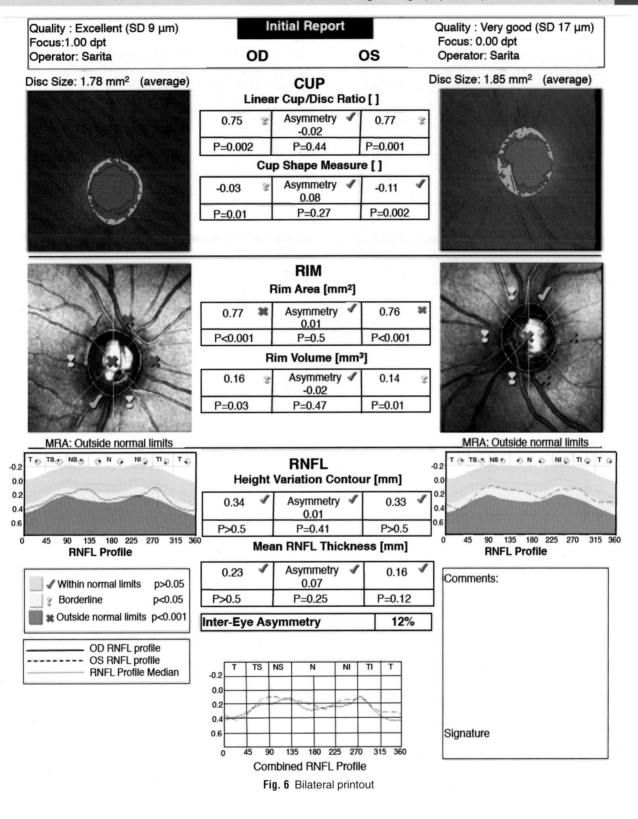

Fig. 6 Bilateral printout

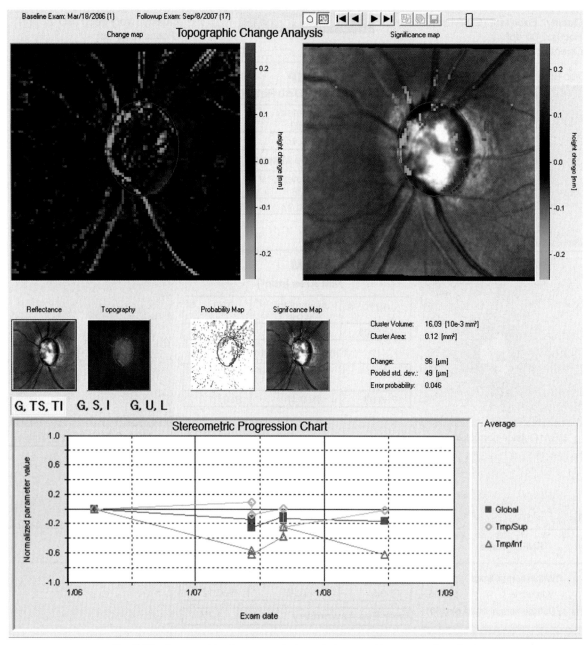

Fig. 7 The topographic change analysis and stereometric progression chart

values of between 25 and 49 μm SD for relative height values and 0.04 to 0.06 mm² for rim or cup area. Several studies have evaluated the utility of CLSO for diagnosis in glaucoma. The sensitivity of HRT as a diagnostic tool has varied from 74 to 92 and of specificity from 81 to 97 in different studies. These are in agreement to that of an expert observer assessing the optic disc on stereoscopic photographs. While abnormal results on HRT suggest structural damage, they should always be considered in association with a patients history and the established methods of clinical assessment of the glaucoma subject and never in isolation. It is not a substitute but an associate of clinical evaluation. The segmentation of the optic disc in sectors may enable one to further identify patterns of glaucoma damage evolution in terms of loss of neuroretinal rim and retinal nerve fiber layer. This may indicate modalities

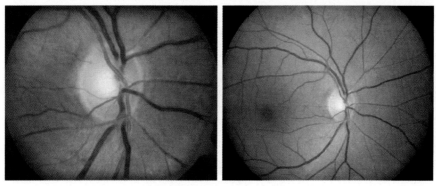

Fig. 8 Optic disc RE of case 1

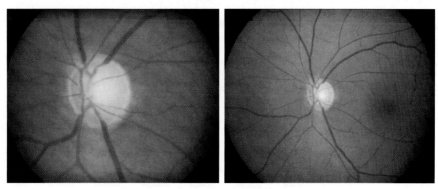

Fig. 9 Optic disc of LE of case 1

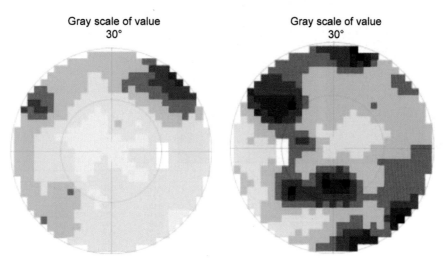

Fig. 10 Visual field of case 1. RE mean defect −0.2 dBs and LE 6.5 dBs

to pre-empt significant loss in areas of greater visual potential. Objective measurements may help us identify and define parameters that constitute normal, suspicious and abnormal and help in the classification of glaucomatous damage. This has implications in standardization of research and clinical findings.

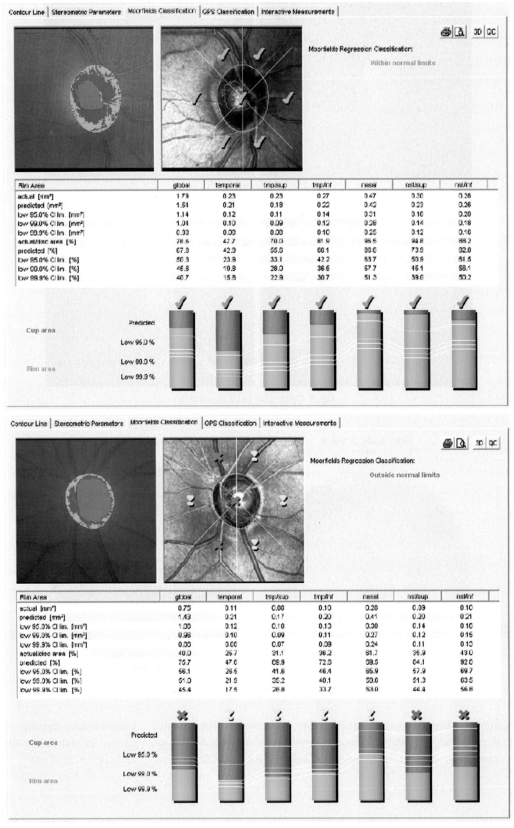

Fig. 11 Moorfields regression for case 1 RE and LE

Table 2 Values for case 2

Parameters (OS)	Global	Parameters (OD)	Global
Disc area [mm²]	2.09	Disc area [mm²]	1.72
Cup area [mm²]	1.38	Cup area [mm²]	1.12
Rim area [mm²]	0.71	Rim area [mm²]	0.6
Cup/disc area ratio	0.66	Cup/disc area ratio	0.65
Cup volume [mm²]	0.51	Cup volume [mm²]	0.47
Mean RNFL thickness [mm]	0.15	Mean RNFL thickness [mm]	0.09
RNFL cross-sectional area [mm²]	0.79	RNFL cross-sectional area [mm²]	0.41
Linear cup/disc ratio	0.81	Linear cup/disc ratio	0.81

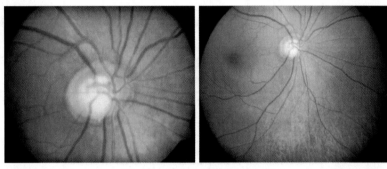

Fig. 12 RE optic disc of case 2

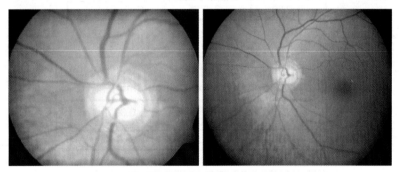

Fig.13 LE optic disc of case 2

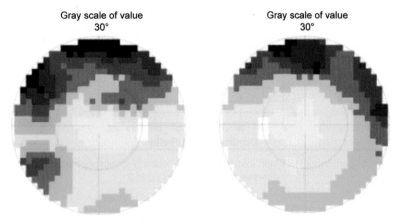

Fig.14 Case 2: Automated perimetry—gray scale

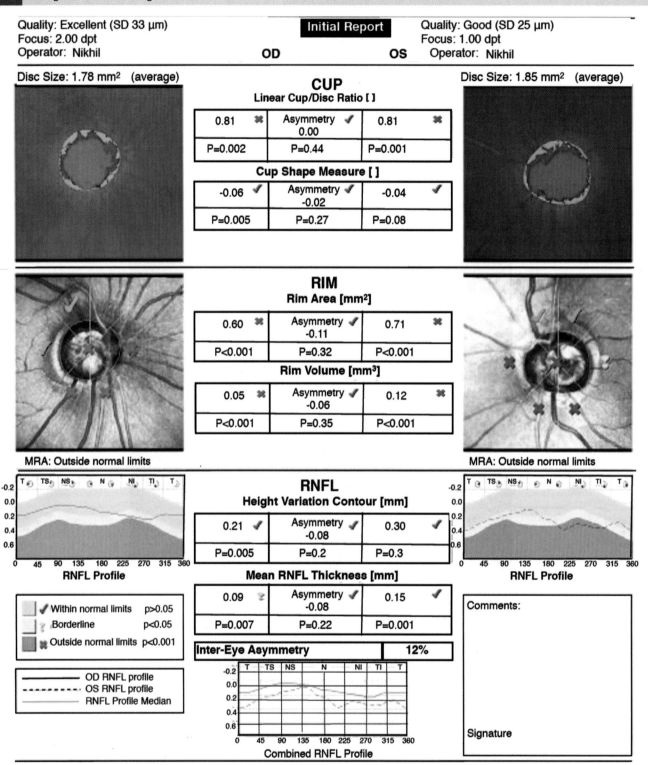

Quality: Excellent (SD 33 µm)
Focus: 2.00 dpt
Operator: Nikhil

Initial Report

OD   OS

Quality: Good (SD 25 µm)
Focus: 1.00 dpt
Operator: Nikhil

Disc Size: 1.78 mm² (average)

Disc Size: 1.85 mm² (average)

CUP
Linear Cup/Disc Ratio [ ]

0.81 ✖	Asymmetry ✓ 0.00	0.81 ✖
P=0.002	P=0.44	P=0.001

Cup Shape Measure [ ]

-0.06 ✓	Asymmetry ✓ -0.02	-0.04 ✓
P=0.005	P=0.27	P=0.08

RIM
Rim Area [mm²]

0.60 ✖	Asymmetry ✓ -0.11	0.71 ✖
P<0.001	P=0.32	P<0.001

Rim Volume [mm³]

0.05 ✖	Asymmetry ✓ -0.06	0.12 ✖
P<0.001	P=0.35	P<0.001

MRA: Outside normal limits

MRA: Outside normal limits

RNFL Profile

RNFL Profile

RNFL
Height Variation Contour [mm]

0.21 ✓	Asymmetry ✓ -0.08	0.30 ✓
P=0.005	P=0.2	P=0.3

Mean RNFL Thickness [mm]

0.09 ⸮	Asymmetry ✓ -0.08	0.15 ✓
P=0.007	P=0.22	P=0.001

| **Inter-Eye Asymmetry** | **12%** |

Combined RNFL Profile

✓ Within normal limits	p>0.05
⸮ Borderline	p<0.05
✖ Outside normal limits	p<0.001

| ——— OD RNFL profile |
| --------- OS RNFL profile |
| ——— RNFL Profile Median |

Comments:

Signature

Fig. 15 Bilateral printout of HRT with information about optic disc morphometric parameters and intereye comparisons of case 2

BIBLIOGRAPHY

1. Fingeret M, Flanagan JG, Liebman JM (Eds). The Essential HRT Primer. Jocoto Advertising Inc. San Ramon by Heidelberg Engineering 2005; 94583.

2. Glaucoma Module. Heidelberg Retina Tomograph. Operating Instructions. Software Version 3.0. Heidelberg Engineering GmbH.

3. Scheuerle AF, Schmidt E. Atlas of Laser Scanning Ophthalmoscopy. Springer Verlag. Berlin Heidelberg; 2004.

4. Sommer et al. Arch Ophthalmol 1991; 109:77-83.

5. Wollstein G, Garway-Heath DF, Hitchings RA. Identification of early glaucoma cases with scanning laser ophthalmoscope. Ophthalmology 1998; 105:1557-63.

21 | Imaging in Glaucoma

— Arijit Mitra, R Ramakrishnan —

CHAPTER OUTLINE

Anterior Segment Optical Coherence Tomography
❖ Principle of Optical Coherence Tomography
❖ ASOCT in Glaucoma
❖ Comparison of Anterior Segment Optical Coherence Tomography Versus Ultrasound Biomicroscopy

Scanning Laser Polarimetry
❖ Principle
❖ Birefringence of the Other Ocular Structures—Anterior Segment Birefringence
❖ Variable Corneal Compensation
❖ Enhanced Corneal Compensation

❖ Clinical Interpretation of the GDx Variable Corneal Compensation Printout
❖ Serial Analysis

Optical Coherence Tomography in Glaucoma
❖ Basic Principles of Optical Coherence Tomography

ANTERIOR SEGMENT OPTICAL COHERENCE TOMOGRAPHY

Optical coherence tomography (OCT) is a cross-sectional, three-dimensional, high-resolution imaging modality that uses low coherence interferometry to achieve axial resolution in the range of 3-20 μm. It can overcome many of the limitations of the current techniques used to image the anterior segment of the eye. OCT is similar to ultrasound except that light is used instead of sound. It is a completely noninvasive technique. As it uses interferometry for depth resolution it can have a long working distance and a wide field of transverse scanning compared to confocal microscopy. OCT has predominantly been used so far for posterior segment imaging of the eye because of various reasons. Anterior segment imaging using OCT (ASOCT) was first demonstrated in 1994 by Izatt et al using light with a wavelength of 830 μm **(Figure 1)**. Not much attention

was paid to anterior segment applications until Lubech described OCT imaging of Laser thermokeratoplasty lesion in 1997 and Maldonado et al reported imaging of LASIK flap in 1998.

The primary limitation of OCT imaging of the anterior segment is speed and penetration. The OCT systems used in commercial retinal scanner have used 830 nm wavelength, with image acquisition time of 1 to 5 seconds.

The wavelength higher than 830 nm in posterior segment had more dissipation in vitreous hence was discarded from posterior segment use, but it found its use in anterior segment. Wavelength 1310 nm allowed deeper penetration even through sclera and cross-sectional imaging of the anterior chamber, including visualization of the angle of the anterior chamber. All of these systems require

image-processing technique to remove artifacts caused by patient motion during data acquisition. A system capable of faster data acquisition would not be affected by involuntary eye movement and would allow real time display.

PRINCIPLE OF OPTICAL COHERENCE TOMOGRAPHY

In a typical optical coherence tomography system **(Figure 2)**, light from a broadband, near-infrared source and a visible aiming beam is combined and coupled into one branch of a fiber-optic Michelson interferometer. Broadband sources include super luminescent diodes, fiber amplifiers, and femtosecond pulse lasers in the wavelength range of 800-1550 nanometers. The light is split into two fibers using a 2 × 2 coupler, one leading to a reference mirror and the second focused into the

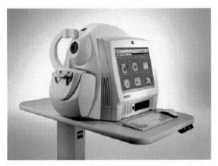

Fig. 1 Anterior segment OCT system (The Visante ASOCT) (Carl Zeiss Meditec, Inc, Dublin, CA, USA)

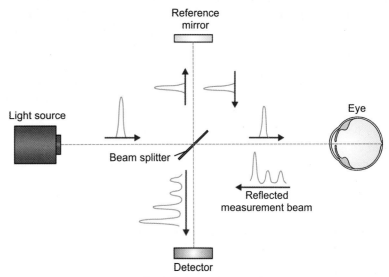

Fig. 2 Principle of OCT

tissue. Light reflects off the reference mirror and is recoupled into the fiber leading to the mirror. Concurrently, light is reflected from index of refraction mismatches in the tissue and recoupled into the fiber leading to the tissue. Reflections result from changes in the index of refraction within the structure of the tissue, for instance between intercellular fluid and collagen fibers. Light that has been back-reflected from the tissue and light from the reference arm recombine within the 2×2 coupler.

Because the broadband source has a short coherence length, only light which has traveled very close to the same time (or optical path length) in the reference and tissue arms will interfere constructively and destructively. By changing the length of the reference arm, reflection sites at various depths in the tissue can be sampled. The depth of resolution of the optical coherence tomography system is determined by the effectiveness of this time gating and hence is inversely proportional to the bandwidth of the source. An optical detector in the final arm of the Michelson interferometer detects the interference between the reference and tissue signals. During optical coherence tomography imaging, the reference-arm mirror is scanned at a constant velocity, allowing depth scans (analogous to ultrasound A-scans) to be made. Either the tissue or the

interferometer optics is mounted on a stage so that the beam can be scanned laterally across the tissue to build up two- and three-dimensional images, pixel by pixel. Majority of the studies published on anterior segment OCT (ASOCT) applications used commercially available retinal scanners. The majority of these studies focused on corneal imaging, with regard to AC angle imaging, however these OCT systems were suboptimal for tissue delineation because 0.8 μm light cannot penetrate the sclera, thereby preventing visualization of the underlying angle structures. In contrast, OCT at 1.3 μm wavelength of light is better suited for AC angle imaging due to two significant properties. First, the amount of scattering in tissue is lower at this wavelength. This enables increased penetration through scattering ocular structures such as the sclera and the iris so that more detailed AC angle morphology is visualized. Second, 1.3 μm wavelength is strongly absorbed by water in ocular media and therefore, only 10 percent of the light incident on the cornea reaches the retina. The reason being that absorption and scattering in most tissue constituents decreases with wavelength in the near

infrared spectrum whereas absorption in water (the primary constituent of vitreous humor) increases sharply, being approximately an order of magnitude higher at 1.3 μm than at 0.8 μm. The improved retinal protection allows for the use of high power illumination that, in turn, enables high-speed imaging. The permissible exposure level at 1.3 μm wavelength is 15 mW according to the current standard set by the American Laser Institute and the American National Standard institute (ANSI 2000). This level is 20 times higher than the 0.7 mW limit at the 0.8 μm wavelength. The high-speed imaging eliminates motion artifacts, reduces examination time, allows for rapid survey of relatively large areas and enables imaging of dynamic ocular events.

In brief, this system uses a semiconductor optical amplifier light source capable of emitting 22 mW of low coherence light with a central wavelength of 1.3 μm wavelength and as spectral bandwidth of 68 mm full width at half maximum. The optical power incident on the eye is 4.9 mW that is well within the permissible levels. The scanning speed is 4000 axial scans per image, giving an image acquisition rate of 8 frames per second. The lateral resolution is 8 μm. The scan geometry is telecentric (rectangular) allowing wide field capability, which is essential for corneal and anterior chamber studies.

Slit lamp adaptation of ASOCT has also been described which use a charged couple device (CCD) camera to visualize the scan area in real time. This can be an ideal device for the immediate postoperative evaluation of filtering blebs and the morphologic features of chamber angle region as it allows noncontact measurements. It may improve detection, documentation and follow-up examination of iris and ciliary body pathological conditions and enable monitoring of ciliary body changes during accommodation.

ASOCT IN GLAUCOMA
- Normal anatomy and physiology
- Screening of angle closure
- Plateau iris
- Malignant glaucoma
- Efficacy of LPI
- Patency of GDD.

Normal Anatomy and Physiology
ASOCT can be used to study the normal anatomy and physiology of the iris and anterior chamber angle structures. It can be used to study the condition in light and dark conditions.

Screening of Angle Closure Glaucoma
Primary angle closure glaucoma is highly prevalent in certain regions of the world. Treating anatomically narrow angles with a laser peripheral iridotomy may prevent development of angle closure. Therefore, early detection of anatomically narrow angle is important. Currently, gonioscopy is the gold standard for evaluating the anterior chamber angle; however it is subjective, semi-quantitative and requires specialized training. Cross-sectional imaging of the anterior

chamber can provide quantitative data and may prove to be less subjective than gonioscopy.

Ultrasound biomicroscopy and Schiempflug photography have been used for quantitative angle evaluation. OCT has the added advantage of being noncontact, devoid of artificial opening of angle and easy to perform. ASOCT can be used to assess angle width. The images obtained are processed using computer to correct image distortion arising from 2 sources. First, the fan shaped scanning geometry of the OCT beam and second, the effect of refraction at the cornea air interface. Due to lower scattering loss at 1.3 μm, highly detailed AC angle imaging is possible, and angle structures including the iris root, the angle recess, the anterior ciliary body, the scleral spur, and in some eyes, the canal of Schlemm can be visualized. Scleral spur particularly is highly reflective and can be easily identified on OCT. Objective assessment of the angle characteristics can also be made from the ASOCT images **(Figures 3 and 4)**. In addition to the AOD (Angle opening distance) andthe ARA (Angle recess area), which have been described previously in UBM studies, two new parameters: the TISA (Trabecular-iris space area) and the TICL (Trabecular-iris contact length) are described for defining AC angle anatomy. The TISA differs from the ARA in that it only measures the filtering area in front of the scleral spur whereas the ARA also includes the nonfiltering angle recess. Thus, the ARA may be less sensitive in identifying a narrow angle in eyes with a relatively deep angle recess. Another advantage of the TISA over the ARA is that identification of the scleral spur is more reliable than the angle recess. This is because the scleral spur is highly reflective and appears bright whereas the recess is less reflective and may be less precisely defined in some eyes.

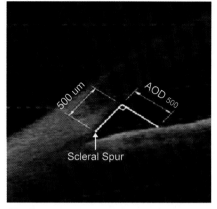

Fig. 3 Angle opening distance at 500 μm (AOD 500)

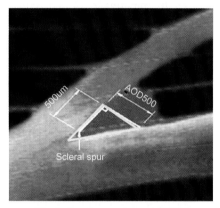

Fig. 4 Angle recess area (ARA)

Other Applications of ASOCT in Glaucoma
Evaluation of the structural causes of angle closure glaucoma such as plateau iris syndrome, malignant glaucoma **(Figure 5)**, and pupillary block glaucoma can be performed. Study of alterations in anatomical configuration of angle structures in response to light and accommodation can be performed. Real time imaging is possible during performance of provocative tests for assessment of angle occludability, such as the dark room and the prone provocative tests.

Other applications of the ASOCT includes its use in the evaluation of the efficacy of various treatments, such as laser peripheral iridotomy **(Figure 6)**, laser iridoplasty or cataract extraction,

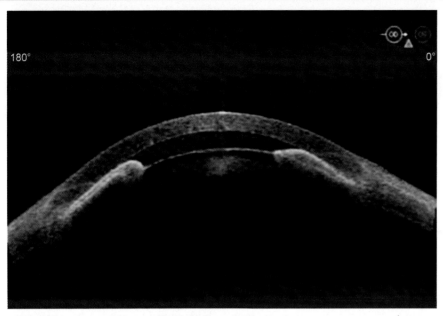

Fig. 5 Malignant glaucoma

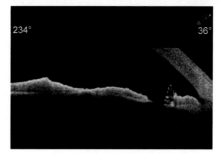

Fig. 6 Evaluation of efficacy of laser peripheral iridectomy

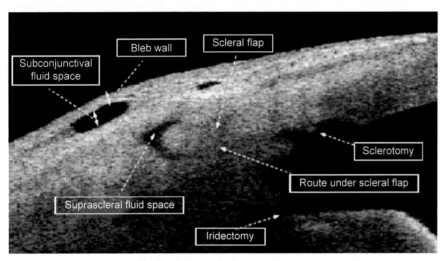

Fig. 7 Bleb morphology on ASOCT

where the angles may be shown objectively to open after such treatment. The patency of iridotomy can be judged well on the ASOCT by viewing the anterior lens capsule behind the full thickness defect created because of PI.

The ASOCT may also be helpful in the assessment of tube patency or position of the glaucoma drainage device in cases of corneal opacity. Noninvasive nature of the OCT allows its safe use in situations where ocular tissue has been lacerated or punctured—in which gonioscopy cannot be performed because of the danger of aqueous leak.

Application in Imaging Trabeculectomy Blebs

Bleb morphology is an important clinical parameter in filtering surgery **(Figure 7)**.

It indicates function of the filtration shunt created by the trabeculectomy procedure and guides in performing interventions such as needling and suture lysis in order to optimize shunt function. ASOCT has been used to image trabeculectomy blebs to provide information about internal structure that is not available at the slit lamp. It is able to provide clear images of the bleb wall, cavity, flap and ostium. Successful blebs display conjunctival thickening as a hallmark of success, regardless of degree of bleb elevation. This reflects facility of transconjunctival aqueous flow.

Highly elevated blebs sometimes display marked conjunctival thickening and only a small cavity. In failed blebs, ASOCT is particularly useful in imaging failed blebs to demonstrate the level of failure. Ostial closure, flap fibrosis and presumed episcleral fibrosis in the absence of the former two situations are all clearly demonstrated. In the early postoperative period, a failing bleb with a closely apposed scleral flap may be resuscitated by suture lysis, resulting in a more expanded bleb. Hence, ASOCT is a useful tool to image trabeculectomy blebs and may aid in postoperative bleb management. It can also image the intrascleral lake and implant used in nonpenetrating glaucoma surgery (deep sclerectomy).

Assessment of Tumors of Iris and Ciliary Body

Accurate localization, measurement of the tumor size, and evaluation of factors such as the depth of penetration and extrascleral extension is a potential application of ASOCT which is still undergoing evaluation.

Others

ASOCT can image upto posterior capsule of lens. Thus it can also show the morphology of lens and its abnormality like developmental cataract, posterior capsular dehiscence in case of posterior polar cataract and subluxated crystalline lenses. It can also be of use in delienating the anterior segment anatomy in cases of opaque corneas, failed grafts, adherent leucomas and help in the surgical planning prior to keratoplasty by preoperatively documenting the potential areas of iris adhesion for which the surgeon should be extra cautious during surgery in order to avoid potential iris trauma during trephination, dissection, etc. It provides information with regard to sites of AC entry during trabeculectomy as well as placement of tube shunts away from the areas of iris adherence.

COMPARISON OF ANTERIOR SEGMENT OPTICAL COHERENCE TOMOGRAPHY VERSUS ULTRASOUND BIOMICROSCOPY

Ultrasound biomicroscopy provides high-resolution images (50 μm lateral resolution in the commercially available system) of the AC angle region, has a depth of penetration of 5 mm in tissue, and is able to image through opaque media. However, it has several limitations. A coupling medium is required such that scanning must be performed through an immersion bath. The procedure is time-consuming and requires a highly skilled operator to obtain high-quality images. There is a risk of infection or corneal abrasion due to the contact nature of the examination. Finally, inadvertent pressure on the eye cup used while scanning

can influence the angle configuration, as demonstrated by Ishikawa et al using a small UBM eyecup. Since the patient is in a supine position, the iris lens diagphragm falls back due to effect of gravity and may lead to artifactual opening up of the angle. ASOCT has several advantages over UBM for the objective assessment of AC angle. It has a higher image resolution than UBM, is totally noncontact, and is easily performed with minimal expertise. The noncontact nature of OCT not only enhances patient comfort and safety but also makes it especially suitable for ocular biometry and AC angle assessment since there is no mechanical distortion of the tissue being imaged. Simultaneous two or four quadrant can be scanned by dual scan and quad scan mode by ASOCT while in UBM only one angle can be imaged at a time.

Advantages of the ASOCT

- It is a noncontact method therefore do not cause indentation of the angle by placement of the scleral cup on the eye (which is required to maintain the water bath in UBM) Also, no possibility of corneal abrasion or punctuate epithelial erosions (possible with UBM).
- It is a more physiological examination as patient is imaged sitting upright. (Lying supine may artificially widen the anterior chamber angle as the iris-lens diaphragm moves posteriorly due to gravity)
- Shorter imaging time. (Patient setup in UBM takes longer. Also, only one angle is imaged at a time with the UBM)
- Rapid image acquisition. Eight frames can be captured per second, allowing operator to choose the best centred image

- Requires less expertise to perform-small learning curve for the operator
- Target may be used to induce accommodation in the eye being imaged.
- More comfortable for the patient, due to noncontact technique, upright position and rapid imaging acquisition
- Less interoperator variability, due to noncontact technique.

Disadvantages of the Anterior Segment Optical Coherence Tomography

At present unable to image structures posterior to the iris as the optical beam cannot penetrate the iris pigment adeqately except in Albinos. Ciliary body imaging cannot be performed unlike the UBM which allows imaging of structures posterior to the iris, in particular, the ciliary body and peripheral retina. In addition, the upper and lower lids come into the field of view and obstruct imaging of the superior and inferior angle, requiring the examiner to manually lift up the eyelids for obtaining a proper view.

SUMMARY

ASOCT using 1.3 μm wavelength is a very helpful tool for non contact anterior segment evaluation. Its measurements correlate well with ultrasound biomicroscopy with various advantages over UBM like noncontact technique, short time, patient friendly, and ability to view dynamic changes. Amongst the limitations of ASOCT are its inability to obtain clear images through opaque media and the iris, obstruction by the eyelids making imaging of the superior and inferior angles difficult and it provides limited visualization of the ciliary body. This imaging modality plays an important role in the fields of refractive surgery, glaucoma and other ophthalmic specialties.

BIBLIOGRAPHY

1. Buchwald HJ, Muller A, Kampmeier J, et al. Optical coherence tomography versus ultrasound biomicroscopy of conjunctival and eyelid lesions. Klin Monatsbl Augenheilkd 2003; 220(12):822-9.

2. Fujimoto JG, Bouma B, Tearney GJ, et al. New technology for high-speed and high-resolution optical coherence tomography. Ann N Y Acad Sci 1998;838:95-107.

3. Fujimoto JG. In: Bouma BE, Tearney GJ, (Eds). Optical coherence tomography: introduction.

4. Handbook of Optical Coherence Tomography. New York, NY: Marcel Dekker Inc; 2002:1-40. of the anterior segment. Graefes Arch Clin Exp Ophthalmol 2000;238(1):8-18.

5. Ishikawa H, Inazumi K, Liebmann JM, Ritch R. Inadvertent corneal indentation can cause artifactitious widening of the iridocorneal angle on ultrasound biomicroscopy. Ophthalmic Surg Lasers 2000;31:342-5.

6. Leung CK, Yick DW, Kwong YY, Li FC, Leung DY, Mohamed S, Tham CC, Chi CC, Lam DS. Analysis of bleb morphology after trabeculectomy with the Visante anterior segment optical coherence tomography. Br J Ophthalmol 2006; 27: [Epub ahead of print].

7. Maberly DA, Pavlin CJ, McGowan HD, et al. Ultrasound biomicroscopic imaging of the anterior aspect of peripheral choroidal melanomas. Am J Ophthalmol 1997;123(4):506-14.

8. Memarzadeh F, Li Y, Francis BA, Smith RE, Gutmark J, Huang D. Optical coherence tomography of the anterior segment in secondary glaucoma with corneal opacity after penetrating keratoplasty. Br J Ophthalmol 2006; [Epub ahead of print].

9. Pavlin CJ, Harasiewicz K, Foster FS. Ultrasound biomicroscopy of anterior segment structures in normal and glaucomatous eyes. Am J Ophthalmol 1992;113:381-9.

10. Pavlin CJ, Sherar MD, Foster FS. Subsurface ultrasound microscopic imaging of the intact eye. Ophthalmology 1990;97:244-5.

11. Radhakrishnan S, Goldsmith J, Huang D, et al. Comparison of optical coherence tomography and ultrasound biomicroscopy for detection of narrow anterior chamber angles. Arch Ophthalmol 2005;123: 1053-9.

12. Radhakrishnan S, Rollins AM, Roth JE, et al. Real-time optical coherence tomography of the anterior segment at 1310 nm. Arch Ophthalmol 2001; 119(8):1179-85.

13. Van den Berg TJ, Spekreijse H. Near infrared light absorption in the human eye media. Vision Res 1997;37(2): 249-53.

14. Wirbelauer C, Karandish A, Haberle H, Pham DT. Noncontact goniometry with optical coherence tomography. Arch Ophthalmol 2005;123: 179-85.

SCANNING LASER POLARIMETRY

The GDx nerve fiber layer analyser is a scanning laser polarimeter.

PRINCIPLE

Infrared Laser light enters the eye at specific orientation. As it goes through the microtubules within the axons it returns at different orientation or axes. The retinal nerve fibre layer (RNFL) is made up of highly ordered parallel axon bundles. The axons contain microtubules, cylindrical intracellular organelles with diameters smaller than the wavelength of light. The highly ordered structure of the microtubules is the source of RNFL birefringence. Birefringence is the splitting of light by a polar material into two components (extraordinary-ray and ordinary-ray) **(Figure 1)**. These components travel at different velocities which creates a relative phase shift. The phase shift is termed retardation. The amount of phase shift or retardation is proportional to the thickness of the RNFL.

The GDx is a confocal scanning laser ophthalmoscope with an integrated ellipsometer to measure retardation. Retinal scanning laser polarimetry (SLP) determines the RNFL thickness, point by point in the peripapillary region by measuring the total retardation in the light reflected from the retina. Polarized light passes through the eye and is reflected off the retina. Because the RNFL is birefringent the two components of the polarized light are phase shifted relative to each other, that is they are retarded. The amount of the retardation is captured by a detector and converted into thickness in microns **(Figure 2)**.

BIREFRINGENCE OF THE OTHER OCULAR STRUCTURES—ANTERIOR SEGMENT BIREFRINGENCE

In addition to the RNFL, the anterior segment (the cornea and the lens) are also birefringent. The total retardation of a subjects eye is the sum of the cornea, lens and RNFL birefringence. Compensation of anterior segment birefringence is necessary to isolate RNFL birefringence. The parameters characterizing anterior segment birefringence are the axis of birefringence and magnitude of retardation. Once these values are known, the anterior segment birefringence can be accurately compensated.

Early scanning laser polarimeters compensated for anterior segment birefringence based on fixed values for the axis and magnitude of the anterior segment birefringence.

VARIABLE CORNEAL COMPENSATION

The GDx variable corneal compensation (VCC) measures and individually compensates for the anterior segment birefringence for each eye **(Figures 3 to 5)**. In order to individually compensate for the anterior segment birefringence, the specific axis and magnitude of the anterior segment birefringence must be known. This is determined by first imaging the eye without compensation. The uncompensated image presents total retardation from the eye and included retardation from the cornea, lens and RNFL. The macular region of the image is then analyzed to determine the axis and magnitude of the anterior segment birefringence. The macular region birefringence is uniform and symmetric due to the radial distribution of Henle's fiber layer. However in uncompensated scans a non uniform retardation pattern is present in the macula due to the birefringence in the anterior segment. The axis and magnitude values from the anterior segment can be computed by analyzing the non-uniform retardation profile around the macula. The axis of

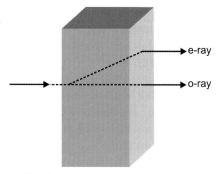

Fig. 1 Birefringence (diagrammatic)

the anterior segment birefringence is determined by the orientation of the "bow-tie" birefringent pattern in the macula and the magnitude of the anterior segment birefringence is calculated by analyzing the circular profile of the birefringence in the macula according to standard equations.

ENHANCED CORNEAL COMPENSATION

CC measurements, however, sometimes exhibit an atypical retardation pattern (ARP), which makes interpretation of the results difficult or impossible. ARP, caused by poor signal to noise ratio, is characterized by irregular patches of elevated retardation values which do not match the expected retardation distribution based on the retinal nerve fibre layer. It is not infrequent among myopic eyes and occurs also in a proportion of emmetropic eyes. A new software based compensation method, called enhanced corneal compensation algorithm (ECC), has been developed to improve signal to noise ratio. A known large birefringence bias is introduced into the measurement beam path to shift the measurement of total retardation into a higher value region. The birefringence bias is determined from the macular region of each measurement and then, point by point, removed mathematically to yield the

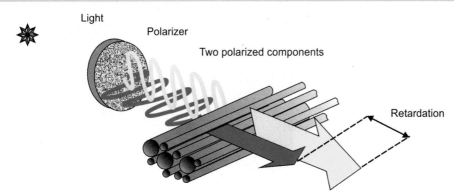

Fig. 2 The amount of retardation from the RNFL is directly proportional to the RNFL thickness

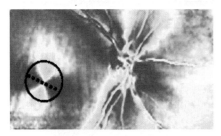

Fig. 3 Bow Tie method

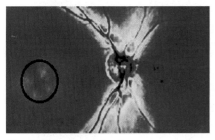

Fig. 4 Alternate method:
- Performed in individuals with macular pathology
- Analyze the refringence pattern over a square area centered on fovea (6° × 6°)
- By averaging the signal from a large area

true RNFL retardation. Thus ECC leads to improvement of TSS.

CLINICAL INTERPRETATION OF THE GDx VARIABLE CORNEAL COMPENSATION PRINTOUT

An age matched comparison is made for each GDx variable corneal compensation scan with the normative database and any significant deviations from the normal limits are flagged as abnormal with a "p" value.

Quantitaive RNFL evaluation is provided through four key elements of the printout:

- Thickness map
- Deviation map
- TSNIT graph
- Parameters.

Thickness Map

It shows the RNFL thickness in a color coded format. RNFL thickness is represented using a color scale that follows the color spectrum going from blue to red. Thick RNFL values are colored yellow, orange and red while thin RNFL values are colored dark blue, light blue and green (**Figure 6**).

Deviation Map

This reveals the location and magnitude of RNFL defects over the entire thickness map. The deviation map analyzes a 128 × 128 pixel region (20° × 20°) centered on the optic disc (**Figures 7A and B**). To reduce the variability due to slight anatomical variations between individuals the 128 × 128 pixel map is averaged into a 32 × 32 square grid where each square is the average of a 4 × 4 pixel region (called super pixels). For each scan the RNFL thickness at each super pixel is compared to the age

matched normative database and the super pixels that fall below the normal range are flagged by colored squares based on the probability of normality. Dark blue squares represent areas where the RNFL thickness is below the 5th percentile of the normative database. This means that there is only a 5 percent probability that the RNFL thickness in this area is within the normal range determined by an age matched comparison to the normative database. Light blue squares represent deviations below the 2 percent level, yellow represents deviations below the 1 percent level and red represents deviations below 0.5 percent. The deviation map uses a grayscale fundus image of the eye as a background and displays abnormal grid values as colored squares over this image.

TSNIT Map

TSNIT stands for Temporal-Superior-Nasal-Inferior-Temporal and displays the RNFL thickness values along the calculation circle starting temporally and moving superiorly, nasally, inferiorly and ending temporally. In a normal eye the TSNIT plot follows the typical double hump pattern with thick RNFL measures superiorly and inferiorly and thin RNFL values nasally and temporally. The TSNIT graph shows the curve of the actual values for that eye along with a shaded area which represents 95 percent normal range for that age. In a healthy eye the TSNIT curve will fall within the shaded area specially in the superior and inferior regions in the center of the printout at the bottom the TSNIT graph for both the eyes are displayed together. In a healthy eye there is good symmetry between the TSNIT graphs of the two eyes and the two curves will overlap. However, in glaucoma, one eye often has more advanced RNFL loss and therefore the two curves will have less overlap.

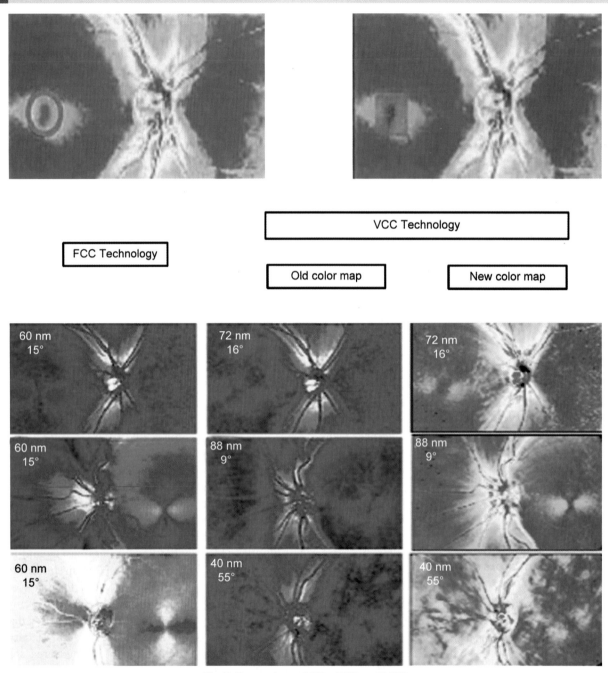

Fig. 5 Comparison of GDx, FCC and VCC

A dip in the curve of one eye relative to another is indicative of RNFL loss.

Parameters

The parameters are displayed in a table in the center of the printout. The TSNIT parameters are summary measures based on RNFL thickness values within the calculation circle **(Figure 9)**. These parameters are automatically compared to the normative database and quantified in terms of probability of normality **(Figures 10 and 11)**. Normal parameter values are displayed in green, abnormal values are color coded based on their probability of normality. The probability levels used are the same as the deviation map.

Calculation Circle

The calculation circle is a fixed circle (a fixed size band) centered on the optic nerve head. The band is 0.4 mm wide and has an outer diameter of

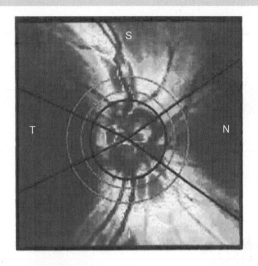

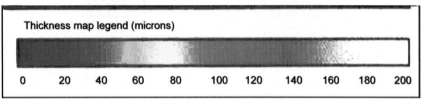

Fig. 6 Thickness map:
- Thick RNFL ◊ Yellow, orange, red
- Thin RNFL ◊ Dark blue, light blue, green
- Blue ◊ Red 120 μ
- Pink and white > 120 μ (uncompensated scan)

3.2 mm and an inner diameter of 2.4 mm **(Figure 9)**.

The TSNIT parameters
- TSNIT average
- Superior average
- Inferior average
- TSNIT standard deviation
- Intereye symmetry
- Nerve fiber indicator.

TSNIT Average
The average RNFL thicness around the entire circle.

Superior Average
The average RNFL thickness in the superior 120° region of the calculation circle.

Inferior Average
The average RNFL Thickness in the inferior 120° region of the calculation circle.

TSNIT Standard Deviation
This measure captures the modulation that is the pea to trough difference of the double hump pattern. A normal eye will have have high modulation in the double hump RNFL pattern while a glaucomatous eye will typically have low modulation in the double hump pattern.

Intereye Symmetry
It measures the degree of symmetry between the right and left eyes by correlating the TSNIT functions from the two eyes **(Figure 8)**. Values range from –1 to +1 where values near 1 represent good symmetry. Normal eyes have good symmetry with values around 0.9.

Nerve Fiber Indicator
The nerve fiber indicator (NFI) is a global measure based on the entire RNFL thickness map. It is calculated using an advanced form of neural network called a support vector machine (SVM). It utilizes information from the entire RNFL thickness map to optimize the discrimination between healthy and glaucomatous eyes. The output of the NFI is a single value that ranges from 1 to 100 with classification based on the ranges:

1-30 → Normal
31-50 → Borderline
51 + → Abnormal.

The TSNIT average, Superior average, Inferior average, TSNIT standard deviation, Intereye symmetry and NFI are abnormal at p < 1 percent level.

They are considered borderline if these are at p < 5 percent level.

The normal values of the TSNIT parameters in the Indian population as per R.P Center database (40–70 yrs) are:

Normal

Glaucoma

Deviation Map

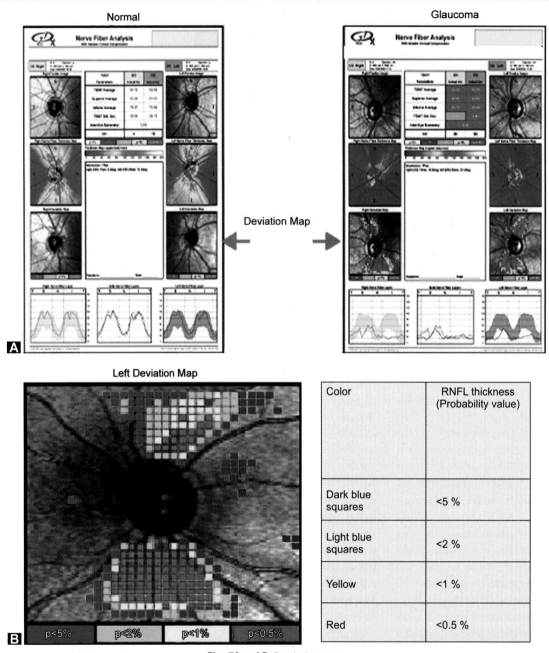

Left Deviation Map

Color	RNFL thickness (Probability value)
Dark blue squares	<5 %
Light blue squares	<2 %
Yellow	<1 %
Red	<0.5 %

| p<5% | p<2% | p<1% | p<0.5% |

Figs 7A and B Deviation map

TSNIT average =
 54.8 ± 4.1 (45.6 – 66.8) microns
Superior average =
 66.8 ± 6.7 (55.1 – 85) microns
Inferior average = 62.1 ± 6.6 (38.9 – 74.3)
NFI = 17.2 ± 6.9 (4 – 35)

The RNFL values are underestimated with the GDx VCC as compared to the OCT and these are values inferred from the retinal birefringence and thus are not absolute values of RNFL thickness.

SERIAL ANALYSIS

The serial analysis printout has 5 elements that should be considered when assessing RNFL change over time:
- Thickness maps
- Deviation maps
- Deviation from reference maps
- Parameters
- TSNIT graphs.

Serial analysis can compare upto 4 exams. The first exam is the baseline or reference exam and all follow-up exams are compared to this baseline exam. A colored rectangle to the left of the thickness map contains the data and quality

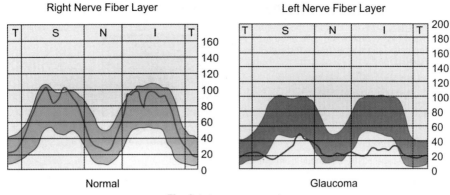

Right Nerve Fiber Layer

Left Nerve Fiber Layer

Normal

Glaucoma

Fig. 8 Intereye symmetry

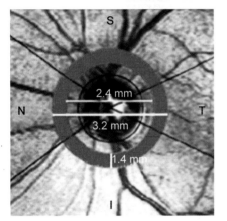

Fig. 9 The calculation circle

score of each exam. The same color is used in the TSNIT graph to indicate which TSNIT curve corresponds to which exam.

The deviation from reference map displays the RNFL difference pixel by pixel of the follow-up exam compared to the baseline exam. If the difference exceeds 20 microns at any pixel the pixel is color coded according to the legend. RNFL change is color coded in 20 micron increments where the first 20 micron change is color coded green, a 40 micron change is color coded light blue and 60 microns is dark blue. The areas of RNFL change shown on the deviation from reference map will frequently correspond to the areas of loss detected by the deviation map. However the correspondence is not always exact because the deviation map shows loss compared to the normative database while the

deviation from reference maps shows RNFL change over time in the same eye.

Adavantages of GDx Variable Corneal Compensation

- Easy to operate
- Does not require pupillary dilatation
- Good reproducibility
- Does not require a reference plane
- Can detect glaucoma at the first exam
- Early detection before standard visual field
- Comparison with age matched normative data.

Limitations

- Does not measure the actual RNFL thickness—Inferred value
- Measures RNFL at different locations for each patient
- Does not differentiate true biological change from variability
- Limited use in moderate/advanced glaucoma.
- Requires a wider database from the Indian population
- 4th Machine prototype—cannot update earlier versions
- Affected by anterior and posterior segment pathology lie:
  ❖ Ocular surface disorder
  ❖ Macular pathology
  ❖ Cataract and refractive surgery
  ❖ Refractive errors—false positive in myopes

❖ Peripapillary atrophy—scleral birefringence interferes with RNFL measurement.

CONCLUSION

GDx VCC is still a relatively new diagnostic tool for RNFL assessment in glaucoma which enables the clinician to pic up preperimetric glaucoma. It provides an objective and quantitative information of the RNFL that is highly reproducible and can discriminate normal from glaucoma with a high degree of accuracy. Clinical interpretation of the results is simple and direct and the procedure is easy to perform without a need for pupillary dilatation. This quantitative RNFL assessment helps in the diagnosis and management of glaucoma and should be used in conjunction with other diagnostic information when making clinical decisions. Treatmnt should not be started based on the GDx VCC parameters alone and the data from other anatomical and functional investigations should be taken into account. An abnormality on the GDx VCC rings an alarm bell and such patients require a closer follow-up to detect progression and confirmation of glaucomatous damage. Nonglaucomatous causes of optic neuropathy must be ruled out by a thorough clinical examination and appropriate investigation. As the technology is relatively new a number of long term studies are required to establish the sensitivity and specificity of GDx VCC in the diagnosis of glaucoma.

TSNIT Parameters

TSNIT Parameters are calculated from within the calculation circle (red band within gray circles)

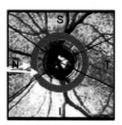

TSNIT Average

- Average RNFL thickness from the entire Calculation Circle (area shown in red)

Superior Average

- Average RNFL thickness in the superior 120° of the Calculation Circle (area in red)

Inferior Average

- Average RNFL thickness in the inferior 120° of the Calculation Circle (area in red)

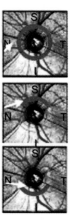

TSNIT Parameters

Inter-Eye Symmetry

- Values near 1 represent good symmetry
- Values near 0 represent poor symmetry

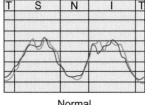

Both Nerve Fiber Layers

Normal
Good Symmetry

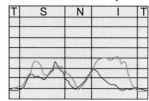

Both Nerve Fiber Layers

Glaucoma
Poor Symmetry

Nerve Fiber Indicator (NFI)

- Based on both focal and diffuse Retinal Nerve Fiber Layer loss

- Utilizes a neural network, trained to discriminate normal from glaucoma

- Is the most sensitive parameter for discriminating normal from glaucoma

- Classification

Normal		Borderline		Abnormal	
1	30	31	50	51	100

TSNIT Parameters	OD Actual Val.	OS Actual Val.
TSNIT Average	48.08	33.27
Superior Average	54.39	46.23
Inferior Average	52.33	28.08
TSNIT Std. Dev.	22.36	14.03
Inter-Eye Symmetry	0.50	
NFI	25	63

p<5%	p>5%	p<2%	p<1%	p<0.5%

Fig. 10 TSNIT parameters

TSNIT Parameters	OD Actual Val.	OS Actual Val.
TSNIT Average	48.08	33.27
Superior Average	54.39	46.23
Inferior Average	62.33	28.06
TSNIT Std. Dev.	22.36	14.83
Inter-Eye Symmetry	0.50	
NFI	25	63

| p>5% | p<5% | p<2% | p<1% | p<0.5% |

Parameters :

• Summary measures based on the calculation circle.

• Values outside normal are color-coded based on probability of normality

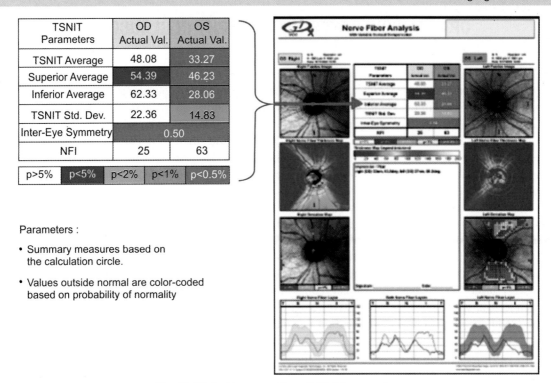

Fig. 11 Clinical interpretation of TSNIT parameters

BIBLIOGRAPHY

1. Dreher AW, Reiter K. Retinal laser ellipsometry: a new method for measuring the retinal nerve fiber thickness distribution. Clinical Vision Sci 1992;7:481-8.

2. Henderson PA, Medeiros FA, et al. Relationship between central corneal thickness and retinal nerve fiber layer thickness in ocular hypertensive patients. Ophthalmology 2005;112(2):251-6.

3. Jonas JB, Hayreh SS. Localized retinal nerve fibre layer defects in chronic experimental high pressure glaucoma in rhesus monkeys. Br J Ophthalmology 1999;83:1291-5.

4. Morgan JE, Waldock A, Jeffery G, Cowey A. Retinal nerve fiber layer polarimetry; Histological and clinical comparison. Br J Ophthalmology 1998;82:684-90.

5. Quigley HA, Atz J, Deric RJ, Gilbert D, Sommer A. An evaluation of optic disc and nerve fiber examination in monitoring progression of early glaucoma damage. Ophthalmology 1992;99:19-28.

6. Reus NJ, Lemij HG. Diagnostic accuracy of the Gdx VCC for glaucoma. Ophthalmology 2004;111(10):1860-5.

7. Shiraashi M, Yaoeda, Fuushima A, Funai S, Funai H, Ofuchi N. Usefulness of GDx VCC in glaucoma detection Eye 2003;20:1019-21.

8. Weinreb RN, Bowd C, Zangwill LM. Glaucoma detection using scanning laser polarimetry with variable corneal compensation; Arch Ophthalmol 2003;121:218-24.

OPTICAL COHERENCE TOMOGRAPHY IN GLAUCOMA

Optical coherence tomography (OCT) is a non-contact noninvasive technology providing high resolution, cross-sectional images of the eye. It is reproducible and correlates with the histological appearance. Its use for glaucoma diagnosis and *in vivo* capabilities of retinal nerve fiber layer (RNFL) and optic nerve head (ONH) analysis has added to the armatarium to help in accurate diagnosis and detecting progression.

Assessment of the optic nerve and retinal nerve fiber layer (RNFL) has been largely subjective. While photographs of the RNFL provide objective information for comparisons, the interpretation of photographs remains subjective, and variation in photographic assessment even among experienced observers is well documented. Furthermore, qualitative assessment of photographs may not be sensitive to small changes over time. It is also difficult to detect diffuse RNFL loss in these photographs.

OCT has an important role in the diagnosis and management of glaucoma.

BASIC PRINCIPLES OF OPTICAL COHERENCE TOMOGRAPHY

Optical coherence tomography is based on the principle of Michelson interferometry. Low-coherence infrared (830 nm) light coupled to a fibroptic travels to a 50/50 beam splitter and is directed through the ocular media to the retina and to a reference mirror, respectively. Light passing through the eye is reflected by structures in different retinal tissue layers. The distance between the beam splitter and reference mirror is continuously varied. When the distance between the light source and retinal tissue is equal to the distance between the light source

and reference mirror, the reflected light from the retinal tissue and reference mirror interacts to produce an interference pattern. The interference pattern is detected and then processed into a signal. The signal is analogous to that obtained by A-scan ultrasonography using light as a source rather than sound. A two-dimensional image is built as the light source is moved across the retina. The image is a series of stacked and aligned A scans to produce a two dimensional cross-sectional retinal image that resembles that of a histological section. This imaging method thus can be considered a form of *in vivo* histology. An infrared-sensitive charge-coupled device video camera documents the position of the scanning beam on the retina. The OCT image can be displayed on a gray or a color scale. Highly reflective structures are shown with bright colors (red and yellow), while those with low reflectivity are represented by darker colors (black and blue). Those with intermediate reflectivity appear green. The Stratus OCT (OCT 3) has a theoretical axial resolution <10 mm.

Optical coherence tomography provides high resolution measurements and cross-sectional imaging of the retina, optic disc and the RNFL. For glaucoma applications, an operator-determined circular or linear path is scanned around the optic disc to generate a series of 100 axial reflectance profiles. From these, a real-time two-dimensional tomographic image is constructed. The first reflection measurement is the vitreous-internal limiting membrane interface. The highly reflective interface posterior to this is the retinal pigment epithelium photoreceptor interface. A threshold of reflectivity between the two is set as the posterior boundary of the RNFL. Retinal nerve fiber layer and retinal thickness

are calculated from these landmarks. Average measurements are given for 12, 30-degree sectors. The depth values of the scans are independent of the optical dimensions of the eye, and no reference plane is required. Useful measurements in glaucoma patients are normally made along a circle concentric with the optic disc.

Clinical Uses

- To evaluate the RNFL for early (preperimetric) glaucoma detection.
- To evaluate optic nerve head tomography in glaucoma patients.
- To detect, study and follow the macular changes in hypotony induced maculopathy after glaucoma surgery.
- To evaluate cystoid macular edema after combined cataract and glaucoma surgery and Use of antiglaucoma medications.

Interpretation of RNFL Thickness Average Analysis

The Stratus OCT 3 offers a variety of RNFL thickness measurement and analysis protocols.

- ***RNFL thickness protocol (3.4 mm):*** Acquires a scan with radius 1.73 mm, centered on the optic disc.
- ***Fast RNFL thickness protocol (3.4 mm):*** Acquires three fast circular 3.4 mm diameter circular scans in rapid succession. Thickness values from these three scans are averaged to generate the RNFL thickness profile. This data is compared with the normative data as well as the other eye (intereye symmetry). This is a time efficient scan alignment and placement is required only once.
- ***Proportional circle:*** This protocol allows measurement of RNFL thickness around the optic disc

along a circular scan, the size of which can be tailored as per individual's need taking into account the size of optic nerve head.

- **Concentric 3 rings:** This protocol enables us to measure RNFL thickness along three equally placed default circular scans of 0.9 mm, 1.81 mm and 2.71 mm radii. However, the scan radius can be altered according to the need.
- **RNFL thickness (2.27X disc):** This circular RNFL thickness scan size is 2.27 times the radius of the optic nerve head. This may help us to measure RNFL thickness with **accuracy is various disc sizes.**
- **RNFL map:** This protocol comprises of six circular scans of 1.44 mm, 1.69 mm, 1.90 mm, 2.25 mm, 2.73 mm, and 3.40 mm radii. This gives an overlay view of the RNFL thickness, around the peripapillary area. Retinal nerve fibre layer measurement with a circular scan of 1.34 mm radius, centered on the optic nerve head has been shown to have a maximum reproducibility. Mean RNFL thickness is calculated using the inbuilt RNFL thickness average analysis protocol.

For understanding purpose the RNFL thickness average analysis printout can be divided into various zones that include:

- *Zone 1:* It is important to check that the patient data has been entered accurately especially the date of birth.
- *Zone 2:* Individual TSNIT curves for each eye presented in comparison with the age matched normative database. The overall RNFL thickness follows a double hump pattern. The green area represents the 5th to 95th percentile of the normal population and profiles of RNFL falling in this area are 'within normal limits'. Yellow represents borderline (1-5th percentile) and red represents 'outside normal limits' (less than 1 percentile). The white indicates more than 95th percentile thickness or 'above normal limits'.
- *Zone 3:* This zone shows the Intereye symmetry. RNFL profiles of both the eyes are overlapped and compared.
- *Zone 4:* This shows a diagram showing quadrant wise and clock hour wise distribution of average RNFL thickness in both eyes.
- *Zone 5 (Data table):* This table shows various ratios, quadrant averages, and difference among quadrants and between the two eyes. Each value is marked in color to show its level of deviation from the normal values.
- *Zone 6:* Red free photograph; photographs of two eyes taken with the infrared camera are present on the printout. These denote the position of scan circle on the fundus with respect to the optic disc center. It is important to check for centration as decentration of the calculation circle can lead to artefacts. The RNFL is thicker closer the optic nerve and thinner areas farther away.
- *Zone 7:* Percentile distribution color coding; A small box denoting the color coding of percentile distribution of normative database is provided.

RNFL Parameters

- **Average thickness:** The average RNFL thickness along the entire circular scan.

S_{avg} **and** I_{avg} **(superior average and inferior average):** The Average RNFL thickness in the respective 90 degrees circular scan.

S_{max} **and** I_{max} **(superior maximum and inferior maximum):** Maximum RNFL thickness recorded in the respective 90° quadrant of the scan.

Max-min: Difference between the maximum and minimum RNFL value along the circular scan. The four ratios provided in the data table are self explanatory. OCT3 also enables us to perform a RNFL thickness serial analysis can serially compare up to 4 scan groups and provide an overview of RNFL thickness change overtime. Interpretation of optic disc scan and optic nerve head analysis.

Stratus OCT3 allows a detailed quantitative evaluation of the optic nerve head. It is provided with two scan protocols

- **Optical disc scan:** It consists of equally placed line scans 4 mm in length, at 30° intervals, centered on the optic disc. The number of lines can be adjusted between 6 and 24 lines.
- **Fast optical disc scan:** It compresses six optical disc scan into one scan and acquire scan in short time of 1.92 seconds. The optic nerve head (ONH) analysis and various ONH parameters are calculated using the inbuilt ONH analysis protocol. This analysis detects the anterior surface of the retinal nerve fibre layer (RNFL) and the retinal pigment epithelium (RPE). The cup is determined by automatic detection of the reference points. The inbuilt algorithm detects and measures all the features of disc anatomy based on anatomical landmarks, (disc reference points), on each side of the disc where the RPE ends. It locates and measures the disc diameter by tracing a straight line between the disc reference points. The cup

diameter is measured on a line parallel to the disc line and offset anteriorly by 150 microns and various optic nerve head parameters are automatically calculated. These parameters include optic disc tomography included average disc area, cup area, rim area (disc area minus the cup area), vertical integrated rim area (VIRA), horizontal integrated rim width (HIRD), cup volume, average cupdisc ratio and horizontal and vertical cup-disc ratios.

Vertical integrated rim area (Volume): This estimates the total volume of RFNL tissue in the rim.

Horizontal integrated rim width (Area): This estimates the total rim area. Rest of the measurements are self-explanatory. The ONH analysis print out can be divided into various zones that include:

- ***Zone 1:*** Patient ID data.
- ***Zone 2:*** Gives the overview of ONH head analysis along with the composite image figure, contructed from all scans and all the important ONH parameters.
- ***Zone 3:*** Individual radial analysis, along with scan image it gives the disc diameter, cup diameter, rim area, and rim length in that partic-

ular meridian. Overlap of TSNIT curve showing a comparison of two eyes.

- ***Zone 4:*** Red free photograph of the optic disc taken with the infrared camera is also available on the printout.

Advantages

- Optical coherence tomography provides objective, quantitative, reproducible measurements of the retina and RNFL thickness.
- Direct measurements of the RNFL are calculated from cross-sectional retinal images.
- Measurements are not affected by refractive status, axial length of the eye, or the presence of early to moderate nuclear sclerotic cataracts.
- No reference plane needs to be determined
- It gives information about the macula, optic disc and retinal nerve fiber layer.

Disadvantages

The presence, of posterior subcapsular and cortical cataracts impairs performance, and pupillary dilation is required to obtain acceptable peripapillary measurements.

Comparison with HRT, GDx and RTA

Other technologies are available for optic nerve head imaging and nerve fibre layer analysis. The past decade has seen the emergence and refinement of Confocal scanning laser ophthalmoscopy (HRT), Scanning laser polarimetry (GDx) and the Retinal thickness analyzer (RTA).

The major limitation of HRT is that the use of a reference plane is required. For this manual tracing of the optic nerve head margin has to be done by a trained technician or ophthalmologist. As compared to HRT II, OCT does not require a trained technician to mark the points for disc margin. The measurements may be affected by blood vessels. The HRT is useful for scanning the optic nerve head and its use for determining RNFL thickness is limited by axial resolution of the CSLO device.

The SLP device, GDx suffers from high variability in readings due to normal anatomical variations in different eyes as well as presence of pathological changes in different individuals. Some of these sources of error, which adversely affect reliability, include ethnicity and age variations, prior corneal surgeries lie LASIK, corneal transplantation, vitreous opacities, motion artifacts and macular structural pathologies.

BIBLIOGRAPHY

1. Bowd C. Zangwill LM, Berry CC, et al. Detecting early glaucoma by assessment of retinal nerve fiber layer thickness and visual function. Invest Ophthalmol Vis Sci 2001;42:1993-2003.
2. Daniel M Stein, Imaging in Glaucoma, Ophthalmology Clinics of North America, Imaging, Joel S. Schuman, Elsevier Saunders 2004;17:41-6.
3. Irene Voo, Clinical applications of OCT, Ophthalmology Clinics of North America, Imaging, Joel S. Schuman, Elsevier Saunders 2004;17:21-31.
4. Jones AL, Sheen NJ, North RV, Morgan JE. The Humphrey optical coherence tomography scanner: quantitative analysis and reproducibility study of the normal human retinal nerve fiber layer. Br J Ophthalmol 2001;85(6):673-7.
5. Quigley HA, Addicks EM, Green WR. Optic nerve damage in human glaucoma. III. Quantitative correlation of nerve fiber loss and visual field defects in glaucoma, ischemic optic neuropathy, papilledema, and toxic optic neuropathy. Arch Ophthalmol 1982;100:135-46.
6. Tewari HK, Wagh VB, Sony P, Venkatesh P, Singh R. Macular thickness evaluation using the optical coherence tomography in normal Indian eyes. Indian J Ophthalmol. 2004;52(3):199-204.
7. Varma R, Steinmann WC, Scott IU. Expert agreement in evaluating the optic disc for glaucoma. Ophthalmology 1992;99:215-21.

PART 3

Glaucoma—Clinical

22 | Classification of Glaucoma

Sandeep Bachu, R Ramakrishnan

There are several systems to classify glaucoma. These include anatomic, gonioscopic, biochemical, epidemiological, genetic and molecular systems of classifications. These systems are arbitrary and none represents an accurate nature of the pathophysiology of glaucoma. Each one has its own advantage and disadvantage and use in a specific situation. As the knowledge of the pathophysiology of glaucoma expands reclassification and redistribution. The various systems commonly used to classify glaucoma are discussed in this chapter. These include:

- Primary and Secondary
- Classification based on etiology or initial event
- Classification based on mechanism of outflow obstruction
- Other mechanisms based on
  - Age
  - Tissue involved
  - Epidemiological classification

We will discuss some of these systems in detail.

PRIMARY AND SECONDARY

Traditionally glaucoma has been classified as primary or secondary. However, with the growing knowledge of pathophysiology this classification is becoming arbitrary.

CLASSIFICATION BASED ON ETIOLOGY OR THE INITIAL EVENT

This classification is based on the initial mechanisms that lead through a staged pathway to change in aqueous humor dynamics and optic nerve damage. This provides an understanding of the pathophysiology and a chance for intervention in the early stage of the disease. The limitation of this classification is that the current knowledge of the disease pathophysiology is still incomplete. Moreover the present treatment is still directed towards lowering the intraocular pressure (IOP).

CLASSIFICATION BASED ON MECHANISM OF OUTFLOW OBSTRUCTION

This is based on the alteration in the angle of the anterior chamber which leads to a change in aqueous humor dynamics and glaucoma. IOP is the only modifiable risk factor in glaucoma. Thus insights into the mechanisms can prove valuable in planning the treatment. Hence, this classification has distinct advantages. Moreover our understanding of the mechanism is more complete than the initial events. The limitations of this system are its focus on IOP. Glaucoma is a disorder involving retinal ganglion cell death and this system is based on IOP which though important is still a risk factor. The non-pressure dependant mechanisms are not included. Moreover multiple mechanisms may coexist.

To simplify, it can be divided into three major systems[1]:
1. Angle closure glaucoma
2. Open angle glaucoma
3. Developmental glaucoma

This is illustrated in **Flow chart 1**.

A similar classification system divides glaucoma into conditions that affect the internal flow, and conditions that affect the outflow of aqueous humor. Internal flow block is caused by such conditions as pupillary block or malignant glaucoma. Outflow block occurs with diseases of the trabecular meshwork (e.g. neovascularization) or that compromise Schlemm's canal, collector channels, and the venous system (e.g. elevated episcleral venous pressure).

Flow chart 1 Classification of glaucoma

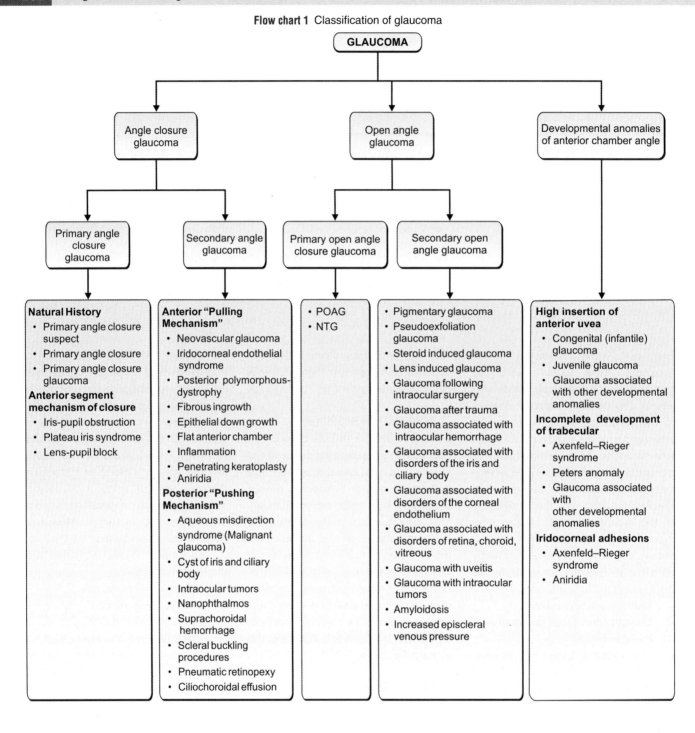

Alternative Classification Systems

Alternative classification systems[2] are based on other features of the disease, including:

1. The site of the outflow obstruction **(Table 1)**, which is divided into diseases that affect the pretrabecular passage of aqueous humor (e.g. posterior synechiae to the lens after ocular inflammation), the trabecular flow (e.g. glaucoma after administration of α-chymotrypsin) and the post-trabecular movement of aqueous humor (e.g. increased episcleral venous pressure from a carotid-cavernous sinus fistula).

2. The tissue principally involved (e.g. glaucoma caused by diseases of the lens or disease of the retina.

3. The proximal initial events (e.g. steroid glaucoma).

4. The age of the patient (e.g. congenital juvenile).

5. POAG has also been subclassified on the basis of:
   - ❖ Optic disc appearance[3]
   - ❖ Extent of visual field defect[4]

CLASSIFICATION OF ANGLE CLOSURE GLAUCOMA[5] (TABLE 2)

Primary Angle Closure Disease

Iridotrabecular contact is the final common pathway of angle closure disease, obstructing aqueous outflow. It can be conceptualized in two ways.

Natural History

a. Primary angle closure suspect.
b. Primary angle closure.
c. Primary angle closure glaucoma.

Anterior Segment Mechanism of Closure

a. Iris-pupil obstruction (e.g. Pupillary block).
b. Ciliary body anomalies (e.g. Plateau iris syndrome).
c. Lens-pupil block (e.g. phacomorphic glaucoma).

Secondary Angle Closure Glaucoma
Anterior "Pulling Mechanism"

The iris is pulled forward by the contraction of a membrane (or) peripheral anterior synechiae:

a. Neovascular glaucoma
b. Iridocorneal endothelial syndrome (e.g. Chandlers syndrome)
c. Posterior polymorphous dystrophy
d. Fibrous ingrowth
e. Epithelial down growth
f. Flat anterior chamber
g. Inflammation
h. Penetrating keratoplasty
i. Aniridia.

Posterior "Pushing Mechanism"

The iris is pushed forward often by anterior rotation of ciliary body.

a. Ciliary block glaucoma (Malignant glaucoma)
b. Cyst of iris and ciliary body
c. Intraocular tumors
d. Nanophthalmos
e. Suprachoroidal hemorrhage
f. Scleral buckling procedures
g. Pneumatic retinopexy
h. Ciliochoroidal effusion.

CLASSIFICATION OF OPEN ANGLE GLAUCOMA
Primary Open Angle Closure Glaucoma

1. Primary open angle glaucoma (POAG).
2. Normal-tension glaucoma (NTG).

Table 1 Open angle glaucoma mechanisms

A. Pretrabecular (membrane overgrowth)
• Fibrovascular membrane (neovascular glaucoma)
• Endothelial layer, often with Descemet-like membrane
• Epithelial downgrowth
• Fibrous ingrowth
• Inflammatory membrane
B. Trabecular (occlusion of intertrabecular spaces)
• Idiopathic
❖ Chronic open angle glaucomas
❖ Steroid-induced glaucoma
• "Clogging" of the trabecular meshwork
❖ Red blood cells
❖ Macrophages
❖ Neoplastic cells
❖ Pigment particles
❖ Protein
• Alterations of the trabecular meshwork
❖ Edema
❖ Trauma
❖ Intraocular foreign bodies (hemosiderosis, chalcosis)
C. Post-trabecular
• Obstruction of Schlemm's canal
❖ Collapse of canal
❖ Clogging of canal
• Elevated episcleral venous pressure
❖ Carotid cavernous fistula
❖ Cavernous sinus thrombosis
❖ Retrobulbar tumors
❖ Thyrotropic exophthalmos
❖ Superior vena cava obstruction
❖ Mediastinal tumors
❖ Sturge-Weber syndrome
❖ Familial episcleral venous pressure elevated

Table 2 Angle closure glaucoma mechanisms

A. Anterior (pulling mechanism)
Contracture of membranes
• Neovascular glaucoma
• Iridocorneal endothelial syndrome
• Posterior polymorphous dystrophy
• Penetrating and nonpenetrating trauma
Contracture of inflammatory precipitates
B. Posterior (pushing mechanism)
With pupillary block
• Pupillary block glaucoma
• Lens induced mechanisms
• Posterior synechiae
Without pupillary block
• Plateau iris syndrome
• Ciliary block glaucoma
• Lens induced mechanisms
• Following lens extraction
• Following scleral buckling
• Following panretinal photocoagulation
• Central retinal vein occlusion
• Intraocular tumors
• Cysts of the iris and ciliary body
• Retrolenticular tissue contracture

Secondary Open Angle Glaucoma

1. Pigmentary glaucoma
2. Pseudoexfoliation glaucoma
3. Steroid induced glaucoma
4. Lens induced glaucoma
   a. Phacolytic glaucoma
   b. Lens particle glaucoma
   c. Phacoanaphylaxis
5. Glaucoma after cataract surgery
   a. α chymotrypsin glaucoma
   b. Glaucoma due to viscoelastic
   c. Uveitis, glaucoma, hyphema (UGH syndrome)
   d. Glaucoma with pigment dispersion and IOL
   e. Glaucoma with vitreous in anterior chamber
6. Glaucoma after trauma
   a. Chemical burns
   b. Electric shock
   c. Radiation
   d. Penetrating injury
   e. Contusion injury
7. Glaucoma associated with intraocular hemorrhage
   a. Ghost cell glaucoma
   b. Hemolytic glaucoma
   c. Hemosiderosis
8. Glaucoma associated with retinal detachment
9. Glaucoma after vitrectomy
   a. Intraocular gas
   b. Intraocular silicon oil
10. Glaucoma with uveitis
    a. Fuchs heterochromic iridocyclitis
    b. Glaucoma cyclitic crisis (Posner-Schlossman syndrome)
    c. Precipitates on trabecular meshwork (trabeculitis)
    d. Herpes simplex
    e. Herpes Zoster
    f. Sarcoidosis
    g. Juvenile rheumatoid arthritis
    h. Syphilis
11. Glaucoma with intraocular tumors
    a. Malignant melanoma
    b. Metastatic lesions
    c. Leukemia and lymphoma
    d. Benign lesions
       - Neuofibromatosis
       - Juvenile xanthogranulomatosis
12. Amyloidosis
13. Increased episcleral venous pressure
    a. Carotid cavernous fistula
    b. Cavernous sinus thrombosis
    c. Retrobulbar tumors
    d. Thyrotropic exophthalmos
    e. Superior, vena cava obstruction
    f. Struge-Weber syndrome
    g. Mediastinal tumors
    h. Familial episcleral venous pressure elevation.

DEVELOPMENTAL ANOMALIES OF ANTERIOR CHAMBER ANGLE (TABLE 3)

1. **High insertion of anterior uvea**
   a. Congenital (infantile) glaucoma
   b. Juvenile glaucoma
   c. Glaucoma associated with other developmental anomalies
2. **Incomplete development of trabecular meshwork/Schlemm's canal**
   a. Axenfeld-Rieger syndrome
   b. Peters anomaly
   c. Glaucoma associated with other developmental anomalies
3. **Iridocorneal adhesions**
   a. Axenfeld-Rieger syndrome
   b. Aniridia.

EPIDEMIOLOGICAL CLASSIFICATION OF GLAUCOMA

Glaucoma is the second largest cause of blindness in the world and the current focus of research. The research is directed towards measuring prevalence, evaluating risk factors and clinical trials. With the varying definitions and classification of glaucoma comparison between various published data becomes difficult and misinterpretation is possible. To overcome this problem, the International Society for Geographical and Epidemiological Ophthalmology provided a framework for classifying cases of glaucoma in cross sectional population based research. It placed emphasis of the diagnosis on glaucomatous optic neuropathy with a reproducible visual field defect, but includes criteria for some eyes in which visual field testing or disc evaluation are impossible make the diagnosis to direct measurements of the structure and function of the optic nerve (**Table 4**). In the public health context, glaucoma can be seen as an optic neuropathy associated with characteristic structural damage to the optic nerve and associated visual dysfunction that may be caused by various pathological processes.

Primary Open Angle Glaucoma

Primary open angle glaucoma (POAG) is optic nerve damage meeting any of the three categories of evidence above, in an eye which does not have evidence of angle closure on gonioscopy, and where there is no identifiable secondary cause

Table 3 Developmental anomalies of anterior chamber angle

A. High insertion of anterior uvea
• Congenital (infantile) glaucoma
• Juvenile glaucoma
• Glaucoma associated with other developmental anomalies
B. Incomplete development of trabecular meshwork/Schlemm's canal
• Axenfeld-Rieger syndrome
• Peters anomaly
• Glaucoma associated with other developmental anomalies
C. Iridocorneal adhesions
• Axenfeld-Rieger syndrome—Broad strands
• Aniridia—Fine strands which contract to close angle

Classification of Glaucoma   295

Table 4 The diagnosis of glaucoma in cross-sectional prevalence surveys
(Three levels of evidence)

Category 1—diagnosis (structural and functional evidence)
Eyes with a CDR or CDR asymmetry >97.5th percentile for the normal population, or a neuroretinal rim width reduced to <0.1 CDR (between 11 and 1 o' clock or 5 and 7 o' clock) that also showed a definite visual field defect consistent with glaucoma.
Category 2—diagnosis (advanced structural damage with unproved field loss)
Glaucoma diagnosed solely on the structural evidence if the subject could not satisfactorily complete visual field testing but had a CDR or CDR asymmetry > 99.5th percentile for the normal population.
In diagnosing category 1 or 2 glaucoma, there should be no alternative explanation for CDR findings or the visual field defect.
Category 3—diagnosis (optic disc not seen and visual field test impossible)
If it is not possible to examine the optic disc, glaucoma is diagnosed if:
• The visual acuity <3/60 and the IOP >99.5th percentile, or
• The visual acuity <3/60 and the eye shows evidence of glaucoma filtering surgery, or medical records were available confirming glaucomatous visual morbidity.

Primary Angle Closure and Narrow Drainage Angles

The acute, symptomatic stage is seen only a minority of patients. The chronic, asymptomatic form of PACG is more predominant. Thus the definition was fully re-evaluated with emphasis placed on visual loss rather than symptomatic disease. It is useful to distinguish between the mechanism by which IOP becomes elevated and the resultant damage that is caused by PACG. According to this, gonioscopic criteria for narrow angles and with evidence of significant obstruction of the functional trabecular meshwork by the peripheral iris would be classified as having primary angle closure (PAC). Those in whom PAC had led to significant glaucomatous damage to the optic nerve would be defined as having PACG. This distinguishes those with and without visual field damage due to glaucomatous optic neuropathy. Thus,

in this new concept, PAC includes both asymptomatic people with occludable angles who have not had an acute attack, and those with PAC who have had an attack that was treated promptly but suffered no detectable nerve damage.

Glaucoma with Secondary Ocular Pathology

Secondary glaucoma is considered to represent those eyes in which a second form of ocular pathology has caused IOP above the normal range, leading to optic nerve damage. The diagnosis of secondary glaucoma is based on the presence of optic neuropathy. These processes may include one of the following:
1. Neovascularization
2. Uveitic
3. Trauma
4. Lens related.

Pigment dispersion syndrome or pseudoexfoliation syndrome as cases

of secondary glaucoma have been omitted from the list.

Many eyes with secondary glaucoma have opaque media, precluding optic disc and visual field examinations. These eyes glaucoma will be diagnosed with the category 3 when optic neuropathy is inferred from reduced visual acuity and a relative afferent pupil defect, in the presence of raised IOP.

Eyes with processes such as exfoliation or uveitis with IOP above the normal range with a normal disc are categorised as secondary ocular hypertensives, or secondary glaucoma suspects.

Glaucoma Suspects

This indicates a suspicion of glaucoma. The various reasons that a person would be considered as a glaucoma suspect are summarized in the **Table 4**.

REFERENCES

1. Stamper RL, Lieberman MF, Drake MV. Introduction and Classification of Glaucomas. Becker-Shaffer's Diagnosis and Therapy of the Glaucomas, 8th edn. Pennsylvania St. Louis, Mosby, 2009.
2. Shields MB, Ritch R, Krupin T. Classification of glaucomas. The glaucomas, 2nd edn. St. Louis, Mosby, 1996.
3. Spaeth GL. A new classification of glaucoma including focal glaucoma. Surv Ophthalmol 1994;38:S9.
4. Mills RP, Budenz DL, Lee PP, et al. Categorizing the stage of glaucoma from pre-diagnosis to end stage disease. Am J Ophthalmol 2006;141:24-30.
5. Foster PJ, Buhrmann R, Quigley HA, Johnson GJ. The definition and classification of glaucoma in prevalence surveys. Br J Ophthalmol 2002; 86(2):238-42.

23 Ocular Hypertension

- ❖ What is Ocular Hypertension?
- ❖ Epidemiology
- ❖ Assessment and Follow-up
- ❖ Baseline Risk Factors that Predict the Conversion to Primary Open Angle Glaucoma
- ❖ Guidelines on Treatment
- ❖ Ocular Hypertension Treatment Study

WHAT IS OCULAR HYPERTENSION?

Ocular hypertension (OHT) is a term reserved for eyes in which the intraocular pressure (IOP) lies above the normal population range. Optic nerve and visual fields show no signs of glaucomatous damage. There is no ocular comorbidity. Excluded from this definition are eyes with raised IOP from demonstrable causes. It has been clearly indicated by most population studies over 40-year age group, that intraocular pressures measured with Goldmann tonometry are distributed in a manner similar to normal distribution (mean 16 mm Hg approximately). *Individuals with IOP greater than two standard deviations above the mean can be labeled as ocular hypertensive.* It decides an upper limit for "normal" IOP in Caucasians of 21 mm Hg. It should be kept in mind that this figure is statistically derived and does not prove that disease is present if measured IOP level exceeds this value.

EPIDEMIOLOGY

The study of epidemiology (the distribution of a disease in a population, and the identifiable conditions that are associated with it) helps us understand some of the factors that alter the risk of ocular hypertension, its progression, and its sequelae. The understanding of OHT has significantly improved in recent years by the application of epidemiologic principles.

Individuals with OHT account for 5 to 6 percent rather than 2.5 percent that would be expected from a true normal distribution. Now it is becoming clearer, that while these values are true for Caucasian population, it might not hold true for other racial groups where the mean IOP is lower (e.g. the Japanese are reported to have a lower mean IOP).

Epidemiological studies have identified those individuals in a population most at risk:

1. *Increasing age:* The prevalence of OHT increases with age. However, one should not have an assumption from this statement that the disease is limited to middle-aged and older individuals; it occurs in young adults as well.
2. *Gender:* Conflicting information exists about the effect of gender on the prevalence of OHT. In several studies, males had a higher prevalence as compared to their counterparts.
3. *Race:* Recent studies have shown conclusively that OHT is more prevalent in individuals of black African or Caribbean origin.
4. Family history of glaucoma
5. Systemic hypertension
6. Diabetes (+/−).

ASSESSMENT AND FOLLOW-UP

Since elevated IOP is the major risk factor for the development of glaucomatous visual loss **(Figure 1)**, finding a "raised" IOP indicates the need for further investigation and management decisions.

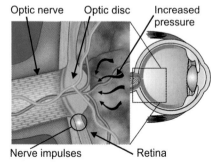

Fig. 1 IOP is a major risk factor for glaucoma

Most ocular hypertensives are detected in routine practice and several scenarios could be possible:

1. An **unconfirmed raised IOP** at screening—a "normal" IOP and no evidence of any other abnormality.

> **Note** *Rule out the various causes of artifactually raised IOP measurements especially "Valsalva"*

2. *Intermittent OHT:* In this condition, raised IOP is confirmed initially but reverts to normal on repeated testing over time and no evidence of other related abnormality detected.
3. **Persistent OHT** where raised IOP is a constant feature.

Assuming an otherwise normal ocular examination, patients in categories 1 and 2 can be advised to seek periodic (e.g. one yearly) re-examination. Patients in category 3 require the ophthalmologist to make a decision regarding follow-up and prophylactic treatment taking into account the associated risk factors.

According to **European Glaucoma Society Guidelines**, follow-up needs to be at intervals of 12 months initially, to be increased if all parameters remain negative with examination of:

- Optic disc
- Visual field
- Intraocular pressure (IOP)
- ONH and RNFL photographs initially and to be repeated every 2 to 3 years.

BASELINE RISK FACTORS THAT PREDICT THE CONVERSION TO PRIMARY OPEN ANGLE GLAUCOMA

Estimates vary as to the conversion rate from OHT to POAG, depending on subject selection and diagnostic criteria. It is likely that approximately 10 percent individuals with persistent OHT will convert to POAG over a ten-year period. Risk factors for the conversion of OHT to POAG can be divided into ocular and systemic factors respectively. The most important are listed below.

Ocular Risk Factors
Highest Recorded IOP

Greater the IOP, greater is the risk. There is general agreement that IOP is the most important known risk factor for progression to open angle glaucoma. Evidence clearly indicates that elevated IOP can cause glaucomatous optic nerve changes in experimental animals. Population surveys also support the increase in prevalence of open angle glaucoma with increasing IOP.

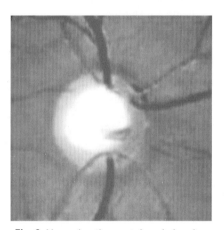

Fig. 2 Normal optic nerve head showing large vertical cup-disc ratio

Cup-disc Ratio

A large vertical cup-disc ratio (**Figure 2**) (indicating reduced neuroretinal rim area/volume) is one of predictive factor identified in various reported population surveys, case-control studies and prospective studies. A patient with a large cup-disc ratio unaltered by glaucoma may be at greater risk for developing POAG.

Cup/Disc (C/D) Ratio Asymmetry

Asymmetry of more than >0.2 between the two eyes provided the disc size is symmetrical (**Figures 3A and B**).

Disc Hemorrhages

These are either flame shaped or blot hemorrhage that can occur at any location around the disc rim. They are usually located within the nerve fiber layer extending across the disc rim into the retina, but they may occur deep in the disc tissue. A cautionary value can be assigned to this ophthalmic finding. The identification of a disc hemorrhage (**Figure 4**) in any eye compels considerations that glaucoma may be present.

Retinal Nerve Fiber Layer Defect

The presence of retinal nerve fiber layer defects in the absence of morphometric optic nerve head changes is an important risk factor. It has been shown that

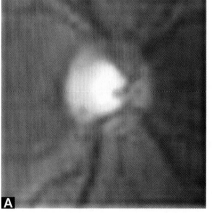 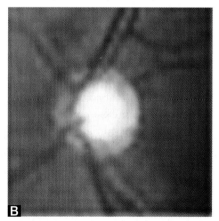

Figs 3A and B Normal optic nerve head showing asymmetry of cup-disc ratio

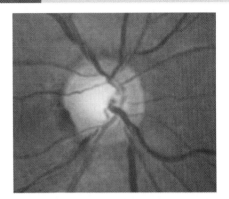

Fig. 4 Disc hemorrhage at the inferior pole of optic disc

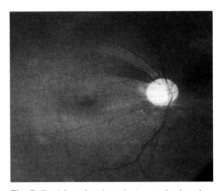

Fig. 5 Red-free fundus photograph showing superior wedge defect. Note good visibility of vessels in that area. Atrophy of the RNFL has unmasked the mottled appearance of the retinal pigment epithelium

as many as 40 percent optic nerve fibers can be lost prior to a standard visual field defect. OHTS has clearly demonstrated that 55 percent of eyes that converted to glaucoma had normal visual fields. Thus, it is of prime importance to evaluate retinal nerve fiber layer **(Figure 5)**.

Thinner than Average Central Corneal Thickness

It is well known that corneal thickness influences the measurement of IOP. Eyes with thicker corneas have a true IOP that is lower than the measured IOP. Conversely, eyes with thin corneas have a true IOP that is greater than measured IOP. Thus, individuals with thicker corneas may be misclassified as having ocular hypertension. Cross-sectional studies have documented that central corneal thickness is greater in individuals with ocular hypertension compared with normotensive individuals. We should also note that excimer laser procedures on the cornea can result in artifactually lowered IOP on measurement.

Systemic Risk Factors

1. Increasing age
2. Family history
3. Individual of African or Caribbean origin.

MANAGEMENT OF OHT
Prophylactic Therapy

A decision to treat any eye with ocular hypertension should be made when the risk factors present in the patient are considered to outweigh the disadvantages of treatment.

GUIDELINES ON TREATMENT

When treating OHT, the aim is to lower the IOP to a level considered safe for the individual patient, and this should be at least a 20 percent reduction. Before initiating treatment, a clinician should carefully evaluate the full implications of treating the individual concerned, including a realistic assessment of the in convenience and potential side effects of such treatment.

A. ***Treating raised IOP without additional risk factors:*** Many specialists would like to treat when the IOP is consistently 28 to 30 mm Hg or over in the absence of other risk factors. The decision to initiate treatment at a lower level of IOP should be based on perceived risk by the ophthalmologist and the patient.

B. ***Treating raised IOP plus other risk factors:*** The ocular hypertension treatment study (OHTS) provides figures for risk, adjusted according to the height of the IOP, the central corneal thickness and the vertical C/D ratio. When these factors combine to give an appreciable 5 year risk of developing a significant optic disc change of visual field defect, the ophthalmologist needs to identify this to the patient and outline the benefits and risks of treatment.

OCULAR HYPERTENSION TREATMENT STUDY
Brief Introduction

It was a prospective, multicenter randomized clinical trial done on 1636 participants who had ocular hypertension, with an IOP between 24 and 32 mm Hg in one eye (minimum 21 mm Hg in the other eye) and no evidence of glaucomatous damage. They were randomized to either observation or treatment with commercially available topical ocular hypotensive medication. The patients were observed for a period of 5 years.

The exclusion criteria included concomitant eye disease, individuals with visual acuity less than 20/40 for any reason, diabetic retinopathy and inability to perform reliable perimetry.

Aim

The aim was to evaluate the safety and efficacy of topical ocular hypotensive therapy in preventing or delaying the onset of visual field loss or optic nerve damage due to primary open angle glaucoma in individuals with ocular hypertension.

Results of OHTS

Although the rate of conversion to primary open angle glaucoma is not likely to be linear, OHTS suggested that untreated ocular hypertensive eyes convert to glaucoma at the rate of 2 percent per year. This study clearly indicated following as risk factors:

1. Increasing age
2. Baseline high IOP
3. Vertical and horizontal cup-disc ratio
4. Pattern standard deviation
5. Central corneal thickness (CCT)

The OHTS was the first study to prospectively document that thinner central corneal measurement predicts the development of POAG. Corneal thickness appeared to be a strong predictive factor for the development of POAG, even after adjusting for the effects of baseline age, IOP, vertical cup-disc ratio, and pattern standard deviation **(Figure 6 and Table 1)**.

An endpoint in OHTS required a confirmed disc or field change, rather than both. **Interestingly, very few of the OHTS converters reached both visual field and disc end points**.

In OHTS, the researchers noted that 4.4 percent of the study participants who received the ocular hypotensive drops developed glaucoma within five years. By comparison, 9.5 percent of the study participants who did not receive the eye drops developed glaucoma. In the medication group, treatment reduced IOP by approximately 20 percent. This modest 20 percent reduction in IOP had significant protective effect in the development of glaucoma.

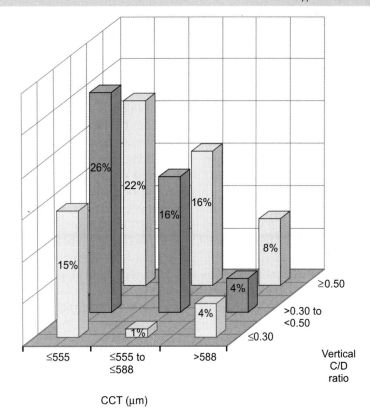

Fig. 6 The percentage of participants in the observation group who developed primary open-angle glaucoma (median follow-up, and ≥0.50 and by central corneal thickness measurements of ≤555 μm, >555 μm, to ≤588 μm and >588 μm 72 months) grouped by baseline vertical cup-disc (VCD) ratios of ≤ 0.30, >0.30 to <0.50

Table 1 Point system for estimating an ocular hypertensive patient's 5-year risk of developing POAG

Baseline predictor	Points for baseline predictor				
	0	1	2	3	4
Age (years)	< 45	45 – < 55	55 – < 65	65 – < 75	≥ 75
Mean IOP (mm Hg)*	< 22	22 – < 24	24 – < 26	26 – < 28	≥ 28
Mean CCT (μm)*	≥ 600	576–600	551–575	526–550	≤ 525
Mean vertical cup-to-disc ratio by contour*	< 0.3	0.3 – < 0.4	0.4 – < 0.5	0.5 – < 0.6	≥ 0.6
Mean PSD (dB)*	< 1.8	1.8 – < 2.0	2.0 – < 2.4	2.4 – < 2.8	≥ 2.8
Sum of points	0–6	7–8	9–10	11–12	> 12
Estimated 5-year risk of POAG	≤ 4.0%	10%	15%	20%	≥ 33%

CCT = Central corneal thickness; dB = Decibels; IOP = Intraocular pressure; PSD – Pattern standard deviation; POAG = Primary open angle glaucoma
*Eye-specific variables are the mean of right and left eyes.

Summary

- OHTS demonstrated a clear relationship between OHT and the development of glaucoma.

- The rate of progression from ocular hypertension with apparently normal optic nerves and visual function to glaucoma is higher than most of us have thought. More individuals with true 'OHT' need to be treated, as the cumulative risk of developing glaucoma depends on level of IOP, with each additional 'mm Hg' increasing the risk.

- Pachymetry has become an integral part of the ophthalmic examination. Understanding corneal thickness as a risk factor needs reliable conversion tables for IOP based upon corneal thickness to be developed. The implication that IOP can be "corrected" with arithmetic, linear "correction" factor of some mm Hg/mm clearly represents an oversimplification of which is undoubtedly a complex and nonlinear relationship between corneal thickness and "true" IOP.

The decision to treat should take into account the patient's life

expectancy and the probability of functional visual loss occurring within the patient's life time. The clinician should always look for the burden of long term treatment i.e., side effects, cost and inconvenience.

The OHTS researchers did put together a risk calculator called STAR II scoring tool for assessing risk. It is based on pooled multivariate Cox proportional hazards. It takes into account following factors:

- Age (30–80 in years)
- Baseline IOP (20–30 mm Hg)
- CCT (475–650 m)
- Pattern standard deviation (0.50 – 3.00 db)
- Vertical CDR (0.000 – 0.80)

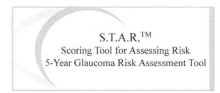

S.T.A.R.™
Scoring Tool for Assessing Risk
5-Year Glaucoma Risk Assessment Tool

Level of Risk over 5 years		Action
Low	<5%	Observe
Moderate	5–15%	Consider treatment
High	>15%	Treat

It is intended to be used in patients with untreated ocular hypertension. It

looks like a regular calculator. We can input patient's data and it gives out the percentage risk that the person would develop POAG in 5 years in percentage. Researchers should make concrete recommendations derived from sound analysis of the presently available results and future studies to provide maximum benefit to our patients and thereby translate the OHTS results into coherent clinical practice.

CONCLUSION

The term "Ocular Hypertension" should be used to indicate that the IOP is consistently outside 2 standard deviations above the mean. Central corneal thickness plays a vital role in the clinical recording of IOP. OHTS conclusively determined that 50 percent of subjects were misclassified as OHT prior to correction for CCT. The management of patients with ocular hypertension accounts for significant proportion of the workload of most ophthalmologists. A modest increase in IOP is not a sufficient reason for treatment.

The clinician should carefully take a decision to treat an eye when risk factors present out weigh the disadvantages of treatment.

BIBLIOGRAPHY

1. Argus WA. Ocular hypertension and central corneal thickness. Ophthalmology 1995;102:1810-2.

2. Brandt JD, Beiser JA, Kass MA, Gordon MO. Central corneal thickness in the Ocular Hypertension Treatment Study (OHTS) Group. Ophthalmology 2001;108;1779-88.

3. Doughty MJ, Zaman ML. Human corneal thickness and its impact on intraocular pressure measures: a review and meta-analysis approach. Surv Ophthalmol 2000;44:367-408.

4. Gordon MO, Beiser JA, Brandt JD, et al. The Ocular Hypertension Treatment Study (OHTS) Group: baseline factors

that predict the onset of primary open angle glaucoma. Arch Ophthalmol 2002;120:714-20.

5. Guidelines for the management of open angle glaucoma and ocular hypertension (2004) by the Royal College of Ophthalmologists, London, UK.

6. Johnson CA, Keltner JL, Cello KE, et al. Baseline visual field characteristics in the ocular hypertension treatment study. Ophthalmology 2002;109: 432-7.

7. Johnson CA, Sample, Trick GL. Short Wavelength Automated Perimetry (SWAP) in the Ocular Hypertensive

Treatment Study (OHTS). Invest Ophthalmol Vis Sci 2002; (ARVO Suppl):86.

8. Klein BEK, Klein R, Sponsel WE, et al. Prevalence of glaucoma: the Beaver Dam Eye Study. Ophthalmology 1992;99:1499-504.

9. Quigley HA, Enger C, Katz J, Sommer A, Scott R, Gilbert D. Risk factors for the development of glaucomatous visual field loss in ocular hypertension. Arch Ophthalmol 1994;112;644-9.

10. Whitacre MM, Stein RA, Hassanein K. The effect of corneal thickness on applanation tonometry. Am J Ophthalmol 1993;115;592-6.

24 | Primary Open Angle Glaucoma

SR Krishnadas

DEFINITION AND INTRODUCTION

Primary open angle glaucoma (POAG) is a chronic, bilateral, asymmetrical, progressive disease in adults characterized by acquired loss of optic nerve fibers accompanied by a characteristic cupping of the optic-discs and matching visual field loss with open iridocorneal angles. It is not associated with any obvious causative ocular or systemic conditions. Elevated intraocular pressure reflecting a reduced aqueous outflow facility is often, though not invariably, associated with POAG as a principal causative risk factor. The mechanism by which intraocular pressure damages the optic nerves is largely unclear, but ischemia of the optic nerves or the nerve fiber layer or mechanical compression of the retinal ganglion cells or a combination of several factors is known to play a role in pathogenesis of optic nerve damage in glaucoma. POAG is the most common form of glaucoma in most communities and accounts for 50 to 60 percent of glaucoma seen in India. Close to 2 million persons worldwide develop this condition every year and about 3 million people are bilaterally blind due to POAG.

EPIDEMIOLOGY

Prevalence and Magnitude—Global and Specific Reference to India

The prevalence of primary open angle glaucoma has been studied extensively worldwide and significantly varies between various races and ethnic groups. In most studies performed in the US and Western Europe,[1] the prevalence of POAG is 0.5 to 1 percent in persons aged over forty. The prevalence of POAG is significantly higher in blacks (4.7%)[2] as compared to whites (1.3%). Hispanics have been found to have a prevalence of over 2.0 percent; whereas in Asians, the prevalence varies widely between populations. Some groups have prevalence rates close to that of Caucasians[3] (Singapore Chinese 2.4%, Japanese 2.6%, Indians 1.7%) but Mongols (0.5%) and Alaskan Inuits (0.1%) have considerably lower rates of prevalence. In Japan, glaucoma appears to be more common than in any other Asian or Caucasian populations. In the Tajimi study,[4] 3.9 percent of those over forty years had POAG with a vast majority of individual having an IOP less than 21 mm Hg. The highest prevalence of POAG is reported in populations in Western Africa. In Ghana,[5] the prevalence of open angle glaucoma is 8 percent in persons aged over forty. Prevalence of open angle glaucoma in Iceland (3%), Australia (4%) and Greece (4%) is also relatively higher as compared to other Caucasian populations. It has, however, been revealed by most population based studies that age has a more significant influence on POAG prevalence than race or ethnicity. POAG is not a common disease before 40 years of age. In a pooled analysis of population based studies, prevalence was seen to increase from 0.6 percent (40-49 years) to 1.5 percent (50-59 years), 2.7 percent (60-69 years), 5.1 percent (70-79 years) and 7.3 percent in those above 80 years and translates to about 10-fold increase in risk as compared to those in the fifth decade of their lives. The age-specific prevalence of primary open angle glaucoma in most Asians and Hispanics is similar to that in the white population.

Prevalence of POAG in India (Table 1)

In India, a wide variation in the prevalence of glaucoma were reported between different studies. The Vellore Eye Study[6] (VES) reported lowest prevalence rates, since, unlike other prevalence studies, this study included patients in the 30 to 60 years age group. The prevalence of POAG increased with age in all the reported studies. There was also a low rate of performance of visual fields in the VES probably underestimating the prevalence of glaucoma in this population as both the optic disc and visual field defect criteria were required to detect glaucoma. The VES also had a high rate of nonresponders (51.5%) in a marked contrast to other prevalence studies, affecting case detection and possible underestimation of the prevalence. The reported prevalence rates of glaucoma in an urban population were significantly higher as revealed in the Chennai Glaucoma Study (CGS)[7] and the Andhra Pradesh Eye Study (APEDS),[8] with the exception of VES. Diabetes and cardiovascular diseases also have reported to have a higher prevalence in rural India. It is speculated that lifestyle changes and cardiovascular disease patterns in urban India may indirectly influence the prevalence of POAG. The proportion of persons with glaucoma who presented with a normal IOP (defined as within two standard deviation from the population mean) were relatively higher in all the studies: 65 percent of persons with POAG in APEDS, 45 percent in ACES (Aravind Comprehensive Eye Survey),[9] 67 percent in CGS (rural) and 82 percent in CGS (urban) had normal IOP at the time of diagnosis. This emphasizes the unreliability of IOP measurement alone in screening for glaucoma, and reinforces careful optic nerve evaluation for accurate diagnosis of glaucoma. Increasing age and higher IOP was a consistent risk factor for glaucoma in all the prevalence studies. ACES reported male gender and myopia to be risk factors for POAG although no other studies observed gender or refractive errors to be associated with increased risk of POAG. Increased incidence of glaucoma with age is a cause for concern since India's population is aging and the prevalence is expected to increase exponentially in the decades to come. A significant proportion of individuals with glaucoma will reside in the Indian subcontinent by 2030. Quigley had projected that number of persons with open angle glaucoma older than 40 years would comprise 18.4 percent of the world's POAG population. In India, despite an inequitable distribution of eye care providers and ophthalmologists in urban areas, the prevalence of primary open angle glaucoma was reported to be twice in an urban population (3.47%) as compared to rural (1.62%).

Incidence of Primary Open Angle Glaucoma

Although several studies that have assessed the prevalence of POAG world-wide have become available, few studies have evaluated the incidence of primary open angle glaucoma in the population. The Barbados Eye Study[10] has reported the four-year incidence of glaucoma over 40 years of age to be 2.2 percent. The risk factors for glaucoma included male gender, African ancestry, higher IOP, and those with suspicious optic nerves. Incidence rate was also observed to be age dependent—increasing from 1.2 percent in the 40 to 49 age group to 4.2 percent in those aged over 70 years. Incidence studies from Framingham, Rotterdam, Australia and Minnesota have reported a similar age dependent incidence rate of primary open angle glaucoma. The Chennai Glaucoma Study is currently prospectively following up a cohort of rural and urban patients from South India for assessing incidence of glaucoma in an Indian population.

RISK FACTORS

- Intraocular pressure (IOP)
- Central corneal thickness (CCT)
- Race
- Age
- Family history

Table 1 Prevalence of POAG in India

Age (years)	APEDS	ACES	CGS (rural)	CGS (urban)	WBGS
40-49	1.27	0.34	0.63	2.26	–
50-59	2.31	1.57	1.62	3.57	2.55
60-69	4.89	1.83	2.58	4.08	2.69
>70	6.32	2.88	3.25	6.42	4.76
Reported prevalence % (95% CI)	2.56 (1.22, 3.91)	1.7 (1.3, 2.1)	1.62 (1.42,1.82)	3.51 (3.04, 4.0)	2.99

APEDS = Andhra Pradesh Eye Disease Study[8]; ACES = Aravind Comprehensive Eye Survey[9]; CGS = Chennai Glaucoma Study[7]; WBGS = West Bengal Glaucoma Study (Rauchaudhri A, et al. Br J Ophthalmol 2005;89:19)

- Suspicious optic nerve head
- Myopia
- Vascular disease.

Intraocular Pressure

Intraocular pressure (IOP) has been consistently demonstrated to be associated with incidence, prevalence and progression of glaucoma. There is strong evidence to support higher mean IOP as a risk factor for development of glaucoma. The evidence for such an observation comes from prospective, randomized clinical trials and also from smaller prospective studies. There is also a strong dose response relationship between IOP and glaucoma that has been consistently proven in prevalence surveys. The Ocular Hypertension Treatment Study (OHTS)[11] has provided the best evidence on the role of IOP as risk factor for development of glaucoma. The average reduction of IOP in the treatment group was 22.5 percent and the cumulative probability of developing POAG was 4.4 percent in the medication group as compared to 9.5 percent in the observation group, with 54 percent relative reduction in development of POAG with treatment. There is also strong evidence in support of higher mean IOP as significant risk factor for progression of disease in glaucoma. The Early Manifest Glaucoma Treatment Study (EMGTS)[12] was specifically designed to study the effect of IOP lowering treatment on progression of glaucoma. The proportion of patients who developed progression was significantly larger in the control as compared to the treatment group (62% versus 45%, respectively). In the analysis of predictive factors for glaucoma progression in the EMGT Study, each 1 mm higher baseline IOP increased risk of glaucoma progression by 5 percent and conversely, each 1 mm Hg reduction of IOP with treatment was associated with a 10 percent risk

reduction in glaucoma progression. In the Collaborative Normal Tension Glaucoma Study,[13] significantly fewer eyes progressed with 30 percent reduction in IOP (12% progression in the treatment group versus 35 percent in the control group). The Advanced Glaucoma Intervention Study (AGIS)[14] results also support a positive relationship between IOP and glaucoma progression. In addition to population based studies and randomized clinical trials, studies have been published that establish link between elevated IOP and apoptosis of optic nerve neurons through blockage of retrograde axonal transport which are proven methods of optic nerve damage in glaucoma.

Central Corneal Thickness

Applanation tonometry described by Goldmann and Schmidt presumed a central corneal thickness of approximately 520 microns. Although it was earlier believed that central corneal thickness (CCT) would influence applanation readings, it was assumed that variations in CCT occurred rarely in the absence of corneal diseases. Following several clinical and epidemiologic studies, it has been observed that CCT even in clinically normal individuals is more variable than was earlier believed. Many persons with ocular hypertension have been observed to have thick corneas leading to overestimation of ocular pressures. In the Ocular Hypertension Treatment Study (OHTS),[11] 24 percent subjects had CCT exceeding 600 microns, thus misclassifying many individuals with normal IOP as ocular hypertensives. The study also revealed that subjects with CCT < 555 microns had three-fold greater risk of developing POAG than participants with CCT > 588 microns, with the conclusion that individuals classified as ocular hypertensives with thinner corneas are at increased risk of conversion to POAG.

Age

In every known population based study and ethnic group,[2,7-9,15-17] the prevalence of POAG increases with age. Prevalence rates roughly tend to double for each decade over 40 (relative risk of 2 for each decade) and is about 10-fold high in >80 age group compared to the 40 to 49 age bracket. The proportion of individuals with optic nerve damage and visual loss from glaucoma increases from 1 percent in persons under 40 years of age to prevalence estimates 3 to 8 times higher in individuals over 70 year of age. The reasons for increasing age contributing to elevated risk of glaucoma could be: elderly individuals are exposed to higher IOP longer, compromise in optic nerve perfusion with age owing to microvascular disease, and possible changes in connective tissue integrity and laminar support in the elderly predisposing to optic nerve excavation and retinal ganglion cell loss.

Race

The prevalence of POAG is 3 to 4 times higher in the African and the ethnic black population in the Americas than Caucasian population.[2] Optic nerve damage tends to occur a decade earlier in blacks, is more severe at the time of diagnosis, and is more refractory to medical and surgical treatment. Higher IOP, vascular abnormalities of the optic nerve and optic nerve head size have been attributed to increased risk of glaucoma prevalence in Africans. POAG seems to develop at earlier age in Africans and has a more rapid progression[18-20] in this ethnic group. The incidence of blindness is estimated to be 8 to 10 times higher in African American[2] patients as compared to Caucasians in the US. In the Hispanics, the prevalence of POAG is estimated to be between that of people of African and European ancestry. The prevalence of POAG in most other ethnic groups is not yet well studied, although in some populations, it is known to be very low: rare in Pacific Islanders, Mongols (0.5%), and certain North American Tribes. The prevalence of POAG in South India[7-9] is close to that of the Caucasians.

Family History

A family history[21,22] of open angle glaucoma has been consistently proven to be a significant risk factor for primary open angle glaucoma. In prevalence surveys, having a first degree relative (parent, sibling or children) with glaucomas has been consistently associated with increased risk of open angle glaucoma. It has also been learnt that the association of risk of glaucoma with family history is stronger when the affected relative is a sibling[23] rather than a parent or child. In a yet another population survey, the estimated lifetime relative risk of glaucoma[24] was 9.2 for first degree relatives with definite glaucoma. In families with multigenerational pedigrees of primary open angle glaucoma, members are at increased risk of glaucoma—17 percent of such family members were detected to have glaucoma in a study in Tasmania.

Refractive Errors—Myopia

Evidence supports myopia to be a risk factor for glaucoma in many studies.[25,26] The Beijing Eye Study[30] reported significantly higher prevalence of open angle glaucoma among subjects with myopia exceeding 6 diopters as compared to those with low myopia or emmetropia.

Fundus Changes Associated with High Myopia

Eyes with myopia tend to have broad, shallow cups with less distinct margins. Visual fields in such eyes tend to reveal baring of blind spot or other refractive scotoma making their interpretation very difficult and unreliable. Low ocular rigidity, thin cornea or sclera

in myopia may also give inaccurate IOP measurements with the various methods of tonometry that are available. It is also known that individuals with myopia and open angle glaucoma tend to have visual field defects closer to fixation and may also progress more rapidly at lower intraocular pressures as compared to emmetropes.

Optic Nerve Head Appearance

Changes in the appearance of the neural rim and the retinal nerve fiber layer define glaucoma and the alterations in the optic nerve head appear to be one of the strongest risk factors in primary open angle glaucoma. However, with significant biologic variability in the appearance of optic nerve head and limitations of the imaging technology available, it is difficult to define the optic disc structural parameters associated with open angle glaucoma. There is strong evidence to support large cup to disc ratio[27] as a significant risk factor in progression to glaucoma. Optic disc hemorrhages were associated with significant risk of progression of glaucoma in the collaborative normal tension glaucoma study[28] and with a six-fold increase in progression of ocular hypertension to glaucoma in the Ocular Hypertension Treatment Study.[29]

Systemic Diseases

Several systemic vascular and endocrine diseases have been associated with increased risk of open angle glaucoma. Several studies have shown high prevalence of diabetes in persons with POAG as well as open angle glaucoma in diabetics. Although the Baltimore Eye Survey or any of the population based studies in India failed to associate glaucoma with increased risk of diabetes mellitus, the Blue Mountain Study, the Rotterdam Eye Study and the Beaver Dam Study supported the association of diabetes mellitus and primary open

angle glaucoma. Although the association and the causes remain unclear, it has been hypothesized that diabetes affects the small vessels of the optic nerve head predisposing to glaucomatous optic nerve damage.

Some investigators have shown a relationship between open angle glaucoma and thyroid disease. A recent report[31] confirmed association of Graves' disease with open angle glaucoma, normal pressure glaucoma and ocular hypertension. Though hypothyroidism has been postulated to be a risk factor in open angle glaucoma by causing increased accumulation of glycosaminoglycans in the aqueous outflow pathway, this claim has not been substantiated in clinical/histopathological studies.

In the Barbados study, baseline systemic hypertension[32] seemed to reduce the risk of open angle glaucoma, while low blood pressure and reduced perfusion pressure in the optic nerves seemed to increase the risk of incident open angle glaucoma. It has long been considered that antihypertensive drugs like beta antagonists that cause a nocturnal dip in systemic blood pressure causes progression of visual fields in glaucoma. Blood flow in and around the eye has been studied to be lower in glaucoma. Statins,[33] the anticholesterol drugs have been shown is some studies to lower the risk of open angle glaucoma and this may be related to the effect of this class of drugs on optic nerve perfusion. The Blue Mountain Eye Study suggests an association between Migraine and open angle glaucoma.

CLINICAL FEATURES
Symptoms

Primary open angle glaucoma (POAG) is usually characterized by insidious, slowly progressive bilateral visual loss from chronic retinal ganglion cell death and midperipheral visual field defects sparing central vision until late in the course of the disease. Most patients with primary open angle glaucoma are asymptomatic. Few patients notice a scotoma while performing monocular visual tasks. Young patients with juvenile open angle glaucoma develop sudden exacerbations in IOP with corneal edema causing colored halos and blurred vision. If not diagnosed until they develop extensive glaucomatous damage, they become symptomatic from loss of fixation or peripheral visual loss in one or both eyes which interferes with routine visual tasks including driving.

Clinical Signs

- Optic disc excavation
- Arcuate nerve fiber layer defects
- Gonioscopically open anterior chamber angles
- Absence of other causes of glaucoma or pressure elevation
- Reduced aqueous outflow.

The eyes with primary open angle glaucoma have characteristic optic nerve damage with excavation and neuroretinal rim loss and thinning with increased cup to disc ratio consequent to loss and degeneration of retinal ganglion cell axons and attenuation and loss of the retinal nerve fiber layer. These individuals have open, uncharacteristic appearing anterior chamber angles on gonioscopic evaluation and arcuate nerve fiber bundle type of visual field defects matching the optic nerve and retinal nerve fiber loss and attenuation. Though bilateral, POAG is usually asymmetric in presentation, with moderate to advanced optic nerve excavation in one eye and minimal to undetectable disc damage in the fellow eye. Intraocular pressure elevation, though an important and most crucial causative risk factor in primary open angle glaucoma in not always found to be elevated, although most patients with POAG have elevated IOP in the range

22 to 40 mm Hg. Few patients invariably have IOP less than 18 mm Hg and are presumed to have a variant of POAG referred to as the normal pressure glaucoma. IOP is subject to diurnal variation and individuals with POAG have wider fluctuation of IOP than normals. Demonstrating diurnal IOP fluctuation may be useful in diagnosing POAG, explaining progressive damage despite apparently normal IOP measurements estimated in the clinicians' office, evaluating efficacy of pressure lowering therapy and distinguishing normal pressure glaucoma from POAG.

An increased resistance to aqueous outflow due to *reduced facility of aqueous outflow* is the basic abnormality contributing to IOP elevation in POAG and consequent optic nerve damage. Outflow facility progressively deteriorates with worsening glaucoma, although measurement of aqueous outflow is not part of a routine clinical evaluation.

A relative afferent pupil defect is characteristic of patients with asymmetric or unilateral glaucoma (Marcus Gunn sign elicited by swinging flashlight test).

Features of Acquired Optic Nerve Damage in Glaucoma

- Progressive thinning of neuroretinal rim
- Vertical optic cup enlargement
- Selective neural rim loss and notching
- Splinter hemorrhages in the disc margin
- Asymmetry between optic cups ≥ 0.2 in discs of equal size
- Neural retinal rim slope
- Optic nerve cupping that exceeds pallor
- Retinal nerve fiber layer defects
- Peripapillary atrophy

DIFFERENTIAL DIAGNOSIS

Glaucomas other than primary open angle mechanisms need to be differentiated carefully by meticulous clinical examination, especially gonioscopy. Intermittent and subacute or chronic

angle closure glaucoma may present with elevated IOP and characteristic optic nerve damage and visual field loss as primary open angle glaucoma, but gonioscopic evaluation reveal narrow anterior chamber angles or peripheral anterior synechiae. Excessively pigmented trabecular meshwork indicates pigmentary or exfoliative glaucoma. Evidence of past ocular trauma, such as angle recession, may signify secondary forms of open angle glaucoma. Prior use of corticosteroids, history of uveitis or trauma could have caused transient IOP elevation and glaucomatous optic disc damage. **Visual field defects** simulating glaucoma are caused by several retinal and optic nerve diseases, including ischemic optic neuropathy and compressive lesions of the optic nerve, chiasma and the visual pathway, which calls for a careful neuro-ophthalmic evaluation. Atypical visual field changes, central visual loss, and pallor of the neuroretinal rim that exceeds cupping are some of the characteristics suggestive of neurological disease simulating glaucoma. Careful retinal evaluation may reveal retinal detachment, chorioretinitis, arterial or venous occlusions, photocoagulation scars or retinoschisis that accounts for the visual field changes. Congenital optic nerve abnormalities, such as optic nerve pits and colobomas are often associated with large cups and occasionally associated with arcuate pattern of nerve fiber bundle type visual field defects, making differentiation from glaucomatous optic nerve difficult. Such field defects tend to be nonprogressive over-time and in case of suspicion, need to be followed-up periodically with baseline visual field evaluation and stereoscopic fundus photographs. *In the absence of raised IOP or other typical features, the diagnosis of POAG needs to be re-evaluated in each visit to exclude other possible causes for progressive visual field loss or change in the appearance of the optic nerve head.*

PATHOLOGY AND PATHOPHYSIOLOGY

A discussion of pathophysiology of primary open angle glaucoma in general addresses two basic issues: Mechanisms of IOP elevation and pathophysiology of optic nerve damage in glaucoma.

Decreased Facility of Aqueous Humor Outflow and Elevation of IOP

Increased IOP seen in most eyes with primary open angle glaucoma is due to a decrease in the facility of outflow of aqueous through the aqueous outflow pathways in the eye. Most resistance to aqueous outflow is seen to exist between the anterior chamber and the lumen of the Schlemm's canal, since incising the trabecular meshwork reduces the resistance to aqueous outflow by about 75 percent.[34,35] Microcannulation and measurement of pressures within trabecular outflow seem to suggest that maximal resistance to aqueous outflow resides in the juxtacanalicular[36,37] tissue. Although alternate hypothesis seems to suggest collapse of Schlemm's canal as a crucial aspect of increase in resistance to aqueous outflow, it has been suggested that such canalicular collapse is possible only under situations of high ocular pressures. There is no evidence to support the view that collapse of Schlemm's canal[38] could occur with an IOP of 25 to 35 mm Hg, as is the situation in most eyes with POAG. Obstruction to intrascleral collector channels has also been hypothesized to cause resistance to aqueous outflow.

Several theories have been put forth that seek to explain the increased resistance to outflow of aqueous humor in the trabecular tissue or the endothelium of Schlemm's canal:

1. Obstruction by extraneous material: Accumulation of pigment, red blood cells, glycosaminoglycans,[39] proteins, amorphous material, collagen, elastin or plaque like material in the trabecular meshwork and juxtacanalicular[40-42] tissue. A normal constituent of the trabecular meshwork that is synthesized excessively or metabolized inadequately is also likely to contribute to outflow resistance.

2. Eyes with glaucoma have fewer trabecular endothelial cells[43,44] than normal eyes. Loss of trabecular cells interferes with normal physiologic functions including synthesis and degradation of macromolecules and phagocytic activity. Phagocytosis in the trabeculum represents a self-cleaning mechanism to rid the outflow pathways of cells and other extracellular materials.

3. A reduction of Giant Vacuoles in the inner wall of endothelium of Schlemm's canal: The giant vacuoles are hypothesized to play a crucial role in transport of fluid from the trabecular meshwork to Schlemm's canal. Reduction of giant vacuolar activity[45,46] is likely to contribute to significant reduction in aqueous humor outflow.

4. A reduction in size and pore density[47] of the inner wall of Schlemm's canal endothelium.

Histopathologic studies of the aqueous drainage pathways, in summary, reveal several abnormalities including alterations in trabecular beams and fragmentation of collagen, narrowed intertrabecular spaces, fused trabecular beams, decreased trabecular endothelial cells, reduced actin filaments, decreased giant vacuoles, narrowing of collector channels and collapse of Schlemm's canal. Some of these changes are observed in eyes of older individuals without glaucoma, and it is surmised that changes in glaucoma are accelerated changes that occur with aging of normal eyes. Moreover, histopathologic changes need to be interpreted with caution since many of these changes could result from long standing IOP elevation, rather than being the cause for elevated intraocular pressures. Most specimens are obtained during glaucoma surgery or from cadaver eyes postmortem, and hence artifacts could be common, making any interpretation of histological changes difficult.

Investigators have proposed several mechanisms to further explain the reasons behind elevated resistance to aqueous outflow. These include alterations in corticosteroid metabolism, dysfunctional adrenergic control, abnormal immunologic processes and role of oxidative stress.

Altered corticosteroid metabolism: It has been proposed that IOP response to topical corticosteroids in susceptible individuals is inherited and is closely linked to the inheritance of POAG. Further research has postulated that endogenous corticosteroids affect trabecular function[48,49] by alteration of prostaglandin and glycosaminoglycan metabolism, synthesis of lysosomal enzymes or cyclic AMP, or inhibition of phagocytosis. Mutations in the trabecular induced glucocorticoid response (TIGR) gene are associated with production of an abnormal, mutant form of glucocorticoid inducible stress response protein called *Myocilin*[50] and are associated with several forms of juvenile open angle glaucoma and a subset of patients with adult onset primary open angle glaucoma.

Abnormal immunologic processes have been postulated to account for the increased outflow resistance to aqueous in POAG. Evidence for immunologic processes in pathogenesis of diminished aqueous outflow include:

- Increased levels of gamma globulins and plasma cells in trabeculum of POAG
- Higher levels of antinuclear antibodies in persons with open angle glaucoma
- Association between POAG and human leukocyte antigens
- Endothelin like immunoreactivity in aqueous of POAG eyes

- Antibodies to heat shock proteins (cell stress proteins) are elevated in POAG serum
- A therapeutic neuroprotective vaccine for treatment of glaucoma based on the hypothesis of immunoreactivity in pathogenesis of POAG has been proposed.

Oxidative damage and influence of other toxins in pathogenesis of glaucoma: Identification of glutathione in the trabecular meshwork of calves has led to the hypothesis that it protects trabecular endothelium from the oxidative insult of hydrogen peroxide and continues to be investigated. It has also been postulated that transforming growth factor β_2 and plasminogen activator inhibitor which have been reported to be significantly increased in concentration in the aqueous of POAG patients as compared to controls may play a role in pathogenesis of increased IOP. To date, no single theory explains trabecular dysfunction in POAG and the precise mechanisms underlying increased outflow resistance remains unclear.

Recently, a new model that describes an *Aqueous outflow pump*[51] has been put forth and explains the aqueous pump failure as a mechanism in primary open angle glaucoma. According to this model, the aqueous outflow system is structured to act as a mechanical pump. The trabecular meshwork actively distends and recoils in response to IOP fluctuation that occurs with ocular pulse, blinking and eye movement. Trabecular flexibility is thus essential for the normal function of the proposed aqueous pump. Aqueous valves transfer aqueous from the anterior chamber to the Schlemm's canal and their normal function requires that trabecular tissues retain their flexibility to recoil from the Schlemm's canal external wall. The aqueous pump provides short-term pressure control by varying stroke volume in response to pressure change and long-term pressure control by regulating trabecular meshwork constituents that control stroke volume. The aqueous pump fails in glaucoma owing to Schlemm's canal apposition and trabecular stiffening. Reversal of pump failure requires Schlemm's canal lumen enlargement. Surgical techniques targeted at the scleral spur and its ciliary body attachment is expected to reverse the structural abnormality restoring the pump failure in open angle glaucoma.

TREATMENT

Data from recently published randomized clinical trials in glaucoma are useful in broadly guiding treatment plans in management of primary open angle glaucoma. Treatment is indicated in all forms of primary open angle glaucoma, with established optic nerve damage and visual field loss attributable to glaucoma irrespective of the level of IOP, since IOP lowering treatment has been proved to be of benefit even in normal pressure glaucoma. Treatment is imperative in younger individuals and those with longer expectancy with demonstrable optic nerve damage and who are likely to go blind in their lifetime. Treatment may be deferred with periodical evaluation in persons with limited life-expectancy and minimal optic nerve damage. However, in instances wherein it is difficult to predict longevity or progression of glaucoma, it is prudent to initiate therapy since several drugs to reduce IOP with significant safety margin are currently available. Development of typical glaucomatous visual field loss, progressive cupping of optic nerve head even in the absence of visual field defects, corneal edema attributable to elevated IOP, vascular occlusion and disc hemorrhages associated with elevated IOP are also definite indications for treatment.

The major goal of glaucoma therapy is to preserve patient's vision for his/her lifetime with as minimal disturbance of the quality of life as possible. Current evidence suggests lowering of IOP by appropriate therapy to a level that will cease progressive retinal ganglion cell loss or visual field progression. The treatment goal is to maximize visual function by stabilization of the course of the disease, and preserve patient's quality of life by minimal adverse events by treatment in the most cost-effective manner as feasible.

Target Intraocular Pressure

Once the decision to treat has been made, treatment goal needs to be set. Target IOP is defined as the level of intraocular pressure below which retinal ganglion cell loss other than due to ageing ceases to occur. Achieving target IOP in persons with glaucoma results in lowering the rate of ganglion cell loss to that of age matched controls and prevents further visual loss. Although there is no well defined methodology to determine target IOP, it is generally believed that more damaged the optic nerve or greater the visual field loss, lower the IOP target needs to be set to prevent progressive loss of visual function. A grading system recommended by the American Academy of Ophthalmology aids in quantifying glaucomatous damage so that an approximate target IOP could be set:

Mild glaucoma: Characteristic optic nerve abnormalities consistent with glaucoma, but visual fields are normal.

Moderate glaucoma: Visual field abnormalities (matching optic disc changes) in one hemifield, but not within five degrees of fixation.

Severe glaucoma: Visual field abnormalities in both hemifields or within five degrees of fixation.

In mild glaucoma, a 20 percent reduction of untreated IOP or an IOP of 17-18 mm Hg is prudent. In moderate glaucoma, a 30 percent reduction or IOP in mid teens (14-16 mm Hg) and in severe glaucoma, 35-40 percent reduction or an IOP less than 12 mm Hg is considered appropriate. Most eyes with advanced glaucoma would require IOP in very low teens or even in single digits to prevent progressive glaucomatous damage. Data from the Advanced Glaucoma Intervention Study (AGIS)[52] also support this view since the study substantiated visual field stability in patients with IOP consistently below 18 mm Hg with a mean IOP of 12.3 mm Hg. Maintaining IOP consistently below 18 mm Hg in a patient with mild to moderate glaucoma and at still lower levels (low teens) in patients with advanced disc damage seems like a reasonable IOP goal. However, individual optic nerves differ in their susceptibility to effect of IOP, and hence, the target IOP determined by these simple guidelines need not be fixed target. If optic nerve excavation or visual field loss progress despite achieving the target pressures so determined, one needs to set the target IOP at a lower level and treatment needs to be more aggressive. Periodical evaluation of glaucoma related damage is mandatory to reset the target IOP to stabilize visual loss.

Achieving low target pressures imply higher treatment costs and treatment related adverse effects due to multiple medications required. Although it is desirable to achieve lowest possible IOPs to stabilize visual loss in glaucoma, this has to be individualized in the light of patients' requirements. If adverse effects of medications or higher cost preclude use of multiple medications, higher IOP than target may be acceptable provided no further optic nerve damage is documented.

Initial Treatment Modality

Once target IOP is determined, treatment modalities available to achieve it is discussed with the patient. Although medical, surgical and laser options as initial treatment is available, medical treatment is generally chosen and if maximal medications do not achieve target IOP, more aggressive modalities are chosen. Although some studies have reported success with initial trabeculectomy surgery, these studies were conducted before the era when newer generations of medications in glaucoma were introduced. Randomized Clinical Trials in glaucoma in general seem to conclude that lowering IOP tends to preserve vision and filtering surgery achieves maximal lowering of IOP as compared to medical or laser treatment. Filtering surgery, is however associated with increased incidence of decline in visual acuity and cataract as compared to other modalities of treatment. Moreover, the Collaborative initial Glaucoma Treatment Study (CIGTS)[53] trial provided data to prove equivalent visual field stability between initial surgery and medical treatment arms over five years. Although medical treatment is relatively safe with only reversible adverse effects, if any, on initial treatment, this modality of treatment has several disadvantages. Long-term medical therapy has adverse outcome on filtering surgery performed subsequently. The failure to adhere to medical treatment regimen is a major issue in failure of treatment. Nonadherence to treatment regimen is a leading cause of blindness from glaucoma and approximately 10 percent of all visual loss in glaucoma is attributable to nonadherence. Escalating cost of drug therapy, adverse effects and complicated dose regimen are crucial factors in determining poor adherence. Physicians also need to ensure that patients follow-up at periodic intervals to monitor efficacy of medical management. Significant barriers to follow-up exist especially in developing societies like India[53,54] and knowledge of these barriers may assist physicians in better management of patients with glaucoma on medical therapy. Laser trabeculoplasty may have a limited role as initial treatment of choice in individuals with poor compliance, although the effects of trabeculoplasty may only be temporary. Even in the western world, only 50 percent of those eyes undergoing trabeculoplasty have effective lowering of IOP in five years. At the other end of the spectrum, primary filtering surgery is an appropriate initial therapy in individuals who have advanced visual field loss or optic nerve damage or significantly elevated IOP wherein target IOP is not considered to be achievable by any other means of treatment modality. A subset of individuals with primary juvenile open angle with high levels of IOP on presentation and considerable optic nerve damage respond poorly to medical treatment and are likely to significantly benefit from initial filtering surgery. However, in most of these individuals, an initial medical treatment is warranted to lower IOP before filtering surgery is contemplated. In a few of these patients, adequate IOP control with medical treatment may obviate the need for initial filtering surgery. Whatever initial therapy is selected, it is crucial to closely follow-up the patients for monitoring of IOP and possible progression. If after adequate trial of one modality, there is insufficient control of IOP or progressive disc or field loss, it is imperative to switch to an alternative treatment modality. In a randomized clinical trial in South India,[55] clinically meaningful IOP reduction was achieved over an intermediate term follow-up with initial medical or surgical treatment of open angle glaucomas and no significant alterations with quality of life were observed in subjects randomized to initial surgery.

Initial Medical Management in POAG

Once the decision to treat POAG with medications is made, the ophthalmologist has to choose the medical therapy that will best suit the individual patient needs and will aim to reduce the IOP to target IOP in the least dosage and in the most cost-effective manner with minimal if any adverse events and minimal effect on quality of life. Prior to initiating therapy, the ophthalmologist has to review the patient's medical history, allergies and any experience with prior glaucoma medications. Documentation of the efficacy or otherwise of any glaucoma medications and adverse outcome of any medications in the past in the patient medical records is mandatory to prevent the likelihood of repeating the similar medications with poor outcome. A careful review of the medical history and a systemic, in particular cardiovascular evaluation is mandated in persons in whom beta blockers are contemplated for reduction of IOP. Beta blockers are contraindicated in patients with bronchial asthma, chronic obstructive pulmonary disease (COPD) or bradycardia. Elderly individuals without overt cardiovascular or respiratory disease, but with poor cardiopulmonary reserve, could become symptomatic with use of nonspecific beta blockers like timolol or levobunolol. Carbonic anhydrase inhibitors have to be used with caution in individuals with calcific kidney disease, metabolic acidosis and sulfonamide allergy. Individuals on prolonged therapy with acetazolamide have to be evaluated frequently to exclude blood dyscrasias due to bone marrow suppression.

Individuals with ocular diseases may also affect the choice of medical therapy in glaucoma. Uveitis, cystoid macular edema and herpes virus infections may be exacerbated or reactivated with the use of prostaglandin analogs. Although currently seldom used, dipiverfin and epinephrine derivatives can cause cystoid macular edema in aphakic eyes and miotics like pilocarpine can decrease visual acuity in persons with cataracts and advanced glaucoma. Stronger miotics and pilocarpine are also cataractogenic and can predispose to retinal breaks and detachments.

In the absence of systemic contraindications like chronic obstructive pulmonary disease (COPD) or congestive heart failure, a nonselective beta blocker is usually an initial choice of treatment of POAG. The beta blockers have been in use for about three decades now, have good ocular and systemic safety profile in individuals with no known cardiac or pulmonary disease, generally well tolerated, inexpensive and effective in a large number of individuals with elevated IOP. A range of beta blockers have been available to choose from, apart from the nonselective beta adrenergic antagonist and the widely preferred timolol. Betaxolol is a nonselective beta$_1$ antagonist which has been proved relatively safe alternative in individuals with COPD. Carteolol, though not available in India, can be used in individuals with coronary artery disease and hyperlipidemias.

Prostaglandin Analogs
In the absence of contraindications, one of the three available prostaglandin analogs Bimatoprost, Latanoprost or Travoprost are excellent initial treatment options in the management of primary open angle glaucoma. They are also the drugs of choice in presence of systemic medical conditions like bronchopulmonary and cardiovascular diseases. These medications are known to have better efficacy than beta blockers in reduction of IOP and require once daily dosage, increasing patient adherence and compliance. IOP fluctuation has been observed to be an independent and significant risk factor in progression of open angle glaucoma.

Prostaglandins offer better diurnal IOP control than other ocular hypotensive medications, making them an obvious first line drug in preference to other glaucoma medications. Several studies have observed differences in the IOP reducing potency of these prostaglandin analogs, but they are of no practical, clinical significance in considering initial medical treatment for glaucoma. Bimatoprost has been considered to be the most cost-effective of these prostaglandin analogs for each mm reduction of IOP, though ocular adverse effects like conjunctival hyperemia, periocular pigmentation and hypertrichosis in general are more common following the use of bimatoprost than other prostaglandins. Latanoprost is effective in lowering IOP with minimal ocular adverse event of all the prostaglandins, but needs to be refrigerated and is of questionable use in many remote, rural regions in the Indian subcontinent. Bimatoprost and travoprost need not be refrigerated and a preservative free latanoprost has recently been made available that makes refrigeration unnecessary and is likely to further improve its adverse effect profile. Availability of generic versions of prostaglandins in India have significantly reduced the cost of medical treatment and have become the widely used drugs in the initial management of primary open angle glaucoma. If there is no adequate response to one prostaglandin, switching to other analogues may be beneficial in obtaining IOP lowering. Prostaglandins and nonselective beta blockers represent most effective[56] ever available in management of open angle glaucoma.

Alpha$_2$ Agonist
In select individuals, brimonidine, an alpha$_2$ selective agonist, is also chosen as an initial drug for reduction of intraocular pressure. Brimonidine reduces aqueous secretion, increases

uveoscleral outflow and is known to be neuroprotective in animal models with optic nerve injury. Patients with cardiopulmonary disease, those with history of ocular inflammation or recently subject to intraocular surgery may benefit from brimonidine as initial therapy.

Carbonic Anhydrase Inhibitors

Topical carbonic anhydrase inhibitors (CAIs) such as dorzolamide or brinzolamide are useful since they reduce IOP without the systemic adverse events of oral CAI like acetazolamide. The IOP lowering efficacy of dorzolamide is lesser than timolol or prostaglandins, though the carbonic anhydrase inhibitors are an effective alternatives in fixed combinations with timolol.

Fixed Combinations

Fixed combinations of timolol with brimonidine, dorzolamide and latanoprost are now widely available for clinical use, and although it is preferable to begin therapy with a single drug and assess its efficacy before trying a combination of drugs, some clinical situations warrant initiation of therapy with a combination of drugs to achieve lower IOP in a shorter time, such as in eyes with advanced optic nerve damage. In such situations, fixed drug combinations as initial therapy offers several advantages. There is increased compliance since there is reduction in the number of medications to be used, and there is lesser exposure to preservatives from multiple drugs, which decreases ocular adverse effects. The cost of therapy is less and compliance significantly enhanced with the use of fixed combination therapy.

Medical therapy is used as first line treatment of primary open angle glaucoma in most practices around the globe and use of trabeculectomy/ filtering surgeries to reduce IOP have declined across the world, including India, owing to the availability of several ocular hypotensive drugs in the last decade. Although the adverse effects of medical treatment could be diverse, they are seldom severe enough to threaten vision or life of the individuals. Most drug side effects are also completely reversible on cessation of therapy. The physician should prescribe the least number of drugs at the safest possible dosage required to control the IOP at the desired level. It is crucial to ensure that patients comply with the prescribed regimen and measure IOP at different times of the day and at different intervals to estimate efficacy of treatment and response to therapy. When one medication lowers IOP, but the reduction is still not sufficient to achieve the desired target IOP goal, a second medication may be added. If the initial therapy with a drug fails to reduce IOP to any significant extent, switching to another class of drug is preferable. Maximum medical therapy currently consists of a prostaglandin analog, beta blocker, topical carbonic anhydrase inhibitor and an alpha receptor agonist. Miotics are also useful in select eyes, as in individuals with glaucoma in aphakia and pseudophakia.

Laser Trabeculoplasty

When medical treatment fails to achieve target IOP, argon or selective laser trabeculoplasty is a viable option in some individuals with POAG. Laser trabeculoplasty (ALT or SLT) could also be a primary treatment in individuals who are unlikely to use medical therapy due to cost, adverse effects or poor adherence to treatment. This technique significantly reduces IOP in 70 to 80 percent of patients, though most individuals continue to require some medications to achieve target IOP. It has, however been possible to substantially reduce the number of medications[57] required in eyes subject to laser trabeculoplasty. Although published data in India is lacking, use of SLT is reported to reduce IOP significantly in 70 to 80 percent of patients with reduction in number of medications required to achieve target IOP. Periodical follow-up is essential since most studies have reported the effects of SLT to be temporary and short lived. Though no prospective studies are available from India on the efficacy of selective laser trabeculoplasty, a five years study of argon laser trabeculoplasty[58] as primary treatment in primary open angle glaucoma revealed mean IOP reduction after laser treatment to be about 7 mm Hg (from a mean pre laser IOP of 25.8 mm Hg to 18.1 mm Hg post laser after five years of follow-up).

Role of Glaucoma Filtering Surgery

If medical treatment and/or laser is insufficient to control progression of POAG, filtering surgery is the only option and has been reported to control IOP in 80 to 90 percent of individuals with POAG. Racial differences are also reported in the response to filtering surgery and the result of the Collaborative Initial Glaucoma Treatment Study (CIGTS)[53] which reported primary medical as well as surgical treatment of primary open angle glaucoma to be equally effective in controlling IOP over intermediate to long-term, may justify primary filtering surgery as a viable option at least in select eyes in the developing world such as India and Africa, adherence to medical treatment may be questionable. It is preferable to use antimetabolite like mitomycin as adjunctive agents to act as pharmacological modulators to prevent or delay conjunctival scarring to enhance longterm filtering success. In a longterm dose response study of mitomycin[59] in India, significant reduction in IOP was achieved with mitomycin, and cataract progression was more frequent in eyes receiving a higher dose of the antimetabolite. Hypotony and other sight threatening complications were relatively infrequent. One needs to be cautious in avoiding adverse effects of antifibrosis agents like mitomycin, and Peng Khaw's modified technique of trabeculectomy[60] is recommended to minimize long term bleb complications from the use of antimetabolite agents in glaucoma filtering surgery. In a long term evaluation of trabeculectomy[62] without antimetabolite in Asian eyes for ten years, surgery appeared to be efficacious in control of IOP and visual field preservation.

If one drainage procedure fails to control IOP or if the risk factors for failure are high, a glaucoma drainage device can be used. A study of Ahmad Glaucoma Valves[61] in India has reported 30 percent IOP lowering with minimal complications in eyes at risk of filtering surgery failure.

Ciliary body ablation to control IOP by reducing aqueous humor formation by trans scleral cycloablation or endocyclophotocoagualiton is reserved for end stage glaucoma.

COURSE AND PROGNOSIS/OUTCOME OF PRIMARY OPEN ANGLE GLAUCOMA

The visual prognosis and outcome in primary open angle glaucoma depends on several factors and include:

- Age
- Severity of optic nerve damage
- The level of IOP
- The vulnerability of optic disc tissue
- Progression of visual field defect
- Response to treatment
- Adherence/compliance to therapy
- Systemic vascular disease.

The St Lucia[63] study, one of the few studies available on the course of untreated primary open angle glaucoma, observed 35 percent of eyes progressing to end stage disease in 10 years and progressive visual field loss observed in 55 percent. On the other hand, progression is slower in treated eyes—approximately a third of patients progressed in nine years longitudinal follow-up. In a yet another retrospective study in Caucasian eyes, 68 percent of patients had progressive visual field deterioration[64] in eight years with an average loss of 1.5 percent per year. The Olmsted County[65] study, yet another retrospective study, detected bilateral progression in 9 percent of treated eyes and unilateral progression in 27 percent in a Caucasian population observed for 20 years. Chen,[66] however had reported that bilateral blindness is uncommon in treated open angle glaucoma and those unilaterally blind were those who had already been blind at the time of diagnosis. The Early Manifest Glaucoma Treatment Study which randomized individuals with early open angle glaucoma to treatment or no treatment, reported 53 percent of recruited individuals to have progressed[67] during the six years of observation. Treatment had reduced the risk of progression of glaucoma by half. Both eyes of the same individual in general respond similarly to IOP rise and to ocular hypotensive treatment. Progression in one eye usually implies more aggressive treatment in both the eyes to limit further progression of disc damage and visual field loss. IOP lowering also needs to be very aggressive with lowest possible target IOP goals in eyes with advanced disc loss or visual field defects since progression to blindness is more likely in eyes with advanced structural and functional loss at diagnosis. Patients with advanced optic nerve damage hence have a worse visual prognosis[68,69] since a damaged optic nerve is more susceptible to further damage even at a lower IOP and hence these eyes require a low normal or even subnormal IOP to stabilize visual function. In a recently published study of predictive factors of progressive damage in chronic open angle glaucoma, the risk factors identified for progression[70] were older age, advanced field loss, smaller neuroretinal rim, and larger area of beta zone peripapillary atrophy.

The response and susceptibility of optic nerve damage to IOP is also highly variable between individuals. While some eyes tolerate elevated IOP for longer periods, others suffer progressive damage at apparently normal levels of IOP and is explained by variable response of the optic nerve tissue to pressure induced damage. Variations in optic nerve perfusion may also play a role in such individual susceptibility to neuronal damage since correlation has been observed between low blood flow velocity in retinal circulation and progression. Control of intraocular pressure, however, remains the only treatable factor in containing progression of glaucomatous nerve damage. Whilst some clinicians subscribe to the to the theory that natural history of glaucoma is not altered by treatment, the consensus of most, based on evidence available from clinical trials, is that control of IOP stabilizes the disease or slows the course of progressive glaucoma[72,73] in most individuals, delaying blindness. Some individuals, though continue to have progressive visual field loss[71] despite marked reduction in IOP by therapeutic intervention. Current evidence, however, favors reduction of IOP as the most appropriate and cost-effective approach[74] to stabilize visual function in individuals with primary open angle glaucoma.

REFERENCES

1. Wilson MR. Primary open angle glaucoma: magnitude of the problem in the US. J Glaucoma 1992;1:64.
2. Tielsch JM, et al. Racial variations in the prevalence of primary open angle glaucoma. The Baltimore Eye Survey. JAMA 1991;266:369.
3. Quigley HA, Broman AT. The number of people with glaucoma worldwide in 2010 and 2020. Br J Ophthalmol 2006; 90(3):262-7
4. Iwase A, Suzuki Y, Araie M, et al. The prevalence of primary open-angle glaucoma in Japanese: the Tajimi Study. Ophthalmology 2004;111:1641-8.
5. Ntim-Amponsah CT, et al. Prevalence of glaucoma in an African population. Eye 2004;18:491.
6. Jacob A, Thomas R, Koshy SP, et al. The prevalence of glaucoma in an urban South Indian population. Ind J Ophthalmol 1998;46:81.
7. Vijaya L, George R, Paul PG, et al. Prevalence of open angle glaucoma in an urban South Indian population in comparison with a rural population. The Chennai Glaucoma Study. Ophthalmol 2008;115:648.
8. Dandona L, Dandona R, Srinivas M, et al. Open angle glaucoma in an urban population in South India: the Andhra Pradesh Eye Disease Study. Ophthalmol 2000;107:1702.
9. Ramakrishnan R, Nirmalan PK, Krishnadas R. Glaucoma in a rural-population of South India: the Aravind Comprehensive Eye Survey. Ophthalmol 2003;110:1484.
10. Leske MC, et al. Incidence of open angle glaucoma: The Barbados Eye Study. Arch Ophthalmol 2001;119:89.
11. Gordon MO, et al. The Ocular Hypertension Treatment Study: baseline factors that predict the onset of primary open angle glaucoma. Arch Ophthalmol 2002;120:714.
12. Bengtsson B, et al. Early Manifest Glaucoma Trial Group: Fluctuation of IOP and glaucoma progression in the Early Manifest Glaucoma Trial. Ophthalmol 2007;114:205.
13. Collaborative Normal Tension Glaucoma Study Group: Comparison of glaucomatous progression between untreated patients with normal tension glaucoma and patients with therapeutically reduced intraocular pressures. Am J Ophthalmol 1998;126:487.
14. The AGIS Investigators: The Advanced Glaucoma Intervention Study (AGIS): 7. The relationship between control of intraocular pressure and visual field deterioration. Am J Ophthalmol 2000;130:429.
15. Hollows FC, Graham PA. Intraocular pressure, Glaucoma, Glaucoma suspects in a defined population. Br J Ophthalmol 1966;50:570.
16. Bengtsson B. The prevalence of glaucoma. Br J Ophthalmol 1981;65:46.
17. Leibowitz, et al. The Framingham Eye Study: Monograph, Surv Ophthalmol 1980; 24(suppl):1.
18. Martin MJ, et al. Race and primary open angle glaucoma. Am J Ophthalmol 1985;99:383.
19. Sommer A, et al. Racial differences in the cause specific prevalence of blindness in East Baltimore. N Engl J Med 1991;325:1412.
20. Racette L, et al. Primary open angle glaucoma in Blacks, a Review. Surv Ophthalmol 2003;48:295.
21. Leske MC, Connell AM, Wu SY, et al. Risk factors for open angle glaucoma. The Barbados Eye Study. Arch Ophthalmol 1995;113:918.
22. Leske MC, Nemesure B, He Q, et al. Patterns of open angle glaucoma in the Barbados Family Study. Ophthalmol 2001;108:1015.
23. Tielsh JM, et al. Family history and risk of primary open angle glaucoma: The Baltimore Eye Survey. Arch Ophthalmol 1994;112:69.
24. Wolfs RC, Klaver CC, Ramrattan RS, et al. Genetic risk of primary open angle glaucoma. Population based familial aggregation study. Arch Ophthalmol 1998;116:1640.
25. Daubs JB, Pitts-Crick R. Effect of refractive error on the risk of ocular hypertension and open angle glaucoma. Trans Ophthalmol Soc UK 1981;101:121.
26. Perkins ES, Phelps CD. Open angle glaucoma, ocular hypertension, low tension glaucoma, and refraction. Arch Ophthalmol 1982;100:1464.
27. Shulzer M, Drance SM, Douglas GR. A comparison of treated and untreated glaucoma suspects. Ophthalmol 1991;98;301.
28. Anderson DR. Collaborative Normal Tension Glaucoma Study. Current Opinion in Ophthalmology 2003;14:86.
29. Budenz DL, Anderson DR, Feuer WJ, et al. Detection and prognostic significance of optic disc hemorrhages during the Ocular Hypertension Treatment Study. Ophthalmol 2006;113:2137.
30. Xu L, Wang Y, Wang S, et al. High myopia and glaucoma susceptibility. The Beijing Eye Study. Ophthalmol 2007;114:216.
31. Ohtsuka K, Nakamura Y. Open angle glaucoma associated with Graves' disease. Am J Ophthalmol 2000;129: 613.
32. Leske MC, et al. Incident open angle glaucoma and blood pressure. Arch Ophthalmol 2002;120:954.
33. McGwin G Jr, et al. Statins and other cholesterol lowering drugs and the presence of glaucoma. Arch Ophthalmol 2004;122:822.
34. Grant WM. Further studies on the facility of flow through the trabecular meshwork. Arch Ophthalmol 1958; 60:523.
35. Peterson BA, Jocson VL, Sears MI. Resistance to aqueous outflow in the Rhesus monkey eye. Am J Ophthalmol 1971;72:445.
36. Johnson MC, Kamm RD. The role of Schlemm's canal in aqueous outflow from the human eye. Invest Ophthalmol Vis Sci 1983;24:320.

37. Bill A, Svedbergh B. Scanning electron microscopic studies of the trabecular meshwork and the canal of Schlemm: an attempt to localize the main resistance to outflow of aqueous humor in man. Acta Ophthalmol 1972;50:295.

38. Moses RA, et al. Schlemm's canal: the effect of intraocular pressure. Invest Ophthalmol Vis Sci 1981;20:61.

39. Segawa K. Electron microscopic changes of the trabecular tissue in primary open angle glaucoma. Ann Ophthalmol 1979;11:49.

40. Rohen JW. Why is intraocular pressure elevated in chronic simple glaucoma? Ophthalmol 1982;90:758.

41. Alvarado JA, Yun AJ, Murphy CG. Juxtacanalicular tissue in primary open angle glaucoma and nonglaucomatous normals. Arch Ophthalmol 1986;104:1517.

42. Lutgen-Drecoll E, Shimiza T, Rohrback M. Quantitative analysis of plaque material in the inner and outer wall of Schlemm's canal in normal and glaucomatous eyes. Exp Eye Res 1986;42:443.

43. Alvarado JA, Murphy CG, Juster R. Trabecular meshwork cellularity in primary open angle glaucoma and nonglaucomatous normals. Ophthalmol 1984;91:564.

44. Grierson I, Howes RC. Age related depletion of the cell population in the human trabecular meshwork. Eye 1987;1:204.

45. Tripathi RC. Ultrastructure of the trabecular wall of Schlemm's canal (a study of normotensive and chronic simple glaucomatous eyes). Trans Ophthalmol Soc UK 1969;89:449.

46. Alvarado JA, Murphy CG. Outflow obstruction in pigmentary and primary open angle glaucoma. Arch Ophthalmol 1992;110:1769.

47. Allingham RR, et al. The relationship between pore density and outflow facility in human eyes. Invest Ophthalmol Vis Sci 1996;33:1661.

48. Bigger JF, Palmberg PF, Becker B. Increased cellular sensitivity to glucocorticoids in primary open angle glaucoma. Invest Ophthalmol 1972; 11:832.

49. Kass MA, Shin DH, Becker B. The ocular hypotensive effect of epinephrine in high and low corticosteroid responders. Invest Ophthalmol 1977;16:530.

50. Stone EM, et al. Identification of a gene that causes primary open angle glaucoma. Science 1997;275:668.

51. Johnstone MA. A New Model describes an Aqueous Outflow Pump and explores cause of pump failure in Glaucoma. Essentials of Ophthalmology (Glaucoma): Springer-Verlag, Berlin Heidelberg; 2006.pp.1-34.

52. The AGIS Investigators: The Advanced Glaucoma Intervention Study (AGIS) 7. The relationship between control of intraocular pressure and visual field deterioration. Am J Ophthalmol 2000; 130:429.

53. Lichter PR, et al. CIGTS Study Group: Intermediate clinical outcomes in the Collaborative Initial Glaucoma Treatment Study comparing initial treatment randomized to medications or surgery. Ophthalmol 2001;108:1943.

54. Lee B, Sathyan P, Rajesh J, Kuldev Singh, Robin AL. Predictors of and Barriers associated with poor follow-up in patients with glaucoma in South India. Arch Ophthalmol 2008; 126(10):1.

55. Congdon NG, Krishnadas R, Robin AL, et al. A Randomized Trial of medicines vs Surgery of Glaucoma in India. Invest Ophthalmol Vis Sci 2006;47: E-Abstract 3430.

56. Vander Valk R, et al. Intraocular pressure lowering effects of commonly used glaucoma drugs: a meta-analysis of randomized clinical trials. Ophthalmol 2005;112:1177.

57. Francis BA, et al. Selective laser trabeculoplasty as a replacement for medical therapy in open angle glaucoma. Am J Ophthalmol 2005;140:524.

58. Agarwal HC, Sihota R, Das C, Dada T. The effect of argon laser trabeculoplasty as primary and secondary therapy in open angle glaucoma in Indian patients. Br J Ophthalmol 2002;86: 733.

59. Robin AL, Krishnadas R, Ramakrishnan, R, et al. A long-term dose response study of mitomycin in glaucoma filtering surgery. Arch Ophthalmol 1997; 115:969.

60. Khaw PT, Shah P. Trabeculectomy: The Moorfields safe surgery system. In: Mermoud A, Shaarawy T (Eds). Englan: Dunitz, Taylor and Frances Group Ltd, textbook of Glaucoma Surgery, 2005.

61. Das JC, Choudhury Z, Sharma P, Bhomaj S. The Ahmad Glaucoma Valve implantation in refractory glaucomas: experience in Indian eyes. Eye 2005;19:183.

62. Sihota R, Gupta V, Agarwal HC. A long term evaluation of trabeculectomy in primary open angle and chronic primary angle closure glaucoma in Asian population. Clin Experiment Ophthalmol 2004;32(1):23.

63. Wilson MR. Progression of visual field loss in untreated glaucoma patients and suspects in St Lucia, West Indies. Trans Am Ophthalmol Soc 2002; 100:365.

64. Kwon YH, et al. Rate of visual field loss and long-term visual outcome in primary open angle glaucoma. Am J Ophthalmol 2001;132:47.

65. Hattenhauer MG, et al. The probability of blindness from open angle glaucoma. Ophthalmol 1998;105:2099.

66. Chen PP. Blindness in patients with treated open angle glaucoma. Ophthalmol 2003;110:726.

67. Leske MC, et al. Early Manifest Glaucoma Trial Group. Factors for glaucoma progression and the effect of treatment: the early manifest glaucoma trial. Arch Ophthalmol 2003;121:48.

68. Perkins ES. Blindness from glaucoma and the economics of

prevention. Trans Ophthalmol Soc UK 1978;98:293.

69. Tezel G, et al. Clinical factors associated with progression of optic disc damage in treated patients. Arch Ophthalmol 2001;119:813.

70. Martus P, et al. Predictive factors for progressive optic nerve damage in various types of chronic open angle glaucoma, Am J Ophthalmol 2005;139:999.

71. Nouri-Mahdavi K, et al. Outcomes of trabeculectomy for primary open angle glaucoma. Ophthalmol 1995; 102;176.

72. Grant WM, Burke JF Jr. Why do some people go blind from glaucoma? Arch Ophthalmol 1982;89:991.

73. Quigley HA, Maumenee AE. Long-term follow-up of treated open angle glaucoma. Am J Ophthalmol 1979; 87:519.

74. Vicente C, et al. Association between mean intraocular pressure, disease stability and cost of treating glaucoma in Canada. Curr Med Res Opin 2004; 20:1245.

25

Normal Tension Glaucoma

Kundan Karan, George V Puthuran

INTRODUCTION

Normal tension glaucoma (NTG) has been one of the most intriguing and diagnostically important forms of glaucoma. It can be considered to be at one end of the spectrum of the open angle glaucomas with primary open angle glaucoma (POAG) being at the other end. The criteria defining NTG over the past 25 years have been highly variable. Though, in general, individuals with optic nerve head and visual field changes akin to glaucoma with open anterior chamber angles and with an IOP which has never been documented above 21 mm Hg are regarded as having NTG.[1] The term "Low tension glaucoma" has also been in vogue, though in NTG, the IOP is either in the 'higher' or 'intermediate' range but never in the 'low' range. Many authors believe that NTG is caused by the same IOP related factors which also lead to primary open angle glaucoma (POAG). However, there is a different school of thought which believes that NTG is caused by additional factors independent of IOP. There is a concept that the pressure in low tension glaucoma (as described by Chandler and Grant[2]) is benign and the disease course is not that unruly. But the disease is mostly progressive pointing to the fact that there might be individual increased susceptibility of the optic disc to intraocular pressures. It has been postulated that the vascular system might also be diseased lending the optic disc vulnerable to even low rise in IOP.[2] Almost all patients with NTG have an IOP-sensitive component. Progression results from this component combined with increased susceptibility of the optic nerve. One non-progressive form of NTG has also been described, but it is very rare.

Sometimes, confusion arises as to the definition of this entity if there has been a single record of IOP that is high. That is to say that when the IOP was consistently lower, whether a single high IOP reading result should be considered POAG or NTG. In such cases it is always safe to consider the diagnosis of NTG because of its aggressiveness. However, it really does not matter what one calls it, as long as it is clear that as for other patients with POAG, exfoliation, and low tension glaucoma, no matter what the IOP, the current level of IOP in the face of clinical progression is too high and therefore, one needs to lower the IOP further.

It can be thought that POAG is a spectrum of disorders where IOP is the predominant causative factor at one end, while other factors that influence glaucomatous optic atrophy predominate at the other end.[1]

Most patients with NTG are asymptomatic and are detected by the ophthalmologist on a routine examination except in case of a scotoma close to fixation. Sometimes, there might also be a credible history of sudden onset. In such cases one has to keep in mind the possibility of anterior ischaemic optic neuropathy (AION). Excluding that, one must observe that in NTG, these patients generally progress without any second episode of sudden onset. Neurological symptoms should be excluded, viz. weakness in extremities, dizziness, headaches, loss of consciousness, diplopia. Moreover, on examination, if the neuroretinal rim shows gross pallor even in the presence of cupping, there should be a detailed neurological examination for the same. The presence of these neurological symptoms in the presence of suspicious cupping but low tension has been termed "LTG-plus."[2]

Sometimes, in cases of POAG or exfoliation glaucoma, the disease progresses further even with low pressure even when the initial damage was caused at high pressures. Their behavior resembles that of NTG and has been termed "LTG equivalent."

The clinical features that are thought to distinguish between POAG and NTG are as follows.

DIFFERENCE BETWEEN PRIMARY OPEN ANGLE GLAUCOMA AND NORMAL TENSION GLAUCOMA
Optic Nerve Head

To start with NTG patients have a thinner neural rim in their optic nerve head as compared to POAG patients. This is even more evident in the inferior or inferotemporal quadrant.[3-5] Some studies, however, did not find any significant difference between the two. In one of the studies it was noted that the cupping in NTG was more sloping, resulting in diminished disc volume alternations.[1] In another study, the only difference noted was that of an "hourglass pattern" to the lamina cribrosa, in which thick connective tissue bundles crossed horizontally between 3 and 9 o' Clock positions, with thinner bundles and larger pores above and below.[6] However, such a difference was not striking enough to segregate high tension from the normal tension group, though it might be conceived that lamina cribrosa architecture might be a causative factor in differentiating the two types. Some studies have also noted larger disc areas in the NTG group while others have refuted it. A study of optic nerve head morphologic characteristics in the high tension and the normal tension groups showed no significant difference in any parameter as measured by laser scanning ophthalmoscopy.[7] Some other factors leading to NTG have been

studied. Some studies suggested that disc hemorrhages were more common in NTG group raising the probability of vascular causative factor for NTG.[8,9] However, some other studies found two subsets in the NTG group—one who had recurrent hemorrhages and another who rarely had any—leading to the possibility of nonvascular factors too as a contributory causative agent. Evidence in some studies suggests that the nerve fiber layer defect is more localized in the NTG group as compared to more diffused loss in the POAG group. It has also been said that the NTG patients have larger parapapillary atrophy as compared to the POAG group, though the appearance was the same when the stage of the glaucomatous damage was taken into consideration. The same school of thought also found that the final appearance of the optic disc is the same in the advanced stages of both the group regardless of the causative factors leading to them.[7]

In one of the studies by Woo et al.[45] which compared the localized nerve fiber layer defect between NTG and POAG, they found that the pattern of localized NFL defects in NTG is different from that in POAG: localized NFL defects in NTG were closer to the fovea and wider in width than those in POAG.

Visual Fields

NTG and POAG may be regarded as two ends of a spectrum. The rate and pattern of visual field loss in POAG has been extensively studied.[31-36] It is unclear whether the same may be seen in NTG. Some studies have addressed this issue. Difference in the visual fields for the same amount of nerve head damage has been noted. It has been found in some studies that the visual field defects are more localized and deep in the NTG group.[4,10-13] However, one study found that this difference or peculiarity is limited to the inferior hemifield only. Other studies, however, found no such peculiarity. One study

found a greater rate of progression in the NTG group, while another study noted a difference in the pattern of progression—the POAG group visual fields progressed first in area and then in depth whereas these two remained constant in the NTG group.[14]

POSSIBLE MECHANISM OF NORMAL TENSION GLAUCOMA
Influence of Intraocular Pressure

Although NTG, by definition is differentiated from POAG by the fact that the intraocular pressures never cross the 21 mm Hg line, however, it has been noted that the pressures do tend to be higher than the normal population.[15] Studies have tried to prove that intraocular pressure levels are directly related to the amount of field loss or ONH changes. However, there are others who claim no difference in the IOP of patients with or without field damage. However, studies including eyes of the same individual with asymmetric IOP do show a faster rate of disease progression in the high IOP group. A randomized trial of treated versus untreated NTG patients has shown that a 30 percent of IOP reduction in the treated group led to sufficient improvement in the disease process, stressing the fact that IOP, specially in the higher range group is an important factor in causing NTG, though there are other factors too which play a role in causing the same. One study also suggested that patients with NTG have a wider diurnal variation than the normal population.

Ocular Vascular Abnormalities

Drance and coworkers[16,17] described two forms of NTG. One is a nonprogressive form, which is usually associated with a transient episode of vascular insufficiency of the optic nerve head. A variety of cardiovascular and hematologic abnormalities are capable of causing both the forms. Hayreh[18] has suggested that NTG differs from anterior ischemic optic neuropathy only in that the latter is a more acute process. Reported associated findings include hemodynamic crises, reduced diastolic ophthalmodynamometry levels and ocular pulse amplitudes, bilateral complete occlusion of the internal carotid artery with reversed ophthalmic artery flow, focal arteriolar narrowing around the optic nerve, and increased vascular resistance of the ophthalmic artery by color Doppler analysis. A study of retinal and choroidal circulation showed that choroidal circulation fills more slowly in patients with NTG than in normal subjects, whereas the retinal circulation was delayed in patients with high-tension POAG compared to normal subjects.

Systemic Vascular Abnormalities

Reports of alterations in systemic blood pressures are conflicting. It has been reported that NTG patients have a significantly greater nocturnal drop in their blood pressure than healthy patients.[19] A twenty-four hours electrocardiographic monitoring showed a significant occurrence of asymptomatic myocardial ischemia (45%) as compared to normal individuals (5%) with many of these ischemic episodes occurring in the night. Visual evoked response during stepwise increasing IOP levels showed aberrations more in the NTG group than the higher tension group, probably indicating a worse and faulty autoregulation in the former group.

Associations of NTG have also been made with frequency of headaches with and without migraine. Though such associations have also been refuted, vasospastic diseases are also thought to be in strong association with NTG. Investigators have described two subsets of open angle glaucoma. One, smaller vasospastic group where there was a highly positive correlation between visual field loss and IOP and second, a larger group with disturbed coagulation and biochemical measurement, suggestive of vascular disease,

with no correlation between field and highest IOP.[20] A study of peripheral vascular endothelial function in NTG patients found impaired acetylcholine-induced peripheral endothelium-mediated vasodilation in comparison to healthy age and gender matched controls.[21] The bulk of the observations, therefore, suggest that vasospastic events are involved in the mechanism of at least some forms of NTG.

DIFFERENTIAL DIAGNOSIS: TENSION GLAUCOMA

Hematological abnormalities have also been found to be associated with NTG in some studies. Some of them being increased blood and plasma viscosity and hypercoagulability states. However, certain other studies have found no clinching evidence for the same. Hypercholesteronemia and MRI evidenced diffuse cerebral ischemia has also been found to be associated with NTG, pointing towards a vascular etiology.

In the conference report of the inaugural meeting of Southeast Asian Glaucoma Interest Group (SEAGIG) in 2000, the prevalence of NTG was thought to be lot higher in Asia as compared to the published data. The risk factors predicting the progression of NTG and the prognosis of the same depend on variable factors including the mean IOP—higher values increase the risk of progression. Many vascular factors were considered to be important risk factors viz. systemic blood pressure, blood viscosity, hemodynamic crisis, carotid and vascular disease, blood coagulation and vasospastic diseases. As for the local factors, disc hemorrhages, peripapillary atrophy and abnormalities in the retinal and choroidal circulation were found to be important risk factors.

Immune mechanism might also play a role in the causation of NTG. Increased incidence of paraproteinemia and autoantibodies including

antirhodopsin antibodies and antiglutathione S-transferase antibodies, has been found in NTG patients. Others include monoclonal gammopathy, serum immunoreactivity to retinal proteins, IgG and IgA deposition in the ganglion cells and in the inner and outer nuclear layers of the retina.

It is likely that NTG also has a genetic basis. Discovery of the Optineurin gene and defects associated with genes of known NTG families might further enhance our knowledge for the same.

Differential Diagnosis

Owing to a wide variety of neurological diseases giving the impression of this condition, it is at times important as well as necessary to do a neuroimaging evaluation depending upon the patient profile and also the nature of ailment. The differential diagnosis of NTG includes:

1. *Congenital disorders:*
   a. Optic nerve anomalies including coloboma, pits, oblique insertion.
   b. Autosomal dominant optic atrophy (Kjer type).
2. *Acquired disorders:*
   a. Past history of steroid use by any route that may have led to elevated intraocular pressure.
   b. Past history of trauma or surgery that may have led to elevated IOP.
   c. Hemodynamic crisis.
   d. Methyl alcohol poisoning
   e. Optic neuritis.
   f. Arteritic ischemic optic neuropathy.
   g. Nonarteritic ischemic optic neuropathy.
   h. Compressive lesions of the optic nerve and tract, (e.g. meningioma, vascular lesion).
   i. Temporal arteritis.
   j. Pituitary or intracranial tumors.
   k. Syphilitic (tertiary) optic neuropahty.

l. Trauma
m. Wide diurnal fluctuations in IOP.

TREATMENT

The treatment of NTG depends essentially on identification of the disease and prompt action. According to the Collaborative Normal Tension Glaucoma Study (CNGTS), aggressive management should be done in these cases aiming to keep the IOP in single digits. However, the condition may still progress even after achieving very low pressures. Here, the possibilities of IOP independent factors must be considered.

An additional aspect of NTG management therefore, includes treating cardiovascular ailments like anemia, congestive heart failure, transient ischemic attacks, and cardiac arrhythmias, to ensure maximal perfusion of the optic nerve head. Studies have shown beneficial effects with calcium channel blockers like nifedipine, verapamil and nimodipine. Nocturnal hypotension should be avoided and antihypertensives should preferably be given in the daytime.

It has been seen that topical administration of verapamil causes a significant reduction of intraocular pressure in ocular hypertensive human subjects.[22] This effect was sustained after topical administration of verapamil three times daily for 2 weeks.[23] However, no prospective controlled studies have been performed. Because in most but not all forms of NTG, outflow function through the trabecular meshwork is not substantially impaired, aqueous suppressants are usually more useful than outflow enhancing drugs. The usual first choice is the beta blockers. Since, in this condition, one starts with "normal" levels of IOP, the clinician usually desires full potency and chooses, if there is no systemic contraindication, a nonselective beta

blocker. If therapy is needed to be added, alpha-two agonists, topical carbonic anhydrase inhibitors, laser trabeculoplasty can be effective in some cases of NTG. However, filtering surgery may be required in most of the cases as the last resort. The bottom line is that many patients with NTG require surgery in most of the cases as the last resort. The bottom line is that many patients with NTG require an IOP in the single numbers that can only be obtained with filtration surgery with the use of antifibrotic agents. But sometimes laser trabeculoplasty with concomitant medical therapy, can be effective to achieve an IOP around ten.[24] The key is to determine if there is sufficient margin in the visual field that can be accurately followed. If there is no margin to follow around central fixation and unless IOP can be lowered to levels achievable with filtration surgery, it is justifiable in such situations to proceed rapidly to filtration surgery. In the words of Chandler: "progressive NTG is not a rare condition. Once the diagnosis has been established by inspection of the optic disc, repeated IOP measurement, and repeated measurement of the visual field, various medical measures are tried in an attempt to bring the IOP to lower levels. If medical treatment fails to lower the IOP significantly, and if repeated measurement of the field demonstrates progressive loss, we must come to a decision as to the future management of the case. If the patient is of advanced age, we may decide to continue with medical treatment (rather than proceeding with filtration surgery) in the hope of preserving some vision during the patient's life time. This is a difficult decision, for our patient might live to an advanced age and eventually become totally blind. When the situation is explained to the patient he may help us in making a decision."[2]

In recent years impressive progress has been made in the molecular genetic

studies of POAG and PACG. These include the discovery of three genes—Myocilin, Optineurin and Cyp1B1—defects in which results in Mendelian transmission of glaucoma. Identification of single nucleotide polymorphisms in multiple other genes that are associated with glaucoma and alteration of drug sensitivity. These discoveries are enriching our knowledge regarding the complex nature of the disease. Hopefully further advancement will help us rein in glaucoma more effectively.

Previously, the Collaborative Normal Tension Glaucoma study group concluded that in NTG, progression is slow. Thirty percent IOP reduction is achieved in approximately 50 percent of patients treated with medical and surgical therapy, surgical treatment does prevent progression in these patients though they are accompanied by complications like cataract and the IOP plays some pathogenetic role in the disease. Yamamoto and Kitazawa[46] from Japan, in their study found that the target IOP in patients with NTG should be somewhere between 10 and 12 mm Hg or less. Such low pressures are difficult to achieve with drugs alone. On the other hand, surgical intervention even with its advancement leads to its own catastrophes including cataract formation, bleb infection, hypotony, maculopathy. As such, they recommended an individual case to case approach in selecting candidates for surgery. Their criteria for surgical intervention included age, visual field, symptoms, pretreatment IOP and the effect of medical management.

RECENT FINDINGS

Normal tension glaucoma (NTG) and primary open angle glaucoma (POAG) represent a continuum of open angle glaucomas, in which a certain level of intraocular pressure (IOP) is the predominant causative risk factor in POAG, while additional IOP-independent factors take increasing importance in NTG.[25] There is considerable overlap between the two conditions, however, and within the population of NTG patients there are subsets in which IOP, blood flow and other factors assume relative importance. In clinical practice, control of IOP remains the mainstay of managing NTG patients, but consideration must also be given to other factors, especially those that may influence perfusion of the optic nerve head. Treatment paradigms are likely to change as researchers continue to investigate the mechanisms of glaucomatous optic neuropathy and search for IOP-independent neuroprotective agents.

In a recent publication, Rohit Varma et al have described about the role of neuroprotection in the management of glaucoma.[44] Glaucoma is no longer diagnosed by elevated IOP levels,[26,27] and it is now recognized as a neuropathy defined by characteristic optic disc and visual field change.[28] The absence of reliance on IOP level

as a diagnostic criteria has occurred because 20 to 30 percent of glaucoma patients have IOP in the normal range.[29,30] Furthermore, the annual progression rate is 9 to 10 percent even in patients treated with IOP-lowering medical, laser, or surgical therapy.[21,37] The Early Manifest Glaucoma Trial[38,39] found that although the mean IOP during follow-up was significantly associated with the risk of progression, this risk was highly variable, and several other baseline factors were significant independent predictors whose combined effect might be as important as IOP. These additional independent predictors included presence of bilateral disease, worse mean deviation, degree of baseline exfoliation, older age, presence of frequent disc hemorrhages, and duration between follow-up visits.[38-40] The Ocular Hypertension; Treatment Study found a relationship between IOP reduction and glaucoma incidence. However, progression was not confirmed in 85 percent of cases.[41] The Collaborative Normal

Tension Glaucoma study found that visual field progression could occur in both treated and untreated normal tension glaucoma patients, and no study analyses detected a relationship between a change in the IOP and visual field progression.[42,43] This clinical evidence of continued disease progression despite IOP management has provided the basis for proposed alternative risk factors and treatment approaches that could modify the clinical course of glaucoma.

CONCLUSION
To conclude, normal tension glaucoma is an important diagnosis that evades detection. Adhering to good and detailed clinical examination will help us detect this condition more and allow an intervention well in advance, at a stage when we can treat the patients more promptly and help keep his vision intact rather than prognosticating him for his loss of vision. This is what will bring satisfaction and smile to the patient and bring us closer to the goal we thrive for.

REFERENCES
1. Shields MB. Shields' Textbook of Glaucoma. Chronic Open Angle Glaucoma and Normal Tension Glaucoma 2005;5:198-207.
2. Chandler and Grant's Glaucoma. Low tension Glaucoma 1997;4:199-211.
3. Caprioli J, Spaeth GL. Comparison of the optic nerve head in high and low-tension glaucoma. Arch Ophthalmol 1985;103:1145.
4. Gramer E, Althaus G, Leydhecker W. Localization and depth of glaucomatous visual field defects in relation to the size of the neuroretinal rim area of the disk in low-tension glaucoma, glaucoma simplex, and pigmentary glaucoma; clinical study with the octopus 201 perimeter and the optic nerve head analyzer. Klin Monatsbl Augenheilkd 1986;189:190.
5. Yamagami J, ARaie M, Shirato S. A comparative study of optic nerve head in low and high-tension glaucomas. Graefes Arch Clin Exp Ophthalmol 1992;230:446.
6. Miller KM, Quigley HA. Comparison of optic disc features in low-tension and typical open-angle glaucoma. Ophthalmic Surg 1987;18:882.
7. Iester M, Mikelberg FS. Optic nerve head morphologic characteristics in high-tension and NTG. Arch Ophthalmol 1999;117:1010.
8. Kitazawa Y, Shirato S, Yamamoto T. Optic disc haemorrhage in low-tension glaucoma. Ophthalmology 1986;93:853.
9. Tezel G, Kass MA, Kolker AE, et al. Comparative optic disc analysis in normal pressure glaucoma, primary open-angle glaucoma and ocular hypertension. Ophthalmology 1996;103:2105.
10. Drance SM, Douglas GR, Airaksinen PJ, et al. Diffuse visual field loss in chronic open-angle and low-tension glaucoma. Am J Ophthalmol 1987;104:577.
11. Chauhan BC, Drance SM, Douglas GR, et al. Visual field damage in NTG and high-tension glaucoma. Am J Ophthalmol 1989;108:636.
12. Gramer E, Althaus G. The impact of intraocular pressure on visual field loss in primary open-angle glaucoma. Klin Monatsbl Augenheilkd 1990;197:218.
13. Hong C, Lee JH, Song KY. Probability of global indices in low tension glaucoma. Korean J Ophthalmol 1995;9:96.

14. Gramer E, Althaus G. Quantification and progression of visual field damage in low–tension, primary open–angle, and pigmentary glaucoma. Klin Monatsbl Augenheilkd 1987;191:184.

15. Gramer E, Leydhecker W. Glaucoma without elevated IOP: a clinical study. Klin Monatsbl Augenheilkd 1985;186:262.

16. Drance SM, Sweeney VP, Morgan RW, et al. Studies of factors involved in the production of low tension glaucoma. Arch Ophthalmol 1973;89:457.

17. Drance SM, Morgan RW, Sweeney VP. Shock-induced optic neuropathy: a cause of nonprogressive glaucoma. N Engl J Med 1973;288:392.

18. Hayreh SS. Anterior ischemic optic neuropathy. New York: Springer-Verlag; 1975. p. 22.

19. Mayer JH, Brandi-Dohrn J, Funk J. Twenty four hour blood pressure monitoring in normal tension glaucoma. Br J Ophthalmol 1996;80:864.

20. Schulzer M, Drance SM, Carter CJ, et al. Biostatistical evidence for two distinct chronic open-angle glaucoma populations. Br J Ophtalmol 1990;74:196.

21. Henry E, Newby DE, Webb DJ, et al. Peripheral endothelial dysfunction in normal pressure glaucoma. Invest Ophthalmol Vis Sci 1999;40:1710.

22. Netland PA, Chaturvedi N, Dreyer EB: Calcium Channel blockers in the management of low-tension and open angle glaucoma. Am J Ophthalmol 1993;115:608-13.

23. Chandler PA: Long-term results in glaucoma therapy. Am J Ophthalmol 1960;49:221-46.

24. Schulzer M. Intraocular pressure reduction in normal tension glaucoma patients. Ophthalmology 1992; 99:1468-70.

25. Shields MB. Normal-tension glaucoma: Is it different from primary open angle glaucoma. Current Opinion in Ophthalmology 2008;19:85-8.

26. American Academy of Ophthalmology, Glaucoma Panel. Primary open-angle glaucoma. Preferred practice pattern. San Francisco, CA: American Academy of Ophthalmology; 2000. pp. 1-36.

27. Sponsel WE. Glaucoma. In: Conn HF, Rakel RE, (Eds). Conn€™s Current Therapy 2001: Latest Approved Methods of Treatment for the Practicing Physician. Philadelphia, PA: Saunders; 2001. pp. 976-9.

28. Walland MJ, Carassa RG, Goldberg I, et al. Failure of medical therapy despite normal intraocular pressure. Clin Exp Ophthalmol 2006;34:827-36.

29. Sommer A, Tielsch JM, Katz J, et al. Relationship between intraocular pressure and primary open-angle glaucoma among white and black Americans. The Baltimore Eye Survey. Arch Ophthalmol 1991;109:1090-5.

30. Friedman DS, Nordstrom B, Mozaffari E, Quigley HA. Glaucoma management among individuals enrolled in a single comprehensive insurance plan. Ophthalmology 2005;112:1500-4.

31. Katz J, Gilbert D, Quigley HA, Sommer A. Estimating progression of visual field loss in glaucoma. Ophthalmology 1997;104:1017-25.

32. Airaksinen PJ, Tuulonen A, Alanko HI. Rate and pattern of neuroretinal rim area decrease in ocular hypertension and glaucoma. Arch Ophthalmol 1992;110:206-10.

33. Zeyen TG, Caprioli J. Progression of disc and field damage in early glaucoma. Arch Ophthalmol 1993;111:62-5.

34. Smith SD, Katz J, Quigley HA. Analysis of progressive change in automated visual fields in glaucoma. Invest Ophthalmol Vis Sci 1996;37:1419-28.

35. Migdal C, Gregory W, Hitchings R. Long-term functional outcome after early surgery compared with laser and medicine in open-angle glaucoma. Ophthalmology 1994;101:1651-7.

36. Gliklich RE, Steinmann WC, Spaeth GL. Visual field change in low-tension glaucoma over a five-year follow-up. Ophthalmology 1989;96:316-20.

37. Eendebak GR, Boen-Tan TN, Bezemer PD. Long-term follow-up of laser trabeculoplasty. Doc Ophthalmol 1990;75:203-14.

38. Heijl A, Leske MC, Bengtsson B, et al. Reduction of intraocular pressure and glaucoma progression: results from the Early Manifest Glaucoma Trial. Arch Ophthalmol 2002;120:1268-79.

39. Leske MC, Heijl A, Hussein M, et al. Factors for glaucoma progression and the effect of treatment: the Early Manifest Glaucoma Trial. Arch Ophthalmol 2003;121:48-56.

40. Leske MC, Heijl A, Hyman L, Bengtsson B, Komaroff E. Factors for progression and glaucoma treatment: the Early Manifest Glaucoma Trial. Curr Opin Ophthalmol 2004;15:102-6.

41. Greenfield DS, Bagga H. Clinical variables associated with glaucomatous injury in eyes with large optic disc cupping. Ophthalmic Surg Lasers Imaging 2005;36:401-9.

42. Collaborative Normal Tension Glaucoma Study Group. Comparison of glaucomatous progression between untreated patients with normal-tension glaucoma and patients with therapeutically reduced intraocular pressures. Am J Ophthalmol 1998;126:487-97.

43. Collaborative Normal Tension Glaucoma Study Group. The effectiveness of intraocular pressure reduction in the treatment of normal-tension glaucoma. Am J Ophthalmol 1998; 126:498-505.

44. Varma R, et al. Disease progression and the need for neuroprotection in glaucoma management. Am J Manage Care 2008;14:S15-9.

45. Woo SJ, Park KH, Kim DM. Comparison of localised nerve fibre layer defects in normal tension glaucoma and primary open angle glaucoma. Br J Ophthalmol 2003;87:695-8.

46. Yamamoto T, Kitazawa Y. Surgical treatment for Normal Tension Glaucoma, Asian Journal of Ophthalmology and Asia Pacific of Ophthalmology 2000;2:6.

26 | Angle-Closure Glaucoma

Ronald SH Chung, Shamira A Perera, Tin Aung

CHAPTER OUTLINE

- ❖ Terminology and Definitions
- ❖ Etiology
- ❖ Patient Assessment
- ❖ Pathophysiology
- ❖ Management of Angle-Closure Glaucoma
- ❖ Acute Primary Angle-Closure

INTRODUCTION

Primary angle-closure glaucoma (PACG) is a major form of glaucoma, affecting 16 million persons worldwide.[1,2] This is a relatively common condition especially in East Asia and a leading cause of bilateral glaucoma blindness in countries such as Singapore, India and China.[3-6] PACG is thought to be more visually destructive than primary open-angle glaucoma (POAG)[7] and patients are commonly asymptomatic until a late stage.

TERMINOLOGY AND DEFINITIONS

The three stages of angle-closure glaucoma, according to the ISGEO classification system, are as follows[8] (**Box 1**):

1. **Primary angle-closure suspect (PACS)** is diagnosed when there is contact between the peripheral iris and posterior trabecular meshwork with no other angle or optic nerve abnormalities.[5,9] The most stringent definition for angle closure requires over 270° of iridotrabecular contact (**diagnosed when the posterior trabecular meshwork is not visible on gonioscopy**). Some

authorities suggest 180° as the cut off because eyes may have a lesser extent of angle-closure but still have peripheral anterior synechiae (PAS).[10]

Such a definition was recently used in population-based surveys in India[11] and Singapore.[12]

2. **Primary angle-closure (PAC)** is present when the peripheral iris obstructs the trabecular meshwork causing raised intraocular pressure (IOP) and/or damage to the anterior segment structures in the presence of a closed angle. The clinical signs include: PAS, increased IOP, iris whorling, glaucomflecken (**Figure 1**), lens opacities or extensive pigment deposition on the trabecular meshwork. There is, however, no glaucomatous optic nerve damage at this stage.

3. **Primary angle-closure glaucoma (PACG)** is PAC with glaucomatous optic neuropathy (GON) and a corresponding visual field defect compatible with glaucoma.

ETIOLOGY

Age

The risk of angle-closure increases with age.[13,14] This is thought to be due to the lens growing in thickness, causing progressive shallowing of the anterior chamber.[15]

Box 1 ISGEO classification of primary angle-closure

Primary angle-closure suspect (PACS)	• Contact between peripheral iris and posterior trabecular meshwork is considered possible
	• Eye otherwise normal
Primary angle-closure (PAC)	• PACS with evidence of trabecular meshwork obstruction by peripheral iris by PAS, raised IOP, iris whorling, glaucomflecken, iris opacities, or excessive pigment deposition on the trabecular surface
	• No optic disc or visual field damage
Primary angle-closure glaucoma (PACG)	• PAC with evidence of glaucomatous optic neuropathy

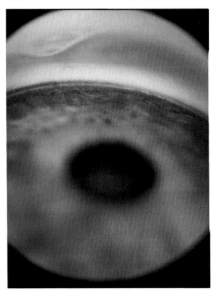

Fig. 1 EyeCam image of a wide open-angle portraying all the angle structures including the ciliary body band

Ethnicity

Inuits have the highest described prevalence of PACG.[16,17] Other populations with a high prevalence of angle-closure include Mongolia,[3] Singapore (Chinese),[13] Myanmar[18] and Hong Kong.[19] However, the rates of angle closure amongst Indians,[6,20] Thais[21] and Malays[13] are lower. Angle-closure glaucoma in Asia is predominantly of the chronic asymptomatic type.

Primary angle-closure glaucoma (PACG) prevalence amongst Caucasians is low, with a prevalence of about 0.1 percent in people over 40 years.[22-24] African-derived persons have PACG prevalence similar to that of Europeans. As both Africans and Asian eyes have brown irides, the development of PACG is not thought to be related to iris color, but more likely to other iris parameters.[29]

Ocular Biometry

Eyes with angle-closure have been shown to have the following characteristics: Shallow central ACD, thick lens, anterior lens position, small corneal diameter and radius of curvature, and short axial length.[25,26] Shallow central ACD may be the most important risk factor since Inuits have the highest prevalence of PACG and the shortest ACDs.[27] Older age groups and females also have a shorter ACD when compared to younger age groups and males.[28] This may explain the increased risk of angle-closure in these groups. The location of the lens is more anterior in PACG eyes and is thicker than normal.[30] Chinese and Indian populations, with higher rates of angle closure, have shorter axial lengths[23] as well. Eyes with extreme short axial lengths may be more affected by acute primary angle-closure (APAC) than by chronic asymptomatic angle closure.[31-33] A more anterior lens position occurs in a greater proportion of angle-closure eyes than normal eyes in a number of studies.[34]

Genetics

Anterior position of the lens, increased lens thickness and shallow ACD are features more commonly seen in close relatives of patients with ACG as compared to the general population.[35-38] The inheritance of PACG is most likely polygenic,[39-42] although both autosomal dominant and autosomal recessive pedigrees exist. Sihota et al[43] found the ACD to be shallowest, the lens thickest and the axial length shortest, in family members having PACG, and these features gradually approach normal values in suspected and unaffected family members. Amongst Chinese twins, additive genetic effects appear to be the major factor in the variation of ACD and relative ACD (defined as ACD/axial length).[44]

No genes have yet been conclusively found for PACG. Primary angle-closure glaucoma subjects have been shown in two studies to carry a mutation in the myocilin gene (MYOC);[45,46] however, another study has not supported this in Chinese patients with chronic PACG.[47] There may be an association between a single nucleotide polymorphism in the matrix metalloproteinase 9 (MMP-9) gene and APAC in Taiwanese[48] **(Box 2)**. However, this was not supported by a study in Singaporean subjects.[49]

CHX10 and MFRP are two genes that regulate ocular size; CHX10 being associated with microphthalmia and MFRP with nanophthalmos. Angle-closure frequently develops in eyes with these conditions and these were logical target genes for investigation.[52,53] However, no association between CHX10, MFRP and PACG was found.

Iris Structure

Characteristics of the iris such as iris thickness, curvature, or volume have been identified as potential risk factors for angle-closure. Recent anterior segment OCT (ASOCT) analysis showed iris curvature, iris volume, and iris thickness are independently associated with the presence of narrow angles, even after controlling for other known ocular risk factors.[54]

Iris volume changes dramatically during pupil dilation. With the help of ASOCT, angle-closure eyes were found to retain more iris volume than normal eyes upon dilation.[55] This may be a result of differences in iris connective tissue in angle-closure eyes. The significance of iris volumetric changes in development of ACG in different racial groups has yet to be fully determined.[55]

Box 2 Risk factors for angle-closure

Increasing age
Female gender
Ethnicity:
Inuit
East Asian
Biometry and ocular anatomy:
Hyperopia
Shallow anterior chamber depth
Shorter axial length
Genetic factors

PATIENT ASSESSMENT
Angle Assessment in Angle-Closure
Gonioscopy

Gonioscopy assesses the angle by the use of a contact lens at the slit lamp **(Figure 1)**. Various grading schemes have been devised to describe the anterior chamber angle. For example, the Spaeth classification assesses the insertion of the iris, the angular width of the angle recess and the configuration of the peripheral iris. The Schaffer classification assesses the risk of closure according to the width of the angle **(Figure 2)**.

Peripheral anterior synechiae (PAS): PAS occurs when the peripheral iris attaches anteriorly in the angle, covering the trabecular meshwork. PAS may be localized or extensive, pinpoint or broad. The ideal method to assess PAS is using dynamic indentation gonioscopy.

New Methods of Angle Imaging
Anterior segment optical coherence tomography (ASOCT) and ultrasound biomicroscopy (UBM): ASOCT and UBM are new anterior segment imaging technologies which are used to assess the angle **(Figures 2 and 3)**. ASOCT examines the angle with infrared light in a noncontact fashion, and like the UBM, semiautomated image analyses can be performed.

Automated analysis depends on accurately identifying the scleral spur, but a recent report revealed that investigators had difficulty identifying the scleral spur in about 30 percent of ASOCT images. This is a major shortcoming for using the ASOCT for angle-assessment with automated analysis.[56] Another report compared ASOCT and the reference standard, gonioscopy in detecting angle-closure in different quadrants of the anterior chamber angle. The highest rates of closed angles, by both methods were in the superior quadrant. ASOCT detected more closed anterior chamber angles than gonioscopy, particularly in the superior and inferior quadrants, but generally showed good agreement.[57] Being a noncontact instrument that can rapidly perform scans of the angles, it could potentially be used as a diagnostic tool for angle-closure. However, studies have shown angle width determined by ASOCT and the extent of PAS, were only weakly correlated.[58]

UBM scanning requires a water bath to be placed on the eye of the supine patient. Research comparing UBM, ASOCT and gonioscopy shows that (time domain) ASOCT and UBM are good at identifying narrow angles, but ASOCT over identifies subjects as having closed angles compared to gonioscopy.[49,50] In another study by Wong HT et al, high definition (or spectral domain) optical coherence tomography coupled with a 60D lens was capable of visualizing the Schwalbe's line and trabecular meshwork in most eyes, thus showing promise as a tool for imaging in angle-closure.[61]

Slit lamp OCT (SL-OCT): This is a slit lamp mounted OCT imaging device. The basic technology is similar to ASOCT. The SL-OCT provides noncontact cross-sectional scans of the anterior segment. Chamber angle, pachymetry, flap thickness, corneal curvature and comprehensive biometric measurements are possible with the instrument, as well as pre- and postsurgical comparisons. A comparison study showed the overall sensitivity and specificity for SL-OCT were 84 percent and 58 percent vs 80 percent and 80 percent for SPAC, using gonioscopy as the reference standard.[59,65]

Scanning peripheral anterior chamber (SPAC) depth analyzer: The SPAC is a noncontact device which rapidly measures the depth of the central and peripheral anterior chamber. These values are compared to a normative database, which produce a risk assessment for angle closure.[51] SPAC is sensitive, but overestimates the proportion of narrow angles relative to both gonioscopy and the modified van Herick grading system for peripheral ACD assessment.[59]

Provocative Testing

Provocation tests try to induce iridotrabecular contact by exposing angle-closure suspects to different examination situations, such as dark room examination, prone positioning examination and postpharmacologic pupil dilation examination. However, these tests have failed to reliably identify patients at risk of angle-closure.[64]

Screening

Detection of anatomically narrow angles (angle-closure suspects) is a key component of any screening program to prevent PACG. Unfortunately, there

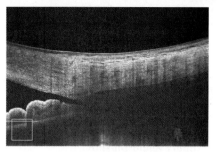

Fig. 2 Cirrus OCT image of a closed angle. There is iridocorneal contact anterior to the level of the scleral spur

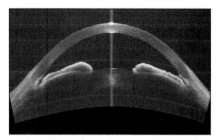

Fig. 3 Anterior segment OCT image showing the iris in close proximity to the angle wall

is no automated imaging device suitable for mass screening at this stage. SPAC, IOL master and ASOCT have each exhibited low specificities when these instruments were used to screen for narrow angles.[68]

PATHOPHYSIOLOGY
Primary Angle-Closure

Ritch et al described the four main mechanisms of angle-closure. Treatments are directed at each of these mechanisms[60] and multiple mechanisms may exist for angle-closure patients **(Box 3A)**.

Level I: Iris and Pupil

Pupillary block is the most common mechanism of angle-closure.[63] Resistance to aqueous flow is increased between the pupil and the anterior

---

Box 3A Mechanisms of primary angle-closure

Levels of block
- Level I: Iris and pupil
- Level II: Ciliary body
- Level III: Lens-induced glaucoma
- Level IV: Malignant glaucoma/ retrolenticular

---

surface of the lens. Pressure builds-up in the posterior chamber which causes anterior bowing of the iris (bombé), and progressive iridotrabecular contact. Laser iridotomy or surgical iridectomy relieves the pressure difference between the anterior and posterior chambers caused by pupil block. Consequently, the iris profile becomes flatter and the iridocorneal angle widens. Quigley suggested that pupil block is a relative concept. Since there is a net forward movement of aqueous, there must be a driving pressure differential for this flow, therefore the pressure is always higher on the posterior than the anterior iris surface, thus all eyes have some degree of pupil block. Increased resistance between lens and pupil margin raises pressure

in the posterior chamber. The higher the posterior chamber pressure, the more anterior the iris position. When the resistance reaches a critical level, the peripheral iris covers the trabecular meshwork and blocks outflow.[29]

Level II: Plateau Iris

The development of plateau iris depends on the location of the ciliary processes. Normal eyes have the junction of iris dilator and the ciliary process close to the posterior limit of the drainage angle and thus close to the scleral spur. Plateau iris develops when this iris-ciliary body junction is placed more centripetal and therefore further from the scleral spur. This leads to an anterior attachment of the iris base, in which the iris remains closer to the meshwork in a plateau configuration, even after iridotomy.[29] About one-third of eyes with narrow angles post PI have plateau iris **(Figures 4)**. Dynamic gonioscopy reveals a double hump sign where the peripheral iris drapes over the ciliary processes. Plateau iris is more common in younger female patients with a family history of PACG and there is usually some component of pupil block. Cataract extraction cannot reliably widen the drainage angles in eyes with plateau iris as iridociliary apposition still occurs.[65,84] Argon laser peripheral iridoplasty may be more effective as long-term treatment.[66,85]

Plateau iris syndrome occurs when angle-closure with raised IOP develops despite a patent iridotomy. Iridociliary cysts, tumors or edema may mimic plateau iris configuration.[64]

A study in Singapore using standardized UBM criteria found plateau iris **(Figure 4)** in about a third of PACS eyes after LPI[65,71] confirming that non-pupil block mechanisms are important in angle-closure in Asians.

However, this may not be pertinent to other populations.[66]

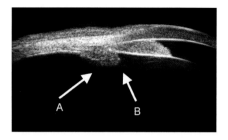

Fig. 4 A UBM image of plateau iris
A. Anteriorly rotated ciliary body
B. Obliteration of the ciliary sulcus and angle-closure

Level III: Lens-induced Glaucoma

A large intumescent lens or an anteriorly subluxed lens[51] may push the iris and ciliary body forward, triggering acute or chronic angle-closure glaucoma (phacomorphic glaucoma) **(Figures 5A and B)**. Treatment involves removing the lens.

Level IV: Malignant Glaucoma/ Retrolenticular

In this condition, aqueous flow is misdirected into the anterior vitreous causing progressive pressure build-up associated with anterior rotation of the ciliary body and forward movement of the lens-iris diaphragm **(Figure 6)**. The iris is pushed against the trabecular meshwork which results in angle-closure. A shallow supraciliary choroidal detachment may be present. At present it is unclear whether this may be the cause of anterior rotation of the ciliary body or a consequence of the process.[51] The ability of the vitreous to conduct fluid may play a significant role. If vitreous allows low resistance passage of aqueous to the posterior chamber then the vitreous will remain in place. But, if aqueous is unable to pass through the vitreous, due to poor vitreous conductivity, the pressure builds-up and triggers malignant glaucoma.[29]

Medical treatment with cycloplegics, hyperosmotic and ocular hypotensive agents may reverse the abnormal anatomy. However, on cessation

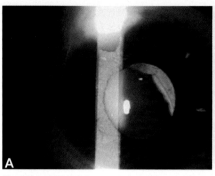 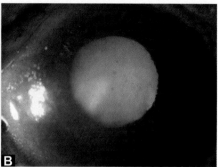

Figs 5A and B (A) Secondary angle-closure glaucoma following traumatic lens subluxation. Trabeculectomy has been done since the pressure was not controlled after laser peripheral iridotomies; (B) Phacomorphic glaucoma

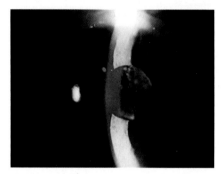

Fig. 6 Aqueous misdirection syndrome. The central and peripheral anterior chamber is shallow. A patent peripheral iridotomy is present

of therapy the condition may recur. In addition, Nd:YAG laser anterior hyaloidotomy or posterior capsulotomy (in pseudophakic patients) may be attempted as well. If laser and medical therapy fails, vitrectomy to create unrestricted flow from the posterior to the anterior chamber is the definitive treatment.

Choroidal effusion: Quigley et al[67] proposed choroidal expansion, a condition which may be associated with scleritis, sulfa drugs and panretinal photocoagulation, as a contributing risk factor for PACG and acute primary angle-closure (APAC). PACG/APAC eyes have been found to have uveal effusions when examined with UBM;[69,70] whether this is a cause or effect of PACG/APAC remains

unknown.[72] Suprachoroidal fluid may accumulate due to rapid changes in IOP, uveal vessel leakage, high IOP induced choroidal congestion or the effect of topical pilocarpine and oral acetazolamide.

Choroidal expansion may contribute to angle-closure by the following sequence of events. Acute choroidal expansion immediately would raise IOP throughout the eye. As aqueous humor leaves via the conventional outflow channels, the normal posterior-anterior pressure differential significantly increases, depending on the level of resistance in the iris-lens channel. An eye that already has high resistance in the iris-lens channel at baseline would have a further increase in resistance due to the channel narrowing. The iris would bow forward and close the angle if critical dimensions were achieved. The degree to which choroidal expansion occurs depends on many variables, including choroidal elasticity and vascular permeability.[29]

Causes of Secondary Angle-Closure (Box 3B)

i. ***Secondary angle closure glaucoma with an anterior pulling mechanism without pupil block:*** This occurs when anterior traction pulls the iris over the trabecular meshwork, usually due to the contraction of abnormal

membranes. Neovascular glaucoma, **(Figures 7A and B)** iridocorneal endothelial syndrome **(Figure 7C)**, surgically induced epithelial in-growth and inflammatory membranes secondary to uveitis are some examples. Rarer causes are aniridia and endothelial posterior polymorphous dystrophy.

ii. ***Secondary angle closure with a posterior pushing mechanism without pupil block:*** Secondary angle-closure may occur when iris tissue is pushed forward to cover the trabecular meshwork. Examples include: iris and ciliary body cysts, silicone oil or expansile gas in the vitreous cavity. A uveal effusion caused by, inflammation, a tightscleral buckle, or retinopathy of prematurity (ROP)[62] may also push the iris over the trabecular meshwork.

MANAGEMENT OF ANGLE-CLOSURE GLAUCOMA
Laser
Laser Peripheral Iridotomy (PI)
Laser PI eliminates pupil block. The iridotomy is usually placed between 11 and 1 o'Clock to minimize visual disturbance. In blue irides, Nd:YAG laser alone is sufficient for PI but in thick brown irides, argon laser is often required to first photocoagulate and thin the iris before applying Nd:YAG laser to enlarge the opening.[61] Prelaser application of brimonidine or apraclonidine is useful for reducing postlaser IOP spikes.[73]

If laser PI is unsuccessful or difficult because of a cloudy cornea,

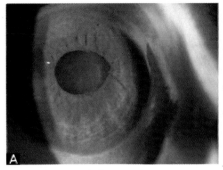 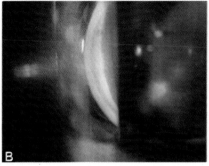 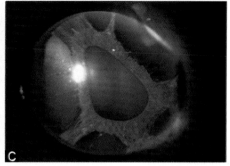

Figs 7A to C (A and B) Neovascular glaucoma with secondary nonpupillary block angle-closure. Note the ectropion uveae corresponding to the peripheral anterior synechiae; (C) ICE syndrome

surgical iridectomy is indicated. There is no difference in visual acuity or IOP outcome between laser PI and surgical iridectomy in a 3-year randomized controlled trial of unilateral APAC.[74]

Up to 58 percent of APAC subjects need further glaucoma treatment post-iridotomy, whilst 32 percent need glaucoma surgery after an APAC attack treated with laser PI. In another study, 90 percent of patients need medications or surgery after laser PI in patients with chronic PACG.[75]

Potential complications of laser PI include: transient IOP spikes, progression of cataract and cornea decompensation,[75-77] iatrogenic injuries to the retina, posterior synechiae and optically induced visual disturbances.[78]

Argon Laser Peripheral Iridoplasty

This may be indicated if the angle remains appositionally closed after a patent PI. Circumferential, low energy laser burns are placed in the peripheral iris to cause the iris to contract and pull it away from the trabecular meshwork, thereby opening up the angle.

Performing iridoplasties in APAC patients, reduces the reliance upon IOP lowering medications,[79] which may have systemic side effects, especially in elderly patients with multiple comorbidities. Medical therapy has a relatively slow onset, and 60 percent of APAC patients treated medically may still develop chronic PACG.[65] In

a randomized controlled trial from Hong Kong, iridoplasty was found to be superior in IOP reduction in the initial two hours after presentation of APAC. Iridoplasties performed in APAC patients lead to a lower percentage of cases with subsequent PAS.[65]

Medical Therapy

Asian patients commonly develop chronic PACG after successful iridotomies. PI only relieves pupil block but other mechanisms, such as progressive lens thickening, plateau iris or a damaged trabecular meshwork may still contribute to development of PACG.[80]

Topical beta blockers, prostagladin analogs, carbonic anhydrase inhibitors and alpha-2-agonists have similar efficacy in angle-closure patients and open-angle glaucoma (POAG) patients and act via a variety of mechanisms. Latanoprost was found to be more effective than timolol in lowering IOP in Asian PACG eyes,[81] even with up to 360º of PAS.[82] Pilocarpine constricts the pupil and pulls the iris away from the trabecular meshwork, but long-term use can result in posterior synechiae and make cataract surgery more difficult. Iridotomies are still necessary in such eyes.

Surgery
Trabeculectomy

Trabeculectomy is indicated when medical or laser treatment fail to control IOP,

or there is progressive visual field loss with glaucomatous optic nerve damage.

Lens Extraction for Angle-Closure

Lens extraction deepens the anterior chamber, decreases angle crowding and relieves pupil block.[85] Lai et al[87] showed that this leads to a decrease in IOP, and a reduced requirement for antiglaucoma medications. Cataract surgery is technically difficult in PACG eyes because of the frequently coexisting shallow anterior chamber, large bulky lens, iris atrophy (secondary to ischemia) and zonular weakness peripheral synechiae may continue to progress even after cataract extraction.[83] Cataract surgery alone as a surgical option may be useful in the setting of mild optic disc damage and medically controlled PACG with coexisting cataract. Tham CC et al, showed that phacoemulsification alone reduced a significant amount of synechial angle-closure as well as increasing anterior chamber depth in patients with PACG.[91]

Combined Lens Extraction and Trabeculectomy Surgery

This combined procedure has similar complication rates when performed in PACG and POAG eyes.[88] Combined surgery has the added advantage of being able to prevent IOP spikes postoperatively **(Box 4)**. In one study of patients with medically uncontrolled PACG, phacotrabeculectomy with MMC reduced IOP to low teens and reduced on average 1.5 glaucoma medications.[93]

Box 4 Management of angle-closure glaucoma

Laser
- Laser peripheral iridotomy
- Argon laser peripheral iriodoplasty

Medical therapy

Surgery
- Trabeculectomy
- Lens extraction for angle-closure
- Combined lens extraction and trabeculectomy surgery

Goniosynechialysis

This procedure strips PAS from the trabecular meshwork using an instrument inserted through a clear corneal incision. The potential problems include IOP spikes, cataract and hyphema. Goniosynechialysis performed concurrently with cataract surgery can be effective when PAS have been present for less than one year, but the relative contribution of each procedure to IOP lowering is still unknown.[89]

ACUTE PRIMARY ANGLE-CLOSURE

Patients with acute primary angle-closure (APAC) present with ocular pain, nausea and vomiting, intermittent blurring of vision with haloes noted around lights and IOP usually greater than 30 mm Hg. Typically, there is marked conjunctival injection, corneal epithelial edema, a mid-dilated unreactive pupil, a shallow peripheral anterior chamber and the presence of a closed angle on gonioscopy.

Management of APAC
Aims of APAC Treatment
- To reduce the IOP
- Reduce inflammation
- Reverse the angle-closure
- Assess and manage the fellow eye.

The patient should be kept supine to encourage posterior movement of the lens and be reassessed regularly. Analgesics and antiemetics are used for symptomatic relief as needed.

Medical Therapy
Medical therapy includes some of the following agents, based on the patient's overall medical status:
- Systemic carbonic anhydrase inhibitors
- Topical miotics
- Topical beta-adrenergic antagonists
- Topical alpha-2-adrenergic agonists
- Systemic hyperosmotic agents.

Hyper osmotic agents such as intravenous mannitol 20 percent or oral glycerol should be used if the IOP remains high despite other medical treatments. Hyperosmotic agents reduce vitreous volume by inducing an osmotic diuresis. In one study, 44 percent of APAC patients required an osmotic agent to reduce IOP[90] sometimes in multiple administrations. Topical steroids should be used to reduce the sometimes marked inflammatory response.

Once, the acute episode subsides, laser PI should be performed to relieve pupil block. The fellow eye of APAC requires prophylactic treatment with a laser PI **(Figure 8)**, since half of these will otherwise suffer an acute attack within 5 years.[92]

Surgery for Acute Primary Angle-Closure
Lens removal will deepen the anterior chamber and open up the drainage angle. There is limited information on whether primary cataract extraction as initial treatment for APAC is superior to other methods, it is, however, an option for refractory cases when pupil block is resistant to medications and lasers.[94] The optimum timing of lens extraction is open to speculation; the risks and technical difficulties of surgery have to be weighed against the need to reduce IOP and prevent PAS formation.[95]

Follow-up Evaluation of Treated PACG/APAC
Regular follow-up with IOP checks and indentation gonioscopy is essential to identify patients who progress to PACG after an APAC attack. Those patients with no signs of developing PACG may still have raised IOP with glaucomatous optic neuropathy. They are managed similarly to those with POAG.

Intraocular Pressure
Eyes with acute PACG or PAC treated with PI may still develop high IOP over time; thus it is essential to have periodic follow-up after iridotomy.

Although PACG is a common form of glaucoma worldwide,[2] data on IOP fluctuation in eyes with PACG is limited. A recent study found that subjects with PACG had the highest diurnal IOP fluctuation, followed by PAC subjects as compared with PACS and normals.[86] The amount of IOP fluctuation in PAC and PACG groups measured approximately 4 to 5 mm Hg with peaks in the early morning, which was similar to studies that found an association of IOP fluctuation with primary open-angle glaucoma.[97-101] Eyes with more advanced disease tend to have greater IOP fluctuation.[86]

Long-term Prognosis after APAC
The long-term prognosis of APAC is guarded. In one study, 4 to 10 years following an APAC attack, 18 percent of eyes were blinded, 48 percent of eyes developed serious glaucomatous optic neuropathy, and 58 percent of eyes had vision worse than 20/40.[96] Patients are thus encouraged to return for periodic follow-up.

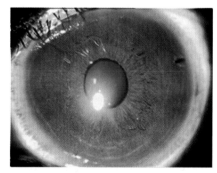

Fig. 8 Laser peripheral iridotomy

REFERENCES

1. Foster PJ, Johnson GJ. Glaucoma in China. How big is the problem? Br J Ophthalmol 2001;85:1277-82.

2. Quigley HA, Broman A. The number of persons with glaucoma worldwide in 2010 and 2020. Br J Ophthalmol 2006;90:151-6.

3. Foster PJ, Bassanhu J, Alsbirk PH, et al. Glaucoma in Mongolia. A population based-survey in Hovsgol Province, northern Mongolia. Arch Ophthalmol 1996;114:1235-41.

4. Foster PJ, Oen FT, Machin D, et al. The prevalence of glaucoma in Chinese residents of Singapore: a cross-sectional population survey of the Tanjong Pagar district. Arch Ophthalmol 2000;118:1105-11.

5. Foster PJ, Johnson GJ. Glaucoma in China. How big is the problem? Br J Ophthalmol 2001;85:1277-82.

6. Dandona L, Dandona R, Mandal P, et al. Angle-closure glaucoma in an urban population in Southern India. The Andhra Pradesh Eye Disease Study. Ophthalmol 2000;107:1710-6.

7. Ang LP, Aung T, Chua WH, Yip LW, Chew PT. Visual field loss from primary angle-closure glaucoma: a comparative study of symptomatic and asymptomatic disease. Ophthalmol 2004;111:1636-40.

8. Foster PJ, Buhrmann R, Quigley HA, Johnson GJ. The definition and classification of glaucoma in prevalence surveys. Br J Ophthalmol 2002;238-42.

9. Aung T, Ang LP, Chan SP, Chew PT. Acute primary angle-closure: long-term intraocular pressure outcome in Asian eyes. Am J Ophthalmol 2001;131:7-12.

10. Foster PJ, Aung T, Nolan WP, Machin, Baasanhu J, Khaw PT, Alsbirk PH, Lee PS, Seah SK, Johnson GJ. Defining "occludable" angles in population surveys: drainage angle width, peripheral anterior synechiae,

and glaucomatous optic neuropathy in East Asian people. Br J Ophthalmol 2004;88:486-90.

11. Vijaya L, George R, Arvind H, et al. Prevalence of angle-closure disease in a rural South Indian population. Arch Ophthalmol 2006;124:403-9.

12. Shen SY, Wong TY, Foster PJ, Loo JL, Rosman M, Loon SC, Wong WL, Saw SM, Aung T. The prevalence and types of glaucoma in Malay people: The Singapore Malay Eye Study. Invest Ophthalmol 2008;49:3846-51.

13. Vijaya L, George R, Arvind H, et al. Prevalence of primary angle-closure disease in an urban South Indian population and comparison with a rural population. The Chennai Glaucoma Study. Ophthalmology 2007;115(4):655-60.

14. Seah SK, Foster PJ, Chew PT, et al. Incidence of acute angle-closure glaucoma in Singapore. An Island-wide survey Arch Ophthalmol 1997;115:1436-40.

15. Markowitz SN, Morin JD. Angle-closure glaucoma: relation between lens thickness, anterior chamber depth and age. Can J Ophthalmol 1984;197:300-2.

16. Alsbirk PH. Primary angle-closure glaucoma. Oculometry, epidemiology, and genetics in a high-risk population. Acta Ophthalmol 1976;54:5-31.

17. Arkell SM, Lightman DA, Sommer A, et al. The prevalence of glaucoma among Eskimos of Northwest Alaska. Arch Ophthalmol 1987;105:482-5.

18. Casson R, Newland H, Muecke J, McGovern S, Durkin S, Sullivan T, Oo T, Aung T , Shein W, Selva D. Prevalence and Causes of Visual Impairment in Rural Myanmar. The Meiktila Eye Study. Ophthalmology 2007;114:2302-8.

19. Lai JS, Liu DT, Tham CC, Li RT, Lam DS. Epidemiology of acute primary

angle-closure glaucoma in the Hong Kong, Chinese population: prospective study. Hong Kong Med J 2001;7:118-23.

20. Vijaya L, George R, Arvind H, Baskaran M, Pradeep G, Paul PG, Ramesh SV, Raju P, Kumaramanickavel G, McCarty C. Prevalence of angle-closure disease in a rural southern Indian population. Arch Ophthalmol 2006;124:403-9.

21. Bourne RRA, Sukudom P, Foster PJ, et al. Prevalence of glaucoma in Thailand: a population based survey in Rom Klao district, Bangkok. Br J Ophthalmol 2003;87:1069-74.

22. Wensor MD, McCarty CA, Stanislavsky YL, et al. The prevalence of glaucoma in the Melbourne Visual Impairment Project. Ophthalmology 1998;105:733-9.

23. Hollows FC, Graham PA. Intraocular pressure, glaucoma and glaucoma suspects in a defined population. Br J Ophthalmol 1966;50:570-86.

24. Coffey M, Reidy A, Wormald R, et al. Prevalence of glaucoma in west of Ireland. Br J Ophthalmol 1993;77:17-21.

25. Raghavan L, Tien-Yin W, David SF, Han TA, Tamuno A, Hong G, Steve KS, Kenji K, Paul JF, Tin A. Determinants of angle-closure in older Singaporeans. Arch Ophthalmol 2008;126:686-91.

26. Lowe RF. Aetiology of the anatomical basis for primary angle-closure glaucoma: biometrical comparisons between normal eyes and eyes with primary angle-closure glaucoma. Br J Ophthalmol 1970;54:161-9.

27. Alsbirk PH. Anterior chamber depth in Greenland Eskimos. A population study of variation with age and sex. Acta Ophthalmol 1974;52:551-64.

28. Foster PJ, Alsbirk PH, Baasanhu J, et al. Anterior chamber depth in Mongolians. Variation with age, sex

and method of measurement. Am J Ophthalmol 1997;124:53-40.

29. Quigley HA. Angle-closure glaucoma—simple answers to complex mechanisms: LXVI Edward Jackson Memorial Lecture. Am J Ophthalmol 2009;148:657-69.

30. Lowe RF. Causes of shallow anterior chamber in primary angle-closure glaucoma. Ultrasonic biometry of normal and angle-closure eyes. Am J Ophthalmol 1969;67:87-93.

31. Lynne LYW, Wang TH, Hung PT. Biometric study of acute primary angle-closure glaucoma. J Formos Med Assoc 1997;96:908-12.

32. Sihota R, Lakshimaiah NC, Agrawal HC, et al. Ocular parameters in the subgroups of angle-closure glaucoma. Clin Exp Ophthalmol 2000;28:253-8.

33. George R, Paul PG, Baskaran M, et al. Ocular biometry in occludable angles and angle-closure glaucoma: a population based survey. Br J Ophthalmol 2003;87:399-402.

34. Friedman DS, Gazzard G, Foster PJ, et al. Ultrasonograghic biomi-croscopy, Scheimpflug photography, and novel provocative tests in contralateral eyes of Chinese patients initially see with acute angle closure. Arch Ophthalmol 2003;121:633-42.

35. Lowe RF. Anterior lens curvature. Comparisons between normal eyes and those with primary angle-closure glaucoma. Br J Ophthalmol 1972;56:409-13.

36. Tomlinson A, Leighton DA. Ocular dimensions in the heredity of angle-closure glaucoma. Br J Ophthalmol 1973;57:475-86.

37. Lowe RF. Primary angle-closure glaucoma. Family histories and anterior chamber depths. Br J Ophthalmol 1964;48:191-5.

38. Alsbirk PH. Anterior chamber depth and primary angle-closure glaucoma. II. A genetic study. Acta Ophthalmol 1975;53:436-49.

39. Wilensky JT, Kaufman PL, Frohlichstein D, Gieser DK, Kass MA, Ritch R, et al. Follow-up of angle-closure glaucoma suspects. Am J Ophthalmol 1993;115:335-45.

40. Alsbrik PH. Anterior chamber depth, gene and environment. Acta Ophthalmol 1982;60:223-34.

41. Lowe RF. Primary angle-closure glaucoma: Inheritence and environment. Br J Ophthalmol 1972;56:13-20.

42. Torniquist R. Chamber depth in primary angle-closure glaucoma. Br J Ophthalmol 1956;40:421-9.

43. Sihota R, Ghate D, Mohan S, Gupta V, Pandey RM, Dada T. Study of biometric parameters in family members of primary angle-closure glaucoma patients. Eye 2008;22:521-7.

44. He M, Wang D, Zheng Y, et al. Heritability of anterior chamber depth as an intermediate phenotype of angle-closure in Chinese: The Guangzhou Twin Eye Study. Invest Ophthalmol 2008;49:81-6.

45. Faucher M, Anctil JL, Rodrigue MA, et al. Founder TIGR/MYOC mutations for glaucoma in the Quebec population. Hum Mol Genet 2002;11:2077-90.

46. Vincent AL, Billingsley G, Buys Y, et al. Digenic inheritance of early-onset glaucoma: CYP1B1, a potential modifier gene. Am J Hum Genet 2002;70:448-60.

47. Aung T, Yong VHK, Chew PTK, et al. Molecular analysis of the Myocilin gene in Chinese subjects with chronic primary angle-closure glaucoma. Invest Ophthalmol Vis Sci 2005;46:1303-6.

48. Wang IJ, Chiang TH, Shih YF, et al. The association of single nucleotide polymorphisms in the MMP-9 genes with susceptibility to acute primary angle-closure glaucoma in Taiwanese patients. Mol Vis 2006;12:1223-32.

49. Radhakrishnan S, See J, Smith SD, et al. Reproducibility of anterior chamber angle measurements obtained with anterior segment optical coherence tomography. Invest Ophthalmol Vis Sci 2007;48:1303-6.

50. Radhakrishnan S, Goldsmith J, Huang D, et al. Comparison of optical coherence tomography and ultrasound biomicroscopy for detection of narrow anterior chamber angles. Arch Ophthalmol 2005;123:1053-9.

51. Kashiwagi K, Abe K, Tsukahara S. Quantitative evaluation of changes in anterior segment biometry by peripheral laser iridotomy using newly developed scanning peripheral anterior chamber depth analyser. Br J Ophthalmol 2004;88:1036-41.

52. Aung T, Yong VH, Lim MC, et al. Lack of association between the rs2664538 polymorphism in the MMP-9 gene and primary angle-closure glaucoma in Singaporean subjects. J Glaucoma 2008;17:257-8.

53. Aung T, Lim MC, Wong TT, et al. Molecular analysis of CHX10 and MFRP in Chinese subjects with primary angle-closure glaucoma and short axial length eyes. Mol Vis 2008;17(14):1313-8.

54. Wang B, Sakata LM, Aung T, et al. Quantitative Iris Parameters and Association with Narrow Angles. Ophthalmology 2009; [Epub ahead of print].

55. Quigley HA, Silver DM, Friedman DS, et al. Iris cross-sectional area decreases with pupil dilation and its dynamic behaviour is a risk factor in angle-closure. J Glaucoma 2009;18:173-9.

56. Sakata LM, Lavanya R, Aung T, et al. Assessment of the scleral spur in anterior segment optical coherence tomography images. Arch Ophthalmol 2008;126:181-5.

57. Sakata LM, Lavanya R, Aung T, et al. Comparison of gonioscopy and anterior segment ocular coherence tomography in detecting angle-closure in different quadrants

of the anterior chamber angle. Ophthalmology 2008;115:769-74.

58. Su DH, Friedman DS, Aung T, et al. Degree of angle-closure and extent of peripheral anterior synechiae: an anterior segment OCT study. Br J Ophthalmol 2008;92:103-7.

59. Baskaran M, Oen FT, Chan YH, et al. Comparison of the scanning peripheral anterior chamber depth analyzer and the modified van Herick grading system in the assessment of angle-closure. Ophthalmology 2007;114:501-6.

60. Ritch R, Lowe RF. In: Ritch R, Shields MB, Krupin T (Eds). Classifications and mechanisms of the glaucomas, The Glaucomas, 2nd edn. S. Louis: Mosby; 1996. p. 752.

61. Wong HT, Lim MC, Aung T, et al. High-definition optical coherence tomography imaging of the iridocorneal angle of the eye. Arch Ophthalmol 2009;127:256-60.

62. Nolan WP, Foster PJ, Devereux JG, et al. YAG laser iridotomy treatment for primary angle-closure in East Asian eyes. Br J Ophthalmol 2000;84: 1255-9.

63. Wong HT, Chua JL, Aung T, et al. Comparison of slit-lamp optical coherence tomography and scanning peripheral anterior chamber depth analyzer to evaluate angle-closure in Asian eyes. Arch Ophthalmol 2009;127:599-603.

64. Foster P, He M, Liebmann J. In: Weinreb RN, Friedman DS (Eds). Angle-closure and angle-closure glaucoma consensus series 3. Kugler Publications; 2006. p. 20.

65. Kumar RS, Bhaskaran M, Chew PT, et al. Prevalence of plateau iris in primary angle closure suspects an ultrasound biomicroscopy study. Ophthalmology 2008;115:430-4.

66. He M, Foster PJ, Johnson GJ, Khaw PT. Angle-closure glaucoma in East Asian and European people. Different diseases? Eye 2006;20:3-12.

67. Quigley HA, Friedman DS, Congdon NG. Possible mechanisms of primary angle-closure and malignant glaucoma. J Glaucoma 2003;12:167-80.

68. Lavanya R, Foster PJ, Aung T, et al. Screening for narrow angles in the Singapore population: evaluation of new noncontact screening methods. Ophthalmology 2008;115:1720-7,e1-2.

69. Kumar RS, Quek D, Lee KY, Oen FT, Sakai H, Koh VT, MohanRam LS, Baskaran M, Wong TT, Aung T. Confirmation of the presence of uveal effusion in asian eyes with primary angle-closure glaucoma: An Ultrasound Biomicroscopy Study. Arch Ophthalmol (in press).

70. Sakai H, Morine-Shinjyo S, Shinzato M, Nakamura Y, Sakai M, Sawaguchi S. Uveal effusion in primary angle-closure glaucoma. Ophthalmology 2005;112:413-9.

71. Kumar RS, Tantisevi V, Aung T, et al. Plateau iris in Asian subjects with primary angle-closure glaucoma. Arch Ophthalmol 2009;127:1269-72.

72. Liebmann JM, Weinreb RN, Ritch R. Angle-closure glaucoma associated with occult annular ciliary body detachment. Arch Ophthalmol 1998;116:731-5.

73. Chen TC, Ang RT, Grosskreutz CL, et al. Brimonidine 0.2% versus apraclonidine 0.5% for prevention of intraocular pressure elevations after anterior segment laser surgery. Ophthalmology 2001;108:1033-8.

74. Fleck BW, Wright E, Fairley EA. A randomized prospective comparison of operative peripheral iridectomy and Nd:YAG laser iridotomy treatment of acute angle-closure glaucoma: 3 years visual acuity and intraocular pressure control outcome. Br J Ophthalmol 1997;81:884-8.

75. Alsagoff Z, Aung T, Ang LP, Chew PT. Long-term clinical course of primary angle-closure glaucoma in an Asian population. Ophthalmology 2000;107:2300-4.

76. Lim LS, Ho CL, Ang LP, Aung T, Tan DT. Inferior corneal decompensation following laser iridotomy in the superior iris. Am J Ophthalmol 2006;142:166-8.

77. Lim LS, Husain R, Gazzard G, Seah SK, Aung T. Cataract progression after prophylactic laser peripheral iridotomy: potential implications for the prevention of glaucoma blindness. Ophthalmology 2005;112:1355-9.

78. Ang LPK, Higashihara H, Sotonzono C, et al. Argon laser iridotomy—induced bullous keratopathy—a growing problem in Japan. Br J Ophthalmol 2007;91:1613-5.

79. Lam DS, Lai JS, Tham CC, et al. Argon laser peripheral iridoplasty versus conventional systemic medical therapy in treatment of acute primary angle-closure glaucoma: a prospective, randomized, controlled trial. Ophthalmology 2002;109:1591-6.

80. Ritch R, Lowe RF. In: Ritch R, Shields MB, Krupin T (Eds). Angle-closure glaucoma: therapeutic overview. The Glaucomas, 2nd edn. S. Louis: Mosby; 1996. pp. 1521-31.

81. Chew PT, Aung T, Aquino MV, Rojanapongpun P. EXACT Study Group. Intraocular pressure-reducing effects and safety of latanoprost versus timolol in patients with chronic angle-closure glaucoma. Ophthalmology 2004;111:427-34.

82. Kook MS, Cho HS, Yang SJ, et al. Efficacy of latanoprost in patients with chronic angle-closure glaucoma and no visible ciliary-body face: a preliminary study. J Ocul Pharmacol Ther 2005;21:75-84.

83. Tran HV, Liebmann JM, Ritch R. Iridociliary apposition in plateau iris syndrome persists after cataract extraction. Am J Ophthalmol 2003; 135:40-3.

84. Ritch R, Tham CC, Lam DS. Long-term success of argon laser peripheral iridoplasty in the management of plateau iris syndrome. Ophthalmology 2004;111:104-8.

85. Roberts TV, Francis IC, Lertusu-mitkul S, Kappagoda MB, Coroneo MT. Primary phacoemulsifica-tion for uncontrolled angle-closure glaucoma. J Cataract Refract Surg 2000;26:1012-6.

86. Kumar MRS, Aung T, et al. Diurnal intraocular pressure fluctuation and associated risk factors in eyes with angle-closure. Ophthalmology 2009 Oct 21 [Epub ahead of print].

87. Lai JS, Tham CC, Chan JC. The clini-cal outcomes of cataract extraction by phacoemulisfication in eyes with primary angle-closure glaucoma (PACG) and co-existing cataract: a prospective case series. J Glaucoma 2006;15:47-52.

88. Aung T. In: Weinreb RN, Friedman DS (Eds). Angle-closure and angle closure-glaucoma Consensus series 3. Kugler Publications; 2006. pp. 27-35.

89. Teekhasaenee C, Ritch R. Combined phacoemulsification and gonio-synechialysis for uncontrolled chronic angle-closure glaucoma af-ter acute angle-closure glaucoma. Ophthalmology 1999;106:669-74; discussion 74-5.

90. Choong YF, Irfan S, Manage MJ. Acute angle-closure glaucoma: an evaluation of a protocol for acute treatment. Eye 1999;13:613-6.

91. Tham CC, Leung DY, Kwong YY, et al. Effects of phacoemulsification ver-sus combined phacotrabeculectomy on drainage angle status in primary angle-closure glaucoma (PACG). J Glaucoma 2009 Apr 15. [Epub ahead of print].

92. Ang LP, Aung T, Chew PT. Acute pri-mary angle-closure in an Asian pop-ulation: long-term outcome of the fellow eye after prophylactic laser pe-ripheral iridotomy. Ophthalmology 2000;107:2092-6.

93. Tham CC, Kwong YY, Lai JS, et al. Phacoemulsification versus combined phacotrabeculectomy in medically uncontrolled chronic angle-closure glaucoma with cataracts. Ophthalmo-logy 2009;116:725-31, e1-3.

94. Harasymowycz PJ, Papamatheakis DG, Ahmed I, Assalian A, Lesk M, Al-Zafiri Y, Kranemann C, Hutaik C. Phacoemulsification and goniosyn-echialysis in the management of un-responsive primary angle-closure. J Glaucoma 2005;14:186-9.

95. Jacobi PC, Dietlein TS, Luke C, et al. Primary phacoemulsification and intraocular lens implantation for acute angle-closure glaucoma. Ophthalmology 2002;109:1597-603.

96. Aung T, Friedman DS, Chew PT, et al. Long-term outcomes in Asians after acute primary angle-closure. Ophthalmology 2004;111:1464-9.

97. Wilensky JT. The role of diurnal pres-sure measurements in the manage-ment of open-angle glaucoma. Curr Opin Ophthalmol 2004;15:90-2.

98. Asrani S, Zeimer R, Wilensky J, et al. Large diurnal fluctuations in intraoc-ular pressure are an independent risk factor in patients with glaucoma. J Glaucoma 2000;9:134-42.

99. Detry-Morel M. Currents on target intraocular pressure and intraocu-lar pressure fluctuations in glau-coma management. Bull Soc Belge Ophthalmol 2008;308:35-43.

100. Saccà SC, Rolando M, Marletta A, et al. Fluctuations of intraocular pressure during the day in open-angle glaucoma, normal-tension glaucoma and normal subjects. Ophthalmologica 1998;212:115-9.

101. Tajunisah I, Reddy SC, Fathilah J. Diurnal variation of intraocular pres-sure in suspected glaucoma patients and their outcome. Graefes Arch Clin Exp Ophthalmol 2007;245:1851-7.

Unilateral Glaucoma

Devendra Maheshwari, R Ramakrishnan

INTRODUCTION

The presence of glaucoma in one eye should alert the ophthalmologist to look more closely for a specific cause. Doing so is important as some types of glaucomas are characteristically unilateral **(Figures 1A to I)**. Glaucoma due a secondary or a known cause may be classified as secondary open-angle and angle closure types. Further, subclassification of the open angle type may delineate those cases caused by the presence of cells or debris in the angle and those due to damaged outflow channels. This chapter is intended to provide a synopsis for differential diagnosis of certain of the unilateral glaucomas, most of which are described individually is greater detail elsewhere in this book.

1. Unilateral angle closure glaucoma
   ❖ Acute primary angle closure attack and primary angle closure glaucoma
   ❖ Unilateral glaucomas due to synechial angle closure
2. Unilateral secondary open angle glaucoma

UNILATERAL ANGLE CLOSURE GLAUCOMAS (TABLE 1)

Primary Acute Angle Closure Glaucoma

In **primary acute angle closure glaucoma**, a closed angle and elevated IOP in only one eye is very common. In the subacute and chronic forms of primary angle closure, unilateral glaucoma is less common. When one finds angle closure and elevated IOP in one eye, in most cases the angle in the fellow eye is narrow and predisposed to closure. Occasionally, the angle in the fellow eye appears of good width on slit lamp examination, and one might conclude that it would not close but this is generally an erroneous conclusion, particularly, if the iris is convex. One may even be misled in a single gonioscopic examination by a transient deepening of the anterior chamber and widening of the angle due to the action of agents such as aqueous humor suppressants or hypertonic agents given systemically for treatment of the contralateral glaucomatous eye. The cases in which one can confidently say that the angle in the fellow eye will not close are those in which there is considerable anatomical asymmetry, such as when one eye is hypermetropic and the other is myopic, or when the cornea is smaller in the affected eye than in the fellow uninvolved eye, and the configuration of the anterior segment is quite different in the two eyes.

Table 1 Causes of unilateral angle closure glaucoma

• Primary acute angle closure glaucoma
• Dislocation of the lens
• Intumescent cataract
• Neovascular glaucoma
• Intraocular tumors
• Central retinal vein occlusion
• Panretinal photocoagulation
• Choroidal hemorrhage
• Massive vitreous hemorrhage
• Scleral buckling surgery
• Orbital venous congestion
• Retrobulbar tumor
• Iris bombe secondary to inflammation
• Iris bombe secondary epithelization
• Pupillary block or malignant glaucoma in aphakia or pseudophakia
• Persistent primary hyperplastic vitreous in childhood

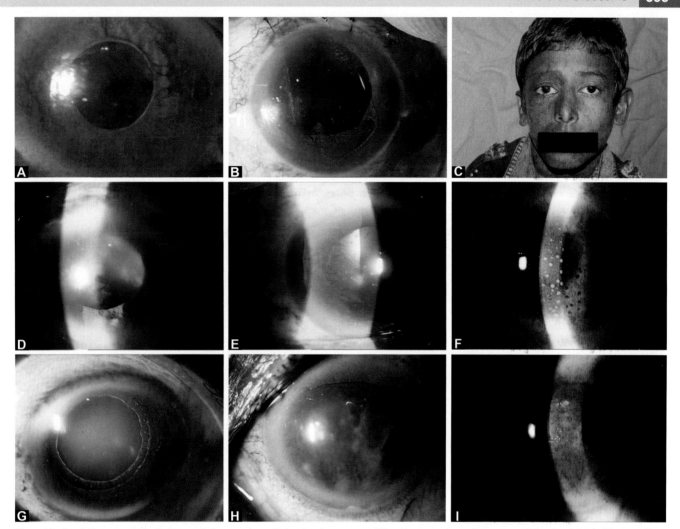

Figs 1A to I Some clinical presentations of unilateral glaucoma: (A) Neovascular glaucoma; (B) Pseudophakic pupillary block; (C) Sturge-Weber syndrome; (D) Lens particle induced glaucoma following cataract extraction; (E) Glaucoma due to postoperative hyphema following cataract extraction with IOL implantation; (F) Uveitic glaucoma; (G) Exfoliation glaucoma; (H and I) Pupillary block glaucoma due to iris cyst

Unilateral Peripheral Synechial Glaucomas

The second broad group of secondary unilateral glaucomas is due to synechial angle closure, associated with peripheral anterior synechiae. These causes are listed in **Table 2**. One of the most common cause is neovascular glaucoma. Rubeosis iridis leads to neovascular glaucoma if the new blood vessels with their fibrous matrix forming on the iris surface extend into the angle and produce angle closure.

Such neovascularization of the iris can be caused by a variety of conditions:

- ***Vascular (nonocular):*** Such as giant cell arteritis, aortic arch syndrome, carotid occlusive disease, carotid ligation, and carotid cavernous fistula (*Ocular:* central retinal vein or artery occlusion).
- ***Inflammatory:*** Uveitis, endophthalmitis, following radiotherapy.
- ***Neoplastic:*** Uveal malignant melanoma, retinoblastoma, metastatic carcinoma.

- ***Embryonal medulloepithelioma*** of the ciliary body.
- ***Retinal diseases:*** Vascular (as discussed above) diabetes mellitus, retinal detachment, Coat's disease, Leber's disease, sickle cell retinopathy, retinopathy of prematurity (retrolental fibroplasis), Eales disease, persistent hyperlastic primary vitreous, and Norrie's disease.

Lacerating trauma to the eye may lead to a fistula that develops from the external surface of the eye to the anterior chamber. This may lead to a flat anterior chamber and peripheral anterior synechiae formation. This also provides a conduit for epithelium to enter the anterior segment. This is an uncommon problem in the setting of microsurgical repair, but must be searched for in eyes that develop, glaucoma at a time remote from the initial lacerating injury.[1] The characteristic slit lamp appearance of a scalloped endothelial membrane is diagnostic for epithelial down growth.

Other possible causes are listed in **Table 2.**

UNILATERAL SECONDARY OPEN ANGLE GLAUCOMAS

In cases in which there is unilateral glaucoma with a clearly open angle and no peripheral anterior synechiae, the diagnosis is aided by special signs in the aqueous humor, on the posterior surface of the cornea, at the pupillary margin, and in the angle **(Table 3)**. These distinguish the following types. Some of them are discussed in detail here.

- Exfoliation glaucoma
- Pigmentary glaucoma
- Glaucoma following blunt trauma
- Hemolytic or ghost-cell glaucoma
- Phacolytic glaucoma
- Extraocular venous congestion and open angle glaucoma
- Steroid induced glaucoma
- Uveitic glaucma (Herpes zoster, Fuchs heterochromic iridocyclitis, Glauco, etc.) and glaucoma
- Glaucomatocyclitic crisis
- Heterochromic cyclitis
- Schwartz's syndrome
- Malignant melanoma.

Open angle unilateral glaucomas may be due to **damage to the outflow channels.**

Trauma

Trauma may produce secondary open-angle glaucoma by a direct effect or a postcontusion angle deformity. The direct effect or trauma on the anterior chamber angle is scarring of the meshwork while postcontusion angle deformity or angle recession is caused by laceration of the anterior face of the ciliary body with posterior displacement of the iris root and pars plicata of the ciliary body except for the longitudinal ciliary muscle. Open angle glaucoma develops in approximately 6 percent of eyes with angle recession, although, with more and more of the angle recessed, glaucoma occurs with a higher frequency. Post-traumatic hyphema is associated with angle recession in 40 to 60 percent of cases.[2] The glaucoma is due to sclerosis and secondary open angle glaucoma, endothelialization of the anterior chamber or secondary angle closure.

One such condition is hemosiderosis bulbi secondary to intraocular hemorrhage or siderosis bulbi due to the retention of an iron-containing foreign body. In both conditions ionized iron may spread to all ocular tissues but is mainly deposited in epithelial cells. Heterochromia and unilateral glaucoma may develop with an associated loss of vision from a toxic affect on the retina. Histopathological examination reveals deposition of iron in the corneal epithelium, iris pigment epithelium, iris dilator and sphincter muscles, both pigmented and non-pigmented ciliary epithelium, lens epithelium, trabecular meshwork, retinal pigment epithelium, and within the sensory retina. The latter may lead to retinal degeneration and gliosis.[3]

Fuchs' Heterochromic Iridocyclitis

Fuchs' heterochromic iridocyclitis is an idiopathic form of low grade iridocyclitis associated with iris stromal atrophy, cataract formation and glaucoma. Because of the diverse number of abnormalities that may be present,

Table 2 Unilateral glaucoma due to peripheral anterior synechiae

- Neovascular glaucoma
- Chronic angle closure glaucoma
- Lens induced (phacomorphic, phacotopic)
- Secondary to flat chamber postoperatively/post-trauma
- Uveitic glaucoma
- Essential iris atrophy
- Chandler's syndrome
- Iris nevus syndrome
- Epithelial invasion of the anterior chamber
- Endothelialization of the anterior chamber
- Malignant melanoma
- Juvenile xanthogranuloma

Table 3 Causes of unilateral secondary open angle glaucoma

- Cells or debris in the angle
- Hyphema
- Uveitis
    - ❖ Iridocyclitis (e.g. Fuchs heterochromic)
    - ❖ Glaucomatocyclitic crisis
- Phacolytic glaucoma
- Following lens rupture
- Hemolytic glaucoma
- Pigmentary glaucoma
- Malignant melanoma
- Exfoliation glaucoma
- Metastatic carcinoma

this may be one of the more difficult uveitis to diagnose. A lack of uniform diagnostic criteria exists. Although Fuchs' HIC typically affects only one eye, it is bilateral in approximately 13 percent of cases. Onset is usually in the third or fourth decade.[4,5] The patient is frequently either asymptomatic or complains of monocular reduced visual acuity on clinical presentation. The eye is white and quiet. Characteristically, there are fine colorless keratic precipitates; some are round, but the most typical are filamentary or star-shaped, scattered over the posterior surface of the cornea. These are best seen by retroillumination. There may be trace flare in the aqueous humor with an occasional white cell. The iris is infiltrated with plasma cells with accompanying degeneration and atrophy. Clinically, atrophy of the iris affects the pupil collarette (transforming it to a hyaline border) and produces hypochromia of the iris stroma with abnormal transillumination of the posterior pigment layer.

Glaucomatocyclitic Crisis (Posner-Schlossman Syndrome)

This idiopathic syndrome was first described by Posner and Schlossman in 1948. This disorder can be characterized as a trabeculitis. The initial episode most commonly occurs between ages 20 or 50 years. Onset of symptoms is usually acute. IOP is often highly elevated. Symptoms are typically unilateral and consist of slight ocular discomfort and blurred vision.[6] The patient may see colored halos around lights secondary to corneal edema. Examination reveals a highly elevated IOP, usually between 40 and 70 mm Hg. The eye is generally quiet with little or no hyperemia. The cornea may have mild to moderate epithelial edema with a few fine keratic precipitates. Keratic precipitates may not be noted for 2 or 3 days after the onset of symptoms and tend to vary in number and position from day to day. Gonioscopy reveals a normal appearing angle, open throughout, with no abnormal pigmentation. Occasionally, one may find a few tiny inflammatory precipitates on the trabecular meshwork. Characteristically, no posterior or anterior synechiae are formed. If tonography is performed, it demonstrates a highly elevated resistance to aqueous outflow in the affected eye but a normal value in the unaffected eye.

This disorder must be distinguished from an acute angle-closure glaucoma attack because treatment is radically different. There are several instances where iridectomy has been performed in an effort to treat this disorder. Iridectomy is of no use in glaucomatocyclitic glaucoma but of course, would be indicated for angle closure glaucoma.

Phacolytic Glaucoma

Phacolytic glaucoma is seen in the setting of a mature cataract. Open angle glaucoma occurs as a results of leakage of high molecular weight proteins through an intact lens capsule.[7] Macrophages also are present in the anterior chamber.

Exfoliation Glaucoma

Pseudoexfoliation of the lens capsule or, as Sugar has termed the condition, "the exfoliation syndrome" is a common disorder with a cosmopolitan distribution. There is some predilection for Scandinavians although the condition is seen in nearly all racial groups. The exfoliation syndrome is most likely an inherited disorder, possibly inherited as an autosomal dominant with incomplete penetrance and invariable expressivity.[8] It occurs in individuals between the ages of 60 and 80 years. And is unilateral in 50 percent of the cases with an associated open angle glaucoma in 70 percent of patients. Clinically, the exfoliated material is present on the pupillary ruff of the iris, anterior iris surface, in the anterior chamber angle, and in a characteristic distribution on the anterior lens capsule. The anterior lens capsule shows a typical central disc surrounded by a clear zone, which is in turn surrounded by a peripheral granular area. Gonioscopy reveals the deposition of pigment (from the iris pigment

epithelium) in the meshwork. There is increases transillumination of the iris near the pupil. Histopathological examination shows of the typical eosinophilic material on the anterior surface of the lens, on the vitreous face and zonular fibers, upon and within the anterior and posterior surfaces of the iris and ciliary body, in the anterior chamber angle and trabecular meshwork, and around conjunctival blood vessels.

Metastatic Carcinoma

Metastatic carcinoma to the iris is unusual but may cause unilateral open angle glaucoma. The hallmark of metastatic carcinoma to the iris is the presence on the iris surface of translucent, gelatinous nodules which may extend to the angle and occlude the meshwork. Occasionally iritis is present, rarely hypopyon.[9] In some instances rubeosis iridis and iris atrophy are present. Rarely, a patient with carcinoma metastatic to the iris presents with a hyphema. Cytological examination of aqueous aspirates may reveal the presence of carcinoma cells. Fluorescein angiography of the iris may show a vascularized lesion which displays leakage in the late phase. Histopathological examination reveals infiltration of the iris and angle structures by tumor cells.[9]

CONCLUSION

Most primary glaucomas are bilateral but may appear as unilateral due to an assymetric presentation. Unilateral Glaucoma is usually secondary and a careful ocular examination is important to look for the cause and start the appropriate management. These are usually associated with a high IOP and if timely intervention is not done, glaucomatous optic neuropathy and blindness can occur.

REFERENCES

1. Friedman AH, Taterka HB, Henkind P. Epithelial implantation onto the iris surface during cataract extraction. A report of two cases. Am J Ophthalmol 1972;71:482-5.

2. Blanton FM. Anterior chamber angle recession and secondary glaucoma. Arch Ophthalmol 1964;72:39-43.

3. Masciulli L, Anderson DR, Charles S. Experimental ocular siderosis in the squirrel monkey. Am J Ophthalmol 1972;74:638-61.

4. Perry H, Yanoff M, Scheie HG. Fuchs heterochromic iridocyclitis. Arch Ophthalmol 1975;93:337-9.

5. Kimura SJ, Hogan MJ, Thygeson P. Fuchs' syndrome of heterochromic cyclitis. Arch Ophthalmol 1955;54:179.

6. Posner A, Schlossman A. Syndrome of unilateral recurrent attacks of glaucoma with cyclitic symptoms. Arch Ophthalmol 1953;39:517-35.

7. Flocks M, Littwin CS, Zimmerman LE. Phacolytic glaucoma. Arch Opthalmol 1955;54:37-45.

8. Sugar HS, Harding C, Barsky D. The exfoliation syndrome. Ann Ophthalmol 1976;8:1165-77.

9. Friedman AH, Freeman T. Metastatic carcinoma of the iris. Am J Ophthalmol 1975;80:947-52.

28 | Exfoliation Syndrome and Exfoliation Glaucoma

Mona Khurana, R Ramakrishnan

INTRODUCTION

Exfoliation syndrome (XFS) is an age-related, generalized disorder of the extracellular matrix, an elastic microfibrillopathy, characterized by progressive production and deposition of abnormal fibrillar material in many ocular and extraocular tissues.[1] **(Figure 1)**. It has been recognized for more than half a century ever since it was first reported by Lindberg in 1917.[2] Initially thought to be a disease of the Scandinavian countries, it has been reported from across the world and is now known to be the most common identifiable cause of open angle glaucoma worldwide.[3-7] Inspite of this, XFS and exfoliation glaucoma (XFG) continue to present a continuum of challenges. It is fascinating with aspect to its varied epidemiology and geographical distribution, it also poses a mystery regarding a definite understanding of its exact composition and pathophysiology. The aggressive nature of exfoliation glaucoma, its resistance to medical management and the increased risk of intraoperative complications make it a distinct entity from primary open angle glaucoma

(POAG). It is a secondary open angle glaucoma. The implications of this disorder are far more than what meets the eye with the ocular findings being only the tip of the iceberg. The disease has been aptly referred to as an *enigma*.[8] The complete implications of its systemic nature are yet to be understood. The discovery of mutations in the *LOXL1* gene that confer susceptibility to exfoliative glaucoma has opened doors for further research.[9-13] This chapter deals with the current concepts, pathogenesis, clinical features and management of glaucoma associated with this disorder.

What's in a Name?

The enigma starts with its name. Although exfoliation syndrome has been recognized for almost a century, there has been a lack of consensus regarding its name. It has been associated with glaucoma by Vogt[14] ever since first reported by Lindberg.[2] Vogt introduced the term '*exfoliation superficialis capsulae anteriores*' assuming that the flocculent material arose as small flecks peeling off from the lens capsule itself. Dvorak

Theobald[15] called it pseudoexfoliation to distinguish it from true exfoliation, the delamination of the lens capsule seen in glass blowers. Other names include senile exfoliation of the lens capsule, senile uveal exfoliation, fibrillopathia epitheliocapsularis and glaucoma capsulare (when associated with glaucoma). More recent studies have again pointed to the lens capsule as one of the sources of the material and have termed it as "Exfoliation syndrome" and "Exfoliation glaucoma" when associated with glaucoma. In the Sigrid Juselius Foundation sponsored

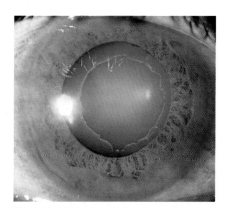

Fig. 1 Exfoliation syndrome is characterized by the deposition of white, flaky, dandruff like material in the anterior segment structures

International Workshop in Finland, the majority favored the name 'exfoliation syndrome' over the alternative, 'pseudoexfoliation syndrome.'[16] Currently, both terms are commonly used in the literature and both have also been used in this book to refer to this condition.

> Exfoliation syndrome (XFS) is an age related, generalized disorder of the extracellular matrix, an elastic micro-fibrillopathy, characterized by progressive production and deposition of abnormal fibrillar material in many ocular and extraocular tissues.

EPIDEMIOLOGY

The epidemiology of XFS and XFG is interesting. Lindbergs first description was in a series of patients from Finland.[2] High prevalence rates continued to be reported from Scandinavia. However it is not unique to the Nordic countries. It is found in almost all parts of the world (with a few exceptions) affecting an estimated 60 to 70 million people worldwide. Yet there are marked geographic differences in prevalence. The reported influences of gender and ethnicity also differ among geographic populations. A high prevalence of XFS has been reported in many populations including Japanese, Indians,[17-22] Australian Aborigines, Bantu tribe of South Africa, Navajos, Peruvian Indians and many European countries. Its prevalence varies from 0 percent in the Inuits of Greenland,[23] 1.6 percent in a south eastern US population,[24] 1.8 percent in the Framingham Eye Study[25] 5 to 25 percent in the Scandinavian countries, and 38 percent in Navajo Indians.[26] In Australia the prevalence of exfoliation was 0.98 percent in the visual impairment project[27] and 2.3 percent in the Blue Mountains Eye Study.[28] The prevalence is more in Caucasians as compared to Africans. The Inuits of

Greenland may be the only population with a very low prevalence rates/no reported prevalence. Low prevalence rates have been reported from southern China. It has also been reported from Ethiopia, South Africa and Gambia where it was pre-viously thought to be rare.

Astrom[29] et al. followed a cohort of 339 individuals for 21 years and found that the prevalence of XFS increased from 23 percent at 66 years of age to 61 percent at 87 years with 1.8 percent annual incidence. Population based data on the prevalence of exfoliation syndrome are available from studies in India.[20-22] It is reported to affect between 3 percent and 6 percent of those aged 40 years or older.

> Marked geographic differences in prevalence.

Racial and Ethnic Variation

The prevalence of exfoliation syndrome varies considerably between countries, within regions or between ethnic groups. This may reflect a true difference due to ethnic causes or climatic variations **(Table 1)**. On the other hand, the differences could be due methodological variations like the age and gender distributions of the populations studied, the clinical criteria used, thoroughness during the examination, examination in dilated or undilated eyes. This makes comparison of results of various studies difficult. Difference among ethnically homogeneous persons or ethnically different people living in close proximity have been reported from studies in France, Crete and New Mexico. The Middle-Norway survey[30] tried to overcome this problem of incomparability. Similar age groups from three different but adjacent areas were examined. The prevalence of XFS in two adjacent towns was almost twice than the third.

Table 1 Causes for variations in prevalence of XFS

True difference in prevalence
Ethnic
Genetic
Geographical
Methodological variations in study design regarding
Age and gender distribution in studies
Studies conducted over a diverse population
Clinical diagnostic criteria used
Variability in definition of glaucoma
Thoroughness of examination
Examination in dilated or undilated eyes

Observations made by a single observer in different populations have also varying rates.[31] Prevalence rates have been noted to be higher in Ireland as compared to its neighboring England. In Nepal, the prevalence of XFS was found to be higher in the Gurung ethnic group as compared to the non Gurung.[32] Uniformly conducted studies would provide a better insight into the true variations in the epidemiology of the disease. Differences among ethnically homogeneous groups or between ethnic groups living in close proximity may be worth exploring and may provide important insights.

Age

The prevalence of exfoliation syndrome is closely linked to age. With increasing mean age, XFS increases in prevalence, reaching a maximum in the seventh to ninth decades of life. Its prevalence in the Framingham study was 0.6 percent in patients younger than 65 years, 2.6 percent in patients between 65 to 74 years and 5.0 percent in patients 75 to 85 years of age. Similar observations have been made in the Indian population.[20-22] Interestingly, a few cases of XFS occurring in individuals less than 40 years have been reported from across the world, the youngest reported case being 17 years old.

Gender

Women have predominated in some series of XFS without glaucoma. Others have found equal or greater prevalence in men. Glaucoma may develop earlier, more frequently, and more severely in men. No gender predilection was reported for the disease in some studies from India while Krishnadas et al.[20] found it to be more prevalent in males. XFS increases the risk of glaucoma four fold in both sexes with no difference in mortality.

Exfoliation Glaucoma
Prevalence of Ocular Hypertension and Glaucoma in XFS

Exfoliation syndrome is associated with ocular hypertension, open angle glaucoma and angle closure glaucoma. Almost all studies have shown an association of XFS with raised IOP and glaucoma. The prevalence of glaucoma in patients with exfoliation syndrome is reportedly 0 to 93 percent. The risk of developing glaucoma is 5 to 10 times more common in eyes with XFS than in those without it. About 25 percent of patients with XFS have elevated intraocular pressure. One-third of these have glaucoma. Patients with XFS and ocular hypertension are twice as likely to convert to glaucoma, whereas patients with XFG are likely to progress more rapidly. The Blue Mountains Eye Study[28] (population-based study with presence of glaucomatous optic nerve head changes as diagnostic criteria), reported a prevalence of 9.3 percent OHT and 14.2 percent glaucoma in patients with XFS. Kozart and Yanoff,[33] studied 100 consecutive patients (clinic based study) with exfoliation and reported 15 percent prevalence of OHT and 7 percent prevalence of glaucoma. Ocular hypertension was present in 4.2 percent of those with XFS in the Aravind comprehensive eye survey (ACES) while 9.3 percent of those with

XFS in the Chennai Glaucoma Study (CGS) were ocular hypertensive. The prevalence of glaucoma among those with exfoliation was reported to be 3.02 percent in the Andhra Pradesh Eye Disease Study (APEDS), 7.5 percent in ACES and 13 percent in of the CGS (the rural cohort).

Prevalence of Exfoliation Syndrome in Open Angle Glaucoma

Surveys of patients in many regions of the world have revealed that 20 to 60 percent of patients with open angle glaucoma may actually have XFG. Prevalence rates of exfoliation in glaucoma cohorts range from as much as 93 percent in Scandinavian countries to 3 to 25 percent in other populations.[24,34-40] Exfoliation glaucoma (XFG) was present in up to two-thirds of individuals with OAG in Ireland and Sweden. Exfoliation was present in 26.7 percent of those identified as primary open angle glaucoma in ACES.[20]

> The distinction between POAG and exfoliation glaucoma is important as it has significant clinical implications. Eyes with XFG have a worse prognosis and more serious course often requiring surgical intervention.

Angle Closure Glaucoma

An association between exfoliation and angle closure glaucoma has been noted with a number of studies showing a higher prevalence of occludable angles in XFS. Ritch[1] found either clinically apparent XFS or exfoliation material on conjunctival biopsy in 17 of 60 (28.3%) consecutive patients with uncomplicated primary ACG or occludable angles. Glaucomatous optic neuropathy was found in 31.3 percent of XFS cases with occludable angles (4.6% of all XFS patients) in a study in South Indian population. Layden and Schaffer[34] reported a 23 percent prevalence of narrow angles in

100 patients with PEX. Wishart[40a] et al. reported 18 percent occludable angles in their study of 76 patients with XFS.

Risk of Glaucoma with Time

Five percent of patients with XFS and no glaucoma at initial visit may develop raised IOP or glaucoma within 5 years and 15 percent experience elevated IOP after 10 years. This clearly indicates that the presence of XFS may be a red flag for the future development of glaucoma.[36,41-44] It must be noted that IOP spikes occur in exfoliation syndrome that may not manifest on a single IOP record. The various risk factors for conversion[45-48] to glaucoma are listed in **Table 2**.

ETIOLOGY AND PATHOGENESIS
Genetics or Geography
Geographical Factors

The exact role of genetic and environmental factors in the pathogenesis of XFS is not clear. The high prevalence rate in Nordic countries suggests that a northern latitude, cold air, and sunlight may contribute but no strong evidence exists. Attempts to link XFS with ultraviolet (UV) rays exposure have been mixed. XFS is more common among Laplanders but rare among Greenland Inuits inspite of a similar latitude.[3] XFS is common in Saudi Arabia where sunlight is more intense than northern latitudes. It is seen to occur at an earlier age in patients living at lower latitude[49] (Greece/Saudi Arabia/Iran).

Table 2 Risk factors for conversion from to exfoliation glaucoma

- Increased intraocular pressure[45]
- Presence of XFM in the angle
- Presence of XFM in the other eye
- Decreased pupillary dilatation[46]
- Increased trabecular meshwork pigmentation[47,48]
- Genetic: LOXL1 SNP
- Geographical factors

Those predominantly involved in outdoor activities were found to be at a greater risk of XFS than those whose occupation was classified as indoor in the APEDS.[22]

Genetic

A genetic role is very likely and is currently the topic of interest. Historically, a genetic basis has always been strongly suspected as both XFS and XFG demonstrate strong familial aggregation that is consistent with inherited disorders. Increased relative risk of XFS in first-degree relatives, in twin studies and transmission through two generation pedigrees has been documented. Patterns like autosomal dominant (AD) inheritance, autosomal recessive, X linked and mitochondrial transmission have been proposed. A clear inheritance pattern has not been demonstrated.

The genetic background as explained above, has always been suspected though the mechanism was not very clear until 2007. Thorleifsson et al[9] identified *single nucleotide polymorphisms* (SNP) associated with XFS in an Icelandic population, replicated in a Swedish cohort. Three single nucleotide polymorphisms in the coding region of the *LOXL1* gene located on chromosome 15q24 were strongly associated with XFS and XFG in these populations (>99% population attributable risk). Two SNPs in the first coding exon and one SNP in the first intron were identified. High risk haplotype of LOXL1 was found to be very common in Icelandic and Swedish population (more than 50 percent of the general population). 25 percent were homozygous. The LOXL1 association with XFS/XFG has been replicated in several other populations including South Indian populations. The rs3825942 variant (Gly1153Asp) was the most prevalent occurring in 94 to 100 percent of XFG, 95 to 100 percent of XFS, and 57 to 88 percent of control individuals.

The second variant, rs1048661 (Arg141 Leu) has not been replicated to the same degree. In fact an inverse relationship has been noted in the Japanese population.

What are SNPs?

- SNPs are variations in single nucleotides resulting in DNA sequence variation that may generate complicated protein changes and may themselves be associated with disease.
- SNPs found in a coding sequence may not always change the amino acid sequence of the protein it is producing due to the degeneracy in the genetic code.
- Synonymous SNPs: Where both lead to the same polypeptide sequence
- Nonsynonymous: Where different polypeptides are produced as in XFS
- SNP not in specific protein coding region may also have consequence for transcription binding factor and gene splicing.

- SNPs in the LOXL1 gene are a major genetic risk factor for XFS and XFG disease with an 80 to 99% population attributable risk in various cohorts
- All XFS patients in the Iceland and Swedish cohort had LOXL1 polymorphism. Similar and high prevalence of LOXL1 variants in XFS and XFG suggests that these variants confer nearly equal risk to developing both the conditions.
- Due to the relative similarity of prevalence in individuals with XFS and XFG, genetic testing is of limited usefulness.

- LOXL1 belongs to the lysyl oxidase or 'LOX' family of extracellular enzymes that have multiple functions, including the oxidative deamination of lysine residues to allow the proper orientation and crosslinking of elastin polymers from tropoelastin.
- LOXL1 and elastin are expressed in the cornea, iris, ciliary body, lens capsule, and optic nerve, TM, zonules
- LOXL1 has a strong biochemical rationale for being associated with XFS and XFG.

Other genes

Studies are currently underway to identify other genes associated with XFS/XFG. Evidence for this is suggested by a second genome-wide association study that has been performed on a Finnish family and demonstrates linkage to 18q12.1-21.33, 2q, 17p, and 19q.[49a]

Multifactorial Etiology

The genetic association has been proven as explained above. A number of nongenetic factors have been hypothesized to be involved in the pathogenesis of exfoliation. As mentioned earlier, these include exposure to ultraviolet light, dietary factors, autoimmunity, infectious agents and trauma. The diagnosis of XFS in younger age group has usually been preceded by ocular trauma, surgery or corneal grafts from elderly donors. This suggests that trauma or surgery may prematurely trigger the development of XFS in a predisposed person. However, many of these hypothesis still need to be proven. Exfoliation syndrome appears to be a complex multifactorial, late onset disease involving multiple genes and nongenetic mechanisms **(Table 3)**.

Etiology of XFS is multifactorial involving genetic and nongenetic mechanisms.

Composition: Fibrils of Unknown Composition?

Microscopic Structure

The exfoliation material pathognomonic for the disease has characteristic light and electron microscopic features. It consists of a tangle of fibrils and filaments embedded in an amorphous matrix. Both large and small fibrils are present. The fibrils are composed of microfibrillar subunits surrounded by an amorphous matrix.

Chemical Structure[50-56]

Despite strikingly characteristic clinical characteristic appearance, the exact

Table 3 Etiology of XFS

Genetic
• Historically, autosomal dominant (AD) inheritance
• LOXL1
Nongenetic
• Exposure to ultraviolet light
• Dietary factors
• Autoimmunity
• Infectious agents
• Trauma
• Oxidative stress

chemical composition of exfoliation material is unclear. This is because the material is difficult to solubilise and different procedures result in different quantities and types of proteins solubilized for mass spectrometry analysis. Moreover the small sample quantity is also a limitation. Current knowledge of its composition is based on indirect histochemical and immunohistochemical methods. Recently, direct analysis with liquid chromatography coupled with tandem mass spectrometry is being used to study the components of XFM.

Basically, it appears to be a complex glycoprotein/proteoglycan structure bearing epitopes of basement membrane and elastic fiber system. It has a protein core surrounded by glycoconjugates, probably glycosaminoglycans which also form the amorphous ground substance. Its *protein components* include both noncollagenous basement membrane components and epitopes of the elastic fiber system. These include elastin, tropoelastin, amyloid P, vitreonectin and components of elastic microfibrils such as fibrillin 1, MAGP-1. Also present as intrinsic components of the XFM are the glycosaminoglycans (GAGs) heparan sulfate and chondroitin sulfate, components of proteoglycans (PGs), the broadly distributed nonprotein constituents of basement

membranes as well as the modulators of extracellular matrix (ECM) formation such as the growth factor TGF-β1 and its latent-form binding proteins LTBP-1 and LTBP-2.

Composition of Exfoliation Material
• Exact chemical composition not clear
• XFM is difficult to solubilize
• Current knowledge is based on indirect histochemical and immuno-histochemical methods and direct analysis with liquid chromatography coupled with tandem mass spectrometry
• A complex glycoprotein/proteoglycan structure
• Protein core surrounded by amorphous substance: glycosaminoglycans
• Contain epitopes of both basement membrane and elastic fiber system

Fibrillin 1, the main component of elastic microfibrils has been demonstrated in exfoliation fibers and their microfibrillar subunits, often in immediate proximity to cellular surfaces. This suggests an excessive production and abnormal aggregation of fibrillin-containing microfibrils in the extracellular matrix in XFS.

The **latent tumor growth factor-beta binding proteins** (LTBP-1 and LTBP-2) have been associated with all exfoliative deposits and co-localized with latent TGF on exfoliation fibers. These LTBPs may have a dual role, both as a structural component of exfoliation fibers and as a means of matrix anchorage of latent TGF β1 to XFM.

The HNK-1 epitope, a carbohydrate moiety also present on many cell adhesion-related glycoproteins, may be involved in the adhesiveness of exfoliation material deposits on intraocular surfaces acting like a glue and binding the various components together and to the ocular structures.[50,51]

Recently, direct analysis with liquid chromatography coupled with tandem mass spectrometry (LC-MS/MS) have been used to study the composition of exfoliative material.

These techniques have shown the presence of elastic microfibril components like of fibrillin 1, fibrillin 2, vitreonectin, proteoglycans syndecan and versecan, the extracellular chaperone, fibulin-2 and desmocollin-2 (glycoproteins). These studies have also unveiled novel components of the XFM, including cell adhesion molecules and ECM proteins, nondescribed PGs, complement proteins, matrix metalloproteases and specific inhibitors, as well as the presence of the multifunctional protein clustering as a major component of the deposits. *New molecules are still being uncovered by biochemical and molecular biological approaches.*

Biochemical Changes in the Aqueous Humor [51,56,56a]

The changes in the aqueous (**Table 4**) require a special mention as most of the experimental work has been done by examining the composition of aqueous due to its easy accessibility during intraocular surgery. Moreover, all the involved ocular tissues are bathed by aqueous. Increased concentration of growth factors, imbalance between TIMP and MMP, increased oxidative stress factors, decrease in protective factors and increase of vasoactive endothelin 1 has been observed.

TGF beta 1: It is a powerful modulator of matrix formation in many fibrotic diseases. High levels have been reported in the aqueous humor of patients with XFS and exfoliative glaucoma along with enhanced mRNA expression. It interacts with lysyl oxidase to influence the formation of elastin. High levels of TGF beta 1 are believed to be both responsible for

Table 4 Changes in aqueous humor

• Reduced outflow
• Increased protein aggregates
• Increased growth factors
• Increased acid phosphatase activity
• Increased homocysteine
• Increased TGF beta 1

overproduction of extracellular matrix and one of the causative factors for the production of exfoliation material.

Matrix metalloproteinases: Extracellular matrix turnover is mediated by matrix metalloproteinases (MMPs). They constitute a large family of endopeptidases that are capable of degrading all extracellular matrix molecules. They are synthesized and secreted as inactive proenzymes and are activated by proteolytic cleavage. TIMPS can inhibit all active MMPs. Decreased levels of activated MMP-2 and the significantly increased concentrations of TIMP-1 and -2 lead to a stoichiometric excess of TIMP-2 over MMP-2 in aqueous humor in XFG. This is related to inappropriate matrix degradation and progressive matrix accumulation. Increased levels of matrix metalloproteinases (MMP) are present in the aqueous humor in XFS. MMP2, MMP3 have been found to be increased in XFS as compared to controls and also their inhibitors TIMP1 and TIMP2. An excess of TIMP2 and decreased endogenous activity of MMP2, along with a decreased MMP2 to TIMP ratio may promote abnormal matrix accumulation. TIMPs also bind to XFM material creating so called *cold spots* for proteolysis.

Homocysteine: Homocysteine is a highly cytotoxic amino acid derived from methionine metabolism. Elevated serum levels result from disturbed methionine metabolism. Increased levels of homocysteine have been observed in the aqueous humor, tear fluid in both XFS and XFG. Lysyl oxidase in vascular endothelia is inhibited by high concentrations of homocysteine. In animal studies hyperhomocysteinemia has been associated with disruption of the elastic fiber component of the extracellular matrix and vascular complications.

Significantly reduced levels of **ascorbic acid**, a free radical scavenger

along with increased levels of 8 isoprostaglandin F2 alpha, a marker of oxidative stress suggest a faulty antioxidative defense mechanism in the pathogenesis.

Pathological Process

The pathological process is characterized by chronic accumulation of abnormal fibrillar matrix product, which is the result of either increased production or decreased degradation or both. Historically, many theories were proposed regarding the pathogenesis of the disease **(Table 5)**.

Pathogenetic Concept and Theories of Pathogenesis

Amyloid Theory

There was an initial positive labelling of XFM with a crude antiamyloid serum suggesting amyloid deposits.[58,59] Sophisticated tests however yielded negative results. Thus this theory could not be substantiated.[60]

Basement Membrane Theory

A frequent association of exfoliative material with basement membranes of various cell types has been observed. This may suggest a disturbed basement membrane metabolism as a possible mechanism. Immunohistochemical studies reveal presence of basement membrane epitopes like laminin, heparin sulfate proteoglycan in XFM aggregates.[61,62]

Elastic Microfibril Theory

This theory was based on the frequent structural association of XFM with components of the elastin system like zonules. Marked localized elastosis of the elastic fibers in lamina cribrosa has also been seen.[57,63] Immunohistochemical demonstration of epitopes of elastin further support this theory.

> Both the basement membrane and elastic microfibril theories appear to describe part of the pathological process.

Table 5 Theories of pathogenesis of XFS

- Stress induced elastosis
- Basement membrane theory
- Elastic microfibril theory
- Protein sink model
- Amyloid theory—not substantiated
- Infectious theory—no conclusive evidence

Infectious Origin

Prevalence of XFM in both partners of married couples, reports of younger patients developing XFS after intraocular surgery or ocular trauma suggested the possibility of an infectious origin.[64-66] Increasing number of younger patients developing XFS after penetrating keratoplasty with grafts from elderly donors also suggested an infectious origin. **However no conclusive evidence is available.[67-69]**

Current Concept

XFS is currently described as a type of stress induced elastosis. It is an elastic microfibrillopathy associated with excessive production of elastic microfibrils by a variety of elastogenic cells. These microfibrils subsequently aggregate into typical exfoliative fibrils. A complex cross linking process is involved in the formation of the XFM. Growth factors especially TGF beta1 and oxidative stress are involved. Other extracellular matrix components, e.g. basement membrane components and glycosaminoglycans may interact and become incorporated into the exfoliation material. Frequent association of XFM with defective basement membranes of various cell types and immunohistochemical evidence of basement membrane epitopes suggest disturbed basement membrane metabolism. An imbalance between MMP and TIMP may be responsible for the incomplete degradation of the newly formed material resulting in accumulation within tissues with deleterious effects over time. An overproduction and abnormal metabolism of glycosaminoglycans has also been suggested to comprise one of the key changes in XFS. This hypothesis is supported by the finding of higher levels of hyaluronan in the aqueous humor of patients with XFS.

> An excessive production, impaired catabolism, and subsequent accumulation of abnormal cross-linked ECM material

Protein Sink Model

A protein sink model has also been proposed. According to this model, soluble proteins normally found in biological fluids change their native conformation and form insoluble structures that accumulate in the form of either intra- and extracellular aggregates or fibrillar lesions.

It has been hypothesized that an aberrant nucleation protein or nucleation protein complex binds to other proteins in the aqueous humor of the eye. These proteins then form a larger and more complex protein matrix that eventually precipitates out of solution and forms the exfoliation material. This material then forms a fine dusting of material on surfaces like the lens capsule and the angle of the anterior chamber and slowly aggregates. The altered blood aqueous barrier allows the entry of proteins present normally in the serum into the aqueous humor. These normal proteins may then interact with nucleation proteins and aid in the formation of the exfoliation material.

Ocular Ischemia

Exfoliation is associated with ocular ischemia, especially iris and anterior segment hypoxia. Ocular and retrobulbar micro and macrovascular blood flow is reduced in patients with and without glaucoma. An increase in the presence of endothelin, a potent vasoconstrictor and decrease in nitric oxide, a vasodilator may cause an imbalance and result in early ischemia. Elevated homocysteine levels may also contribute to ischemia.

To Summarize

The nature of the molecules forming the XFM indicates an excessive production, impaired catabolism and subsequent accumulation of abnormal cross-linked ECM material. Matrix proteolytic imbalances, low-grade inflammatory processes, and the presence of ischemia/hypoxia, together with dysregulated cellular and oxidative stress mechanisms, also appear to be significant contributors to the pathobiology of XFS.

Source of the Exfoliative Material

Intraocular: The characteristic fibrils are produced at multiple sites by various intraocular cells including pre-equatorial lens epithelium, non-pigmented ciliary epithelium, trabecular endothelium, vascular endothelium and virtually all types of iris cells. Active fibrillogenesis is accompanied by a destruction of the cells' normal basement membrane.

Extraocular Sites and Systemic Association

Aggregates of exfoliation fibers have been identified in conjunctiva, orbital tissue, skin and in autopsy specimens of heart, lung, liver, kidney, gallbladder, and cerebral meninges. These deposits were focally present in the interstitial fibrovascular connective tissue septa of these organs, frequently adjacent to elastic fibers, elastic microfibrils, collagen fibers, fibroblasts, and the walls of small blood vessels (**Table 6**).

A large number of systemic associations have been reported with exfoliation syndrome and exfoliation glaucoma (**Table 7**). XFS correlated positively with a history of hypertension, angina, myocardial infarction, or stroke, suggestive of vascular effects of the disease.[28] Transient ischemic attacks, sensorineural deafness, Alzheimer's and aneurysms

XFM Production

Ocular: XFM is produced by	Systemic: XFM is found in close proximity to
Pre-equatorial lens epithelium	Fibroblasts
Non-pigmented ciliary epithelium	Smooth and striated muscle cells
Trabecular endothelium	Vascular walls
Vascular endothelium	Cardiac muscle
Virtually all types of iris cells	

Table 6 Extraocular and systemic sites of XFM deposits

Extraocular sites
• Conjunctiva
• Orbital tissue
Systemic sites
• Skin
• Visceral organs
• Heart
• Lung
• Liver
• Kidney
• Gallbladder
• Meninges
• Blood vessel walls

Table 7 Systemic associations of XFS*

- Cardiovascular disorders
- Aneurysms of abdominal aorta
- Sensorineural deafness
- Reduced carotid blood flow
- Transient ischemic attacks
- Alzheimers

*No increase in mortality rate has been reported

of the abdominal aorta have been associated with XFS. However, no increase in mortality rate has been reported in patients with XFS.

PATHOGENESIS OF GLAUCOMA

Glaucoma may develop in up to 50 percent of eyes with XFS and is different and more difficult to control than POAG. The following are the proposed mechanisms (**Table 8**).

Outflow Obstruction and IOP Elevation

The glaucoma associated with XFS is a **secondary open angle glaucoma** associated with an increase in outflow resistance. One-fifth of the patients may also have narrow angles which serves as an additional mechanism. The primary cause of chronic pressure elevation is the active participation of the

trabecular endothelial cells especially the endothelial cells of the Schlemm's canal in the production of exfoliation material. Locally produced as well as passively deposited exfoliation material in the juxtacanalicular tissue clogs the trabecular meshwork causing outflow obstruction. Over a period of time the exfoliative material leads to subsequent degenerative changes in the TM and especially in the Schlemm's canal. A study of aqueous humor dynamics suggests a higher resistance to aqueous flow and a decreased uveoscleral outflow. Blockage of the aqueous veins due to perivascular aggregation may also contribute to the IOP elevation. The amount of XFM can be correlated to the IOP level and axon count. Other sources of outflow obstruction include melanin granules and increased aqueous protein concentration. XFM aggregates in TM may also act as a nidus for deposition of albumin derived from a deranged blood aqueous barrier.

Occasionally, another mechanism noted in some eyes is the formation of a pretrabecular membrane. This results from a migration and proliferation of corneal endothelial cells as a result of

anterior chamber hypoxia and may be responsible for the variable response to treatment in some cases.

Pigment Dispersion

There is increased pigment dispersion in exfoliation syndrome and exfoliative glaucoma. The degree of pigmentation of the trabecular meshwork correlates with the level of IOP. However the pigmentation is patchy unlike pigment dispersion syndrome (PDS) and pigmentary glaucoma (PG). Pigment granules are larger and are present within the endothelial cells, preferentially in the innermost part of the uveoscleral meshwork in contrast to the deeper involvement in PDS. Thus pigment dispersion and accumulation does not play a major role in chronic pressure elevation but causes acute and transient rise of pressure. This has an additional effect on the metabolically compromised cells and may lead to additional glaucomatous damage and an acute and transient IOP rise especially after pupillary dilatation.

Non-IOP Related Factors
Vascular Factors

Factors apart from the mechanical component may contribute to the glaucomatous damage. Perivascular accumulation of XFM with elastotic degeneration in the walls of iris vessels, ciliary arteries, aqueous veins, vortex veins and central retinal artery has been noted in eyes with XFS and XFG.

Structural Factors

The lamina cribrosa undergoes a site specific elastosis suggesting abnormal synthesis and/or degradation of elastin. These changes may increase the susceptibility to mechanical and ischemic damage.

Angle Closure Glaucoma

Eyes with XFS may have narrow anterior chamber angles, smaller anterior

Table 8 Pathogenesis of Glaucoma in Exfoliation Syndrome

Secondary open angle glaucoma
- Exfoliation material produced locally in TM and passive accumulation via the aqueous
- Leads to disorganization and degeneration of the JCT and Schlemm's canal. Focal collapse of the canal occurs leading to decreased aqueous outflow and increased intraocular pressure (IOP)
- Pigment
- Responsible for IOP spikes especially postpupillary dilatation
- Acute elevation of IOP with open angles mimicking angle closure

Non-IOP dependant mechanisms
- Degeneration of vascular endothelial cells and pericytes
- Exfoliation material in the walls of posterior ciliary arteries and vortex veins, central retinal vessels
- Elastosis of lamina cribrosa

Angle closure glaucoma
- Zonular weakness and forward movement of lens causing pupillary block
- Aggravated by miotic therapy
- Posterior synechiae

Neovascular glaucoma
- Secondary to CRVO

chamber volumes, especially in prone position along with a minimal subluxation of lens (owing to the presence of zonular weakness). This predisposes to the development of a pupillary block. The formation of posterior synechiae, breakdown of blood aqueous barrier, and a rigid iris also contribute to the development of angle closure glaucoma. These eyes tend to be more myopic in the presence of a normal axial length than their fellow eyes. This is due to a forward shift in the lens or a progression of nuclear sclerosis. This is an important distinguishing factor from primary angle closure glaucoma and also in assessing the zonular status. In rare cases, aqueous misdirection syndrome can occur due to marked zonular laxity and anterior subluxation of lens and marked contraction of the ciliary muscles.

CLINICAL FEATURES

Early Features: The Red Flags

To a careful examiner, diagnosis of exfoliation in a fully dilated pupil should pose no difficulty. The classical picture of dandruff or flake like deposits on the anterior lens surface represents, however, a very late stage of the disease, *which is preceded by a long, chronic, preclinical course.* Early subtle signs **(Table 9)** can easily be missed. They can be present in the absence of an elevated IOP or full blown features

Table 9 Early signs of XFS

- Exfoliation material on the ciliary process seen on indirect ophthalmoscopy with indentation
- Exfoliation material on or behind the pupillary margin
- Precapsular deposits on anterior lens surface
- Absence of pupillary ruff
- Excessive pigment dispersion after pupillary dilatation
- Pigmentation of trabecular meshwork
- Poor mydriasis

and can be detected by **careful clinical examination in a dilated eye**. One should keep in mind that exfoliation syndrome is *essentially bilateral with marked asymmetry.*

The Most Striking Early Features

The pupillary margin: XFM is present on the pupillary margin providing the first clue even before dilation **(Figures 2A to D)**. In a small pupil, the XFM may be hidden behind the pupillary margin. In such cases it is detected by gonioscopy by looking under the pupillary margin.

The lens (precapsular stage): A precapsular stage has been described as a precursor of exfoliation deposits. A uniform, homogeneous or ground glass appearance of the anterior lens surface as compared to the other eye is seen. By thorough biomicroscopic examination, this diffuse-matte homogeneous film on the surface of the anterior lens capsule can be observed prior to the formation of typical deposits **(Figure 3)**. To visualize these early changes on slit lamp examination it has been suggested to place the slit beam at 45 degree to the axis of observation, reducing the light source, and focus temporally to highlight the subtle deposits on the lens surface.

The pupil and iris: Additional red flags comprise pupillary atrophy of the iris pigment epithelium, absence of pupillary ruff, pigment dispersion after pupillary dilatation, increased trabecular pigmentation and poor mydriasis **(Figure 4)**. Fellow eyes of unilateral cases with signs of pigment dispersion and loss of pupillary ruff without clinically detectable exfoliation material are called 'exfoliation suspects'.

The ciliary processes: One of the earliest sites for observing exfoliation is the ciliary processes and not the more easily accessible and viewed lens surface. Deposits of exfoliation material have been reported to occur

earliest on the ciliary processes and can be seen by indirect ophthalmoscopy in the fellow 'normal' eyes.

In the absence of the crystalline lens: In addition XFM can be seen on the anterior vitreous face, PCIOL, posterior capsule in pseudophakic eyes **(Figures 5A to D)**.

Laterality: Unilateral or Highly Asymmetrical

Patients can present with unilateral disease or bilateral involvement with a marked asymmetry. Unilateral involvement is often regarded as a precursor to bilateral disease. Conversion rates from unilateral to bilateral may vary from 15 to 40 percent within 5 years. The terms unilateral and monocular may actually be misleading. Early pigment related signs have been found in the fellow "normal" eyes and XFM has been found following conjunctival biopsy in virtually all normal fellow eyes. These eyes have been referred to as **exfoliation 'suspects'**. Thus histopathologically both eyes have been found to be involved. These fellow eyes often show abnormal aqueous humor dynamics or glaucoma. Immunohistochemical studies using antibodies against HNK 1 and LTBP 1 show presence of exfoliative material in iris vessels and dilator vessels bilaterally support the concept of a bilaterally asymmetrical disease.

> The presence of exfoliation in one eye should prompt one to look for these subtle signs in the fellow eye.

Clinical Features of Established XFS (Table 10)

Exfoliation material (XFM): The hallmark of exfoliation syndrome is the appearance of a white, flaky dandruff like material on the anterior lens capsule in a characteristic pattern. XFM can be seen on the iris, corneal endothelium, anterior lens surface, lens zonules and ciliary processes.

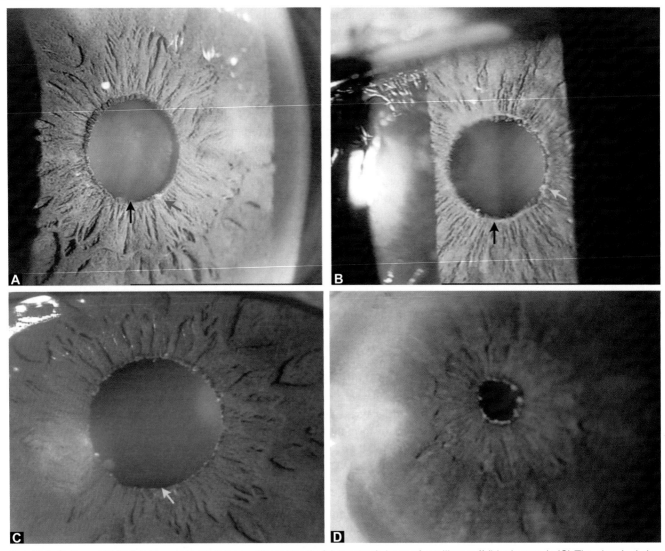

Figs 2A to D (A and B) Exfoliative material at the pupillary margin (blue arrow). Loss of pupillary ruff (black arrow); (C) The classical sign of XFS—exfoliation material on the pupillary margin; (D) Exfoliative material on the pupillary margin. Note that the pupil is miotic

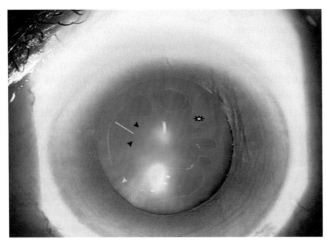

Fig. 3 Formation of the intermediate zone. The three zone pattern (central disc, clear intermediate zone and peripheral zone) is seen in most areas (arrow heads). Early clefts are present in the starred area where the intermediate zone has not formed completely

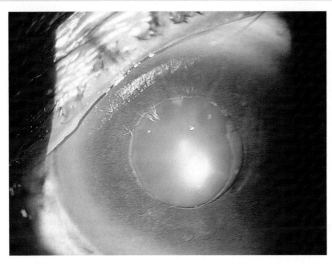

Fig. 4 Poor pupillary dilation in XFG

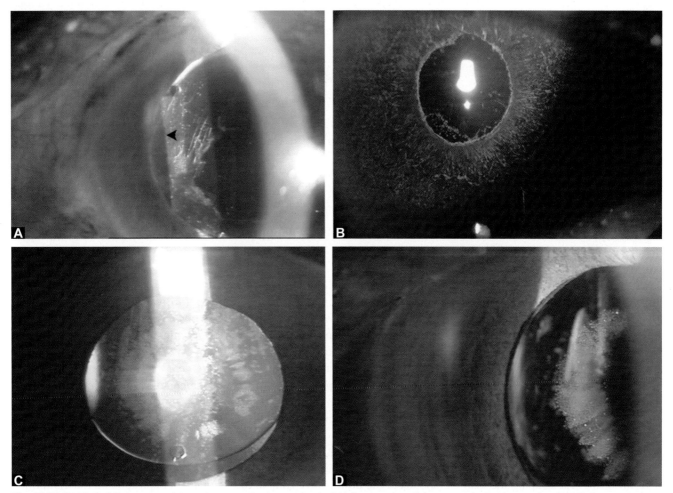

Figs 5A TO D (A) Exfoliation material on the posterior lens capsule (black arrow head) in a pseudophakic eye post-Nd:YAG capsulotomy; (B) Exfoliation material on the broken anterior vitreous face dotting the vitreous strands in an aphakic eye. There is a loss of pupillary ruff with XFM on the pupillary margins with diffuse pigmentary changes in the iris; (C and D) The process of deposition of XFM continues even after cataract extraction. The same pattern is seen on the surface of a posterior chamber intraocular lens

Table 10 Clinical signs of exfoliation syndrome and exfoliation glaucoma

Cornea	Scattered flakes and pigments on endothelial surface
	Occasional pattern of Krukenberg spindle
	Altered endothelial cell count and morphology related to degree of pigment dispersion
	CDK in men
	Distinct type of keratopathy with thickening of DM with deposition of XFM onto or within DM
Iris	Deposits of exfoliation material on pupillary margin and iris sphincter:
	Transillumination defects in peripupillary area (Starry sky appearance)
	Increased iris rigidity and poor mydriasis
	Iris vascular abnormalities and ischemia
	Blood aqueous barrier dysfunction and posterior synechiae
	Pigment dispersion evenly on iris surface (larger granules)
Zonules	Frayed/broken with tendency for subluxation of lens
	Exfoliation material detected earliest on ciliary processes and zonules
Lens	Exfoliation material on anterior lens surface
	Subluxation and dislocation
	Cataract
	Pigments on anterior lens surface
Intraocular pressure	Normal/high
	More IOP spikes and diurnal fluctuations
	Postpupillary dilation IOP spikes
Angle of anterior chamber	XFS material in angle
	Patchy TM pigmentation
	Sampaolesi line
	Narrow angles seen in 14-23%
Optic nerve head and retina	Mean disc area smaller than normal
	Diffuse cupping is seen in exfoliation glaucoma
	Larger area of pallor of optic nerve head in exfoliation glaucoma
	Thinner RNFL on OCT
	CRVO

- Central disc
  - Homogeneous matted fibrillar layer with rolled up edges (loose attachment)
  - Underlying lens capsule and epithelium are essentially normal
- Intermediate zone
  - 1-2 mm wide, devoid of XFM, normal lens capsule
- Peripheral granular zone
  - Nodular aggregates on a fibrillar layer, rolled up edges, melanin granules
- Pre-equatorial zone
  - Hidden by iris, nodular excrescences, pathological alterations of lens zonules and capsule

Phacodonesis

Phacodonesis is common and spontaneous subluxation or dislocation of the lens can occur. This is primarily due to a weakness in the zonules and is more likely to be present in advanced cases with dense XFS.

Cataract

XFS syndrome has been known to be associated with a greater prevalence of cataract though the exact etiology of this association is not known. Ocular ischemia and oxidative damage have been proposed as causes of cataract. **A higher rate of nuclear and subcapsular cataract has been reported.**

Iris

Exfoliation Material

Deposition of the exfoliation material is prominent at the pupillary margin.

Pigment

Pigment loss from the iris and its deposition on the anterior segment structures is an important feature. It gives rise to characteristic transillumination defects (TID) at the pupillary margin, loss of pupillary ruff and diffuse pigment deposition on the iris surface. The pigment particles are larger than those found in pigment dispersion syndrome and tend to be deposited

Lens

Exfoliation Material

Deposits of XFM on the lens are the most important and consistent feature of XFS. The classical pattern consists of 3 zones or the 'Bull's eye' visible clearly after dilatation **(Figure 6C)**. It includes: a **central disc** corresponding roughly to the diameter of the pupil; a granular, often layered, peripheral zone, and a 1 to 2 mm clear area between them (the intermediate zone) that forms as a result of the iris scraping the exfoliation material from the surface of the lens during pupillary movement **(Figures 6A and B)**. The central disc is a homogeneous white sheet with rolled up edges. It may be absent in 20 to 60 percent cases. The peripheral zone is always present. It is granular in the periphery and frosty centrally with radial striations. It extends equatorially as tongue shaped projections which merge into the normal capsule before reaching the anterior insertion of the zonules.

The **pre-equatorial zone** is clinically hidden by the iris and corresponds to the proliferative zone of the lens epithelium. It consists of abundant nodular excrescences covering the zonules and their attachments.

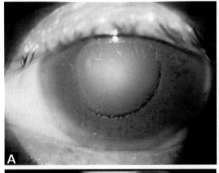

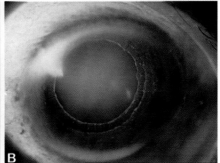

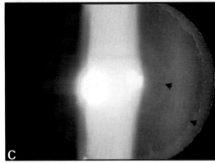

Figs 6A to C (A) Exfoliative material on the pupillary margin and the anterior lens surface seen after pupillary dilatation. Note that the mydriasis is poor; (B) The three zones seen on the anterior lens surface; (C) Three zones or Bull's eye pattern seen on the anterior lens capsule on retroillumination (arrow head)

evenly on the iris surface. Pigment release and dispersion in the anterior segment occurs after pupillary dilation.

Vascular

The lumen of blood vessels in the iris is often narrowed and may become obliterated. In advanced stages, the vascular wall cells degenerate completely. Fluorescein angiographic studies have shown partial occlusion of radial iris capillaries associated with hypoperfusion, microneovascularization, a reduced number of vessels, and diffuse, patchy fluorescein leakage, especially in the pupillary region. Indocyanine green angiography provides better recognition of iris hypoperfusion and anastomotic vessels.

Blood Aqueous Barrier

Fluorescein angiography studies have demonstrated impairment in the blood aqueous barrier. This is primarily localized to the iris and to some extent to the ciliary body. The impairment has a direct bearing on the early postoperative period making these eyes more prone to a transitory fibrinoid

reaction. It may also lead to formation of posterior synechiae, pupillary block glaucoma and neovascularization of the iris (NVI).

Pupil

Eyes with XFS dilate poorly. The pupil of the involved eye may be smaller as compared to the uninvolved eye. At the same time, the constriction with pilocarpine is also less. This can be attributed to fibrotic and degenerative changes in the iris sphincter and dilator muscles. This is significant during the surgical management. The exfoliation material can be seen on the pupillary margin with loss of pupillary ruff. XFS predisposes to the formation of posterior synechiae even in the absence of miotic therapy. This is due to an impaired blood aqueous barrier.

> A profuse pigment release from the posterior pigment epithelium followed by a marked IOP rise is seen 1 to 2 hours after pupillary dilatation. Thus it is a good practice to check postdilatation IOP especially in already compromised eyes with glaucomatous damage.

Cornea
Exfoliation Material and Pigment

Flakes of exfoliation material may be present on the endothelium. A diffuse, nonspecific pigmentation of the central endothelium may be seen, occasionally having the pattern of a Krukenberg spindle. In the angle of the anterior chamber, the pigment is characteristically deposited on Schwalbe's line and sometimes as a wavy line or lines anterior to Schwalbe's line (Sampaolesi line).

Specular Microscopy

Specular microscopy demonstrates a significantly decreased endothelial cell density along with morphological changes in both the involved and uninvolved fellow eye.

Cornea
Central Corneal Thickness

The central corneal thickness is also increased in eyes with XFS reflecting early corneal dysfunction.

Corneal Degeneration

A greater frequency of cornea guttata and a significant association with climatic droplet keratopathy has been observed. A patient with lattice degeneration of the cornea with XFS has also been described. Clinical and histopathologic evidence of a distinct keratopathy in XFS, different from Fuchs' endothelial dystrophy has also been observed. It is characterized by a diffuse, irregular thickening of Descemet's membrane, focal accumulations of exfoliation material on or within Descemet's membrane, and a pronounced melanin phagocytosis by the endothelial cells. Exfoliation material can also be produced by corneal endothelial cells.[70] The resulting corneal endotheliopathy predisposes to early corneal endothelial decompensation at only moderate rises of IOP or after cataract surgery.[71]

Corneal endothelial changes may help in early diagnosis, especially in fellow eyes of presumed 'unilateral cases' in asymmetric cases. It is also important to assess these endothelial changes preoperatively as they affect the outcome of the surgery.

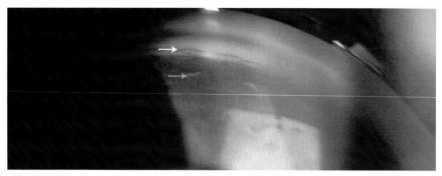

Fig. 7 Gonioscopic view of exfoliative material in the angle peripheral iris (blue arrow) and Sampaolesi's line (white arrow)

Zonules and Ciliary Body

Exfoliation material is detected earliest on the ciliary processes and zonules. Cycloscopy in the uninvolved eye of unilateral cases revealed XFM on the ciliary processes in 77 percent cases. XFM deposits are present on zonules which may be frayed or broken. This explains the tendency for lens subluxation. The process continues over time, even after cataract surgery and IOL implantation and may lead to late decentration, subluxation or dislocation of posterior chamber intraocular lens.

Anterior Chamber Angle

Increased trabecular pigmentation is a prominent sign seen on gonioscopy. The pigmentation is typically patchy in contrast to the homogeneous mascara line seen in PDS. It may be an early diagnostic sign preceding the development of XFM on the lens or iris. It is denser in the involved eye in unilateral cases. A strong correlation appears to exist between elevated IOP and the degree of meshwork pigmentation.[72] Pigment is deposited on the Schwalbe's line and also anterior to it in a wavy form (Sampaolesi's line) **(Figure 7)**. XFM may be seen in the angle. Narrow angles occur in a significant proportion of patients.

Optic Nerve Head and Retinal Nerve Fiber Layer

The mean optic disc area has been reported to be smaller in eyes with XFS and exfoliative glaucoma. In eyes with exfoliative glaucoma, cupping tends to be more diffuse as compared to POAG. The percentage area of optic disc pallor in XFS patients may be greater than controls. A relatively smaller disc is diagnostically important as early changes may be easily overlooked. The RNFL has been found to be significantly thinner in XFS eyes.[73]

Other Ocular Structures

After cataract extraction, XFM may be found on the anterior vitreous face, vitreous strands of the broken anterior vitreous face in aphakic eyes and on the posterior capsule and the posterior chamber intraocular lens. The characteristic zones may be seen on the anterior surface of the posterior chamber intraocular lens.

Exfoliation and CRVO

A possible association of CRVO and exfoliation syndrome and exfoliation glaucoma has been suggested.

EXFOLIATION GLAUCOMA
Secondary Open Angle Glaucoma

Exfoliation glaucoma (XFG) is a **secondary open angle glaucoma** occurring due to the deposition of exfoliative material in the trabecular meshwork. It mimics primary open angle glaucoma in many forms and may many a times go undetected. Yet it is a distinct entity **(Table 11)** and it is important to differentiate the two. Recognition requires a

Table 11 Differentiating features of XFG from POAG

More aggressive
Worse prognosis
Higher mean IOP
More diurnal fluctuations with marked pressure spikes
Marked optic nerve damage
Rapid visual field loss
Poor response to medications
Frequent need for surgical intervention
Asymmetric presentation
Postmydriasis IOP spikes
Pigmentation in anterior chamber
Steroid response similar to normal population
Greater rate of conversion from ocular hypertension
Histological: TM essentially normal except for the deposition of XFM
Evidence of IOP independent mechanisms
SNPs

meticulous examination. When open angle glaucoma is encountered with considerable cupping, elevated IOP, field loss in one eye with no evidence of glaucoma in the other eye, the most common finding is exfoliative material in the affected eye. The clinical importance is that exfoliative open angle glaucoma is more likely to go out of control, with more inter visit spikes and requires faithful and frequent follow ups. Early failure of medical therapy and late failure of laser trabeculoplasty is common and these cases may require an early surgery. Surgery is associated with an increased risk of intra and early postoperative complications.

'Normal Tension' Exfoliation Glaucoma

Pressure-independent risk factors may contribute to glaucomatous changes of the optic nerve head. A higher maximum IOP level, a greater IOP fluctuation within normal range could be significant risk factors for development of glaucomatous ONH changes in eyes with exfoliation in the presence of a normal pressure.[74] Non-IOP dependant factors include impaired ocular and retrobulbar perfusion and abnormalities of elastic tissue of the lamina cribrosa. This is supported by the ultrastructral and immunohistochemical demonstration of the exfoliation fibers in the vortex veins, ophthalmic artery, central retinal vein and iris stroma. Iris neovascularization and patchy occlusion of normal iris vasculature has been observed. Significant hemodynamic alterations in retrobulbar, ONH and peripapillary vasculature have been noted. In addition, a widespread elastosis of the vessels has been seen. The disturbed autoregulation related to microvascular alterations or changes in lamina cribrosa might result in an increased vulnerability with minor pressure changes within normal IOP ranges.

- The exfoliative process as a risk factor for optic disc changes independent of IOP
- Normotensive eyes with exfoliation should also be followed up on a regular basis
- Higher maximum IOP levels and greater IOP fluctuations may be valuable indicators for upcoming glaucomatous damage.

Acute Open Angle Glaucoma

Dispersion of pigment granules and XFM in the anterior chamber is common after diagnostic pupillary dilation and may lead to marked rise in IOP sometimes causing diffuse corneal edema producing a deceptive clinical picture of acute primary angle closure glaucoma. Such pressure peaks may even mimic acute pupillary block with a red eye, corneal edema, pressure rise of more then 50 mm Hg in spite of an open angle. There is a positive correlation between the degree of IOP rise and pigment release, both reaching a maximum two hours following mydriasis and going back to normal after 12 to 24 hours. It is important to distinguish it from acute angle closure as a peripheral iridotomy may worsen the situation by increasing the pigment load. In rare cases, spontaneous subluxation of the lens into vitreous may induce a phacolytic glaucoma.

Clinical Presentations of XFG
- Secondary open angle glaucoma
- Normal tension glaucoma
- Acute open angle glaucoma
- Angle closure glaucoma
- Neovascular glaucoma

Angle Closure Glaucoma

An association between exfoliation and angle closure glaucoma has been observed. These eyes as mentioned earlier may have a narrow anterior chamber angle, smaller anterior chamber volume, especially in prone position along with a minimal subluxation of lens which predisposes to pupillary block. A rigid iris also contributes to the development of angle closure glaucoma. These eyes tend to be more myopic in the presence of a normal axial length due to a forward shift in the lens or a progression of nuclear sclerosis. Other mechanisms for angle closure glaucoma include formation of posterior synechiae due to a deranged blood aqueous barrier leading to pupillary block and neovascularization of the iris. In rare cases, aqueous

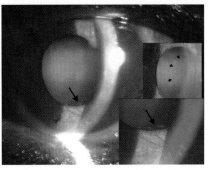

Fig. 8 Neovascular glaucoma postcentral retinal vein occlusion in an eye with exfoliation. The arrows point to the exfoliative membrane on the anterior lens capsule. (high magnification in inset)

misdirection syndrome can occur due to marked zonular laxity and anterior subluxation of lens and marked contraction of the ciliary muscles.

Neovascular Glaucoma

CRVO is more common in patients with exfoliation. Thus neovascular glaucoma can occur in these eyes **(Figure 8)**.

The Overlap

- Patients with diagnosed exfoliation glaucoma and open angle may develop a superimposed angle closure with the passage of time as the zonular weakness increases. This emphasizes the need for a regular gonioscopy especially if the glaucoma is progressing. A laser iridotomy may be useful in such a situation.
- Exfoliation glaucoma has been known to occur in patients with pigmentary glaucoma and cause a rapid progression in these cases (It is discussed in detail the subsequent chapter on pigmentary glaucoma).[75]

Occasionally the conditions may coexist and patients with PDS and PG may develop XFG at a later age. This is known as the overlap syndrome.[75]

DIFFERENTIAL DIAGNOSIS (TABLE 12)

Table 12 Differential diagnosis

- Pigment dispersion syndrome and pigmentary glaucoma
- Other disorders associated with melanin dispersion in the anterior segment
  - ❖ Uveitis
  - ❖ Trauma
  - ❖ Surgery
  - ❖ Diabetes
- True exfoliation of the lens
- True exfoliation with angle closure disease
- Fibrin and amyloid deposits on the anterior lens capsule

True Exfoliation of the Lens

It is a rare condition which typically results from exposure to extremely high temperature. It has also been seen after trauma and exposure to radiation. Idiopathic cases have also been reported. In contrast to exfoliation syndrome, where a newly formed material is deposited on the surface of intact lens capsule, true lens exfoliation is characterized by a splitting and delamination of the anterior lens capsule. It presents as a clear diaphanous membrane with its free edge floating in the aqueous. In some cases, the two conditions may coexist.

Pigment Dispersion Syndrome and Pigmentary Glaucoma

Pigment dispersion syndrome and pigmentary glaucoma is also characterized by pigment deposition on the anterior segment structures and the trabecular meshwork (**Figures 9A to C**). The pigment accumulates in the trabecular meshwork leading to trabecular dysfunction and glaucoma. However, both the conditions can be distinguished based on the following:

- PG is autosomal dominant
- Affects a younger age group
- Krukenberg spindle

- Typical location of TID in mid periphery
- Concave iris configuration
- Uniform dense pigmentation of TM

Uveitis

In uveitic eyes, synechiae, fibrin or a cyclitic membranes may involve the pupillary border and the anterior lens capsule. However it lacks the homogeneous appearance and the characteristic white flakes.

Amyloidosis

Systemic amyloidosis may produce similar ocular picture including the deposition of white flakes resembling exfoliation material in the anterior segment. Glaucoma may also occur. However it is fairly uncommon and is associated with characteristic systemic findings and a characteristic histological picture.

Primary Open Angle Glaucoma

Primary open angle glaucoma (POAG) can be considered as a differential

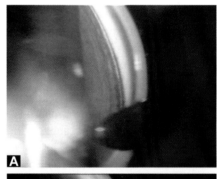
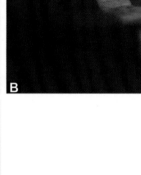
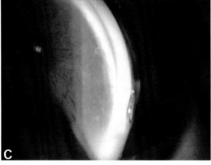

Figs 9A to C (A and B) Gonioscopic photographs showing the characteristic concave iris configuration and dense homogeneous pigmentation of the trabecular meshwork in pigment dispersion syndrome in contrast to XFS seen in (C)

diagnosis. POAG progresses more slowly as compared to XFG.

MANAGEMENT

Distinguishing exfoliation glaucoma from POAG is important as IOP is difficult to control and refractory to medical therapy in XFG. Reduction and stabilization of IOP is more important. Patients should be examined regularly with detailed examination of the optic disc and visual fields. IOP measurements should take into account the central corneal thickness (CCT) values.

The peak levels of IOP occur outside office hours, indicating that a single snapshot value is not reliable. Once diagnosed XFG requires initial medical management, many a times combination therapy with a frequent follow-up and diurnal IOP monitoring.

Medical Management
Medications

While the approach to the medical management is same as POAG, a more aggressive treatment and frequent follow-up is required. A target pressure of less than 17 mm Hg has been found to prevent or slow progression. However, the target IOP depends on the degree of damage and many other factors and needs to be evaluated and reset periodically. In many cases it is difficult to reach the target IOP with monotherapy and combination therapy may be required. This, along with diurnal pressure monitoring and frequent follow-ups forms an integral part of management. The aim should be to decrease both mean IOP and its fluctuations.

The drugs currently available include beta blockers, prostaglandin analogs, alpha agonists, carbonic anhydrase inhibitors and pilocarpine.

Medical Management

- Poor response to medical therapy
- IOP often cannot be controlled with monotherapy
- More IOP spikes and fluctuations (outside office hours)
- Frequent follow-up is required
- Pilocarpine may decrease IOP by increasing trabecular outflow. It also decreases pigment and XFM liberation by immobilizing the pupil. Use is limited by its side effects.
- Prostaglandin analogs increase the uveoscleral outflow and may also decrease aqueous TGF beta levels
- Carbonic anhydrase inhibitors should be avoided in paients with compromised corneal endothelium
- Response to laser trabeculoplasty is good but short lived. Postlaser IOP spikes are common and should be managed promptly. Use of a lower energy setting is recommended.

Aqueous Suppressants

Beta blockers are effective in controlling IOP. Despite initial IOP reductions by beta blockers, significant diurnal fluctuations have been noted in XFG in contrast to POAG. Dorzolamide is almost as effective as timolol and also has an additive action in combination therapy.[76,77] In patients with compromised corneal endothelium carbonic anhydrase inhibitors should be avoided. Alpha adrenergic agonists like brimonidine may also be used. Some authors have suggested that decreasing aqueous production can lead to worsening of the trabecular function.

Prostaglandin Analogs

Prostaglandin analogs, increasing the aqueous outflow via the uveoscleral pathway have been found to be effective in lowering IOP in exfoliation glaucoma. Latanoprost has been shown to provide a better control of diurnal fluctuation as compared to timolol.[78] Both latanoprost and travoprost have been found to reduce IOP at each time point in a 24 hour study. A 3 months crossover trial comparing latanoprost to bimatoprost showed a statistically greater IOP reduction for all time points and mean diurnal curve with bimatoprost (35% vs 31%).[79,80] Latanoprost has also been found to lower the aqueous levels of certain proposed pathogenetic factors like TGF-β1 in eyes with exfoliative glaucoma suggesting that it may confer a beneficial effect on the abnormal matrix process despite normalization of IOP.[81] Information regarding the long-term results is limited.

Pilocarpine

Cholinergic agents lower the IOP by increasing the aqueous outflow. This may enable clearing of the trabecular meshwork. Additionally, by limiting the pupillary movement iridolenticular friction and pigment release is prevented.

Despite good pressure lowering effects and several potential benefits of pilocarpine, there are many hazards to its use like aggravation of the blood aqueous barrier dysfunction, development of posterior synechiae by restricting pupillary movement, aggravation of lens opacities and ciliary block glaucoma in eyes with marked zonular instability.

A multicentric 12 years prospective trial, the Inter-national Collaborative Exfoliation Syndrome Treatment (ICEST) study examined treatment with latanoprost and pilocarpine vs timolol vs fixed-combination timolol/dorzolamide in eyes with exfoliation syndrome and elevated IOP. They found that the latanoprost and pilocarpine arm had lower IOP and improved aqueous outflow.[82] Additional studies may provide further insights.

Lasers

Eyes with XFG respond well to laser trabeculoplasty. With higher baseline IOP, the drop in IOP after ALT is greater in these eyes than in non-XFG eyes.[83-85] The success rate varies from 70 to 90 percent with IOP reduction upto 30 percent. It has been suggested that the increased response is related both to the high baseline IOP as well as the heavily pigmented trabecular meshwork.[86] However, postlaser complications are more common. Inflammatory reaction and IOP spikes are frequently seen.[87] The patients require a careful follow-up along with IOP lowering and anti-inflammatory medications in the early post laser period. The initial significant effect on IOP may gradually decline, (approximately 10% per year) more so than in eyes without XFS.[88] A number of studies have reported a success rate of up to 50 percent after 5 years. A dramatic lowering of IOP followed by a creeping up of pressure on follow-up visits even within the acceptable range should alert the examiner as these eyes are more prone to a late failure of laser treatment presenting with high IOP, unexpected disc damage and visual field progression. Continuously accumulating XFM and pigment granules producing a functional blockade may be responsible for the high failure rate.

Selective laser trabeculoplasty (SLT) is similar in principle to ALT. It uses a Q switched laser which selectively targets the intracellular melanin granules in the trabecular meshwork cells. Most studies have focused on a mixed population of POAG and XFG. Just like ALT, the energy settings in XFG should be lower to avoid pressure spikes which are common. Success rates are similar to ALT. IOP reduction is more pronounced if prelaser IOP is high. It is theoretically repeatable and can be done after failed ALT.

Close monitoring is required for one eyed patients, patients with advanced damage, high prelaser IOP and repeat trabeculoplasty. In XFG with narrow angles, in which the lens is displaced anteriorly, laser trabeculoplasty should be preceded by peripheral iridoplasty in order to widen the distance between the iris and the trabecular meshwork.[89]

Peripheral laser iridotomy is performed when angle closure is present along with exfoliation (**Figures 10A and B**). However, angle closure caused by anterior lens movement or subluxation may not be cured by iridotomy alone and may require argon laser iridoplasty to mechanically pull the iris away from the trabecular meshwork.[90]

Surgical Management
Glaucoma Surgery
Surgery may be necessary earlier and more frequently as compared to other forms of glaucoma due to the early failure of medical and laser treatment. The decision for filtering surgery should be

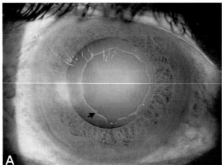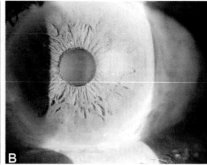

Figs 10A and B Exfoliative material on the anterior surface (intermediate zone) seen after pupillary dilatation (black arrow)

made on an individual basis considering the risk benefit ratio.

Trabeculectomy
Trabeculectomy with antimetabolites is the surgery of choice. The results are comparable to those in eyes with POAG.[91-93] However, perioperative and early postoperative complications are more common. The surgical technique of trabeculectomy is similar to that used in POAG with the concomitant use of antimetabolites. Following trabeculectomy patients may progress less frequently as compared to POAG. Theoretically, more complications can be expected during trabeculectomy in XFG, because higher preoperative IOP indicates an increased risk of choroidal hemorrhage or effusion. Furthermore, there is a risk of hemorrhage owing to iris vasculopathy when peripheral iridectomy is performed. In the case of loose zonules and anterior movement of the lens, vitreous may obliterate the trabeculectomy opening and the lens may be damaged inadvertently. The risk of a fibrinous reaction in the early postoperative period is increased and cataract formation occurs more frequently after trabeculectomy in XFG patients.[94] These can be attributed to

the breakdown of an already compromised blood aqueous barrier which results in an inflammatory response, fibrin formation and posterior synechiae. Intraocular pressure fluctuations are also commonly encountered.

Nonpenetrating Glaucoma Filtering Surgeries
New surgical modalities which bypass the functional blockage of the trabecular meshwork have also been tried in XFG. These techniques may avoid the unfavorable bleb related complications. The fact that the anterior chamber is not entered in nonpenetrating filtering procedures may be of benefit in these eyes when iris vasculopathy and an abnormal blood-aqueous barrier are taken into account.

Tanihara et al[95,96] reported better results in XFG than in POAG patients after trabeculotomy ab externo by putting a probe into Schlemm's canal. However, in deep sclerectomy, the success rates in XFG and POAG eyes 3.5 years after surgery appear to be similar.[97] Rekonen et al[98] also found similar results after deep sclerectomy in XFG and POAG patients. However, the trabeculo-Descemet's membrane seems to be more fragile in

XFG eyes than in eyes without exfoliation. In a study comparing XFG and POAG eyes in which deep sclerectomy had been performed, no patients in either group developed postoperative inflammation.[99]

Trabecular Aspiration

Trabecular aspiration has been tried in XFG on the grounds that it removes XFM aggregates and opens up the trabecular meshwork.[100,101] The trabecular debris is aspirated with a suction force of 100 to 200 mm Hg with a modified intraocular aspiration probe. As a primary procedure it resulted in a mean intraocular pressure reduction of 49 percent at 15 months. However, when combined with cataract surgery, this method has proved less successful than the combined phacotrabeculectomy procedure.[102] Further studies are needed to elucidate the role of this procedure in XFG patients.

> Since XFG is a difficult form of glaucoma, a low target IOP is required. Trabeculectomy should be considered as the treatment of choice. NPGS can be considered in cases with less damage where a less IOP reduction is needed due to a favorable side effect profile.

Combined Cataract and Glaucoma Surgery

Patients with exfoliation syndrome are at increased risk of developing cataracts. Moreover since the prevalence of XFS increases with age one frequently encounters coexistent cataract and XFG. When visually significant cataract is present, trabeculectomy can be combined with cataract extraction preferably phacoemulsification with posterior chamber IOL combined with trabeculectomy has been found to

effectively control IOP.[103] Alternatively, manual small incision cataract surgery combined with trabeculectomy is another option, especially in the developing countries.

However certain points must be kept in mind. Eyes with XFS dilate less and have greater incidences of spontaneous lens displacement, capsular rupture, zonular dehiscence, and vitreous loss.[104-106] Pupillary diameter and zonular fragility have been suggested as the most important risk factors for capsular rupture and vitreous loss. Posterior capsular opacification is increased in eyes with XFS compared with those without it.[107] The incidence of vitreous loss with incarceration of vitreous in the ostium is higher than in eyes with non-XFG. Late postoperative decentration of intraocular lenses and capsular bags, capsular contraction syndrome **(Figure 11)** is greater in eyes with XFS.

Cataract Surgery

Cataract surgery may alone be sufficient in eyes with little or no glaucoma damage or in eyes with well controlled glaucoma on minimal medications. It must be kept in mind that these eyes are more prone to complications at the time of cataract extraction as mentioned above.

Strategies for Success

With phacoemulsification cataract surgery in patients with exfoliation has become much safer. However some issues need to be addressed to reduce the risk of intra- and postoperative complications.

Preoperative Assessment

A good preoperative assessment is half the battle won. The pupillary

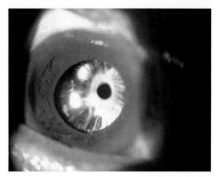

Fig. 11 Capsular contraction in a patient with exfoliation glaucoma after a phaco-trabeculectomy

dilation, presence of phacodonesis, control of glaucoma and zonular status should be carefully noted. Indicators of weak zonules[108] are a shallow anterior chamber and myopia despite a normal axial length. It should be noted that the clinical signs of weak zonules, such as distinct phacodonesis, iridodonesis, vitreous prolapse and lens subluxation, may not always be found. However, slight phacodonesis and / or an iridolenticular gap may be seen. Prostaglandin analogs may be stopped preoperatively to prevent postoperative inflammation. Proper preoperative patient counseling is also of utmost importance.

Intraoperative

The pupil: The small pupil can be managed in several ways, including stretch pupilloplasty, iris hooks and rings. Mechanical pupil stretching works quite well with the fibrotic pupillary margins. Iris hooks can be used to maximize exposure if there are multiple other risk factors, such as a brunescent cataract, a crowded anterior chamber, or weak zonules. The Beehler dilator, a two- or three-pronged device, gives a symmetrical stretch. Akman

> **Surgical Management of Combined Cataract and Glaucoma Surgery: Strategies for Success**
> 1. Assess risk factors preoperatively
>   - Pupillary dilatation
>   - Zonular status
>   - Specular microscopy—for corneal endothelial abnormalities predisposing to post-operative corneal decompensation
> 2. Prepare for small pupils
> 3. Careful CCC
> 4. Appropriate phacoemulsification technique and machine parameters for minimal intra operative stress on zonules.
> 5. Capsular tension ring and segments
> 6. Prepare for postoperative inflammation

et al[109] compared the methods of pupil dilatation in eyes with exfoliation and concluded that all of them were useful. The iris retractor hooks and pupil dilator are both good at keeping the pupil dilated during surgery. The dilator ring causes the least iris trauma.

Capsulorhexis (CCC): It requires special attention as it is the prerequisite for phacoemulsification and capsular tension ring (CTR) insertion if required. The capsule is pseudoelastic and controlling the capsulorhexis is difficult especially in the presence of weak zonules. It is important to avoid overinflating the anterior chamber with viscoelastics when loose zonular support is suspected. Capsular wrinkling indicates the presence of zonular weakness. A good practice is to initiate it in the area of intact zonules which provide a counter traction. Capsular retractors may be used for additional counter traction in the area of weak zonules. Iris hooks can be used in eyes with small pupils to aid in the capsulorhexis. The CCC should be neither too small, nor too large. Too small a diameter will add further stress to loose zonules during manipulation of the nucleus in the bag, whereas too large a diameter may engage the zonular attachments. It may be better to err on the side of a small CCC to maximize

control and avoid a radial tear. However, a small CCC is prone to marked shrinkage in the postoperative period (capsular contraction syndrome). To avoid this, the small CCC can be enlarged after implanting the PCIOL or alternatively small relaxing cuts can be given at the CCC edge.

Hydroprocedures: The degree of hydrodissection must be balanced and aggressive hydrodissection must be avoided. It is performed very carefully whenever loose zonules are suspected and in every case of advanced XFS.

Zonules: Weak zonules present a serious challenge during surgery. One of the major risk factors for surgical complications is the development or presence of zonular laxity or loss. Care should be taken to exert minimal stress on the zonules during the surgery. A cortical cleaving hydrodissection, hydrodelineation and chopping techniques are preferred. A lower bottle height minimizes the stretch on the zonules. It is important to achieve free nucleus rotation and use phaco chop because it avoids directing aspiration forces to the peripheral capsule. Several mechanical devices can be used intraoperatively to minimize further zonular loss if zonular loss occurs.

Severe zonular deficiency with phacodonesis or lens subluxation poses a particular challenge and special hooks, attached to the CCC edge may be used to stabilize the capsular bag during phacoemulsification, followed by suturing a modified or using a CTS (capsular tension segment) to the scleral wall. A hook especially designed for stabilization of the capsule has been described.

Capsular tension ring: When the zonules are loose, a capsular tension ring (CTR) may be useful. The stage of the surgery at which a CTR is implanted should be evaluated individually in every case. It can be inserted at the beginning of the surgery or later. Some

surgeons prefer to insert the ring after hydrodissection in order to support the zonular apparatus and stabilize the capsular bag during phacoemulsification.[110] The advantage is that if the capsular bag gets decentered, the CTR will center it during surgery. A capsular tension segment (CTS) can also be placed in case of localized zonular dehiscence. Others prefer to insert the ring after the epinucleus and cortical remnants have been removed, thereby avoiding entrapment of cortical material by the CTR against the capsular bag. It must be kept in mind that early CTR insertion may itself create further zonular damage. Insertion of a CTR does not prevent postoperative capsular phimosis, late subluxation or dislocation of the whole complex.

Phacoemulsification: In cases with inadequate pupil dilatation, hard lens nucleus, endothelial cell abnormalities or reduced zonular support, gentle manipulation of the nucleus in phacoemulsification is mandatory. Chopping techniques are preferred as they place minimum stress on the zonules (all forces are directed to the center of the nucleus). Vacuum and flow rate should be reduced. While aspirating the cortex, stripping the cortex tangentially places less stress on the zonules.

Intraocular lens: Weak zonules can lead to capsule contraction syndrome and delayed bag-IOL dislocation postoperatively. Implantation of an acrylic posterior chamber intraocular lens with stiff haptics may be preferred to minimize anterior capsular fibrosis.

Postoperative

IOP: The IOP decline over time may be greater in XFG patients as compared to POAG. The proposed mechanism for reduction in IOP is the improved outflow as a result of the clearing of deposits of exfoliation material by high flow states during surgery. However in the early postoperative period these eyes are at a greater risk for developing an immediate elevation of IOP. Care should be taken to remove all the viscoelastic from the eye intraoperatively. Postoperative IOP monitoring is important especially in patients with advanced visual field defects or severe ONH damage. Any spikes should be promptly treated.

Inflammation: Postoperative breakdown of blood aqueous barrier, inflammation and fibrinoid reaction, cellular deposits on the IOL and posterior synechiae is significantly increased in eyes with XFS and XFG. This is due to the compromised blood aqueous barrier in eyes with exfoloiation. The increased inflammation may partly be due to increased manipulation when the nucleus is extruded through a small pupil in case extracapsular cataract extraction (ECCE) or manual small incision cataract surgery is performed. With phacoemulsification, the risk of an inflammatory response developing after cataract surgery has dramatically reduced. The patients need to be maintained on topical steroids for a longer time.

Even with uneventful surgery, decentration or dislocation of the IOL within the bag can occur many years postoperatively due to progressive zonular disintegration and capsular shrinkage. Capsular phimosis may occur in the late postoperative period as weak zonules result in decreased centrifugal force. Assymetric capsular contraction forces may cause decentration of the PCIOL. In addition to reduced capsular tension counteracting its contracture, the coexistence of anterior capsule contraction and instability of the blood-aqueous barrier may contribute to the contraction. In cases of pronounced fibrosis and shrinkage of the anterior capsule without decentration of an in-the-bag IOL, Nd:YAG laser radial anterior capsulotomy is recommended numerous methods of

securing a subluxated IOL to either the sclera or the iris have been reported. If a complete dislocation of the encapsulated IOL occurs, a vitreoretinal approach is necessary.

RECENT ADVANCES

Genetics

In a breakthrough genome-wide association study done in an Icelandic population, replicated in a Swedish population, the genetic etiology of XFS and XFG was unravelled. Polymorphisms in the coding region of the *LOXL1* gene located on chromosome 15q24.1 were found to be strongly associated with XFS and XFG in these populations. *LOXL1* gene is a member of the lysyl oxidase gene family. The prototypic member of the family is essential for the biogenesis of connective tissue and encodes for an extracellular copper-dependent amine oxidase that catalyzes the first step in the formation of crosslinks in collagens and elastin. These results have been replicated in many populations including India. The search for more genes continues. Different mutations may lead to greater or lesser disease severity and these need to be explored, much as has been done with myocilin mutations.

Modifiable Risk Factors

An increasing number of systemic associations have been reported recently. There may be some evidence of modifiable risk factors.

Homocysteine: High levels of Homocysteine, a highly cytotoxic amino acid derived from disturbed methionine metabolism have been noted in plasma, aqueous humor, and tear fluid in patients with XFS and XFG. Hyperhomocysteinemia is associated with nearly all of the systemic associations of XFS mentioned and raises the question as to whether it

might be a modifiable risk factor for XFS. Treatment with folic acid and vitamins B_6 and B_{12} reduce homocysteine concentrations in patients with coronary artery disease. There may be a possibility that these patients may benefit from lowering of plasma homocysteine levels.[111]

A decreased serum concentration of vitamins B_6 and B_{12} and folate has recently been reported in patients with XFS.[112]

Transforming growth factor β1 (TGF-β1) interacts with lysyl oxidase to influence the formation of elastic tissue and is believed to be both responsible for overproduction of extracellular matrix and an important causative factor for the production of exfoliation material. Levels of TGF-β1 are significantly elevated in the aqueous humor of eyes with XFS. Latanoprost reduces the concentration of TGF-β1 in eyes with exfoliative glaucoma and may play an additional role in the management of XFS and XFG.

UNANSWERED QUESTIONS

Study of this disease is certainly intriguing and leaves many questions unanswered.

- Exact composition and mechanism of production of exfoliation fibers
- Prediction of development of XFG in patients with XFS and the severity
- Is it possible to predict whether the prediction of inheritence?
- Identification and modulation of modifiable risk factors and their effect
- What are the systemic implications?

These and many more questions are now open to further exploration in an attempt to manage this very common and severe yet fascinating and challenging secondary open angle glaucoma.

REFERENCES

1. Ritch R, Schlotzer-Schrehardt U, Exfoliation syndrome. Surv Ophthalmol 2001;45:265-315.

2. Lindberg J, Kliniska undersokningar over depigmentering av pupillarranden och genomlysbarket av iris vid fall av alderstarr samit i normala ogon hos gamla personer [clinical studies of depigmentation of the pupillary margin and transillumination of the iris in cases of senile cataract and also in normal eyes in the aged] [MD]. Helsingfors 1917 Thesis. 1917.

3. Forsius H. Exfoliation syndrome in various ethnic populations. Acta Ophthalmol S 1988;184:71-85.

4. Krause U. Frequency of capsular glaucoma in central Finland. Acta Ophthalmol (Copenh), 1973;51:235-40.

5. Krasue U, Alanko H, Karna J. Prevalence of exfoliation syndrome in Finland. Acta Ophthalmol 1988; 184S:120-2.

6. Sveinsson K. The frequency of senile exfoliation in Iceland. Fibrillopathy or pseudoexfoliation. Acta Ophthalmol (Copenh) 1974;52:596-602.

7. Ritch R. Exfoliation syndrome: the most common identifiable cause of open angle glaucoma. J Glaucoma, 1994;3:176-8.

8. Shields M, Ritch R. The enigma of exfoliation syndrome. Acta Ophthalmol Scand 85:470-1.

9. Thorleifsson G, et al. Common sequence variants in the LOXL1 gene confer susceptibility to exfoliation glaucoma. Science 2007;317:1397-400.

10. Fingert JH, et al. LOXL1 mutations are associated with exfoliation syndrome in patients from the midwestern United States. Am J Ophthalmol 2007;144:974-5.

11. Challa P, et al. Analysis of LOXL1 polymorphisms in a United States population with pseudoexfoliation glaucoma. Mol Vis 2008;14:146-9.

12. Chen H, et al. Ethnicity-based subgroup meta-analysis of the association of LOXL1 polymorphisms with glaucoma. Mol Vis 2010;16:167-77,

13. Ramprasad V, et al. Association of non-synonymous single nucleotide polymorphisms in the LOXL1 gene with pseudoexfoliation syndrome in India. Mol Vis 2008.pp.318-22.

14. Vogt A, Ein neues S. Abschilferung der Linsenvorderkapsel als wahrscheinliche Ursache von senilem chronischem Glaukom. Schweiz med Wschr 1926;75:1-12.

15. Dvorak-Theobald G, Pseudoexfoliation of the lens capsule: relation to true exfoliation of the lens capsule as reported in the literature, and role in the production of glaucoma capsulocuticulare. Trans Am Ophthalmol Soc 1953;51:385-407.

16. Tarkkanen A. HAO Forsius Exfoliation syndrome. Acta Ophthalmol 1988;66:1-150.

17. Sood GC, et al. Capsular exfoliation syndrome. Br J Ophthalmol 1973;57:120-4.

18. Sood N, Ratnaraj A. Pseudoexfoliation of the lens capsule. Orient Arch Ophthalmol 1968;6:62.

19. Lamba P, Giridhar A. Pseudoexfoliation syndrome (prevalence based on random survey hospital data). Indian J Ophthalmol 1984;32:169-73.

20. Krishnadas R, et al. Pseudoexfoliation in a rural population of southern India: the Aravind Comprehensive Eye Survey. Am J Ophthalmol 2003;135:830-7.

21. Arvind H, et al. Pseudoexfoliation in South India. Br J Ophthalmol 2003; 87:1321-3.

22. Thomas R, Nirmalan P, Krishnaiah S. Pseudoexfoliation in Southern India: the Andhra Pradesh Eye Disease Study. Invest Ophthalmol Vis Sci 2005;46:1170-6.

23. Forsius H. Prevalence of pseudoexfoliation of the lens in Finns, Lapps, Icelanders, Eskimos and Russians. Trans Am Acad Ophthalmol UK 1979;99:296.

24. Cashwell LF, Jr Shields MB. Exfoliation syndrome. Prevalence in a southeastern United States population. Arch Ophthalmol 1988; 106:335-6.

25. Hiller R, Sperduto R, Krueger D. Pseudoexfoliation, intraocular pressure, and senile lens changes in a population based survey. Arch Ophthalmol 1982;100:1080-7.

26. Faulkner HW. Pseudoexfoliation of the lens among the Navajo Indians. Am J Ophthalmol 1971;72:206-7.

27. McCarthy C, Taylor H. Pseudoexfoliation syndrome in Australian adults. Am J Ophthalmol 2000;129:629-33.

28. Mitchell P, Wang JJ, Hourihan F. The relationship between glaucoma and pseudoexfoliation: the Blue Mountains Eye Study. Arch Ophthalmol 1999;117:1319-24.

29. Astrom S, Stenlund H, Linden C. Incidence and prevalence of pseudoexfoliations and open-angle glaucoma in northern Sweden: II. Results after 21 years of follow-up. Acta Ophthalmol (Copenh) 2007;85:470-1.

30. Ringvold A, et al. The prevalence of pseudoexfoliation in three separate municipalities of Middle-Norway. A preliminary report. Acta Ophthalmol (Copenh) 1987;65:S17-20.

31. Aasved H. Prevalence of fibrillopathica epitheliocapsularis (pseudoexfoliation) and capsular glaucoma. Trans Am Acad Ophthalmol Soc UK 1975;99:293-5.

32. Shakya S, Dulal S, Maharjan I. Pseudoexfoliation syndrome in various ethnic population of Nepal. Nepal Med Coll J 2008;10:147-50.

33. Kozart DM, Yanoff M. Intraocular pressure status in 100 consecutive patients with exfoliation syndrome. Ophthalmology 1982;89:214-8.

34. Layden WE, Shaffer RN. Exfoliation syndrome. Am J Ophthalmol 1974;78: 835-41.

35. Roth M, Epstein D. Exfoliation syndrome. Am J Ophthalmol 1980; 89:477.

36. Aasved H. The frequency of fibrillopathia epitheliocapsularis (so-called senile exfoliation or pseudo-exfoliation) in patients with open-angle glaucoma. Acta Ophthalmol (Copenh) 1971;49:194-210.

37. Shimizu K, Kimura Y, Aoki K. Prevalence of exfoliation syndrome in the Japanese. Acta Ophthalmol Suppl 1988;184:112-5.

38. Sziklai P, Suveges I. Glaucoma capsulare in patients with open-angle glaucoma in hungary. Acta Ophthalmol 1988;66:90.

39. Valle O. Prevalence of simple and capsular glaucoma in the Central Hospital District of Kotka. Acta Ophthalmol Suppl 1988;184:116-9.

40. Cashwell LF, Jr Shields MB. Exfoliation syndrome in the southeastern United States. I. Prevalence in open-angle glaucoma and non-glaucoma populations. Acta Ophthalmol Suppl 1988;184:99-102.

40a. Wishart PK, Spaeth GL, Poryzees EM. Anterior chamber angle in exfoliation syndrome. Br J Ophthalmol 1985;69: 103-7.

41. Henry JC, et al. Long-term follow-up of pseudoexfoliation and the development of elevated intraocular pressure. Ophthalmology 1987;94: 545-52.

42. Brooks A, Gillies W. The presentation and prognosis of glaucoma in psedoexfoliation of the lens capsule. Ophthalmology 1988;95:271.

43. Crittendon JJ, Shields MB. Exfoliation syndrome in the southeastern United States. II. Characteristics of patient population and clinical course. Acta Ophthalmol Suppl 1988;184: 103-6.

44. Klemetti A. Intraocular pressure in exfoliation syndrome. Acta Ophthalmol Suppl 1988;184:54-8.

45. Grodum K, Heijl A, Bengtsson B. Risk of glaucoma in ocular hypertension with and without pseudoexfoliation. Ophthalmology 2005;112:386-90.

46. Puska PM. Unilateral exfoliation syndrome: conversion to bilateral exfoliation and to glaucoma: a prospective 10-year follow-up study. J Glaucoma 2002;11:517-24.

47. Shuba L, Nicolela MT, Rafuse PE. Correlation of capsular pseudoexfoliation material and iridocorneal angle pigment with the severity of pseudoexfoliation glaucoma. J Glaucoma 2007;16:94-7.

48. Schlotzer-Schrehardt U, Kuchle M, Naumann GAO. Electron-microscopic identification of pseudoexfoliation material in extrabulbar tissue. Arch Ophthalmol 1991;109:565.

49. Summanen P, Tonjum AM. Exfoliation syndrome among Saudis. Acta Ophthalmol Suppl 1988;184:107-11.

49a. Lemmela S, Forsman E, Sistonen P, et al. Genome-wide scan of exfoliation syndrome. Invest Ophthalmol Vis Sci 2007;48:4136-42.

50. Kubota T, et al. Immunoelectron microscopic localization of the HNK-1 carbohydrate epitope in the anterior segment of pseudoexfoliation and normal eye. Curr Eye Res 1997.pp. 231-8.

51. Lamari F, et al. Profiling of the eye aqueous humor in exfoliation syndrome by high-performance liquid chromatographic analysis of hyaluronan and galactosamino-glycans. J Chromatogr B Biomed Sci Appl 1998;709:173-8.

52. Schlötzer-Schrehardt U, et al. Increased extracellular deposition of fibrillin-containing fibrils in pseudoexfoliation syndrome. Invest Ophthalmol Vis Sci 1997;38:970-84.

53. Schlötzer-Schrehardt U, et al. Latent TGF-1 binding protein (LTBP-1): a new marker for intra- and extraocular PEX deposits 2000;216:412-9.

54. Streeten B, et al. Pseudoexfoliative material contains an elastic micro-fibrillar-associated glycoprotein. Trans Am Acad Ophthalmol Soc 1986;84:304-20.

55. Streeten B, Trends N. Aberrant synthesis and aggregation of elastic tissue components in pseudo-exfoliative fibrillopathy: a unifying concept. New Trends Ophthalmol 1993;8:187-96.

56. Koliakos GG, et al. Prooxidant-antioxidant balance, peroxide and catalase activity in the aqueous humour and serum of patients with exfoliation syndrome or exfoliative glaucoma. Graefes Arch Clin Exp Ophthalmol 2008;246:1477-83.

56a. Johnson TV, Fan S, Camras CB, Toris CB. Aqueous humor dynamics in exfoliation syndrome. Arch Ophthalmol 2008;126:914-20.

57. Pena J, et al. Elastosis of the lamina cribrosa in glaucomatous optic neuro-pathy. Exp Eye Res 1998;67:517-24.

58. Ringvold A, Husby G. Pseudo-exfoliation material—an amyloid-like substance. Exp Eye Res 1973;17: 289-99.

59. Streeten B, et al. Comparison of components in pseudoexfoliation fibers and Alzheimer's disease plaques. Invest Ophthalmol Vis Sci 1996;37:S90.

60. Dark A, Streeten B, Corniwall C. Pseudoexfoliative disease of the lens: A study in electron microscopy and histochemistry. Br J Ophthalmol 1977;61:462-72.

61. Dickson D, Ramsey S. Fibrillopathia epitheliocapsularis. Review of the

nature and origin of pseudoexfoliative deposits. Trans Am Acad Ophthalmol Soc UK 1979;99:284-92.

62. Eagle RJ, Font RL, Fine B. The basement membrane exfoliation syndrome. Arch Ophthalmol 1979;97:510-5.

63. Netland PA, et al. Elastosis of the lamina cribrosa in pseudoexfoliation syndrome with glaucoma. Ophthalmology 1995;102:878-86.

64. Horven I, Hutchinson BT. Exfoliation syndrome. Case reports of 31 and 35-year-old patients. Acta Ophthalmol (Copenh) 1967;45:294-8.

65. Konstas AG, et al. Exfoliation syndrome in a 17-year-old girl. Arch Ophthalmol 1997;115:1063-7.

66. Ringvold A, et al. The Middle-Norway eye-screening study. I. Epidemiology of the pseudoexfoliation syndrome. Acta Ophthalmol 1988;66:652-7.

67. Konstas AG, Williamson TH. Co-existence of exfoliation syndrome, previous iris surgery, and heterochromia. Acta Ophthalmol (Copenh) 1993;71:850-2.

68. Küchle M, Naumann G. Occurrence of pseudoexfoliation following penetrating keratoplasty for keratoconus. Br J Ophthalmol 1992;76:98-100.

69. Sampaolesi R, Casiraghi J, Geria R. The occurrence of exfoliation syndrome after penetrating keratoplasty: a report of three cases (abstract). Klin Monatsbl Augenheilkd 1995;206: S8-9.

70. Schlötzer-Schrehardt U, Dörfler S, Naumann G. Corneal endothelial involvement in pseudoexfoliation syndrome. Arch Ophthalmol 1993; 111:666-74.

71. Naumann G. Schlötzer-Schrehar, Keratopathy in pseudoexfoliation syndrome as a cause of corneal endothelial decompensation. A clinicopathologic study. Ophthalmology 2000;107:1111-24.

72. Moreno-Montañés J, et al. Pseudo-exfoliation syndrome: clinical study of the anterior chamber angle. J Fr Ophthalmol 1990;13:183-8.

73. Yuksel N, Altintas O, Celik M, Ozkan B, Caglar Y. Analysis of retinal nerve fibre thickness in patients with exfoliation syndrome using OCT. Ophthalmologica 2007;221:229-304.

74. Koz GO, Turkcu MF, Yarangumeli A, et al. Normotensive glaucoma and risk factors in normotensive eyes with pseudoexfoliation syndrome. J Glaucoma 2009;18:684-8.

75. Ritch R, Mudumbai R, Liebmann JM. Combined exfoliation and pigment dispersion: an overlap syndrome. Ophthalmology 2000;107:1004-8.

76. Heijl A, Strahlman E, Sverrisson T, et al. A comparison of dorzolamide and timolol in patients with pseudo-exfoliation and glaucoma or ocular hypertension. Ophthalmology 1997; 104:137-42.

77. Konstas AGP, Maltezos A, Bufidis T, et al. Twenty-four hour control of intraocular pressure with dorzolamide and timolol maleate in exfoliation and primary open-angle glaucoma Eye 2000;14:73-7.

78. Konstas AGP, Mylopoulos N, Karabatsas CH, et al. Diurnal intraocular pressure reduction with Latanoprost 0.005% compared to timolol maleate 0.5% as monotherapy in subjects with exfoliation glaucoma. Eye 2004;18:893-9.

79. Konstas AGP, Kozobolis VP, Katsimpris IE, et al. Efficacy and Safety of latanoprost versus travoprost in exfoliative glaucoma patients. Ophthalmology 2007;114:653-7.

80. Konstas AGP, Hollo G, Irkee M. Diurnal IOP control with bimatoprost vs latanoprost in exfoliative glaucoma: a crossover observer masked three centre study. Br J Ophthalmol 2007;91:757-60.

81. Konstas AGP, Koliakos GG, Karabatsas CH, et al. Latanoprost therapy reduces the levels of TGF beta 1 and gelatinases in the aqueous humour of patients with exfoliative glaucoma. Exp Eye Res. 2006;82(2):319-22.

82. Angelilli A, Ritch R, Krupin T, Konstas AGP, Liebmann JM, Ilitchev E, Marmor M, ICEST Study Group. The International Collaborative Exfoliation Syndrome Treatment (ICEST) Study: Results. E-2474.

83. Tuulonen A. Laser trabeculoplasty as primary therapy in chronic open-angle glaucoma. Acta Ophthalmol (Copenh) 1984;62:150-5.

84. Psilas K, et al. Comparative study of argon laser trabeculoplasty in primary open-angle and pseudoexfoliation glaucoma. Ophthalmologica 1989;198: 57-63.

85. Threlkeld AB, et al. Comparative study of the efficacy of argon laser trabeculoplasty for exfoliation and primary open-angle glaucoma. J Glaucoma 1996;5:311-6.

86. Bergea B. Some factors affecting the intraocular pressure reduction after argon laser trabeculoplasty in open-angle glaucoma. Acta Ophthalmol (Copenh) 1984;62:696-704.

87. Leung K, Gillies W. The detection and management of the acute rise in intraocular pressure following laser trabeculoplasty. Aust N Z J Ophthalmol 1986;14:259-62.

88. Svedbergh B. Argon laser trabeculoplasty in capsular glaucoma. Acta Ophthalmol (Copenh) 1988;184:S141-7.

89. Ritch R. Schlo U. Schlötzer-Schrehardt, Exfoliation syndrome. Surv Ophthalmol 2001;45:265-315.

90. Ritch R, Podos S. Laser trabeculoplasty in the exfoliation syndrome. Bull N Y Acad Med 1983;59:339-44.

91. Jerndal T, Kriisa V. Results of trabeculectomy for pseudoexfoliative glaucoma. A study of 52 cases. Br J Ophthalmol 1974;58:927-30.

92. Konstas A, Jay J, Marshall G. Prevalence, diagnostic features,

and response to trabeculectomy in exfoliation glaucoma. Ophthalmology 1993;100:619-27.

93. Popovic V, Sjostrand J. Course of exfoliation and simplex glaucoma after primary trabeculectomy. Br J Ophthalmol 1999;83:305-10.

94. Vesti E, Raitta C. A review of the outcome of trabeculectomy in open-angle glaucoma. Ophthalmic Surg Lasers 1997;28:128-32.

95. Tanihara H, et al. Surgical effects of trabeculotomy ab externo on adult eyes with primary open angle glaucoma and pseudoexfoliation syndrome. Arch Ophthalmol 1993;111:1653-61.

96. Tanihara H, et al. Long-term surgical results of combined trabeculotomy ab externo and cataract extraction. Ophthalmic Surg 1995;26:316-24.

97. Drolsum L. Long-term follow-up after deep sclerectomy in patients with pseudoexfoliative glaucoma. Acta Ophthalmol Scand 2006;84:502-6.

98. Rekonen P, et al. Deep sclerectomy for the treatment of exfoliation and primary open-angle glaucoma. Acta Ophthalmol Scand 2006;84:507-11.

99. Drolsum L. Deep sclerectomy in patients with capsular glaucoma. Acta Ophthalmol Scand 2003;81:567-72.

100. Jacobi PC, Dietlein TS, Krieglstein GK, Bimanual trabecular aspiration in pseudoexfoliation glaucoma: an alternative in nonfiltering glaucoma surgery. Ophthalmology 1998;105:886-94.

101. Jacobi PC, Krieglstein GK. Trabecular aspiration. A new mode to treat pseudoexfoliation glaucoma. Invest Ophthalmol Vis Sci 1995;36:2270-6.

102. Jacobi PC, Dietlein TS, Krieglstein GK. Comparative study of trabecular aspiration vs trabeculectomy in glaucoma triple procedure to treat pseudoexfoliation glaucoma. Arch Ophthalmol 1999;117:1311-8.

103. Landa G, et al. Graefes Arch Clin Exp Ophthalmol. Results of combined phacoemulsification and trabeculectomy with mitomycin C in pseudoexfoliation versus non-pseudoexfoliation glaucoma 2005;243:1236-40.

104. Skuta G, et al. Zonular dialysis during extracapsular cataract extraction in pseudoexfoliation syndrome. Arch Ophthalmol 1987;105:632-4.

105. Zetterström C, Olivestedt G, Lundvall A. Exfoliation syndrome and extra-capsular cataract extraction with implantation of posterior chamber lens. Acta Ophthalmol 1992;70:85-90.

106. Moreno-Montañés J, et al. Pseudoex-foliation syndrome: clinical factors related to capsular rupture in cataract surgery. Acta Ophthalmol 1993;71:181-4.

107. Küchle M, et al. Pseudoexfoliation syndrome and secondary cataract. Br J Ophthalmol 1997;81:862-6.

108. Küchle M, et al. Anterior chamber depth and complications during cataract surgery in eyes with pseudoexfoliation syndrome. Am J Ophthalmol 2000;129:281-5.

109. Akman A, et al. Comparison of various pupil dilatation methods for phacoemulsification in eyes with a small pupil secondary to pseudoexfoliation. Ophthalmology, 2004;111:1693-8.

110. Bayraktar S, et al. Capsular tension ring implantation after capsulorhexis in phacoemulsification of cataracts associated with pseudoexfoliation syndrome. Intraoperative complications and early postoperative findings. J Cataract Refract Surg 2001;27:1620-8.

111. Vessani RM, et al. Plasma homo-cysteine is elevated in patients with exfoliation syndrome. Am J Ophthalmol 2003;136:41-6.

112. Roedl JB, Bleich S, Reulbach U, et al. Vitamin deficiency and hyper-homocysteinemia in pseudoexfolia-tion glaucoma. J Neural Transm 2007;114:571-5.

29 | Pigment Dispersion Syndrome and Pigmentary Glaucoma

Mona Khurana, Manju Pillai, R Ramakrishnan

INTRODUCTION

Pigment dispersion syndrome (PDS) and pigmentary glaucoma (PG) are fascinating ocular conditions that have been recognized for over 60 years. They occur because of the liberation of pigment from the iris pigment epithelium into the anterior chamber. Pigment dispersion syndrome (PDS) is characterized by disruption of pigment and deposition of these pigment granules in the anterior segment. Pigmentary glaucoma is a secondary open angle glaucoma in which in addition to these changes there are optic nerve head changes and visual field changes characteristic of glaucoma.

HISTORY

Krukenberg in 1899 was the first to describe a spindle shaped pigment deposition on the cornea.[1] In 1901, von Hippel postulated that increased intraocular pressure (IOP) could be caused by the pigment obstructing the outflow system.[2] Levinson suggested the iris pigment epithelium (IPE) as the source of this pigment.[3] In 1949, Sugar and Barbour described 2 young, myopic men with Krukenberg spindles,

trabecular hyperpigmentation, and open angles, whose IOP increased with mydriasis and decreased with pilocarpine.[4] They described it as a distinct form of glaucoma naming it *pigmentary glaucoma*. In 1966, Sugar reviewed 147 cases, and observed additional features like bilaterality, frequent association with myopia, greater incidence in men than in women, and a relatively young age at onset.[5] These features were confirmed by Scheie and Cameron.[6] In 1979, Campbell proposed a hypothesis for the pathogenesis of pigment dispersion.[7]

EPIDEMIOLOGY AND GENETICS

The incidence of PDS is thought to be 4.8/100,000 and PG is 1.4/100,000 (western populaton).[8] The prevalence of PDS in a population screening was 2.45 percent (Caucasian).[9] PDS is a risk factor for the development of glaucoma. Pigmentary glaucoma may account for 1.5 percent of glaucomas worldwide.

Age: Pigment dispersion begins in the teens or twenties and continues until about the mid-40s in most people. Although pigmentary glaucoma typically occurs in young adults it may also

be seen in older individuals. Young people are more prone due to greater degree of pigment regeneration and pronounced accommodation.

Race: Pigment dispersion syndrome is common in the Caucasian population mostly affecting the age group between 20 and 45 years. It is relatively less common in Africans and Asians. This may be because of a thinner iris stroma in the Caucasians as compared to the Africans or an underdiagnosis in Africans. Although pigmentary glaucoma is more common in Caucasians, it has also been reported in Africans, Mullatos and Asians. Even though PDS is less common in Africans, once people of African ancestry develop PDS they are more likely to convert to PG.

Gender: Men and women are equally affected by PDS. However men develop glaucoma three times more often than women and at a younger mean age.[10-12]

Laterality: It is a bilateral condition. The presentation may be asymmetric.

Refractive error: The most common refractive error encountered is mild to moderate myopia and 60 to 80 percent of patients with PDS and PG are myopic.[5,6] A higher degree of myopia may be associated with an early development of glaucomatous optic nerve damage. The remaining 20 to 40 percent may be emmetropic and rarely hyperopic also. The enlarged ciliary body ring in myopes may lead to iridolenticular and iridozonular contact, resulting in pigment dispersion.

Genetics
Inheritance is autosomal dominant with an incomplete penetrance.[13] In 1961 Stankovic reported four generations with pigmentary glaucoma.[14] PDS and PG has been observed in three generations.[15] Some families with PDS have been linked to a genetic markers found on chromosome 7q35-q36.[16] Studies in mice with iris transillumination defects and PG have revealed mutations in two genes involved in the melanosomal melanin production. However these mutations are not present in humans with PG. The spectrum of clinical presentations suggests that iris pigment epithelial defects and glaucoma may be represented by two independent gene loci located close together on the same chromosome and, thus, tend to be inherited together.[17]

> **Pearls**
> - Family screening is important
> - Closer follow-up in Africans with PDS and PG [20,21]

ATYPICAL PRESENTATIONS
Krukenberg spindles have been noted during pregnancy in black women.[18] Pigment dispersion has been described in 20 black patients with an average age of 73 years, hyperopia, with female preponderance and a flat iris insertion.[19]

CLINICAL FEATURES (TABLE 1)
Symptoms
The patients with PDS and PG are mostly asymptomatic. However, they may experience blurring of vision, pain and occasionally colored haloes around light after pupillary dilatation or exercise which triggers active pigment dispersion and causes an acute rise in IOP.

> **Pearls**
> *Record at each visit:*
> - Postdilated IOP
> - Postexercise IOP (if possible)
> - Degree of pigmentation
> - Gonioscopy is a must

Signs
The clinical features of PDS and PG are due to the liberation of pigment granules and their distinct distribution in the anterior segment. The characteristic features of PDS include a triad of transillumination defects of the iris, Krukenberg spindles and increased pigmentation of the trabecular meshwork. There is a spectrum of patients with severe transillumination defects without glaucoma at one end, and patients with mild transillumination defects with glaucoma at the other end.

Table 1 Clinical signs of pigment dispersion syndrome

Cornea	Krukenberg spindle
Iris	• Transillumination defects • Diffuse pigment deposition with a velvety appearance • Heterochromia in asymmetric cases • Concave configuration and posterior insertion of iris (on gonioscopy)
Lens/Zonules	Pigment at insertion of posterior lens zonules (pathognomonic)
Anterior chamber	• Deep anterior chamber • Pigments in anterior chamber
Angle of anterior chamber	• Wide open angle • Large ciliary body band • Posterior iris insertion with concave configuration • Homogeneous and heavily pigmented trabecular meshwork (4+) • Sampaolesi's line

However, the presence of transillumination defects is not necessary to make a diagnosis of PDS.

Krukenberg Spindle
Krukenberg spindle is the name given to corneal endothelial pigment deposition (**Figure 1**). It is usually in the form of a vertical band or spindle about 6 mm in length and 3 mm in width being broader inferiorly. This is attributed to aqueous convection currents. The pigment is phagocytized by endothelial cells without compromise in their function. Although polymorphism and polymegathism has been noted, no changes are seen in endothelial cell density or corneal thickness.[22]

> **Note** The Krukenberg spindle though seen in 95% of the patients with PDS is not pathognomic and can be present in other conditions also.

Transillumination Defects
Iris transillumination defects (TID) are one of the clinical signs used in the diagnosis of PDS and may be present in 86 percent cases at the time of diagnosis. However they may not always be present and their presence is not essential for the diagnosis of PDS. They are radial, present in the mid periphery ranging from dot-like to V shape. They usually increase with time, may coalesce and in advanced cases the periphery of the lens can be visualized through the iris. In some cases, they

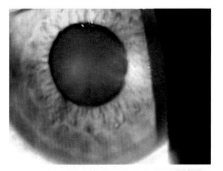

Fig. 1 Krukenberg spindle in a patient with pigmentary glaucoma

may also involve the peripheral and the peripupillary iris. Their position usually corresponds to the anterior packet of zonules. However, these can be difficult to detect in highly pigmented iris with thick stromas. Thus they are not always essential in making a diagnosis of PDS. Infrared imaging techniques are the most sensitive for the clinical diagnosis in such cases.[23] Moreover, defects may fill up in older patients. Their number or clock hours must be monitored.

Other Changes in the Iris

The dispersed pigment particles tend to deposit on the iris surface preferably aggregating in the furrows giving it a dark velvety appearance.[5,22] This is seen more often in eyes with brown iris as compared to TIDs (**Figure 2**). In extreme cases with marked asymmetry, heterochromia may be seen.

The Triad
- Krukenberg spindle
- Iris transillumination defects
- Characteristic gonioscopy findings of dense homogenous trabecular pigmentation.

Iris contour: A prominent iris concavity is present, especially in the midperiphery. It has been extensively studied with ultrasound biomicroscopy and will be discussed further ahead in the chapter.

Gonioscopy

The angle is wide open with a concave iris configuration more so in the midperiphery (**Figure 3**). There is a dense, homogeneous band like pigmentation of the pigmented trabecular meshwork like a 'mascara line' (**Figure 4**). Pigment is also present on and anterior to the Schwalbe's line (Sampaolesi's line), zonules, anterior hyaloid face and posterior lens capsule at the

insertion of the zonules (**Scheie Stripe or Zentmayer line**). The pigment on the zonules and posterior capsule is pathognomic and can be seen on slit-lamp examination in a dilated pupil or during gonioscopy in an eye with a fully dilated pupil. It persists even after the disappearance of the Krukenberg spindle, the filling of the TIDs and the clearing of pigment from the TM.

Pigment reversal sign is seen in the regression phase of PDS or PG. With age and clearing of pigment from the angle, the pigment may become lighter and limited to the filtering part of the meshwork (**Figures 5A and B**). The normal pigment pattern may thus reverse with the pigment band in the superior angle being darker than the inferior one.

Note In older patients pigment reversal sign may be the only finding suggestive of previous pigment dispersion distinguishing it from normal tension glaucoma.

Other Pigments

Eggert's line: Pigment on the hyaloid capsular ligament.
Pigments can be seen in filtration blebs in eyes with PG.

Anterior Chamber

The anterior chamber is deep both centrally and peripherally more so in the mid periphery with the iris assuming a

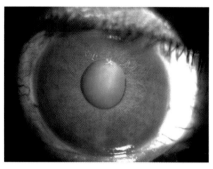

Fig. 2 Absence of the pupillary ruff and velvety appearance of the iris. Transillumination defects are not seen in brown eyes with thick stroma

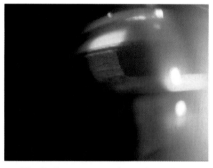

Fig. 3 Concave configuration of the peripheral iris seen on gonioscopy

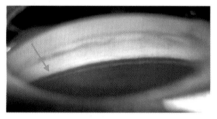

Fig. 4 Homogeneous (4+) pigmentation of the trabecular meshwork in a patient of pigmentary glaucoma

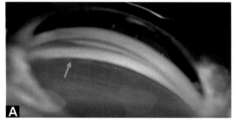
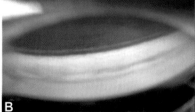

Figs 5A and B (A) With the passage of time the pigments clear from the trabecular meshwork giving it a patchy appearance (blue arrow shows the inferior angle from which pigment has started clearing after the treatment was started). Compare with the homogeneous pigmentation in the superior angle in (B)

concave configuration.[24] Pigments may be seen floating in the anterior chamber especially postdilatation and exercise. Careful slit-lamp examination with a high power slit beam may help detect them and to distinguish them from white blood cells and RBCs.

Pupil

Anisocoria may be seen in asymmetric cases with the larger pupil corresponding to the more severely affected eye. This may be due to the hyperplasia of the dilator muscle. The pupil may be distorted to the side with the maximal transillumination defects where iris dilator muscle hyperplasia is also seen.[25,26]

> **Pearls**
> - Regular retinal examinations
> - Dilate with caution: Record postdilated IOP

Optic Nerve Head

Optic nerve head changes in pigmentary glaucoma are similar to those seen in primary open angle glaucoma. The beta zone may be slightly smaller.[27]

Retina

PDS is associated with a high incidence of retinal detachment about 6 to 8 percent irrespective of miotic therapy.[6] Lattice degeneration is also common.[28,29]

> **Note** Retinal examinations at regular intervals have been suggested owing to the increased risk of retinal tears in PDS patients. Dilatation, however, should be done with care knowing that dilation causes extensive dispersion of pigment with an acute rise in IOP.[30]

NATURAL HISTORY

The mean age of onset of PDS is around mid 20s but it can start as early as mid teens. A clinical spectrum has been proposed. First is the inactive pigment dispersion with a stable IOP. Second, clinically detectable active pigment dispersion with a stable IOP. The third is a clinically detectable active pigment dispersion, elevated IOP followed by progressive optic nerve head changes and progression of glaucoma. Lastly, inactive pigment dispersion with progression of glaucoma.[31] The clinical course can be divided into two phases.

ACTIVE PHASE

During the active phase there is an active and increased release of iris pigment which accumulates in the anterior segment. There is also an increase in the transillumination defects and trabecular meshwork pigmentation. It is asymptomatic and initially the IOP may remain normal throughout the day. Increase in pigment dispersion may be noted after exercise and pharmacological mydriasis.

Conversion to ocular hypertension and glaucoma may occur during this phase. IOP spikes are common after pupillary dilatation and exercise. The reported rates of conversion from PDS to PG of 11.5 percent at 27 months, 35 percent at 17 years and 38.8 percent at 4 years.[12,31,32]

Risk Factors for Progression

The risk factors for progression to pigmentary glaucoma are:[12,31-33]
- IOP greater than 21 mm Hg at presentation
- IOP fluctuations
- Male gender
- Black race
- Presence of Krukenberg spindles
- Signs of active dispersion of pigment
- Greater TM pigmentation
- Myopia.

The risk of developing PG from PDS in the general population is probably lower than 10 percent at 5 years, increasing to 15 percent by 15 years.[33]

REGRESSION PHASE

Interestingly, the severity of both PDS and PG decreases in middle age, when pigment liberation ceases in a majority of patients. The pigment starts clearing and passes out of the trabecular meshwork with age.[34] Thus, the trabecular meshwork pigmentation decreases and becomes more patchy. The "pigment reversal sign" is seen when the pigment band becomes darker in the superior angle than inferiorly. Transillumination defects disappear with time and IOP may become normal. With the reduction of IOP over time, glaucoma medications may be reduced or discontinued depending upon the extent of trabecular meshwork damage which has occurred during the active phase of the disease. This lowering or 'normalization' of IOP can often be misleading and lead to a misdiagnosis of POAG or normal tension glaucoma as the eye clearly has a glaucomatous optic nerve head with a normal IOP.[35] This stage is also referred to as "burnt out glaucoma."

> **What does the natural history teach?**
> Careful documentation of changes in pigmentation
> **Document during the Active Phase**
> - Size of spindle
> - Degree of angle pigmentation
> - Pattern of pigmentation.
> **Regression Phase**
> - "Pigment reversal" sign
> - Burnt out glaucoma

Why Regression?

The regression can be attributed to both the loss of accommodation and the lens enlargement which occurs with increasing age. With age, the pupil also becomes smaller. This leads to more iris-lens touch and makes it more difficult for the aqueous to flow from the posterior to the anterior chamber.

This trapped aqueous in the posterior chamber pushes the iris forward off the zonules. In other words a relative pupillary block occurs, decreasing the iridozonular contact which in turn decreases the dispersion of pigment. The trabecular endothelial cells gradually remove the pigment, giving the appearance of primary open-angle glaucoma patient. The pigment reversal sign on gonioscopy is particularly helpful in differentiating from normal tension glaucoma although it is not specific for PG and can be seen whenever pigment spontaneously clears from the angle.

> **Note** Always look for subtle signs of PDS in an elderly patient with NTG. It may signify that the damage to the ONH discovered in the old age actually occurred at a younger age and may have bearing on management.

PATHOPHYSIOLOGY

In the 1950s, the discovery of iris transillumination defects led to the concept that the trabecular pigment originated from the IPE.[36,37] Focal atrophy of iris epithelium and hypertrophy of the iris dilator was noted in iris specimens. Congenital atrophy or degeneration of the IPE was suggested as a cause of loss of iris pigment. In 1979, Campbell[7] proposed the pathogenesis of PDS to involve mechanical damage to the IPE during rubbing of the posterior iris against the anterior zonular bundles during physiologic pupillary movement.

Ultrasound biomicroscopic studies have helped in gaining insights into the pathophysiology of PDS. The pathophysiology can be discussed under the following categories:

- Pathophysiology of pigment release
- Pathophysiology of increased IOP and glaucoma

Pigment Release

Mechanical, genetic and environmental factors contribute to the pathogenesis of pigment dispersion. Out of the various theories of pathogenesis which have been proposed, Campbell's theory is the most accepted one.[7]

Campbell's Theory

Mechanical rubbing between the peripheral iris and the anterior zonular packets leads to pigment release from the iris. The iris is concave and the fact that the transillumination defects correspond to anterior zonular packets support this theory[38] **(Figure 6)**. The released pigment granules move into the anterior chamber via the aqueous humor and undergo phagocytosis and become trapped within the trabecular meshwork causing a reduced outflow facility and a rise in the IOP. The reason for the concave iris configuration is the '*reverse pupillary block*' due to the relatively higher pressure in the anterior chamber as compared to the posterior chamber resulting in the iris bowing backwards.[39]

Certain structural features account for the deep anterior chamber measured peripherally and centrally. These include a larger iris size as compared to the anterior segment, a greater iris-trabecular meshwork distance and a posterior iris insertion. These features have been confirmed by UBM studies which reveal a posterior iris insertion and a concave configuration resulting in a deeper peripheral anterior chamber. A floppier iris stroma with a lower resistance to dynamic forces has also been observed.

However, the anatomical features do not completely explain the posterior bowing of the iris. A pressure gradient is required to trigger the process. This pressure gradient is created during blinking and accommodation.

Blinking: Campbell proposed that during a blink transient indentation of the cornea pushes iris back against the lens acting as a mechanical pump. This creates a transient pressure gradient between anterior and posterior chambers and promotes aqueous flow from posterior to anterior chamber against

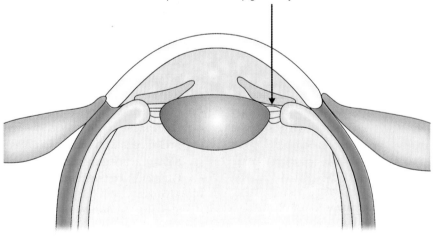

Campbell's theory
Mechanical rubbing between the peripheral iris and the anterior zonular packets causes pigmentary loss from the iris

Fig. 6 Campbell's theory

a pressure gradient. The pressure wave created acts on the iris pushing it posteriorly towards the lens zonular complex. An abnormally greater iris lens contact in eyes with pigment dispersion prevents pressure equilibrium between the anterior and the posterior chamber causing a pronounced iris concavity. This results in a 'reverse pupillary block', an increased iridizonular contact and pigment dispersion. Prevention of blinking has been seen to reverse the concavity due increase in volume and pressure of the posterior chamber as a result of continued aqueous formation.[40] When PDS patients are permitted to blink and rescanned with UBM, the concave iris configuration returns in all eyes. Chew et al demonstrated that during blinking of the nictitating membrane in the chick eye, the cornea indents in a wave form from the periphery to the centre and that the anterior chamber depth similarly decreases.[40]

Accommodation: Accommodation causes an increased iris concavity. Contraction of the ciliary ring leads to shallowing of the anterior chamber, anterior lens movement and increased iridolenticular contact. Aqueous in the anterior chamber is forced into the angle recess and the peripheral iris becomes more concave. As accommodation is relaxed, the iris resumes its initial configuration.

In addition to posterior iris bowing during accommodation, the pupil constricts. Relaxation of accommodation accompanied by pupillary dilation might result in additional iridozonular friction.[41-43]

Exercise

Movements, especially abrupt may cause the zonules to rub against the back of the iris. It is more with exercises involving jumping and jarring like basketball or volleyball. The pigment release associated with pupillary dilation is another contributing factor. Another theory is that exercise causes increased systolic volume changes of the choroidal vasculature. This may be one of the mechanisms that the aqueous anteriorly from posterior chamber and increases iridolenticular contact leading to reverse pupillary block.[44]

Dilation of the pupil leads to additional pigment release and IOP spikes.

Altered electro oculograms of the retinal pigment epithelium-photoreceptor complex hint towards indicate the role of congenital or structural abnormalities of the iris pigment epithelium in the pathogenesis of the disease.[29]

An abnormal persistence of the marginal bundle of Drault might lead to an abnormality of zonular position.[45] Long anterior lens zonules (LANZ) may insert onto the anterior lens capsule centrally causing a mechanical disruption of IPE more centrally. This may be genetic.

Ultrasound Biomicroscopy Studies

Ultrasound biomicroscopy (UBM) studies reveal an increased iris concavity in patients with PDS and PG. Iridolenticular contact distance is also greater in PDS eyes than control eyes.[40,42] The size of the iris is large relative to that of the anterior segment. This may be the basic anatomic cause of the midperipheral iris concavity and predisposition to iridozonular contact.

When compared with normals, patients with PDS were found to have a greater mean iris-trabecular meshwork distance.[46] Thus, iridozonular contact appears to be facilitated by a congenitally more posterior iris insertion.

Ultrasound biomicroscopy during accommodation in eyes with PDS shows iridozonular contact at the lens margin, consistent with the usual position of iris transillumination defects.

Anatomical Considerations

Iridozonular contact could be exacerbated by a more posterior than usual insertion of iris into the ciliary body or by more anteriorly placed zonular packets.

Wide variations in anterior chamber depth and a flatter keratometry have also been reported in patients with PDS.[47,48] PDS patients had flatter keratometry of up to approximately two diopters than age-matched myopic patients.

At a histopathological level, atrophy and dysplasia of the iris epithelium, poor differentiation of the dilator muscles of the iris and abnormalities in iris stroma have been reported, and suspected as the primary abnormality in PDS.[49-51]

Immunological abnormalities may contribute to the development of PDS. No conclusive evidence is currently available.

Pathogenesis of Raised Intraocular Pressure and Pigmentary Glaucoma

The development of PG from PDS is related to more than just a consequence from the release of melanin granules from iris pigment epithelium with subsequent obstruction of the trabecular meshwork.[47] Pigment particles from the iris and ciliary body of donor monkey eyes when injected into the anterior chamber of healthy eyes of live monkeys resulted in only a short-term increase in IOP and outflow resistance returning to normal after one week. The pigment released has been found to accumulate in trabecular endothelial cells, connective tissue cells and endothelium lining the outer wall of Schlemm's canal.[50] The obstruction of the aqueous drainage pathways appears to be a result of a combination of factors. The pigment is phagocytized by trabecular endothelial cells and macrophages. The pigment-laden trabecular endothelial cells die due to the phagocytic overload. They detach from the trabecular sheets and with pigment-laden macrophages partially obstruct the intertrabecular spaces. The denuded corneoscleral and uveoscleral trabecular sheets collapse and disintegrate further obstructing the intertrabecular spaces. These changes have been documented in enucleated human eyes with PDS. Eventually, the outermost terminations of aqueous channels that abut the internal boundary of the juxtacanalicular tissue are affected by reduction in surface area, further increasing outflow resistance[52-54] **(Flow chart 1)**. These factors compromise the outflow facility, resulting in increased IOP. As a result, even when the pigment release decreases or stops, the IOP may remain high due to the permanent dysfunction of the trabecular meshwork and reduction in outflow facility.

> **Note** Observations that the degree of trabecular damage may not relate to the development of pigmentary glaucoma suggest that a developmental anomaly of the angle may also be present.

Multifactorial

In many cases, PDS progresses to high IOP and PG. However a significant number of cases of PDS do not progress to high IOP. This signifies the role of additional factors. These have been listed in **Table 2**. It is likely that a genetic susceptibility of the trabecular meshwork tissue to damage by the pigment/cell debris is required for the conversion to and progression of glaucoma. Mouse model experiments provide a strong evidence for such susceptibility.[55,56]

DIFFERENTIAL DIAGNOSIS

Many ocular conditions with increased TM pigmentation or iris transillumination defects due to release of pigment from the uveal tissue can resemble pigment dispersion syndrome and pigmentary glaucoma. However each condition possesses specific differentiating features. These conditions include exfoliation syndrome and exfoliation glaucoma, uveitis and any form of iris trauma. Disorders associated with signs of pigment dispersion are listed in **Table 3**. These conditions also include the disruption of melanoma cells (e.g. melanomalytic dispersion), cysts of the iris and ciliary body, postoperative conditions and diabetes. They often occur unilaterally.

Pseudophakic Secondary Pigment Dispersion

Cases of pigment dispersion and pigmentary glaucoma secondary to chaffing of iris by square edge posterior chamber intraocular lenses that were implanted in the ciliary sulcus, requiring lens repositioning, lens exchange with/without glaucoma surgery have been reported.[57-59] Close contact between the edge of the IOL and

posterior pigmented iris epithelium has been documented by UBM. The clinical findings along with pigment dispersion include raised IOP, iris transillumination defects (according to the position of optic/haptic) uveitis, spontaneous hyphema. Recently, it has been reported even 'in the bag' lenses.[60]

Phakic intraocular lenses can also result in PDS and PG. In these conditions, trabecular pigmentation is often less dense and is usually unevenly distributed throughout the circumference of the meshwork.

Uveitis

Occasionally, pigment granules in the anterior chamber may be confused with inflammatory cells, leading to a misdiagnosis of uveitis.

Exfoliation Glaucoma

Although sometimes associated with pigment dispersion, exfoliation glaucoma is a distinct secondary open angle glaucoma. The two conditions can be easily differentiated by a detailed clinical examination **(Table 4)**. The age of onset for exfoliation glaucoma is usually older than 60 years, and onset

Table 2 Multifactorial etiology of pigment dispersion syndrome and pigmentary glaucoma

• Campbell's theory and frictional contact between the concave peripheral iris and anterior zonules leading to lysis of IPE and pigment release
❖ Reverse pupillary block
❖ Mechanical obstruction of the TM by pigment (reversible damage)
❖ Permanent damage of TM
• Myopia
• Blinking
• Accommodation
• Exercise
• Pupillary dilation
• Posterior iris insertion and/or anterior zonular insertion
• Developmental angle anomaly
• Larger and thinner iris
• Inherent tendency of IPE dispersion
• Inherent genetic susceptibility of TM to damage by pigment
• Low grade inflammation

Flow chart 1 Pathogenesis of increased IOP in pigmentary glaucoma

```
                          ┌──────────┐
                          │ Pigment  │
                          └──────────┘
                               │
                               ▼
                  ┌──────────────────────────┐
                  │ Engulfed by trabecular cells │
                  └──────────────────────────┘
                               │
                               ▼
                     ┌────────────────┐
                     │    Partial      │
                     │ degeneration of │
                     │  melanoprotein  │
                     └────────────────┘
```

Macrophages   Free radical production

Trabecular beams denuded

Vulnerable to fusion

Obliteration of outflow channels
and increased resistance to aqueous outflow

Increase IOP

Table 3 Differential diagnosis of pigment dispersion

- Exfoliation syndrome
- Uveitis
- Pseudophakia
- Iris cysts
- Trauma
- Intraocular surgery
- Following laser procedures like iridotomy, trabeculoplasty
- Pigmented intraocular tumors
- Rhegmatogenous retinal detachment
- Diabetes mellitus

Table 4 Comparison between exfoliation and pigmentary glaucoma

	XFS	PG
Age	60-70 years	40-50 years
Transillumination defects	Pupillary ruff, periupillary	Midperipheral
Trabecular pigmentation	Patchy	Homogeneous, uniform, dense (4+)
XFS material	Present	Absent
Pigment on posterior corneal surface	Usually diffuse, rarely Krukenberg spindle may be present	Krukenberg spindle
Anterior chamber	Normal/shallow	Deep
Response to medication	Poor	Good
Laser iridotomy	Only when associated with occludable angles	Only in cases with UBM proven irido zonular touch
Intraoperative complications	More common	Same as for POAG
Postoperative course	More inflammation in early postoperative period	More prone to hypotony (usually young myopes). More chance of failure of trabeculectomy

is rare in persons younger than 40 years. Trabecular meshwork pigmentation in exfoliation glaucoma is patchy as compared to PDS and PG. Iris transillumination characteristically begins at the pupillary border and not the midperiphery. Unlike PDS it is a unilateral or highly asymmetrical disease. The presence of white flakes of exfoliation material at the pupillary border and on the anterior lens surface is diagnostic of exfoliation syndrome.

Schwartz Syndrome

Rhegmatogenous retinal detatchment may rarely be associated with pigment dispersion and a high IOP. This rare condition was described by Schwartz. These patients owing to the RD may have varying amounts of pigment dispersion in the anterior chamber and on anterior segment examination may be misdiagnosed as pigmentary glaucoma. The diagnosis of Schwartz syndrome can be made after a detailed posterior segment examination. Moreover one must bear in mind that both pigmentary glaucoma and retinal detachment may also coexist.

The Overlap Syndrome

The overlap concept was first introduced in 1990, in a report of five middle-aged patients with increasingly uncontrollable IOP.[61] All patients had both XFS and pigment dispersion syndrome. Ritch et al identified 26 such patients in a retrospective chart review.[62,63] While there can be other overlap combinations, PDS/XFS was chosen as a paradigm for the syndrome because of the ease of diagnosis and its prevalence.

Presence of Asymmetry

PDS typically is a bilateral disease, although asymmetry may occur. A correlation exists between the amount of pigment lost from the posterior surface of the iris, increased degree of

pigmentation in the trabecular meshwork, and degree of dysfunction in the trabecular meshwork as evidenced by elevation of the IOP. The size and density of the Krukenberg spindle does not necessarily correlate with trabecular meshwork damage. However, the amount of pigment that is presented to the trabecular meshwork does play a role in the elevation of the IOP. Markedly asymmetric disease is usually due to an additional factor such as anisometropia, trauma or the development of exfoliation. Such causes should be looked for in a patient with marked asymmetry or if a previously stable and adherent patient progresses suddenly.

MANAGEMENT

PDS is a risk factor for the development of ocular hypertension, all patients should undergo periodic eye examinations especially during the pigment liberation phase.

Principles of Treatment
Treating the Primary Cause: Iridozonular Contact

Eliminating the iris concavity and iridozonular contact may prevent progression of the disease and the development of glaucoma by immobilizing the pupil and may allow a reversal of previously existing damage.

Principles of treatment
- Decrease pigment liberation and dispersion
- Elimination of iris concavity and iridozonular contact
- Decrease the IOP
- Prevent disease progression

The Reversal of Iridozonular Contact

Keeping in mind the pathogenesis of pigment dispersion, consideration should be given to directing therapy toward eliminating acute pigment release, rather than just treating elevated IOP.

Miotics

The reversal of iridozonular contact may be achieved by using pilocarpine. Scanning with UBM following administration of topical pilocarpine showed resolution of the iris concavity and iridozonular contact in all eyes producing a convex rather than a planar configuration.[64] Pilocarpine thus reduces pigment liberation and also decreases the IOP by increasing trabecular outflow. However, since most of the patients are young and myopic they may not tolerate it well. In such a case *Pilocarpine Ocuserts* are a reasonable option. Their use on the other hand adds to the pre existing risk of retinal detachment. Moreover, they are currently unavailable.

Alpha 1 receptor antagonists like thymoxamine and dapiprazole are other options for avoiding physiological mydriasis. They spare the ciliary muscle and relax the dilator. However their long-term efficacy is controversial and adverse effects like burning, hyperemia have been reported. Dapiprazole is expensive and has a shorter shelf life after reconstitution.[65]

Laser Iridotomy

Laser PI can be performed to relieve the reverse pupillary block of PDS in UBM proven cases. It results in an equalization of pressure in the anterior and posterior chamber and morphological changes that more closely resemble normal iris shape and iridolenticular contact.[66-69] It relieves reverse pupillary block by allowing aqueous to flow from the anterior to the posterior chamber and produces a planar iris configuration.

Miotics vs Laser Iridotomy

The exercise-induced release of pigment and elevation of IOP can be blocked by pilocarpine.[64,65] Whereas pilocarpine completely inhibits exercise-induced pigment release and IOP elevation, iridotomy does so incompletely.[70-72] Laser iridotomy causes the iris to flatten whereas pilocarpine makes it convex.

Lowering the IOP

Progressive glaucomatous optic neuropathy in PG is primarily pressure dependent and reduction of IOP is the mainstay of therapy. Sequential ophthalmic examinations should include IOP monitoring, gonioscopy to assess the degree and progression of trabecular pigmentation, stereoscopic evaluation and photography of the optic nerve, and perimetry.

Each of these parameters must be evaluated to determine the proper course of intervention.

MEDICAL MANAGEMENT
Beta-Adrenergic Antagonists

Since a long time beta blockers have been the main stay of initial medical therapy for PG. They cause suppression of aqueous humor production and have a relatively easy dosing schedule with minimal ocular side effects.

Prostaglandin Analogues

Aqueous outflow enhancers are preferred considering the mechanism of the disease. Prostaglandin analogues, which lower IOP by increasing the pigment laden aqueous outflow via the uveoscleral (the alternate) pathway and bypassing the diseased TM are quite effective in treating PG and offer the advantage of once daily administration and may be more effective than aqueous suppressants. The iris surface color change that may occur during therapy appears to involve increased melanin production by iris melanocytes and is not known to affect the IPE or result in pigment dispersion.

Parasympathomimetics

As learnt from the natural history of the disease, treatment directed at increasing relative pupillary block should relieve iridozonular contact and diminish pigment liberation. This can be achieved by parasympathomimetics like pilocarpine. The relief of iridozonular contact following miotic therapy has been demonstrated with UBM. Pupillary miosis increases resistance to aqueous flow from the posterior chamber, past the lens surface, and through the pupil into the anterior chamber. This increased resistance allows aqueous pressure to build within the posterior chamber (i.e. relative pupillary block), and forces the iris to move anteriorly, away from the zonules, and assume a convex configuration. In addition to this, it also lowers the IOP by increasing the trabecular outflow and makes the pupil immobile. However, strong miotics in young individuals rarely are tolerated because of the associated spasm of accommodation and blurring of vision.

Low-dose pilocarpine, in the form of Ocusert, often provides enough miosis to create pupillary block, without disabling side effects. These are currently unavailable. A pilocarpine gel can be used.

> **Note** A careful peripheral retinal examination should be performed before and after the institution of or change in miotic therapy because of the higher incidence of retinal breaks and detachment in these patients.

Alpha-Adrenergic Agonists

Alpha-agonists can be used as second line of treatment in combination with other aqueous suppressants or prostaglandin analogues. The limiting factor is the development of allergy on prolonged use in about 50% patients.

Carbonic Anhydrase Inhibitors

Topical carbonic anhydrase inhibitors (CAIs) are effective in lowering IOP in PG and are generally well tolerated. They cause additional IOP lowering when given in combination with beta blockers, prostaglandin analogs and alpha agonists. Systemic CAIs are used to treat IOP spikes seen post dilation or post laser procedures. The can also be used temporarily to lower IOP preoperatively.

LASER TRABECULOPLASTY

Argon or selective laser trabeculoplasty can be done for PG.[73,74] Although the initial result is often good the effect is short lived in a large proportion of patients when compared to patients with POAG. Contrary to primary or juvenile open-angle glaucoma, younger patients show a good response to trabeculoplasty. These eyes with pigmentary glaucoma require less energy than usual because of the increased trabecular pigmentation.

Post-laser spikes are common and need to be managed promptly. There have been reports of sustained post IOP elevations requiring trabeculectomies.[75]

Laser Peripheral Iridotomy

Laser iridotomy causes equalization of pressures between the anterior and posterior chambers. The iris becomes flat, thereby decreasing iridozonular contact. This prevents continued pigment liberation. The effect has been found to be more pronounced in younger patients with a well documented concave iris configuration. However, long-term lowering of IOP and stabilization of glaucomatous optic neuropathy and visual field loss have not been demonstrated conclusively. The iridotomy does not completely reverse exercise induced rise in intraocular pressure. Laser iridotomy should be used with caution because of the lack of data regarding its long-term efficacy of this procedure. Moreover the pigment liberated due to the iridotomy poses an additional risk so the risk benefit ratio must be considered. It may be useful in patients less than 45 years with a well documented iris concavity, active pigment dispersion especially following mydriasis and an adequately functioning trabecular meshwork.

The Dilemma: *The effectiveness and indications of Laser PI is a subject of debate. It is not the ideal choice in at least two groups of patients: PDS without ocular hypertension with minimal risk of progression to PG. Patients with advanced glaucomatous damage on multiple medications where LPI induced pigment release and IOP spike can add to the pre-existing damage. Presently it is done only in UBM documented cases.*

SURGICAL MANAGEMENT
Filtering Surgery

The surgical management is on the same principles as POAG. Surgery is indicated when there is progression of visual field defects or optic nerve head changes despite medical/laser therapy. The progression in the optic nerve head damage along with visual field defects should be the principal guidelines used in deciding whether surgery is needed. Cases not controlled with maximum medications require surgery. The procedure of choice is trabeculectomy. Since most patients tend to be young, they are at an increased risk of failure. Antimetabolites, however should be used with caution as these young myopic males are at a greater risk of hypotony. No unusual problems are encountered intraoperatively. The long-term prognosis is usually good and irreversible vision loss occurs in relatively few eyes.

Nonpenetrating Glaucoma Surgery

NPGS is a potential therapy for pigmentary glaucoma. It targets the site of pathology—the pigment-laden trabecular meshwork—which can be reconditioned to establish filtration.

Trabecular Aspiration

Trabecular aspiration achieves a good short-term effect in the reduction of

IOP but it does not appear to be suitable for long-term IOP reduction.

PDS AND EXERCISE

Patients with PDS are usually of a younger age group for whom exercise may be a part of their lifestyle or profession. Non jarring exercises usually are not known to produce IOP spikes whereas IOP spikes have been seen after exercises involving jumping (basketball, volleyball, etc). So it is a good practice to check for post exercise IOP in such patients and manage accordingly.

To summarize, treatment should begin early in order to prevent the development of glaucomatous damage and should be designed to prevent progression of the disease rather than merely lower IOP. Miotic treatment produces a convex iris configuration, completely inhibiting pigment liberation, while laser iridotomy produces a planar configuration and may not completely inhibit pigment liberation. Aqueous suppressants theoretically may negatively impact the course of the disease and PG analogs may be preferred. Laser trabeculoplasty produces better results in younger patients than older ones because of the location of the pigment in the trabecular meshwork. However the postlaser spikes are common and the effect is short lived. Surgery is the treatment of choice when maximum medical therapy fails. One should look out for hypotony and MMC related complications in the post operative period.

CONCLUSION

PDS is an inherited disorder of abnormal iridozonular contact which is exaggerated by physiologic pupillary movement, blinking and accommodation. This contact results in disruption of the IPE cells and liberation of pigment, which is deposited on structures throughout the anterior segment. Pigment liberation can be triggered

by exercise and by pupillary dilation. Myopia predisposes to the phenotypic expression of the disorder, which affects men and women equally, but men develop glaucoma two to three times as often as women and at an earlier age. Pigment dispersion begins in the teens or twenties and continues until about the mid-40s in most people, at which time a combination of relative pupillary block and presbyopia lead to gradual cessation of pigment liberation. After this, the visible signs of pigment loss can reverse and IOP control can improve. Older patients presenting for the first time with glaucomatous damage and normal IOP may be misdiagnosed as having normal-tension glaucoma.

Campbell's mechanical theory is the most accepted for the pathogenesis but does not explain the process completely. UBM also do not always demonstrate an iridozonular contact. Asymmetric pigment dispersion and pigmentary glaucoma has been reported in the literature. Study of the anatomical and physiological differences between such eyes is an interesting option to look into the unanswered questions. Studies using UBM and the Pentacam to investigate found a larger back radius of corneal curvature, a more posterior iris insertion of the iris root, an increased iris concavity and increased iridozonular contact in eyes with a greater degree of pigment loss. Genetic susceptibility of the drainage tissue to pigment/cell debris induced damage is being investigated. Laser peripheral iridotomy relieves the pupil block of pigment dispersion syndrome and reduces aqueous pigment, but the benefits in preventing or treating glaucoma are still controversial. Prospective studies and randomized control trials are warranted. Advances in technology and molecular and genetic studies will help shed more light on the pathogenesis and management of the disease.

REFERENCES

1. Krukenberg F. Beiderseitige ange-borene Melanose der Hornhaut. Klin Monatsbl Augenheilkd 1899;37:254-8.

2 von Hippel E. Zur pathologischen Anatomie des Glaukom. Arch Ophthalmol 1901;52:498.

3. Levinsohn G. Beitrag zur patholo-gische Anatomie und Pathologie des Glaukoms. Arch Augenheilkd 1909; 62:131-54.

4. Sugar HS, Barbour FA. Pigmentary glaucoma: a rare clinical entity. Am J Ophthalmol 1949;32:90.

5. Sugar HS. Pigmentary glaucoma: a 25-year review. Am J Ophthalmol 1966;62:499-507.

6. Scheie HG, Cameron JD. Pigment dispersion syndrome: a clinical study. Br J Ophthalmol 1981;65:264-9.

7. Campbell DG. Pigmentary dispersion and glaucoma: a new theory. Arch Ophthalmol 1979;97:1667-72.

8. Siddiqui Y, Ten Hulzen RD, Cameron JD, Hodge DO, Johnson DH. What is the risk of developing pigmen-tary glaucoma from pigment disper-sion syndrome? Am J Ophthalmol 2003;135:794-9.

9. Ritch R, Steinberger D, Liebmann JM. Prevalence of pigment disper-sion syndrome in a population under-going glaucoma screening. Am J Ophthalmol 1993;115:707-10.

10. Lotufo D, Ritch R, Sperling M, et al. Pigmentary and primary open angle glaucoma in young patients. Invest Ophthalmol Vis Sci 1986; 27(suppl):166.

11. Becker B, Podos SM. Krukenberg's spindles and primary open-angle glaucoma. Arch Ophthalmol 1966; 70:635.

12. Migliazzo CV, Shaffer RN, Nykin R, Magee S. Long-term analysis of pigmentary dispersion syndrome and pigmentary glaucoma. Ophthalmo-logy 1986;93:1528-36.

13. Bovell AM, Damji KF, Dohadwala AA, Hodge WG, Allingham RR. Familial occurrence of pigment dispersion syndrome. Can J Ophthalmol 2001; 36:11-7.

14. Stankovic J, Ein Beitrag zur Kenntnis der Vererbung des Pigmentglaucom. Klin Monatsbl Augenheilkd 1961; 139:165.

15. Allen TD, Ackerman WG: Hereditary glaucoma in a pedigree of three generations. Arch Ophthalmol 1942; 27:139-157

16. Andersen JS, Pralea AM, DelBono EA, et al. A gene responsible for the pigment dispersion syndrome maps to chromosome 7q35-q36. Arch Ophthalmol; 115:384-8.

17. Fine BS, Yanoff M, Sheie HG. Pigmentary 'glaucoma': a histologic study. Trans Am Acad Ophthalmol Otolaryngol 1974;78:314-25.

18. Duncan TE. Krukenberg spindles in pregnancy. Arch Ophthalmol 1974;91:355-8.

19. Semple HC, Ball SF. Pigmentary glau-coma in the black population. Am J Ophthalmol 1990;109:518.

20. Wilelnsky JT, Buerk KM, Podos SM. Krukeknberg's spindles. Am J Ophthalmol 1975;79:220.

21. Farrar SM, Shields MB. Current concepts in pigmentary glaucoma. Surv Ophthalmol 1993;37:233.

22. Murrell WJ, Shihab Z, Lamberts DW, et al. The corneal endothelium and central corneal thickness in pigmen-tary dispersion syndrome. Arch Ophthalmol 1986;104:845-6.

23. Alward WL, Munden PM, Verdick RE, et al. Use of infrared videography to detect and record iris transillu-mination defects. Arch Ophthalmol 1990;108:748-51.

24. Davidson JA, Brubaker RF, Ilstrup DM. Dimensions of the anterior cham-ber in pigment dispersion syndrome. Arch Ophthalmol 1983;101:81-3.

25. Feibel RM, Perlmutter JC. Anisocoria in the pigmentary dispersion syndrome. Am J Ophthalmol 1990; 110:657-60.

26. Feibel RM. Anisocoria in the pigmen-tary dispersion syndrome: further cases. J Glaucoma 1993;2:37-8.

27. Jonas JB, Ditchtl A, Budde WM, Lang P. Optic disc morphology in pigmentary glaucoma. Br J Ophthalmol 1998;82: 875-9.

28. Weseley P, Liebmann J, Walsh JB, et al. Lattice degeneration of the retina and the pigment dispersion syndrome. Am J Ophthalmol 1992;114:539-43.

29. Greenstein VC, Seiple W, Liebmann J, Ritch R. Retinal pigment epithelial dysfunction in patients with pigment dispersion syndrome: implications for the theory of pathogenesis. Arch Ophthalmol 2001;119:1291-5.

30. Küchle M, Mardin CY, Nguyen NX, Martus P, Naumann GO. Quantification of aqueous melanin granules in primary pigment disper-sion syndrome. Am J Ophthalmol 1998;126:425-31.

31. Richter CU, Richardson TM, Grant WM. Pigmentary dispersion syndrome and pigmentary glaucoma: a prospec-tive study of the natural history. Arch Ophthalmol 1986;104:211-5.

32. Farrar SM, Shields MB, Miller KN, Stoup CM. Risk factors for the devel-opment and severity of glaucoma in the pigment dispersion syndrome. Am J Ophthalmol 1989;108:223-9.

33. Siddiqui Y, Ten Hulzen RD, Cameron JD, Hodge DO, Johnson DH. What is the risk of developing pigmen-tary glaucoma from pigment disper-sion syndrome? Am J Ophthalmol 2003;135:794-9.

34. Lichter PR, Shaffer RM. Diagnostic and prognostic signs in pigmen-tary glaucoma. Trans Am Acad Ophthalmol Otolaryngol 1970;74:984.

35. Ritch R. Nonprogressive low-tension glaucoma with pigmentary dispersion. Am J Ophthalmol 1982;94:190-6.

36. Bick MW. Pigmentary glaucoma in females. Arch Ophthalmnol 1957; 58:483.

37. Scheie HG, Fleischhauer HW. Idiopathic atrophy of the epithelial layers of the iris and ciliary body: a clinical study. Arch Ophthalmol 1958;59:216-28.

38. Campbell DG, Schertzer RM. Pathophysiology of pigment dispersion syndrome and pigmentary glaucoma. Curr Opin Ophthalmol 1996;6:96-101.

39. Karickhoff JR. Pigmentary dispersion syndrome and pigmentary glaucoma: a new mechanism concept, a new treatment, and a new technique. Ophthalmic Surg 1992;23:269-77.

40. Chew SJ, Tello C, Wallman J, Ritch R. Blinking indents the cornea and reduces anterior chamber volume as shown by ultrasound biomicroscopy. Invest Ophthalmol Vis Sci 1994;35:1573.

41. Pavlin CJ, Macken P, Trope G, et al. Accommodation and iridotomy in the pigment dispersion syndrome. Ophthalmic Surg Lasers 1996;27:113-20.

42. Carassa RG, Bettin P, Fiori M, et al. Nd:YAG laser iridotomy in pigment dispersion syndrome: an ultrasound biomicroscopic study. BJ Ophthalmol 1998;82:150-3.

43. Balidis MO, Bunce C, Sandy CJ, Wormald RP, Miller MH. Iris configuration in accommodation in pigment dispersion syndrome. Eye 2002;16:694-700.

44. Jensen PK, Nissen O, Kessing SV. Exercise and reversed pupillary block in pigmentary glaucoma. Am J Ophthalmol 1995;120:110-2.

45. Barishak YR. Embryology of the Eye and Its Adnexae. Basel, Karger, 1992 (Straub W, edn, Developments in Ophthalmology; vol 24).

46. Sokol J, Stegman Z, Liebmann JM et al. Location of the iris insertion in pigment dispersion syndrome. Ophthalmology 1996;103:289-93.

47. Lord FD, Pathanapitoon K, Mikelberg FS. Keratometry and axial length in pigment dispersion syndrome: a descriptive case-control study. J. Glaucoma 2001;10:383-5.

48. Yip LW, Sothornwit N, Bekowitz J, Mikelberg FS. A comparison of interocular differences in patients with pigment dispersion syndrome. J Glaucoma 2009;18:1-5.

49. Kupfer C, Kuwabara T, Kaiser-Kupfer M. The histopathology of pigmentary dispersion syndrome with glaucoma. Am J Ophthalmol 1975;80:857-62.

50. Fine BS, Yanoff M, Sheie HG. Pigmentary 'glaucoma': a histologic study. Trans Am Acad Ophthalmol Otolaryngol 1974;78:314-25.

51. Kaiser-Kupfer MI, Kupfer C, McCain L. Asymmetric pigment dispersion syndrome. Trans Am Ophthalmol Soc 1983;81:310-24.

52. Kampik A, Green WR, Quigley HA, Pierce LH. Scanning and transmission electron microscopic studies of two cases of pigment dispersion syndrome. Am J Ophthalmol 1981; 91:573-87.

53. Richardson TM, Hutchinson BT, Grant WM. The outflow tract in pigmentary glaucoma: a light and electron microscopic study. Arch Ophthalmol 1977; 95:1015-25.

54. Alvarado JA, Murphy CG. Outflow obstruction in pigmentary and primary open angle glaucoma. Arch Ophthalmol 1992;110:1769-78.

55. Anderson MG, Libby RT, Mao M, et al. Genetic context determines susceptibility to intraocular pressure elevation in a mouse pigmentary glaucoma. BMC Biol 2006;4:20.

56. Lynch S, Yanagi G, DelBono E, Wiggs JL. DNA sequence variants in the tyro-sinase-related protein 1 (TYRP1) gene are not associated with human pigmentary glaucoma. Mol Vis 2002; 8:127-9.

57. Micheli T, Cheung LM, Sharma S, Assaad NN, Guzowski M, Francis IC, Norman J, Coroneo MT. Acute haptic-induced pigmentary glaucoma with an AcrySof intraocular lens. J Cataract Refract Surg 2002;28:1869-72.

58. Wintle R, Austin M. Pigment dispersion with elevated intraocular pressure after AcrySof intraocular lens implantation in the ciliary sulcus. J Cataract Refract Surg 2001;27:642-4.

59. Boutboul S, Letaief I, Lalloum F, Puech M, Borderie V, Laroche L. Pigmentary glaucoma secondary to in-the-bag intraocular lens implantation. J Cataract Refract Surg 2008; 34:1595-7.

60. Rhéaume MA, Duperré J, Harasymowycz P, Thompson P. Pigment dispersion and recurrent hyphema associated with in-the-bag lens implantation. J Cataract Refract Surg 2009;35:1464-7.

61. Layden WE, Ritch R, King DG, Teekhasaenee C. Combined exfoliation and pigment dispersion syndrome. Am J Ophthalmol 1990; 109:530-4.

62. Mudumbai R, Liebmann JM, Ritch R. Combined exfoliation and pigment dispersion: an overlap syndrome. Trans Am Ophthalmol Soc. 1999;97: 297-314.

63. Ritch R, Mudumbai R, Liebmann JM. Combined exfoliation and pigment dispersion: paradigm of an overlap

syndrome. Ophthalmology 2000;107:1004-8.

64. Potash SD, Tello C, Leibmann J, Ritch R. Ultrasound biomicroscopy in pigment dispersion syndrome. Ophthalmology 1994;101:332-9.

65. Mastropasqua L, Carpineto P, Ciancaglini M, Gallenga PE. The effectiveness of dapiprazole, an alpha adrenergic agent in pigmentary glaucoma. Ophthalmic Surg Lasers 1996;27:806-9.

66. Breingan PJ, Esaki K, Ishikawa H, et al. Iridolenticular contact decreases following laser iridotomy for pigment dispersion syndrome. Arch. Ophthalmol 1999;117:325-28.

67. Küchle M, Nguyen NX, Mardin CY, Naumann GO. Effect of neodymium:YAG laser iridotomy on number of aqueous melanin granules in primary pigment dispersion syndrome. Graefes Arch Clin Exp Ophthalmol 2001;239:411-5.

68. Gandolfi SA, Vecchi M. Effect of a YAG laser iridotomy on intraocular presure in pigment dispersion syndrome. Ophthalmology 1996;103(10):1693-5.

69. Reistad CE, Shields MB, Campbell DG, Ritch R, Wang JC, Wand M; American Glaucoma Society Pigmentary Glaucoma Iridotomy Study Group. The influence of peripheral iridotomy on the intraocular pressure course in patients with pigmentary glaucoma. J. Glaucoma 2005;14:255-9.

70. Haynes WL, Alward WL, Tello C, et al. Incomplete elimination of exercise-induced pigment dispersion by laser iridotomy in pigment dispersion syndrome. Ophthalmic Surg Lasers 1995;26:484-6.

71. Pavlin CJ, Macken P, Trope G, et al. Accommodation and iridotomy in the pigment dispersion syndrome. Ophthalmic Surg Lasers 1996;27:113-20.

72. Jampel HD. Lack of effect of peripheral laser iridotomy in pigment dispersion syndrome.

73. Ritch R, Liebmann J, Robin A et al. Argon laser trabeculoplasty in pigmentary glaucoma. Ophthalmology 1993;100:909-13.

74. Harasymowycz PJ, Papamatheakis DG, Latina M, De Leon M, Lesk MR, Damji KF. Selective laser trabeculoplasty (SLT) complicated by intraocular pressure elevation in eyes with heavily pigmented trabecular meshworks. Am J Ophthalmol 2005;139:1110-3.

75. Birt CM. Intraocular pressure spike after YAG iridotomy in patients with pigment dispersion. Can J Ophthalmol 2004;39:234-9.

30 | Lens-induced Glaucoma

R Venkatesh, Kavitha Palanisamy

CHAPTER OUTLINE
- Classification
- Phacomorphic Glaucoma
- Phacolytic Glaucoma
- Glaucoma Associated with Ectopia Lentis
- Lens Particle Glaucoma
- Phacoanaphylaxis

INTRODUCTION

Blindness affects an estimated 12.5 million people in India, with cataract as the cause in 50 to 80 percent of this group. This, together with social and economic factors, often results in delayed presentation until advanced stages such as intumescent, mature, and hypermature cataracts. Hence, complications such as lens induced glaucoma are more common.[1-4]

CLASSIFICATION

Lens induced glaucoma can be subdivided into two major categories:
1. Open angle glaucoma
   a. Phacolytic
   b. Phacoanaphylactic
   c. Phacotoxic
2. Closed angle (pupillary block) glaucoma
   a. Phacomorphic glaucoma
   b. Ectopia lentis

Studies indicate a higher incidence of phacomorphic (3:1) than phacolytic glaucoma.

PHACOMORPHIC GLAUCOMA

Phacomorphic glaucoma is a common entity in developing countries like India owing to decreased awareness of the cataract and delay in its removal. It is seen in eyes with a swollen cataractous lens.

Mechanism of Glaucoma

The cataract progresses enough to become intumescent with an increased anteroposterior length. Swelling of the lens leads to a progressive reduction in the iridocorneal angle. Angle closure may be secondary to a pupillary block mechanism or it may be due to forward displacement of the lens-iris diaphragm. Pupillary block glaucoma is caused by changes in the size of the crystalline lens and its relatively anterior position.

Predisposing Factors

Certain factors predispose to the development of phacomorphic glaucoma. These include:
- Intumescent cataract
- Traumatic cataract
- Rapidly developing senile cataract
- Phacomorphic glaucoma is more common in smaller hyperopic eyes with a larger lens and a shallower AC.

An angle-closure attack can be precipitated by pupillary dilation in dim light. The dilation to midposition relaxes the peripheral iris so that it may bow forward, coming into contact with the trabecular meshwork, setting the stage for pupillary block. Angle closure is also facilitated by the pressure originating posterior to the lens and the enlargement of the lens itself.

- Zonular weakness secondary to exfoliation, trauma, or age can play a part in causing phacomorphic glaucoma.

Clinical Features
Symptoms

More often, phacomorphic glaucoma presents as acute angle closure glaucoma characterized by eye pain, headache, blurred vision, perception of haloes around light and also nausea, vomiting, bradycardia and diaphoreses due to vasovagal response. These symptoms usually occur at night because mid dilated pupil during sleep aggravates pupillary block.

Signs

Clinical examination reveals reduced visual acuity, conjunctival congestion, corneal edema, reduced anterior chamber depth, cells and flare, mid dilated pupil, intumescent cataractous lens and significantly elevated intraocular pressure **(Figure 1)**.

> **Note** Fellow eye may show anatomically predisposed features and probably a cataract.[5]

Management

The treatment focuses on the following objectives:

- Lowering the intraocular pressure as soon as possible
- Preventing both the diseased and fellow eye from another episode.[6]
- Cataract extraction is the only definitive treatment for an intumescent cataract.

Medical Management

Initially, antiglaucoma medications are used to decrease the intraocular pressure. Topical beta blockers, alpha agonists, carbonic anhydrase inhibitor and hyperosmotic agents (intravenous mannitol) are the mainstay of treatment. Pilocarpine tends to aggravate the pupillary block.[7]

Lasers

If intraocular pressure is not lowered with medical therapy, the following can be tried:[8,9]

- Argon laser gonioplasty
- Argon laser coreoplasty.

Prophylactic laser iridotomy in the fellow eye if it is anatomically predisposed.[11]

Surgical Management

Surgery for phacomorphic glaucoma is challenging due to white intumescent cataracts. This intumescence and swelling leads to increased convexity of lens causing a shallow anterior chamber and difficult capsulorhexis.[29]

Preoperative: Successful postoperative outcome is more likely when surgery is performed in quiet eye. B-scan ultrasonography is essential to rule out any posterior segment pathology. Assessment of corneal endothelial count to determine risk of corneal decompensation is optional.

Intravenous mannitol 20 percent preoperatively, and ocular massage following block may help decompress the eye and help anterior chamber to deepen.

Surgical Technique

A shallow anterior chamber with elevated IOP complicated multiples surgical steps. Choice of surgical technique depends on various considerations. Extracapsular cataract extraction (ECCE) requires a large incision in a globe with very high IOP, which increases the risk of sight threatening complications such as expulsive hemorrhage.[3,4] The surgical steps are technically more challenging and may be complicated by iris tissue prolapse through the large limbal wound.

Small incision cataract surgery (SICS) in our experience significantly faster, less expensive, and less technology dependent than phacoemulsification. Phacoe-mulsification in phacomorphic glaucoma is more challenging. Continous curvilinear capsulorhexis (CCC) is technically more difficult owing to increased convexity of anterior capsule (due to increased intracapsular pressure) leading to extension of tear. The risk of endothelial cell loss is also greater because of close proximity of the phacotip during the nucleus emulsification as well as by the reduced endothelial reserve count. The chances of suprachoroidal hemorrhage are high due to rapid fluctuation of IOP during the procedure. Overinfusion of any OVDs increase the risk of iris prolapse.

Intraoperatively, small gauge vitrectomy may be used as an adjuvant to deepen the anterior chamber.[27,28] The limitations of this technique are that direct visual control is often not possible because of the dense cataracts and there is a small risk for retinal detachment, as

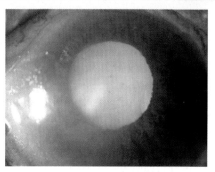

Fig. 1 Phacomorphic glaucoma

reported after small-gauge vitrectomy for various posterior segment disorders. Phacoemulsification with a biplanar valved incision has the advantage of maintaining a deep anterior chamber and avoiding iris prolapse in these eyes. Needle puncture of the capsule with aspiration of liquid cortex under counter pressure of viscoelastic prevents tear in the anterior capsule during capsulorhexis. Alternatively a bent needle attached to a syringe of balanced salt solution may be used to perform the capsulorhexis through a paracentesis. BSS is used to maintain pressure inside the anterior chamber and dilute the liquid cortex.[30] High molecular weight viscoelastics can also be used to deepen shallow anterior chamber, but are effective only after positive pressure has been relieved through vitrectomy. Viscoat (combination of sodium hyaluronate and chondroitin sulfate) and chilled BSS Plus can be used to protect corneal endothelium during phacoemulsification.

Combined surgery: Trabeculectomy combined with cataract surgery may be required in patients with long duration of glaucoma, with more likelihood of developing peripheral anterior synechiae.[31] If the intraocular pressure has been elevated for long time with complete synechial closure of the angle and IOP not controlled by medical treatment a combined procedure—phacotrabeculectomy, trabeculectomy with small incision cataract surgery or extracapsular cataract extraction in conjuction with trabeculectomy may be indicated to control IOP. Adjunctive use of antimetabolites must be used if a combined surgery is planed. Patient should be explained about risk of surgery and prognosis for visual outcome.

Glaucoma drainage devices: Ahmed glaucoma valve has also been implanted along with cataract surgery due to concern over failure of trabeculectomy in an inflamed eye with phacomorphic glaucoma in patients with late presentation. Good intraocular pressure control in teens during follow-up has been reported.[21,32]

PHACOLYTIC GLAUCOMA

The term 'phacolytic glaucoma' was coined by Flocks at in 1955.[12] First clinical description of the condition was by Gifford in 1900.[11] It is characterized by an acute rise in intraocular pressure in eyes which advanced cataract, associated with aqueous flare and cells.[10]

Pathogenesis

Earlier, it was thought that phacolytic glaucoma is due to obstruction of intertrabecular spaces by macrophages distended with engulfed lens material and morgagnian fluid that escaped from the lens.[13] Currently, direct obstruction of outflow pathway by leaking heavy molecular weight soluble proteins is found to be more specific than macrophage response in pathogenesis of phacolytic glaucoma.[13,17-19] With age and cataract progression these proteins get accumulated in the liquid cortex of the lens and additional microscopic changes in lens capsule allow release of these proteins into anterior chamber.

Clinical Features
Symptoms
The patient presents with a history of gradual decline in visual acuity, acute

onset pain, redness and watering. The vision may be reduced to perception of light at the time of presentation.

Signs
Clinical examination reveals conjunctival congestion, corneal edema, deep anterior chamber with heavy flare and cells, mature or hypermature cataract with or without soft white spots on the anterior capsule **(Figures 2A and B)** and a sterile hypopyon which may blood stained. Engorged iris stromal vessels may be seen. The anterior chamber angle is open on gonioscopy and the intraocular pressure is raised. The fellow eye shows a normal anterior chamber.

Posterior segment evaluation may show retinal perivasculitis due to leaking lens proteins. The material may also leak from the lens into the vitreous cavity.[25] A mature cataract may dislocate into vitreous and cause a rare presentation of subacute type phacolytic glaucoma due to intermittent leakage of proteins.[20]

Management
The principles of management are to control intraocular pressure and inflammation. This is achieved by topical steroids and aqueous suppressants like beta blockers, alpha adrenengic agonist, topical or systemic carbonic anhydrase inhibitors or hyperosmotic agents. Removal of the lens is the definitive treatment.

Preoperative care: All attempts should be made to reduce intraocular pressure and inflammation prior to surgery. Intravenous mannitol 20 percent may be administered intravenously prior to surgery if there are no medical contraindications. Digital massage, may be employed to help reduce IOP following a block. Retrobulbar or peribulbar anesthesia is preferred to topical or can be combined with general anesthesia in order to decrease orbital vascular congestion.[22]

Surgical Management
Cataract Extraction
The goal of surgery is to remove the lens which is source high molecular weight proteins thus decreasing obstruction of trabecular meshwork and reducing IOP. Methods of cataract extraction may be:

- Extracapsular cataract extraction (ECCE)
- Manual small incision sutureless cataract surgery (SICS)
- Phacoemulsification.

In our experience manual small incision sutureless cataract surgery with trypan blue staining of the anterior capsule is a safe and effective method of cataract extraction for patients with phacolytic glaucoma.

Combined Surgery
Trabeculectomy 'with antimetabolites' (as the eyes are inflamed) combined with cataract extraction is an option in

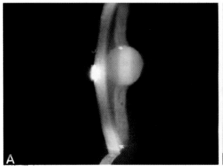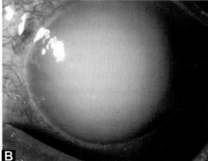

Figs 2A and B Phacolytic glaucoma

patients with long history of phacolytic glaucoma or with preoperative uncontrolled ocular hypertension.[10]

Operative Technique

Capsular staining with trypan blue facilitates capsulotomy or capsulorhexis, which is otherwise difficult in these white morgagnian cataracts. Capsule may be fibrotic and is prone to tear with the initial puncture of CCC due to increased pressure from liquefied cortex. Filling the bag with viscoelastics after the initial puncture and aspiration of liquid cortex gives good control during capsulorhexis in these cases. For manual small incision cataract suurgery, a Sinskey hook can then be used to lever out one pole of the nucleus outside the capsular bag, and the rest of the nucleus is rotated out into the anterior chamber. The nucleus may be delivered using an irrigating vectis followed by aspiration of the residual cortex and IOL implantation.[14-16]

Phacoemulsification is difficult to perform in such cases due to poor view resulting from corneal edema and inflammation.[23]

For phacolytic glaucoma secondary to a dislocated cataract in the vitreous cavity, pars plana vitrectomy and lensectomy is the approach of choice.

Postoperative care: Topical antibiotic and steroids as in standard cataract surgery should be started.

Topical antiglaucoma medications may be required till inflammation subsides.[23]

Complications

Posterior capsule rupture due to increased capsular fragility can occur. Removal of remnant lens material and anterior vitrectomy should be done.[23] Persistent inflammation and cystoid macular edema postoperatively may occur.[24] Vitreous opacities postoperatively may be related to inflammation and resolve with conservative treatment.[26]

GLAUCOMA ASSOCIATED WITH ECTOPIA LENTIS[35]

Subluxation or dislocation of the lens can occur due to the following reasons:
- Post-traumatic **(Figures 3A to C)**
- Ectopia lentis et pupillae
- As a part of the following conditions:
  - Marfan syndrome **(Figures 4A to C)**
  - Homocystinuria
  - Weill-Marchesani syndrome **(Figure 5)**
  - Ehler-Danlos syndrome
  - Hyperlysinemia
  - Aniridia
  - Buphthalmos
  - Megalocornea

Clinical Features
Symptoms

Symptoms vary according to the individual state of the lens. Minimum subluxation may be asymptomatic. If the lens is shifted within the pupillary axis then monocular diplopia may occur. Loss of zonular support results in difficulties with accommodation and near vision. When dislocation results in pupillary block and angle closure glaucoma is present, the patient experiences a red and painful eye, decreased visual acuity and sometimes headache, nausea and vomiting.

Signs

The clinical signs include phacodonesis, iridodonesis and shallowing of the anterior chamber. Gonioscopically, the iris may be seen to assume the shape of a volcano with the pupil forming the central crater. This is the result of the anterior movement of the lens and increased contact with the middle-third of the iris. The entire lens may be seen in the anterior chamber in case of anterior dislocation of the lens **(Figures 3A and B)**. Ultrasound biomicroscope (UBM) can be used to image areas of stretched or absent zonules.

Mechanism of Glaucoma
Management

The extraction of a subluxated lens is associated with increased surgical risks and should usually be avoided unless the lens is in anterior chamber or lens extraction is required to relieve the glaucoma or improve vision. Therapeutic approach depends on the

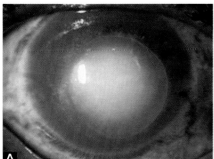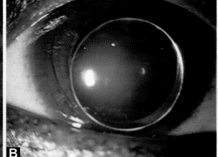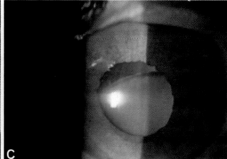

Figs 3A to C (A) Post-traumatic subluxation of the cataractous lens; (B) Clear lens into the anterior chamber; (C) Traumatic inferior subluxation of the crystalline lens. Note the sphincter tears at the pupillary margin

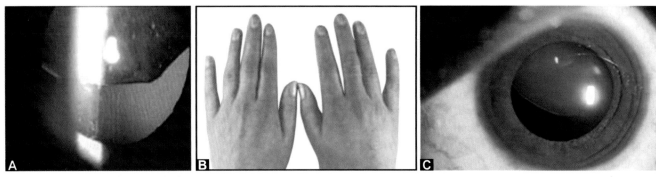

Figs 4A to C Marfan syndrome: The lens is subluxated superiorly. Lens equator and zonules can be seen

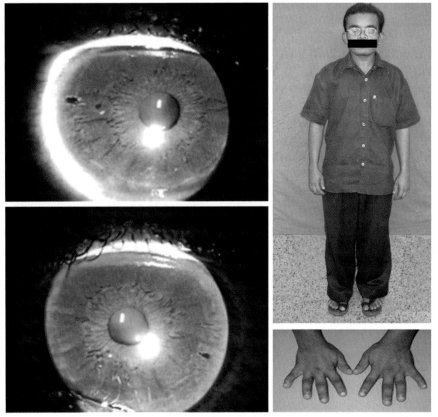

Fig. 5 Weill-Marchesani syndrome: Secondary angle closure with anterior subluxation of the lens. Note the typical systemic features—short stature and stubby fingers; Peripheral laser iridotomy has been done in both eyes of the patient

degree of dislocation and the symptoms. In cases of partial subluxation within the pupillary space that does not cause significant visual impairment or pupillary block, a conservative nonintervention strategy could be followed. When the previous condition is accompanied by pupillary block, then a laser peripheral iridectomy is the

appropriate solution **(Figure 5)**. Total anterior dislocation requires removal of the lens. Dislocation in the vitreous cavity may be followed carefully as long as the cataract is not hypermature and no inflammation or glaucoma is noticed. However the patient should be followed up closely as inflammation and glaucoma may develop any

time. If any of these factors are present, removal of the lens is indicated.

LENS PARTICLE GLAUCOMA

It is associated with a grossly ruptured lens capsule and resultant liberated lens material which obstructs the trabecular meshwork.[11]

The onset of IOP elevation usually occurs soon after the primary event and is generally proportional to the amount of "fluffed-up" lens cortical material in the anterior chamber. Uncommon clinical variations include an onset of glaucoma many years after capsular disruption or after a spontaneous rupture in the lens capsule.[13]

Clinical Features
Symptoms

It is characterized by significant pain, redness and decreased vision.

Signs

Clinical examination shows corneal edema, heavy cells and flare and chunky white material in the aqueous humor. Fluffy cortical matter, peripheral anterior synechiae and posterior synechiae may be present in long standing cases.

Management
Medical

Elevated intraocular pressure and inflammation are treated medically with antiglaucoma medications and steroids. Miotics should be avoided.

Surgical

Surgical management includes removal of the residual lens material to avoid complications such as corneal decompensation, posterior synechiae, peripheral anterior synechiae, cystoid macular edema, and retinal detachment.

PHACOANAPHYLAXIS

It is an uncommon condition. Usually there is a history of either a penetrating injury or disruption of the lens capsule by extra capsular cataract extraction.[33,34]

Clinical Features

Typically, it is a chronic, relentless, granulomatous type of inflammation that centers on lens material in the primary involved eye or in the fellow eye after it had undergone extracapsular cataract extraction or phacoemulsification. Occasionally the inflammation involves the trabecular meshwork leading to a rise in intraocular pressure.

Phacoanaphylaxis is treated with antiglaucoma medications and steroids to control intraocular pressure and reduce inflammation. Any residual lens matter must be removed.

REFERENCES

1. Murthy GV, Gupta SK, Bachani D, et al. Current estimates of blindness in India. Br J Ophthalmol 2005;89:257-60.
2. Dandona L, Dandona R, Naduvilath T, et al. Is the current eye-care policy focus almost exclusively on cataract adequate to deal with blindness in India. The Lancet 1998;74:341-3.
3. Jose R. National programme for control of blindness. Indian J Community Health 1997;3:5-9.
4. Minassian D, Mehra V. 3.8 million blinded by cataract each year: projections from the first epidemiological study of incidence of cataract blindness in India. Br J Ophthalmol 1990;74:341-3.
5. Spalton DJ, Hitchings RA, Hunter PA. Atlas of clinical ophthalmology, Philadelphia, PA, JB Lippincott and Co, 1984.
6. Hoskins H, Kass M. Beckar Shaffer's Diagnosis and Therapy of Glaucoma 6th edn, Stouis MD, CV Mosby Co, 1989.
7. Kramer P, Ritch R. The treatment of acute angle closure glaucoma revisited, Ann ophthalmology 1984;16:1101-3.
8. Ritch R, et al. Argon laser treatment for medically unresponsive attacks of angle closure glaucoma Am J Ophthalmol 1982;94:197-204.
9. Koster HR, Liehmann J, Ritch R, Herdok S. Acute angle closure glaucoma in a patient with AIDS successfully treated with argon laser peripheral iridoplasty. Ophthalmic surgery 1990;21:501-2.
10. Andrew breganza, et al. Management of phacolytic glaucoma: experience of 135 cases Indian J Ophthalmol 1998; 46:139-43.
11. Gifford H. The danger of the spontaneous cure of senile cataract. Am J Ophthalmol 1900;17:289-93.
12. Flock's M, Litterin CS, Zimmerman LE. Phacolytic glaucoma a clinico-pahthologic sutdy of 138 cases of glaucoma assosicated with hypermature cataract. Arch Ophthalmol 1955; 54:37-45.
13. Epstein DL, Jedzhiok JA, Grant WM. Identification of heavy molecular wieight soluble proteins in aqueous humor is human phacolytic glaucoma. Invest Ophthalmol Vis Sci 1978; 17;398-402.
14. Rengaraj Venkatesh, Veena K, Ravindran RD. Capsulotomy and hydroprocedures for nucleus prolapsed in manual small incisional cataract surgery. Indian J Ophthalmology 2009;57:15-8.
15. Venkatesh R, Murulikrishnan R, Balent LC, Prakash SK, Prajna NV. Outcomes of high volume cataract surgeries in a developing country. Br J Ophthalmol 2005;89:1079-83.
16. Rengaraj Venkatesh, Colin S, Tan H, Kumar TT, Ravindran RD. Safety and efficacy of manual small incision cataract surgery for phacolytic glaucoma. Br J Ophthalmol 2007;91:279-81.
17. Epstein Dl, Jedzinaik JA, Gant WM. Obstruction of aqueous outflow by lens particle and by heavy molecular weight soluble lens proteins. Invest Ophthalmol Vis Sci 1978;17:272.
18. Epstein DL. Diagnosis and management of lens induced glaucoma. Ophthalmology 1982;89:227.
19. Pradhan D, Hennig A, Kumar J. Fester A. Prospective study of 413 cases of lens induced glaucoma in Nepal. Indian J Ophthalmol 2001;49:103-7.
20. Pollard ZF. Phacolytic glaucoma secondary to ectopia uveitis Am J Ophthalmol 1975;7:999-1001.
21. Goldberg MF. Cytological diagnosis of Phacolytic glaucoma utilizing milipore filteration of the aqueous. Br J Ophthalmol 1967;51:847.
22. Ritcher C. Lens Induced Open Angle Glaucoma. In: Ritch R, Shields MB, Kurupin T, (eds). The glaucomas 2nd et St. Louis Mosby 1996;1023-6.
23. MC Kibben M. Cataract extraction and intraocular lens implantation in eyes with phacomorphic or phacolytic glaucoma. J Cataract Refract Surgery 1996;22:633-6.
24. Prajna NV, Ramakrishnan R, Krishnadas R, Manoharan N. Lens indcued glaucoma – visual result and

risk factors for final visual acuity. Indian J Ophthalmol 1996;44:149-55.

25. Thomas R, Breganza A, George T, et al. Vitreous opacities in phacolytic glaucoma. Ophthal Surg Lasers 1996;27:839-43.

26. Rao SK, Capsulorhexis in white catracts. J Cataract Refract Surgery 2000;26:477-8.

27. Chang DF, Pars plana vitreous tap for phacoemulsification in crowed eye. J Cataract and Refract Surg 2001;27:1911-4.

28. Dada T, et al. Suture less single port transconjunctival pars plana limited vitrectomy combined with phacoemulsification for management of Phacomorphic glaucoma. J Cataract and Refract Surgery 2007;33:9511-55.

29. Rao SK, Padmanaban P. Capsulorhexis in eyes with Phacomorphic glaucoma. J Cataract Refract Surgery 1998;24:882-4.

30. Chan DD, et al. Continuous curvilinear capsulorhexis in intumescent or hypermature cataract with liquefied cortex. J Cataract refract surg 2003: 29:431-4.

31. Angna SK, Pradhan R, Garg SP. Cataract induced glaucoma an insight into management. Indian J Ophthalmol 1991;39:97-101.

32. Chandra DJ, et al. Combined extracapsular cataract extraction with Ahmed glaucoma valve implantation in phacomorphic glaucoma. Indian J Ophthalmol 2002;50:25-8.

33. Peartman EM, Albert DM. Clinically unsuspected phacoanaphylaxis after ocular trauma. Arch Ophthalmol 1995;244:1977.

34. Ellant JP, Obstbaun SA. Lens induced glaucoma. Doc Ophthalmol 1992;81: 317.

35. Dimitris P, Ilias G, Nikos K, Augustine K, Andreas D, Chrysanthi K, Gerasimos G. Lens-induced glaucoma in the elderly. Clin Interv Aging 2009;4:331-6.

31 | Glaucoma in Aphakia and Pseudophakia

Sandhya Reddy, Venkat Reddy, R Ramakrishnan

CHAPTER OUTLINE

❖ Pathogenesis of Glaucoma in Aphakia and Pseudophakia
❖ Clinical Conditions
❖ Management

INTRODUCTION

Glaucoma can occur after intraocular surgeries. The terms aphakic and pseudophakic glaucoma have been previously used in literature. Currently, this terminology is not preferred. Glaucoma in pseudophakia and aphakia refer to conditions that cause increased intraocular pressure (IOP) soon after surgery as well as to those conditions that occur much later. A transient rise in IOP has been reported in 33 percent to almost 100 percent of eyes after cataract extraction. This pressure rise may be undetected because it occurs several hours after surgery, and the pressure may return to near normal levels by the next morning or whenever the patient is seen for the first postoperative visit. The ocular hypertension may be sufficient to cause pain, nausea and vomiting and corneal edema. Optic nerve damage may occur in patients with pre-exisiting glaucoma. The elevated IOP usually abates spontaneously over 2 to 4 days.

Glaucoma in aphakia and pseudophakia can be classified according to the mechanism of glaucoma and the time of presentation (Table 1).

Glaucoma in Aphakic and Pseudophakic Eyes

Incidence: This depends on the type of surgery done, extracapsular cataract extraction or phacoemulsification. It varies and an incidence of 12 percent was noted by Duke Elder in 1969.[1] Declining incidence has been reported these days due to improved microsurgical techniques, instrumentation and fine sutures.[2,3] A higher incidence is noted with congenital cataract surgeries.[4]

PATHOGENESIS OF GLAUCOMA

The cause of glaucoma post ocular surgeries has been attributed to various factors namely mechanical factors, inflammatory factors, surgical factors and implant factors.

Mechanical Factors

Pseudophakic pupillary block can be associated with all types of intraocular lenses (Figures 1A and B). Risk factors include excessive inflammation causing posterior synechiae (e.g. in case PCIOL and iris fixated IOLs), to direct insult of the trabecular meshwork (e.g. by an ACIOL). It has been noted that the incidence of pupillary block is sufficiently low as to not warrant routine iridectomy with cataract surgery.[5,6] However, iridectomy should be considered when excessive inflammation is expected, using iris-fixation lens or rigid uniplanar anterior chamber IOL, or in combination with filtering procedures. Diabetics are associated with increased inflammation and increased thickness of the iris and ciliary body, which may increase the risk of pupillary block. Even a successful iridectomy can be occluded by vitreous, intraocular lens rotation, inflammatory membrane, or lens remnants, and can cause pupillary block. Angle closure glaucoma can occur without pupillary block in a pseudophakic eye due to formation of peripheral anterior synechiae due to multiple reasons (Figures 1C and D).

Inflammatory Factors

Inflammation and hemorrhage are inevitable consequences of surgery, and they may lead to fibrosis and anatomical distortion when excessive. Inflammation is more common in certain patients (e.g. diabetes, uveitis), with certain types of IOLs (e.g. ACIOL, iris fixated), and complications

Table 1 Mechanism of Glaucoma in aphakia and pseudophakia

Open-angle glaucoma	Angle-closure glaucoma
A. Early Onset Glaucoma	**A. With pupillary block**
• Pre-existing chronic open-angle glaucoma	• Anterior hyaloid face
• Chymotrypsin-induced glaucoma	• Posterior lens capsule
• Hyphema/debris	• Intraocular lens
• Viscoelastic material	• Posterior synechiae
• Diopathic pressure elevation	• Silicone oil
B. Intermediate onset (after first postoperative week)	**B. Aqueous misdirection (malignant glaucoma)**
• Pre-existing chronic open-angle glaucoma	
• Vitreous in the anterior chamber	
• Hyphema	
• Inflammation	
• Lens particle glaucoma	
• Corticosteroid-induced glaucoma	
• Ghost-cell glaucoma	
C. Late onset (more than 2 months postoperatively)	**C. Without pupillary block**
• Pre-existing chronic open-angle glaucoma	• Pre-existing angle-closure glaucoma
• Ghost-cell glaucoma	• Inflammation/hyphema
• Neodymium:yttrium-aluminum-garnet (Nd:YAG) laser capsulotomy	• Prolonged anterior chamber shallowing
• Vitreous in the anterior chamber	• Iris incarceration in cataract incision
• Late-occurring hemorrhage	• Intraocular lens haptics
• Chronic inflammation	• Neovascular glaucoma
• Endothelial proliferation	• Epithelial ingrowth
• Proliferation of iris melanocytes across the trabecular meshwork	• Fibrous ingrowth

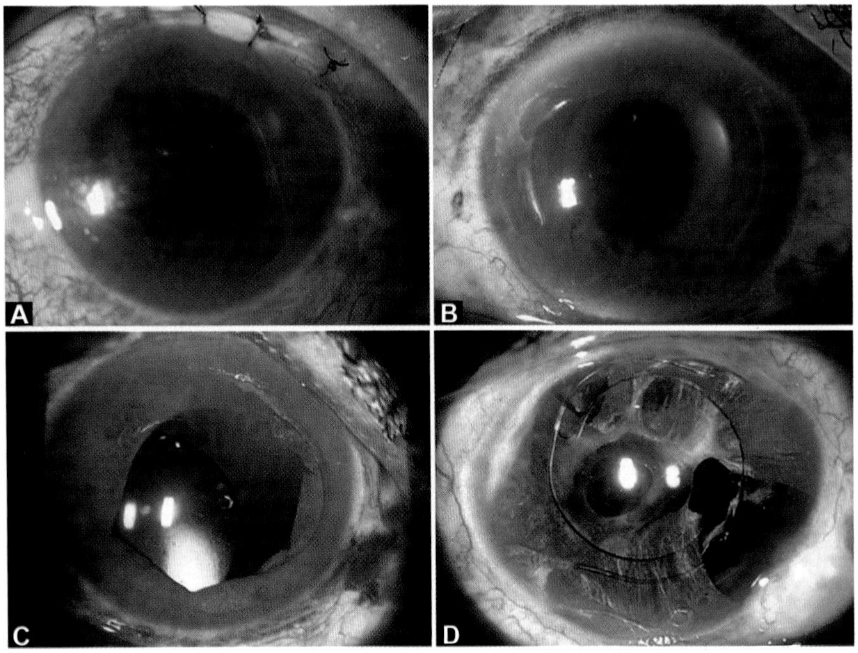

Figs 1A to D (A and B) Pseudophakic pupillary block glaucoma following extracapsular cataract extraction with anterior chamber intraocular lens implantation; (C and D) Angle closure without pupillary block

like retained lens nucleus fragment, retained cortical matter and hyphema **(Figures 2 to 4)**.

UGH Syndrome

The clinical triad of uveitis, glaucoma, and hyphema, especially associated with early ACIOLs, has been well described as UGH syndrome.[7-9] Glaucoma is believed to be caused by movement of the IOL against the iris causing the release of inflammatory and red blood cell debris that obstruct the trabecular meshwork. The haptic may cause direct damage to the trabecular meshwork, thus contributing to the glaucoma. Uveitis is particularly common if metal clip lenses are used. A similar condition may be seen with certain posterior chamber acrylic lens implanted in the sulcus instead of the capsular bag.

Surgical Factors

Incomplete cortical aspiration, **(Figure 3)** insufficient removal of visco-elastic agents, retained air bubble and nucleus drop into vitreous have been associated with glaucoma.

Implant Factors

Poor IOL quality, biodegradation of implant, toxic lens syndrome and forward movement of iris-implant diaphragm have been implicated in the mechanism of glaucoma.

The mechanism of glaucoma is multifactorial, either open angle or angle closure. The onset can be early, intermediate or late.

CLINICAL CONDITIONS
Pupillary block in aphakia

This condition is rarely seen, except in aphakic patients undergoing additional procedures. Apposition of the intact anterior hyaloid face to the pupil or iridectomy site presenting as iris bombé is the main mechanism for pressure elevation. Predisposing factors include a prolonged period

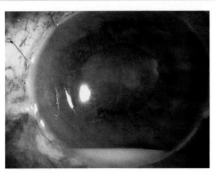

Fig. 2 Postoperative uveitis

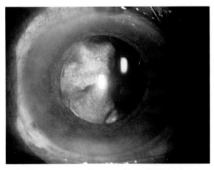

Fig. 3 Lens particle induced glaucoma due to residual cortical matter following cataract extraction with IOL implantation

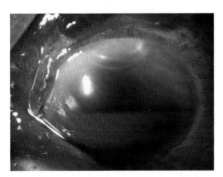

Fig. 4 Hyphema in the early postoperative period can lead to raised intraocular pressure

of flat chamber, severe postoperative inflammation, and failure of peripheral iridectomy. Posterior vitreous detachment also is a predisposing factor. Eventually, posterior synechiae may develop between the posterior iris surface and the anterior hyaloid face and lead to complete pupillary block.

Clinical Signs

Clinical signs of pupillary block include the following:

1. Increased shallowing of the peripheral anterior chamber,
2. Segmental block/irregular shallowing of the anterior chamber (e.g. loculation of the vitreous behind the iris), and overall shallowing of the AC. The central AC is deep and forward bowing of the peripheral iris occurs distinguishing it from malignant glaucoma.

Some authors include increased IOP in their classic description of the clinical findings, others assert that IOP is not a reliable indicator because 50 percent of patients with aphakic pupillary block may have IOP less than 21 mm Hg. It is postulated that IOP in the reference range can be achieved by concurrent conditions, which decrease the IOP, such as uveitis, wound leak, and choroidal detachment.

Aphakic pupillary block can occur anytime after surgery, and an increased incidence after congenital cataract extraction has been noted.[10-15] This may be associated with the increased strength of the anterior hyaloid in this population. Medical treatment includes aggressive dilation, aqueous suppression, cycloplegics, and hyperosmotic agents. Iridotomy and anterior hyaloidotomy ultimately may be required. Pupillary block has also been described in aphakic eyes which have undergone surgery for retinal detachment with intraocular silicone oil injection.

Non pupillary block mechanisms include alpha chymotrypsin induced glaucoma which was seen in the earlier days and ghost cell glaucoma.

Pupillary Block in Pseudophakia

As mentioned previously pseudophakic pupillary block can be associated with all types of IOLs. Risk factors include excessive inflammation causing posterior synechiae.

The clinical presentation is similar to pupillary block due to other etiologies. IOP is normal unless the patient has concurrent angle closure. A decreased peripheral anterior chamber depth is seen. Further investigative methods may include ultrasound biomicroscopy, Scheimpflug video imaging, and optical coherence tomography may be done for confirming the diagnosis.

Aqueous Misdirection Syndrome

First described by von Graefe in 1869, malignant glaucoma denotes a process involving a shallow central AC associated with increased IOP.[16] Although typically occurring early in the postoperative period, it can be delayed by weeks or years. Classically, it was seen after glaucoma surgeries,[16-18] non phakic malignant glaucoma is seen after cataract surgery in eyes with or without pre-existing glaucoma.[19]

Mechanisms like apposition of the ciliary process against the lens or vitreous, posterior diversion of aqueous, and iris abutting against the AC angle by forward displacement of the lens have been proposed. A small middle segment, sudden hypotony, inflammation, hyaloid abnormality, sudden blockage of posterior to anterior flow of aqueous may initiate it. In patients with ACIOL, the mechanism probably involves posterior displacement of the iris against the anterior hyaloid face by the IOL.

Complicating 0.6 to 4 percent of eyes following surgical intervention for acute angle-closure glaucoma, it also has been associated with the addition of a miotic[20,21] or cessation of a mydriatic. Malignant glaucoma has been associated in both aphakia and pseudophakia. Pupillary block, choroidal detachment, and suprachoroidal hemorrhage are considered in the differential diagnosis.

Management

Historically, the importance of disrupting the vitreous was noted first by Chandler in 1950 when lens removal as treatment for aqueous misdirection was not curative unless vitreous was lost during the procedure.[17] Today, medical therapy may be curative and includes aqueous suppression, cycloplegia, and hyperosmotic agents. Hyperosmotics decrease the pressure exerted by the vitreous, whereas cycloplegics pull the lens back by tightening the zonules. If the condition persists, YAG capsulotomy and anterior hyaloidotomy to disrupt the anterior hyaloid face and the posterior capsule may be needed.[22-25] Vitrectomy with anterior chamber deepening may be required.

IOP Elevation After Capsulotomy[26-29]

Production of fibrous matrix and contraction of the capsule caused by migrated lens epithelial cells cause visually significant posterior capsular opacification necessitating Nd:YAG capsulotomy. In a study involving 49 capsulotomies, increased IOP was noted in 37 eyes (75%) with pressure peak at 3 hours and average return to baseline at 1 week. Further, patients with pre-existing glaucoma were at a higher risk of developing elevated IOP. This has been postulated to be caused by the obstruction of outflow by capsular debris, inflammatory cells, and heavy molecular weight protein. Pressure elevation at 1 hour usually correlates with the ultimate pressure elevation.

Distortion of AC Angle

Distortion of the angle of the anterior chamber has been observed following cataract surgery, especially ECCE. The presence of a white ridge resembling an inverted snowbank in the early postoperative period, which protruded into the AC from the region of the internal lips of the cataract incision has been noted. Whether this represents corneal stromal edema or tight corneoscleral suture remains debated. However, Kirsch showed that this structure was associated with peripheral anterior synechiae, vitreous adhesion, **(Figure 5)** and hyphema, all of which could cause elevated IOP.[30] Other mechanisms include fibrous ingrowth and epithelial downgrowth. Angle closure glaucoma without pupillary block can occur due to prolonged shallowing of the anterior chamber following cataract surgery due to wound leak.

MANAGEMENT

Preoperative Considerations

In preparing for a cataract surgery, there are certain considerations that may help to minimize the risk of postoperative complications related to glaucoma, particularly in eyes with pre-existing glaucoma.

IOP reduction: Many surgeons prefer to reduce the vitreous volume and IOP by applying external pressure to the globe before surgery to maintain a deep anterior chamber and to minimize the potential complications of vitreous loss and expulsive hemorrhage. The external force may be accomplished by digital pressure, a rubber ball with an elastic band around the head, or a pneumatic rubber balloon (i.e. a Honan IOP reducer). Although the IOP does not correlate directly or linearly with the pressure in the Honan balloon, it is safe in normotensive eyes, especially when the instrument is set at 30 mm Hg for 5 minutes. However, the induced IOP rise is a function of the initial ocular tension, and marked pressure elevations may occur in eyes

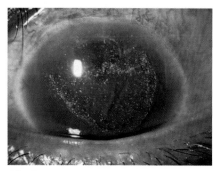

Fig. 5 Vitreous in anterior chamber in an aphakic eye

with initial levels above 30 mm Hg, indicating the need for extreme caution in these cases.

Selection of intraocular lens: Posterior chamber intraocular lens implantation in association with extracapsular cataract extraction and phacoemulsification, although not devoid of potential glaucoma-related complications, is generally associated with a slight reduction in postoperative IOP and is well-tolerated even in eyes with advanced pre-existing glaucoma. Anterior chamber lenses, however, are more problematic, and preoperative glaucoma or anterior chamber angle abnormalities are relative contraindications to their use.

Intraoperative Considerations

Attention to gentle handling of tissues, hemostasis, and minimal intraocular manipulation may reduce the risk of postoperative IOP rise associated with hemorrhage or excessive inflammation or pigment dispersion. The technique of wound closure (specifically a sutureless sclerocorneal tunnel incision) and the surgeon's experience are more important than prophylactic medications in preventing IOP elevation after phacoemulsification. Judicious use of intraocular agents such as viscoelastic substances and thorough irrigation to remove the material at the end of the case, especially in eyes with pre-existing glaucoma, may help to minimize the risk of postoperative glaucoma complications.

Another class of agents often injected into the eye during cataract surgery are the miotics, acetylcholine and carbachol, which are used to constrict the pupil, especially after posterior chamber intraocular lens implantation. Acetylcholine, compared with balanced salt solution, is associated with insignificant lower IOPs at 3 and 6 hours postoperatively, although the difference was not statistically significantly different at 24 hours. The combination of preoperative acetazolamide and intraoperative acetylcholine may be more effective than either drug alone in controlling postoperative IOP elevation. Carbachol has been found to be associated with lower postoperative pressures compared with acetylcholine or balanced salt solution at 24 hours, 2 days, and 3 days postoperatively. The intracameral use of carbachol therefore may be helpful in avoiding early IOP rises, especially in eyes with preexisting glaucoma.

Early Postoperative Period

The IOP can rise within 6 to 7 hours after routine cataract extraction and generally returns to normal within 1 week. However, high pressures may cause pain and disruption of the corneoscleral wound. Eyes with advanced glaucomatous optic nerve damage may have further nerve damage with even short pressure elevation. Anterior ischemic optic neuropathy has been reported to occur during these periods of IOP elevation.

The management is by IOP lowering medication like timolol, acetazolamide and alpha adrenergic agents. The use of pilocarpine drops is limited by the fact that it significantly

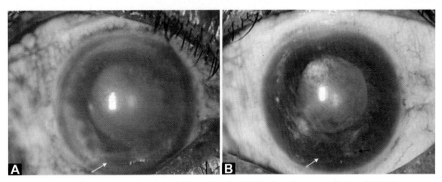

Figs 6A and B Pseudophakic pupillary block: (A) Before laser peripheral iridotomy; (B) After laser peripheral iridotomy

increases postoperative inflammation. Epinephrine is generally avoided because of the macular edema. Steroids may be helpful in controlling the IOP when inflammation is excessive. Indomethacin has been also been shown to reduce the postoperative rise, presumably by inhibiting prostaglandin. When uveitis and glaucoma are associated with retained lens fragments in the vitreous, pars plana vitrectomy is reported to yield good results.

Late Postoperative Period

Uveitis, glaucoma, and *hyphema* may be managed with mydriatics. Miotics may occasionally be used to minimize iris movement against the lens in mild cases. In more severe cases, steroids should be employed for the iritis and a carbonic anhydrase inhibitor or topical beta-blocker or alpha agonist for the glaucoma. Rarely, argon laser photocoagulation may be effective in controlling the hemorrhage if the bleeding sites are visible. Recurrent hyphema and glaucoma is usually an indication to remove the lens. When glaucoma and hyphema are associated with vitreous hemorrhage, pars plana vitrectomy is recommended. Pigment dispersion in pseudophakia can usually be controlled medically in most cases. Removal or redialing of the lens may be required in some cases.

Pupillary block in aphakia may initially be treated with an iridotomy. To be effective, the iridotomy must be over a pocket of aqueous behind the iris.

Management is dependent on the mechanism of the glaucoma. In both aphakic/pseudophakic pupillary block, the initial treatment is mydriasis. This is used to either break the block or enlarge the pupil beyond the edges of the ACIOL. Temporizing measures include aqueous suppressants and hyperosmotics. Miotics can help in the long-term management after the acute phase. Ultimately, iridotomy usually is needed in both cases **(Figures 6A and B)**. In aphakia, the iridotomy must be placed over a pocket of aqueous behind the iris, and this may require multiple attempts.

Surgical Management of Glaucoma in Aphakia and Pseudophakia

Filtering procedures and glaucoma drainage devices (valved and non valved) are the surgical options available in case the medical and laser procedures fail to control the glaucoma. Due to the increased chances of complications and failure rate following trabeculectomy in aphakic eyes, glaucoma drainage devices are a preferred option with a reasonably good success rate.

REFERENCES

1. Duke-Elder S. Disease of the lens and vitreous: glaucoma and hypotony. In: System of Ophthalmology 1969;11:11.

2. Stark WJ, Worthen DM, Holladay JT, et al. The FDA report on intraocular lenses. Ophthalmology 1983;90:311-7.

3. Hoskins HD Jr. Management of pseudophakic glaucoma. In: Greve EL, ed. Surgical Management of Coexisting Glaucoma and Cataract, 1987.

4. Urban B, Bakunowicz-Lazarczyk A. Aphakic glaucoma after congenital cataract surgery with and without intraocular lens implantation. Klin Oczna 2010;112:105-7.

5. Chulze RR, Copeland. Posterior chamber intraocular lens implantation without peripheral iridectomy—a preliminary report. Ophthalmic Surg 1982;13:567.

6. Simel PJ. Posterior chamber implants without iridectomy. Am Intraocular Implant Soc J 1982;8:141-3.

7. Percival SBP, Das K. UGH syndrome after posterior chamber lens implantation. Am Intraocular Implant Soc J 1983;9:200.

8. Van Liefferinge T, Van Oye R, Kestelyn P. Uveitis glaucoma-hyphema syndrome: a late complication of posterior chamber lenses. Bull Soc Belge Ophthalmol 1994;252:61.

9. Ellingson FT. The uveitis-glaucoma-hyphema syndrome associated with the Mark-VII Choyce anterior chamber lens implant. Am Intraocular Implant Soc J 1978;4:50.

10. Chrousos GA, Parks MM, O'Neill JF. Incidence of chronic glaucoma, retinal detachment and secondary membrane surgery in pediatric aphakic patients. Ophthalmology 1984;91:1238.

11. Egbert JE, Wright MM, Dahlhauser KF, et al. A prospective study of ocular hypertension and glaucoma after pediatric cataract surgery. Ophthalmology 1995;102:1098.

12. Simon JW, Mehta N, Simmons ST, et al. Glaucoma after pediatric lensectomy/vitrectomy. Ophthalmology 1991;98:670.

13. Asrani SG, Wilensky JT. Glaucoma after congenital cataract surgery. Ophthalmology 1995;102:863.

14. Vajpayee RB, Angra SK, Titiyal JS, et al. Pseudophakic pupillary-block glaucoma in children. Am J Ophthalmol 1991;111:715.

15. Lee AF, Lee SM, Chou JC, et al. Glaucoma following congenital cataract surgery. Zhonghua Yi Xue Za Zhi (Taipei) 1998;61:65.

16. Von Graefe A. Beitrage zur pathologie und therapie des glaucoms. Arch Fur Ophthalmol 1869;15:108.

17. Chandler PA, Simmons RJ, Grant WM. Malignant glaucoma: medical and surgical treatment. Am J Ophthalmol 1968;66:495.

18. Lowe RF. Malignant glaucoma related to primary angle closure glaucoma. Aust J Ophthalmol 1979;7:11.

19. Reed JE, Thomas JV, Lytle RA, et al. Malignant glaucoma induced by an intraocular lens. Ophthalmic Surg 1990;21:177.

20. Pecora JL. Malignant glaucoma worsened by miotics in a post-operative angle-closure glaucoma patient. Am J Ophthalmol 1979;11:1412.

21. Rieser JC, Schwartz B. Miotic-induced malignant glaucoma. Arch Ophthalmol 1972;87:706.

22. Risco JM, Tomey KF, Perkins TW. Laser capsulotomy through intraocular lens positioning holes in anterior aqueous misdirection. Arch Ophthalmol 1989;107:1569.

23. Weber PA, Henry MA, Kapetansky FM, et al. Argon laser treatment of the ciliary processes in aphakic glaucoma with flat anterior chamber. Am J Ophthalmol 1984;97:82.

24. Epstein DL, Steinert RF, Puliafito CA. Neodymium: YAG laser therapy to the anterior hyaloid in aphakic malignant (ciliovitreal block) glaucoma. Am J Ophthalmol 1984;98:137.

25. Melamed S, Ashkenazi I, Blumenthal M. Nd:YAG laser hyaloidotomy for malignant glaucoma following one-piece 7 mm intraocular lens implantation. Br J Ophthalmol 1991;75:501.

26. Channell MM, Beckman H. Intraocular pressure changes after Nd:YAG laser posterior Capsulotomy. Arch Ophthalmol 1984;102:1024.

27. Keates F, et al. Long term follow-up of Nd: YAG laser posterior Capsulotomy. Am Intraocular Implant Soc J. 1984; 10:164.

28. Kurata F, et al. Progressive glaucomatous visual field loss after Neodymium:YAG laser Capsulotomy. Am J Ophthalmol 1984;98:632.

29. Flohr MJ, Robin AL, Kelley JS. Early complications following Q-switched Neodymium:YAG laser posterior capsulotomy. Ophthalmology 1985;92:360.

30. Kirsch RE, Levine O, Singer JA. Ridge at internal edge of cataract incision. Arch Ophthalmol 1976;94:2098-104.

32 | Uveitic Glaucoma

SR Rathinam

INTRODUCTION

Uveitis is a complex intraocular inflammatory disorder which includes a number of varying etiologies. Visual loss in uveitis is mainly because of glaucoma, cataract, retinal atrophy, retinal detachment, macular scarring and optic atrophy. Uveitic glaucoma is a common complication and its management can prove to be a challenge for both uveitis and glaucoma specialists.[1-3] Either the inflammation or postinflammatory structural damage or use of steroids results in uveitic glaucoma. Mechanism and pathogenesis of glaucoma varies according to the etiology of uveitis.[1] Likewise, the management is tailored for each patient. Management protocol includes meticulous initial assessment, follow-up for inflammatory as well as intraocular pressure control and also for iatrogenic complications. Prognosis depends on the severity and sequelae of uveitis with which the patient presents, and on good compliance with treatment by the patient.

PREVALENCE OF UVEITIC GLAUCOMA

The prevalence of uveitic glaucoma is reported to be between 5 percent and 19 percent.[3] This prevalence varies depending upon age at onset of uveitis, anatomical location of inflammation, etiology, severity, chronicity and on treatment of uveitis. In general, anterior uveitis, older age at presentation, chronic inflammation and prolonged steroid use are related to a higher prevalence of uveitic glaucoma. *Clinically speaking certain types of uveitis, such as herpetic keratouveitis, uveitis associated with Juvenile Idiopathic Arthritis, toxoplasmosis and sarcoidosis are associated with a higher prevalence of secondary glaucoma.*[4-6] There is inherent selection bias in the reported

> **Uveitic ocular hypertension and Uveitic glaucoma**
> *Uveitis related ocular hypertension* refers to temporary IOP elevation without optic nerve head damage.
> *Uveitic glaucoma* is used for cases with optic nerve head damage and/or visual field defects.

prevalence studies as they are from uveitis clinic population and it may be different from the prevalence in a glaucoma clinic and general ophthalmic clinic patient population.

MECHANISM OF INTRAOCULAR PRESSURE VARIATION IN THE COURSE OF UVEITIS

Intraocular pressure (IOP) variations depend upon multiple factors including cellular, biochemical and morphological alterations **(Table 1)**. Initial IOP can be decreased, normal or increased. Usually acute uveitis patients may come with low intraocular pressure due to ciliary shock and reduced aqueous production which slowly improves with control of inflammation. Very low tension on presentation is also seen in ciliary detachment, ciliary atrophy and serous retinal detachment in cases of Vogt-Koyanagi-Harada syndrome and sympathetic ophthalmia. Normalization of pressure is possible with control of inflammation in above conditions. Intraocular pressure fails to return to

Table 1 Etiopathogenesis of glaucoma in uveitis

1. Alteration in aqueous humor
i. Inflammatory cells
ii. Inflammatory mediators, cytokines prostaglandins
iii. Proteins
iv. Red blood cells in hyphema
v. Lens protein in phacolysis
2. Morphological changes in angle
i. Peripheral anterior synechiae
ii. Trabeculitis
3. Drug induced
4. Combined mechanism

normal in cases of chronic, progressive inflammation and atrophy of the ciliary body which eventually result in hypotony and phthisis.[7]

Open Angle Glaucoma

Despite lowered aqueous production in acute uveitis, intraocular pressure gets elevated resulting in either ocular hypertension or glaucoma because of disproportionate increase in outflow resistance.[1] There are several causes for outflow resistance as given in **Table 1**. Ocular inflammation results in increased vascular permeability and elevated proteins in aqueous humor. Simple mechanical effect of high viscosity increases the outflow resistance. Presence of inflammatory cells, red blood cells, lens protein and inflammatory mediators also contributes in increasing the outflow resistance resulting in elevation of intraocular pressure. Lens protein uveitis is a unilateral, granulomatous uveitis that occurs in response to retained lens fragments following cataract surgery, following trauma to the lens capsule, or in the setting of a leaking hypermature lens.[2] Presence of trabeculitis may result in increased resistance to outflow and an elevated IOP. Elevated IOP because of trabeculitis parallels the course of the inflammation. The most common conditions causing trabeculitis are herpetic anterior uveitis,

cytomegalovirus infection, sarcoidosis, toxoplasmosis, syphilis, and Posner Schlossman syndrome.[1-6]

Angle Closure Glaucoma

Morphologic changes in the anterior chamber angle can result in acute uveitic angle closure and an elevated IOP. *Acute uveitic angle closure can be caused by either pupillary block or non-pupillary block mechanisms.*

Pupillary block occurs in uveitis when the pupil becomes secluded by 360 degrees posterior synechiae or by an inflammatory pupillary membrane. Iris bombe and peripheral anterior synechiae may develop from chronic apposition of iris to the outflow tissues if pupillary block is not promptly corrected **(Figure 1)**. The second type is a nonpupillary block angle closure glaucoma that occurs in ciliochoroidal effusion and forward movement of the lens iris diaphragm. Understanding the mechanism of angle closure is very important in establishing the diagnosis as well as its treatment. Ciliochoroidal effusions are more common in certain uveitic conditions such as Vogt-Koyanagi-Harada disease, scleritis and sympathetic ophthalmia. Treatment varies accordingly.[8] In pupillary-block angle closure, iris bombe may be seen and the recommended treatment is a laser peripheral iridotomy. On the other hand, in nonpupillary block glaucoma, iris bombe will not be seen. Cycloplegia and systemic corticosteroids are the mainstay of treatment.

Drug Induced Glaucoma
Corticosteroids

Treatment of uveitis with corticosteroids can result in elevated outflow resistance and thereby increase the IOP in steroid responders. Glucocorticoids elevate IOP exclusively by an elevation in outflow resistance and reduction in aqueous outflow. Wide-ranging effects have been observed in the trabecular

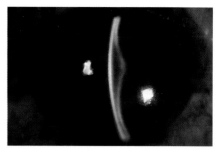

Fig. 1 Iris bombe and corneal edema in a patient with uveitic glaucoma

meshwork (TM) and they are likely to be mediated by more than one mechanism.[9,10] An interesting effect of TM exposure to glucocorticoids is the induction of myocilin mRNA expression. This protein is intimately involved with TM outflow resistance, although its exact function is unknown.

Elevated intraocular pressure (IOP) can occur as a result of systemic or ocular (topical, periocular or intravitreal) administration of corticosteroids.[11-14] Risk factors associated with corticosteroid-induced IOP rise include primary open angle glaucoma, glaucoma suspects, family history of glaucoma, children, patients with connective tissue disease, high myopia and type 1 diabetes mellitus.[10] IOP elevation tends to occur days to weeks after the onset of uveitis and initiation of treatment with corticosteroids. The extent of IOP elevation depends on the potency of the corticosteroid, the dose and duration of treatment, the route of administration, and the patient's susceptibility to corticosteroid-induced ocular hypertension.[15] When treated with topical corticosteroids for 4 to 6 weeks, 5 percent of the population demonstrates

Effect of corticosteroids on TM[2]
- Alterations in cell size
- Cytoskeletal organization
- Extracellular matrix deposition
- Matrix metalloproteinase expression
- Na-K-Cl cotransport system
- Induction of myocilin mRNA expression.

a rise in IOP > 16 mm Hg, and 30 percent have a rise of 6 to 15 mm Hg.[16] With the increasing use of intravitreal corticosteroids, more patients with uveitis will require medical and surgical management of corticosteroid-induced elevated intraocular pressure. Most patients with IVTA-induced IOP elevation require only topical medications for IOP control whereas in the FA implant study 37 percent required IOP lowering surgery.[14]

Combined Mechanism

Chronic, combined mechanism may also be seen in patients with chronic inflammation who may have angle closure as well as steroid induced glaucoma.

Combined mechanism glaucoma is seen in the following forms of uveitis:

Chronic uveitis

Juvenile idiopathic arthritis

Sarcoidosis,

*Sympathetic ophthalmia and VKH syndrome

*(Prone for angle closure with or without steroid induced glaucoma)

Significance of Anatomical Location of Primary Inflammation

Clinical signs indicate the specific uveitic diagnosis (**Table 2**). Anterior uveitis is relatively mild and easy to treat when it is compared with pan uveitis, however, the prevalence of glaucoma is high in anterior uveitis because of frequent use of topical steroids, higher occurrence of posterior and peripheral anterior synechiae and associated trabaculitis. Herpes virus-associated uveitis, Fuchs' heterochromic iridocyclitis, Juvenile idiopathic uveitis are common anterior uveitis usually result in glaucoma (**Table 3**).

In **herpetic keratouveitis**, IOP elevation is common on presentation. It is characterized by corneal stromal keratitis, central pigmented keratic precipitates, Descemet's folds,

iris atrophic patches and an elevated pressure. Iris stromal atrophy caused by virus induced ischemia is a unique finding that differentiates herpetic uveitis from other causes (**Figure 2**).

Posner Schlossman syndrome, or glaucomatocyclitic crisis patients are generally young and present with pain and blurred vision. The inflammation is characteristically mild and appears out of proportion to the rise in IOP. It is characterized by recurrent, unilateral, acute uveitis with an elevated IOP. Viral etiology has been attributed in some studies.

Fuchs' heterochromic cyclitis patients are asymptomatic for a longer period, till they develop secondary glaucoma or cataract. Fuchs iridocyclitis is characterized by a chronic, usually unilateral, mild uveitis with diffusely distributed white stellate keratic precipitates, and iris heterochromia.[1] Posterior synechiae are uncommon despite chronic inflammation. Vitreous

cellular infiltrates and cataract are seen in this form of uveitis obscuring the fundus view. Cataract surgery carries good prognosis while management of glaucoma remains a challenge.

Juvenile idiopathic arthritis (JIA) is a heterogeneous group of chronic arthritis diseases in childhood that is frequently accompanied by a vision-threatening uveitis. Clinically silent uveitis in a white eye is a typical presentation. The complications include cataract, glaucoma, band keratopathy, macular edema and ocular hypotony. Angle closure as well as steroid induced glaucoma are common in this entity. Children pose unique challenges in management (**Table 4**).

Posterior uveitis is less commonly associated with glaucoma or ocular hypertension. Sarcoidosis, Vogt-Koyanagi-Harada syndrome and sympathetic ophthalmia are the leading causes of glaucoma in posterior/pan uveitis.[1]

Table 2 Clinical signs in etiological diagnosis in cases of uveitic glaucoma

Investigations	Signs	Diagnosis
Slit-lamp	Central Kps Descemet's folds Iris atrophy	Viral uveitis
	Granulomatous keratic precipitates	Sarcoid, VKH, sympathetic ophthalmia
	Iris heterochromia	Fuchs' hetrochronic uveitis
	Iris bombe, peripheral anterior synechiae	Chronic uveitis, VKH, sympathetic ophthalmia
	Leaking Morgagnian cataract	Lens induced uveitis and glaucoma
Indirect ophthalmoscopy	Retinochoroiditis	Toxoplasmosis
	Exudative retinal detachment	VKH, sympathetic ophthalmia
	Retinal vasculitis, vitreous reaction	Sarcoidosis
Gonioscopy	Peripheral anterior synechiae	Chronic recurrent uveitis
	Angle recession foreign body Hyphema	Traumatic uveitis
	Hyphema presence of angle vessels	Fuchs' hetrochronic uveitis
	Lens matter in anterior chamber	Lens protein uveitis
	Silicone oil	Post-RD surgery glaucoma
	Granulomatous angle keratic precipitates	Sarcoidosis
UBM	Ciliary body tumor	Masquerade syndrome

Table 3 Mechanism of glaucoma in different types of uveitis

Anatomical classification of uveitis	Etiological diagnosis	Type of glaucoma		
		Open angle	Closed angle	Steroid induced glaucoma
Anterior uveitis	Fuchs' heterochromic uveitis	√		
	Lens protein uveitis	√		
	PS syndrome	√		
	Juvenile ideopathic arthritis and uveitis		√	√
	HLA B27 related		√	
	Postoperative uveitis		√	
Chronic intermediate uveitis		√		√
Pan uveitis	ARN	√		
	Sarcoidosis	√	√	
	Masquerade syndrome	√		
	Viral uveitis	√		
	VKH syndrome		√	√
	Sympathetic opthalmia		√	√
	Sarcoidosis		√	√
Posterior uveitis	Toxoplasmosis	√		

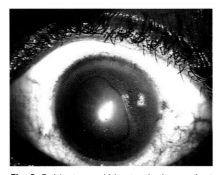

Fig. 2 Sphincter and iris atrophy in a patient with herpetic anterior uveitis

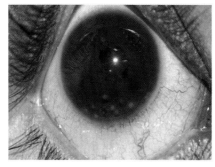

Fig. 3 Granulomatous keratic precipitates in a patient with sarcoidosis

Sarcoid uveitis is characterized by the presence of granulomatous keratic precipitates, Bussaca nodules vitritis, pars plana snowbanking, periphlebitis, perivascular sheathing and occasionally optic nerve involvement (**Figure 3**).

VKH syndrome and sympathetic ophthalmia are bilateral granulomatous uveitis with uveal thickening and serous retinal detachment. As discussed earlier, all three types can cause angle closure glaucoma as well as steroid induced glaucoma while sarcoid uveitis also causes open angle glaucoma probably because of trabeculitis. Histopathologic studies performed on eyes with sarcoid uveitis have demonstrated the presence of inflammatory debris and cells within the trabecular meshwork.

CLINICAL WORK-UP IN UVEITIC GLAUCOMA

Etiological diagnosis of uveitis is essential to understand the possible mechanism of glaucoma. A **complete history** and uveitis work-up should be

Table 4 Challenges of diagnosis and treatment in uveitis glaucoma

Clinical scenario	Challenges
Presence of corneal opacity in sclero-keratits	Difficulty in gonioscopy, optic disc measurement
Small pupil Complicated cataract Opaque vitreous	Difficulty in optic disc measurement
Chronic recurrent uveitis	Closure of PI
	Failure of filtering surgery
	Prostaglandin analogs contraindicated
Pediatric uveitis	Lack of history
	Asymptomatic uveitis, hence late diagnosis
	Difficulty in examination, may need anesthesia
Failure to control uveitis	Failure of surgical treatment

performed in all patients with uveitic glaucoma. Detailed slit-lamp examination, gonioscopy, applanation tonometry, visual fields and ultrasound bio microscopy and ultrasonogram are essential **(Table 2)**.

Detailed slit lamp examination can assess important clinical signs associated with uveitic glaucoma including corneal dendrites, keratic precipitates, Descemet's folds, angle depth, posterior synechiae, peripheral anterior synechiae, iris bombe, hypopyon and hypermature cataract **(Figure 4)**. The fundus should also be examined carefully for any evidence of toxoplasmic retinochoroiditis or for clinical signs of sarcoid, VKH syndrome and sympathetic ophthalmia. Patients with Posner-Schlossman syndrome can be especially challenging to diagnose as the inflammatory response can be very subtle and the eye is typically normal between attacks. The IOP elevation reverses with treatment. Patients with herpetic keratouveitis may present with blisters on the forehead **(Figure 5)**. They can develop a chronic relapsing remitting course and corneal edema may challenge the fundus examination.

Gonioscopy is essential in every patient of uveitic glaucoma to differentiate between an open and closed angle as both types are common in several uveitic entities. In the acute phase of angle closure, appositional closure of the angle may be found on indentation gonioscopy. Prompt identification and timely iridotomy will prevent peripheral anterior synechiae and chronic angle closure. In addition to angle assessment, gonioscopy may also reveal the cause of the IOP rise, such as retained lens cortex in the angle after cataract surgery or a microscopic silicone oil hyperoleum in the superior angle. Forward movement of the lens iris diaphragm due to ciliochoroidal effusion can also result in non-pupillary block

angle closure by a "pushing" mechanism. Iris bombe is not seen in these patients.

B-scan ultrasonography, high frequency ultrasound biomicroscopy and anterior segment optical coherence tomography may be required to demonstrate the nonpupillary block acute uveitic angle closure glaucoma. The presence of choroidal thickening, supraciliary effusions and forward rotation of the ciliary body are diagnostic. Ultrasonogram (B-scan) is done in cases of very low tension, to rule out retinal detachment.

Uveitic glaucoma may be a diagnostic as well as a management challenge. The elevation of intraocular pressure may either be transient or persistent and severely damaging. On the other hand, exacerbation of uveitis may cause shutdown of the ciliary body and lead to hypotony, hence an IOP reading at one point of time may miss the elevated pre-ssure. The ophthalmologic examination of small children with uveitic glaucoma is more challenging starting from history, uveitis diagnosis, visual fields recording or examination of chamber angle till the follow-up.

MANAGEMENT OF ELEVATED IOP IN PATIENTS WITH UVEITIS

General principles: In general, the inflammation has to be brought under control for better prognosis of both uveitis and uveitic glaucoma. The timing of IOP elevation can also help in management. Patient with acute rises in IOP observed only during acute inflammation can probably be managed adequately with medical therapy alone, whereas a patient with postinflammatory structural damage and chronic glaucoma is more likely to require surgical intervention. In patients who develop ocular hypertension in response to corticosteroids, alternative therapy with weaker corticosteroids or immunosuppressive therapy may be considered. However,

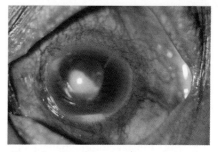
Fig. 4 Leaking Morgagnian cataract with hypopyon causing lens induced uveitis

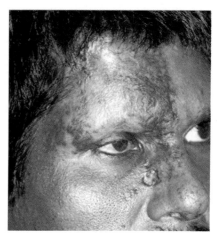
Fig. 5 Herpetic skin lesions

weaker corticosteroids are usually not strong enough to control moderate to severe inflammation. In resistant uveitis, use of long-acting depot corticosteroid preparations is undertaken with caution. Frequent follow-up for IOP elevation in such cases is mandatory.

First Line of Therapy

• Aqueous suppressants
• Beta-blockers followed by carbonic anhydrase inhibitors and alpha agonists. Prostaglandin analogues are avoided. Rarely, if used in cases with resolved uveitis extreme caution must be exercised.[1,2]

Medical Management

The choice of IOP lowering treatment depends on the state of the inflammation and the extent of optic nerve damage. Topical hypotensive therapy for raised IOP in uveitis is similar to treatment for POAG. Beta-blockers are usually the first line of management for raised IOP in uveitis. The choice of a second-line agent in uveitic glaucoma depends on the level of the IOP. With high IOP levels, the second-line therapy may be a systemic carbonic anhydrase inhibitor (CAI) such as acetazolamide followed by topical alpha agonists. Prostaglandin analogs may have a proinflammatory effect. There are few case reports on exacerbation of pre-existing iridocyclitis, and recurrences of herpetic keratitis or kerato-uveitis, and formation of cystoid macular edema.[17,18] When used in rare cases of resolved or controlled uveitis, extreme caution must be exercised.

Medications that are definitely pro-inflammatory and must be avoided in patients with active uveitis include pilocarpine, prostaglandin analogues, epinephrine, and epinephrine prodrugs.[1,2]

In patients with corticosteroid-induced ocular hypertension/glaucoma use of steroid is avoided when ever possible. In selected cases, removal of a periocular or intraocular depot of corticosteroid may result in successful resolution of the IOP elevation. Nonsteroidal immunosuppressive therapy is usually considered for patients requiring long-term use of oral corticosteroids to control inflammation. It is important to note that it takes several weeks to produce an effective anti-inflammatory effect with immunosuppressive agents and patients must be maintained on corticosteroids until then. Most patients with corticosteroid-induced ocular hypertension can be managed with topical medications, the exception being patients with IOP elevation due to the intravitreal steroid implants.

Laser Procedures

Laser peripheral iridotomy: Laser peripheral iridotomy is the treatment of choice for acute angle closure due to pupillary block. The inflammatory response following laser iridotomy in patients with uveitis tends to be more severe and prolonged than in patients with primary angle closure, hence prelaser and postlaser corticosteroids treatment is essential. In addition, as there is a higher rate of closure of the iridotomy, performing at least two iridotomies is recommended.[19]

Laser trabeculoplasty: In general, laser trabeculoplasty is contraindicated in the management of elevated IOP in uveitis. However, some have found SLT effective in corticosteroid induced ocular hypertension/glaucoma in a quiet eye.

Cyclophotocoagulation

Cyclophotocoagulation must be used with extreme caution in uveitic glaucoma for two reasons. Firstly, the procedure can exacerbate inflammation. Secondly, there is a greater risk of atrophy in a ciliary body that has already sustained damage from recurrent inflammation; this can eventually lead to hypotony and/or phthisis.

- Uveitic glaucoma is an imbalance between reduced aqueous production and even lower outflow
- Cyclodestructive procedure to an already damaged ciliary body may precipitate a profound drop in IOP
- Cyclodestruction in uveitis may potentially exacerbate the inflammation or precipitate phthisis.

Surgical Management

Irrespective of the type of surgical intervention, uveitis should be under control for a minimum of three months before surgery in an ideal situation. In patients with recurrent uveitis, perioperative course of systemic corticosteroid (e.g. 0.5 to 1 mg/kg/day of oral prednisolone) is started to prevent inflammatory damage and failure of surgery. If the patient is already on steroids, he is advised to continue topical or systemic corticosteroids in the perioperative period.

Decision to perform surgery depends on:
- Control of inflammation
- Mechanisms of IOP elevation
- Presenting intraocular pressure
- The degree of nerve damage
- Response to medical therapy
- Tolerance to medical therapy
- Compliance

Trabeculectomy

Trabeculectomy is indicated in uveitis when the IOP is uncontrolled despite maximum tolerated medical therapy. Trabeculectomy without antifibrosis agents has a relatively lesser chance of survival in patients with uveitis[20-22] therefore use of either 5-fluorouracil or mitomycin-C is recommended. Uveitic eyes are particularly at risk for postoperative hypotony, therefore the scleral flap is sutured tightly. If hypotony is noted postoperatively with shallowing of the anterior chamber, cycloplegia can help to move the lens-iris diaphragm posteriorly. The frequency of postoperative corticosteroid therapy is determined based on the balance between the need to control active inflammation and the need to accelerate healing. Topical corticosteroids are generally used for 6 to 8 weeks postoperatively and may need to be tapered slowly.

Aqueous Drainage Devices

Failure of a trabeculectomy with antifibrotic agents is an indication for the use of aqueous drainage devices. Both the valved Ahmed and the nonvalved Baerveldt implant have been used for IOP control in such patients although Ahmed Glaucoma Valve is preferred. There are a few studies that have reported outcomes of aqueous drainage device implantation in uveitic patients.[23-27] Success rate is not comparable because of varying study design, however it varies between 77 and 92 percent in 2 years.[24,25] Complications include flat anterior chamber, hypotony, choroidal effusion, cystoid macular edema and phthisis.

Other Surgical Procedures

Goniotomy, viscocanalastomy and trabeculodialysis have all been reported for the treatment of uveitic glaucoma with varying success rates[1,2] However, these procedures are not in widespread use and trabeculectomy and aqueous drainage devices remain the mainstay of surgical treatment. Trabectome[28] has recently been developed for ab-interno trabeculectomy. Although, there is no data yet on its efficacy in patients with uveitic glaucoma, it may be a better option in patients with well-controlled inflammation and mild optic nerve damage. Management of elevated IOP can be challenging in patients with active inflammation and structural damage; however, adequate control of inflammation and good compliance by the patient results in good prognosis.

REFERENCES

1. Joseph R. Zelefsky, MD, Emmett T. Cunningham, Jr, Evaluation and Management of Elevated Intraocular Pressure in Patients with Uveitis. AAO Focal Points (In press).

2. Kok H, Barton K. Uveitic glaucoma. Ophthalmol Clin N Am 2002;15:375-87.

3. Moorthy RS, Mermoud A, Baerveldt G, et al. Glaucoma associated with uveitis. Surv Ophthalmol 1997;41:361-94.

4. Westfall AC, Lauer AK, Suhler EB, Rosenbaum JT. Toxoplasmosis retinochoroiditis and elevated intraocular pressure. J Glaucoma 2005;14:3-10.

5. Kwon YH, Dreyer EB. Inflammatory glaucomas. Int Ophthalmol Clin 1996;36:81-9.

6. Sung VCT, Barton K. Management of inflammatory glaucomas. Curr Opin Ophthalmol 2004;15:136-40.

7. Tran VT, Mermoud A, Herbort CP. Appraisal and management of ocular hypotony and glaucoma associated with uveitis. Int Ophthalmol Clin 2000;40:175-203.

8. Rathinam SR, Namperumalsamy P. Angle closure glaucoma as a presenting sign of Vogt-Koyanagi Harada syndrome. Br J Ophthalmol 1997;81:608-9.

9. Wordingera RJ, Abbot FC. Effects of glucocorticoids on the trabecular meshwork: towards a better understanding of glaucoma. Prog Retin Eye Res 1999;18:629-67.

10. Jones R, Rhee DJ. Corticosteroid-induced ocular hypertension and glaucoma: a brief review and update of the literature. Curr Opin Ophthalmol 2006;17:163-7.

11. Becker B. Intraocular pressure response to topical steroids. Invest Ophthalmol 1965;4:198-205.

12. Levin DS, Han DP, Dev S, et al. Subtenon's depot corticosteroid injections in patients with a history of corticosteroid-induced intraocular pressure elevation. Am J Ophthalmol 2002;133:196-202.

13. Rhee DJ, Peck RE, Belmont J, et al. Intraocular pressure alterations following intravitreal triamcinolone acetonide. Br J Ophthalmol 2006;90:999-1003.

14. Goldstein DA, Godfrey DG, Hall A, et al. Intraocular pressure in patients with uveitis treated with fluocinolone acetonide implants. Arch Ophthalmol 2007;125:1478-85.

15. Clark A. Steroids, ocular hypertension, and glaucoma. J Glaucoma 1995;4:354-69.

16. Armaly MF. Statistical attributes of the steroid hypertensive response in the clinically normal eye. I. The demonstration of three levels of response. Invest Ophthalmol 1965;4:187-97.

17. Warwar RE, Bullock JD, Ballal D. Cystoid macular edema and anterior uveitis associated with Latanoprost use: experience and incidence in a retrospective review of 94 patients. Ophthalmol 1998;105:263-8.

18. Wand M, Gilbert CM, Liesegang TJ. Latanoprost and herpes simplex keratitis. Am J Ophthalmol 1999;127:602-4.

19. Spencer NA, Hall AJ, Stawell RJ. Nd:YAG laser iridotomy in uveitic glaucoma. Clin Experiment Ophthalmol 2001;29:217-9.

20. Towler HM, McCluskey P, Shaer B, et al. Long-term follow-up of trabeculectomy with intraoperative 5-fluorouracil for uveitis-related glaucoma. Ophthalmol 2000;107:1822-8.

21. Noble J, Derzko-Dzulynsky L, Rabinovitch T, Birt C. Outcome of trabeculectomy with intraoperative mitomycin C for uveitic glaucoma. Can J Ophthalmol 2007;42:89-94.

22. Katz GJ, Higginbotham EJ, Lichter PR, et al. Mitomycin C versus 5-fluorouracil in high-risk glaucoma filtering surgery. Ophthalmol 1995;102:1263-9.

23. DaMata A, Burk SE, Netland PA, et al. Management of uveitic glaucoma with Ahmed glaucoma valve implantation. Ophthalmology 1999;106:2168-72.

24. Papadaki TG, Zacharopoulos IP, Pasquale LR, et al. Long-term results of Ahmed glaucoma implantation for uveitic glaucoma. Am J Ophthalmol 2007;144:62-9.

25. Ceballos EM, Parrish RK 2nd, Schiffman JC. Outcome of Baerveldt glaucoma drainage implants for the treatment of uveitic glaucoma. Ophthalmology 2002;109:2256-60.

26. Hill RA, Nguyen QH, Baerveldt G, et al. Trabeculectomy and Molteno implantation for glaucoma associated with uveitis. Ophthalmology 1993;100:903-8.

27. Valimaki J, Airaksinen PJ, Tuulonen A. Molteno implantation for secondary glaucoma in juvenile rheumatoid arthritis. Arch Ophthalmol 1997;115:1253-6.

28. Minckler D, Baerveldt G, Ramirez MA, et al. Clinical results with the Trabectome, a novel surgical device for treatment of open-angle glaucoma. Trans Am Ophthalmol Soc 2006;104:40-50.

33 | Neovascular Glaucoma

Nidhi Gupta, SR Krishnadas

CHAPTER OUTLINE

- Pathogenesis
- Conditions Commonly Associated with Neovascular Glaucoma
- Stages of Neovascular Glaucoma
- Clinical Picture
- Differential Diagnosis
- Management
- Future Therapeutic Options

INTRODUCTION

Neovascular glaucoma (NVG) is a devastating ocular disease, often caused as an end stage complication of retinal ischemia. It is caused by a fibrovascular membrane that develops over the surface of iris and angle. At first, the membrane merely covers the angle but then, it contracts to form peripheral anterior synechiae. Neovascular glaucoma rarely, if ever, occurs as a primary condition but it is always associated with other abnormalities, most commonly some form of ocular ischemia.

Neovascular glaucoma was first described in 1866 following central retinal vein occlusion. In 1906, Coats described new vessel formation on the iris in the eyes with central retinal vein occlusion.[1] Nettleship and Salus noted the association of neovascular glaucoma and diabetes mellitus. Various terms have been proposed on the basis of clinical features for this type of glaucoma; hemorrhagic glaucoma, congestive glaucoma, thrombotic glaucoma. However, the term 'neovascular glaucoma' proposed by Weiss and coworkers better fits with the physiology of this condition and has become the accepted one.

PATHOGENESIS

The most accepted theory on the pathogenesis of NVG is that ischemia of retina liberates an angiogenic factor that diffuses forward and causes new vessel formation on iris and angle.[2] Capillary occlusion or ischemia appears to be the initiating event in this process. A number of substances have been proposed as the angiogenic factors which include vascular endothelial growth factor (VEGF), fibroblast growth factor (FGF), transforming growth factor-alpha (TGF-α), transforming growth factor-beta (TGF-β), tumor necrosis factor-alpha (TNF-α), insulin like growth factor (IGF), interleukin-6 and platelet derived growth factor (PDGF) **(Table 1)**. This process stimulates a cascade leading to activation, proliferation and migration of endothelial cells with the formation of new, leaky, fragile blood vessels. VEGF seems to be the leading candidate if a single factor is sought. Müller cells are thought to represent a significant source of VEGF under the conditions of retinal hypoxia.[3] Elevated levels of VEGF have been found in concentration 40 to 100 times normal in aqueous humor of patients with NVG.[4]

Stages of Angiogenesis and Mediating Factors

The other theory states that the formation of new vessels in the eye is affected to a large extent by the homeostatic balance between VEGF, the other proangiogenic factors, and the antiangiogenic factor, pigment epithelium derived factor (PEDF).[5,6] PEDF is naturally occurring and extremely potent inhibitor of angiogenesis that not only targets new vessel growth but also has a neuroprotective activity. Observation of reduced PEDF levels in the vitreous of patients with active diabetic retinopathy compared with inactive retinopathy further supports the theory of a VEGF-PEDF homeostatic equilibrium.[7,8]

CONDITIONS COMMONLY ASSOCIATED WITH NEOVASCULAR GLAUCOMA

Neovascular glaucoma is associated with a number of diseases and conditions **(Table 2)**. Diabetes mellitus

Table 1 Stages of angiogenesis and mediating factors

Stages	Mediating factors
1. Increased endothelial cell permeability	Vascular endothelial growth factor (VEGF)
2. Breakdown of basement membrane and extracellular matrix	Fibroblast growth factor (FGF)
3. Endothelial buds through basement membrane and extracellular matrix	VEGF, FGF, proteinases
4. Endothelial cell migration and mitosis	VEGF, FGF
5. Endothelial cell branching and lumen formation	FGF

Table 2 Disease and conditions associated with neovascularization iris and neovascular glaucoma

Ocular vascular disease	Trauma
Central retinal vein occlusion	Essential iris atrophy
Central retinal artery occlusion	Neurofibromatosis
Branch retinal vein occlusion	Lupus erythematosus
Branch retinal artery occlusion	Marfan's syndrome
Sturge-Weber syndrome with choroidal hemangioma	Recurrent hemorrhages
Leber's miliary aneurysm	Vitreous wick syndrome
Sickle cell retinopathy	
Diabetes mellitus	
Extraocular disease	**Ocular neoplasms**
Carotid artery disease	Malignant melanoma
Ocular ischemia	Retinoblastoma
Aortic arch syndrome	Optic nerve glioma associated with venous stasis
Carotid cavernous fistula	Metastatic carcinoma
Giant cell arteritis	Reticulum cell carcinoma
Pulseless disease	Medulloepithelioma
	Squamous cell carcinoma conjunctiva
	Angiomatosis retinae
Assorted ocular disease	**Ocular inflammatory disease**
Retinal detachment	Chronic uveitis

is associated with about one-third of cases of NVG, central retinal vein occlusion with another one-third, and a variety of conditions with the last third—ocular ischemic disease being the most common in the last group.

Diabetes Mellitus

Diabetes mellitus is one of the most common causes of NVG accounting for approximately one-third of cases. Rubeosis iridis is seen in 1 to 17 percent of diabetic eyes and 33 to 64 percent of eyes with PDR.[9,10] NVG is usually seen in the eyes with proliferative diabetic retinopathy and nonproliferative diabetic retinopathy if there are large areas of capillary nonperfusion. The prevalence of NVG is related to the duration of disease and presence of other vascular disease such as hypertension. Intracapsular cataract surgery in patients of diabetic retinopathy has been associated with an increased risk of postoperative rubeosis iridis and NVG.[11,12] It is common for NVG to appear within 6 months of vitrectomy in diabetic patients, especially in aphakic eyes; the reason being, the lens and the vitreous may act as a mechanical barrier to the forward movement of angiogenic factors elaborated by retina.

The vitreous may act as an endogenous inhibitor of angiogenic stimuli.

Central Retinal Vein Occlusion

It is one of the most common cause of neovascular glaucoma. It is estimated that 30 percent of patients who suffer from central retinal vein occlusion (CRVO) develop NVG. NVG can present from 2 weeks to 2 years following CRVO. However, the conditions often presents about 3 months after CRVO and has been called as **100-day glaucoma**.

Younger patients with CRVO often have associated vascular diseases such as hypertension and collagen vascular disease. Older patients with CRVO often have associated glaucoma or elevated intraocular pressures.

Elevated intraocular pressure or glaucoma has been reported in 10 to 23 percent of eyes that develop CRVO.[13,14] Green and coworkers proposed that posterior bowing of lamina cribrosa in glaucoma creates a mechanical obstruction that impedes the venous outflow and contributes to venous occlusion. In most cases, the underlying glaucoma is open angle or exfoliative in nature but CRVO following angle closure glaucoma can also be seen in few cases. The presence of preexisting glaucoma increases the risk of neovascular glaucoma after CRVO and may make neovascular glaucoma more refractory to treatment.

> The underlying glaucoma is often masked because these eyes may have low IOP for weeks to months following vein occlusion due to transient poor perfusion of the ciliary body.

Ocular Ischemic Syndrome

Ocular ischemic syndrome is the third most common cause of neovascular glaucoma. Seventy-five percent of cases of ocular ischemic syndrome are caused by carotid artery stenosis[15] but it can also occur as a result of aortic arch disease, e.g. syphilis, Takayasu arteritis, dissecting aneurysm; in which case presentation may be bilateral. Symptoms include a dull periocular pain that can be secondary to ischemia. Vision may vary from 20/20 to no light perception. IOP can be elevated secondary to NVG or it can be decreased secondary to ciliary body hypoperfusion or normal as a result of both processes. Midperipheral intraretinal hemorrhages are seen in contrast to diabetic retinopathy and CRVO where hemorrhages are seen in the posterior pole. Other signs include corneal decompensation, iritis, iris atrophy, cataract and spontaneous arterial pulsation. Intravenous fluorescein angiogram demonstrates prolonged choroidal filling and increased arteriovenous transit time.[16,17]

STAGES OF NEOVASCULAR GLAUCOMA

The clinical and histological events that lead from a predisposing factor through rubeosis iridis to advanced neovascular glaucoma may be thought of in three stages:

1. Rubeotic stage.
2. Secondary open angle glaucoma stage.
3. Secondary angle closure glaucoma stage.

These stages generally follow each other. Rubeotic and secondary open angle glaucoma stages are usually taken as early stages of neovascular glaucoma whereas secondary angle closure glaucoma stage is included under advanced stage of neovascular glaucoma.

Preglaucoma Stage (Rubeosis Iridis)

The preglaucoma stage is characterized by normal IOP unless pre-existing glaucoma is present. Slit lamp biomicroscopy reveals dilated tufts of capillaries and fine, randomly oriented

vessels on the surface of iris near the pupillary margin **(Figure 1)**. The new vessels are characterized by leakage of fluorescein. Neovascularization is most commonly seen on peripupillary iris although it may be seen in anterior chamber angle in patients with diabetes and CRVO. It may also be seen at the margins of any pre existing peripheral iridectomy. Gonioscopy may therefore reveal a normal anterior chamber angle or a variable amount of angle neovascularization. According to a report, the new vessels developing after central retinal vein occlusion are larger in diameter and more irregular than those associated with diabetes mellitus.

Neovasular glaucoma does not invariably follow the development of rubeosis iridis and the latter condition may rarely resolve spontaneously. The reported incidence of neovascular glaucoma following diabetes with rubeosis iridis ranges from 13 to 41 percent; whereas, those associated with CRVO is probably significantly greater.

Secondary Open Angle Glaucoma Stage

The rubeosis iridis in this stage is more florid. By gonioscopy, the angle is still open, but the neovascularization may be intense. IOP is elevated and may rise suddenly, causing the patient to present with acute onset glaucoma. Biomicroscopic examination of aqueous often reveals an inflammatory reaction.

The hallmark of this stage is a fibrovascular membrane that covers the anterior chamber angle and anterior surface of iris and may even extend up to the posterior iris surface. The glaucoma in this stage results from obstruction of trabecular meshwork by this fibrovascular membrane, with variable contribution from the inflammation and hemorrhage.

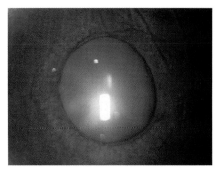

Fig. 1 Neovascularization of the iris is more prominent near the pupillary margin

Secondary Angle Closure Glaucoma Stage

In this stage, the fibrovascular membrane in the angle eventually contracts and pulls the vessels taut, bridging the angle initially and then tenting the iris toward the trabecular meshwork. As these peripheral anterior synechiae coalesce, synechial angle closure occurs. The radial traction along the surface of iris pulls the posterior pigment layer of iris around the pupillary margin onto the anterior surface, resulting in *ectropion uveae* **(Figures 2A to D)**. When one sees ectropion uveae in NVG, usually synechial angle closure is present in the same quadrant **(Figure 2E)**. As the synechiae coalesce, angle closure becomes total. In advanced neovascularization of the iris, new vessels can advance onto a cataractous lens via the posterior synechiae.

The picture of a very smooth, zippered up, line of iridocorneal adhesion is almost pathognomic. Once this end stage of NVG is reached, there is often a remarkable decrease in number of new vessel visible in the angle.

CLINICAL PICTURE

Having presented this orderly picture of progressive neovascularization, it should be noted that great variability in the presentation and rate of progression is the rule rather than the exception. It would be difficult to miss the full-blown picture of NVG. The eye is often

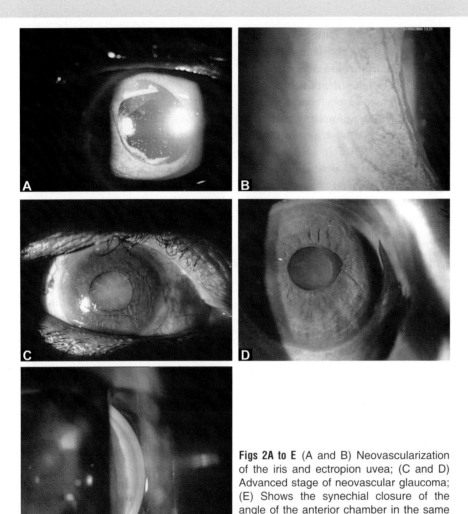

Figs 2A to E (A and B) Neovascularization of the iris and ectropion uvea; (C and D) Advanced stage of neovascular glaucoma; (E) Shows the synechial closure of the angle of the anterior chamber in the same quadrant as ectropion uveae

In some cases of NVG, such as carotid artery obstructive disease, the pressure may be normal or subnormal.

In the late stages of NVG, patients usually have a painful eye with bullous keratopathy, moderate anterior chamber reaction with or without hyphema and severe rubeosis. Pupil is mid-dilated, distorted and fixed; ectropion uveae is present. At this stage, new vessels may be much less visible especially in the angle because of synechial angle closure.

DIFFERENTIAL DIAGNOSIS

In the differential diagnosis, there are two stages to consider: open angle stage and close angle stage.

In the open angle stage, neovascular glaucoma should be differentiated from glaucoma associated with acute iridocyclitis, Fuchs' heterochromic iridocyclitis and exfoliation syndrome. It should be remembered that eyes with uveitis may have dilatation of normal iris vessels that can be confused with neovascularization.

In the angle closure stage of neovascular glaucoma, the new vessels can be less apparent. A differential diagnosis includes other causes of iris distortion and peripheral anterior synechiae such as acute angle closure glaucoma and iridocorneal endothelial syndrome and trauma.[18]

MANAGEMENT

Despite advances in medical and surgical management of glaucoma, the visual prognosis of patients with NVG remains poor. The principle goals in treating NVG include:

1. Controlling ischemia and halting production of angiogenic factors.
2. Finding alternative outflow channel.
3. Decrease aqueous production.
4. Controlling painful blind eye.

painful and photophobic with tearing and blurred vision. Usually, the vision is extremely poor because of edematous cornea and primary disorder underlying the NVG. Sometimes, visual acuity may be remarkably good, 20/40 or even better, if cornea is clear and primary retinal disorder does not remarkably affect the macula. When first seen, the affected eye may have ciliary injection, a steamy cornea from epithelial edema, moderate flare and new vessels in the iris and angle. Clinically, new vessels are first detected as small tufts at pupillary margin. An early sign of rubeosis iridis is increased permeability of

blood vessels at pupillary border as detected by fluorescein angiography or fluorophotometry. At times it may be difficult to distinguish new vessels from normal iris vessels, especially in the inflamed eyes. Normal iris vessels have a uniform size and radial course and they don't branch within the iris. In contrast, new vessels have an irregular size and irregular course and they branch frequently. New vessels also lie on the iris surface rather than the stroma as normal vessels do.

IOP is usually high (in the range of 60s), when a fibrovascular membrane covers a substantial portion of trabecular meshwork.

Recognizing the etiology of NVG is imperative for treatment to decrease the production of angiogenic factors. Visual outcomes will only be improved with early detection of NVI/NVA and the prompt initiation of therapy that targets the underlying disease process along with IOP control.

Medical Management

The management of NVG is approached through four stages that reflect the progression of this disease: prophylactic treatment, early stage treatment, advanced stage treatment and end stage treatment.

Prophylactic Treatment

In high-risk patients or patients who have early NVI with normal IOP, prevention of NVG is the single most important aspect in management. Reducing the amount of viable retina is known to inhibit and reverse new vessel formation in anterior segment. In the majority of patients with NVG secondary to PDR, wherein retinal ischemia is the underlying etiology, the ablation of peripheral retina is the first line therapy to counter the angiogenic cascade. In most cases, panretinal photocoagulation (PRP) with argon laser is the treatment of choice.[19,20]

Panretinal Photocoagulation

Panretinal photocoagulation can be delivered in three ways: slit lamp delivery system, indirect laser, endolaser at the time of vitrectomy. The amount of PRP required varies.

Although the efficacy of prophylactic PRP in preventing NVG is well documented in patients with diabetic retinopathy, a 10 years prospective study of eyes with CRVO undergoing PRP revealed no significant difference in the incidence of subsequent NVG compared to eyes without PRP. In the CVOS, prophylactic PRP in patients with ischemic CRVO but without manifest rubeosis iridis did not completely prevent the development of NVI/NVA. The CVOS investigators recommended performing PRP promptly **when two clock hours of NVI and/or any NVA is observed**.

There is also a higher success rate of glaucoma filtering surgery when PRP is performed initially, because it eliminates or reduces the active anterior segment neovascularization.[21] PRP may reverse IOP elevation in open angle stage and in some cases of early angle closure NVG.[22]

Anterior Retinal Cryotherapy

When adequate PRP is not possible because of cloudy media, physician should consider other retinal ablation modality that is anterior retinal cryotherapy. This may be combined with diode transcleral cyclophotocoagulation if required.

Goniophotocoagulation

It is a form of laser therapy which involves the direct application of argon laser to new vessels in the anterior chamber angle. This is most effective when used in early stages of the disease to prevent progressive angle closure and eventual intractable neovascular glaucoma. Although no longer commonly used, it may be beneficial in patients with high risk of developing NVG when PRP has not been successful or possible.

Early Stage Treatment

This stage is characterized by the development of a fibrovascular membrane across part of the angle or the entire angle and an increase in IOP.

With secondary open angle glaucoma, treatment is identical to prophylactic therapy and includes PRP (fill in PRP if already performed initially), anterior retinal cryotherapy, cyclophotocoagulation and antiglaucoma therapy. An additional option for peripheral retinal ablation is pars plana vitrectomy with laser endophotocoagulation, which can be combined with the direct laser coagulation of the ciliary processes for prompt IOP control.

Medical Therapy

The most important medical therapy for this stage includes antiglaucoma medication, topical atropine 1 percent to decrease ocular congestion and topical steroids to decrease inflammation. Standard antiglaucoma medication to treat elevated IOP includes topical beta blockers, topical alpha-2 agonists, topical carbonic anhydrase inhibitor.

Topical pilocarpine and prostaglandin analogs are contraindicated because they may increase inflammation.

Advanced Stage Treatment

This stage is characterized by synechial angle closure and elevated IOP. PRP is still the initial and most important treatment, both to prevent further NVI/NVA and angle closure and to prepare the eye for surgical intervention.

Medical therapy is indicated with topical steroids, cycloplegics and anti-glaucoma medications to make the eye quiet and decrease IOP as discussed earlier. IOP is usually not controlled in this stage despite of medical management because of extensive synechiae, so residual glaucoma is treated with surgical options (discussed later).

End Stage Treatment

This stage is characterized by complete angle closure by peripheral anterior synechiae with no remaining useful vision.

The primary goal of treatment in this stage is pain control. The medical therapy includes topical steroids, atropine 1 percent and antiglaucoma medications. If pain persists despite of medical management then cyclodestructive procedures are used. Various cyclodestructive procedures used are: cyclocryotherapy, trans-scleral Nd:YAG cyclophotocoagulation and diode laser cyclophotocoagulation. Few studies indicates that diode laser cyclophotocoagulation **(Figure 3)** provides less postoperative inflammation and better IOP control than Nd:YAG cyclophotocoagulation and has become the surgical procedure of choice for NVG when surgical procedure like trabeculectomy is not indicated.[23] Complications of cyclodestructive procedures like sympathetic ophthalmia, anterior segment ischemia and phthisis bulbi should always be kept in mind.

Retrobulbar alcohol injection is indicated after all medical and surgical options have been explored and patient does not want enucleation. Enucleation is the last resort when intractable pain is not relieved by any other treatment modality.

Surgical Care

Surgical care is indicated in patients with useful vision and regressed NVI and when IOP is not controlled with maximum medical therapy. Preoperative care is fundamental to the postoperative success of any surgical intervention. Before surgery, adequate PRP should be completed to reduce vasoproliferative stimulus. Atropine and steroids are indicated to decrease inflammation and antiglaucoma medication to decrease

IOP. After PRP, it is preferable to wait for 3 to 4 weeks to allow the eye to quiet down.

Anti-VEGF agents can also be administered preoperatively.

Surgical modalities include:
- Trabeculectomy with/without antifibrotic agents
- Glaucoma drainage devices.

Trabeculectomy with Antimetabolites

Incisional filtering surgery in patients with active NVG is associated with a high incidence of intraoperative bleeding and postoperative progression of fibrovascular membrane.[21] Either 5-fluorouracil (50 mg/ml) for 5 minutes or mitomycin-C (0.2-0.4 mg/ml) for 3 to 5 minutes can be used to increase the success rate **(Figure 4)**. Mitomycin-C used intraoperatively has been shown to be more effective than 5-fluorouracil in routine trabeculectomies.[24]

Glaucoma Drainage Devices

Implanting glaucoma drainage devices (GDDs) is another modality of treatment which is indicated when trabeculectomy fails, in refractory NVG, and in cases of extensive conjunctival scarring (where standard filtering procedure is difficult to perform). Molteno, Kruplin, and Ahmed valve implants **(Figure 5)** are more commonly used. In addition, improved success rate has been reported in patients with refractory NVG when drainage tube is implanted through the pars plana route and combined with pars plana vitrectomy.[25,26]

FUTURE THERAPEUTIC OPTIONS

Several treatments for NVG in eyes with intractable glaucoma are

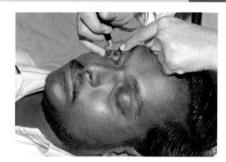

Fig. 3 Diode cyclophotocoagulation being done

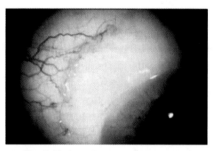

Fig. 4 Trabeculectomy in a case of neovascular glaucoma

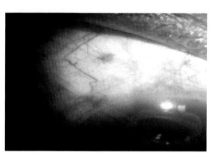

Fig. 5 Ahmed valve implant in a case of neovascular glaucoma

under investigation. One option is to perform surgical retinectomy[27,28] (to reroute the aqueous drainage through the choroidal circulation) at the time of pars plana vitrectomy but it is associated with risk of complications like retinal detachment, proliferative vitreoretinopathy and phthisis bulbi.

Researchers have also suggested using photodynamic therapy with verteporfin to occlude new iris vessels without damaging adjacent tissue or normal iris vessels, but no results on the progression of rubeosis or NVG have yet been reported.[29] Additionally, the intravitreal injection of crystalline triamcinolone has been studied as a potential treatment to cause a regression of iris neovasculature.[30]

Novel anti-VEGF compounds, which include bevacizumab and, small interfering RNA (siRNA) directed against VEGF receptor 1, and VEGF trap are being considered.[31] In particular, intravitreal bevacizumab has been used. It leads to resolution of active retinal and iris neovascularization, and thus a significant regression of rubeosis iridis and a concurrent reduction in IOP.[32]

In a primate model of rubeosis iridis, systemic treatment with alpha-interferon, a polypeptide that inhibits the proliferation and migration of endothelial cells and new vessel growth, resulted in the regression of the rubeosis.[33] Troxerutin improves microvascular flow by inhibiting platelet and erythrocyte aggregation, increasing erythrocyte deformability, and reducing blood viscosity.[34]

Recent studies suggest that PEDF induces prosurvival genes through cyclic adenosine monophosphate-responsive element binding protein and nuclear factor-kappa B activation.[35] In this regard, PEDF may have the additional advantage of helping to preserve the integrity of retinal neurons that are damaged from both the underlying retinal ischemia and the resultant elevated IOP in NVG.

SUMMARY

Neovascular glaucoma is a devastating ocular condition often associated with poor prognosis. Medical or surgical treatment is not associated with high success rate. Retinal ablation which reduces levels of retinal ischemia and further angiogenic cascade remains the most effective treatment. The best hope for preventing the blindness associated with NVG is continued research into angiogenesis pathway and development of newer pharmacological agents which prevent the neovascularization. Such therapeutic approaches may become the mainstay in prevention and treatment of neovascular glaucoma.

REFERENCES

1. Coats G. Further cases of thrombosis of the central vein. Roy Lond Ophthal Hosp Rep 1906;16:516.
2. Patz A, Lutty G, Coughlin WR. Inhibitors of neovascularisation in relation to diabetic and other proliferative retinopathies. Trans Am Ophthalmol Soc 1978;76:102.
3. Tsai JC, Shields MB. Neovascular glaucoma. In: Tombran-Tink J, Barnstable CJ, (Eds). Ophthalmology: Ocular Angiogenesis: Diseases, Mechanisms, and Therapeutics. Totowa, NJ: Humana Press Inc: In press.
4. Tripathi RC, et al. Increased level of vascular endothelial growth factor in aqueous humor of patients with neovascular glaucoma, Ophthalmology 1998;105:232.
5. Tombran-Tink J, Barnstable CJ. Therapeutic prospects for PEDF: more than a promising angiogenesis inhibitor. Trends Mol Med 2003;9:244-50.
6. Tombran-Tink J, Barnstable CJ. PEDF: a multifaceted neurotrophic factor. Nat Rev Neurosci 2003;4:1-10.
7. Ogata N, Tombran-Tink J, Nishikawa M, et al. Pigment epithelium-derived factor in the vitreous is low in diabetic retinopathy and high in rhegmatogenous retinal detachment. Am J Ophthalmol 2001;132:378-82.
8. Ogata N, Nishikawa M, Nishimura T, et al. Unbalanced vitreous levels of pigment epithelium-derived factor and vascular endothelial growth factor in diabetic retinopathy. Am J Ophthalmol 2002;134:348-53.
9. Ohrt V. Glaucoma due to rubeosis iridis diabetic. Ophthalmologica 1961; 142:356.
10. Madsen PH. Ocular findings in 123 patients with diabetic retinopathy. Doc Ophthalmol 1970;29:331.
11. Aiello LM, Wand M, Liang G. Neovascular glaucoma and vitreous hemorrhage following cataract surgery in patients with diabetes mellitus. Ophthalmology 1983;90:814.
12. Beasley H. Rubeosis iridis in aphakic diabetics. JAMA 1970;213:128.
13. Bertelsen TI. The relation between thrombosis in the retinal vein and primary glaucoma. Acta Ophthalmol Scand Suppl 1961;39:603.
14. Dryden RM. Central retinal vein occlusion and chronic simple glaucoma. Arch Ophthalmol 1965;73:659.
15. Mizener JB, Hayreh SS. Ocular ischemic syndrome. Ophthalmology 1997;104:859.
16. Sturrock, Mueller. Chronic ocular ischemia. Br J Ophthalmol 1984;68:716.
17. Brown GC, Magargal LE. Ocular ischemic syndrome: clinical, fluorescein angiographic and carotid angiographic features. Int Ophthalmol 1988;11:239.
18. Shields MB. Textbook of Glaucoma. 4th edn. 1998;269-86.
19. Tasman W, Magargal LE, Augsburger JJ. Effects of argon laser photocoagulation on rubeosis iridis and angle neovascularization. Ophthalmology 1980;87:400-2.
20. Striga M, Ivanisevic M. Comparison between efficacy of full- and mild-scatter (panretinal) photocoagulation on the course of diabetic rubeosis iridis. Ophthalmologica 1993;207:144-7.

21. Allen RC, Bellows AR, Hutchinson BT, Murphy SD. Filtration surgery in the treatment of neovascular glaucoma. Ophthalmology 1982;89:1181-7.

22. Jacobson DR, Murphy RP, Rosenthal AR. The treatment of angle neovascularization with panretinal photocoagulation. Ophthalmology 1979;86:1270.

23. Bloom, Tsai JC, Sharma K. Trans sclera diode laser photocoagulation in the treatment of advanced refractory glaucoma. Ophthalmology 1997:104;508.

24. Tsai JC, Feuer WJ, Parrish RK II, Grajewski AL. 5-fluorouracil filtering surgery and neovascular glaucoma. Long-term follow-up of the original pilot study. Ophthalmology 1995;102:887-92.

25. Scott IU, Alexandrakis G, Flynn HW Jr, et al. Combined pars plana vitrectomy and glaucoma drainage implant placement for refractory glaucoma. Am J Ophthalmol 2000;129:334-41.

26. Luttrull JK, Avery RL. Pars plana implant and vitrectomy for treatment of neovascular glaucoma. Retina 1995;15:379-87.

27. Kirchhof B. Retinectomy lowers intraocular pressure in otherwise intractable glaucoma: preliminary results. Ophthalmic Surg 1994;25:262-7.

28. Joussen AM, Walter P, Jonescu-Cuypers CP, et al. Retinectomy for treatment of intractable glaucoma: long term results. Br J Ophthalmol. 2003;87:1094-102.

29. Muller VA, Ruokonen P, Schellenbeck M, et al. Treatment of rubeosis iridis with photodynamic therapy with verteporfin—a new therapeutic and prophylactic option for patients with the risk of neovascular glaucoma? Ophthalmic Res 2003;35:60-4.

30. Jonas JB, Hayler JK, Sofker A, Panda-Jonas S. Regression of neovascular iris vessels by intravitreal injection of crystalline cortisone. J Glaucoma 2001;10:284-7.

31. Adamis AP, Shima DT, Tolentino MJ, et al. Inhibition of vascular endothelial growth factor prevents retinal ischemia-associated iris neovascularization in a nonhuman primate. Arch Ophthalmol 1996;114:66.

32. Avery RL. Regression of retinal and iris neovascularization after intravitreal bevacizumab (Avastin) treatment. Retina 2006;26:352-4.

33. Miller JW, Stinson WG, Folkman J. Regression of experimental iris neovascularization with systemic alpha-interferon Ophthalmology 1993;100:9.

34. Glacet-Bernard A, Coscas G, Chabanel A, et al. A randomized, double-masked study on the treatment of retinal vein occlusion with troxerutin. Am J Ophthalmol 1994;118:421-9.

35. Yabe T, Kanemitsu K, Sanagi T, et al. Pigment epithelium-derived factor induces prosurvival genes through cyclic AMP-responsive element binding protein and nuclear factor kappa B activation in rat cultured cerebellar granule cells: implication for its neuroprotective effect. Neuroscience. 2005;133:691-700.

34 | Ocular Trauma and Glaucoma

Mohan Kumar, R Ramakrishnan

INTRODUCTION

The term traumatic glaucoma incorporates variety of post-traumatic mechanisms that lead to a rise in intraocular pressure. It usually occurs following a blunt injury that causes anterior segment deformation during the impact. It can also occur following penetrating injuries. Transient or prolonged elevations in intraocular pressure and damage to trabecular meshwork and other structures predispose traumatized eyes to the development of glaucomatous optic nerve loss. Each trauma case is unique, but ocular injury tends to occur in certain patterns. An understanding of these patterns allows one to accurately predict the risk of glaucoma development and the type of glaucoma likely to occur. Another point to be considered is that the adjunctive treatment for traumatic glaucoma like steroid therapy or scleral buckling can cause increase in intraocular pressure. Patients with ocular trauma must be carefully counseled on life long risk of glaucoma. Close follow-up is recommended with specific attention to any early signs of glaucomatous changes.

MECHANISM OF GLAUCOMA FOLLOWING OCULAR TRAUMA

Glaucoma Following Blunt Injury

Early Onset

- Iritis
- Hyphema
- Traumatic lens subluxation and dislocation
- Traumatic intumescence of lens.

Delayed Onset

- Angle recession glaucoma
- Ghost cell glaucoma.

Glaucoma Following Penetrating Injury

- Epithelial/Stromal down growth
- Siderosis
- Peripheral anterior synechiae (PAS).

Other Situations

- Chemical injury
- Ocular surgery.

Glaucoma Following

- Cataract surgery
- Penetrating keratoplasty
- Vitreoretinal procedures
- Aqueous misdirection syndrome.

Incidence

The lifetime prevalence of ocular trauma is estimated to be 19.8 percent with a 5 years incidence of 1.6 percent.[1] The incidence of traumatic hyphema is 17/100, 000 and 30 to 94 percent of these patients exhibit angle recession.[2,3] A typical patient is a male, younger than 30 years of age. 20 to 30 percent of the reported patients with ocular trauma may have traumatic glaucoma or intraocular pressure more than 21 mm Hg. A 10 years prospective study revealed 9 percent incidence of traumatic glaucoma with 6 percent of the cases being late onset.[3] Late-onset glaucoma from blunt trauma ranges from 1.3 to 20 percent in other studies. Similar findings have been reported in the Indian population.

PATHOGENESIS OF TRAUMATIC GLAUCOMA

Pathogenesis of Glaucoma in Blunt Trauma

Blunt trauma to the eye is a common injury and each case must be considered as risk factor for the development of glaucoma. Ideally, these patients should be made aware of their risk for glaucoma and receive appropriate follow-up.

During blunt trauma, at initial impact of an object to the eye, the cornea and anterior sclera are rapidly displaced posteriorly with a compensatory expansion at the equator of the eye. The expansion causes tears in various parts of anterior segment that are affected by hemorrhage, inflammation and scarring and referred to **as seven anterior rings of tissue by Campbell**. These include:[4-6]

1. Radial tears of **sphincter pupillae**
2. Tear at the iris base **(iridodialysis)**
3. Tear of anterior ciliary body **(angle recession)**
4. Tear at the attachment of ciliary body and scleral spur **(cyclodialysis cleft)**
5. Tear at the level **of trabecular meshwork**
6. Tear of the **zonules: Zonulodialysis**
7. Detachment of the retina at the **Ora serrata: Retinal dialysis**.

Early-Onset Glaucoma

Although aqueous production may be temporarily reduced by the inflamed post-traumatic ciliary body, outflow channels are also affected, which may lead to rise in intraocular pressure. Outflow channels may be damaged by the actual tear or blocked by hemorrhage, platelets, inflammatory cells, ghosts cells, fibrous ingrowth or scar tissue.

In addition, **subluxation** and dislocation of the lens (**Figures 1A to C**) in blunt and penetrating trauma can lead to glaucoma due to variety of mechanisms. Traumatic rupture of the lens capsule can release lens proteins and cause **phacoanaphylactic uveitis**, leading to uveitic glaucoma. This inflammation can also cause peripheral anterior synechiae closing the angle. Pupillary block can occur with posterior synechiae, anterior subluxated lens or traumatic lens swelling.[7]

Late-Onset Glaucoma

It is usually related to significant amount of trabecular meshwork damage or PAS formation. With an already damaged meshwork or a partially closed angle, there is an inadequate healthy tissue to compensate for this change. Interestingly there is increased risk of developing primary open angle glaucoma (50%) in the other eye, showing that there may be already impaired outflow facility. Less commonly, penetrating injuries with metal foreign bodies can cause **siderosis** or **chalcosis** leading to open angle glaucoma.

CLINICAL FINDINGS

Symptoms

In case of an acute rise in intraocular pressure, symptoms of headache, nausea, blurry vision, or photophobia may be present. Late-onset glaucoma from gradual intraocular pressure rise in usually asymptomatic. Therefore, a detailed history of the event should be taken.

> **Note** A ruptured globe or penetrating injury should be ruled out. Some critical signs that aid in diagnosis are 360° chemosis, shallow anterior chamber (AC) and scleral show on indirect examination, and limitation of eye movement. Pressure on the globe should be avoided until surgical intervention is taken. Once a ruptured globe has been ruled out or repaired, accurate intraocular pressure readings may be taken. Then, critical signs suggesting equatorial expansion of the globe should be evaluated by slit lamp examination.

Signs

Hyphema: A hyphema results from torn anterior ciliary or iris stromal arteries and is graded by the fraction of blood in the anterior chamber.

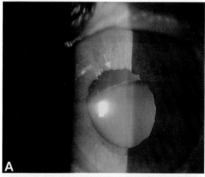
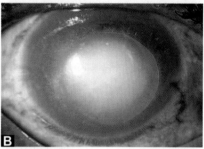
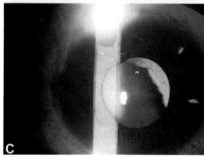

Figs 1A to C (A) Traumatic inferior subluxation of the crystalline lens. Note the sphincter tears at the pupillary margin. (arrow); (B) Traumatic dislocation of the cataractous lens into the anterior chamber; (C) Secondary angle closure glaucoma following subluxation of lens. Trabeculectomy was done

Rebleeding: It may be obvious or subtle with bright red blood layered over red blood. This is easily confused with the bright red color of a dissolving clot at the periphery. Rebleeding is associated with a poor prognosis related to the increased risk of intraocular pressure rise and corneal blood staining.[8]

Microhyphema vs traumatic iritis: Circulating pigmented red blood cells should be differentiated from inflammatory cells because of the 7 percent rebleeding rate noted in children with no frank hyphema.[9]

Vossius ring: Pigment on the anterior lens capsule would indicate compression of the pupillary margin onto the anterior capsule.

Adherent leukoma: Iris adherent to the cornea.

Sphincter tears: Fine radial tears at the pupillary margin or sphincter dysfunction with **traumatic mydriasis.**

Iridodialysis: A tear at the iris base and is seen as a separation of the iris at the limbus exposing zonular fibers below.

Anterior displaced lens: It can cause a relative pupillary block and narrow angle.

Cyclodialysis cleft: The internal scleral wall is seen because the ciliary body is torn from the scleral spur. Intraocular pressure may be low. Cyclodialysis cleft usually effects less than 90° of the angle.

Angle recession: It is a tear between the longitudinal and circular muscles of the ciliary body. If the tear is shallow, then the ciliary body band appears darker and the scleral spur appears whiter than the fellow eye. In deeper tears, there is unevenness in the width of the ciliary band on gonioscopy especially when compared with the uninvolved fellow eye.

Trabecular meshwork damage: These findings are subtle. Torn iris processes at the angle, prominent white scleral spur, and the glistening back wall of the canal may be apparent if the tear extends through the corneoscleral meshwork.[5] In addition debris, pigment, PAS and blood can be present in the angle.

Traumatic Iritis

Initially intraocular pressure in case of traumatic iritis is often low due to decreased aqueous production by a stunned ciliary body. Later, it rises due to swelling and clogging of trabecular meshwork by inflammatory debris. The intraocular pressure elevation is mild and easily controlled.[10] Recommended treatment for traumatic iritis includes cycloplegia and topical steroids. These alone can reduce intraocular pressure to acceptable range. If hypotensive agents are used, β-blockers and carbonic anhydrase inhibitors are usually the first range. Prostaglandin analogs and pilocarpine are usually avoided as they can exacerbate inflammation and risk of posterior synechiae.

Hyphema

Blood in the anterior chamber, whether microscopic or layered is a common finding after ocular trauma **(Figure 2)**. Acute elevation in intraocular pressure in eyes with hyphema is caused by mechanical obstruction of trabecular meshwork by blood products and fibrin. The hyphema can be graded by the volume of the anterior chamber filled with blood after layering of the red blood cells **(Table 1)**. They may also be graded on the basis of actual height in millimeters of blood layering in the anterior chamber. In small anterior chamber bleeds without actual layering of blood but with evidence of suspended red blood cells on slit-lamp examination, the hyphema is termed as microscopic.

Chronic IOP elevation is due to permanent damage to meshwork either by direct trauma with or without visible angle recession or rarely by secondary fibrosis and descemetization of angle.[11] Therefore, unless anterior chamber fibrotic changes are evident on examination and gonioscopy, patients with history of hyphema who go on to develop glaucoma are usually approached as an angle recession patient, even in absence of discernable recession on examination.

Two subgroups of hyphema patients warrant special attention: **Sickle cell patients** and those with **rebleed.** The rate of rebleed after a traumatic hyphema has been

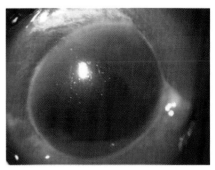

Fig. 2 Traumatic hyphema

Table 1 Grading of hyphema

Grade I	Less than one-third of the anterior chamber
Grade II	One-third to one-half of the anterior chamber
Grade III	One-half to nearly total
Grade IV	Total (eight ball)

variably reported from 3.5 to 3.8 percent.[12] Rebleed is usually more severe and more damaging than initial hyphema. Sickle cell patients are not only at higher risk for rebleed but also more likely to develop glaucomatous nerve damage even with moderate IOP elevations.[13]

Patients with hyphema need to be followed daily for 3 to 5 days to monitor for rebleed and for IOP check up. Eye rest and shielding throughout this period is important. IOP > 25 mm Hg should be treated. Surgical washout of AC is usually reserved for cases with elevated IOP uncontrolled by medical therapy or evidence of corneal blood staining.

A careful and deliberate gonioscopic examination of both eyes will reveal sometimes visually unimpressive changes of angle recession.[14] Gonioscopy is typically performed 3 to 6 weeks after injury to minimize the risk of causing a rebleed. Regardless of what is observed during this examination, it is an ideal opportunity to educate the patient about the injury the eye has sustained and lifelong risk for glaucoma. Baseline visual fields and disc photos should be obtained.

Angle Recession

Secondary open angle glaucoma associated with angle recession represents one of the most common form of trauma related glaucoma. Angle recession seen by gonioscopy is not responsible for outflow obstruction but represents a visible marker of invisible damage sustained by trabecular meshwork.

Clinical Features

Usually the IOP rises a few months after the initial injury. The anterior chamber is deep or of irregular depth. Sphincter tears at the pupillary margin are usually present indicating trauma in the past. These form a valuable clinical sign when the patient gives a negative history of trauma. A rossette shaped cataract, trabecular meshwork pigmentation, iridodialysis may be present **(Figures 3 to 5)**. On gonioscopy, angle recession is seen.

Usually 5 to 20 percent patients will go on develop glaucoma.[15] Persons who have 180° or more AR have more chances of developing glaucoma.[16] Of these, up to 50 percent will eventually develop glaucoma in fellow eye. This suggests that these patients might have a predisposition to glaucoma and that trauma can predispose to the initiation of the cascade of glaucomatous damage.

Initial treatment of angle recession glaucoma is medical. If it fails, glaucoma filtering surgery the next choice. Trabeculectomy with antimetabolites is associated with the greatest reduction of IOP and fewest postoperative glaucoma medication. Laser trabeculoplasty tends to be relatively ineffective.[17] Cyclodestructive procedures are reserved for patients with limited visual potential but can offer effective and long lasting IOP control in refractory cases.

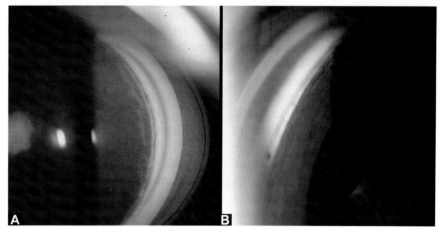

Figs 3A and B Gonioscopic view of angle recession

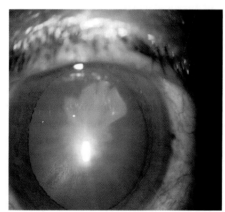

Fig. 4 Traumatic cataract (Rosette shaped)

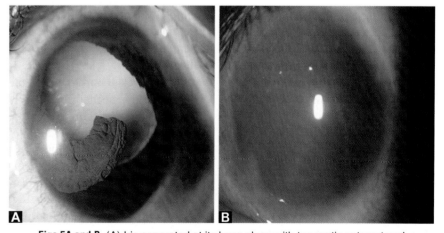

Figs 5A and B (A) Iris separated at its base along with traumatic cataract and subluxation of the lens; (B) Traumatic aniridia

Ghost Cell Glaucoma

Fresh red blood cells present in hyphema are pliable and easily percolate through the trabecular meshwork but the same is not possible with degenerated ghost cell erythrocytes. These rigid, khaki colored cells over the course of several weeks can raise IOP, obstructing the meshwork.[18]

The resulting ghost cell glaucoma occurs, however 2 to 3 weeks after vitreous hemorrhage with rupture of the anterior hyaloid face. It can occur after any intraocular hemorrhage, even if no vitreous hemorrhage or disruption of the hyaloid occurs. The ghost cells can be observed flowing freely in the anterior chamber or as a tan stripe in a back ground of red cells, creating so called **candy stripe sign**.

Definitive diagnosis is made by microscopic examination of an anterior chamber specimen.[19] On light microscopy, the ghost cells appear as rigid spheres with small dense adherent spots on their surface called **Heinz bodies**. Medical treatment mostly is sufficient to control IOP. Certain cases where IOP is not adequately controlled by medical therapy may require anterior chamber wash or vitrectomy procedures to aid in pressure control.

Glaucoma Secondary to Penetrating Injury

Here, the glaucoma can occur due to multiple factors. Mechanisms associated with blunt trauma such as hyphema, angle recession and ghost cell glaucoma can also coexist.

Any penetrating injury can initiate inflammation that eventually leads to uveitic glaucoma. Thus, inflammation should be carefully controlled and cycloplegia is usually recommended during acute postinjury phase. Any glaucoma patient with a history of trauma must be examined for PAS.

Long-term use of corticosteroids is common and this can lead to elevated IOP. The rise in IOP tends to occur 2 to 3 weeks after initiation of therapy and is dose dependent.[20] Even after cessation of steroid treatment patients require life long IOP control, due to irreversible changes in the trabecular meshwork.

Siderosis

Iron is toxic to the **epithelial tissues** of the eye. Excess Iron either from retained foreign body or from chronic intraocular hemorrhage (hemosiderosis) can lead to a pattern of tissue damage in the eye termed as siderosis. Up to 40 percent of open globe injuries retain some amount of intraocular foreign body.[21]

Clinical findings include iris heterochromia with darkening of iris in the affected eye, a dilated and poorly reactive pupil, rust like deposits on the corneal endothelium and anterior lens surface, optic nerve head edema, raised IOP and pigmentary retinopathy. Degenerative changes in the trabecular meshwork including sclerosis and loss of intertrabecular spaces have been found in siderotic eyes. Any eye with retained metallic foreign body or long standing intraocular hemorrhage must be followed closely for glaucoma and for ERG changes associated with this condition.[22]

Glaucoma Secondary to Chemical Injury

Both acid and alkali burns can acutely raise the IOP. The mechanism is poorly understood and thought to be due to contraction of anterior tissues of the eye[23] causing a slow progressive increase in IOP. Acutely, topical steroids and aqueous suppressants can be helpful in managing the pressure. Cases that progress to sterile corneal ulceration typically have the most extensive anterior segment damage

and are more likely to develop glaucoma and eventful phthisis.[24]

Glaucoma Following Ocular Surgery

This can be due to the following factors:
- Malignant glaucoma (aqueous misdirection syndrome)
- Glaucoma in aphakia and pseudophakia
- Glaucoma following penetrating keratoplasty
- Glaucoma following vitreoretinal surgery
(The above are discussed in detail in a separate chapters).

Diagnostic Features

The diagnosis of traumatic glaucoma is mainly clinical and includes a detailed history of the mechanism of injury, slit lamp examination, IOP measurements, gonioscopy, optic nerve head, and nerve fiber analysis. Most importantly, patients with a history of blunt trauma (especially in those with documented angle recession or hyphema) should have yearly examination for life to look for late-onset glaucoma. These patients are similar to glaucoma suspects. Thus, if they have other risk factors such as high IOP and suspicious cup-to-disc ratios, baseline disc photos, a baseline visual field and a structural test which may be helpful in demonstrating nerve fiber loss before visual field loss should be considered.

Black patients have an 8 percent risk for having sickle cell disease and are a subset of patients that may need a sickle cell preparation and hemoglobin electrophoresis in the presence of hyphema.

These patients will produce sickled cells that may not easily pass through the trabecular meshwork and lead to rapid increases in IOP. Laboratory tests in patients with a history of a bleeding disorder should also be considered: Platelet counts, liver function tests prothrombin time, and partial thromboplastin time.[9]

MANAGEMENT

Principle of management: Treatment of traumatic glaucoma involves lowering IOP or precluding its rise to prevent optic nerve damage. Treatment also depends on the cause of the unstable IOP and the amount of time after the traumatic event.

Medical Management

Acutely, the increase in IOP is usually caused by blockage of the angle with hyphema, debris, and inflammatory cells. These patients are usually young, they can tolerate acute increase in IOP without nerve damage. Treatment with aqueous suppressants such as beta blockers, alpha-2 agonists, and carbonic anhydrase inhibitors (CAIs) is recommended. CAIs should not be used in patients with sickle-cell disease or trait. Parasympathomimetics and prostaglandin analogs are associated with increased inflammation and should be avoided. Cycloplegics and topical steroids should also be used for up to 6 weeks to decrease inflammation and cellular infiltration of the damaged angle.

Rebleeding

Another concern in the acute phase of traumatic hyphema is the risk of rebleeding (usually in the first 2 to 5 days), which increases the risk of IOP rise and the development of total hyphema. First-line of management includes no use of anticoagulation or nonsteroidal anti-inflammatory drugs such as aspirin, no exertional activities, head elevation of 30° and the use of an eye shield at all times. Hospital admission in hyperactive children, those with a large hyphema or high IOP, and those with sickle cell disease or a

bleeding disorder should be considered, though this is controversial given the variable cost and effectiveness. In patients with a bleeding disorder such as hemophilia, clotting factors should be administered as soon as possible.

Controversy exists regarding the use of antifibrinolytic agents to prevent rebleeding. Tranexamic acid and Aminocaproic acid have been shown to significantly reduce the incidence of rebleeding by stabilizing the fibrin clot. However, more recent studies do not show an improvement in visual outcome and thus these drugs have fallen out of favor. Furthermore, these patients have to be monitored closely for the many side effects of these drugs such as dizziness, hypotension, and vomiting. It is also contraindicated in patients with renal or hepatic insufficiency or hemophilia. A topical preparation of aminocaproic acid with promising results has been developed though it is not yet available commercially. Topical and oral steroids, drugs commonly used in eye trauma, may also help to prevent rebleeding by inhibiting fibrinolysis and stabilizing the blood ocular barrier.[8] If rebleeding occurs, an IOP check will help evaluate further treatment options, which may include the use of an antifibrinolytic drug.

Surgical Management

In the subacute period, a persistent IOP rise of more than 50 mm Hg for 5 days, an IOP more than 35 mm Hg for greater than 7 days, or a persistent hyphema for more than 10 days on maximal medical therapy may require an anterior chamber (AC) washout. This is meant to decrease the rate of optic nerve damage, PAS formation,

and corneal blood staining, respectively. In those with sickle cell, an anterior chamber (AC) washout should be considered if IOP is more than 30 mm of Hg for more than 24 hours.[8]

An AC washout includes creating two paracentesis incisions with saline irrigation through one incision and a depression of the posterior lip of the second paracentesis. This technique allows for easy transition to bimanual irrigation/aspiration or cutting to further control bleeding.

Numerous studies report different treatment options for late-onset glaucoma. Many patients may need life-long treatment with topical medications. In those refractory to medical therapy, argon laser trabeculoplasty and trabeculectomy without antimetabolite have yielded disappointing results.[21,25] Failure may be due to increased fibroblast proliferation in younger patients or a change in their aqueous humor after trauma. The use of mitomycin C and 5-fluorouracil has decreased the rate of trabeculectomy failure. Also, glaucoma drainage devices in eyes with past failed filtering procedures have been shown to control IOP.[5,26]

CONCLUSION

Glaucoma is a common and often devastating consequence of ocular injury, whether from accidental trauma or intentional surgical interventions. A thorough knowledge of the risk factors for post-traumatic glaucoma and careful examination is required for rapid identification of affected patients. Patient education, careful examination and early intervention provide patients with the best chance for long-term vision preservation.

REFERENCES

1. Wong T, Klein B, Klein R. The prevalence and 5-year incidence of ocular Trauma – The Beaver Dam Eye Study. Ophthalmology 2000;107:2196-202.

2. Sihota R, Sood NN, Agarwal HC. Traumatic glaucoma. Acta Ophthalmol Scand 1995;73:252-4.

3. Kaufman JH, Tolpin DW. Glaucoma after traumatic angle recession. A ten-year prospective study. Am J Ophthalmol 1974;74:648-54.

4. Campbell, DG. Traumatic glaucoma. In: Shingleton BG, Hersh PS, Kenyon KR (Eds). Eye Trauma. St. Louis, Mo: Mosby Year Book 1991;117-25.

5. Chi TS, Netland PA. Angle-recession glaucoma. Int Ophthalmol clin 1995; 35:117-24.

6. Campbell D. Traumatic glaucoma. In: Shingleton B, Hersh p, Kenyon K (Eds). Eye Trauma. St. Louis: Mosby Year Book 1991.pp.117-25.

7. Irvin JA, Smith RE. Lens injuries. In: Shingleton BG, Hersh PS, Kenyon KR, (Eds). Eye Trauma. St.Louis, Mo: Mosby Year Book 1991.pp.127-8.

8. Walton W, Von Hagen S, Grigorian R, Zarbin M. Management of traumatic hyphema. Surv Ophthalmol 2002;47:297-334.

9. Shingleton BJ, Hersh PS. Traumatic hyphema. In: Shingleton BG, Hersh PS, kenyon KR (Eds). Eye Trauma. St.Louis, Mo:Mosby Year Book 1991;107.

10. De Leon-Ortega JE, Girkin C. Ocular trauma-related glaucoma. Ophthalmol Clin N Am 2002;15:215-23.

11. Shingleton B, Hersh P, Kenyon K. Eye trauma St. Louis: Mosby Year Book 1991.pp.104-16.

12. Volpe Nj, Larrison WI, Hersh PS, et al. Secondary hemorrhage in traumatic hyphema. Am J Ophthalmol 1991; 112:507-13.

13. Goldberg MF. Sickled erythrocytes, hyphema, and secondary glaucoma: I. The diagnosis and treatment of sickled erythrocytes in human hyphemas. Ophthalmic Surg 1979;10:17-31.

14. Filipe JA, Barros H, Castro-Correia J. Sports-related ocular injuries: a three year follow-up study. Ophthalmology 1997;104:313-8.

15. Salmon JF, mermoud A, Ivey A et al. The detection of post-traumatic angle recession by gonioscopy in a population-based glaucoma survey. Ophthalmology 1994;101:1844-50.

16. Alper M. contusion angle deformity and glaucoma. Arch Ophthalmol 1963;69:77-89.

17. Goldberg I. Argon laser trabeculoplasty and the open angle glaucomas. Aust N Z J Ophthalmol 1985;13:243-8.

18. Campbell DG. Ghost cell glaucoma following trauma. Ophthalmology 1981;88:1151-8.

19. Cameron J, Havener VR. Histologic confirmation of ghost cell glaucoma by routine light microscopy. Am J Ophthalmol 1983;96:251-2.

20. Polansky JR, Weinreb RN. Steroids as anti-inflammatory agents. In: Sears ML (Ed.). Pharmacology of the Eye. Berlin: Springer-Verlag. Handbook of Experimental Pharmacology 1984;69: 460-538.

21. De Juan E, Sternberg P Jr, Michels R. Penetrating ocular injuries. Ophthalmology 1983;90:1318-22.

22. Schechner R, Miller B, Merksamer E, et al. A long-term follow-up of ocular siderosis: quantitative assessment of the electroretinogram. Doc Ophthalmol 1990;76:231-40.

23. Paerson CA, Eakins EA, Paterson E, et al. The ocular hypertensive response following experimental acid burns in the rabbit eye. Invest Ophthalmol Vis Sci 1979;18:67.

24. Kuckelkorn R, Kottek A, Reim M. Intraocular complications after severe chemical burns-incidence and surgical treatment. Klin Monatsbl Augenheilkd 1994;205:86-92.

25. Robin AL, Pollack IP. Argon laser trabeculoplasty in secondary forms of open angle glaucoma. Arch Ophthalmol 1983;101:382-4.

26. Mermoud A, Salmon JF, Barron A, Straker C, Murray AD. Surgical management of post-traumatic angle recession glaucoma. Ophthalmology 1993;100:634-42.

35 | Steroid-induced Glaucoma

Ankit Gupta, R Ramakrishnan

CHAPTER OUTLINE
- Steroid Responders and Corticosteroid Sensitivity
- Routes of Administration and Pressure Response
- Clinical Presentation
- Mechanism of Glaucoma
- Prevention
- Management

INTRODUCTION

A substantial percentage of the population responds to chronic steroid therapy, given by any of the routes of administration available today, with a variable increase in the intraocular pressure (IOP). This elevation in the IOP can lead to glaucomatous optic nerve damage and subsequent loss of vision. Such an outcome of steroid usage is referred to as *steroid-induced glaucoma*.

STEROID RESPONDERS AND THEIR CORTICOSTEROID SENSITIVITY

Prospective studies of topical steroid response in both general population and POAG populations have been performed to assess their steroid responsiveness. The researchers have used a potent topical corticosteroid such as 0.1 percent betamethasone or 0.1 percent dexamethasone for 3 to 6 weeks.

Becker et al and Armaly et al described the trimodal distribution of pressure response to corticosteroids in general population.[1-3] POAG populations have been shown to have a greater number of individuals with an elevated IOP response to topical corticosteroids.[1-3] The actual percentage of high responders varies according to the criteria used to define this group.[1-3]

Schwartz et al[4] could not confirm the trimodal distribution of steroid responders and Palmberg et al demonstrated the lack of reproducibility of the intraocular pressure response to dexamethasone.[5] Studies differ on whether ocular hypertensives do[6] or do not[7] have a greater incidence of high steroid response than the general population.

The differential distribution of the corticosteroid sensitivity in the various groups in population has been controversially attributed to inheritance by some[1,8,9] and an acquired etiology by others.[4,10-14] Becker et al[1,8] postulated an autosomal recessive mode for corticosteroid response whereas Armaly[9] proposed a polygenic inheritance for POAG, with the gene for the topical corticosteroid response being one of the genes involved. Suggestions that nongenetic factors play a major role were supported by a twin heritability study of monozygotic and like-sex dizygotic twins which revealed a low estimate of heritability.[4,10-12]

The Culprits: Corticosteroids

Corticosteroids are primarily used for their anti-inflammatory properties, and the pressure inducing side effect is considered to be in direct proportion to the anti-inflammatory potency of the various steroid formulations.

Kitazawa et al demonstrated that the pressure inducing potency of the corticosteroids is related to the dosage of the drug. In their study with high topical steroid responders, 0.01 percent betamethasone caused significantly less pressure elevation than a 0.1 percent concentration.[15]

Studies conducted on animals have shown that the formulations may also have varying pressure inducing and anti-inflammatory effects, with a 0.1 percent dexamethasone acetate preparation having a better anti-inflammatory effect than 0.1 percent dexamethasone alcohol or a sodium phosphate and both acetate and sodium phosphate having the same effect on IOP.

Flurandrenolide, a less commonly used corticosteroid, has also been reported to cause steroid induced glaucoma.[16]

ROUTES OF ADMINISTRATION AND PRESSURE RESPONSE

Topical therapy: In the form of drops or ointment steroids applied directly to the eye or to the skin of the eyelids are associated with an increase in IOP.[17,18] This is more often associated with an IOP rise than with systemic therapy.[19-21]

Periocular therapy: Subconjunctival, subtenon's, or retrobulbar injections of steroids,[22-26] particularly the long acting corticosteroids are the most potent route of administration in regards to steroid induced glaucoma. The patients acceptance of an earlier topical corticosteroid therapy is not a correct predictor of the nature of response to the periocular therapy.[25] The repository preparations are particularly dangerous because of their long duration of action and the future need for a surgical excision of the remaining drug before the pressure are brought under control.[24-27] The repositories should therefore be always injected in an inferior quadrant so as to facilitate an easy excision if required and also not to compromise the superior site for a future filtering surgery should the need arise.

Intraocular therapy: Intravitreal injections of triamcinolone acetonide, for the treatment of intraocular neovascular or inflammatory disease, have been documented to cause an elevation in the IOP by several mm Hg in most cases. This spike is seen usually within 3 to 4 weeks of initiating treatment.[28-30]

Systemic therapy: Systemic absorption of the corticosteroids is the least likely form of steroid administration to cause an increase in the IOP.[26-35] Of the systemic routes besides oral administration even **inhalation and nasal corticosteroids and skin applications at areas remote from the eye[34-38] can also increase the IOP.**

CLINICAL PRESENTATION

Typically raised IOP is seen with topical, periocular, or oral steroid therapy.

IOP usually gets elevated within a few weeks of potent topical ocular corticosteroid or in months with weaker steroid preparations. The patient is asymptomatic at presentation and the diagnosis is made on the basis of clinical findings corroborating with a history of steroid usage. The picture resembles that of open angle glaucoma with normal appearing anterior chamber and open angles on gonioscopy.[40,41] The IOP is elevated with the optic disc showing glaucomatous damage, the extent depending on the duration of elevated IOP before diagnosis. An intensive systemic steroid therapy can result in an acute presentation with the pressure rise seen within hours after steroid administration,[39] this being the rarer type of presentation.

Children especially less than 6 years of age have been shown to be greater steroid-responders as compared with adults. Incidents of increased IOP in children on treatment of external diseases with nasal or inhalational steroids have been reported.[42]

IOP elevation in the first few weeks after a glaucoma filtering surgery despite a good filtering bleb has been attributed to influence of topical steroid therapy.[43] Concomitant use of postoperative steroids after laser refractive surgery can lead to advanced optic nerve damage as a result steroid induced elevated IOP misdiagnosed as normal IOP due to decreased central corneal thickness, changes in ocular rigidity and corneal edema.[44-49]

MECHANISM OF GLAUCOMA

There is a uniform consensus amongst researchers that the IOP elevation due to steroid administration results from reduction in facility of aqueous outflow.[50-52] The dispute is with regards to the precise mechanism responsible for the reduction in outflow. Studies on cultured human trabecular cells and rabbit eyes[53-56] suggest that the

trabecular and anterior uveal tissue have a high concentration of glucocorticoid receptors and probably represent the target tissue in the steroid induced mediation of reduced aqueous outflow facility.

Influence on Phagocytosis

TM cells are actively phagocytic and help in the removal of debris, pigment and other materials from the aqueous outflow drainage pathway. A decrease in phagocytic activity has been proposed in the pathogenesis of steroid-induced glaucoma. Corticosteroids are known to suppress this phagocytic activity, resulting in deposition of debris in TM. This is supported by ultra structural studies showing marked depositions of amorphous material in TM.[57,58] Glucocorticoid receptor beta (GRbeta), can block dexamethasone (DEX) responsiveness in TM cells. The lower expression of GRbeta in glaucomatous TM cells may contribute to the altered phagocytic function of TM cells, and may lead to the increased aqueous humor outflow resistance mediated by glucocorticoids.[59]

Influence on Extracellular Matrix

The trabecular extracellular matrix contains glycosaminoglycans which are hyaluronidase sensitive. Hyaluronidase from lysosomes depolymerizes hyaluronate, resulting in breakdown of polymerized GAGs. The corticosteroids stabilize the lysosomal membrane leading to an accumulation of polymerized GAGs in the trabecular meshwork. Francois[60-62] postulated that GAGs in the polymerized form become hydrated, producing a 'biologic edema' that may increase resistance to aqueous outflow. Dexamethasone induced ocular hypertension has been produced in perfusion cultured human eyes, in which morphologic changes in the trabecular meshwork were similar to those reported in steroid-induced glaucoma and POAG.[63]

Dexamethasone also has been shown to increase the expression of the extracellular matrix protein fibronectin in cultured human TM cells,[64] a finding also seen in the outflow pathways of patients with POAG. It also caused the formation of cross linked actin network in the TM cytoskeleton.[65]

Genetic influences: Studies implicating POAG cases and their relatives as high responders to steroid therapy[1-3] and the subsequent discovery that the mutations in the genes for myocilin (MYOC) and optineurin (OPTN) proteins are associated with familial POAG have kindled interest in the search for the involvement of these genes in the human and in animal models of steroid induced glaucomas.

PREVENTION

The patient: Identification of at risk individuals is important.

- Individuals with POAG
- Family history of POAG
- Diabetics[66]
- Cases with connective tissue disorders[67]
- High myopes

General measures to be applied in all cases:

- Avoid steroids when a safer drug will suffice
- Use the least amount of steroid necessary
- Establishing a baseline IOP before initiating therapy
- Monitor the IOP closely for the entire duration of corticosteroid therapy.

MANAGEMENT
Use of Alternative Drugs
Usage of alternative drugs to corticosteroids in susceptible individuals. These include:

Nonadrenal Steroids
These constitute a group of drugs related to progesterone has been shown to have useful anti-inflammatory properties with significantly less pressure inducing effects than most corticosteroids. Medrysone has been describes as causing no IOP elevation,[68,69] but because of its limited corneal penetration, it is primarily used to treat extraocular diseases. Fluoromethalone (0.1%) though having a substantially less anti-inflammatory potency than corticosteroids.[70-72] is more efficacious than Medrysone in treating inflammation of the anterior segment. However, some conflicting reports even show a significant rise in IOP with Fluoromethalone therapy. The acetate derivative of Fluoromethalone has been found to be as effective as 1 percent prednisolone acetate.[71] Rimexolone 1 percent is a recent potent anti-inflammatory glucocorticoid with a reduced propensity to raise IOP. Like fluoromethalone it lacks a hydroxyl substitute at C21 position of its chemical structure. The anti-inflammatory efficacy is comparable to that of prednisolone acetate but is more similar to FML in its lesser effect on IOP elevation.[73]

Nonsteroidal Anti-inflammatory Drugs
Topical NSAIDS, acting through their inhibition of cyclo-oxygenase pathway, are effective in treating anterior segment inflammation, probably by reducing the breakdown of blood-aqueous barrier. Experiences with flurbiprofen[74] and biclofenac[75] indicate that these NSAID agents do not cause an elevation of IOP.

BOL-303242-X is a novel selective glucocorticoid receptor agonist under clinical evaluation for the treatment of inflammatory skin and eye diseases. Data from *in vitro* and *in vivo* studies suggest an improved side-effect profile of this compound compared to classical glucocorticoids.[76]

Discontinuation of Steroids
Discontinuation of the steroid is sometimes the only modality required. The more common chronic forms of steroid-induced elevation of IOP resolve in 1 to 4 weeks, and the acute forms within days of stopping the steroid.[41] François et al showed that in patients with a family history of glaucoma who were on steroid therapy, glaucoma persisted despite stopping all steroids.[40] Espildora et al demonstrated that the duration of steroid therapy also plays a role in reversal of IOP post steroid cessation, with all cases on steroid therapy for less than 2 months showing reversal of IOP on stopping steroids. IOP remained chronically elevated in all patients who used the steroid for more than 4 years.[77] If continued steroid therapy is essential, control of IOP by additional use of antiglaucoma medications or changing to a steroid with a lesser potential for IOP rise can be substituted.

In all cases where depot steroids appear to be responsible for the rise in IOP, excision of the depot steroid is indicated if medical management fails.[24-27] If the depot steroid cannot be removed because it is deemed essential or because of its location, filtering surgery may be indicated.

Management of Glaucoma
The medical management of these cases is essentially on the same lines as POAG.

Although published data were promising regarding the efficacy of Anecortave acetate (a cortisone, a synthetic molecule derived from cortisol acetate with angiostatic properties but devoid of glucocorticoid activity) for steroid-induced OHT, the decision to suspend trials for the treatment of POAG means that, at least for now, this therapeutic option is no longer being widely investigated. Filtering surgery or a glaucoma drainage device is indicated when glaucoma is uncontrolled on maximum tolerable medication.

Laser trabeculoplasty is not usually successful in lowering IOP.

REFERENCES

1. Becker B, Hahn KA. Topical corticosteroids and heredity in primary open-angle glaucoma. Am J Ophthalmol 1964;57:543.

2. Armaly MF. The heritable nature of dexamethasone-induced ocular hypertension. Arch Ophthalmol 1966; 75:32.

3. Armaly MF. Inheritance of dexamethasone hypertension and glaucoma. Arch Ophthalmol 1967;77:747.

4. Schwartz JT, Reuling FH, Feinleib M, et al. Twin study on ocular pressure after topical dexamethasone. 1. Frequency distribution of pressure response. Am J Ophthalmol 1973;76: 126.

5. Palmberg PF, Mandell A, Wilensky JT, et al. The reproducibility of the intraocular pressure response to dexamethasone. Am J Ophthalmol 1975;80:844.

6. Dean GO Jr, Deutsch AR, Hiatt RL. The effect of dexamethasone on borderline ocular hypertension. An Ophthalmol 1975;7:193.

7. Levene R, Wigdor A, Edelstein A, et al. Topical corticosteroid in normal patients and glaucoma suspects. Arch Ophthalmol 1967;77:593.

8. Becker B. The genetic problem of chronic simple glaucoma. Ann Ophthalmol 1971;3:351.

9. Schwartz JT, Reuling FH, Feinleib M, et al. Twin heritability study of the effect of corticosteroids on intraocular pressure. J Med Genet 1972;9:137.

10. Schwartz JT, Reuling FH Jr, Feinleib M, et al. Twin heritability study of the corticosteroid response. Trans Am Acad Ophthalmol Otol 1973;77:126.

11. Schwartz JT, Reuling FH, Feinleib M, et al. Twin study on ocular pressure following topically applied dexamethasone. Arch Ophthalmol 1973;90:281-6.

12. Akingbehin AO. Corticosteroid induced ocular hypertension. An acquired form. Br J Ophthalmol 1982;66:541.

13. Spaeth GL. Traumatic hyphema, angle recession, dexamethasone hypertension, and glaucoma. Arch Ophthalmol 1967;78:714.

14. Akingbehin AO. Corticosteroid-induced ocular hypertension. II. An acquired form. Br J Ophthalmol 1982;66:541-5.

15. Kitazawa Y. Increased intraocular pressure induced by corticosteroids. Am J Ophthalmol 1976;82:492.

16. Brubaker RF, Halpin JA. Open angle glaucoma associated with topical administration of fluandrenolide to the eye. Mayo Clin Proc 1975;50:322.

17. Cubey RB. Glaucoma following the application of corticosteroid to the skin of the eyelids. Br J Dermatol 1976;95:207.

18. Zugerman C, Sauders D, Levit F. Glaucoma from topically applied steroids. Arch Dermatol 1976;112:1326.

19. Vie R. Glaucoma and amaurosis associated with long-term application of topical corticosteroids to the eyelids. Acta Derm Venereol 1980;60:541.

20. Kalina RE. Increased intraocular pressure following subconjunctival corticosteroid administration. Arch Ophthalmol 1969;81:788.

21. Nozik RA. Periocular injection of steroids. Trans Am Acad Ophthalmol Otol 1972;76:695.

22. Herschler J. Intractable intraocular hypertension induced by repository triamcinolone acetonide. Am J Ophthalmol 1972;74:501.

23. Herschler J. Increased intraocular pressure induced by repository corticosteroids. Am J Ophthalmol 1976; 82:90.

24. Ferry AP, Harris WP, Nelson MH. Histopathologic features of subconjunctivally injected corticosteroids. Am J Ophthalmol 1987;103:716.

25. Akduman L, Kolker AE, Black DL, et al. Treatment of persistent glaucoma secondary tto periocular corticosteroids. Am J Ophthalmol 1996; 122:275.

26. Wingate RJ, Beaumont PE. Intravitreal triamcinolone and elevated intraocular pressure. Aust N Z J Ophthalmol 1999;27:431.

27. Bakri SJ, Beer PM. The effect of intravitreal triamcinolone acetonide on intraocular pressure. Ophth Surg Lasers Imaging 2003;32:386.

28. Jonas JB, Kressing I, Degenring R. Intraocular pressure after intravitreal injection of triamcinolone acetonide. Br J Ophthalmol 2003;87:24.

29. Stern JJ. Acute glaucoma during cortisone therapy. Am J Ophthalmol 1953;36:389.

30. Covell LL. Glaucoma induced by systemic steroid therapy. Am J Ophthalmol 1958;45:108.

31. Godel V, Feiler-Ofry V, Stein R. Systemic steroids and ocular fluid dynamics. I. Analysis of the sample as a whole: influence of dosage and duration of therapy. Acta ophthalmol 1972;50:655.

32. Godel V, Feiler-Ofry V, Stein R. Systemic steroids and ocular fluid dynamics. II. Systemic versus topical steroids. Acta Ophthalmol 1972;50:664.

33. Adhikary HP, Sells RA, Basu PK. Ocular complications of systemic steroid after renal transplantation and their association with HLA. Br J Ophthalmol 1982;66:290.

34. Opatowsky I, Feldman RM, Gross R, et al. Intraocular pressure elevation associated with inhalation and nasal corticosteroids. Ophthalmology 1995;102:177.

35. Schwartzenberg GW, Buys YM. Glaucoma secondary to topical use of steroid cream. Can J Ophthalmol 1999;34:222.

36. Spaeth GL, Rodrigues MM, Weinreb S. Steroid induced glaucoma. (A) Persistent elevation of intraocular pressure. (B) Histopathological aspects. Trans Am Ophthalmol Soc 1977;75:353.

37. Mitchell P, Cumming RG, Mackey DA. Inhaled corticosteroids, family history, and risk of glaucoma. Ophthalmology 1999;106:2301.

38. Francois J. Corticosteroid glaucoma. Ann Ophthalmol 1977;9:1075.

39. Weinreb RN, Polansky JR, Kramer SG, et al. Acute effects of dexamethasone on intraocular pressure in glaucoma. Invest Ophthalmol Vis Sci 1985;26:170.

40. Biedner B, David R, Grudsky A, et al. Intraocular pressure response to corticosteroids in children. Br J Ophthalmol 1980;64:430.

41. Gnad HD, Martenet AC. Congenitals Glaucoma and cortisone. Klin Monatsbl Augenheilkd 1973;162:86.

42. Desnoeck M, Casteels I, Casteels K. Intraocular pressure elevation in a child due to the use of inhalation steroids—a case report. Bull Soc Belge Ophthalmol 2001;280:97.

43. Wilensky JT, Snyder D, Gieser D. Steroid induced ocular hypertension in patients with filtering blebs. Ophthalmology 1980;87:240.

44. Morales J, Good D. Permanent glaucomatous visual loss after photorefractive keratectomy. J Cataract Refract Surg 1998;24:715.

45. Shaikh NM, Shaikh S, Singh K, et al. Progression to end stage glaucoma after laser in situ keratomileusis. J Cataract Refract Surg 2002;28:356.

46. Damji KF, Muni RH, Munger RM. Influence of corneal variables on accuracy of intraocular pressure measurement. J Glaucoma 2003;12:69.

47. Najman-Vainer J, Smith RJ, Maloney RK. Interface fluid after LASIK: misleading tonometry can lead to end stage glaucoma. J Cataract Refract Surg 2000;26:471.

48. Knorz MC. Flap and interface complications in LASIK. Curr Opin Ophthalmol 2002;13:242.

49. Hamilton DR, Manche EE, Rich LF, et al. Steroid induced glaucoma after LASIK associated with interface fluid. Ophthalmology 2002;109:659.

50. Armaly MF. Effect of corticosteroids on intraocular pressure and fluid dynamics. II. The effect of dexamethasone in the glaucomatous eye. Arch Ophthalmol 1963;70:492.

51. Miller D, Peczon JD, Whitworth CG. Corticosteroids and functions in the anterior segment of the eye. Am J Ophthalmol 1965;59:31.

52. Kupfer C, Ross K. Studies of aqueous humor dynamics in man. I. Measurements in young normal subjects. Invest Ophthalmol 1971;10:518-22.

53. Tchernitchin A, Wenk EJ, Hernandez, et al. Glucocorticoid localization by radioautography in the rabbit eye following systemic administration of 3H-Dexamethasone. Invest Ophthalmol 1980;19(10):1231-6.

54. Weinreb RN, Bloom E, Baxter JD, et al. Detection of glucocorticoid receptors in cultured human trabecular cells. Invest Ophthalmol Vis Sci 1980;19:1231.

55. McCarty GR, Schwartz B. Increased concentration of glucocorticoid receptors in rabbit iris-ciliary body compared to rabbit live. Invest Ophthalmol Vis Sci 1982;23:525.

56. Southren AL, Dominguez MO, Gordon GG, et al. Nuclear translocation of the cytoplasmic glucocorticoid receptor in the iris-ciliary body and adjacent corneoscleral tissue of the rabbit following topical administration of various glucocorticoids. Invest Ophthalmol Vis Sci 1983;24:147.

57. Rohen JW, Linner E, Witmer R. Electron microscopic studies on the trabecular meshwork in two cases of corticosteroid glaucoma. Exp Eye Res 1973;17:19.

58. Roll P, Benedikt O. Electron microscopic investigation of the trabecular meshwork in cortisone glaucoma. Klin Monatsbl Augenheilkd 1979;174:421.

59. Zhang X, Ognibene CM, et al. Dexamethasone inhibition of trabecular meshwork cell phagocytosis and its modulation by glucocorticoid receptor beta. Exp Eye Res 2007;84:275-84.

60. Francois J, Victoria-Troncoso V. Mucopolysaccharides and pathogenesis of cortisone glaucoma. Klin Monatsbl Augenheilkd 1974;165:5.

61. Francois J. The importance of the mucopolysaccharides in intraocular pressure regulation. Invest Ophthalmol 1975;14:173.

62. Francois J. Tissue culture of ocular fibroblasts. Am Ophthalmol 1975;11:1551.

63. Clark AF, Wilson K, de Kater AW, et al. Dexamethasone induced ocular hypertension in perfusion cultured human eyes. Invest Ophthalmol Vis Sci 1985;26:1093.

64. Steely HT, Browder SL, Julian MB, et al. The effects of dexamethasone on fibronectin expression in cultured human trabecular meshwork cells. Invest Ophthalmol Vis Sci 1992;33:2242.

65. Clark AF, Wilson K, McCartney MD, et al. Glucocorticoid induced formation of cross linked actin networks in cultured human trabecular meshwork cells. Invest Ophthalmol Vis Sci 1994;35:281.

66. Becker B. Diabetes mellitus and primary open angle glaucoma. Am J Ophthalmol 1966;62:1039.

67. Gaston H, Absolon MJ, Thurtle OA, et al. Steroid responsiveness in connective tissue diseases. Br J Ophthalmol 1983;67:487.

68. Bedrossian RH, Eriksen SP. The treatment of ocular inflammation with Medrysone. Arch Ophthalmol 1969;99:184.

69. Leibowitz HM, Ryan WJ Jr, Kupferman A. Comparative anti-inflammatory efficacy of topical corticosteroids with low glaucoma inducing potential. Arch Ophthalmol 1992;110: 118.

70. Mindel JS, Travitian HO, Smith H Jr, et al. Comparative ocular pressure elevation by medrysone, fluorometholone, and dexamethasone phosphate. Arch Ophthalmol 1980; 98:1577.

71. Morrison E, Archer DB. Effect of fluorometholone on the intraocular pressure of corticosteroid responders. Br J Ophthalmol 1984;68:581.

72. Stewart RH, Kimbrough RL. Intraocular pressure response to topically administered fluorometholone. Arch Ophthalmol 1979;97:2139.

73. Leibowitz HM, Bartlett JD, Rich R, et al. Intraocular pressure raising potential of 1% rimexolone in patients responding to corticosteroids. Arch Ophthalmol 1996;114:933-7.

74. Gieser DK, Hodapp E, Goldberg I, et al. Flurbiprofen and intraocular pressure. Ann Ophthalmol 1981;13:831.

75. Strelow SA, Sherwood MB, Broncato LJB, et al. The effect of diclofenac sodium ophthalmic solution on intraocular pressure following cataract extraction. Ophthalmic Surg 1992;23:170.

76. Zhang JZ, Cavet ME, VanderMeid KR, Salvador-Silva M, et al. Bol- 303242-X, a novel selective glucocorticoid receptor agonist with full anti-inflammatory properties in human ocular cells. Mol Vis 2009;15:1606-16.

77. Espildora J, Vicuna P, et al. Cortisone induced glaucoma: a report on 44 affected eyes. J Fr Ophthalmol 1981; 4:503.

36 | Glaucoma Associated with Penetrating Keratoplasty

Oswald Rondón

INTRODUCTION

Glaucoma in the setting of a corneal transplant may not be as common as other glaucomas, but it is nonetheless of noteworthy importance. Glaucoma is one of the most serious complications after penetrating keratoplasty (PK) **(Figure 1)** because of its significant incidence and severity, and the difficulty in its diagnosis and treatment. Postkeratoplasty glaucoma represents the 2nd leading cause of graft failure after graft rejection.

THE CHALLENGE

The 1st challenge in post-PK glaucoma management is accurate determination of the intraocular pressure (IOP). Goldmann applanation tonometry is the accepted gold standard of IOP measurement, but in patients with PKs Goldmann applanation can be difficult due to the irregular astigmatism that is often present postoperatively. The irregular astigmatism can make interpretation of the mires problematic. Two alternatives to Goldmann applanation are pneumatic tonometry and the Tonopen®. Pneumatic tonometry and the Tonopen® can be effective because they do not depend on a uniform cornea for accurate measurements. If the latter two

are not options then two-finger tension tono-metry is always an option, especially if the patient's fellow eye is normal and thus can be used as a standard (Other techniques have been mentioned in detail in the chapter on tonometry).

EPIDEMIOLOGY

The incidence of post-PK glaucoma is quite important. Reported incidences of IOP elevation in both early and late postoperative periods vary considerably. Karesh et al reported the incidence of early and late (greater than 3 months postoperative) IOP elevation at 31 and 23 percent, respectively.[1] Foulks et al reported incidences of immediate and chronic (persistently elevated after 2 days requiring medical treatment) IOP elevation of 9 percent and 18 percent, respectively.[2] França et al reported an incidence of 21.5 percent.[3]

RISK FACTORS

Unfortunately, there are many risk factors for the development of post-PK glaucoma. The following have been identified as risk factors **(Box 1)**. One could reasonably argue that almost every patient that undergoes penetrating keratoplasty has a risk factor for the development of glaucoma!

MECHANISM OF GLAUCOMA
Early Postoperative Period

Early in the postoperative course, glaucoma after PK can have the same pressure elevating mechanisms as that are associated with other intraocular procedures: uveitis, hemorrhage,

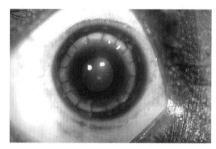

Fig. 1 Penetrating keratoplasty

Box 1 Risk factors for post-PK glaucoma

- Age greater than 60
- Aphakia
- Pre-existing glaucoma
- Bullous keratopathy
- Herpetic keratitis
- Trauma
- Keratoconus
- Repeat PK
- Combined CE/PK (ICEE>ECCE)
- Vitrectomy at time of surgery
- Anterior segment reconstruction at time of surgery

pupillary block and steroid-induced glaucoma.

Late Postoperative Period

Late in the postoperative course glaucoma can be caused by peripheral anterior synechiae (PAS) formation and rarely epithelial downgrowth. However, there are two additional mechanisms of glaucoma that can occur that are unique to eyes that have undergone PK: collapse of the trabecular meshwork and compression of the anterior chamber angle.

Collapse of the Trabecular Meshwork

Collapse of the trabecular meshwork may result from loss of anterior support due to the incision in Descemet's membrane, which may be compounded in aphakia by reduction in posterior support from loss of zonular tension. This hypothesis has been supported by observation in one study that through-and-through suturing was associated with better outflow facility in autopsy eyes than conventional suturing.[4] Other studies, in contrast, have shown lower postoperative IOPs with superficial sutures. **The norm today by most corneal specialists is relatively superficial and not through-and-through suturing**.

Compression of AC Angle

The 2nd post-PK-specific mechanism leading to glaucoma is that of compression of anterior chamber (AC) angle. This occurrence may be caused by conventional techniques of PK, causing an early postoperative IOP rise and subsequent chronic glaucoma due to peripheral anterior synechiae.

Graft Size

Based on mathematical models it has been postulated that the following factors may minimize angle compression and also improve trabecular

support: donor graft that is larger than recipient trephine, looser or shorter suture bites to minimize tissue compression, smaller trephine size, thinner peripheral host cornea and larger host corneal diameter. Of the aforementioned donor graft size has been studied extensively. Reports have been conflicting as to whether an oversized corneal donor graft improves outflow and reduces postoperative glaucoma. A perfusion study with autopsy eyes did not reveal an improvement outflow facility, and the use of 0.5 mm oversized grafts in one clinical series did not afford any protection against postoperative glaucoma.[5] However, other studies have shown that oversized grafts are associated with deeper anterior chambers, lower incidence of progressive angle closure, and lower postoperative IOPs compared with eyes with same sized grafts.

MEDICAL MANAGEMENT

Medical treatment should always be tried first, unless a specific, treatable condition, such as pupillary block, is apparent. The standard topical antiglaucoma regimen is generally accepted keeping in mind that antiglaucoma medications can cause surface toxicity.

A topical medication of particular interest is dorzolamide. Case reports have stated that dorzolamide may cause corneal decompensation in patients with compromised endothelial function.[6] The long-term effect of dorzolamide on endothelial function is still under study.

SURGICAL MANAGEMENT

In the realm of surgical management the 1st option is laser trabeculoplasty. Laser trabeculoplasty can be quite effective but it requires a clear graft and an open anterior chamber angle.

The other step in management is incisional surgery. No glaucoma operation has been found to be entirely suitable for controlling IOP and preserving graft clarity.

If the superior conjunctiva is sufficiently mobile and there is good visual potential then trabeculectomy is the initial surgery of choice. The most recent study showed that when trabeculectomy with mitomycin-C (MMC) was performed after PK there was a 73 percent (19/26) success rate.[7] Success was defined as IOP ≤ 21 with or without medications. The graft clarity rate was 69.2 percent (18/26). Mean follow-up was 22.3 months. When concomitant PK/Trab with MMC was studied, one series of 24 eyes found that the cumulative probability of corneal graft survival was 85 percent at 1 year and 60 percent at 2 years.[8] The cumulative probability of adequate IOP control was 67 percent at 3 months, 55 percent at 12 months, and 50 percent at 24 months.

If the health of the superior conjunctiva is not optimal enough for a trabeculectomy but there is good visual potential a glaucoma drainage implant (GDI) is the surgery of choice. However, placement of a GDI into the AC may be complicated by tube cornea touch with subsequent endothelial decompensation. In one series 70 percent and 55 percent of PKs survived at 2 and 3 years, respectively after GDI placement into the AC.[9] A retrospective review of simultaneous PK and GDI showed 92 and 50 percent graft success and 92 and 86 percent IOP control at 1 and 3 years, respectively.[10] Pars plana insertion is a reasonable option (GDI with PPV). This approach avoids complications related to AC placement but the trade-off is introduction of posterior segment complications. In a study of 34 patients complete success at 1 year and 2 years, respectively, after both GDI and PK were 63 percent and 33 percent.[11] Success rates for IOP control and corneal graft clarity were 85 and 62 percent, and 64 percent and 41 percent, respectively. One or more posterior segment complications occurred in 15 (44%) patients.

For patients with poor visual potential or for those who cannot undergo surgery transcleral ciliary body ablation is the procedure of choice.

Cyclocryotherapy was once the most commonly used surgical procedure for glaucoma after PK. Because of the high incidence of serious complications transcleral cyclophotocoagulation (CPC) has largely replaced cryotherapy. In one series of 39 patients, 77 percent had a final IOP between 7 and 21 mm Hg, but 44 percent of those with clear grafts before CPC had graft decompensation.[12] Interestingly, in a study which compared trabeculectomy with MMC, GDI, and CPC in the management of intractable glaucoma after PK no differences were found among the three glaucoma procedures with respect to controlling IOP and graft failure.[13] There was a trend for patients treated with CPC to have a higher incidence of graft failure, hypotony, and visual loss by more than one line, although this was not statistically significant.

Surgical options
• Trabeculectomy (with antimetabolites)
• Glaucoma drainage Implants
• Trans scleral ciliary body ablation
• Cyclocryotherapy
• Cyclophotocoagulation

CONCLUSION

In conclusion, glaucoma is one of the most serious complications after a penetrating keratoplasty. Its incidence and severity is substantial. There are many therapeutic medical and surgical options for management but despite the many treatment options available postoperative glaucoma can be difficult to manage.

REFERENCES

1. Karesh JW, Nirankari VS. Factors associated with glaucoma after penetrating keratoplasty. Am J Ophthalmol 1983;96:160.

2. Foulks GN. Glaucoma associated with penetrating keratoplasty. Ophthalmology 1987;94:871.

3. França ET, Arcieri ES, Arcieri RS. A study of glaucoma after penetrating keratoplasty. Cornea 2003;22:91.

4. Zimmerman TJ, Waltman SR, Sachs U. Intraocular pressure after aphakic penetrating keratoplasty "through-and-through" suturing. Ophthalmic Surg 1979;10:49.

5. Zimmerman TJ, Krupin T, Grodzki W. Size of donor corneal button and outflow facility in aphakic eyes. Am Ophthalmol 1979;11:809.

6. Konowal A, Morrison JC, Brown SV. Irreversible corneal decompensation in patients treated with topical dorzolamide. Am J Ophthalmol 1999;127:403.

7. Ishioka M, Shimazoki J, Yamagami J, Fyshima H. Trabeculectomy with mitomycin-C for postkeratoplasty glaucoma. British J Ophthalmol 2000;84:714.

8. WuDunn D, Alfonso E, Palmberg PF. Combined penetrating keratoplasty and trabeculectomy with mitomycin-C. Ophthalmology 1999;106:396.

9. Kwon YH, Taylor JM, Hong S. Long-term results of eyes with penetrating keratoplasty and glaucoma drainage implant. Ophthalmology 2001;108:272.

10. Al Torbak A. Graft survival and glaucoma outcome after simultaneous penetrating keratoplasty and Ahmed glaucoma valve implant. Cornea 2003;22:194.

11. Sidoti PA, Mosny AY, Ritterband DC, Seedor JA. Pars plana tube insertion of glaucoma drainage implants and penetrating keratoplasty in patients with glaucoma and corneal disease. Ophthalmology 2001;108:1050.

12. Threlkeld AB, Shields MB. Non- contact transcleral Nd:YAG cyclophotocoagulation for glaucoma after penetrating keratoplasty. Am J Ophthalmol 1995;120:569.

13. Ayyala RS, Pieroth L, Vinals AF, Schuman JS, Netland PA, Dreyer EB, Cooper ML, Mattox CG, Frangie JP, Wu HK, Zurakowski D. Comparison of mitomycin-C trabeculectomy, glaucoma drainage implant, laser neodymium: YAG cyclophotocoagulation in management of glaucoma after penetrating keratoplasty. Ophthalmology 1998;105:1550.

37

Glaucoma in Corneal Disorders

Ashish Bacchav, R Ramakrishnan

CHAPTER OUTLINE

❖ Iridocorneal Endothelial Syndrome
❖ Posterior Polymorphous Dystrophy
❖ Fuchs Endothelial Dystrophy
❖ Peters Anomaly

INTRODUCTION

Corneal disorders and glaucoma may coexist in many conditions. These may be grouped under three categories:

- Common anterior segment abnormalities.
- Corneal endothelial abnormalities resulting from glaucoma.
- A primary corneal abnormality.

We shall discuss the most common disorders.

IRIDOCORNEAL ENDOTHELIAL SYNDROME

Terminology

The term iridocorneal endothelial syndrome was suggested by Eagle and Yanoff[1-3] to denote a spectrum of disease that is characterized by a primary corneal endothelial abnormality leading to the formation of a membrane over the anterior surface of the iris and angle. It comprises corneal edema, anterior chamber angle changes, alterations in the iris and secondary angle closure glaucoma without pupillary block.

Variations within the ICE syndrome have been classified primarily on the basis of changes in the iris.

Essential Iris Atrophy

Described by Harms[4] in 1903, it is characterized by atrophy of the iris with hole formation. Also called as progressive iris atrophy.

Chandler Syndrome

It differs from essential iris atrophy in that changes in the iris are limited to slight corectopia and mild stromal atrophy.[5] Corneal edema, often with normal intraocular pressure in seen.

Cogan-Reese Syndrome

Described by Cogan and Reese in 1969,[6] it is characterized by nodular pigmented lesions of the iris associated with some features of ICE syndrome.

General Features

The ICE syndrome usually is clinically unilateral, however, subclinical abnormalities of the corneal endothelium can be seen in the fellow eye. Bilateral clinical manifestations, though rare, have been reported.

It usually presents in third to fifth decade and is more common in women. Familial cases are rare and there are no associated systemic diseases.

The most common presenting manifestations are abnormalities of the iris, reduced visual acuity, and pain.[7-9]

Clinical Features
Corneal Changes

Corneal endothelial abnormalities may be seen by slit-lamp biomicroscopy as a fine hammered-silver appearance of the posterior cornea.

There may be corneal edema with variable degrees of reduced vision and pain. Corneal edema occurs at normal IOP or at slightly elevated levels.

Specular microscopy shows diffuse abnormality of the corneal endothelial cells, with various degrees of pleomorphism in size and shape, dark areas within the cells, and loss of the clear hexagonal margins. These typical endothelial cells are called ICE cells.[10-13]

These endothelial cells appear dark by specular microscopy except for a light central spot and a light peripheral zone. Cells clustered together, forming a continuum are called as ICE tissue. This gives the appearance of a negative of normal corneal endothelium.

Varied and complex alterations of cells lining multilayered collagenous tissue posterior to Descemets membrane have been seen on electron microscopy in advanced cases.[14]

On histology, the ICE cells are rounded and hexagonal with numerous microvilli on the apical surface, tonofilaments in the cytoplasm, and indentations on the basal surface containing clumps of fibrillar collagenous material. Some studies have found their structure similar to epithelial cells.[15]

Anterior Chamber Angle

Peripheral anterior synechiae, usually extending to or beyond Schwalbe's line are characteristic. These are produced due to the contraction of the cellular membrane that extends down from the cornea to the angle of the anterior chamber and iris. Initially, it may cover an open angle in some areas with PAS in other parts. Slowly the PAS progress and close the entire angle. The IOP rises proportionally.

Iris

Iris changes constitute the primary basis for distinguishing the different variations of ICE syndrome.

Essential Iris Atrophy

It is characterized by diffuse iris atrophy, corectopia, polycoria and hole formation. The holes are of two types— **stretch holes and melting holes (Figure 1)**. In stretch holes, the iris is markedly thinned in the quadrant away from the direction of pupillary distortion, and the holes develop within the area that is being stretched.[7,15] In other eyes, melting holes develop without associated corectopia or thinning of the iris. This is due to a cellular membrane on portions of the anterior surface of the iris which is similar to and continuous with that seen over the anterior chamber angle. The membrane is most often found in the quadrant toward which the pupil is distorted.

Cogan-Reese Syndrome

It is by the presence of pigmented, pedunculated nodules on the surface of the iris with variable atrophy of the iris tissue **(Figure 2)**. The nodular lesions have an ultrastructure similar to that of the underlying stroma of the iris.[6]

Chandlers Syndrome

It is characterized by minimal corectopia and mild atrophy of the stroma of the iris.[5]

Pathogenesis of ICE Syndrome

Campbell et al[16] proposed a membrane theory, according to which, the abnormality of the corneal endothelium is the primary defect in the ICE syndrome. The endothelial defect is responsible for corneal edema. It also leads to the proliferation of the cellular membrane across the anterior chamber angle and on the surface of the iris.

Contraction of this cellular membrane causes the formation of peripheral anterior synechiae, corectopia, and ectropion uvea. Stretching of the iris in the direction away from the corectopia, especially when the iris is anchored by peripheral anterior synechiae on both sides, contributes to the atrophy and hole formation, although additional factors, such as ischemia may also be involved. The cellular membrane is also believed to be responsible for the development of nodular lesions of the iris in Cogan-Reese syndrome, possibly by encircling and pinching off portions of the iris stroma to form the nodules. The associated glaucoma results from a secondary angle closure due to the formation of PAS. Additionally, the membrane may lead to a trabecular meshwork obstruction. The underlying condition that leads to the corneal endothelial changes is not known. A

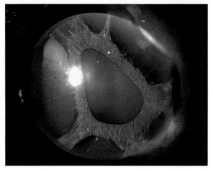

Fig. 1 Essential iris atrophy. Thinning of the iris with stretch holes and melting holes

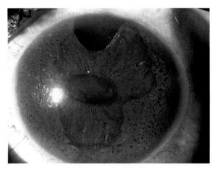

Fig. 2 Cogan-Reese syndrome. Characteristic pigmented, pedunculated nodules in the iris. Trabeculectomy has been done

viral etiology,[17,18] especially Epstein-Barr virus and Herpes Simpex virus has been postulated.

Differential Diagnosis

Fuchs endothelial dystrophy and posterior poymorphous dystrophy can be distinguished from ICE syndrome by the absence of characteristic iris and angle changes.

The Axenfeld-Rieger syndrome can be distinguished from ICE syndrome by its bilaterality, congenital nature and associated systemic findings.

Management

Patients require treatment for corneal edema and associated glaucoma.

Medical management of glaucoma involves reducing aqueous production. Drugs such as timolol maleate and carbonic anhydrase inhibitors have been tried successfully.

Topical carbonic anhydrase inhibitors should be avoided in case of low endothelial counts.

Filtering with antimetabolites is successful, although late failure may occur because of endothelialization of the filtering bleb. When medical treatment or conventional filtration surgery fails, glaucoma drainage implants appear to be an effective method for lowering IOP.

Corneal edema can be controlled by the use of hypertonic saline solutions and soft contact lenses. Irreversible chronic corneal edema requires penetrating keratoplasty once the glaucoma has been controlled.

POSTERIOR POLYMORPHOUS DYSTROPHY

Clinical Features

It is a bilateral, familial disorder of the corneal endothelium. Posterior polymorphous dystrophy (PPD) typically remains asymptomatic until adulthood. The inheritance pattern is usually autosomal dominant, and there is no race or sex predilection. The gene for *PPD, VSX1,* has been identified on chromosome 20.

Corneal Changes

Corneal changes are characterized by an appearance of vesicles on the posterior aspect of cornea at the level of the Descemet's membrane. They may be linear or present in groups, surrounded by an aureole of gray haze. There may be bandlike thickenings at the level of Descemet's membrane.[19]

On slit-lamp biomicroscopy and specular microscopy, two patterns of endothelial abnormality are seen. In one form, there are localized vesicular and band patterns resembling craters or doughnut-like lesions, with snail tracks. The cornea remains clear. In the other type of pattern, there is a geographic pattern with associated haze of Descemet's membrane and deep corneal stroma. It may be associated with iridocorneal adhesions and glaucoma.

Anterior Chamber Angle and Iris Changes

Broad peripheral anterior synechiae extending to or beyond Schwalbe's line, which may be associated with corectopia, ectropion uvea, and atrophy of the iris may be seen in some patients.

Pathogenesis

A membrane theory has been proposed for cases of PPD with iridocorneal adhesions.[20-22] It is postulated that a dystrophic endothelium, producing a basement membrane-like material, extends across the anterior chamber angle and onto the iris and subsequently, causes the synechiae formation and changes in the iris. The glaucoma may be caused by the iridocorneal adhesions in these cases. In many cases, the adhesions may bridge an open trabecular meshwork without obstructing the outflow. In the eyes with open angles, a high insertion of the anterior uvea may be present due to a developmental anamoly of the anterior chamber angle, similar to that seen in several of the developmental glaucomas and may be responsible for the subsequent collapse of the trabecular meshwork and glaucoma. In other cases, the mechanism of aqueous outflow obstruction may be the abnormal membrane covering the trabecular meshwork in an open angle.

Differential Diagnosis

These include Fuchs' endothelial dystrophy, congenital hereditary corneal dystrophy, and posterior amorphous corneal dystrophy. In PPD, there are diffuse gray-white, sheet like opacities of the posterior corneal stroma, with fine iris processes extending to Schwalbe's line, various abnormalities of the iris, but no glaucoma. In the presence of iridocorneal adhesions, Axenfeld-Rieger syndrome and the ICE syndrome should be considered as differential diagnosis.

Management

Most cases of PPD are asymptomatic and do not require any treatment.

Chronic corneal edema can be treated with hyperosmolar agents. Long standing corneal edema can be treated with keratoplasty.

The glaucoma may respond to drugs that lower aqueous production. Laser trabeculoplasty is not likely to be successful in these cases, and filtering surgery, generally is indicated when medical therapy is no longer adequate.

FUCHS ENDOTHELIAL DYSTROPHY

This clinical entity was described by Fuchs[27] in 1910 and the association with a dystrophy of the corneal endothelium was subsequently recognized.

It is a bilateral disorder occuring more commonly in women with an onset between 40 to 70 years of age.

There is a strong familial tendency, and an autosomal dominant inheritance pattern has been described.[28]

The gene for Fuchs' dystrophy, *COL8A2,* was identified on chromosome lp.

Clinical Features

Cornea guttata is a common condition, the incidence of which increases significantly with age.[23] Slit-lamp biomicroscopy reveals a beaten silver appearance of the central posterior cornea, similar to that seen in the ICE syndrome. Corneal stromal edema may be seen in some cases.

Specular microscopy shows enlarged endothelial cells with dark areas that overlap the cell borders.[24]

Histopathology and Pathogenesis

The primary pathology is an alteration in the corneal endothelium that leads to a deposition of collagen on the posterior surface of Descemet's membrane. Histologically, this may appear as warts or excrescences.

In some cases, focal accumulations may be covered by additional basement membrane or there may be a uniform thickening of the posterior collagen layers.[25,26] Edema of the corneal stroma and endothelium is seen.

Most of Fuchs' corneal endothelial dystrophy patients have a high incidence of angle-closure glaucoma due to the high incidence of axial hypermetropia and shallow anterior chambers. It was thought to be caused by a gradual thickening of the cornea and an eventual closure of the anterior chamber angle. However, later studies revealed an association between axial hypermetropia and shallow anterior chamber depth.

10 to 15 percent of patients with Fuchs' endothelial dystrophy have open-angle glaucoma.

Management

Glaucoma is usually not present in eyes with Fuchs' endothelial dystrophy. Treatment is directed towards the reduction of IOP. Even further reduction of a normal IOP may sometimes help to decrease the corneal edema.

Laser iridotomy is done in case of angle closure disease. Filtering procedures are done when medical therapy fails to control the IOP.

PETERS ANOMALY

Originally described by Peters in 1906,[29] it is characterized by bilateral central corneal opacities with adhesions from the iris to this defect.

The pattern of inheritance is autosomal recessive.

Clinical Features

It is usually present since birth. It is characterized by a central defect in

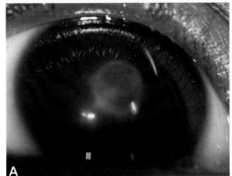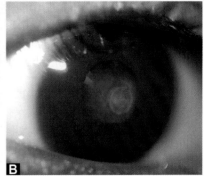

Figs 3A and B Peters anomaly

the Descemet's membrane and the endothelium with thinning and opacification of the corresponding area of corneal stroma **(Figures 3A and B)**. Iris adhesion extend to this defect. It may be associated with or without cataract and Axenfeld-Rieger syndrome. Over 50 percent of patients present with glaucoma, most commonly at birth.

Systemic Associations

Peters plus syndrome is a multiple malformation syndrome characterized by Peters anomaly of the eye and other extraocular defects including cleft palate, congenital heart defects, developmental delay, cleft lip and rarely meningoencephalocele and congenital hypothyroidism.[29-33]

Mechanism of Glaucoma

The mechanism of glaucoma is not clearly understood.

Anterior chamber dysgenesis in which abnormal cleavage of the anterior chamber occurs, may be responsible for glaucoma. Some cases may have presence of peripheral anterior synechiae which can cause glaucoma.

Differential Diagnosis

It must be distinguished from bilateral corneal opacities in infants. These include primary congenital glaucoma, mucopolysaccharidoses, congenital hereditary endothelial dystrophy and birth trauma.

Management

Children with bilateral corneal opacities must be screened for glaucoma.

Medical therapy can be tried initially before surgical intervention.

Surgical management includes trabeculectomy and trabeculotomy. These help maintain the IOP in milder forms. A drainage implant procedure is necessary when IOP is not controlled by the above measures.

Corneal opacities require penetrating keratoplasty, the results of which are often poor. Intractable glaucoma cases require cyclodestructive procedures such as diode laser cyclophotocoagulation.

Systemic examination and treatment of associations are often necessary.

AXENFELD RIEGER SYNDROME

Firstly, described by Axenfeld in 1902,[34] a case with prominent anteriorly displaced Schwalbe's line and tissue strands extending from it to this prominent line.

In 1932, Rieger[34-36] described similar cases in addition to iris atrophy, corectopia, polycoria and hole formation. These changes may be associated with developmental defects of the teeth and bones.

Axenfelds anomaly refers to presence of posterior embryotoxon on the cornea. Riegers anomaly includes peripheral abnormalities with additional changes of the iris like corectopia, polycoria and hole formation. Riegers syndrome includes ocular anomalies plus systemic developmental defects. Currently, the term Axenfeld-Rieger Syndrome is used for all clinical variations within this spectrum of developmental disorders.

Clinical Features

Inherited as an autosomal dominant trait, it presents as a bilateral developmental disorder of the eyes, with no gender and racial predilection. It has a high incidence of glaucoma. It may also be associated with systemic developmental defects.

Ocular Features

It usually involves the peripheral cornea, anterior chamber angle and the iris.

Cornea: Characteristically, it shows a prominent anteriorly displaced Schwalbe's line **(Figure 4)**. It may either be complete or just involve the temporal quadrant. Gonioscopy can also be done to visualize it. The cornea is otherwise normal.

Anterior Chamber Angle

The angle is open with few tissue strands bridging the angle from the peripheral iris to the Schwalbe's line. These iridocorneal adhesions are similar in color and texture to the iris tissue. These strands range from a few to many that may involve the entire circumference of the angle. The trabecular meshwork is visible, but the scleral spur is typically obscured by the peripheral iris which inserts into the posterior portion of the meshwork.

Iris

The iris features range from mild stromal thinning to marked atrophy, corectopia, polycoria and hole formation. In the presence of corectopia, the pupil is usually displaced towards a prominent peripheral tissue strand. The atrophy and hole formation occur in the quadrant away from the direction of the corectopia.

Glaucoma: More than 50 percent of the patients with Axenfeld-Rieger syndrome develop glaucoma. The clinical presentation most commonly is seen in childhood. The presence of iris defects and iridocorneal endothelial strands does not correlate to the presence and severity of glaucoma.

Developmental Defects

These include deformities of the teeth and facial bones. The dental anomalies include microdontia, hypodontia and oligodontia. The most common teeth are the anterior maxillary primary and permanent central incisors.[37-39] Facial anomalies include maxillary hypoplasia, flattening of midface, receeding upper lip and a prominent lower lip. Hypertelorism, telecanthus, micrognathia and mandibular prognathism have also been described.[40,41] Other occasional associations include pituitary anomalies, redundant periumblical skin, hypospadias, heart defects and skeletal disorders.

Pathogenesis

A developmental arrest of certain neural crest cells occurring late in the gestation has been postulated as the mechanism of A-R syndrome.[42] There is an abnormal retention of the primordial endothelial layer on the portions of the iris and anterior chamber and alterations in the aqueous outflow structures. The retained endothelium with associated basement membrane is believed to form an iridocorneal membrane, the contraction

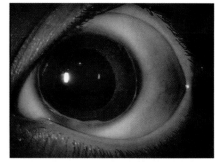

Fig. 4 Posterior embryotoxon in Axenfeld-Rieger syndrome

of which leads to iris changes and glaucoma.

The neural crest cells also gives rise to most of the mesenchyme related to the forebrain and pituitary gland, bones of the facial part.

Differential Diagnosis

Iridocorneal endothelial syndrome: It is unilateral, absence of family history, onset in young adulthood distinguish ICE from A-R syndrome.

Peters anomaly: Peters anamoly almost always involves the central cornea, however, rarely the two can coexist.

Aniridia: Presence of partial iris tissue and anterior chamber abnormalities may help distinguish it from A-R syndrome.

Management

Glaucoma management is the prime concern in A-R syndrome.

Almost 50 percent of these patients develop glaucoma, which develops in childhood or early adulthood.

Medical management includes drugs that reduce aqueous production. Beta blockers, carbonic anhydrase inhibitors have been tried.

Surgical management includes goniotomy, trabeculotomy and trabeculectomy. Trabeculectomy has been tried with good success.

REFERENCES

1. Eagle RC Jr, Font RL, Yanoff M, et al. Proliferative endotheliopathy with iris abnormalities: the iridocorneal endothelial syndrome. Arch Ophthalmol 1979;97:2104.

2. Yanoff M, Shields MB, McCracken JS, Klintworth GK, et al. Corneal edema in essential iris atrophy. Ophthalmology 1979;86:1549.

3. Yanoff M. Iridocorneal endothelial syndrome: unification of a disease spectrum. Surv Ophthalmol 1979;24:1.

4. Harms C. Einseitige spontane Luckenbildung der Iris durch Atrophie ohne mechanische Zerrung. Klin Monatsbl Augenheilkd 1903;41:522.

5. Chandler PA. Atrophy of the stroma of the iris: endothelial dystrophy, corneal edema, and glaucoma. Am J Ophthalmol 1956;41:607.

6. Cogan DG, Reese AB. A syndrome of iris nodules, ectopic Descemet's membrane, and unilateral glaucoma. Doc Ophthalmol 1969;26:424.

7. Wilson MC, Shields MB. A comparison of the clinical variations of the iridocorneal endothelial syndrome. Arch Ophthalmol 1989;107:1465.

8. Shiellds MB, Campbell DG, Simmons RJ. The essential iris atrophies. Am J Ophthalmol 1978;85:749.

9. Shield MB. Progressive essential iris atrophies, Chandlers syndrome and iris nevus syndrome: a spectrum of disease: Surv Ophthalmol 1979;24:3.

10. Setala K, Vannas A. Corneal endothelial cells in essential iris atrophy. A specular microscopic study. Acta Ophthlamol 1979;57:1929.

11. Hirst LW, Quigley HA, Stark WJ, Shields MB. Specular microscopy of iridocorneal endothelial syndrome, Am J Ophthalmol 1980;89:11.

12. Neubauer L, Lund O-E, Leibowitz HM. Specular microscopic appearance of the corneal endothelium in iridocorneal endothelial syndrome. Arch Ophthalmol 1983;101:916.

13. Bourne WM. Partial corneal involvement in the iridocorneal endothelial syndrome. Arch Ophthalmol 1982;94:774.

14. Rodrigues MM, Stulting RD, Waring GO III. Clinical, electron microscopic and immunohistochemical study of the corneal endothelium and Descemets membrane in the iridocorneal endothelial syndrome. Am J Ophthalmol 1986;101:16.

15. Lee WR, Marshal GE, Kirkness CM. Corneal endothelial cell abnormalities in an early stage of the iridocorneal endothelial syndrome. Br J Ophthalmol 1994;78:624.

16. Campbell DG, Shields MB, Smith TR. The corneal endothelium and the spectrum of essential iris atrophy. Am J Ophthalmol 1978;86:317.

17. Tsai CS, Ritch R, Strauss SE, et al. Antibodies to Epstein-Barr virus in iridocorneal endothelial syndrome. Arch Ophthalmolo 1990;108:1572.

18. Alvarado JA, Underwood JL, Green WR, et al. Detection of Herpes simplex viral DNA in the iridocorneal endothelial syndrome. Arch Ophthalmol 1994;112:1601.

19. Cibis GW, Tripathi RC. The differential diagnosis of Descemets Tears (Haabs striae) and posterior polymorphous dystrophy bands. A clinicopathologis study. Ophthalmology 1982;89:614.

20. Cibis GW, Krachmer JA, Phelps CD, Weingeist TA. The clinical spectrum of posterior polymorphous dystrophy. Arch Ophthalmol 1977;95:1529.

21. Krachmer JH. Posterior polymorphous corneal dystrophy: a disease characterised by epithelial like endothelial cells which influence management and prognosis. Trans Am Ophthalmol Soc 1985;83:413.

22. Threlkeld AB, Green WR, Quigley HA, et al. A clinicopathologic study of posterior polymorphous dystrophy: implications of pathogenetic mechanism of associated glaucoma. Tr Am Ophthalmol Soc 1994;92:133.

23. Laing RA, Leibowitz HM, Oak SS, et al. Endothelia mosaic in Fuchs dystrophy. A qualitative evaluation with the specular microscope. Arch Ophthamol 1981;99:80.

24. Lorenzetti DWC, Uotila MH, Parikh N, Kaufman HE. Central cornea guttata. Incidence in the general population. Am J Ophthalmol 1967;64:1155.

25. Mangovern M, Beauchamp GR, McTigue JW, et al. Inheritance of Fuchs combine dystrophy. Ophthalmology 1979;86:1879.

26. Rodrigues MM, Krachmer JH, Hackett J, et al. Fuchs' corneal dystrophy. A clinicopathologic study of the variation in corneal edema. Ophthalmology 1986;93:789.

27. Fuchs E. Dystrophis epithelialis corneal. Arch Ophthalmol 1910;76:478.

28. Mangovern M, Beauchamp GR, McTigue JW, et al. Inheritance of Fuchs combine dystrophy. Ophthalmology 1979;86:1879.

29. Hirst LW, Waring GO III. Clinical specular microscopy of posterior polymorphous endothelial dystrophy. Am J Ophthalmol 1983;95:145.

30. Kivlin JD, Fineman RM, Crandall AS, Olson RJ. Peters anomaly as a consequence of genetic and nongenetic syndromes. Arch Ophthalmol 1986;194:61.

31. Van Schooneveld MJ, Delleman JW, Beemer FA, Bleeler-Wagemakers EM. Peters plus: a new syndrome: Ophthalmolo Pediatr Genet 1984;4:141.

32. Traboulsi EI, Maumenee IH. Peters anomaly and associated congenital malformations. Arch Ophthalmol 1992;110:1739.

33. Sullivan TJ, Clarke MP, Heathcote JG, et al. Multiple congenital contractures in association with Peters anomaly and chorioretinal colobomata. J Peditr Ophthalmol Strabismus 1992;29:370.

34. Rieger H. Demonstration von cwei: Fallen von Verlagerung and Schlitzform der Pupille mit Hypoplasie des Irisvorderblattes an beinden Augen einer 10 und 25 jahrigen Patientin. Z Augenheilk 1934; 84:98.

35. Rieger H. Beitrage zur Kenntnis seltener Missbildungen der Iris. II. Uber Hypoplasie des Irisvorderblattes mit Verlangerung and Entrundung der Pupille. Grefes Arch Clin Exp Ophthalmol 1935;133:602.

36. Rieger H. Dysgenesi mesodermalis Corneae et Iridis. Z Augenheik 1935; 86:333.

37. Mathis H. Zahnunterzahl and Missbildungen der Iris. Z Stomatol 1936;34:895.

38. Rieger H. Erbfragen in der Augenheilkunde. Graefes Arch Clin Exp Ophthalmol 1941;143:277.

39. Wesley RK, Baker JD, Golnick AL. Riegers syndrome clinical features and report of an isolated case. J Peditr Ophthalmolo Strabismus 1978;15:67.

40. Alkemade PPH. Dysgenesis Mesodermalis of the iris and the Cornea. Assen, Netherlands, Charles C Thomas, 1969.

41. Piper HF, Schwinger E, Von Dormarus H. Dysplasia of the limbus cornea, the mesodermal iris layer and the facial skeleton in one family. Klin Monastsbl Augenheillkd 1985;186:287.

42. Sheilds MB. Axenfeld-Rieger syndrome. A theory of mechanism and distinctions from the iridocorneal endothelial syndrome. Trans Am Ophthalmol Soc 1983;81:736.

38 Glaucoma Associated with Intraocular Tumors

Ashish Kumar, R Ramakrishnan

CHAPTER OUTLINE

- Tumors of the Primary Uveal Melanomas
- Benign Tumors of the Anterior Uvea
- Systemic Malignancies
- Ocular Tumors of Childhood
- Phacomatosis
- Management of Tumor Induced Glaucoma

A variety of intraocular tumors and pseudotumors can give rise to glaucoma.[1] The most common tumors include uveal melanoma, uveal metastasis, and retinoblastoma. Patients with these tumors are often treated for the glaucoma, while the underlying neoplasm remains unsuspected, causing a delay in diagnosis that may have serious consequences.

Tumor-induced glaucomas are almost always unilateral and the mechanism can vary with the size and extent of the tumor. For patients with an intraocular malignancy, the emphasis shifts from the prevention of blindness to the preservation of life, while care must be taken in eyes with benign lesions to avoid loss of vision from unnecessary treatment. In one survey of 2597 patients with intraocular tumors, five percent of the tumor containing eyes had tumor-induced elevated intraocular pressure (IOP) at the time of diagnosis of the tumor.[1]

TUMORS OF THE UVEAL TRACT
Primary Uveal Melanomas
Melanomas of the uveal tract, the most common primary intraocular malignancy, are frequently associated with

glaucoma with an overall prevalence of 20 percent.[2] Anterior uveal melanomas lead to IOP elevation more frequently than posterior melanomas, with reports of 41[2] and 45 percent[3] in two series, while choroidal melanomas with 14 percent in one study.[2] A clinical series from an oncology service in which 3 percent of 2111 eyes with uveal melanomas had associated IOP elevation, including 7 percent with iris melanomas, 17 percent with ciliary body melanomas, and 2 percent with choroidal melanomas.[1]

Clinical Presentations
Iris Melanoma[4]
Usually, it appears as a well-circumscribed variably pigmented, stationary or slowly growing lesion that does not significantly alter IOP. However, it can occupy enough of the trabecular meshwork to produce glaucoma. Much less common is the diffuse iris melanoma, which characteristically produce a classic syndrome of unilateral acquired hyperchromic heterochromia and ipsilateral glaucoma. Slit lamp and gonioscopic examinations reveal a slightly elevated, brown mass, diffuse or patchy pigmented lesion on the iris stroma. However, some may be

amelanotic, often associated some with secondary vasculature.

Ciliary Body Melanoma
Melanomas of the anterior uveal tract most often arise from the ciliary body and tend to attain a fairly large size before diagnosis. They may be difficult to visualize directly, often presenting as a smooth-domed elevation of the overlying iris. Wide dilatation, however, may allow gonioscopic visualization, which is typically seen as a chocolate-brown mass between the iris and lens, sometimes with anterior displacement of the peripheral iris in the anterior chamber angle.

Choroidal Melanoma
Clinically, choroidal melanomas appear as a variably pigmented mass that can produce a secondary nonrhegmatogenous retinal detachment. A rather specific clinical feature in many cases is the *mushroom* shape, which occurs when the tumor breaks through Bruch's membrane. The finding of a retinal detachment and glaucoma in the same eye, therefore, should alert the clinician to the possibility of an underlying malignant melanoma.

Pathology of Uveal Melanoma

Most circumscribed iris melanomas are composed of spindle-shaped melanoma cells with occasional epithelioid cells in contrast to diffuse ones which have a greater proportion of more malignant epithelioid cells and carry a worse systemic prognosis.

Ciliary body melanomas contain both spindle and epithelioid cells, but the proportion of epithelioid cells is greater than in iris melanomas. Choroidal melanomas can be composed of spindle cells, epithelioid cells or any combination of the two.

Mechanism of Glaucoma

Melanomas of the anterior uvea may lead to glaucoma by either open angle or angle closure mechanism, with the former being more common. Aqueous humor outflow in the open anterior chamber angle can be obstructed by the direct extension of the tumor, or by seeding of tumor cells or melanin granules.

In some eyes, the melanoma may arise either from iris, ciliary body or the iridociliary junction and spread circumferentially, creating a **ring melanoma**. It may extend posteriorly, causing a retinal detachment and mimick a choroidal tumor. Macrophages containing melanin from a necrotic melanoma may obstruct the trabecular meshwork, condition referred to as **melanomalytic glaucoma**.[5]

Most common mechanism of glaucoma for both types of iris melanoma is direct invasion of the trabecular meshwork by tumor tissue.

Another variation of anterior uveal melanoma associated with glaucoma is **tapioca melanoma**. This rare melanoma of the iris creates a nodular appearance resembling tapioca pudding.[6] Another reported mechanism of IOP elevation with an iris melanoma is neovascular glaucoma.[7]

Choroidal melanomas may present with acute angle closure glaucoma due to the forward displacement of the lens-iris diaphragm by a large posterior tumor, commonly associated with a total retinal detachment. Other reported mechanism of IOP elevation in association with choroidal melanomas include neovascular glaucoma (56%) and pigment dispersion in the vitreous with melanomalytic glaucoma.[8]

Differential Diagnosis

The changes associated with melanoma may mask the underlying melanoma, while other mass lesions may simulate an anterior uveal melanoma.

Iritis: Iritis may appear to be present in some cases of glaucoma and melanoma, usually representing tumor cells in the anterior chamber.[3] While other eyes may have primary iritis with inflammatory nodules simulating malignancy.

Primary cyst of the iris: Most common lesion to be confused with melanoma.

Iris nevi: Especially difficult to distinguish not only clinically, but also, histologically.

> **Note** Choroidal melanomas may be masked by conditions presenting as intraocular inflammation and hemorrhage due to necrosis of the tumors.

Diagnostic Adjuncts
Ultrasonography

It is useful for differentiating ciliary body melanoma or choroidal melanoma when masked by retinal detachment, vitreous hemorrhage or other opacity in the ocular media, but, not with other masses of the posterior ocular segment.

Radioactive Phosphorus Uptake

The P[32] test helps in differentiating benign from malignant lesions of the choroid.

Fluorescein Angiography of the Iris

Used for differentiating melanomas from benign lesions of the iris.

Cytopathologic Studies

Useful for differentiating a primary or metastatic malignancy. It is performed by aspiration of aqueous or vitreous and then, a histopathological study is done. A fine needle aspiration biopsy may also be used to obtain material for cytopathologic study.

Frozen Section Diagnosis

It is helpful in identifying a tumor of the iris and in determining the surgical resection margin of the lesion.

Prognosis

Uveal melanomas associated with glaucoma usually have worse prognosis. In one study, three of four patients with a primary melanoma of the ciliary body and glaucoma died of metastatic disease within 2½ years after enucleation.[3]

Histopathologic studies of eyes with ciliary body melanoma and glaucoma often reveal tumor cell in the aqueous outflow system, which is a potential route of extraocular metastasis. Patients with choroidal melanomas and glaucoma also have a more guarded prognosis, because the tumor is usually large by the time the glaucoma has developed. Melanomas of the iris[9,10] in general have a better prognosis due to earlier detection and small size at the time of detection, however metastases have been reported to occur.[11,12]

Management

Iris melanoma: In most cases, initial management consists of periodic observation and medical management of any associated glaucoma. Tumor growth or uncontrolled glaucoma warrant aggressive management. This consists of complete excision by sector iridectomy, photocoagulation or enucleation.

Ciliary body melanoma: Small ones can be managed by periodic observation until growth is documented. Somewhat, larger tumors can be man-aged by local resection or episcleral plaque radiotherapy. Larger ones are generally managed by enucleation. *Choroidal melanoma:* They can be managed by simple observation, photocoagulation, radiotherapy, local resection, enucleation and even orbital exenteration.

Filtering surgery should be avoided, since seeding of iris melanoma cells through trabeculectomy site into the filtering bleb with extraocular dissemination and fatal metastases have been documented. When surgical intervention is required, especially in eyes with iris melanoma, a cyclodestructive procedure is probably the procedure of choice.

BENIGN TUMORS OF THE ANTERIOR UVEA

Several benign lesions should be considered in the differential diagnosis of anterior uveal tumors. There include nevi, cysts, melanocytoses, melanocytoma, adenomas and leiomyomas .

Nevi of the Iris

It is not uncommon to find one or more nevi on the stromal surface usually recognized as small, discrete, flat or slightly elevated lesions of variable pigmentation. In retrospective clinicopathologic study, lesions of the anterior uvea that were originally diagnosed as melanomas, 80 percent were reclassified as nevi of several cell types.[13] However, five clinical variables were associated with a higher risk of malignancy:

a. Diameter > 3 mm
b. Pigment dispersion
c. Prominent tumor vascularity
d. Elevated IOP
e. Tumor related ocular symptoms.

Glaucoma usually occurs by direct extension of the nevi across the trabecular meshwork.[13,14] Diffuse nevi of the iris associated with progressive synechial closure of the angle and subsequent intraocular pressure elevation is known as **iris nevus syndrome**. A subset of ICE syndrome, the Cogan-Reese syndrome has a similar clinical appearance. The benign lesions of the iris in both of these conditions have been mistaken for malignant melanomas, which has led to enucleation in some patients.

Cysts

Primary cysts arising from the epithelial layers of the iris and ciliary body or less often from iris stroma, are usually stationary, rarely progressing or causing visual complications **(Figures 1A to C)**. Glaucoma causing mechanisms may be angle closure[15] pigment dispersion[16] or a mucus-producing epithelial cyst of the iris stroma of unknown origin.[17]

Secondary cysts of the iris may result from surgery, trauma or neoplasia and are more likely than primary to lead to inflammatory glaucoma.[18,19] UBM has been shown to be a useful diagnostic adjunct for both primary and secondary ones. Iris cysts have been successfully treated by laser cystotomy.[15,20]

Melanocytomas

Clinically, they appear as darkly pigmental lesion, usually on the optic nerve head and less often in the choroid, ciliary body or iris. The latter ones cause glaucoma either by direct spread into the anterior chamber or[21] dispersion of pigment into the angle from a necrotic melanocytoma.[22]

Melanoses

Melanoses iridis is characterized by verrucous-like elevations of the surface of a darkly pigmented, velvety iris. Usually, unilateral or sometimes sectorial or bilateral.[23] Melanosis oculi has additional hyperpigmentation of the episclera, choriod or both and causes glaucoma through hyperpigmentation of the trabecular meshwork.[24]

Adenomas

Benign adenomas like Fuchs' adenoma[25] may arise from the epithelium of the ciliary body predominantly in adults. In children they may be associated with hyperplastic primary vitreous.[26] They must be differentiated from anterior uveal cysts and melanomas.[27]

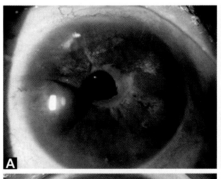
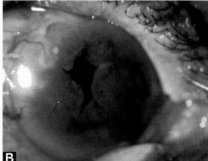
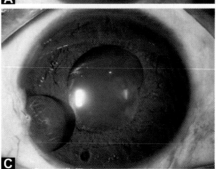

Figs 1A to C Various presentations of iris cysts

Leiomyomas

Rare leiomyomas may appear as a slow-growing grayish, white, vascularized nodule on the surface of the iris. Glaucoma is not a typical complication.

SYSTEMIC MALIGNANCIES
Metastatic Carcinomas

Tumors from the distant primary sites can metastasize to the uvea through hematogenous route. Retinal and optic nerve metastases are rather rare.

The most common primary sites for metastasis to the eye are lung and breast. Studies have shown the incidence of ocular metastases from lung to be between 6 and 6.7 percent, although results differed for metastases from the breast which was 37 and 9.7 percent. Other sites are gastrointestinal tract, kidney, thyroid and skin.

The most common site of ocular metastasis is the posterior uvea. Choroidal metastases produce glaucoma only when large, whereas iris and ciliary body metastases frequently do so because of their tendency to involve the angle structures.

Iris and Ciliary Body Metastases

These can occur as solid or as diffuse multinodular lesions,[28] often associated with rubeosis iridis, iridocyclitis or hyphema. They may seed into the aqueous, producing a pseudohypopyon, composed of tumor cells layered inferiorly because the tumor cells are frequently loosely cohesive and friable.

Glaucoma is usually due to seeding into the anterior chamber angle and trabecular meshwork, mechanically blocking the aqueous outflow. Angle closure glaucoma can occur due to compression of the iris from the tumor or by peripheral anterior synechiae.

Slit lamp examination, gonioscopy and clinical awareness usually can suggest the diagnosis. In case of doubt, transocular fine needle aspiration biopsy can be helpful. Serologic tumor markers have also been useful.

Primary management consists of systemic chemotherapy and radiotherapy. Enucleation is usually reserved for blind, painful eyes. Glaucoma should be controlled medically whenever possible.

Choroidal Metastases

Appear as single, multiple elevated or diffuse lesions often associated with a secondary nonrhegmatogenous retinal detachment. Characteristically, they have a cream yellow color.

Rarely, they produce glaucoma until and unless diffuse involvement of posterior uvea occur leading to intractable glaucoma. Mechanism is usually due to angle closure because of an anterior displacement of lens-iris diaphragm secondary total retinal detachment.

It is managed by external beam radiotherapy combined with chemotherapy. In severe cases, enucleation is done.

Metastatic Melanomas

Although ocular melanomas are nearly always primary malignancies, metastatic melanomas have been reported and may occasionally cause glaucoma.[29] Cutaneous malignant melanoma which has metastasized to the eye becomes necrotic possibly in response to immunotherapy or irradiation, resulting in hypopyon of tumor cells and pigment laden macrophages has been also called black hypopyon and are associated with glaucoma.

Leukemias

In a survey, the incidence of leukemic infiltrates in the ocular tissues was 28 percent.[30] In an other series of childhood leukemias, the 5-year survival rate in patients with ocular manifestations was 21.4 percent, compared to 45.7 percent for those without.[31]

Leukemic infiltration of the anterior ocular segment leads to glaucoma in some cases, which may present in association with hyphema and hypopyon.[32] Both acute and chronic leukemias in adult, may also have ocular involvement with reported cases presenting variously as bilateral hypopyon[33,34] or a massive subretinal hemmorhage with acute angle closure glaucoma.[35] For relapsing phase, it may be necessary to study aqueous aspirates as well as for the diagnosis. Treatment usually includes irradiation and chemotherapy.

OCULAR TUMORS OF CHILDHOOD

There are certain childhood tumors in which the ocular involvement is a primary part of the disorders. These are retinoblastoma, juvenile xanthogranuloma and medulloepithelioma.

Retinoblastoma

It is the most common malignant intraocular tumor of childhood. Although glaucoma is not recognised clinically, but, histopathologic studies suggest that it is a frequent complication of the disease. In one study, it was found that glaucoma inducing mechanism was present in 50 percent of cases although clinically recorded only in 23 percent.[36]

Mechanism

Neovascularization of iris is the most commonm cause of associated glaucoma. Both, rubeosis iridis and neovascular glaucoma are frequently overlooked clinically and should be considered in all cases of retinoblastoma.

Other causes are angle closure due to massive exudative[36] retinal detachment as well as obstruction of the anterior chamber angle by inflammatory cells or necrotic tumor tissue.[37]

Management

Physician should be familiar with the clinical variations of the tumor and the differential diagnosis for the appropriate diagnosis and management. When glaucoma is present, the tumor is usually quite advanced and enucleation is considered the treatment of choice.

Juvenile Xanthogranuloma

Although its not a true neoplasm, it can cause an iris mass and secondary glaucoma.[38] Its a benign, self-limiting disease of infants and young children[39] characterized by discrete, yellow, papular cutaneous lesions primarily of the head and neck, as well as salmon colored to lightly pigmented lesions of the iris.[40,41] Glaucoma may occur from invasion of the anterior chamber angle with histiocytes or from hyphema or secondary uveitis.

Treatment consists of systemic and local corticosteroids and medical treatment of the associated glaucoma. Invasive surgery should be avoided, if possible.

Medulloepithelioma

Also known as Diktyoma, it is an embryonic tumor that becomes clinically apparent in the first few years of life.[42,43] It arises most often from non pigmented ciliary epithelium. Grossly, the tumor appears as a yellow or pink solid or cystic mass of the iris or ciliary body. Glaucoma can result from iris neovascularization or from direct invasion of the angle structures.

As most intraocular medulloepitheliomas are relatively benign, an attempt at local resection by iridocyclectomy is generally appropriate for smaller ones. Unfortunately complete removal is extremely difficult and recurrence is common, eventually requiring enucleation.

PHACOMATOSIS

The term was coined by Van der Hoeve in 1932, meaning "mother spot" or "birthmark". They are characterised by the formation of hamartias and hamartomas in the eye, central nervous system, skin and viscera. Other system may be involved to a lesser degree, including pulmonary, cardiovascular, gastrointestinal, renal and skeletal. In some cases, the anomalies are present at birth, while others become manifest later in life.

Glaucoma is common in some phacomatoses, rare in others. The following discussion is limited to those phacomatoses which frequently or occasionally may have associated with glaucoma (Phacomatosis are discussed in detail in a separate chapter).

Glaucoma in the Phacomatoses

Commonly Associated with Glaucoma
- Encephalotrigeminal angiomatosis (Sturge-Weber syndrome)
- Klippel-Trenaunay-Weber syndrome (Combined form)
- Oculodermal melanocytosis (Nevus of Ota)

Occasionally Associated with Glaucoma
- Neurofibromatosis (von Recklinghausen's disease)
- Angiomatosis retinae (von Hippel-Lindau syndrome)

Rarely Associated with Glaucoma
- Basal cell nevus syndrome
- Tuberous sclerosis (Bourneville's disease)
- Klippel-Trenaunay-Weber syndrome (pure form)
- Diffuse congenital hemangiomatosis
- Racemose angioma of the retinae (Wyburn-Mason syndrome)
- Unassociated with glaucoma
- Ataxia-telangiectasia (Louis-Bar syndrome)

Encephalotrigeminal Angiomatosis (Sturge-Weber Syndrome)
General Features

The hamartoma in this condition arises from vascular tissue and are characterized by facial cutaneous angioma (nevus flammeus, port wine stain), which is present at birth, usually unilateral, and involves the region of distribution of the first and second divisions of the trigeminal nerve **(Figure 2)**.[44,45] Bilateral cases occur in 10 to 30 percent of cases.[46,47]

Ocular Features

Hemangiomas may affect the lid, episclera, conjunctiva, iris and ciliary body. Anderson's rule states that when the hemangioma involves the upper lid, there is ipsilateral involvement. If the upper lid is spared, the ipsilateral eye is spared. Exceptions may occur.[48] Slit lamp examination typically reveals dense episcleral vascular plexus and occasional ampulliform dilation of conjunctival vessels. Some patients, also have a choroidal hemangioma (40%).[49] Iris hyperchomia occurs in 7 to 8 percent of cases.[50] NVI also has been reported.[51]

Theories of Glaucoma Mechanism

One-third of patients with the syndrome have increased intraocular pressure[52] usually when the hamangioma involves lid, tarsus and conjunctiva. Vascular or mechanical causes offer the most plausible mechanism for glaucoma. Mechanical theories are based on occlusion of anterior chamber angle, leading to blockage of aqueous humor outflow.

Numerous authors have believed that glaucoma occurs because of developmental anomalies that result in anterior chamber angle malformations.

Hemorrhage from the choroidal hemangioma may result in subretinal hemorrhage and retinal detachment, with forward displacement of the iris

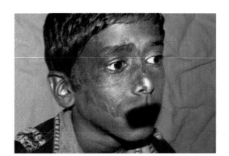
Fig. 2 Sturge-Weber syndrome

and angle closure secondary to PAS formation either on a mechanical basis or due to neovascularization. Most of the eyes coming to pathologic examination have had this severe outcome.

The vascular theories relate the elevation of intraocular pressure to the presence of vascular malformations that might increase aqueous humor production, decrease aqueous outflow, or actually change the components of aqueous fluid or interfere with extrascleral drainage.

Many authors have postulated vascular hypertrophy as the cause for glaucoma. An increase in the number or size of choroidal vessels has been postulated as the cause of choroidal congestion with increased transudation, decreased outflow of aqueous humor, or both.[53] The absence of glaucoma in most eyes with choroidal hemangioma refutes this theory. Furthermore, choroidal hemangiomas often are associated with anterior segment structural anomalies, which themselves may result in glaucoma.

The most likely cause of elevated intraocular pressure seems to be a combination of developmental angle anomalies and elevated episcleral venous pressure,[54] which may result in alterations of the meshwork similar to those found with aging. The relative contribution of each depends on the individual case. Careful gonioscopy, tonography, and measurement of episcleral venous pressure are useful in determining the cause.

Management
Medical therapy may suffice to control the glaucoma that occurs in later life, while the infantile form usually requires surgical intervention. Success has been reported with a trabeculectomy in children and adults.[55,56]

However, filtering surgery in these patients is commonly associated with intraoperative choroidal effusion and occasionally with expulsive hemorrhage.[57] It is advisable to perform prophylactic sclerotomy in order to reduce this complication. In one study of 30 patients, goniotomy was not associated with these complications and may be the first choice in most cases. Since it may not be certain whether the glaucoma is due to an anterior chamber angle anomaly or elevated episcleral venous pressure, a combined trabeculotomy-trabeculectomy may improve the chances of success, by treating both possible sources of elevated IOP,[58] although it does not reduce the potential for serious complications. Another alternative to reduce the risk of massive choroidal effusion and expulsive hemorrhage is a cyclodestructive procedure.

Von Recklinghausen's Neurofibromatosis
Primarily a neuroectodermal dysplasia characterized by tumor like formation derived from the proliferation of peripheral nerve elements.

General Features
The principal systemic lesions in this condition involve the skin and include

Café au lait spots, which are flat, hyperpigmented lesions with well-circumscribed borders, and neurofibromas, that appear as soft, flesh-colored, pedunculated masses. The latter lesions arise from Schwann cells. Central nervous system involvement is uncommon, although neurofibromas may develop from cranial nerves, especially the acoustic nerve. Two subsets of neurofibromatosis have been distinguished: *Peripheral* (Von Recklinghausen's), characterized by the skin lesions, and *central*, characterized by bilateral acoustic Schwannomas.[59] Both are inherited by an autosomal dominant mode with variable expressivity. Genetic analysis of a kindred with von Recklinghausen's neurofibromatosis indicated that the responsible gene is located near the centromere on chromosome 17.[60]

Ocular Features
In the peripheral form, the eyelids, conjunctiva, iris, ciliary body, and choroids may be involved with the neurofibromas. The hamartomatous lesions of the iris are called *Lisch nodules* (**Figure 3A**).[61] They are usually bilateral and characterized by well-defined, clear to yellow, or brown, dome-shaped, gelatinous elevations on the iris stroma. An ultrastructural study indicates that

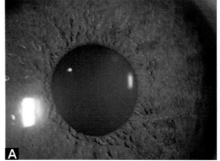 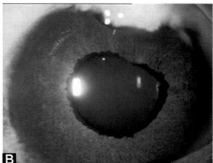

Figs 3A and B (A) Lisch nodules; (B) Ectropion uveae in neurofibromatosis (trabeculectomy has been done)

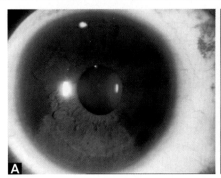 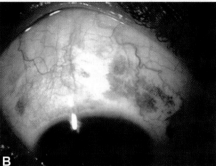

Figs 4A and B Nevus of OTA

they are of melanocytic origin. Lisch nodules are a nearly constant feature of von Recklinghausen's neurofibromatosis, occurring in 92 percent of one series of 77 patients.[62] In another study of 64 patient, the nodules were seen in 95 percent and in all patients aged 16 years or older.[63] In addition, chorioretinal hamartomas and gliomas of the optic nerve are occasionally present. Ectropion uveae may also be present **(Figure 3B)**. A fluorescein angiographic study of the choroidal lesions revealed avascular patches of hypofluorescence similar to multiple small choroidal nevi. The central form of neurofibromatosis does not typically have ocular findings, other than present posterior subcapsular or nuclear cataracts.

Intraocular pressure elevation is more likely to occur in neurofibromatosis when the lids are involved with neurofibromas. The several possible mechanisms of glaucoma include:

a. Infiltration of the angle with neurofibromatous tissue
b. Closure of the anterior chamber angle due to nodular thickening of the ciliary body and choroids
c. Fibrovascular membrane resembling neovascular glaucoma
d. Failure of normal anterior chamber angle development.[64]

Management

The choice of treatment depends on the severity of the glaucoma, the patient's age at onset, and the mechanism of glaucoma. Congenital glaucoma should be managed surgically. Medical treatment may be initiated in juvenile or adult-onset glaucoma.

Von Hippel Lindau Disease

It is also known as angiomatosis retinae. This phakomatosis is characterized by angiomatosis of the retina and, in a small percentage of cases, the cerebellum. Most cases are not familial. Glaucoma may occur as a late sequelae due to rubeosis iridis or iridocyclitis.

Nevus of OTA (Oculodermal Melanocytosis)

It is characterized by deep dermal pigmentation, usually, unilateral on the distribution of the first and second divisions. **(Figures 4A and B)** and occasionally, the mandibular division of the trigeminal nerve.[65] Patients with melanosis oculi or ocular melanocytosis do not demonstrate skin involvement.

Mechanism of Glaucoma

Acute angle closure and open angle glaucomas have been reported. Other studies have reported melanocytic infiltration of the anterior chamber angle. Elevated IOP, with or without glaucomatous damage, was seen in 10 percent of one series.[65] The involved eye typically has unusually heavy pigmentation of the trabecular meshwork and histopathologic studies have revealed melanocytes in the meshwork.[66,67]

Management

Medical management as with other form of open angle glaucoma, should be tried first. Where this fails, laser trabeculoplasty (with lower energy settings) may be effective[24] although filtering surgery will most likely be required.

MANAGEMENT OF TUMOR INDUCED GLAUCOMA

Patients with primary neoplasm should be evaluated for metastatic disease.

Local treatment of nonmetastatic primary ocular tumors: Total removal, resection, destruction.

A. **Resection:** Total surgical removal with defined tumor margins is done for iris, iridociliary and and uveal melanomas. Since, filtering surgery is contraindicated, cyclodestruction can be combined with tumor removal.
B. Radiation
C. Chemotherapy.

Radiation

Radiation therapy alone can cure tumour induced glaucoma, in some cases, especially, in case of leukemia and lymphoma induced glaucoma. These are extremely sensitive to low doses of external beam radiation therapy (EBRT). Moderate dose of EBRT is also useful for treating anterior uveal metastasis with angle rotation.

In many cases, treatment of the tumour leads to resolution of the glaucoma.

When the tumor removal is not feasible, the IOP is controlled medically. Trabeculectomy and glaucoma drainage devices are contraindicated as they provide a portal of exit for the malignant cells. One must keep in mind that the aim is to first save the patient's life. The pharmacological reduction of IOP can be achieved by beta blockers, alpha agonists and carbonic anhydrase inhibitors. Prostaglandin analogs and pilocarpine are avoided as, theoretically by increasing the aqueous outflow they may promote metastasis.

Refractory Glaucoma

Once the intraocular tumor or its treatment affects the vision, the treatment is directed towards reducing the pain rather than the IOP management.

Evaluate for metastasis
Assess systemic prognosis
Control IOP medically
Treat the tumor with/without concurrent cyclodestruction:
- Resection
- Radiation
- Chemotherapy

If resection is not possible:
- Medical management
- Cyclodestruction
- Enucleation

REFERENCES

1. Shields CL, Shields JA, Shields MB, Augsburger JJ. Prevalence and mechanisms of secondary intraocular pressure elevation in eyes with intraocular tumors. Ophthalmology 1987;94:839.
2. Yanoff M. Glaucoma mechanisms in ocular malignant melanomas. Am J Ophthalmol 1970;70:898.
3. Shields MB, Klintworth GK. Anterior uveal melanomas and intraocular pressure. Ophthalmology 1980; 87:503.
4. Shields JA, Sanborn GE, Augsberger JJ. The differential diagnosis of iris melanomas. Ophthalmology 1983;90:716.
5. Yanoff M, Scheie HG. Melanomalytic glaucoma. Report of a case. Arch Ophthalmol 1970;84:471.
6. Reese AB, Mund ML, Iwamoto T. Tapioca melanoma of the iris. Part I. Clinical and light microscopy studies. Am J Ophthalmol 1972;74:840.
7. Shields MB, Proia AD. Neovascular glaucoma associated with an iris melanoma. A clinicopathologic report. Arch Ophthalmol 1987;105:672.
8. EL Baba F, Hagler WS, De La Cruz A, Green WR. Choroidal melanoma with pigment dispersion in vitreous and melanomalytic glaucoma. Ophthalmology 1988;95:370.
9. Rones B, Zimmerman LE. The prognosis of primary tumors of the iris treated by iridectomy. Arch Ophthalmol 1958; 60:193.
10. Dunphy EB, Dryja TP, Albert DM, Smith TR. Melanocytic tumor of the anterior uvea. Am J Ophthalmol 1978;86:680.
11. Sunba MSN, Rahi AHS, Morgan G. Tumors of the anterior uvea. I Metastasizing malignant melanoma of the iris. Arch Ophthalmol 1980;98:82.
12. Charteris DG. Progression of an iris melanoma over 41 years. Br J ophthalmol 1990;74:566.
13. Jakobiec FA, Silbert G. Are most iris "melanomas" "really nevi? A clinicopathologic study of 189 lesions. Arch Ophthalmol 1981;99:2117.
14. Nik NA, Hidayat A, Zimmerman LE, Fine BS. Diffuse iris nevus manifested by unilateral open angle glaucoma. Arch Ophthalmol 1981;99:125.
15. Vela A, Rieser JC, Campbell DG. The heredity and treatment of angle closure glaucoma secondary to iris and ciliary body cysts. Ophthalmology 1983;91:332.
16. Alward WLM, Occoining KC. Pigment dispersion secondary to cysts of the iris pigment epithelium. Arch Ophthalmol 1995;113:1574.
17. Albert DL, Brownstein S, Kattleman BS. Mucogenic glaucoma caused by an epithelial cyst of the iris stroma. Am J Ophthalmol 1992;114:222.
18. Shields JA, Kline WM, Augsburger JJ. Primary iris cysts a review of the literature and report of 62 cases. Br J Ophthalmol 1984;68:152.
19. Finger PT, McCormick SA, Lombardo J, et al. Epithelial inclusion cyst of the iris. Arch Ophthalmol 1995;113:777.
20. Bron AJ, Wilson CB, Hill AR. Laser treatment of primary ring shaped epithelial iris cyst. Br J Ophthalmol 1984;68:859.
21. Nakazawa M, Tamai M. Iris melanocytoma with secondary glaucoma. Am J Ophthalmol 1984;97:797.
22. Shields JA, Annesley WH Jr, Spaeth GL. Necrotic melanocytoma of iris with secondary glaucoma. Am J Ophthalmol 1977;84:826.
23. Traboulsi EI, Maumenee IH. Bilateral melanosis of the iris. Am J Ophthalmol 1987;103:115.
24. Goncalves V, Sandler T, O'Donnell, FE Jr. Open angle glaucoma in melanosis oculi. Response to laser trabeculoplasty. Ann Ophthamol 1985;17:33.
25. Lieb WE, Shields JA, Eagle RC Jr, et al. Cystic adenoma of the pigmented ciliary epithelium. Clinical, pathologic

and immunohistopathologic findings. Ophthalmology 1990;97:1489.

26. Doro S, Werblin TP, Haas B, et al. Fetal adenoma of the pigmented ciliary epithelium associated with persistent hyperplasia primary vitreous. Ophthalmology 1986;93:1343.

27. Shields CL, Shields JA, Cook GR, et al. Differentiation of adenoma of the iris pigment epithelium from iris cyst and melanoma. Am J Ophthalmol 1985; 100:678.

28. Shields JA, et al. Metastatic tumors to the iris. Personal experience with 40 cases. The 1994 JD Allen Lecture (submitted).

29. Char DH, Schwartz A, Miller TR, Abele JS. Ocular metastases from systemic melanoma. Am J Ophthalmol 1980; 90:702.

30. Nelson CC, Hertzberg BS, Klintworth GK. A histopathologic study of 716 unselected eyes in patients with cancer at the time of death. Am J Ophthalmol 1983;95:788.

31. Leonardy NJ, Rupani M, Dent G, Klintworth GK. Analysis of 135 autopsy eyes for ocular involvement in leukemia. Am J Ophthalmol 1990;109:436.

32. Zakka KA, Yee RD, Shorr N, et al. Leukemic iris infiltration. Am J ophthalmol 1980;89:204.

33. Santoni G, Fiore C, Lupidi G, Bibbiani U. Recurring bilateral hypopyon in chronic myeloid leukemia in blastic transformation. A case report. Graefes Arch Clin Exp Ophthalmol 1985;223: 211.

34. Ayliffe W, Foster CS, Marcoux P, et al. Relapsing acute myeloid leukemia manifesting as hypopyin uveitis. Am J Ophthalmol 1995;119:361.

35. Kozlowski IMD, Horose T, Jalkh AE. Massive subretinal hemorrhage with acute angle closure glaucoma in chronic myelocytic leukemia. Am J Ophthalmol 1987;103:837.

36. Fraser D, Font RL. Ocular inflammation and hemorrhage as initial manifestations of uveal malignant melanoma. Incidence and prognosis. Arch Ophthalmol 1979;97:1311.

37. Yoshizumi MO, Thomas JV, Smith TR. Glaucoma inducing mechanisms in eyes with retinoblastoma. Arch Ophthalmol 1978;96:105.

38. Shields CL. Treatment of nonresectable malignant iris tumors with custom-designed plaque radiotherapy. Br J Ophthalmol 1995;79:306.

39. Bruner WE, Stark WJ, Green WR. Presumed juvenile xanthogranuloma of the iris and ciliary body in an adult. Arch Ophthalmol 1982;100:457.

40. Zimmerman L. Ocular lesions of juvenile xanthogranuloma. Trans Am Acad Ophthalmol Otol 1965;69:412.

41. Schwartz LW, Rodrigues MM, Hallett JW. Juvenile xanthogranuloma diagnosed by paracentesis. Am J Ophthalmol 1974;77:243.

42. Broughton WL, Zimmerman LE. A clinicopathologic study of 56 cases of intraocular medulloepitheliomas. Am J Ophthalmol 1978;85:407.

44. Ehrlich LM. Bilateral glaucoma associated with unilateral nevus flammeus. Arch Ophthamol 1941;25: 1002.

45. Yamanaka R. Naevus flammeus mit gleicheitigem Glaukom, Klin Monatsbl Augenheilkd 1927;78:372.

46. Duke-Elder S. System of ophthalmology, Vol 11, Diseases of the lens and vitreous glaucoma nadhypotony, St Louis, 1969, Mosby.

47. Shaffer RN, Weiss DI. Congenital and paediatric glaucomas, St Louis 1970. Mosby.

48. Walsh FB, Hoyt WF. Clinical Neurophthalmology, 3rd edn, Baltimore 1969, Williams and Wilkins.

49. Duke-Elder S. System of Ophthalmology, vol II, Diseases of the lens and vitreous: glaucoma and hypotony, St Louis, 1969, Mosby.

50. Alexander GL. The Sturge-Weber syndrome. In: Vinken PJ, Bruyn GW, (Eds). Handbook of clinical neurology, Vol 14, The phakomatoses, Amsterdam, 1972, North Holland Publising.

51. Verma L, et al. Iris Neovascularization in Sturge-Weber Syndrome, Indian J Ophthalmol 1991;39:82.

52. Alexander GL, Norman RM. The Sturge-Weber Syndrome, Bristol, John Wright and Sons, 1960.

53. Dunphy EB. Glaucoma accompanying nevus flammeus, Am J Ophthalmol 1935;18:709.

54. Jorgenson JS, Guthoff R. Sturge-Weber syndrome: glaucoma with elevated episcleral venous pressure, Klin Monatsbl Augenheilkd 1987;191: 275.

55. Ali MA, Fahmy IA, Spaeth GL. Trabeculectomy for glaucoma associated with Sturge-Weber syndrome. Ophthalmic Surg 1990;21:352.

56. Iwach AG, Hoskins HD Jr, Hetherington J Jr, Shaffer RN. Analysis of surgical and medical management of glaucoma in Sturge-Weber syndrome. Ophthalmology 1990;97:904.

57. Theodossiadis G, Damanakis A, Koutsandrea C. Expulsive choroidal effusion during glaucoma surgery in a child with Sturge-Weber syndrome. Klin Monatsbl Augenheilkd 1985;186: 300.

58. Agarwal HC, Sandramouli S, Sihota R, Sood NN. Sturge-Weber syndrome management of glaucoma

with combined trabeculotomy-Trabeculectomy. Ophthalmic Surg 1993;24:399.

59. Pearson-Webb MA, Kaiser-Kupfer MI, Eldridge R. Eye findings in bilateral acoustic (central) neurofibromatosis: Association with presenile lens opacities and cataracts but absence of Lisch nodules. N Engl J Med 1986; 315:1553.

60. Barker D, Wright E, Nguyen K, et al. Gene for von Recklinghausen neurofibromatosis is in the pericentromeric region of chromosome 17. Science 1987;236:1100.

61. Lubs M-L-E, Bauer MSA, Formas ME, Djokic B. Lisch nodules in neurofibromatosis type. I. New Eng J Med 1991;324:1264.

62. Lewis RA, Riccardi VM, Von Recklinghausen neurofibromatosis. Incidence of iris hamartomata. Ophthalmology 1981;88:348.

63. Huson S, Jones D, Beck L. Ophthalmic manifestations of neurofibromatosis, Br J Ophthalmol 1987;71:235.

64. Grant WM, Walton DS. Distinctive gonioscopic findings in glaucoma due to neurofibromatosis. Arch Ophthalmol 1968;79:127.

65. Teekhasaenee C, et al. Ocular findings in oculodermal melanocytosis, Arch Ophthalmol 1990;108:1114.

66. Sugar HS. Glaucoma with trabecular melanocytosis. Ann Ophthalmol 1982;14:374.

67. Futa R, Shimizu T, Okura F, Yasutake T. A case of open angle glaucoma associated with nevus Ota-electron microscopic study of the anterior chamber angle and iris. Folia Ophthalmol Jpn 1984;35:501.

39 | Developmental Glaucoma— An Overview

Anil K Mandal, Debasis Chakrabarti, Raka (Chatterjee) Chakrabarti

DEFINITIONS

Buphthalmos is a general term [Greek *bous*=ox and *ophthalmos*=eye] that describes the marked ocular enlargement arising from any type of infantile/childhood glaucoma. In *congenital glaucoma*, the glaucoma exists at birth, and usually before birth. *Infantile glaucoma* occurs after birth and until 3 years of age. *Juvenile glaucoma* occurs after the age of three to teenage years.

Primary congenital glaucoma (PCG) or developmental glaucomas result from maldevelopment of the aqueous outflow system (isolated trabeculodysgenesis).

Secondary developmental glaucomas result from damage to the aqueous outflow system, secondary to maldevelopment of some other ocular structure.

In this chapter, we will discuss PCG in some detail and some secondary developmental glaucomas in brief.

CLINICAL FEATURES

PCG is the most common form of developmental glaucomas, occurring in about one in 10,000 livebirths. The condition is typically bilateral (unilateral in 25-30% of cases). The classic triad of symptoms[1] include epiphora (excessive tearing), photophobia (hypersensitivity to light) and blepharospasm (squeezing of eyelids). However, enlarged eyeball and corneal haziness seem to be the more common presenting features in the Indian subcontinent **(Figure 1)**.[2] Rarely, the condition may present as a 'red eye', mimicking conjunctivitis.

The Cardinal Signs

Refraction: Myopia and astigmatism are commonly seen.

Ocular enlargement: The neonatal globe is distensible and is stretched by the increased intraocular pressure. Pressure-induced corneal enlargement predominantly occurs before the age of 3 years, but the sclera may be deformable until approximately 10 years, hence the increase in axial length.

Corneal changes: The normal neonatal horizontal corneal diameter is approximately 10 to 10.5 mm, increasing by an additional 0.5 to 1.0 mm in the first year of life.[3] Enlargement of the corneal diameter to greater than 12 mm in the first year of life is highly suspicious of developmental glaucoma. *Haab's striae*

refer to the stretch-induced breaks in the Descemet's membrane **(Figure 2)**. They are typically horizontal and linear when they occur centrally, but, parallel or curvilinear to the limbus when they occur peripherally in the cornea. The initial corneal edema in PCG is simple epithelial edema due to elevated IOP. Persistence and progression may lead to

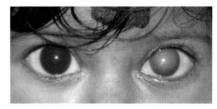

Fig. 1 A six-month-old child with infantile glaucoma in left eye

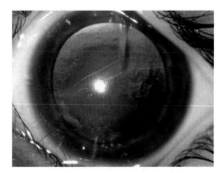

Fig. 2 Haab's striae

permanent stromal edema, stromal scarring and irregular corneal astigmatism.

Scleral changes: Scleral expansion and thinning causes a 'blue-sclera' appearance due to increased visibility of underlying uveal tissue.

Optic nerve cupping: Optic nerve head cupping may occur rapidly in infants but in many cases, it is fortunately, reversible with normalization of IOP.

Increased IOP

Late sequel: In untreated eyes, there may be corneal ulceration and lens subluxation (due to stretching and rupture of the zonules). Blunt trauma in these susceptible eyes can lead to hyphema, retinal detachment, globe rupture and phthisis bulbi.

DIFFERENTIAL DIAGNOSIS

Several clinical entities may share some of the clinical features of PCG, but none exhibit all of the cardinal features like tearing, photophobia, blepharospasm, generalized ocular enlargement, corneal haziness, optic nerve head cupping and raised IOP.

Conditions with Epiphora and Red Eye

The most common cause of epiphora in the infant is *congenital nasolacrimal duct obstruction* (CNLDO). There may be fullness of the sac area and chronic mucopurulent discharge. Other signs of PCG are typically absent.

Conjunctivitis can present with redness and tearing.

Meesman's and Reis-Buckler corneal dystrophies may present with ocular irritation and tearing, but have characteristic corneal lesions.

Congenital hereditary endothelial dystrophy (CHED) may present with tearing, photophobia and corneal edema.

Rubella keratitis may also present with pain, redness and watering.

Conditions with Corneal Enlargement

High axial myopia can present with large eyes, including large corneas. A myopic fundus with tilted optic disc, peripapillary scleral halo and choroidal mottling are characteristic.

Megalocornea is a condition of marked corneal enlargement, often to diameters of 14 to 16 mm. Families have been reported in which some members have megalocornea and others have PCG.

Conditions with Corneal Haziness

Sclerocornea is typically bilateral (90%) and is characterized by opaque scleral tissue, usually accompanied by vessels, extending into the cornea.

Obstetric trauma can cause rupture of the Descemet's membrane with resultant corneal edema. These traumatic breaks are said to be vertically oriented (however, they may be curvilinear or run diagonally across the cornea as well) while those caused by increased IOP are horizontal, usually unilateral, more commonly affects the left eye (because of higher incidence of left occipito-anterior position of fetus) and may be accompanied by periorbital bruises.

Ocular herpes in the newborn may present with conjunctivitis, epithelial keratitis, stromal immune reaction, cataract and necrotizing chorioretinitis.

Congenital syphilis may present with bilateral interstitial keratitis.

Certain **metabolic conditions** present with corneal clouding. These include mucopolysaccharidoses, e.g. Hurler's syndrome (mucopolysaccharidosis I-H), cystinosis, amyloidosis.

Conditions with Elevated IOP

Rubella syndrome may cause an angle anomaly and glaucoma virtually indistinguishable from PCG. Look carefully for other signs like cataract, cardiac anomalies (PDA, ASD, VSD) and mental retardation. However, rubella viremia in the third trimester can cause isolated anterior chamber angle involvement and glaucoma.

WORK-UP

History: The following questions need to be addressed:
- Age of onset of symptoms?
- Birth history?
- Forceps delivery?
- Family history?
- Consanguineous marriage?
- Antenatal history (maternal rubella?
- Any other systemic anomaly noticed by parents?

Initial examination: A gentle torchlight examination and digital IOP estimation can often make the diagnosis. If necessary, a mild sedative such as chloral hydrate syrup (25 to 50 mg/kg body wt.) can be used. In older children, a complete evaluation including refraction, slit-lamp examination, applanation tonometry, gonioscopy and fundus evaluation may be possible.

Examination under anesthesia (EUA): A physician's and anesthetist's clearance is mandatory before taking up the child for EUA. For measuring the IOP, we prefer the hand-held Perkins applanation tonometer and use it at the earliest stage of inhalation anesthesia before intubation, to reduce errors related to anesthesia. Remember that most anesthetics, particularly halothane, can reduce the IOP. An exception is ketamine hydrochloride, which may increase IOP. The normal IOP in an infant under halothane anesthesia is said to be approximately 9-10 mm Hg and a pressure of 20 mm Hg or more should arouse suspicion. The mean IOP in unanesthetized newborns is said to be about 11.4+/-2.4 mm Hg. *White-to-white* horizontal corneal diameter is measured with calipers. A detailed ocular examination is performed using a portable hand-held slit-lamp or under the operating microscope, looking carefully for corneal details (edema, scarring, Haab's striae), iris details (abnormal iris vessels, aniridia), and lens (cataract). Gonioscopy is performed using a Koeppe goniolens. Characteristic gonioscopic features in PCG include an anterior (and usually flat) insertion of the iris directly into the trabecular meshwork (whereas, in a normal newborn eye, the iris usually inserts posterior to the scleral spur and the ciliary body is seen as a distinct band). Other gonioscopic features include the **Loch Ness Monster phenomenon** (loops of vessels from the major arterial circle seen above the iris) and **Lister's morning mist** (a fine, fluffy tissue covering the peripheral iris). Fundus is examined using 20D lens, or a 90D lens using the illumination of the microscope, or a direct ophthalmoscope. Mydriasis can be obtained using a drop of 2.5 percent phenylephrine and one percent cyclopentolate. If surgery is contemplated, fundus should be seen without dilation. Note disc size, cupping and neuroretinal rim abnormalities. A cup-disc ratio greater than 0.3 is rare in normal infants and must be considered suspicious.

USG A-Scan and B-Scan

A-scan reveals increased axial length and AC depth, but reduced lens thickness. The normal axial length is about 17 mm at 40 gestational weeks and increases to about 20 mm at one year of age. B-scan helps to detect cupping and to rule out any posterior segment pathology in eyes with opaque media.

TREATMENT

Definitive treatment is surgical. Anti-glaucoma medications only play a supportive role to reduce the IOP temporarily, to clear the cornea and to facilitate surgical intervention. Beta-blockers, e.g. timolol 0.25 or 0.5 percent may be used after excluding pulmonary and cardiac problems. Topical carbonic anhydrase inhibitors, e.g. dorzolamide 2 percent is well-tolerated. Prostaglandin analogues, e.g. Latanoprost 0.005 percent, Bimatoprost 0.03 percent and Travoprost 0.004 percent are useful in some cases but long-term safety profile is unavailable. **Alpha-2 agonist (brimonidine 0.125% or 0.2%) is absolutely contraindicated in children below 5 years of age because of the risk of life-threatening apnea.** Cholinergic drugs, e.g. pilocarpine are not very effective in developmental glaucoma because of the abnormal insertion of ciliary muscle into the trabecular meshwork.

Surgery

Early surgical intervention is of prime importance in the management of patients with developmental glaucoma. Goniotomy can be performed in children with mild or moderate corneal edema. In our subcontinent, children mostly present with cloudy corneas where goniotomy is difficult; combined external trabeculotomy with trabeculectomy is our preferred surgical approach.[4] The surgical details are discussed in the subsequent chapter. Because of potentially serious complications, we personally prefer to avoid use of intraoperative anti-metabolites like Mitomycin C in primary surgery and reserve its use only in refractory cases like previously failed surgery. Other options for refractory cases are glaucoma drainage implants like Ahmed Glaucoma Valve and cyclodestructive procedures like trans-scleral cyclo-photocoagulation (TSCPC).

FOLLOW-UP

Postoperatively, the child is examined next day, after one week and after one month and thereafter at 4 to 6 months interval. Visual acuity measurement by age-appropriate techniques, refraction, glass prescription, amblyopia correction and IOP estimation are important issues. EUA is performed as and when deemed necessary. Lifelong follow-up at regular intervals combined with adequate social support allow the best possible outcome for the child.

SECONDARY CONGENITAL GLAUCOMAS

Axenfeld-Rieger Syndrome

Ocular defects in Axenfeld-Rieger syndrome are typically bilateral. Family history is often positive. The structures more commonly involved are the peripheral cornea, anterior chamber angle and the iris. A prominent, anteriorly displaced Schwalbe's line, which appears on the slit-lamp as a white line in the posterior cornea near the limbus, is an important finding. Gonioscopy reveals tissue strands bridging the angle from the peripheral iris to the prominent Schwalbe's line. Apart from the peripheral changes, iris may be normal or may exhibit mild stromal thinning to marked atrophy with hole formation, corectopia and ectropion uvea. There may be associated systemic anomalies including dental anomalies (microdontia, hypodontia, oligodontia) and facial anomalies (maxillary hypoplasia with flattening of the midface). The most important differential diagnosis is iridocorneal endothelial (ICE) syndromes, which are typically unilateral, more commonly seen in young females, rarely familial and are marked by corneal endothelial abnormalities, but not prominent Schwalbe's line. Glaucoma occurs in slightly more than half of patients with A-R syndrome

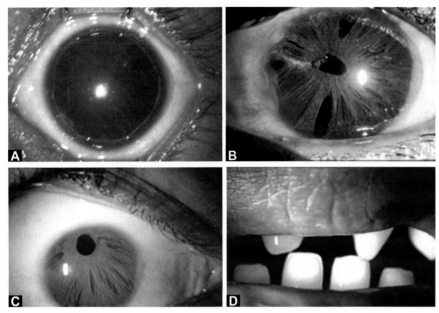

Figs 3A to D (A) Axenfeld-Rieger anomaly with prominent Schwalbe's line; (B to D) Axenfeld-Rieger syndrome

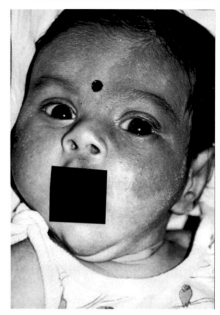

Fig. 4 A young girl with Sturge-Weber syndrome

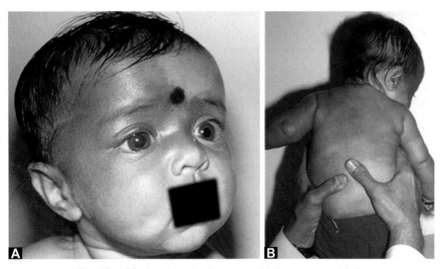

Figs 5A and B A child with phacomatosis pigmentovascularis

and is typically difficult to control. Glaucoma most commonly develops between childhood and early adulthood, but may appear in infancy or late in life. For this reason, patients must be monitored throughout life. Medical therapy with beta-blockers or carbonic anhydrase inhibitors may be beneficial. If surgery is contemplated, trabeculectomy is the procedure of choice.

Peter's Anomaly

The condition is present at birth and usually bilateral. The hallmark is a central defect in the descemet's membrane and endothelium with thinning and opacification of the corresponding area of corneal stroma. Adhesions may extend from the borders of this defect to the iris. Some cases are associated with keratolenticular contact or cataract. Approximately half of the patients will develop glaucoma, which is frequently present at birth. Initial trabeculectomy may offer the best chances of success. Penetrating keratoplasty is also frequently necessary.

Aniridia

Aniridia is a bilateral, uncommon, panocular disorder which may have a variety of features including cataract, glaucoma, limbal stem cell deficiency, nystagmus, strabismus, ectopia lentis, optic nerve hypoplasia and poor foveal reflex. A rudimentary iris is often visible on gonioscopy. Congenital glaucoma is rare, but the reported incidence of

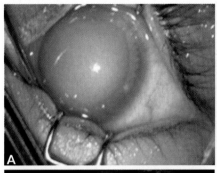
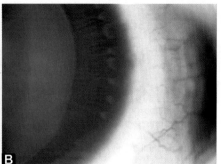
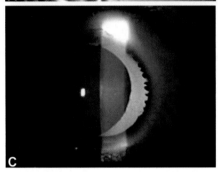

Figs 6A to C Congenital glaucoma with aniridia

glaucoma later in childhood is reported as 65 to 75 percent. Medical therapy may be initially helpful, but surgery is eventually required in up to half of the patients. Goniotomy, trabeculotomy, combined trabeculotomy + trabeculectomy, and trabeculectomy with MMC are the surgical options. It is important to advise an ultrasound of abdomen to rule out any associated Wilm's tumor.

Other Secondary Developmental Glaucomas

Secondary glaucomas can also occur in conditions like phakomatoses (e.g. Sturge–Weber syndrome, neurofibromatosis, etc.), oculocerebrorenal syndrome of Lowe, homocystinuria, PHPV, ROP, broad-thumb (Rubenstein-Tayabi) syndrome (**Figures 3 to 6**).

REFERENCES

1. Hoskins HD Jr, Kass MA. Becker-Shaffer's diagnosis and therapy of the glaucomas, 6th edn. CV Mosby: St. Louis; 1989.
2. Mandal AK, Chakrabarti D. Presenting symptoms and signs in Indian children with primary developmental glaucoma. Poster presented in Asia ARVO 2009.
3. Kwitko ML. The pediatric glaucomas. Int Ophthalmol Clin 1981;21:199-222.
4. Mandal AK, Netland PA. The pediatric glaucomas, 1st edn. Elsevier (Butterworth Heinemann), 2006.

40 Primary Congenital Glaucoma—Pathogenesis, Clinical Features, Diagnosis, Differential Diagnosis and Management

Anil Kumar Mandal, Debasis Chakrabarti, Raka (Chatterjee) Chakrabarti

CHAPTER OUTLINE
- ❖ Pathology and Pathogenesis
- ❖ Clinical Presentation
- ❖ Factors Influencing Therapeutic Decisions
- ❖ Therapy
- ❖ Follow-up
- ❖ Role of Genetic Study and Genetic Counseling

INTRODUCTION

Developmental glaucoma refers to glaucoma associated with developmental anomalies of the eye that are present at birth. These include both primary congenital glaucoma (isolated trabeculodysgenesis) and glaucomas associated with systemic developmental anomalies or those of the eye. It is an uncommon disease and its impact on visual development is extreme. The **primary objective** in the management of developmental glaucomas is to normalize and permanently control the intraocular pressure thereby preventing loss of visual acuity; to preserve the visual field and ocular integrity; and to stimulate the development of binocular stereoscopic vision. Clinicians should be familiar with the pathology, pathogenesis and the clinical course of the ailment before they can treat it. The aim of this chapter is to highlight current concepts in the diagnosis and management of developmental glaucomas. We will discuss mainly about primary developmental glaucomas **(Figure 1)**.

PATHOLOGY AND PATHOGENESIS

The embryologic basis of all developmental glaucomas is fetal maldevelopment of the iridocorneal angle, called goniodysgenesis. Trabeculodysgenesis refers to maldevelopment of the trabecular meshwork, iridodysgenesis refers to maldevelopment of the iris and corneodysgenesis refers to maldevelopment of the cornea. These may appear either singly or in combination. Isolated trabeculodysgenesis is the hallmark of primary developmental glaucoma.

Barkan (1955) initially assumed that a thin imperforate membrane covering the anterior chamber angle of the eyes prevents aqueous humor outflow and leads to increased intraocular pressure.[1] The presence of "Barkan's membrane" was subsequently championed by Worst in 1966.[2,3] However, light microscopy as well as electron microscopic studies provided no evidence of a membrane in any of the specimens.[4-10]

Based on the clinical and histopathological observations of the current concepts of normal anterior segment development, the mechanism of developmental glaucomas has been attributed to a developmental arrest, late in gestation, of certain anterior segment structures derived from neural crest cells (Angular neuro-cristopathies).[11]

Anderson (1981) provided histopathological proof that in eyes with primary congenital glaucoma, the iris and ciliary body have the appearance of an eye in the seventh or eighth month of gestation rather than one which is at full term development. The iris and ciliary body fail to recede posteriorly

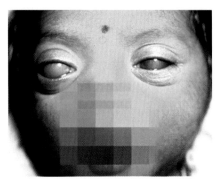

Fig. 1 Primary congenital glaucoma

and the iris insertion and ciliary body overlap the posterior portion of the trabecular meshwork. He believed that in infantile glaucoma, the thickened trabecular beams prevent the normal posterior migration of the ciliary body and iris root. Observations suggest that the developmental immaturity of the outflow system renders it functionally incompetent.[12]

High intraocular pressure causes corneal clouding, rapid enlargement of the globe and limbal stretching. The corneal diameter can enlarge upto as much as 16 to 17 mm. There may be stretching of the descemet's membrane, the corneal endothelium resulting in linear ruptures (Haab's striae), which can lead to corneal stromal and epithelial edema as well as corneal scarring if the problem is chronic. Sclera also expands slowly under the influence of increased intraocular pressure and the associated scleral thinning brings about increased visibility of the underlying uveal tissue in neonates and causes the sclera to appear blue. Thus, in the advanced stages of the disease, the eye is enlarged in all dimensions, resembling an ox eye (Buphthalmos). The optic nerve head in neonates and children is more vulnerable to increased intraocular pressure than adults and in advanced stages of the disease, the disc may show complete cupping. However, optic disc cupping may be reversible with normalization of intraocular pressure particularly in the early stage. Such reversal is very unusual in adults with intraocular pressure induced optic disc damage.

CLINICAL PRESENTATION

The classical clinical triad consists of epiphora, photophobia and blepharospasm. However, our clinical experience shows that this may not be true for our population. Corneal haziness and enlargement of the eyeball seem to be the most common complaints of the parents. In a prospective evaluation of 43 children with PCG, we found that the most common symptom was hazy cornea (47.2%) and large eyes (37.8%).[13]

Examination Under Anesthesia (EUA)

Most of the children require examination under anesthesia (EUA). The following is the protocol for evaluation:

External Examination

It is important to detect and exclude the other conditions associated with epiphora, photophobia and blepharospasm.

The most common cause of epiphora in the newborn and the infant is blocked tear duct or congenital nasolacrimal duct occlusion (CNLDO). Photophobia is not associated with this problem. CNLDO is differentiated from congenital glaucoma in that the former condition is associated with fullness of the lacrimal sac which is often accompanied by chronic muco-purulent discharge.

Corneal Assessment

The cornea is examined to document the presence or absence of breaks in Descemet's membrane (Haab's striae) and corneal enlargement in order to distinguish the glaucomatous signs from other corneal abnormalities.

Conditions associated with neonatal corneal clouding include the following and can be easily remembered using the mnemonic STUMPED:

STUMPED
1. **S**clerocornea
2. **T**ears in Descemet's membrane (developmental glaucoma, obstetric trauma)
3. **U**lcers
4. **M**etabolic diseases, e.g. mucopolysacchardoses
5. **P**eter's anomaly

6. **E**ndothelial dystrophies, e.g. posterior polymorphous dystrophies, congenital hereditary endothelial dystrophies
7. **D**ermoid (central corneal dermoid).

Conditions associated with congenital corneal enlargement
1. Axial myopia
2. Megalocornea
3. Anterior megalophthalmos

The corneal diameter is measured with calipers, from white to white along the horizontal meridian, as the vertical meridian is artifactiously narrowed by encroachment of sclera at the superior limbus.

The normal neonatal horizontal corneal diameter is approximately 10 to 10.5 mm, increasing by 0.5 to 1 mm in the first year. Enlargement of corneal diameter to more than 12 mm in the first year of life is highly indicative of developmental glaucoma.[13]

Corneal enlargement due to increased intraocular pressure predominantly occurs before the age of three year, but the sclera may be deformable until about 10 years.[14-20]

Increased intraocular pressure also stretches the corneal endothelium and Descemet's membrane, resulting in breaks in these layers known as Haab's striae.[21] These are typically horizontal and linear when they occur centrally in the cornea, but parallel and curvilinear to the limbus when they occur in the periphery. Birth trauma (forceps injury) may also cause tears in Descemet's membrane with resultant corneal edema and clouding mimicking primary infantile glaucoma. It has been stated that Descemet's membrane breaks resulting from birth trauma are oblique or vertically oriented.[21-24] Obstetrical corneal trauma is usually unilateral and more commonly affects the left eye because of higher incidence of left occiput anterior presentation of the infant's head at birth. There are attendant signs of periorbital skin changes as a result of trauma (bruising), normal intraocular pressure and no corneal enlargement.

Refraction

Refraction should be done whenever media clarity permits. Most children are myopic; however, the amount of myopia expected from axial length considerations may actually be less because of nature's "emmetropization mechanisms" like flattened cornea, decreased lens thickness and deep anterior chamber.[24]

Tonometry

All anesthetics alter intraocular pressure of patients with infantile glaucoma, seemingly in the plane of anesthesia and as a direct effect on the cardiovascular tonus. A rapid lowering of intraocular pressure occurs particularly with halothane (fluothane) and readings 15 to 20 mm below the true measurement can be obtained. Agents which achieve only light anesthesia and those that induce deeper anesthesia only slowly such as diethylether, cyclopropane or ketamine, allow the intraocular pressure to be measured somewhere between the artificially elevated intraocular pressure of the "excitement" stage of anesthesia or the actual intraocular pressure elevating effect of cyclopropane or succinyl choline (atleast transiently), and the artificially lowered intraocular pressure of deep anesthesia, especially with halothane. Standardization of anesthesia for intraocular pressure measurement for diagnosis and follow-up of infantile glaucoma is obviously highly desirable and inconsistent readings should always be interpreted, considering the patient's general stage of anesthesia and the specific anesthetic used.

The normal intraocular pressure in an infant under halothane anesthesia is said to be approximately 9 to 10 mm Hg and a pressure of 20 mm Hg or greater should arouse suspicion.[25] The most reliable method of measuring intraocular pressure is probably with the child awake and cooperative. The Perkins tonometer has been found to be particularly suitable in this situation. In one study, the mean intraocular pressure in unanesthetized newborns was 11.4 ± 2.4 mm Hg.[26]

There is no ideal method to measure intraocular pressure. Our preference is the hand-held Perkins applanation tonometer used at the earliest stage of inhalation anesthesia before intubation to reduce errors related to anesthesia, relying on the rest of the examination to interpret the importance of the intraocular pressure reading.

Slit-lamp Examination or Examination under Microscope

This portion of the examination is best performed with a portable hand held slit lamp or binocular operating microscope. The corneal findings are judged under magnification and stereopsis. The anterior chamber in primary congenital glaucoma is characteristically deep, especially, when the globe is distorted. The iris is typically normal, although it may have stromal hypoplasia with loss of the crypts. Other developmental glaucomas are characterized by a spectrum of changes in the anterior segment structures.

Gonioscopy

Evaluation of the anterior chamber angle is essential for the accurate diagnosis of developmental glaucoma. The Koeppe (14-16 mm) lens provides the surgeon with the appropriate view of the angle. If corneal clouding is marked, it could preclude a view of the angle. Anterior chamber angle in childhood differs significantly from that of adults. In the normal newborn eye, the iris usually inserts posterior to the scleral spur. Trabecular meshwork appears more transluscent than that of the adult. Gonioscopy of the eye with primary congenital glaucoma reveals an anterior insertion of the iris directly into the trabecular meshwork. Iris insertion is most commonly flat, although a concave insertion may also be seen. The surface of the trabecular meshwork may have a stippled appearance and the meshwork may appear thicker than normal. Sometimes, loops of blood vessels from the major arterial circle and fine fluffy tissue may be seen in the angle on gonioscopy.

Ophthalmoscopy

The optic nerve head in normal newborn is typically pink, but may have slight pallor and a small physiological cup is usually present. A cup-disc ratio > 0.3 or asymmetry between the two eyes is suggestive of developmental glaucoma.

Ultrasonography

Ultrasonic ocular biometry[27] has been recommended by some investigators for routine use in diagnosis and follow-up of congenital glaucoma. Normal axial length in an infant ranges from 17.5 to 20 mm and increases to 22 mm in length by one year of age. Results confirm the clinical value of echographic biometry for both the diagnosis of developmental glaucoma in cases with borderline intraocular pressure, and that of glaucoma in the fellow eye of patients with presumed unilateral disease. The method has proved its efficiency in the follow-up of patients with developmental glaucoma who had undergone surgery.

FACTORS INFLUENCING THERAPEUTIC DECISIONS
Structural Defects
Isolated Trabeculodysgenesis

It is the hallmark of primary developmental glaucoma and is highly responsive to goniotomy and trabeculotomy ab externo.

Irido-Trabeculodysgenesis

When other defects are associated with trabeculodysgenesis, the success rate of goniotomy and/or trabeculotomy is lowered. In iridodysgenesis, where the only iris defect is hypoplasia of the anterior stroma, good response to surgery has been reported. However, when the iris defect is associated with abnormal vessels that appear to wander, somewhat irregularly across the surface of the iris, then the prognosis is extremely grave. In such cases, multiple surgeries are usually needed.

Irido-Corneo-Trabeculodysgenesis

In patients with Axenfeld-Rieger's anomaly, surgical therapy does not have good prognosis and medical therapy is used initially. Often, medical therapy too is unsuccessful; therefore, surgical intervention becomes necessary. In such cases, surgery should be tailored to the specific cause.

Age

The age of the child at the onset of glaucoma is also a factor in choosing appropriate therapy. In general, children under the age of three years are best treated surgically. Children over three years of age deserve a trial of medical therapy unless a specific defect of trabeculodysgenesis is seen.

Corneal Clarity

In situations, where corneal clouding prevents adequate visualization of the trabecular meshwork, goniotomy is technically impossible and trabeculotomy ab externo has to be performed as the initial surgical procedure.[28]

Corneal Diameter

Corneal enlargement is a poor prognostic factor in the management of the developmental glaucoma. It is generally accepted that the success of goniotomy is not as good in eyes with significant buphthalmos. Barkan[29] felt that eyes with corneal diameter greater than 15 mm are not suitable for goniotomy. We feel that in patients with a significant increase in corneal diameter, goniotomy is technically difficult to perform and ab externo combined trabeculotomy cum trabeculectomy should be the initial procedure of choice.

Severity of Glaucoma

In advanced cases of developmental glaucoma, we prefer to perform ab externo combined trabeculotomy cum trabeculectomy, because it offers the highest success rate in such a situation.

Systemic Syndromes
Sturge-Weber Syndrome

When glaucoma is present in infancy, developmental anomalies that obstruct the aqueous outflow are thought to predominate and goniotomy or trabeculotomy is the surgical procedure of choice. When glaucoma in Sturge-Weber syndrome has its onset in later life, it is thought to be predominantly because of elevated episcleral venous pressure. Angle defect is less severe and, sometimes, minimal. In such patients, medical therapy should be tried first. If medical therapy fails, surgery should be performed on these eyes.[30] We prefer to use a technique combining ab externo trabeculotomy and trabeculectomy in such cases. We feel, that a combined surgical approach offers the best hope of success in such a condition.

Lowe's Syndrome

Hemorrhage frequently accompanies surgery, therefore, medical therapy should be tried initially. If it fails, surgery may be attempted, but prognosis is poor.[31]

THERAPY
Medical Therapy

Developmental glaucoma is essentially a surgical entity. Medical therapy is used only as a temporary measure till surgery is performed. Topical Timolol 0.25 or 0.5 percent and topical Dorzolamide 2 percent are usually safe and well tolerated. The technique of punctal occlusion must be explained to the parents to decrease the systemic absorption of the drug.

During the last few years, there has been an explosion of knowledge regarding the medical therapy for glaucoma, with the invention of effective antiglaucoma medications. Although, regulatory agencies worldwide usually do not include children in antiglaucoma drug approval studies, clinicians have found these medications useful in children with elevated intraocular pressure. For the medical therapy of pediatric glaucoma, clinicians should have a balanced view about indications and contraindications of different antiglaucoma medications in children.

> We caution that when using topical glaucoma medications, children may be at increased risk of systemic side effects compare to adults, due to reduced body mass and blood volume for drug distribution.

Surgery

Although medical treatment may delay the need for surgery in some pediatric glaucomas, most patients require surgical intervention.

Goniotomy

After the introduction of clinical gonioscopy, Otto Barkan (1936) modified the de Vincentiis' operation (1892) by using a specially designed glass contact lens to visualize the angle structures while using a knife to create an internal cleft in the trabecular tissue. He called the operation "goniotomy".[32]

The objective of goniotomy is to incise the obstructing tissue that causes the retention of aqueous and thereby, restore the access of aqueous to Schlemm's canal, thus, maintaining the physiological direction of the flow.

Results of goniotomy reported by various authors show a near uniform success rate of 80 percent in primary infantile glaucoma.[33] Goniotomy appears to be as effective as external trabeculotomy in this condition. It appears that goniotomy is most successful in patients in whom glaucoma is recognized early and treated between one month and one year of age. Early diagnosis and prompt treatment are important if good results are to be obtained. The severity of the filtration angle defect must also be considered in determining success with goniotomy.

Trabeculectomy Ab Externo

Trabeculectomy ab externo or external trabeculotomy as practiced today, is an alternative to goniotomy for the surgical treatment of congenital and childhood glaucomas. It can be used even when corneal haze prevents an adequate gonioscopic view which is a prerequisite for performing goniotomy.

Simultaneously and independently described by Buriani and Smith in 1960, trabeculotomy ab externo has given results better than goniotomy.

Our preferred operation is trabeculotomy ab externo, which has a number of major advantages[34] over the alternative operation of goniotomy.

Advantages

i. A trabeculotomy is anatomically more precise in rupturing the inner wall of the Schlemm's canal and trabecular meshwork, creating continuity between the anterior chamber and Schlemm's canal.

ii. Trabeculotomy is easier for a well-trained micro surgeon because it does not require the introduction of sharp instruments across the anterior chamber.

iii. There is no need for the surgeon to adapt the visual distortion produced by the operating gonioprism.

iv. Success of trabeculotomy depends only on the type of angle anomaly and not on the severity of glaucoma, the size of the cornea or the presence of corneal edema, all of which have been reported to influence the success of goniotomy.

v. Trabeculotomy produces less surgical trauma as the anterior chamber is entered only briefly. There is lower incidence of postoperative cataract and fewer postoperative complications.

vi. Trabeculotomy has a higher documented success rate than goniotomy.

In patients with a scarred and edematous cornea, the goniotomist has the choice of either operating with no view of the operation site or doing a trabeculotomy. Most surgeons would prefer to do a trabeculotomy than operate "blind". Thus, the goniotomist, who may have little experience with trabeculotomy, uses this procedure in difficult eyes. This is an argument for using trabeculotomy in all cases and gaining experience with the procedure in easier and more predictable operations.

The popularity of trabeculotomy ab externo, as an initial procedure in the surgical management of developmental glaucoma, has been championed by a number of authorities.[34,35]

Combined Trabeculotomy cum Trabeculectomy (Combined Trab-Trab)

We prefer to use a technique combining ab externo trabeculotomy with trabeculectomy in most of the cases of developmental glaucoma.

The trabeculotomy is performed to remove the possible obstruction to the aqueous outflow by a congenital angle deformity while the trabeculectomy is included to bypass the episcleral venous system. In other words, the combined procedure is designed to deal with both possible mechanisms associated with some forms of developmental glaucoma, e.g. the Sturge-Weber syndrome.

In our observation, compared to the Western population, a larger number of Indian patients present with corneal clouding and edema in which goniotomy is technically impossible. External trabeculotomy is the initial procedure of choice. Another important consideration is that while most patients have symptoms suggestive of congenital glaucoma at birth or within six months of birth, patients usually present late because of poverty, illiteracy, ignorance and inadequate eye care facilities in remote corners of the country. In such advanced cases, we prefer to perform combined trabeculotomy cum trabeculectomy which offers the best hope of success.

Surgical Technique
Combined Trabeculotomy cum Trabeculectomy (Combined Trab-Trab)
The surgical technique[25] is described in detail:

The patient is usually a child and general anesthesia is required.

After the child is anesthetized, the operative field is prepared with antiseptic solution.

A surgical microscope designed for ophthalmic surgery is a must.

i. A limbus-based conjunctival flap is raised (7 mm from the limbus) with blunt-tipped westcott scissors and plain forceps and the dissection is usually done in the episcleral plane. Hemostasis is meticulously maintained throughout the dissection of the conjunctival flap. We use a bipolar underwater cautery in an effort to minimize trauma to the tissue.

ii. Retracting the conjunctival flap gently towards the pupil, light cautery is applied on the sclera.

iii. A one-half thickness scleral incision is then made with a BP blade along the V outlined by cautery. Here, we must bear in mind that the sclera in a buphthalmic child is usually much thinner than the adult eye (**Figure 2**).

iv. A partial thickness scleral flap is then dissected toward the limbus using a No. 15 blade. The flap is held with Pierse-Hoskins forceps during the dissection.

v. We prefer a triangular flap, as it allows adequate exposure of the Schlemm's canal and involves less scleral dissection than a rectangular flap. Care should be taken to maintain the same plane while dissecting the scleral flap, especially near the limbus.

vi. Surgical landmarks and anatomy of the limbal region should be carefully identified before one can proceed to the next step.

Closest to the limbus is a transparent band of deep corneal lamellae. Behind that is a narrow grayish blue band, which represents the trabecular meshwork, following which is the white, opaque sclera. The junction of the posterior border of the trabecular band and the sclera is the external landmark to the scleral spur and the landmark to the canal of Schlemm. In most of the eyes, this is situated between 2 and 2.5 mm behind the surgical limbus.

vii. A 2 × 2 mm trabeculectomy flap is outlined without penetrating the anterior chamber (**Figure 3**). A central radial incision is then made across the scleral spur. The objective of this radial incision is to cut the external wall of Schlemm's canal and to avoid entering the anterior chamber. It is important to bear in mind that Schlemm's canal is separated from the anterior chamber only by the trabecular meshwork.

This is the most delicate step in the operation and demands the most micro surgical skill. Under high magnification, the radial incision is gradually deepened with a razor blade-chip until it is carried through the external wall of Schlemm's canal, at which point there is gush of aqueous, occasionally, mixed with blood. In our experience, a drop of aqueous is more common than a drop of blood. The dissection is carefully continued through the external wall until the inner wall of the canal becomes visible. The inner wall is characteristically slightly pigmented and is composed of crises-crossing fibers. Some surgeons confirm passage into the canal by passing a 6-0 nylon suture into the canal, as described by Smith.[36]

The internal arm of the trabeculotome is introduced into the canal using the external parallel arm as a guide.

Once 90 percent of the trabeculotome is within the canal, it is rotated into the anterior chamber and rotation is continued until 75 percent of the probe arm length has entered the chamber. Then, the rotation is reversed and the instrument is withdrawn. About 2 to 2 1/2 clock hours of the internal wall of Schlemm's canal and trabecular meshwork are disrupted by the movement of the trabeculotome into the anterior chamber. The trabeculotome is then passed into the Schlemm's canal on the other side of the radial incision and rotated into the anterior chamber. In total, about 100° to 120° of trabecular meshwork is ruptured by this technique (**Figures 4 to 7**).

It is important that no force should be used when introducing the probe into the canal, as this will create a false passage. If the probe does not slip easily down the canal, it should be withdrawn and dissection of the outer canal continued until the surgeon is satisfied that all fibers of the outer wall are removed. The probe is then reintroduced into the canal. As the probe passes into the anterior chamber, rupturing the inner wall of the canal, there should be some slight resistance and there may be a little intracameral bleeding from the inner wall. This bleeding is typical and perhaps even a favorable sign indicating that communication has been created between canal of Schlemm and the anterior chamber. This bleeding is innocuous and almost always clears by the following day.

The important point is that the probe should pass with ease along the canal and from the canal into the anterior chamber without forcing it.

The probe is swept in a plane parallel to the iris. As the probe is swung from the canal into the anterior chamber, the surgeon should carefully watch the iris for movement, particularly, if the probe passes easily. Movement of the iris or a totally unresisted passage of the probe implies that the probe is in the anterior chamber and touching the iris root. If not corrected, this may cause an iridodialysis. The probe should be immediately withdrawn without continuing its entry into the anterior chamber and replaced, keeping the tip of the probe slightly anterior, so that, it does not prematurely rupture the inner wall.

The cornea should also be carefully monitored to ensure that the probe does not rip through the sclera, cornea and Descemet's membrane. This is easy to detect because small air bubbles appear in the cornea, as the probe ruptures through corneal lamellae. In case this occurs, the probe needs to be repositioned, pushing the tip a little posteriorly. The trabeculotomy has been completed and now trabeculectomy has to be performed. The incision into the anterior chamber is deepened by careful dissection with the microblade until the opening is large enough to introduce a straight or angled Vannas scissors, with which the anterior incision is completed. Then, the radial incision and finally, the posterior incision just anterior to the scleral spur and parallel to the limbus are made, and the trabecular block is removed **(Figure 8)**. The iris blocks the trabecular opening maintaining the anterior chamber, which should remain formed throughout the procedure.

An iridectomy is then made **(Figure 9)**. It is imperative that the base of the iridectomy opening is wider than the trabeculotomy opening to prevent the iris pillars from being pushed into this opening postoperatively:

The scleral flap is then closed with three 10-0 nylon suture, one at the apex and one each side **(Figure 10)**.

The conjunctiva and Tenon's capsule are then closed with a running

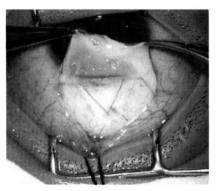
Fig. 2 Partial thickness triangular scleral flap delineated

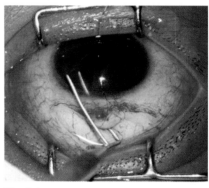
Fig. 5 The probe rotated into AC from the left side

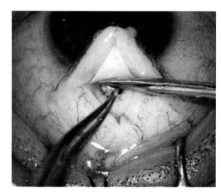
Fig. 8 The deeper trabecular block removed

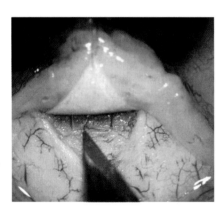
Fig. 3 Anatomy of the limbal region identified and Schlemm's canal explored

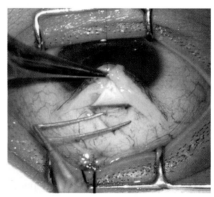
Fig. 6 Trabeculotomy probe introduced into the right side of the radial incision

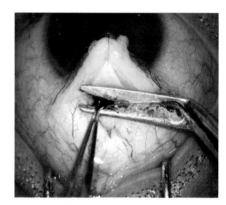
Fig. 9 Iridectomy done

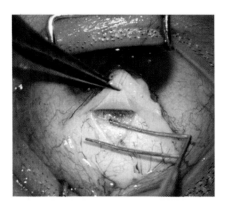
Fig. 4 Trabeculotomy probe introduced into the left side of the radial incision

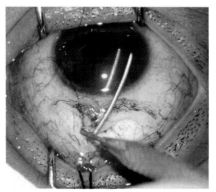
Fig. 7 Trabeculotomy probe rotated into AC from the right side

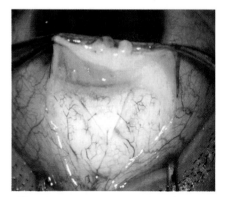
Fig. 10 Closure of the triangular scleral flap with 10-0 nylon

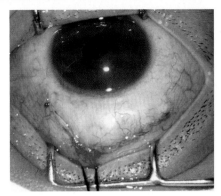

Fig. 11 Closure of the conjunctival incision with 8-0 vicryl

suture of absorbable material (e.g. 6-0 vicryl) **(Figure 11)**.

In highly buphthalmic eyes, the Schlemm's canal may not be located with certainty. In such cases, it is possible to convert the procedure to a trabeculectomy by removing a block of deep limbal tissue beneath the scleral flap.

Some surgeons prefer to perform a paracentesis opening with a beveled corneal incision at the beginning of the surgery. In such a situation, the anterior chamber is reformed with BSS, and 'patency' of the trabeculectomy can be tested at the conclusion of the surgery. We, however, do not favor a paracentesis opening for possible cataractogenic effect of fluid injection in AC.

Results

There are several published reports on primary combined trabeculotomy-trabeculectomy in different types of developmental glaucomas **(Figures 12 to 18)**.[37-44] We recently published our results of combined trabeculotomy-trabeculectomy (CTT). Six hundred and twenty-four eyes of 360 consecutive patients who underwent primary CTT for primary developmental glaucoma from January 1990 to June 2004 were studied.[44] Mean IOP reduced from 28.1+/-7.5 mm Hg to 14.9+/-5.9 mm Hg (P<0.0001). Probability of success

(IOP<21 mm Hg) was 85.2 percent, 80.4 percent, 77.2 percent, 72.6 percent, 66.2 and 57.5 percent at first, second, third, fourth, fifth and sixth years respectively. Data on Snellen visual acuity was available in 27.8 percent children. At the final follow-up visit, 42 percent children had visual acuity>/=20/60. In multivariate analysis, failure increased by three-fold in the presence of preoperative IOP>35 mm Hg (HR=3.12, 95% CI=1.4-6.7) and two-fold in cases with a history of prior glaucoma surgery (HR=2.57, 95% CI=1.1-6.0). There were no major intraoperative complications.

In refractory cases of developmental glaucoma, trabeculectomy with mitomycin C may be a useful option.[45,46]

Glaucoma Drainage Implants

The use of glaucoma drainage implants in pediatric patients was first described by Molteno and his colleagues in 1973. Since then, clinical experience has been gained and modifications have been made in surgical methods and designs. Glaucoma drainage implants[47] are indicated when other surgical treatments have a poor prognosis for success, prior conventional surgery fails, or significant conjunctival scarring precludes filtration surgery.[47] Available types of drainage implants can be characterized as open-tube, (nonrestrictive) e.g. Molteno and Baerveldt implant or valved (flow-restrictive) devices, e.g. Krupin and Ahmed valves. The Ahmed glaucoma valve is a popular choice in pediatric patients because the flow-restrictive device reduces the risk of hypotony and its associated complications. The success rate of IOP control with various types of implants reported in various studies ranges from 54 to 95 percent, depending on the patient age, definition of success, length of follow-up and other factors.[47] In most of these

studies, medical therapy and other surgical procedures had already failed before implant surgery, and there were few other options for IOP control. In these refractory conditions, surgical results of glaucoma drainage implants for pediatric patients are encouraging.

Cyclodestructive Procedures

These procedures constitute a valuable adjunct in the surgical armamentarium for refractory cases or when the surgeon wishes to avoid incisional surgery, such as in eyes with poor visual potential. These include cyclocryotherapy and trans-scleral cyclophotocoagulation (TSCPC) utilizing Nd:YAG laser or diode laser.

FOLLOW-UP

The responsibility of the surgeon does not stop with surgery, and it is also very important not to be lulled into a false sense of security by surgical control of intraocular pressure. Visual rehabilitation is as important in the management of the disease as is intraocular pressure control. Visual rehabilitation involves correction of refractive errors, correction of opacities in the media such as corneal scarring and cataract, and orthoptic treatment to stimulate the development of binocular stereoscopic vision. Anisometropia and amblyopia must also be aggressively managed to give the best chance to these children for good vision in both eyes. These should be undertaken at as early an age as possible. A properly functioning visual rehabilitation department plays an important role in the integrated management of children with congenital glaucoma.[51]

An attempt should be made to familiarize the parents with the protracted nature of the illness, the prognosis, the frequent necessity for repeated surgery and the lifelong need for continued examinations.[52]

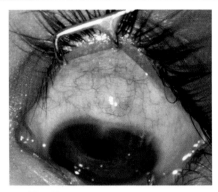

Fig. 12 Three years postoperative appearance of the bleb

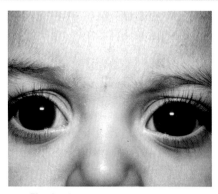

Fig. 15 Six months postoperative appearance of clear cornea

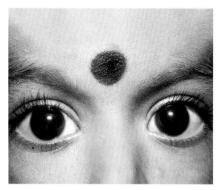

Fig. 18 Four years postoperative appearance showing normal corneal clarity

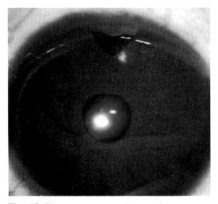

Fig. 13 Three years postoperative appearance of anterior segment showing clear cornea with Haab's striae

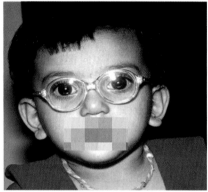

Fig. 16 Three years postoperative appearance of the same child with normal vision

in five PCG families from India and devised PCR-based RFLP methods to rapidly screen these mutations.[48] We further screened 138 PCG cases and found that 30.8 percent of these cases were positive for any of the previously identified 6 mutations and that R368H happened to be the most prevalent mutation in the Indian population.[49] We also studied 260 unrelated PCG cases from different ethnic background and found that *CYP1B1* was involved in approximately 38 percent of cases. A total of 17 different mutations were observed, of which nine were novel.[50]

SUMMARY

Pediatric glaucomas are relatively rare, but potentially blinding diseases. Early diagnosis and meticulous surgery are crucial in proper management. In our experience, combined trabeculotomy with trabeculectomy has good results. An integrated approach, combining surgical facilities with visual rehabilitation facilities and genetic study facilities provides maximum benefit to the patients.[51]

Continued clinical monitoring combined with adequate support from the parents and family members along with adequate social support should allow the best possible outcome for the affected children.[52]

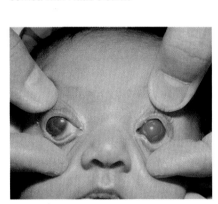

Fig. 14 Primary congenital glaucoma operated at the age of one week

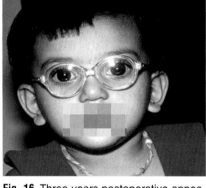

Fig. 17 Simultaneous bilateral primary trabeculotomy-trabeculectomy at the age of three days

ROLE OF GENETIC STUDY AND GENETIC COUNSELING

An autosomal recessive mode of inheritance is well-documented for PCG. Even though three different loci

have been mapped for PCG, mutations in the *CYP1B1* gene (GLC3A locus) is the most predominant and is reported in most ethnic backgrounds. We have reported the involvement of *CYP1B1*

REFERENCES

1. Barkan O. Pathogenesis of congenital glaucoma. Gonioscopic and anatomic observation of the angle of the anterior chamber in the normal eye and in congenital glaucoma. Am J Ophthalmol 1955;40:1-11.

2. Worst JGF. The pathogenesis of congenital glaucoma. Assen. Netherlands, Royal Van Gorcum: Springfield, Illinois, Charles C Thomas, 1966.

3. Worst JGF. Congenital glaucoma. Remarks on the aspect of the chamber angle: Ontogenic and pathogenic background and mode of action of goniotomy: Invest Ophthalmol Vis Sci 1968;7:127-34.

4. Anderson DR. The development of the trabecular meshwork and its abnormality in primary infantile glaucoma. Trans Am Ophthalmol Soc 1981;79:45-485.

5. Hannson HA, Jerndal T. Scanning electron microscopic studies of the development of the irido corneal angle in human eyes. Invest Ophthalmol Vis Sci 1971;10:252-65.

6. Maul E, Strozzi L, Munoz C, Revs C. Outflow pathways in congenital glaucoma. Am J Ophthalmol 1980;89:667-75.

7. Maumenee AE. The pathogenesis of congenital glaucoma: a new theory. Trans Am Ophthalmol Soc 1958;56:507-70.

8. Maumenee AE. The pathogenesis of congenital glaucoma: a new theory. Am J Ophthalmol 1959;47:827-59.

9. Maumenee AE. Further observations on the pathogenesis of congenital glaucoma. Trans Am Ophthalmol Soc 1962;60:140-62.

10. Maumenee AE. Further observations on the pathogenesis of congenital glaucoma. Am J Ophthalmol 1963;55:1163-76.

11. Kupfer C, Kaiser-Kupfer MI. Observations on the development of the anterior chamber angle with reference to the pathogenesis of congenital glaucomas. Am J Ophthalmol 1979;88:424-6.

12. Tawara A, Inomata H. Developmental immaturity of the trabecular meshwork in congenital glaucoma. Am J Ophthalmol 1981;92:508-25.

13. Chakrabarti D, Mandal AK, et al. Prospective evaluation of symptoms and signs in primary developmental glaucoma. Paper accepted in the annual meeting of The Glaucoma Society of India, 2007.

14. Hoskins HD Jr, Kass MA. Becker - Shaffer's diagnosis and therapy of the glaucomas. St Louis: CV Mosby Co, 6 edn, 1989.

15. Walton DS. Glaucoma in infants and children. In Harley RD (Ed) Paediatric ophthalmology, (2nd Edn) WB Saunders Co; 1983.pp.585-98.

16. Kwitko ML. The paediatric glaucomas, in Shin DH (Ed): Glaucoma surgery, International ophthalmology clinics. Boston Little Brown 1981;21(1):199-222.

17. Kwitko ML. Glaucoma in Infants and children. New York, Appleton - Century-Crofts, 1973.

18. Shaffer RN, Weiss DI. The congenital and pediatric glaucoma. St Louis, CV Mosby, 1970.

19. Morin JD, Merin S, Sheppard RW. Primary congenital glaucoma: a survey. Can J Ophthalmol 1974;9:17-28.

20. deLuise VP, Anderson DR. Primary infantile glaucoma (congenital glaucoma). Surv Ophthalmol 1983;28:1-19.

21. Waring GO, Laibson PR, Rodriguez M. Clinical and pathological alteration of Descemet's membrane. Surv Ophthalmol 1974;18:325.

22. Mann I: Developmental abnormalities of the eye. Philadelphia: JB Lippincott, 1957.

23. Maumenee AE. Further observations on the pathogenesis of congenital glaucoma. Am J Ophthalmol 1963;55:1163.

24. Duke - Elder S. System of ophthalmology Vol III, Part 2, congenital deformities, St Louis: CV Mosby Co, PP 1969;548-65.

25. Mandal AK. Current Concepts in the Diagnosis and Management of Developmental Glaucomas. Indian J Ophthalmol 1993;41:51-70.

26. Radtke MD, Cohen BE. Intraocular pres-sure measurement in the newborn. Am J Ophthalmol 1974;78:501-4.

27. Reibaldi A. Biometric ultrasound in the diagnosis and follow-up of congenital glaucoma. Ann Ophthalmol 1982;14:707-8.

28. Hoskins HD, et al. Goniotomy vs trabeculotomy. J Paediatric Ophthalmol Strabismus 1984;21:158.

29. Barkan O. Goniotomy for the relief of congenital glaucoma. Br J Ophthalmol 1948;32;701-25.

30. Phelps CD. The pathogenesis of glaucoma in Sturge-Weber syndrome. Ophthalmology 1978;85:276-86.

31. Curtin VT, et al. Ocular pathology in oculo-cerebro-renal syndrome of Lowe. Am J Ophthalmol 1967;64:533.

32. Barkan O. Technique of goniotomy. Arch Ophthalmol 1938;19:217-21.

33. Barkan O. Surgery of congenital glaucoma review of 196 eyes operated by goniotimy. Am J Ophthalmol 1953;36:1523-34.

34. Luntz MH. The advantages of trabeculotomy over goniotomy. J Pediatric Ophthalmol Strabismus 1984;21:150-3.

35. Mcpherson SD Jr, et al. Goniotomy vs external trabeculotomy for developmental glaucoma. Am J Ophthalmol 1983;95:427-31.

36. Smith R. A new technique for opening the canal of Schlemm. Br J Ophthalmol 1963;44:370-3.

37. Mandal AK. Micro Surgical Technique combines Trabeculotomy and trabeculectomy to Treat Developmental Glaucoma, Ocular Surgery News, International Edition 1994;5(8):38-43.

38. Mandal AK, Naduvilath TJ, Jayagandan A. Surgical Results of Combined Trabeculotomy-Trabeculectomy for Developmental Glaucoma. Ophthalmology 1998;105:974-82.

39. Mandal AK. Primary combined trabeculotomy-trabeculectomy for early-onset glaucoma in Sturge-Weber syndrome. Ophthalmology 1999;106:1621-7.

40. Mandal AK, Bhatia PG, Gothwal VK, et al. Safety and efficacy of simultaneous bilateral primary combined trabeculotomy-trabeculectomy for developmental glaucoma. Indian J Ophthalmol 2002;50:13-9.

41. Mandal AK, Gothwal VK, Bagga H, et al. Outcome of surgery on infants younger than one month of age with congenital glaucoma. Ophthalmology 2003;110:1909-15.

42. Mandal AK, Bhatia PG, Bhaskar, A, Nutheti R. Long-term surgical and visual outcomes in children with developmental glaucoma operated within 6 months of birth. Ophthalmology 2004;111:283-90.

43. Mandal AK, Bhende J, Nutheti R, Krishnaiah S. Combined trabeculotomy and trabeculectomy in advanced primary developmental glaucoma with corneal diameter of 14mm or more. Eye 2006;20:135-43.

44. Mandal AK, Gothwal VK, Nutheti R. Surgical outcome of primary developmental glaucoma: a single surgeon's long-term experience from a tertiary eye care center in India. Eye 2007;21:764-74.

45. Mandal AK, Walton DS, John T, Jayagandan A. Mitomycin C-Augmented Trabeculectomy in Refractory Congenital Glaucoma. Ophthalmology 1997;104:996-1003.

46. Mandal AK, Prasad K, Naduvilath TJ. Surgical results and complications of mitomycin C-augmented trabeculectomy in refractory developmental glaucoma. Ophthalmic Surg Lasers 1999;30:473-80.

47. Ishida K, Mandal AK, Netland PA. Glaucoma drainage implants in pediatric patients. Ophthalmol Clin N Am 2005;18:431-42.

48. Panicker SG, Reddy ABM, Mandal AK, et al. Identification of novel mutations causing familial primary congenital glaucoma in Indian pedigrees. Invest Ophthalmol Vis Sci 2002;43:1358-66.

49. Reddy ABM, Panicker SG, Mandal AK, et al. Identification of R368H as a predominant-CYP1B1 allele causing primary congenital glaucoma in Indian patients. Invest Ophthalmol Vis Sci 2003;44:4200-3.

50. Panicker SG, Mandal AK, Reddy ABM, Gothwal VK. Correlations of genotype with phenotype in Indian patients with primary congenital glaucoma. Invest Ophthalmol Vis Sci 2004;45:1149-56.

51. Mandal AK, Netland PA, Gothwal VK. Advances in the in the management of the developmental glaucoma. Recent Advances in Ophthalmology, Vol. 8, Editors: Nema HV and Nema N by New Delhi: Jaypee Brothers Medical Publishers, Chapter 5; 2006.pp.83-129.

52. Mandal AK, Netland PA. "The Pediatric Glaucomas" published by Elsevier Science in 2006.

41 | Glaucoma in Phacomatosis

Kavitha Palanisamy, R Venkatesh

CHAPTER OUTLINE
- ❖ Sturge-Weber Syndrome
- ❖ Von Recklinghausen's Neurofibromatosis (NF1)
- ❖ Von Hippel-Lindau Disease (Angiomatosis Retinae)
- ❖ Tuberous Sclerosis
- ❖ Nevus of Ota
- ❖ Phakomatosis Pigmentovascularis
- ❖ Cutis Marmorata Telangiectatica Congenital

DEFINITION

Phakomatosis (*Greek: Phakos, a lentil*) is a group of hereditary disorders characterized by the presence of hamartias and hamartomas involving different organ system derived from all the three embryonic layers. The term was coined by van der Hoeve in 1932[1] to unify the diverse manifestations of tuberous sclerosis and neurofibromatosis, both of which involve multiple organs and could present either early or late in life. Because of the inborn nature of the tumors, they were called phacomata from the Greek *phakos*, meaning "mother spot".

Hamartias—nontumorous growths on the skin and mucous membranes that arise from cells, normally found in the tissue at the involved site, e.g. congenital vascular malformations of ataxia telangiectasia.

Hamartomas—localized tumors arising from cells, normally found at the site of growth, e.g. glial tumors of tuberous sclerosis: tumorous malformations of hamartias are hamartomas. Hamartomas primarily involve the eye, skin and nervous system, but can also involve to a lesser degree; pulmonary, cardiovascular, gastrointestinal, renal and skeletal systems.

The conditions that are frequently or occasionally associated with glaucoma are von Hippel-Lindau syndrome (Angiomatosis retinae), Von Recklinghausen's neurofibromatosis, tuberous sclerosis (Bourneville's disease) and Sturge-Weber syndrome (encephalotrigeminal angiomatosis). Sturge-Weber syndrome is not as clearly hereditary as the three classical phacomatoses; the vascular tumors in Sturge-Weber are generally present at birth, rather than arising *de novo* in later life, and malignant transformation is rare.[2] The other conditions are Klippel-Treanaunay-Weber syndrome (in its pure form), diffuse congenital hemangiomatosis, basal cell nevus syndrome, Wyburn-Mason syndrome (racemose angioma of the retina), nevus of Ota (Oculodermal Melanocytosis), Ataxia telangiectasia (Louis-Bar syndrome).

STURGE-WEBER SYNDROME

Sturge described an association of facial angioma, ipsilateral congenital glaucoma and hemiparetic epilepsy. Sturge observed that patients with unilateral facial Port-wine stains (nevus flammeus) regularly had seizures and hemiparesis of the contralateral side- and speculated correctly that this was the result of an intracranial hemangioma. Weber described the characteristic 'railroad track' linear calcification seen on skull X-rays.

Sturge-Weber syndrome is classified into *complete trisymptomatic Sturge-Weber syndrome* when all three organ systems are involved, *incomplete bisymptomatic Sturge-Weber syndrome* when the involvement is either oculocutaneous or neurocutaneous, and *incomplete monosymptomatic Sturge-Weber syndrome* when only neural or cutaneous involvement is noted. In a review of 51 patients, the condition was recognized before 24 months of age in more than half the cases.[3]

> **Note** Patients with no cutaneous involvement appear to be spared from the ocular manifestations of the syndrome.

Clinical Features
- Convulsive disorders (89%)
- Facial angioma (86%)
- Abnormal X-ray findings (63%)

- Mental retardation (54%)
- Ocular abnormalities (37%)
- Hemiplegias (31%).

The hallmark of Sturge-Weber syndrome is a facial cutaneous venous dilation, also referred to as nevus flammeus or port-wine stain, **(Figures 1A and B)** which is present in as many as 96 percent of patients and is visible at birth. The facial venous dilation appears as one or several dull red patches of irregular outline, along, but not limited to, the distribution of one or more divisions of the trigeminal nerve.

A leptomeningeal congenital venous angiomatosis may be present. It is usually ipsilateral to the facial lesion and located most commonly in the meninges overlying the occipital and posterior parietal lobes.

Ocular Involvement

Ocular involvement may include:

- Eyelid hemangioma like superficial changes (which on histology demonstrate only venous dilation)
- Glaucoma
- Conjunctival and episcleral hemangiomas
- Diffuse choroidal hemangiomas
- Heterochromia of the irides
- Tortuous retinal vessels with occasional arteriovenous communications.

Glaucoma

Glaucoma occurs in approximately one-half of the cases in which the port-wine stain involves the ophthalmic and maxillary divisions of the trigeminal nerve. **Anderson's rule** says that when nevus flammeus involves the upper lid, there is ipsilateral intraocular involvement.[4] Bilateral cases are rare and may occur when vascular malformation is widespread.

A corneal diameter of more than 12 mm during the first year of life, corneal edema, tears in the descemet membrane (Haab striae), unilateral or bilateral myopic shift, optic nerve cupping greater than 0.3, or any cup asymmetry associated with intraocular pressure above the high teens, may indicate the presence of infantile glaucoma.

Conjunctival and Episcleral Hemangiomas

Increased conjunctival vascularity **(Figure 2)** can be seen on slit lamp examination or as a pinkish discoloration seen by the naked eye. The abnormal plexus of episcleral vessels may be hidden by the overlying tissue of the tenons in infancy and only appreciated clinically in later childhood. These prominent tortuous conjunctival and episcleral vascular plexuses affect as many as 70 percent of patients with Sturge-Weber syndrome and often correlate with increased episcleral venous pressure, probably resulting from arteriovenous shunts within the episcleral hemangiomas.

Iris heterochromia occurs in approximately 10 percent of patients with Sturge-Weber syndrome. The more deeply pigmented iris usually is ipsilateral to the port-wine stain, signifying an increase in melanocytes number or activity.

Diffuse Choroidal Hemangioma

Diffuse choroidal hemangioma appears on indirect binocular ophthalmoscopy as a salmon orange, elevated mass with indistinct margins. The diffuse thickening of the choroid caused by the hemangioma produces a deep red color in the posterior fundus, the "tomato ketchup" fundus, which is obvious when compared to an uninvolved eye.

The overlying retinal vessels may be affected, demonstrating dilation and tortuosity as well as peripheral arteriovenous communications.

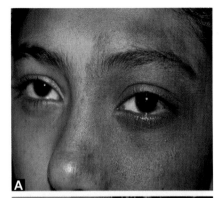

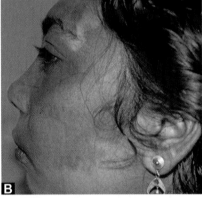

Figs 1A and B Unilateral facial Port-wine stains in Sturge-Weber syndrome

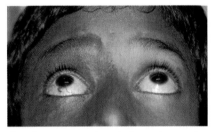

Fig. 2 Unilateral facial Port-wine stains and prominent tortuous conjunctival and episcleral vessels in Sturge-Weber syndrome

Cutaneous Features

Nevus Flammeus or Port-wine Stain

The facial cutaneous venous lesion is usually the first component of the syndrome to be observed because it is visible at birth. It may be very pale at first. Although, it does not increase in extent, it usually becomes darker with age. Although not a medically threatening condition in and of itself, the cosmetic deformity that the port-wine stain imposes may carry a psychological impact.

Mechanism of Glaucoma: Theories

Weiss[5] described two mechanisms, the more common of which occurs in infants, with a developmental anomaly of the anterior chamber angle similar to that of congenital glaucoma. One histopathologic report described a partial developmental anomaly of the anterior chamber angle[6] and another study revealed neovascularization in the trabecular meshwork.[7] Cibis and associates[8] found aging changes, similar to those seen in chronic open-angle glaucoma in the trabecular meshwork of three eyes with Sturge-Weber syndrome.

The other mechanism of glaucoma appears later in life and is associated with an open anterior chamber angle and small arteriovenous fistulas in the episcleral vessels. Phelps[9] observed episcleral hemangiomas in all cases and elevated episcleral venous pressure whenever this parameter could be studied, but saw no abnormalities of the anterior chamber angle. He thought that elevated episcleral venous pressure was the most common glaucoma mechanism in all ages of patients with the Sturge-Weber syndrome.

Differential Diagnoses

- **Klippel-Trenaunay-Weber syndrome** consists of port-wine stains of the extremities and face, as well as hemihypertrophy of soft and bony tissues, in addition to all the characteristics of Sturge-Weber syndrome. This syndrome is sporadic as is Sturge-Weber syndrome. Also, in Klippel-Trenaunay-Weber syndrome, an association is noted between hemihypertrophy and solid visceral tumors, most commonly affecting the kidney, adrenal gland, or liver.
- **Beckwith-Wiedemann syndrome** consists of a facial port-wine stain, macroglossia, omphalocele, and visceral hyperplasia. A risk of visceral neoplasia is also noted. Severe hypoglycemia resulting from pancreatic islet-cell hyperplasia is very common and may be life-threatening.

Work-up

This includes:
- Skull X-ray
- CT
- MRI
- A-scan and B-scan ultrasonography
- Fluorescein angiography.

A-scan and B-scan ultrasonography are useful in the diagnosis of diffuse choroidal hemangioma. B-scan ultrasonography characteristically shows a solid echogenic mass, whereas, A-scan ultrasonography demonstrates high internal reflectivity.

Fluorescein angiography may reveal only an exaggerated background choroidal fluorescence early in the disease, widespread and irregular areas of hyperfluorescence secondary to diffuse leakage of dye from the surface of the tumor during the later stages of angiography, or even a diffuse multiloculated pattern of fluorescein accumulation in the outer retina characteristic of polycystic degeneration and edema in more advanced disease.

Management

Medical therapy may suffice to control the glaucoma that occurs in later life, whereas, the infantile form usually requires surgical intervention.[5] In most cases of glaucoma associated with elevated episcleral venous pressure, medical therapy has limited efficacy, and this appears to be true for prostaglandins.[9] Success has been reported with a trabeculectomy in children and adults.[10,11] However, filtering surgery in these patients is commonly associated with intraoperative choroidal effusion,[11-13] and occasionally with expulsive hemorrhage.[11-14] In one study of 30 patients, goniotomy was not associated with these complications and was the investigator's first choice in most cases.[11] Because, it may not be certain whether the glaucoma is caused by an anterior chamber angle anomaly or elevated episcleral venous pressure, a combined trabeculotomy-trabeculectomy may improve the chances of success, by treating both possible sources of elevated IOP,[12,15] although it does not reduce the potential for serious complications.

Some surgeons prefer to perform one or more prophylactic posterior sclerotomies just before filtration surgery or any other intraocular procedure to reduce the risk of choroidal or retinal effusion and expulsive hemorrhage. Another surgical approach to reduce pressure in these patients while minimizing intraocular complications, is a valved or nonvalved aqueous drainage device. One case series reported good outcomes after a two-staged Baerveldt glaucoma implant.[16] A final technique that may be considered is a cyclodestructive procedure that avoids incisional surgery.

VON RECKLINGHAUSEN'S NEUROFIBROMATOSIS (NF1)

The principal systemic lesions in this condition involve the skin and include cafe-au-lait spots, which are flat, hyperpigmented lesions with well-circumscribed borders, and neurofibromas, which appear as soft, flesh-colored, pedunculated masses. The latter lesions arise from Schwann cells. Central nervous system involvement is uncommon, although neurofibromas may develop from cranial nerves, especially the acoustic nerve. Two subsets of neurofibromatosis have been distinguished: *peripheral* (von Recklinghausen's neurofibromatosis), characterized by the skin lesions, and *central*, characterized by bilateral acoustic schwannomas.[17] Both are inherited by an autosomal dominant mode with variable expressivity. Genetic analysis of a kindred with von Recklinghausen's neurofibromatosis indicated that the responsible gene is located near the centromere on chromosome 17.[18]

Neurofibromatosis-1: According to the NIH consensus statement, diagnosis of neurofibromatosis-1 is established if two or more of the characteristics **(Table 1)** are present.

Systemic Features

- ***Cutaneous involvement:*** The cutaneous manifestations of neurofibromatosis-1 are a prominent aspect of this disorder. They include hyperpigmentation, hypopigmentation, and cutaneous neurofibromas.

- ❖ Hyperpigmentation can occur in focal or diffuse forms.
  - ◆ Focal hyperpigmentation: Café-au-lait spots are a distinct area of hyperpigmentation due to an increased number of melanocytes, as well as giant pigment granule (macromelanosome) production by melanocytes. Focal hyperpigmentation also includes axillary and inguinal freckling.
  - ◆ Diffuse hyperpigmentation: Diffuse or generalized hyperpigmentation is not well characterized, but often it is noticed by an astute physician or family member.

- ❖ Hypopigmentation can occur in patients with neurofibromatosis-1.
  - ◆ Hypomelanotic macules
  - ◆ Punctate hypopigmented lesions
  - ◆ Local areas of skin hypopigmentation.
- ❖ Cutaneous neurofibromas
  - ◆ Small, pink to skin-colored, dome-shaped papules **(Figures 3A and B)**
  - ◆ May enlarge, becoming immense soft-tissue masses
  - ◆ Can occur anywhere on the body
  - ◆ Histologically, indistinguishable from the solitary neurofibroma, they appear as well-circumscribed, nonencapsulated spindle-cell tumors of the dermis.

- ***CNS involvement:*** CNS involvement in neurofibromatosis-1 is multifaceted. Abnormalities of CNS development are common. Similarly, functional problems are often noted, and benign and malignant tumors of the CNS occur at a greatly increased incidence in neurofibromatosis-1.
  - ❖ Abnormalities of CNS development
    - ◆ Simple megalencephaly is common and generally harmless. Its main features, brain matter and skull circumference are increased
    - ◆ Hydrocephalus may present at any age and is symptomatic (vomiting, irritability, lethargy, papilledema). If it is not due to a tumor, it is usually treated with a shunt
    - ◆ Vascular occlusions
    - ◆ Dural ectasia

Table 1 NIH criteria for diagnosis of neurofibromatosis

Neurofibromatosis -1
• Six or more café-au-lait spots, 15 mm or larger, in an adult; 6 or more café- au-lait spots, 5 mm or larger, in a child (before puberty)
• Two or more neurofibromas of any type or 1 plexiform neurofibroma
• Freckling of the axillary or inguinal region, an optic pathway glioma, 2 or more Lisch nodules
• Characteristic osseous lesions, such as sphenoid dysplasia
• A first-degree relative with neurofibromatosis-1 (as defined by the above criteria)
Two or more of the above characteristics should be present
NIH criteria for diagnosis of neurofibromatosis-2 (definite, presumptive and suggestive)
Definite neurofibromatosis-2:
Bilateral vestibular schwannomas (VS), also known as acoustic neuroma
Presumptive (probable) neurofibromatosis-2:
• Family history of neurofibromatosis-2 (first-degree family relative) PLUS
• Unilateral vestibular schwannomas (VS) or any two of the following:
❖ Meningioma
❖ Glioma
❖ Schwannoma
❖ Juvenile posterior subcapsular lens opacity
❖ Juvenile cortical cataract
Suggestive (requiring evaluation) neurofibromatosis-2:
• Unilateral vestibular schwannomas plus at least two of any of the following:
❖ Meningioma
❖ Glioma
❖ Schwannoma
❖ Juvenile posterior subcapsular lenticular opacities/juvenile cortical cataract
• Multiple meningiomas (2 or more) plus unilateral vestibular schwannoma or any two of the following:
❖ Glioma
❖ Schwannoma
❖ Juvenile posterior subcapsular lenticular opacities/juvenile cortical cataract

- ◆ Absence of the sphenoid wing
- ◆ Lambdoid suture defect.
- ❖ Functional problems include seizures (which affect as many as 5 percent of patients with neurofibromatosis-1), learning disabilities, and emotional/behavioral disturbances.
- ❖ Benign and malignant tumors of the CNS
    - ◆ Nerve root and spinal cord neurofibromas can lead to deficits depending on location.
    - ◆ Gliomas are more common in neurofibromatosis-2, but can also be associated with neurofibromatosis-1. Incidence of optic nerve and optic chiasm gliomas has been estimated at 1 percent in neurofibromatosis-1 in a population-based series; however, incidence may be as high as 15 percent.
    - ◆ Meningiomas are more common in patients with neurofibromatosis-2, but can occur in patients with neurofibromatosis-1.
- • *Skeletal involvement (Figure 3C)*
    - ❖ Progressive kyphoscoliosis may lead to paraparesis without intervention.
    - ❖ Deformities of long bones include pseudoarthroses, hypertrophy/destruction associated with plexiform neurofibromas, and lytic metaphyseal and diaphyseal defects.
    - ❖ Short stature is very common.
- • *Visceral involvement*
    - ❖ Neurofibromas of the GI tract
    - ❖ Pheochromocytomas, which are 10 times more frequent in patients with neurofibromatosis (Approximately 5-10% of all pheochromocytomas

are in patients with neurofibromatosis.)
- ❖ Reports of associations with other soft-tissue tumors.

Ocular Features

- • *Cornea*—'Lignes grises', representing hyperplastic intrastromal nerves[19]
- • *Conjunctiva*—small localized elevated tumors 1 to 3 mm in diameter. They are firm, non tender, fixed in position and covered by normal epithelium.
- • *Uveal Tract*—iris may be sparsely or diffusely peppered with small "Lisch spots" which are lightly pigmented, almost gelatinous lesions resembling nevi[20] **(Figure 3D)**. Microscopy indicates they are of melanocytic origin.[21] Lisch nodules are a nearly constant feature of von Recklinghausen's neurofibromatosis,

occurring in 92 percent of one series of 77 patients.[22] Chorioretinal hamartomas and gliomas of the optic nerve are occasionally present. A fluorescein angiographic study of the choroidal lesions revealed avascular patches of hypofluorescence similar to multiple small choroidal nevi.[23] The central form of neurofibromatosis does not typically have ocular findings, other than presenile posterior subcapsular or nuclear cataracts.[17]

- • *Retinal and optic nerve lesions*—retinal hamartomas which are rare are identical to those seen in tuberous sclerosis. Congenital medullation of nerve fiber layer is a more frequent finding.
- • *Eyelid and orbital lesions*—eyelid may show plexiform neuroma, fibroma molluscum, schwannoma, and café-au-lait spots. The

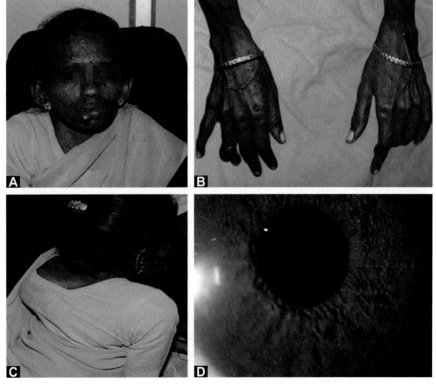

Figs 3A to D (A to C) Cutaneous and skeletal features of neurofibromatosis-1.
(D) Lisch nodules

hypertrophied nerves of plexiform neuroma feels like a bag of worms and knotted cords.

Mechanism of Glaucoma

Possible mechanisms of glaucoma include infiltration of the angle with neurofibromatous tissue, closure of the anterior chamber angle caused by nodular thickening of the ciliary body and choroid, fibrovascular membrane resembling neovascular glaucoma, and failure of normal anterior chamber angle development.[24,25]

Mangement

Management requires a multidisciplinary approach. In treating the glaucoma, medical measures should be attempted first, because surgical approaches are often not satisfactory. Management is usually along the lines of congenital glaucoma.

VON HIPPEL-LINDAU DISEASE (ANGIOMATOSIS RETINAE)

A retinal hemangioma was illustrated for the first time by Panas and Remy in1879. Progression of retinal angiomas was described by von Hippel (1904) and later Lindau (1926) described cerebellar angiomas.[26] The combination of these two is referred to as Von Hippel-Lindau disease.

The inheritance pattern is autosomal dominant with incomplete penetrance and delayed expression. The responsible gene is on chromosome 3 (3p25-p26). This gene behaves as a typical tumor suppressor gene, as defined in Knudson's theory of carcinogenesis. A nonhereditary form also exists. The disease usually presents in the 2nd or 3rd decade.

Systemic Features

Hemangioblastomas (capillary hemangiomas) of the brain and spinal cord, renal cell carcinoma and pheochromocytoma are present. The classical CNS

lesions are solid and cystic cerebellar hemangioblastomas,[27] which occur in about 40 percent of affected individuals by the age of 30 years and in about 70 percent of them by the age of 60 years.[28] The component cells in these tumors appear benign by histology. Similar vascular lesions also occur in the medulla and spinal cord in 10 to 15 percent of the patients who have von Hippel-Lindau disease.

Ocular Features

The classic ocular lesion is the retinal capillary hemangioma which is present in 50 to 60 percent of patients with von Hippel-Lindau syndrome. The ocular changes occur in the following steps:

1. Early stage of angioma formation with development of feeder and draining vessels
2. Stage of exudation, hemorrhage and retinal detachment
3. Destruction of the eye with secondary glaucoama and phthisis bulbi.

The earliest fundus sign is a fullness of retinal veins in one segment which become dilated and tortuous, these vessels feed the angiomatous formations in the far periphery, especially in the temporal side. As the tumor grows, the angioma becomes larger and the afferent and efferent vessels become thick, tortuous and dilated. Usual direction of growth is towards the vitreous, but occasionally, it can also grow towards the choroid. In addition to vascular anomalies and retinal angiomas, there is massive exudation of lipids into and beneath the retina. This can also at times lead to the formation of a macula star.

Glaucoma may occur as a late sequalae of rubeosis iridis or iridocyclitis.

Work-up
General work-up include:
- Vanillylmandelic acid levels in urine
- CT scan of brain with contrast

- MRI of brain (posterior fossa emphasis)
- Abdominal CT scan (to look for pheochromocytoma)
- Ophthalmic ultrasound
- Ocular color Doppler sonography
- FFA
- OCT.

Treatment
- *Argon laser photocoagulation* is effective in treating angiomatosis retinae. Treatment consists of a large spot size, with low-intensity, long-duration burns directed at the angioma.
  - Repeated laser treatment is required, except for small tumors. Obliteration of the tumor is confirmed by clinical observation and fluorescein angiograph.
  - If the tumor turns yellowish, photocoagulation becomes difficult because of the poor penetration of laser light.
- *Cryotherapy*, a repetitive freeze/thaw technique, may be used to treat anterior angiomas and larger posterior angiomas.
  - To minimize the risk of hemorrhage, no more than 2 or 3 freeze/thaw cycles should be used per session. Multiple sessions generally are needed to arrest tumors.
  - Resolution of the macular edema and improved visual acuity are common results of tumor eradication by cryotherapy.
- *Scleral buckle and fluid drainage methods* may be needed to treat larger tumors, tumors associated with retinal detachment, angiomas resistant to cryotherapy, or tumors involving subretinal exudation. Large tumors may develop surface membranes and vitreous traction, leading to vitreous hemor-

rhage or rhegmatogenous retinal detachment. Such complications may require treatment by vitreous surgery, endodiathermy, or scleral buckling techniques.

- *Penetrating diathermy* under a lamellar scleral bed is an effective treatment of larger angiomas.
- *Endodiathermy* may be used, instead of vitreous surgical techniques or scleral buckling procedures, to treat vitreous hemorrhage or retinal detachment.
- *Radiation*, applied in various forms, is another field among future directions in the care for this incessant pathology.

TUBEROUS SCLEROSIS

It is a multiorgan tumor syndrome that is characterised by multifocal, bilateral retinal astrocytic hamartomas, astrocytic tumors of the CNS, several unusual cutaneous lesions, mental retardation, seizures, and a variety of cysts and tumors of other organs.

Prevalence in general population has been estimated to be around one per 10,000 persons.[29] About one-third are familial and two-third are sporadic. Signs and symptoms usually begin by the time, when the patient is six years of age.

Tuberous Sclerosis genes have been identified on loci on the long arm of chromosome 9 *(9q32-34)*, on long arm of chromosome 11, on the short arm of chromosome 16 *(16p13)*, and on the long arm of chromosome 12 *(12q22-24)*.

- Comprehensive diagnostic criteria were set out first by Dr Manuel R Gomez; they now exist in revised form as set forth in a consensus statement from the Diagnostic Criteria Committee of the National Tuberous Sclerosis Association (USA).
  - ❖ *Major features*
    - ◆ Facial angiofibromas or forehead plaque
    - ◆ Nontraumatic ungual or periungual fibroma
    - ◆ Hypomelanotic macules (>3)
    - ◆ Shagreen patch (connective tissue nevus)
    - ◆ Multiple retinal nodular hamartoma
    - ◆ *Cortical tuber:* When cerebellar cortical dysplasia and cerebral white matter migration tracts occur together, they should be counted as one rather than two features of tuberous sclerosis.
    - ◆ Subependymal nodule
    - ◆ Subependymal giant cell astrocytoma
    - ◆ Cardiac rhabdomyoma, single or multiple
    - ◆ *Lymphangioleiomyomatosis:* When both lymphangioleiomyomatosis (LAM) and renal AMLs are present, other features of tuberous sclerosis should be present before a definite diagnosis is assigned. As many as 60 percent of women with sporadic LAM (and not TSC) may have a renal or other AMLs.
    - ◆ *Renal AML:* When both LAM and renal AMLs are present, other features of tuberous sclerosis should be present before a definite diagnosis is assigned (see previous remarks).
  - ❖ *Minor features*
    - ◆ Multiple randomly distributed pits in dental enamel[5]
    - ◆ *Hamartomatous rectal polyps:* Histologic confirmation is suggested.
    - ◆ *Bone cysts:* Radiographic confirmation is sufficient.
    - ◆ *Cerebral white matter radial migration lines:* Radiographic confirmation is sufficient. One panel member felt strongly that three or more radial migration lines should constitute a major sign.
    - ◆ Gingival fibromas
    - ◆ Nonrenal hamartoma: Histologic confirmation is suggested.
    - ◆ Retinal achromic patch
    - ◆ "Confetti" skin lesions
    - ◆ Multiple renal cysts.
  - ❖ *Diagnostic criteria*
    - ◆ *Definite TSC:* Either two major features or one major feature plus two minor features
    - ◆ *Probable TSC:* One major plus one minor feature
    - ◆ *Possible TSC:* Either one major feature or two or more minor features.

Systemic Features

Skin Lesions

Adenoma sebaceum—usually seen between 2 to 5 years. It is considered as a pathognomonic lesion of tuberous sclerosis, seen in atleast 90 percent of all patients. It consists of multiple small reddish brown nodules distributed over the nose and cheeks in a butterfly pattern which tends to enlarge until puberty. Telangiectatic vessels are common over the nose. Histologically, the lesions are angiofibromas.

Ash leaf spots of depigmentation—hypopigmented macular or patch lesions, pathologically achromic nevi, which are evident under ultraviolet illumination (woods lamp), and may be present at birth.

Periungual and subungual fibromas are seen at puberty in about 40 percent all patients and begin as small nodules at the margin of or beneath the nails of the fingers and toes and enlarge and cause pain.

Central Nervous System (CNS)

Cerebrum, cerebellum, medulla and spinal cord are involved. The CNS hamartomas are of two types, i.e cortical foci (tubers) and subependymal nodules along with the ventricular system. These hamartomas are composed of typical astrocytes. Patients have mental retardation and convulsive disorders.

Visceral Involvement

Hamartomas may involve any organ. Cardiac hamartomas may lead to fatal arrythmias. Three-fourth of patients have renal hamartomas, which cause urinary tract symptoms. Two-third patients have cystic lesions of the pulmonary parenchyma that show a honeycomb appearance on radiological examination.

Ocular Features

Characteristic lesion is retinal hamartoma. More than 50 percent patients have bilateral lesions. Morphologically, they are divided into three types:[30]

TYPE 1—relatively flat, soft looking and semitransparent lesions. They may be single or multiple, seen at posterior pole. They have gelatinous indistinct boundaries of light gray or faint yellow and are slightly elevated.

TYPE 2—elevated, nodular, and solid-appearing masses. Usually elevated ½ to 4 disc diameters, achromic and multinodular, often occurring near or along the disc margins and also in the retinal midperiphery. They resemble tapioca, white mulberries or salmon eggs. It is currently believed that type 1 lesions evolve into type 2.

TYPE 3—combination of type 1 and 2. The fundi of patients with tuberous sclerosis can exhibit midperipheral depigmented lesions with a surrounding rim of pigment proliferation.

Histology: They are composed of a felt-like network of atypical astrocytes and small blood vessels located in the superficial layers of the retina and optic nerve head.

Glaucoma

Rare iris abnormalities have been reported and include focal areas of stromal depigmentation and atypical colobomata. hamartomas of the IPE and ciliary epithelium occur in some patients and may be the cause of clinically apparent iris abnormalities.

Rubeosis iridis and neovascular glaucoma has been reported to occur in these eyes.

Treatment

The treatment is symptomatic and aimed at potentially treatable problem such as cardiac rhabdomyomas, cysts and tumors of the kidney, and enlarging CNS astrocytomas.

NEVUS OF OTA

The nevus of Ota (i.e. oculodermal melanocytosis) is not included in all reported classifications of the phakomatoses, but it does fit the broader definition of the disease group.

General Features

The hamartoma, histologically, is composed of melanocytes in ocular tissues, especially the episclera, the skin in the distribution of the trigeminal nerve, **(Figures 4A and B)** and occasionally, the nasal or buccal mucosa. In a study of 194 patients, 67 had only dermal involvement, 12 had only ocular involvement, and 115 had both.[31] It is nearly always unilateral with a preponderance of females and a tendency toward races with darker pigmentation.[32] Degeneration to malignant melanomas may occur in white patients, but rarely in nonwhites.[33-36]

Glaucoma

Evidence of chronic glaucoma has been observed in patients with the nevus of Ota.[37-41] Elevated IOP, with or without glaucomatous damage, was seen in 10 percent of one series.[25] The involved eye typically has unusually heavy pigmentation of the trabecular meshwork, and histopathologic studies have revealed melanocytes in the meshwork.[39,40]

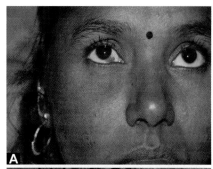
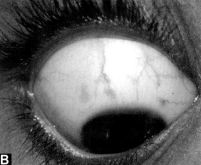

Figs 4A and B Nevus of Ota (Oculodermal melanocytosis)

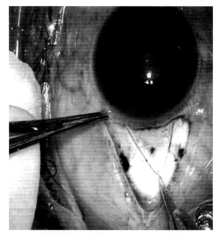

Fig. 5 Trabeculectomy being done in a patients with secondary glaucoma due to nevus of Ota

Management

Medical management, as with other forms of open-angle glaucoma, should be tried first. If this fails, laser trabeculoplasty may be effective,[42] although filtering surgery will most likely be required **(Figure 5).**

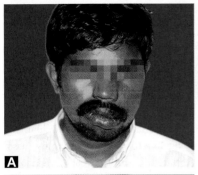
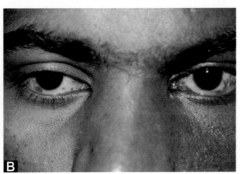
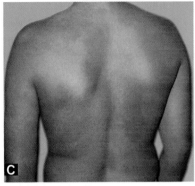

Figs 6A to C Phacomatosis pigmentovascularis

PHAKOMATOSIS PIGMENTOVASCULARIS

It represents an overlap between oculo-dermal vascular malformation (nevus flammeus) oculodermal melanocystosis **(Figures 6A to C)**. Present together and involving the globe extensively, they can cause congenital glaucoma when there is a partial involvement of the globe IOP elevation occurs later in life. They have a more important role in predisposition to glaucoma.

CUTIS MARMORATA TELANGIECTATICA CONGENITAL

It involves periocular vascular anomalies associated either with regional or generalized cutaneous marbling. It is associated with infantile trabeculo-dysgenic glaucoma and intraoperative suprachoroidal hemorrhage.

REFERENCES

1. Van der Hoeve J. Eye symptoms in phakomatoses. Trans Ophthalmol Soc UK 1932;52:380.
2. Cruen AF. Tuberous Sclerosis and the eye. In Ryan SJ (Ed). Retina, St. Louis: CV Mosby Company 1989;1:571-9.
3. Sullivan TJ, Clarke MP, Morin JD. The ocular manifestations of the Sturge-Weber syndrome. J Pediatr Ophthalmol Strabismus 1992;29:349.
4. William P, Boger 111, Robert A Peterson. Pediatric ophthalmology: In: Manual of Ocular Diagnosis and Therapy (4th edn). Little Brown and Company 1992;p.286.
5. Weiss DI. Dual origin of glaucoma in encephalotrigeminal haemangio-matosis. Trans ophthalmol soc UK 1973:93:477.
6. Christensen GR, Records RE. Glaucoma and expulsive hemorrhage mechanisms in the Sturge-Weber syndrome. Ophthalmology 1979;86:1360.
7. Mwinula JH, Sagawa T, Tawara A, et al. Anterior chamber angle vascularization in Sturge-Weber syndrome: report of a case. Graefes Arch Clin Exp Ophthalmol 1994;232:387.
8. Cibis GW, Tripathi RC, Tripathi BJ. Glaucoma in Sturge-Weber syndrome. Opthalmology 1984;91:1061.
9. Altuna JC, Greenfield DS, Wand M, et al. Latanoprost in glaucoma associated with Sturge-Weber syndrome: benefits and side-effects. J Glaucoma 1999;8:199.
10. Ali MA, Fahmy IA, Spaeth GL. Trabeculectomy for glaucoma associated with Sturge-Weber syndrome. Ophthalmic Surg 1990; 21:352.
11. Iwach AG, Hoskins HD Jr, Hetherington J Jr, et al. Analysis of surgical and medical management of glaucoma in Sturge-Weber syndrome. Ophthalmology 1990;97:904.
12. Board RJ, Shields MB. Combined trabeculotomy-trabeculectomy for the management of glaucoma associated with Sturge-Weber syndrome. Ophthalmic Surg 1981;12:813.
13. Bellows AR, Chylack LT Jr, Epstein DL, et al. Choroidal effusion during glaucoma surgery in patients with prominent episcleral vessels. Arch Ophthalmol 1979;97:493.
14. Theodossiadis G, Damanakis A, Koutsandrea C. Expulsive choroidal effusion during glaucoma surgery in a child with Sturge-Weber syndrome. Klin Monatsbl Augenheilkd 1985; 186:300.
15. Agarwal HC, Sandramouli S, Sihota R, et al. Sturge-Weber syndrome: management of glaucoma with combined trabeculotomy-trabeculectomy. Ophthalmic Surg 1993;24:399.
16. Budenz DL, Sakamoto D, Eliezer R, et al. Two-staged Baerveldt glaucoma implant for childhood glaucoma associated with Sturge-Weber syndrome. Ophthalmology 2000;107:2105.
17. Pearson-Webb MA, Kaiser-Kupfer MI, Eldridge R. Eye findings in bilateral acoustic (central) neurofibromatosis: association with presenile lens

opacities and cataracts but absence of Lisch nodules. N Engl J Med 1986;315: 1553.

18. Barker D, Wright E, Nguyen K, et al. Gene for von Recklinghausen neurofibromatosis is in the pericentromeric region of chromosome 17. Science 1987;236:1100.

19. Retinoblastomas, leucocoria and phakomatose. In: Apple DT, Rabb MF (Eds). Ocular pathology, St Louis: The CV Mosby company 1985;905-29.

20. Lubs M-L E, Bauer MSA, Formas ME, et al. Lisch nodules in neurofibromatosis type I. N Engl J Med 1991;324:1264.

21. Perry HD, Font RL. Iris nodules in von Recklinghausen's neurofibromatosis: electron microscopic confirmation of their melanocytic origin. Arch Ophthalmol 1982;100:1635.

22. Lewis RA, Riccardi VM. Von Recklinghausen neurofibromatosis: incidence of iris hamartomata. Ophthalmology 1981;88:348.

23. Huson S, Jones D, Beck L. Ophthalmic manifestations of neurofibromatosis. Br J Ophthalmol 1987;71:235.

24. Grant WM, Walton DS. Distinctive gonioscopic findings in glaucoma due to neurofibromatosis. Arch Ophthalmol 1968;79:127.

25. Wolter JR, Butler RG. Pigment spots of the iris and ectropion uveae: with glaucoma in neurofibromatosis. Am J Ophthalmol 1963;56:964.

26. Weiss JS, Ritch R. Glaucoma in the Phakomatosis. In: Ritch R, Shields B, Krupin T (Eds). Glaucomas. St Louis: The CV Mosby Company 1989;pp.905-29

27. Neumann HP, Eggert HR, Scheremet R, et al. central nervous system lesions in von Hippel-lindau syndrome. J neurol neurosurg psychiatry. 1992;55:889-901.

28. Maher ER, Yates JR, Harries R, et al. clinical features and natural history of von hippel-lindau disease. Q J Med. 1990;77:1151-63.

29. Northrup H. Tuberous Sclerosis Complex: genetic aspects. J Dermatol. 1992;19:914-9.

30. Asdourian GK, Lewis RA. The phakomatosis. In peyman GA, sanders DR, Goldberg MK (Eds). Principles and practice of ophthalmology. Philidelphia: WB Saunders company 1980;pp.1186-204.

31. Teekhasaenee C, Ritch R, Rutnin U, et al. Ocular findings in oculodermal melanocytosis. Arch Ophthalmol 1990;108:1114.

32. Mishima Y, Mevorah B. Nevus Ota and nevus Ito in American Negroes. J Invest Dermatol 1961;36:133.

33. Albert DM, Scheie HG. Nevus of Ota with malignant melanoma of the choroids: report of a case. Arch Ophthalmol 1963;69:774.

34. Font RL, Reynolds AM, Zimmerman LE. Diffuse malignant melanoma of the iris in the nevus of Ota. Arch Ophthalmol 1967;77:513.

35. Sabates FN, Yamashita T. Congenital melanosis oculi: complicated by two independent malignant melanomas of the choroid. Arch Ophthalmol 1967;77:801.

36. Velazquez N, Jones IS. Ocular and oculodermal melanocytosis associated with uveal melanoma. Ophthalmology 1983;90:1472.

37. Fishman GRA, Anderson R. Nevus of Ota: report of two cases, one with open-angle glaucoma. Am J Ophthalmol 1962;54:453.

38. Foulks GN, Shields MB. Glaucoma in oculodermal melanocytosis. Ann Ophthalmol 1977;9:1299.

39. Sugar HS. Glaucoma with trabecular melanocytosis. Ann Ophthalmol 1982;14:374.

40. Futa R, Shimizu T, Okura F, et al. A case of open-angle glaucoma associated with nevus Ota—electron microscopic study of the anterior chamber angle and iris. Folia Ophthalmol Jpn 1984;35:501.

41. Khawly JA, Imami N, Shields MB. Glaucoma associated with the nevus of Ota. Arch Ophthalmol 1995;113: 1208.

42. Goncalves V, Sandler T, O'Donnell FE Jr. Open angle glaucoma in melanosis oculi: response to laser trabeculoplasty. Ann Ophthalmol 1985; 17:33.

PART 4

Glaucoma—Therapeutics

42 | Medical Management of Glaucoma

Ankit Gupta, Mona Khurana, R Ramakrishnan

Glaucoma is the second largest of cause of blindness worldwide. Management of glaucoma is challenging as the aim is to preserve quality of life by slowing or halting the progressive visual field loss. Although glaucoma is an optic neuropathy, the treatment currently is directed towards lowering the only modifiable risk factor, i.e. the intraocular pressure (IOP). This has been supported by various randomized control trials. Neuroprotection and neuroregeneration are current areas of research and in the future may be able to address the optic nerve pathology directly.

Options available for lowering the IOP are medications, lasers and surgery. Collaborative Initial Glaucoma Treatment Study (CIGTS) showed that surgery and medicine are equally effective in preserving vision.[1] Currently medications are commonly used to lower the IOP in most situations. The management of a glaucoma patient is essentially a customized treatment for the patient and tailored to the individual. No two patients are alike and the approach may vary. However certain guidelines need to be kept in mind while starting treatment. The efficacy, side effects and adherence should govern the clinical approach.

THE NEED FOR TREATMENT

At the outset, it must be kept in mind that once started the treatment of glaucoma is lifelong. Glaucoma is a condition where both under-diagnosis and over-treatment are quite common. Under-diagnosis can lead to progression of visual field loss and irreversible blindness. Overdiagnosis also has its own implications. One often comes across patients with no or early glaucoma who are overtreated and patients with advanced glaucoma who are undertreated. In a clinical scenario it is not unusual to see patients with normal optic disc and visual fields on multiple antiglaucoma medications. Usually there is a reluctance of the clinician to stop or decrease the number of medications in such patients. Over-treatment or unnecessary treatment affects the quality of life, subjects patients to the risks of side-effects and has economic implications. Thus initiation of therapy should not be taken lightly. It is essential to ascertain the need of therapy before starting it. It is important to distinguish early glaucoma from glaucoma suspects. Elderly patients with ocular hypertension should be treated less aggressively. The risk of side effects of medications used for aggressive IOP lowering outweighs their benefit in such a situation.

Establish a Baseline

Before starting treatment it is essential to obtain a good baseline. Decisions to initiate or change therapy and judgments of therapeutic benefit of medications may depend upon the baseline characteristics. This includes the pretreatment IOP range, the status of the anterior chamber angle by gonioscopy, optic nerve head and retinal nerve fiber layer (RNFL) changes and visual field status. The following baseline measurements need to be taken:

- **Baseline IOP:** When assessing IOP, there is no substitute for an adequate baseline. This should ideally include multiple IOP readings at various times of the day.
- Baseline gonioscopy to document the status of the angle of the anterior chamber

- Baseline structural and functional tests for assessing and documenting optic nerve head damage
- Central corneal thickness (CCT)

Though time consuming it is extremely helpful in planning the manage-ment. In case of patients already on treatment this may be obtained from their previous records or treating clinician.

SETTING A TARGET PRESSURE

The treatment of glaucoma is lifelong and setting a target pressure is useful.[2-4] Target pressure is defined as *a range of IOP* enough to limit the progression of visual field loss to a rate that will preserve his/her visual function and maintain daily pattern without affecting quality of life. In other words it is an estimate of mean IOP obtained with treatment that is expected to prevent further glaucomatous change. It may be a percentage reduction or an absolute reduction from baseline IOP. Life expectancy, severity of glaucoma, baseline or highest recorded IOP should be taken into account while setting the target. Its concept is debated[5,6] and the level may need to be reassessed and modified over time.

The adequacy of the target pressure is reassessed periodically by comparing optic nerve status (by optic disc appearance, quantitative assessments of the disc and nerve fiber layer, and visual field tests) with previous examinations. If progression occurs at the target pressure, undetected IOP fluctuations and adherence to therapy should be re-evaluated before adjusting the target IOP. Target pressure is an estimate, and all treatment decisions must be individualized according to the needs of the patient. Decisions must be based on risk versus benefits which tend to change over time.

Factors Influencing Target IOP

Many factors must be taken into account when deciding the target IOP. These include extent of visual damage already present, the threat of visual field damage to visual performance (such as proximity to fixation), the presence of risk factors for further damage, the pre-treatment IOP level, family history and the patient's estimated life expectancy.[7] The severity of glaucomatous damage is one of the most important factors for setting target IOP. It is assessed by optic disc evaluation and extent of visual fields loss. Eyes with visual field defects closer to fixation require a lower target IOP. With increasing age there is a steady decrease in the number of nerve fibers in the optic nerve head (4-5% per decade after 50 years) which is accelerated in glaucoma. A young patient with mild glaucomatous optic nerve head damage may require a lower target pressure than an elderly patient with a similar amount of damage but less life expectancy. The target IOP also depends upon the baseline IOP at which the damage occurred. Glaucomatous optic nerve hypoplasia (ONH) changes occurring at a lower IOP require a more aggressive IOP lowering.

Estimation Methods
- **Percentage Drop in IOP**
- **Absolute Reduction.**

Clinical trials have used certain formula to set the target IOP in the study population to achieve a uniform lowering of IOP (**Box 1**). These need to be interpreted with reference to the clinical situations as patient characteristics may be different as compared to the study population. The most common and simplest method for setting the target IOP is to aim for a percentage drop from the baseline IOP of 30-50%. The drop should be at least 20% to account for the diurnal fluctuation and inaccuracies in current IOP measurement techniques. This technique has its limitation, e.g. if baseline is 40 mm Hg a target of 50% would mean lowering the IOP to 20 mm Hg, which may not be enough, as per AGIS report. Therefore IOP based on the severity of glaucoma may also be considered. The best approach would be a combined approach of percentage IOP drops and absolute levels.

A grading system has been recommended by the **American Academy of Ophthalmology** by quantifying glaucomatous damage so that an approximate target IOP could be set.

- *Mild glaucoma:* Characteristic optic nerve abnormalities consistent with glaucoma, but with visual normal fields. Recommended target pressure 20% reduction of untreated IOP or an IOP of 17-18 mm Hg.
- *Moderate glaucoma:* Visual field abnormalities matching optic disc changes in one hemi field, but not within five degrees of fixation. A 30% reduction or IOP in mid teens (14-16 mm Hg) is recommended.

Box 1 Formulae for Target IOP

1. *Jampel's formula:*
   Target range = {initial IOP × [I − initial IOP/100} − Z + Y ± 1 mm Hg}
   Z = Optic nerve damage severity factor
   Y = Burden of therapy factor
2. *Zeyen's Simpler version:*
   Target IOP = Maximum IOP − Maximum IOP% - Z
   Z = Optic nerve damage severity factor
   (Y factor was excluded as it was difficult of quantify)
3. *CIGTS formula[1]:*
   Target IOP = [1 − {reference IOP + VF score}/100] × [reference IOP]

- *Severe glaucoma:* Visual field abnormalities in both hemifields or within five degrees of fixation. 35–40% reduction or an IOP less than 12 mm Hg is considered appropriate.

Eyes with advanced glaucoma may require IOP in very low teens or even in single digits to prevent progressive glaucomatous damage. Visual field stability is seen in patients with IOP consistently below 18 mm Hg with a mean IOP of 12.3 mm Hg. Maintaining IOP consistently below 18 mm Hg in a patient with mild to moderate glaucoma and at still lower levels (low teens) in patients with advanced disc damage seems like a reasonable IOP goal. However, periodical evaluation of glaucoma related damage is mandatory to reset the target IOP to stabilize visual loss.

MONOCULAR TRIAL

The clinical management of glaucoma would be simple if all the patients responded well and in a similar manner to antiglaucoma medications (AGM). On initiation of therapy one needs to confirm its efficacy in the patient. This is not as easy considering the dynamic nature of IOP which changes not only with the time of the day but also with posture, season, hydration and numerous other factors. Thus a single IOP measurement is not as useful as multiple IOP measurements. Ideally, IOP variation must be characterized before and after starting the treatment.

The monocular trial also known as the 'uniocular' or the 'one eye trial' has for long been the gold standard to determine both the IOP lowering effect and the side effects of IOP lowering medications and has been a standard practice since many years. It was developed to help distinguish between therapeutic and spontaneous IOP components of variation.

One eye is started on an anti glaucoma medication whereas the untreated fellow eye serves as a control. This helps distinguish between the intraocular pressure lowering effect of a newly-initiated medication and the diurnal variations in IOP. Thus, it gives an estimate of the contribution. Following a successful monocular trial, the drug is then applied bilaterally assuming a similar control in both eyes.

Put simply, IOP is measured in both the eyes and treatment is started in one eye, preferably in the eye with the higher pressure. The patient is called 4–6 weeks later at the same time of the day and the IOP is measured in both eyes. The change in IOP in the trial eye represents a sum of therapeutic and spontaneous IOP change. The IOP change in the untreated eye represents a purely spontaneous change. The true therapeutic IOP change attributable to treatment is calculated by subtracting the IOP change in the untreated eye from the change in the treated eye.

The basis of this trial are the following assumptions

These include:

1. IOP variation is symmetric between fellow-eye pairs so that the untreated eye can serve as a control for the treated eye.
2. There is no or minimal crossover effect of the antiglaucoma medications, i.e. treatment of one eye does not affect the IOP of the untreated fellow eye.
3. The IOP lowering effect of the drug is similar in both eyes.

Questioning the monocular trail:

However, recent developments have questioned the above assumptions and raised a few concerns about the monocular trial.[8] The fact that IOP does not vary symmetrically between eyes has challenged this practice. Moreover some drugs may lower IOP in the contralateral eye when instilled monocularly causing underestimation of the IOP lowering effect in the treated eye (1.5 mm Hg in beta blockers).

Bilateral simultaneous trials suggest that both eyes respond similarly to the same medication.

Conclusions based on the monocular trial can lead to continued use of an ineffective medication, or worse, discontinuation of an effective medication. A different method of evaluating efficacy of the antiglaucoma medication is to compare the mean of several pre-treatment IOP readings to the mean of several on-treatment IOP readings. The tendency to switch treatments if the first on-treatment IOP is not at target should be avoided. A monocular trail may not be done if a good baseline IOP has been established or if the AGM has a high likelihood of causing a good reduction in IOP. It may be more useful when adding a second or third agent. It may also be useful in stopping therapy, i.e. **reverse uniocular trials**. When the target IOP is no longer being maintained with a particular regimen, one often thinks about replacing or adding medications to the current drugs. A reverse uniocular trial by temporarily discontinuing a drop in one eye, may help to indicate whether the rising pressure is caused by loss of drug efficacy or worsening of the glaucoma.

INITIATING TREATMENT

Monotherapy

In most patients a single drug may be adequate to lower the IOP to the target IOP. For many years beta blockers have been the drug of choice for the first line of therapy. They are effective and also well tolerated topically in healthy individuals. The systemic side effects are a limiting factor. Over the past few years, there has been an increasing trend towards the use of prostaglandin analogues as the first line of treatment. Sufficient IOP reduction may not be possible with monotherapy. The indicators would be progression even at target IOP, target IOP not achieved or not maintained.

The options available are:
- Switching to new drug (New monotherapy)
- Adding medications (Adjunctive therapy)

Switching /New Monotherapy
- Medications that do not lower the IOP must be stopped.
- If the IOP lowering is ≤ 10% the medication should be stopped and changed.
- If the IOP lowering is 10–20% the medication should be switched. However this must be documented in the patients' records as the drug may be used later on as an adjunct.

> **Note** Do not use a single IOP reading to asses the effect of treatment.

The new mediation can be from a different class of medications are from this same class. Switching with in the same class is only done for prostaglandin analogue.

Adjunctive Treatment
A second agent is added if the initial treatment has not lowered the IOP adequately. Usually a drug from a different class of medication is added. The efficacy depends upon the mechanism of action. Usually drugs with different mechanisms of action act as an effective combination therapy.

Prostaglandin analogues or beta blockers are usually the first line of therapy and most medications provide additional IOP lowering when added. Fixed combinations are widely available and will be discussed in a different section in detail.

Maximal Medical Therapy
At one time this included every AGM available. Over the past years many new antiglaucoma medications have become available. It is difficult to get an additional IOP lowering when adding a second agent to a prostaglandin and the third agent likely adds less than the second. Optimal medical therapy or maximal tolerated medical therapy has now replaced the concept of MMT.[9]

The Non Responders
Non responders to treatment have been observed with both Latanoprost and Timolol. The mechanisms for which remain largely unknown. Determination of response to medication is not easy considering the dynamic nature of IOP and errors in IOP calculation.

Pharmacogenomics may help predict the IOP lowering response in a patient and avoid prescribing drugs expected to have low efficacy. It is based on a candidate gene approach mainly involving beta 1 blockers and prostaglandin analogues.

SYSTEMIC MEDICATION AND SYSTEMIC STATUS
Interactions of antiglaucoma medications with systemic drugs must be considered before starting treatment. Carbonic anhydrase inhibitors may cause hypokalemia if used in conjunction with thiazide diuretics. For example, topical beta blockers may be less effective in patients on systemic beta blockers.

Many antiglaucoma medications have systemic side effects. They may exacerbate pre-existing systemic conditions and even prove life threatening in some cases. Age is one more factor which needs to be considered while instituting therapy. An elderly patient with a good visual field reserve may not be treated as aggressively as a younger patient with a longer life expectancy where any decline in visual function is unacceptable.

EDUCATING THE PATIENT
Prescribing the medication is not enough and the patient needs to be educated on many points:

How to Instil Eye Drops (Figures 1A to C)
The success of treatment of glaucoma directly depends upon the eye drops reaching the intended place. It can be a limiting factor even in patients adherent to the treatment. Thus teaching the patient (in case of self administration

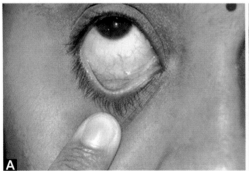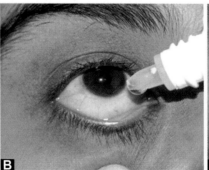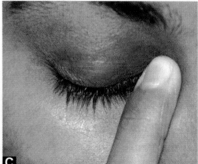

Figs 1A to C Proper technique for eye drops instillation of drops) or attendant the correct technique is important.

A stepwise approach can be followed:
- Wash hands prior to putting eye drops
- Open the bottle and be careful not to contaminate the cap
- The patient (or attendant) pulls down the lower lid with the index finger of one hand.
- With the other hand one drop is placed in the inferior cul–de–sac.
- Avoid touching the tip of the dropper to the conjunctiva, lashes, or skin.
- Tilting the head back slightly may be helpful.
- Close his eyes for 3-5 minutes.
- ***Digital NLO (Naso Lacrimal Occlusion)*** should be encouraged to decrease systemic side effects. Occluding the nasolacrimal ducts, either by pinching them closed or by simple eyelid closure increases the amount of medication delivered to the eye. It also decreases the amount of medication delivered to the systemic circulation by two-thirds. All glaucoma patients must be instructed in the techniques and told to occlude the nasolacrimal system for 3-5 minutes after each drops.
- ***Spacing of eye drops***: If a second medication needs to instilled a gap of 5-10 minutes is essential. This prevents the additional drop from diluting and washing out the first drop before it gets absorbed
- Ointments or gels should be instilled last
- Agonist are instilled before antagonist.

Written Instructions
Glaucoma patients are usually elderly and may be on multiple medications. This can be confusing for them as they may also be taking systemic medications. Thus it is important to write clear instruction and the time of instillation of antiglaucoma medications to avoid confusion.

Warning About Side Effects
The patients should be told about both minor and common side effects which may be expected with the treatment. This will not cause alarm and also help in increasing adherence. It is important also to alert the patient regarding major side effects which need to be reported to the physician immediately. This ensures safety of the patient.

Lifestyle
One must consider the patients lifestyle before prescribing AGM. This concerns adressing issues like dosing schedules in patients with fixed hour working shifts or may be related to their side effects as a limiting factor, e.g. pilocarpine for individuals driving at night. More the patient may also need some lifestyle modifications. Sirsasana, playing certain musical instruments, drinking large quantities of water are related to a transient rise in IOP. The patient needs to be warned about this possibility.

Cost
The treatment of glaucoma being life long, cost is a major concern. Factors influencing treatment cost are
- Price of the drug
- Amount wasted during instillation

GENERICS
Many generic products are available in the market. These contain the same active ingredient, are identical in strength and have a similar dose frequency as the branded drug. Moreover they are cheaper and easily available. However preservatives pH, antioxidants, viscosity agents and buffers may differ. There are concern regarding:
- Efficacy
- Changes in comfort
- Side effects due to change in inactive ingredients.

ADHERENCE AND PERSISTENCE
It is a common saying that 'drugs work in patients who take them.' Thus ensuring and monitoring adherence is an integral and critical part of the medical management of glaucoma. *Adherence* is the extent to which the patient continues the agreed-upon mode of treatment. The term compliance is not preferred as it indicates passive behavior on part of the patient. Persistency is the total time for which the patient correctly takes the appropriate medication. *Persistency* is thought in part to represent the patient's satisfaction with the agent's tolerability as well as the physician's satisfaction with the agent's clinical efficacy.[10-12] Poor adherence can be present with respect to medication regime or to follow up.

Poor adherence to medication regimens accounts for substantial worsening of disease and increased healthcare cost. When patients are without symptoms, they may not realize the importance of daily adherence. Various clinical trials have reported average adherence rates of 43–78% among patients receiving treatment for chronic conditions. Generally for most clinical trials, adherence of 80% is considered acceptable. The most commonly sited reasons by patients include forgetfulness, lack of information and emotional factors.[13]

The following factors are related to non-adherence:
- Glaucoma is an asymptomatic disease
- Self-administering drops requires coordination, manual dexterity, eye hand coordination and good vision

(all of which tend to decrease in aging glaucoma patients).

- Adding a second medication and/or increasing the complexity of glaucoma therapy is associated with a statistically significant decrease in adherence[14]
- Side effect of drops
- Cost of medication
- Comorbidities
- Barriers to follow up: The most prevalent barriers to follow-up are the belief that there is no problem with one's eyes and lack of escort to accompany the patient during their clinic visit.[15,16]
- Many of the factors associated with poor adherence to medication are found to be associated with poor follow-up to clinic visits.

It is difficult for the clinician to judge the adherence.

Non-adherence can be in the form of:

- Taking an incomplete/incorrect dose
- Taking medication at wrong time
- Forgetting to take medication
- Poor adherence to follow-up regime

Adherence should be assessed at each visit mainly by indirect methods in the form of patient self reports or the clinical assessment (monitoring of the optic nerve head and visual fields is essential). The physician must be alert and able to predict patients with poor adherence. One should be aware of certain behavioral patterns, e.g. improvement in adherence with medication a few days before and after their appointment with their physician. Finally, methods to improve adherence must be used. A multicomponent approach to improve adherence includes:

- A good patient provider relationship
- Better patient education about the disease, medication schedule and side effects
- Behavioral reinforcement

- Enlisting social support
- Individual tailoring (e.g. to lifestyle)
- Simplifying treatment schedule or prescribing more 'forgiving' medications.

GENERAL PHARMACOLOGIC PRINCIPLES

IOP reduction has been validated to slow the progression of the disease. For the medical treatment, six classes of drugs are available **(Box 2)**. The more commonly used are the prostaglandin analogue and beta blockers. Cholinergics are the least used. The ideal agent should cause maximum IOP lowering, minimal side effects, least frequency of daily dosing and also affordable. An additional non-IOP lowering effect, e.g. increased ocular blood flow or neuroprotection is an added advantage. The agents are discussed in detail in the subsequent sections.

Pharmacokinetics of Topical Drugs

The average drop of medication has an approximate volume of 20 to 50 μl whereas the tear lake holds approximately 7 to 10 μl, (20% of one drop). Most of the instilled one drop is lost because of the overflow. Some elderly patients with lax lids can hold more than the normal amount of medications in their tear lakes. Only 42% is still present after 5 minutes (at a tears turn over rate 15% per minute). Due to a short contact time, the drug concentration in the drop is high. To increase contact time and efficacy, some medications are delivered in gels, ointments or other viscous materials. The penetration of topically applied medication into the eye is proportional to the concentration of the drug that comes in contact with the cornea overtime, which gets diluted by tears and gets washed out into the lacrimal drainage system.

Box 2 Antiglaucoma drugs

Topical
1. *Adrenergic antagonists:*
   - *β blockers:* Timolol, levo-bunolol, betaxolol, carteolol, metipronolol.
2. *Adrenergic agonists:*
   - *Non-selective:* Epinephrine, dipivefrin.
   - *Alpha 2 selective:* Brimonidine, apraclonidine.
3. *Parasympathomimetics:*
   - *Direct parasympathomimetics:* Pilocarpine
   - *Indirect (anticholinesterase agents):* Ecothiophate iodide, demecurium bromide, iso-flurophate, physostigmine, neostigmine.
4. *Prostaglandin analogues:*
   - Latanoprost
   - Bimatoprost
   - Travoprost
   - Unoprestone tafluprost.
5. *Carbonic anhydrase inhibitors:*
   - Dorzolamide
   - Brinzolamide

Systemic
1. *Hyperosmotic agents:*
   Intravenous:
   - Mannitol, urea
   Oral:
   - Glycerol
   - Isosorbide.
2. *Carbonic anhydrase inhibitors:* Acetazolamide, dichlorphenamide, methazolamide.

The cornea has both a lipid barrier (i.e. epithelium and endothelium) and a water barrier (i.e. stroma). In order to enter the eye, topical medications are designed to overcome these natural barriers. Medication must be soluble in both lipids and water, although lipid solubility is more important than water solubility as the lipid content of the epithelium and the endothelium is 100 times more than that of stroma. Because of the dual nature of the corneal barriers, drugs possessing both lipid and water solubility penetrate the cornea more readily. Topical drugs sometimes need help penetrating the cornea. Preservatives such as benzalkonium chloride increase the penetration of medications through the corneal epithelium, e.g. benzalkonium chloride increases carbachol penetration twentyfold. Sometimes inflamed eyes will also demonstrate increased penetration.

If the drop is irritating, it can cause reflex tearing, which can wash the drug away and decrease its effectiveness. There are many enzymes which metabolize the drugs in the cornea. This metabolic capability is used by the prodrugs like dipivefrin and latanoprost.

Once in the anterior chamber the drugs are eliminated with the bulk flow of the aqueous humor via the trabecular meshwork or the uveoscleral out flow. Part of the medications are eliminated through the limbal, conjunctival and scleral vessels. One must keep in mind that the drugs are directly absorbed into the systemic circulation without any first pass metabolism and hence the systemic side effects. Some medications are bound to uveal pigment and require higher doses in patients with dark pigmentation.

REFERENCES

1. Lichter PR, Musch DC, Gillespie BW, Guire KE, Janz NK, Wren PA, et al. Interim clinical outcomes in the collaborative initial glaucoma treatment study (CIGTS) comparing initial treatment randomized to medications or surgery. Ophthalmology 2001;108:1943-53.

2. Coleman AL, Caprioli J. The logic behind target intraocular pressure. Am J Ophthalmology 2009;147:379-80.

3. Jampel HD. Target pressure in glaucoma therapy. J Glaucoma 1997;6:133-8.

4. Goldberg I. Stepping up glaucoma management: when and how? Open Ophthalmol J 2009;17:67-9.

5. Singh K, Shrivastava A. Intraocular pressure fluctuations: how much do they matter? Curr Opin Ophthalmol. 2009;20:84-7.

6. Singh K, Spaeth G, Zimmerman T, Minckler D. Target pressure-glaucomatologists' holey grail. Ophthalmology 2000;107:629-30.

7. European Glaucoma Society: Terminology and Guidelines for Glaucoma: Flowcharts VI: Target IOP.3. Savona: Editrice Dogma; 2008.

8. Realini TD. A prospective, randomized, investigator-masked evaluation of the monocular trial in ocular hypertension or open-angle glaucoma. Ophthalmology 2009;116:1237-42.

9. Singh K, Shrivastava A. Medical management of glaucoma: Principles and practice. Indian J Ophthalmol. 2011 January; 59(Suppl 1): S88-S92.

10. Robin AL, Grover DS. Compliance and adherence in glaucoma management. Indian J Ophthalmol. 2011; 59(Suppl1): S93-S6.

11. Schwartz GA, Quigley HA. Adherence and persistence with glaucoma therapy. Surv Ophthalmol 2008;53 (Suppl 1): S57-S68.

12. Schwartz GF. Compliance and persistency in glaucoma follow-up treatment. Curr Opin Ophthalmol 2005; 16:114-21.

13. Osterberg L, Blaschke T. Adherence to medication. N Engl J Med 2005;353:487-97.

14. Robin AL, Covert D. Does adjunctive glaucoma therapy affect adherence to the initial primary therapy. Ophthalmology 2005;128:198-204.

15. Lee BW, Sathyan P, John RK, Singh K, Robin AL. Predictors of and barriers associated with poor follow-up in patients with glaucoma in South India. Arch Ophthalmol 2008;126: 1448-54.

16. Robin AL, Nirmalan PK, Krishnadas R, Ramakrishnan R, Katz J, Tielsch J, et al. The utilization of eye care services by persons with glaucoma in rural South India. Trans Am Ophthalmol Soc 2004;102:47-55.

PARASYMPATHOMIMETIC AGENTS

CHOLINERGIC OR PARASYMPATHOMIMETIC AGENTS

Cholinergic agents were the first to be used for the management of glaucoma. Since they *mimic the action of acetylcholine they are called cholinergic agents. They are a*lso referred to as ***parasympathomimetics, cholinergic agonists or stimulators, or Miotics*** (due to their effecton the pupil).

Physostigmine, a cholinesterase inhibitor derived from the calabar bean (seed of physostigma venosum) was introduced by Laquer in 1876. One year later Weber treated glaucoma using pilocarpine derived from the leaves of Pilocarpus microphyllus, a South American shrub. These two agents were used in the management of glaucoma for many years. They *were the first line drugs* in the long term management of open angle glaucomas despite their use being limited by their side effects. In the recent times with the advent of newer drugs, the cholinergic agents are now used as *second line agents* in the management of glaucomas, though however they do maintain a preferential position in the management of selected type of cases.

MECHANISM OF ACTION

Cholinergic agents mimic the action of acetylcholine, a neurotransmitter present at the postganglionic parasympathetic endings, some postganglionic sympathetic endings, autonomic ganglia, somatic nerve endings and CNS. Acetylcholine activates cells by binding to cholinergic receptors. Acetylcholinestrase, an enzyme present at the nerve endings hydrolyzes it in order to limit its action. The cholinergic agents act directly by mimicking acetylcholine at the neuromuscular junction or indirectly by inhibiting the acetylcholinestrase thus retarding the degradation of acetylcholine and prolonging its action.

In the eye the parasympathetic nervous system innervates the ciliary body and the iris sphincter. These agents cause the contraction of the longitudinal muscle of the ciliary body which leads to increased aqueous outflow whereas contraction of the circular muscle leads to increased accommodation and contraction of the iris sphincter leads to miosis.

Cholinergic Receptors

They are of two types of cholinergic receptors: Nicotinic and Muscarinic. M1, M2, M3 are the receptor subtypes abundantly present in the eye. M4 and M5 have not been seen in the ciliary body.

Topical agents include:

- Pilocarpine
- Carbachol
- Ecothiophate (indirectly acting agent)

PILOCARPINE

It is the most commonly used and extensively studied parasympathomimetic. It is a directly-acting cholinergic agonist which acts on the muscarinic receptors located in the smooth muscles. It may also have some an indirect effect by activating acetylcholine production. It is more potent at muscarinic than at nicotinic receptor sites.

Mechanism of Action

It has multiple effects on the physiology of the eye.[1-10] The following ocular effects of pilocarpine are generally applicable to all the miotics.

Ciliary Muscle Contraction

- Pilocarpine *stimulates* ciliary muscle contraction by acting on the *m3 muscarinic receptor subtype* which is prominently located in the human ciliary muscle cells and iris sphincter.

- The ciliary muscle has attachments to the scleral spur and the contraction generates *traction causing posterior displacement of the spur. This causes further traction on the trabecular meshwork*. Alteration in the configuration of the trabecular meshwork (separation of trabecular sheets), or Schlemm's canal (prevented from collapsing), or both lead to an increased aqueous outflow facility.

- Another action of pilocarpine is due to the effect of ciliary muscle contraction on the lens. Associated relaxation of the zonules causes changes in lens diameter and curvature resulting in accommodative myopia.

Pupil Constriction

Pilocarpine directly stimulates the cholinergic receptors and acts on the muscarinic receptors (M3) found on the iris sphincter muscle. Miosis is the result of *constriction of the iris sphincter* muscle from direct stimulation of its muscarinic receptors.

This is useful in angle closure disease as it pulls the iris root away from the trabecular meshwork. It *improves outflow* in eyes with angle closure due to pupillary block.

It also changes the anatomy of peripheral iris in cases of plateau iris. The effect is independent of the pupillary size.

Decrease in Uveoscleral Outflow

Pilocarpine *decreases uveoscleral outflow*, which may have clinical significance in eyes with markedly reduced conventional outflow, as pilocarpine may cause a paradoxical rise in IOP.[11]

Pharmacokinetics and Dosage[12-16]

- Pilocarpine is available in a concentration of 0.25-10%. It is manufactured as a water soluble, hydrochloride or nitrate and is stable at a slightly acidic pH. *IOP lowering is dose related and is seen upto a concentration of 4%.* It is usually used in a concentration of 2%. Pilocarpine binds to the melanin in iris and ciliary body. Thus iris color may influence the IOP response and in darkly pigmented eyes higher concentrations 4% or 6% may produce additional pressure reduction. Higher concentration may increase the duration of the effect without additional pressure lowering. This increase duration must be weighed against the increase side effects.

- Pilocarpine penetrates the cornea well. It has a rapid onset of action with the IOP lowering effect starting within minutes of administration lasting for 4-8 hours. *Maximum response is seen within 2 hours, lasting for 8 hours.* Therefore traditionally it is *given in a dose of 4 times a day. The IOP reduction is around 20%* at peak time with a 10-15% reduction at 12-15 hours after instillation.

Alternative Drug Delivery Systems

The amount of pilocarpine delivered by commercial droppers is significantly in excess of that needed to produce the desired response. The result is an initial overdosing with the associated side effects, followed by an underdosing before the next instillation.[17,18]

Using vehicles for drug delivery that can prolong the duration of the therapeutic effectiveness, thereby decreasing the frequency of instillation and hence lesser side effects.

Delivery systems are:

1. ***Pilocarpine gel:*** Pilocarpine hydrochloride in high viscosity acrylic vehicle applied *once at bedtime* and it prolongs and enhances drug penetration.[19-23] *It has the advantage of* less induced myopia and impaired nocturnal visual fields. However, a subtle, diffuse, superficial though reversible corneal haze is seen in 20-28% cases. The IOP control with pilocarpine gel starts to decline after 12 hours, hence IOP monitoring is required to confirm the diurnal IOP control.

2. ***Membrane-controlled delivery system (ocusert):*** Pilocarpine is also formulated in a polymeric membrane delivery device for a constant release of 20 and 40 micrograms of drug every hour.[24,25] The lower rate gives an IOP reduction comparable to 1% pilocarpine drops administrated 4 times a day where as the higher rate gives a reduction comparable to 2-4% drops. It induces less miosis, less myopic shift and provides better diurnal control of IOP. Occasionally an 'ocusert burst' may cause intense miosis and myopic shift. It is useful and young patients. Unfortunately it is no longer available.

Soluble insert devices impregnated with pilocarpine, stiffened paper strip with pilocarpine incorporated into a water soluble polyvinyl alcohol film, and a soft contact lens soaked in pilocarpine have also been tried.[26,27] None of these vehicles have been recommended for general use.

Drug Interactions

The effect of pilocarpine is additive to most available antiglaucoma medications.[28-31] It produces additional IOP reduction with epinephrine. In combination with brimonidine IOP reduction achieved may be better than individual drugs used alone. Formulations containing pilocarpine and Timolol have been reported to be synergistic with an additional reduction of 3-4 mm in IOP as compared to either drug used alone. Some studies have shown that it produces additional IOP lowering with Prostaglandin analogues although the amount of lowering is unpredictable. The timing of administration is also important. It can be used effectively with carbonic anhydrase inhibitors. With other miotics it fails, produce additional the IOP lowering. When used in combination with other antiglaucoma medications it can be used in a dose of 3 or even two times a day.

USES

Angle Closure Glaucoma

Topical pilocarpine is used to treat an attack of acute angle closure and also facilitate laser iridotomy. It must be noted that high IOP can cause iris sphincter ischemia and render it unresponsive to the effect of pilocarpine. In such a situation, the IOP must be lowered by other agents before starting pilocarpine. Frequent instillation of pilocarpine in such a situation may not lower the IOP and lead to systemic side effects.

Peripheral Iridotomy

It is used to achieve miosis before iridotomy. Usually 2% pilocarpine is used.

Plateau Iris Syndrome

In plateau iris syndrome, the iris remains in contact with the trabecular meshwork despite a patent iridotomy. In such cases pilocarpine can be used to open the angle and prevent formation of synechiae.

Pigmentary Glaucoma and Pigment Dispersion Syndrome

Pilocarpine induced miosis can change the concave iris configuration in pigment dispersion syndrome by causing a relative pupillary block. This decreases the iridozonular contact and decreases pigment release. However most patients are young and myopic and may not tolerate the drug. Pilocarpine gel may be used especially prior to any strenuous activity such cases. A careful retinal examination is also mandatory to rule out any peripheral breaks before starting therapy with pilocarpine.

Exfoliation Glaucoma

Studies are under way to use pilocarpine in exfoliation glaucoma as it increases the outflow facility. It also immobilizes the pupil thus decreasing the pigment release. The altered blood aqueous barrier is one disadvantage.

Counter Productive Effects

Though used in the management of angle closure glaucoma counter productive effects in angle closure glaucoma may occur. Increased anteroposterior lens diameter may decrease the anterior chamber depth. In patients with zonular laxity it may aggravate the laxity resulting in anterior lens displacement further shallowing the anterior chamber. These effects can exacerbate or precipitate an acute attack in predisposed eyes.

> **Note** Numerous paradoxical effects of miotics have been reported in literature. So it is important to differentiate primary from secondary causes of angle closure. Careful history and examination is essential before starting these agents. Routine gonioscopy is a must to rule out development of miotic induced angle closure.

Contraindications

It is contraindicated where miosis is undesirable as in uveitis. Since it causes a breakdown of blood aqueous barrier it is not used in eyes with uveitis and in some secondary glaucomas. If used in secondary angle closure glaucomas like lens induced glaucomas it may worsen the condition by causing forward movement of the lens iris diaphragm. It should not be used in case of hypersensitivity to any of its components. The contraindications are listed below:

Ocular

- Active anterior uveitis
- Rubeosis iridis
- Extensive angle closure with little reserve of conventional outflow. Treatment may produce a paradoxical rise in IOP by decreasing the uveoscleral outflow
- High myopia
- History of retinal detachment
- Peripheral retinal degeneration.

Systemic

- Severe pulmonary disease.
- Peptic ulcer
- Parkinson's disease
- Bradycardia
- Hypotension
- Myasthenia gravis

Side Effects
Systemic[32-34]

Systemic side effects are rare with the usual doses of pilocarpine used in chronic management of glaucoma. The danger comes when large doses are given within a short period of time as in pupillary block cases. These agents can produce muscarinic like systemic side effects. Muscarinic receptors are present in smooth muscles and glands. The side effects occur as a result of its action on these receptors and the subsequent smooth muscle contraction. These include nausea, vomiting, diarrhea, abdominal cramping, salivation, sweating, bradycardia, hypotension, bronchospasm, muscle weakness and central nervous system stimulation.

Pilocarpine is not advisable in patients with asthma or chronic obstructive pulmonary diseases.[32] Other organs affected by smooth muscles contraction include the ureters, urinary bladder, gall bladder and the capsular muscle of the spleen, which may cause leukocytosis.

Atrioventricular block may occur in predisposed patients. Patients with

Alzheimer diseases are more sensitive to cholinergic agents and may develop progressive cognitive dysfunction.[33] These side effects and the dosing schedule may affect adherence.[34]

Ocular Side Effects

Ocular side effects are common with pilocarpine. They interfere with the quality of life thus affecting the compliance. These include conjunctival injection, ocular and periocular pain (headache), twitching of the eyelids, fluctuating myopic shift in refraction, and decreased vision in dim illumination.

Ciliary Muscle Contraction

Headache and browache are common especially in young patients. *This is due to ciliary muscle contraction which produces a spasm.* It usually subsides with continued therapy.

Myopic Shift

Young patients complain of a fluctuating myopic shift in refraction upto 12-15 D. This is due to axial thickening and forward shift of the lens causing myopia.[35-37] It starts in 15 min, peaking in an hour and lasting upto 2 hours of instillation. Pilocarpine gel may be a better option in such patients.

Cataractogenic Effect

Cataract development may be faster especially older patients. Small anterior subcapsular vacuoles are noted in the initial stages. It is more common with echothiophate. Older patient with lens opacities complain of decreased vision in dim illumination following pilocarpine use and should be cautioned against driving at night.

Rhegmatogenous Retinal Detachment (RD)

RD is presumed to be a result of vitreous traction induced retinal tears.[38,39] A definite cause and effect relationship has not been established. Pre-existing retinal pathology is a risk factor so perform peripheral fundus exam before pilocarpine therapy.

Miosis

Miosis leads to dimness of vision and a constriction of visual fields. The problem is more pronounced in patients with posterior subcapsular cataracts.

Blood Aqueous Barrier

Parasympathomimetics cause an increase in the blood aqueous barrier permeability in a dose dependent manner.[40] They should be discontinued 3-4 weeks before intraocular surgery. They are contraindicated in cases with uveitis or rubeosis iridis.

Cicatricial pemphigoid has been reported in some patients.

Hypersensitivity and toxic reactions[41] seen involving the eyelids and conjunctiva may occur. In most of the cases preservative has been implicated as the culprit.

CARBACHOL[42-47]

It is a parasympathomimetic with a dual mechanism of action. It produces direct motor end plate stimulation and indirect parasympathomimetic action by inhibiting acetyl cholinesterase.

Dose

It is used in a dosage of 1.5-3% 3 times a day. This is more potent and has a prolonged pressure lowering effect than 2% pilocarpine given four times a day. However it causes more accommodative spasm and pain. It has poor corneal penetration requiring adjuvants like benzalkonium chloride to achieve effective aqueous levels.

Clinical Use

Currently intracameral carbachol to achieve miosis at the end of cataract surgery. It also provides better IOP control in early postoperative period.

INDIRECTLY ACTING PARASYMPATHOMIMETICS
Echothiophate Iodide[48-52]

It is the stronger pure inhibitor of acetyl cholinesterase (true and pseudo) and acts by extending the life of acetylcholine at the neuromuscular junction. It is a parasympathomimetic and organophosphate. It binds irreversibly to cholinesterase. It is hydrolyzed by cholinesterase very slowly, thus it has a prolonged duration of action (lasting for 1 week) with peak in 4-6 hours enabling a twice daily regime. In some patients it is more effective than pilocarpine and may be used in pseudophakics and aphakics.

Dose

Ecothiophate 0.06% given two times a day produces a maximal effect equivalent in the peak effect to 4% pilocarpine within 24 hours which last upto 2 weeks. It produces intense and prolonged miosis. It is manufactured as a white crystalline solid, i.e. mixed with a diluent at the time of dispensing. Because of limited stability, solution of the drug should be refrigerated.

Side Effects

Its benefits are limited by the ocular and systemic side effect.

Systemic

Its systemic side effects are a limiting factor for its use. They are similar but more severe than pilocarpine. Additionally, toxic reactions to anesthetic agents metabolized by pseudo cholinesterase are seen. It depletes both true and pseudo cholinesterase which begins in 2 weeks peaking at 5-7 weeks and stays for several weeks after discontinuing the drug. After general anesthesia, a prolonged respiratory paralysis may occur in patients on echothiophate if succinylcholine is used as muscle relaxant, as it is metabolized by pseudo cholinesterase. Thus it should be stopped 6 weeks before general anesthesia with succinylcholine. The antidote for echothiophate iodide toxicity is pralidoxime chloride.

Pseudo cholinesterase depletions in newborns may occur if mothers treated with echothiophate late in pregnancy.

Ocular
Cataract

A cataractogenic effect has been observed with long term use of echothiophate.[51,52] Fine anterior sub capsular vacuoles have been described. The exact mechanism is unclear.

Iris Cysts

Iris cysts near the pupillary margin have been seen reported in children receiving echothiophate for the treatment of accomodative esotropia.

Other ocular side effects include:

- Ocular pemphigoid and contact dermatitis.
- Corneal epithelial toxicity

Physostigmine

Physostigmine is one of the oldest drugs and was successfully used for the treatment of glaucoma in 1864. Also known as eserine it is a parasympathomimetic, more specifically a reversible cholinesterase inhibitor obtained from the Calabar bean. It helps prolong the activity of acetylcholine and by interfering with the metabolism of acetylcholine, physostigmine indirectly stimulates both nicotinic and muscarinic receptors. It causes a constriction of the pupil more marked than in the case of any other known drug and stimulates the fibers of the ciliary muscle.

Demecarium Bromide

It is a potent, stable, long acting cholinesterase inhibitor with considerable specificity for acetylcholinesterase. It is less effective than echothiophate. However, it is effective in patients who do not respond adequately echothiophate. It is no longer manufactured.

Isoflurophate

It is a potent cholinesterase inhibitor with the greater action against pseudocholinesterase. It is available as an ointment (0.025%) given every 12-72 hours or a solution of 0.01-0.1% in anhydrous peanut oil. This oil causes allergy and must be refrigerated. It is hydrolysis

very rapidly and may get inactivated even during application.

Neostigmine

It is a short acting anticholinesterase given in a 3-5% aqueous solution every 4-6 hours. It is more stable and potent than physostigmine causing less vascular congestion and conjunctival follicular hypertrophy. However, its corneal penetration is poor.

Summary

Pilocarpine is available since 1870. Given the newer agents, its use has decreased. It is still useful in controlling IOP both short-term and long-term

especially in angle closure glaucoma and plateau iris.

- All cholinergic agents lower the IOP by increasing the aqueous outflow.
- They differ in how they stimulate the ciliary body
- Pilocarpine stimulates the cholinergic receptors directly
- Cholinesterase inhibitors inhibit acetylcholinestrase, prolonging the duration of action of endogenous acetylcholine.
- Carbachol acts both directly and indirectly
- Ocular and systemic side effects limit their use
- Have a role in selected glaucomas and clinical situations.

REFERENCES

1. Mindel JS, Kharlamb AB. Alteration of acetylcholine synthesis by pilocarpine. In vivo and in vitro studies. Arch ophthalmol 1984;102:1546.
2. Van Buskirk Em. Changes in the facility of aqueous outflow induced by lens depression and intraocular pressure in excised human eyes. Am J Ophthalmol 1976;82:736.
3. Moses RA, Grodzki WJJ. Choroid tension and facility of aqueous outflow. Invest Ophthalmol Vis Sci 1977;16:1062.
4. Cairns JE. Goniospasis: a method designed to relieve canalicular blockade in primary open angle glaucoma. Ann Ophthalmol 1976;8:1417.
5. Kaufman PL, Barany EH. Loss of acute pilocarpine effect on outflow facility following surgical disinsertion and retrodisplacement of the ciliary muscle from the scleral spur in the cynomolgus monkey. Invest Ophthalmol 1976;15:793.
6. Kaufrman PL, Bill A, Barany EH. Formation and drainage of aqueous humor following total iris removal and ciliary muscle disinsertion in the cynomolgus monkey. Invest Ophthalmol Vis Sci 1977;16:226.

7. Lutjen-Drecoll E, Kaufman PL, Barany EH. Light and electron microscopy of the anterior chamber angle structures following surgical disinsertion of the ciliary muscle in the cynomolgus monkey. Invest Ophthalmol Vis Sci 1977;16:218.
8. Grierson I, Lee WR, Abraham S. Effects of pilocarpine on the morphology of the human outflow apparatus. Br J Ophthalmol 1978;62:302.
9. Grierson I, Lee WR, Abraham S. The effects of topical pilocarpine on the morphology of the human outflow apparatus of the baboon (Papio Cynocephalus). Invest Ophthalmol Vis Sci 1979;18:346. Br J Ophthalmol 1978;62:302.
10. Bill A, Phillips CI. Uveoscleral drainage of aqueous humor in human eyes. Exp Eye Res 1971;12:275.
11. Bleiman BS, Scheartz Al. Paradoxical intraocular pressure response to pilocarpine: A proposed mechanism and treatment. Arch Ophthalmol 1979;97:1305.
12. Doane MG, Jensen AD, Dohlman CH. Penetration routes of topically applied eye medications. Am J Ophthalmol 1978;85:383.

13. Krohn DL, Breitfeller JM. Transcorneal flux of topical pilocarpine to the human aqueous. Am J Ophthalmol 1979; 87:50.
14. Drance SM, Nash PA. The dose response of human intraocular pressure to pilocarpine. Can J Ophthalmol 1971;6:9.
15. Drance SM, Bensted M, Schulzer M. Pilocarpine and intraocular pressure: duration of effectiveness of 4 percent and 8 percent pilocarpine instillation. Arch Ophthalmol 1974;91:104.
16. Harris LS, Galin MA. Effect of ocular pigmentation on hypotensive response to pilocarpine. Am J Ophthalmol 1971;72:923.
17. Patton TF, Francoeur M. Ocular bioavailability and systemic loss to topically applied ophthalmic drugs. Am J Ophthalmol 1978;85:225.
18. File RR, Patton TF. Topically applied pilocarpine: human pupillary response as a function of drop size. Arch Ophthalmol 1980;98:112.
19. March WF, Stewart RM, Mandell AI, et al. Duration of effect of pilocarpine gel. Arch Ophthalmol 1982;100: 1270.
20. Goldberg I, Ashburn FSJ, Kass MA, et al. Efficacy and patient acceptance

of pilocarpine gel. Am J Ophthalmol 1979;88:843.

21. Johnson DH, Epstein DL, Allen RC, et al. A one year multi centre clinical trial of pilocarpine gel. Am J Ophthalmol 1984;97:723.

22. Johnson DH, Kenyon KR, Epstein DL, et al. Corneal changes during pilocarpine gel therapy. Am J Ophthalmol 1986;101:13.

23. Place VA, Fisher M, Herbet S, et al. Comparative pharmacologic effects of pilocarpine administered to normal subjects by eye drops or by ocular therapeutic systems. Am J Ophthalmol 1975;80:706.

24. Quigley HA, Pollack IP, Harbin TSJ. Pilocarpine Ocuserts: long-term clinical trials and selected pharmacodynamics. Arch Ophthalmol 1975;93:771.

25. Bensinger R, Shin DH, Kass MA, et al. Pilocarpine ocular inserts. Invest Ophthalmol 1976;15:1008.

26. Kelly JA, Molyneux PD, Smith SA, et al. Relative bioavailability of pilocarpine from a novel ophthalmic delivery system and conventional eye drops formulations. Br J Ophthalmol 1989;73:360.

27. Ruben M, Watkins R. Pilocarpine dispensation for the soft hydrophilic contact lens. Br J Ophthalmol 1975;59:455.

28. Kronfeld PC. The efficacy of combinations of ocular hypotensive drugs. A tonographic approach. Arch Ophthalmol 1967;78:1407.

29. Harris LS, Mittag TW, Galin MA. Aqueous dynamics of pilocarpine -treated eyes; the influence of topically applied epinephrine. Arch Ophthalmol 1971;86:1.

30. Keates EU. Evaluation of timolol maleate combination therapy in chronic open angle glaucoma. Am J Ophthalmol 1976;88:565.

31. Kass MA, Gordon MO, Hoff MR, et al. Topical timolol administration reduces the incidence of glaucomatous damage in ocular hypertensive individuals. A randomized double – masked, long term clinical trial. Arch Ophthalmol 1989;107:1590.

32. Curti PC. Renovanz HD/ (The effect of unintentional over doses of pilocarpine on pulmonary surfactant in mice.) (German) Klin Monatsbl Augenheilk 1981;179:113.

33. Reyes PF, Dwyer BA, Schwartzman RJ, et al. Mental status changes induced by eye drops in dementia of the Alzheimer type. J Neurol Neurosurg Psychiatry 1987;50:113.

34. Granstrom PA, Norell S. Visual ability and drug regimen: relation to compliance with glaucoma therapy. Acta Ophthalmol (Copenh) 1983;61: 206.

35. Abramson DH, Chang S, Coleman DJ, et al. Pilocarpine induced lens changes: an ultrasonic biometric evaluation of dose response. Arch Ophthalmol 1974;92:464.

36. Francois J, Goes F. Ultrasonographic study of the effect of different miotics on the eye components. Ophthalmologica 1977;175:328.

37. Abramson DH, Franzen LA, Coleman DJ. Pilocarpine in the presbyope: demonstration of an effect on the anterior chamber and lens thickness. Arch Ophthalmol 1973;89:100.

38. Pape LG, Forbes M. Retinal detachment and mitotic therapy. Am J Ophthalmol 1978;85:558.

39. Beasley H, Fraunfelder FT. Retinal detachments and topical ocular miotics. Ophthalmology 1979;86:95.

40. Mori M, Araie M, Sakurai M, et al. Effects of pilocarpine and tropicamide on blood aqueous barrier permeability in man. Invest Ophthalmol Vis Sci 1992;33:416.

41. Jackson WB. Differentiating conjunctivitis of diverse origins (review). Surv Ophthalmol 1993;38 (Suppl):91.

42. O'Brien CS, Swan KC. Carbaminoylcholine chloride in the treatment of glaucoma simplex. Arch Ophthalmol 1942;27:253.

43. Francois J, Goes F. Ultrasonographic study of the effect of different miotics on the eye components. Ophthalmologica 1977;175:328.

44. Ruiz RS, Rhem MN, Prager TC. Effects of carbachol and acetylcholine on intraocular pressure after cataract extraction. Am J Ophthalmol 1989;107:7.

45. Hollanda RH, Drance SM, House PH, et al. Control of intraocular pressure after cataract extraction. Can J Ophthalmol 1990;25:128.

46. Linn DK, Zimmerman TJ, Nardin GF, et al. Effect of intra-cameral carbachol on intraocular pressure after cataract extraction. Am J Ophthalmol 1989;107:133.

47. Wood TO. Effect of carbachol on postoperative intraocular pressure. J Cataract Refract Surg 1988;14:654.

48. Ellis PP, Esterdahl M. Echothiophate iodide therapy in children: effect upon blood Cholinesterase levels. Arch Ophthalmol 1967;77:598.

49. Ellis PP, Littlejohn K. Effects of topical anticholinesterases on procaine hydrolysis. Am J Ophthalmol 1974;77:71.

50. Birks DA, Prior VJ, Silk E, et al. Echothiophate iodide treatment of glaucoma in pregnancy. Arch Ophthalmol 1968;79:283.

51. Axelsson U, Holmberg A. The frequency of cataract after miotic therapy. Acta Ophthalmol (Copenh) 1966;44:421.

52. Thoft RA. Incidence of lens changes in patients treated with ecothiophate iodide. Arch Ophthalmol 1968; 80:317.

β-ADRENERGIC RECEPTOR ANTAGONISTS

Beta receptor antagonists are the most frequently used ocular hypotensive agents because they are effective in most types of glaucomas and have relatively few ocular side effects. The lowering of IOP through intravenous or oral administration of propranolol, a non-selective ß blocker in glaucoma patients was first reported in 1967.[1] Potential development of propranolol as a topical IOP lowering drug was limited by its unwanted corneal anesthetic property. Following this, the development of another topical non-selective ß blocker, timolol, for lowering IOP took place.[2]

CLASSIFICATION

ß blockers can be characterized as selective or non-selective based on the relative affinities for the specific receptors subtypes. The selectivity however is not absolute. At high concentration selective ß blockers can bind with other ß receptors subtypes. Most ß blockers have a low affinity for the ß-3 receptor subtype.

BETA RECEPTORS

- There are three subtypes of ß-adrenergic receptors;[3,4] ß-1, ß-2, and ß-3 receptors. ß-1 receptors are located mainly in the heart and their stimulation increases the heart rate and force of cardiac contraction.
- ß-2 receptors are located in the bronchial, vascular, gastrointestinal, and genitourinary smooth muscles. Stimulation of these ß-2 receptors causes relaxation of smooth muscles.
- ß-3 receptors are found in adipose tissues and they are involved in lipolysis.

Ocular ß adrenergic receptors largely consist of the ß-2 receptor subtype.

MECHANISM OF ACTION OF BETA BLOCKERS

The main mechanism of action of topical beta blockers is suppression of aqueous humor formation by about 30-50%. Resistance to aqueous humor outflow does not appear to be affected by this class of drugs.

Normally beta receptor agonists stimulate G Protein (a regulatory protein) to activate the enzyme adenylate cyclase.[5] This catalyzes the conversion of ATP to cAMP. cAMP acts as "Second messenger" to trigger a cascade of biochemical events. It regulates the ion channels and enzymes in the ciliary epithelium responsible for aqueous humor production.

Despite their being in use for a long time, the exact mechanism of action of beta blockers is not completely known and various mechanisms have been proposed. These include:

Blockade of β₂ Receptors in the Ciliary Processes

Beta blockers act on the ß₂ subtype of the ß receptor family which are located in the ciliary processes and cause inhibition of catecholamine (mainly adrenaline) stimulated synthesis of cyclic AMP, which is essential for a resting physiological sympathetic tone in the ciliary processes. This results in a decrease in the aqueous humor synthesis. This also possibly affects the local capillary perfusion to reduce ultra filtration.

Other Mechanisms

The standard beta-receptors model does not entirely explain how they affect IOP. A simple effect on cAMP levels does not completely explain the receptor mediated response to beta blockers.

The endogenous catecholamines may be bloodborne as well as released from sympathetic neurons terminating in the ciliary body. The ß2 receptors are present in the blood vessels of the ciliary body. Blockage of these receptors in the ciliary artery may result in unopposed alpha-receptors mediated vascular constriction and reduced blood supply to the ciliary body and ciliary epithelium. This could reduce capillary perfusion pressure and a decrease in ultrafiltration and aqueous formation.[6,7] There may be antagonism of noradrenaline released from the synaptic terminals.

It is interesting to see that why a ß1 selective antagonist (Betaxolol) should lower IOP if the receptors responsible for mediating aqueous humor production are of ß2 type. One explanation may be that betaxolol is only relatively ß1 selective and at high concentrations also blocks ß2 receptors to some extent. This also explains its less IOP lowering effect. It has been found to acheive a higher local concentration at adrenoreceptors which may compensate for its lower ß2 binding capacity.[8]

At the same time it may be possible that part of the effect is due to other mechanisms. They could act by interfering with chloride conductance, or calcium channels blockage (betoxolol) or involvement of serotonergic receptors (5HT 1A) present in the ciliary epithelium.[9]

Non IOP Lowering Effects

Non specific beta blockers cause vasoconstriction (by an unopposed alpha adrenergic action) but since the number of beta receptors at back of eye are few, this may be of no consequence. Studies on short term and long term use of timolol have controversial results showing a decrease or no difference.

Vasodilation due occurs to calcium channel blockage (CCB) independent of beta blocking activity may occur. This is seen especially with propranolol and betaxolol. Betaxolol has weak CCB activity. Some studies have reported an increased effect on ocular and ONH circulation bur without effects on microvascular calibre of anterior ONH. Indirect evidence that betaxolol may improve hemodynamics needs to be interpreted with caution. Betaxolol has also been proposed to have a role in neuroprotection. Calcium channel blocking activity of betaxolol also antagonizes the excitotoxic damage mediated by calcium overload in neurons. *In vitro* studies have shown that it also reduces Na^+ entry into the cells. *In vivo* effect on retinal ischemia is seen only in animal models.

> **Note** Beta blockers have a very little effect on the already slow aqueous humor formation during the sleep period as the catecholamine tone is already low. Thus they do not significantly reduce night time IOP.

Pharmacokinetics

The serum half life of absorbed topical beta blockers is only a few hours (betaxolol 12-20 hours), their ocular availability is prolonged due to melanin binding.

DRUGS IN CLINICAL USE
Timolol Maleate
It was approved for clinical use in 1978. It is a potent nonselective beta blocking agent.

Dose
It is available in a concentration of 0.25% and 0.5% and more recently 0.1%. Both 0.25% and 0.5% concentrations of Timolol provide an equal lowering of IOP, although the latter provides a longer duration of action.

The mechanism of action is by about a 50% reduction in aqueous humor production at daytime.[10,11]

Timolol causes a rapid decline in IOP within one hour after topical application with the peak concentration of the drug in aqueous and hence the peak IOP lowering occurring in two hours post instillation. The preferred concentration by most is 0.5% given twice a day. When given in children a lower concentration is preferred. Digital punctal occlusion is advisable to avoid systemic side effects. Timolol is partially metabolized in the liver and excreted mainly by the kidneys.

To reduce systemic side effects and improve the therapeutic index, formulations of Timolol in a gel-forming solution have been introduced in 0.1%, 0.25% and 0.5% concentrations for once daily use. The more viscous formulation increases corneal contact time, increases ocular bioavailability. Timolol gel produces an additional 1 to 2 mm IOP lowering than the solution during 24 hours after instillation.

> **Note** The optimum frequency is twice daily; studies are underway regarding the efficacy of a once daily regime. Some formulations for once a day dosing are also available.

IOP Reduction[12,13]
It causes a reduction in IOP within 30 minutes to 1 hour of its topical application with a peak reduction after 2 hours. A significant IOP lowering effect can persist for 12 hours with a measurable effect for 24 hours. Both concentrations produce the same peak IOP lowering effect though their trough effect may differ. IOP lowering is between 19 and 29%. In a meta-analysis the mean percentage reduction in IOP by Timolol was 26.9% at 3 months.[14,15]

- ***Twenty-four-hour IOP control:*** It appears to be less effective during the night.[16-18] This is because of the little inhibitory effect on nocturnal aqueous secretion which is already reduced. Moreover sympathetic activity is reduced at night. Since these agents compete with endogenous adrenaline for the beta receptors this may add to the decreased nocturnal effect.

- ***Long term IOP control:*** The initial reduction however may not be sustained and many patients may lose this maximum IOP lowering effect within 1 year. This may be due to:
  - ❖ *Tachyphalxis:* IOP lowering efficacy may decrease over time
  - ❖ *Short term escape:* IOP lowering efficacy may decrease with in period of weeks due to up regulation of local ß adrenergic receptors.
  - ❖ *Long term drift:* The effect of timolol can taper off in some patients over a longer period of months or years. Aqueous humor flow has been found to be slightly higher after a year's treatment. A receptor or intracellular alteration may be responsible for this. It may partly be attributed to the progression of glaucoma.

Non Responder Rate
The non responder rate with timolol is about 20%. (IOP reduction less than 6 mm Hg or IOP more than 20 mm Hg).

Washout Period
On discontinuation after a long therapy, aqueous flow does not increase significantly until the fourth day and the IOP effect is still seen by 14 days. Washout period is four weeks.

Contralateral IOP Lowering
Topical timolol can cause IOP lowering in the contralateral eye of about 1.5 mm Hg due to systemic absorption.[19]

Interactions with Systemic Drugs

- In patients who are already on the therapy with oral ß blockers, timolol eye drops may produce little IOP lowering effect.[20]
- Timolol can elicit bradycardia or cardiac arrhythmia when used along with drugs like:
  - Antiarrhythmic agents like digitalis, digoxin.
  - Sodium channel blockers like quinidine, procainamide, lidocaine.
  - Calcium channel blocker like verapamil and diltiazem.

Interaction with Topical Drugs

- Combined action of beta blockers with epinephrine or dipivefrin is poor
- Effective combination with all other antiglaucoma medication producing additional IOP lowering effect.

Formulations

It is preferable to use timolol in the lowest possible concentration which is effective in order to minimize systemic side effects.

Timolol is also available in an anionic heteropolysaccharide gellan gum, which prolongs the residence time of the drug in the tear film. Given once a day it has an efficacy equivalent to twice a day timolol maleate.

Gels have the advantage of an increased ocular contact time. This enhances the drug delivery to the eye. The systemic complications are also less due to decreased absorption.[21,22] Moreover preparations with a concentration of 0.1% are also available. They are generally given in once a day dose and have a comparable IOP lowering effect to the twice a day timolol solution. This improves adherence to therapy. 0.1% gel both preserved and unpreserved is available.

Preservative Free Formulations

Preservative free formulations in the form of unit dose or special bottles with one way valves and antimicrobial coatings are available. However, cost is a limiting factor. The preservative free formulations produce less conjuctival inflammation.

Timolol Hemihydrate

The safety and efficacy of timolol hemihydrate 0.5% a lipophilic, non-selective beta blocker solution, is comparable to timolol maleate 0.5%.

Generic Preparations

An increasing number of generic beta blocker preparations have appeared on the market. The duration of action and tolerability (ocular and system) of these new products may differ depending on their non medicinal constituents.

Fixed Combinations

Timolol is present in majority of the fixed combinations currently available. The effect is additive with most other groups except dipivefrin and epinephrine. The fixed combinations are effective and have the additional advantage of increasing adherence, decreasing cost and less exposure to preservatives.

Adverse Effects

Systemic:[23,24] Systemic side effects include fatigue, coldness of extre-mities, paraesthesia, GI symptoms, skin rash, alopecia, dry mouth, bradycardia. Potentially fatal side effects include: heart failure, heart block, bronchospasm, respiratory failure.

Ocular: Ocular side effects include blurred vision, burning, stinging, ocular irritation, decreased corneal sensitivity, visual disturbances, diplopia, ptosis, cystoid macular edema, pseudopemphigoid, choroidal detachment following filtration surgery.

Main Points

- Non-selective ß1 and ß2 blocking agent
- Lacks intrinsic sympathomimetic activity and membrane stabilizing properties
- Does not cause corneal anesthesia and its subsequent side effects as was the case with propranolol.[25]
- Reduces IOP without any effect on the visual acuity, accommodation and pupil size.
- The IOP lowering of the contra-lateral eye is suggestive of a systemic absorption and subsequent action.
- Binds to melanin and not metabolized by ocular tissue, thus a higher concentration may be required in eyes with dark colored iris.
- Does not have much effect on nocturnal IOP.

BETAXOLOL[26,27]

Betaxolol is a lipophilic, selective ß1 adrenergic antagonist. It was introduced in early 1980's as a cardioselective beta blockers. Although a ß1 selective blocker, receptor occupancy studies of human aqueous from betaxolol treated eyes suggest a role of ß2 receptor blockade.

Dose

It is available as 0.5% solution or 0.25% microsuspension given in a dose of two times a day.

IOP Reduction

IOP reduction is slightly less than timolol, with a 20 to 30% lowering of IOP.[28]

Non IOP Related Effects

Some studies have found that on long-term follow-up betaxolol treated patients showed more favorable course regarding retinal sensitivity as measured by static automated perimetry. This may be is explained by its:

- Proposed neuroprotective action
- Beneficial effect on optic disc blood flow.

Systemic Side Effects

The main feature which distinguishes it from other topical non–selective ß blockers is the *apparent* lack of systemic side effects. Betaxolol has a more favorable pulmonary side effect profile than non-selective, ß blockers. In patients with known reactive airway disease, the use of betaxolol is considered *relatively safer* than the non-selective ß blocker. Cases and controls with COPD, asthma and chronic bronchitis have shown no changes in pulmonary function with betaxolol. Although a ß1 blocker would be suspected to have some cardiac effect, ophthalmic betaxolol is unable to offer systemic blockade with no effect on pulse rate.

Interaction with Other Anti Glaucoma Medications

It is additive to pilocarpine, carbonic anhydrase inhibitors and alpha agonists.

LEVOBUNOLOL[29-32]

It is an analogue of propranolol. It is a lipophilic, non-selective ß1 and ß2 adrenergic antagonist. On instillation it is converted *in vivo* into an equipotent metabolite dihydrobunolol (DHB). It also has a weak alpha 1 antagonistic and calcium channel blocking action.

Dose

It is available as 0.25% and 0.5% concentration. 0.5% once a day provides good IOP control in some patients. Its action starts within the first hour post instillation, peaks at 3 (2-6 hours) hours, lasting upto 24 hours. Its prolonged action is due to its binding and slow release from ocular melanin along with its metabolism to

dihydrobunolol which also has beta blocking activity. The metabolite of levobunolol, dihydrobunolol, has ß blockers activity and may also add to the sustained effect of levobunolol. Levobunolol is equivalent to Timolol in efficacy and superior to betaxolol. Once a daily dosage is a significant advantage in terms of both compliance and cost. Clinical trials show it to be well tolerated by patients, with no significant difference in the incidence of side effects when compared to Timolol. It is a potent ocular hypotensive agent and like Timolol is safe in patients without cardiac or pulmonary complications.

CARTEOLOL

Carteolol is a nonselective hydrophilic ß-adrenergic antagonist with intrinsic sympathomimetic activity (ISA). This produces an early, transient adrenergic agonist response that is not found in the other topical ß blockers.

Dose

Carteolol 1%, used twice daily produces a mean IOP reduction of 23%. The ocular hypotensive efficacy and duration of action are comparable to Timolol. In contrast levobunolol has shown to have a greater age-adjusted IOP lowering effect than Carteolol. The once daily Carteolol alginate shows equivalent IOP lowering to that of the standard formulation.

Carteolol causes less ocular irritation than timolol in the first few minutes after instillation.

In theory, Carteolol's ISA should be advantageous in decreasing the respiratory and cardiovascular effects from ß blockade after systemic absorption. This sympathomimetic activity does not seem to protect against cardiovascular effects such as reduced BP and pulse. Carteolol decreases systolic and diastolic blood pressure and heart rate.

It is however less likely than timolol to induce nocturnal bradycardia and cause cardiovascular adverse events overall. Also, ISA protects against the cardiovascular risks associated with cholesterol abnormalities.[33] ISA may also be helpful locally by maintaining or improving ocular blood flow through vasodilatation or minimization of vasoconstriction.

METIPRANOLOL

Metipranolol 0.3% (OptiPranolol) is another non-selective lipophilic ß blocker available since 1991. Its affinities for the ß1 and ß2 adrenergic receptors are about equal.

The IOP lowering efficacy is similar to other non-selective ß blockers. Onset of action is within 30 minutes, the maximal effect appears at two hours, and a detectable IOP–lowering effect persists for 24 hours. Like levobunolol, an active metabolite of metipranolol, deacetylmetipranolol, may contribute to the prolonged IOP lowering effect.

DRUG INTERACTIONS

- IOP lowering with combination of Timolol and miotics is greater than either of the drugs used alone, although less than the arithmetic sum of the effects of individual drugs.
- It is additive with apraclonidine, brimonidine.
- Oral carbonic anhydrase inhibitors are effective as a second drug with Timolol. Topical CAIs are not as effective but have fewer side effects.
- Topical prostaglandin agents are effective in conjugation with Timolol. Fixed dose combination of prostaglandin analogue with timolol is available.
- Concurrent use of systemic and topical ß blockers lowers the IOP lowering efficacy of the latter.

SIDE EFFECTS
Ocular
Adverse ocular reactions are usually low with topical ß blocker therapy. These include:

- Tear film is altered in cases with low baseline tear flow.
- *Burning and conjunctival hyperemia:* They occur occasionally but are frequently associated with superficial punctuate keratopathy and corneal anesthesia.
- Beta blockers do not stimulate cell proliferation directly in the Tenon's fibroblasts, but do so indirectly by chronic inflammation from the irritating effects of the antiglaucama medications or preservatives.
- Granulomatous anterior uveitis has been seen with metipranolol therapy.[34]
- A side effect under the influence of ß blockers on ocular blood flow is currently under investigation.
- Clinically available ß blockers do not cause corneal anesthesia. Longer blur is expected for a gel-forming preparation. Patients may be hypersensitive to certain components in the drug formations.

Systemic Side Effects
Beta receptors exist in organs throughout the body and their non therapeutic blockade can cause pulmonary, cardiovascular, neurological and metabolic side effects. Systemic side effects are reported more often than ocular reactions and potentially constitute the more significant adverse effect of the topical ß blocker therapy.

Systemic Absorption
Topically applied drugs are absorbed via the nasal mucosa into the systemic circulation. They attain sufficient serum levels via absorption into conjunctival, nasal, oropharyngeal and gastrointestinal mucosa to have systemic effects. Starting with lower concentration and

using nasolacrimal occlusion techniques may decrease systemic side effects. Measurable plasma levels of Timolol are present within 8 minutes or less of topical application. A careful review of the patient's medical history is essential before prescribing a ß blocker.

Respiratory Effects
ß2 receptor blockage produces contraction of bronchial smooth muscle, which may cause bronchospasm and airway obstruction, especially in asthmatics. The non-selective beta blockers are thus contraindicated in asthamatics, patients with COPD. Carteolol has an ISA which may make it a safer option theoretically. However there is no clinical support for this in literature. Betaxolol, specific for ß1 receptors, may be a safer alternative as compared to non-selective agents and has been used in mild asthma.[35] However, several reports suggest that it may compromise breathing in patients with pulmonary disease as it may not be completely selective in its action. If started it should be in consultation with the medical specialist or an alternative class of topical antiglaucoma drugs may be prescribed.

Cardiovascular Effects
- ß1 receptor blockage results in slowing of the pulse rate and weakens myocardial contractility. This reduces the cardiac output and lowers the blood pressure. In most healthy patients, these effects are of no consequence. They usually cause a minor decrease in resting heart rate and decreases exercise induced tachycardia. However healthy individuals may be at risk under certain circumstances, such as the stress of surgery.
- *Cardiac conduction defects:* Beta blockers have been associated with severe bradycardia, arrhythmias in patients with pre-existing

sinus bradycardia and arrhythmia (second and third degree atrio-ventricular block). This is due to the ß1 receptor blockage. Betaxolol has lesser tendency to produce conduction defects.
- Syncope may result from hypoperfusion to the brain.
- Decreased perfusion to the heart can lead to angina or myocardial infarction and may prove fatal.
- Blood flow to other organs may be reduced due to the vasoconstriction mediated by the unopposed action of circulating norepinephrine on alpha receptors. This vasospasm may not be long lasting and produces no change in vascular resistance.
- Selecting another glaucoma drug class is important because of the potential for serious complications in patients with pre-existing cardiac conditions such as sinus bradycardia and greater than first-degree heart block.

Central Nervous System Effects
Depression is commonly seen. Beta blockers may cause or increase the pre-exisiting depression associated with glaucoma. The topical drug may gain access to the CNS by their lipophilic nature and transport across blood brain barrier. Other CNS side effects which may be seen are anxiety, confusion, dysarthria, hallucinations, lightheadedness, drowsiness, weakness, fatigue, dissociative behavior and emotional liability. They aggravate muscle weakness in pre-existing myasthenia gravis. However with the association of glaucoma with depression it is difficult to attribute it to the drug only. Because of potential effects of beta-adrenergic blocking agents relative to blood pressure and pulse, these agents should be used with caution in patients with cerebrovascular insufficiency. If signs or symptoms suggesting reduced cerebral blood flow are observed,

consideration should be given to discontinuing these agents.

Muscle Weakness
Blockade of beta-adrenergic receptors has been reported to potentiate muscle weakness consistent with certain myasthenic symptoms (e.g. diplopia, ptosis, and generalized weakness). Timolol has been reported rarely to increase muscle weakness in some patients with myasthenia gravis or myasthenic symptoms.

Cholesterol Metabolism
ß blockers have harmful effects on lipid metabolism. The mechanism involves inhibiting the enzymes of cholesterol metabolism, which results in an increase in serum triglycerides and a reduction in the high-density lipoprotein (HDL) levels. Systemic beta blockers are contra indicated in patients with history of dyslipoproteinemia-related

cardiac events. Carteolol may be used in such cases.

Response to Hypoglycemia
Adrenergic outflow and betablockers contribute to the symptoms and physiological response to hypoglycemia. Blockade of the symptoms and signs of low blood sugar level could seriously delay the physiological response to an insulin reaction. For this reason, oral beta blockers are relatively contraindicated when treatment cardiovascular disease in diabetics.

Other Reactions
These include gastrointestinal distress like nausea, diarrhea and cramping, dermatologic disorders and impotence.

Contraindications
Non-selective topical ß blockers are contraindicated in patients with

asthma, chronic obstructive pulmonary disease (emphysema and bronchitis), sinus bradycardia and heart block and some cases of congestive heart failure. They should be avoided in patients on antiarrhythmic drugs as these have a narrow therapeutic index.

Summary
Rapid acceptance of timolol and other beta blockers is due to their convenient dose schedule, lack of significant ocular side effects and cost. It was drug of choice for lowering IOP for until the introduction of prostaglandin analogues. It is a popular drug for the initial therapy as well as adjunctive therapy to lower IOP. It is useful in virtually all forms of glaucoma and is additive to other available antiglaucoma medications. The main drawback is the systemic side effects.

REFERENCES

1. Philips CI, Howitt G, Rowlands DJ. Propranolol as ocular hypertensive agent. Br J Ophthalmol 1967;51:222-6.
2. Katz IM, Hubbard WA, Getson AJ, Gould AL. Intraocular pressure decrease in normal volunteers following timolol ophthalmic solution. Invest Ophthalmol 1976;15:489-92.
3. Westfall TC, Westfall DP. Neurotansmission, the autonomic and somatic motor nervous systems. In: Brunton LL, Lazo JS, Parker KL (Eds.). Goodman and Gilman's The pharmacological Basis of Therapeutics. 10th ed. McGraw-Hill, New York 2006;137-81.
4. Henderer JD, Rapuano CJ. Ocular pharmacology. In: Brunton LL, Lazo JS, Parker KL (Eds.). Goodman and Gilman's The pharmacological Basis of Therapeutics. 10th ed. McGraw-Hill, New York 2006; 1707-37.
5. Brubaker RF. Flow of aqueous humor in humans. Invest Ophthalmol Vis SCi 1991;32:3145-66.
6. Nyborg NC, Nielson PJ. Beta-adrenergic receptors regulating vascular smooth muscle tone are only localized to the intraocular segment of the long posterior ciliary artery in bovine eye. Survey of Ophthalmology 1995;39:S66-S75.
7. Watanabe K, Chiou GC. Action mechanism of timolol to lower the intraocular pressure in rabbits. Ophthalmic Res 1983;15:160-7.
8. Santafé J, Martínez de Ibarreta MJ, Segarra J, Melena J, Garrido M. A complex interaction between topical verapamil and timolol on intraocular pressure in conscious rabbits. Naunyn Schmiedebergs Arch Pharmacol. 1996;354:198-204.
9. Osborne NN, Chidlow G. Do beta-adrenoceptors and serotonin 5-HT1A receptors have similar functions in the control of intraocular pressure in the rabbit? Ophthalmologica 1996;210:308-14.
10. Coakes RL, Brubaker RF. The mechanism of timolol in lowering intraocular pressure. In the normal eye. Arch Ophthalmol 1978;96:2045-8.
11. Yablonski ME, Zimmerman TJ, Waltman SR, Becker B. A fluorophotometric study of the effect of topical timolol on aqueous humor dynamics. Exp Eye Res. 1978;27:135-42.
12. Zimmerman TJ, Kaufman HE. A beta-adrenergic blocking agent for the treatment of glaucoma. Arch Ophthalmol. 1977;95:601-4.
13. Zimmerman TJ, Kaufman HE. Dose response and duration of action. Arch. Ophthal 1977;95:605-7.
14. Zhang WY, Po AI, Dua HS, et al. Meta-analysis of randomised controlled trials companing latanoprost with timolol in the treatment of patients with open angle glaucoma or

ocular hypertension. Br J Ophthalmol 2001;85:890-981.

15. van der Valk R, Webers C, Schouten J, et al. Intraocular pressure lowering effect of all commonly used glaucoma drugs. Ophthalmology 2005;112:1177-85.

16. Topper JE, Brubaker RF. Effecta of timolol, epinephrine and acetazolamide on aqueous flow during sleep. Invest Ophthalmol Vis Sci 1985;26:1315-9.

17. Claridge KG, Smith SE. Diurnal variation in pulsatile ocular blood flow in normal and glaucomatous eyes. Surv Ophthalmol 1994;38:S198-S205.

18. Liu JHK, Mederios FA, Slight JR, Weinreb RN. Comparing diurnal and nocturnal effects of brinzolamide and timolol on intraocular pressure in patients receiving latanoprost monotherapy. Ophthalmology 2009;116:449-54.

19. Kwitko GM, Shin DH, Ahn BH, Hong YJ. Bilateral effects of long-term monocular timolol therapy. Am J Ophthalmol 1987;104:591-4.

20. Blondecu, P, Cote M and Tetrault L. Effect of Timolol eye drops in subjects receiving systemic propranolol Therapy. Can J Ophthalmol 1983;18: 18-21.

21. Shedden A, Laurence J, Tipping R, the Timoptic XE 0.5% study group. Efficacy and tolerability of timolol maleate ophthalmic gel-forming solution versus timolol ophthalmic solution in adults with open angle glaucoma or ocular hypertension; a six month, double masked, multicenter study. Clin Ther 2001;23:440-50.

22. Sheddon AH, Laurence J, Barrish A, Olah TV. Plasma timolol concentrations of timolol maleate: timolol gel-forming solution (Timoptic-XE) once daily versus timolol maleate ophthalmic solution twice daily. Doc Ophthalmol 2001;103:73-9.

23. Lama PJ. Systemic adverse effects of beta-adrenergic blockers: an evidence-based assessment. Am J Ophthalmol 2002;134:749-60.

24. Leier CV, Baker ND, Weber P. Cardiovascular effects of ophthalmic timolol. Ann Intern Med 1986;104:197-9.

25. Kitazawa Y, Tsuchisaka H. Effects of timolol on corneal sensitivity and tear production. Int Ophthalmol 1980;3:25-9.

26. Reiss GR, Brubaker RF. The mechanism of betaxolol, a new ocular hypotensive agent. Ophthalmology 1983;90:1369-72.

27. Allen RC, Hertzmark E, Walker AM, Epstein DL. A double-masked comparison of betaxolol vs timolol in the treatment of open-angle glaucoma. Am J Ophthalmol1986;101:535-41.

28. Feghali JG, Kaufman PL, Radius RL, Mandell AI. A comparison of betaxolol and timolol in open angle glaucoma and ocular hypertension. Acta Ophthalmol (Copenh) 1988;66: 180-6.

29. Levobunolol. A four-year study of efficacy and safety in glaucoma treatment. The Levobunolol Study Group. Ophthalmology 1989;96:642-5.

30. Boozman FW 3rd, Carriker R, Foerster R, Allen RC, Novack GD, Batoosingh AL. Long-term evaluation of 0.25% levobunolol and timolol for therapy for elevated intraocular pressure. Arch ophthalmol 1988;106: 614.

31. Rakofsky SI, Melamed S, Cohen JS, Slight JR, Spaeth G. A comparison of the ocular hypotensive efficacy of once-daily and twice-daily levobunolol treatment. Ophthalmology 1989;96:8-11.

32. Derick RJ, Robin AL, Tielsch J, Wexler JL, Kelley EP, Stoeckerl JF. Once-daily versus twice-daily levobunolol (0.5%) therapy: a crossover study. Ophthalmology 1992;99:424-9.

33. Freeman SF, Friedman NJ, Shields MB, et al. Effects of ocular carteolol and timolol on plasma high density cholesterol lipoprotein level. Am J Ophthalmol 1993;116:600.

34. Beck RW, Moke P, Blair RC, Nissenbaum R. Uveitis associated with topical beta-blockers. Arch Ophthalmol 1996;114:1181-2.

35. Diggory P, Heyworth P, Chau G, McKenzie S, Sharma A, Luke I. Improved lung function tests on changing from topical timolol: nonselective beta-blockade impairs lung function tests in elderly patients. Eye (Lond) 1993;7:661-3.

ADRENERGIC AGONISTS

Adrenergic agonists agents can be classified as non selective (acting on alpha and beta receptors) and selective (alpha receptors).

The Alpha Adrenergic Receptors

Alpha-adrenergic receptors are widely distributors in the human body. There are three alpha one adrenoceptor subtypes (α1A, α1B, α1D) and three alpha two adrenoceptor subtypes (α2A, α2B, α2D). α1A and α2A are the common subtypes found in ocular tissues.[1] Beta receptors have been discussed in the previous section.

NON-SELECTIVE (ALPHA AND BETA) AGONISTS

Non selective alpha agonist used for the treatment of glaucoma include epinephrine and dipivefrin (prodrug).

Mechanism of Action

The mechanism of IOP reduction by non selective adrenergic agonists is controversial. Ideally a balance between both alpha and beta receptors is responsible for a norma aqueous formation and outflow. The alpha stimulation causes vasoconstriction in the ciliary process and reduces the ultrafiltration pressure, reducing aqueous formation. Beta stimulation in the ciliary epithelium increases aqueous formation. Non–selective adrenergic agonists increase both conventional[2] and uveoscleral outflow.[3]

Triphasic Action[4]

Phase 1: Decreased aqueous production occurs within minutes of instillation of the drug, due to the alpha adrenergic induced vasoconstriction, which reduces the ultrafiltration of plasma into the stroma of the ciliary processes.

This phase is however very transient and not of sufficient magnitude to significantly influence IOP. However it may be effective in controlling IOP spikes.

Phase 2: Early increase in outflow facility is due to the adrenergic induced increase in true outflow facility. The effect is divided into two parts. The first is the early increase in outflow and the second component which continues hours after administration when the vasoconstrictor and mydriatic effects of the drug are gone.

Phase 3: Late increase in outflow facility takes place for weeks to months after continued administration of epinephrine.

The possible mechanisms for phase 3 are:

- Activation of lysosomal hyaluronidase by epinephrine which in turn increases glycosaminoglycan metabolism in trabecular meshwork.
- Development of super sensitivity to epinephrine.
- Gradual release of the agent from pigment binding sites.

Onset of action occurs at 1 hour with a peak effect at 4 hours lasting for 12 hours. A twice daily dosing schedule is recommended. Treatment should be started with the lower concentration and increased if required.

Epinephrine[5,6]

It is available in a concentration of 0.5%, 1%, 2% in the form of 3 salts:

- Epinephrine hydrochloride – pH 3.5 hence irritating
- Epinephrine borate - pH 7.4 (less ocular irritation)
- Epinephrine bitartarate - low pH (more ocular irritation).

The IOP lowering *starts* in 1 hour, *peaks* in 2-6 hours and is back to *baseline* in 12-24 hours.

Dipivefrin[7-9]

It is dipivalyl epinephrine (2 pivalic acid groups added to parent drug). It is a prodrug form of epinephrine in which two pivalyl acid chains are esterified with epinephrine to increase the lipophilicity of the molecule. It gets converted to epinephrine by esterase enzyme in the cornea. It is 600 times more lipid soluble, thus its the passage through the cornea into the anterior chamber is 17 times higher than epinephrine. External and systemic side effects are few due to its lipophilicity.

It is the only available form of epinephrine. It is used in a concentration of 0.1% every 12-24 hours. The IOP starts to fall in 30-60 min with a peak effect seen in 1-4 hours and returning back to baseline in 12-24 hours.

Drug Interactions[10-15]

- Epinephrine compound + Miotics/carbonic hydrase inhibitors = IOP reduction significantly more than either drug used alone.
- Epinephrine compound + timolol (non-selective beta blocker) = significant additional pressure reduction for the first few weeks, after which the pressure lowering effect of the combination is only slightly greater than with timolol alone. Both the drugs act on the same receptor but in opposite directions.
- Epinephrine compound + betaxolol (cardioselective beta1 blocker) = greater additional pressure lowering effect than addition to timolol, but betaxolol alone has

less pressure lowering efficacy than non-selective timolol.

- Epinephrine + non-selective beta blocker = little/No IOP lowering
- Epinephrine + Betaxolol = significant additive IOP reduction.
- Epinephrine + Prostaglandin analogues = Significant additive IOP reduction

At least 50% of glaucoma patients with use of topical epinephrine become intolerant to the therapy due to its side effects.

Side Effects[16-25]

They are more common with epinephrine than dipivefrin.

Ocular Side Effects

Ocular Surface

- Conjunctival hyperemia—it is delayed due to initial vasoconstriction followed by rebound vasodilation.
- Burning sensation, tearing
- Hypersensitivity blepharoconjunctivitis with lid erythema, lichenification, chemosis and follicular hypertrophy.
- Adenochrome deposits:
  - ❖ Epinephrine undergoes oxidation and polymerization to form adenochrome.
  - ❖ Adenochrome is commonly deposited in lower tarsal conjunctiva where it may be mistaken for a foreign body
  - ❖ Deposits in the upper tarsal conjunctiva may cause recurrent corneal erosions
  - ❖ Deposits in the corneal epithelium, in the presence of increased IOP and bullous keratopathy, produces a black cornea.
  - ❖ Deposits in lacrimal sac and NLD may cause chronic epiphora.

- Deposits may stain a senile scleral plaque. It may give the appearance of a malignant melanoma.
- Epidermalization of puncta/punctual stenosis. It may lead to severe epiphora.
- Corneal epithelial haze even with IOP control. It is reversible on stopping the drug.
- Corneal epithelial erosions from adenochrome deposits.

Intraocular

- Decreased endothelial count on prolonged use.
- Mydriasis, a standard response to epinephrine, may precipitate angle-closure in the predisposed eye.
- Visual disturbance/blurred vision.
- Epinephrine maculopathy
  - ❖ A form of cystoid macular edema (CME), which occurs in some aphakic eyes receiving topical epinephrine.
  - ❖ Occurs months to years after starting treatment.
  - ❖ Presents with gradual loss of vision.
  - ❖ Reversible on stopping drug.
  - ❖ A petaloid pattern is seen on fundus fluorescein angiography (FFA).
  - ❖ Epinephrine induced synthesis of prostaglandins which in turn cause distruption of blood ocular barrier resulting in CME.

Systemic Side Effects

- Headache/browache—attributed to their vasoconstrictive action.
- Anxiety/nervousness/faintness/tremors
- Elevated blood pressure/palpitations/tachycardia/dysrhythmia/ hypertension/arrhythmias/cerebro vascular accident.[26]

Indications

- Used only rarely for glaucoma management in the present time.
- Used only in cases where there is intolerance to first and second line drugs, especially in combination either miotics and topical CA Inhibitors.

Contraindications

- Severe hypertension/cardiac disease
- Thyrotoxicosis
- MAO inhibitor therapy
- Children and pregnant females
- Eyes with occludable angles
- Aphakic eyes.

SELECTIVE ALPHA ADRENERGIC AGONISTS

These agents differ from the non-selective alpha agonists by their binding affinity for the alpha receptors. These are the target receptors for glaucoma. Three medications (clonidine, apraclonidine, brimonidine) have been used. These medications are relatively selective for alpha 2 receptors with some amount of alpha 1 activity. Out of these brimonidine has the least alpha 1 activity. Clonidine was introduced in 1966, Brimonidine in 1974, and Apraclonidine in 1978.

Mechanism of Action

- Reduction in aqueous humor production[27,28]
- Other mechanisms of IOP reduction include:
  - ❖ Reduced episcleral pressure (clonidine)[29,30]
  - ❖ Increased outflow facility
  - ❖ Increased uveoscleral outflow (brimonidine)[31,32]

Neuroprotection:[33-35] Selective alpha agonists especially brimonidine have been found to be neuroprotective. This effect has been demonstrated in experimental cases of optic nerve crush injury models, ocular hypertensive rat models of glaucoma and, rat models of ischemia-induced injury. Increased RGC survival was seen in these models. This action may be mediated via alpha 2a receptors. The proposed mechanism was inhibition of proapoptotic signalling and activation of antiapoptotic pathways. The neuroprotective effect has not been demonstrated in clinical trials in humans.

CLONIDINE

This was the first alpha2 agonist to be used. It causes IOP lowering after systemic or topical administration by reducing aqueous humor production. This is caused by constriction of the blood vessels in the ciliary process. Studies have demonstrated a significant reduction in IOP with both concentrations of clonidine (0.25% and 0.125%) with a slightly more reduction seen with 0.25%. The duration of action with 0.125% concentration is 6 hours and 8 hours with 0.25% clonidine. A maximum reduction of 4.4+/- 6.1 mm Hg has been observed. A small reduction in IOP in the fellow eye has also been observed.[36,37]

However its clinical used its limited by the fact that it penetrates the blood brain barrier even after topical administration causing episode of significant hypotension.

APRACLONIDINE

It is a derivative of clonidine, produced by adding an amino group in para position of the benzene ring. Apraclonidine is more polar and less lipophilic than clonidine. This probably allows less penetration into both the posterior segment of the eye and systemic circulation, allowing for an excellent therapeutic index. It has a less ability to penetrate the blood brain barrier as compared to the parent compound, clonidine so has less systemic side effects.

Mechanism of Action

- It lowers IOP by stimulation of alpha 2 receptors and hence inducing vasoconstricton in the vessels of the uveal tract resulting in decreased aqueous production.
- Apraclonidine also increases uveoscleral outflow.

Dosage

It is available in a concentration of 1%, 0.5%, 0.25% concentrations and is given twice daily.

IOP Reduction

- 27%-37% IOP reduction is seen with the above concentrations at a twice daily dose. This is at par with topical beta blockers at BD dosage. Onset of action is within 1 hour with a peak reduction of 6.5 +/-4.3 mm Hg at 3-5 hours after administration. The trough effect is also significant with 20-30% IOP reduction from baseline after 12 hours of therapy.
- Unlike timolol it causes an effective 27% lowering of nocturnal IOP.

Indications

Apraclonidine's effect on the prevention of IOP spikes post laser procedures like ALT and argon or Nd: YAG Iridotomy has been well documented.[38-42] However benefits with long term treatment with this drug are not proven.

Apraclonidine 0.5% used three times a day lowers IOP in glaucoma and ocular hypertension. Certain factors limit its chronic use. These include:
- Tachyphylaxis
- High incidence of side effects like follicular conjunctivitis.

BRIMONIDINE

Brimonidine tartrate is much more selective for alpha 2 receptors than apraclonidine. Mechanism of IOP lowering and efficacy is same as apraclonidine. It acts by suppressing aqueous production, and increasing uveoscleral outflow. It has an additional property of potential neuroprotection which still needs to be established in humans.

Significant systemic absorption of topical brimonidine occurs in adults, peak plasma concentrations occurring within 1-4 hours with a half-life of approximately 2.5 hours. Systemic metabolism of brimonidine is primarily by the liver and urinary excretion is the major route of elimination of the drug and its metabolites.

The increased sensitivity of infants to brimonidine could be because of the weight (no dose adjustment is made), excessive systemic absorption, immature metabolism and excretion (hepatic phase I reactions do not reach maturity until 6 months of age), an immature blood–brain barrier, or increased receptor sensitivity.

Randomized trials comparing 0.2% brimonidine versus 0.5% timolol have shown that brimonidine produces a sustained mean reductions in IOP. It was found that while the peak IOP reduction was greater with brimonidine the mean IOP decrease at trough was greater with timolol.[43,44]

It is effective when used in combination with beta blockers.[45]

Dosage

- 0.2% three times a day when given as monotherapy
- The dose is twice a day if used in combination.
- Formulations with the concentration of 0.15% and 0.1% with a different preservative are also available. They have a similar IOP lowering effect with fewer side effects
- Brimonidine has a good additive effect with beta blockers, carbonic anhydrase inhibitors and miotics. It is available in a fixed combination with timolol 0.5%.
- It can be used as a solo agent in patients in whom beta blockers are contraindicated or patients who are intolerant or unresponsive to other first line medications.

Ocular Side Effects of Selective Alpha Agonists

Ocular side effects are commonly seen with these agents.[46,47] Being relatively more selective for the alpha-2 receptors, side effects are seen least with brimonidine. Conjunctival blanching occurs immediately after instillation due to vasoconstriction. However on a long-term use conjunctival hyperemia and allergic conjunctivitis may be seen. Lid retraction may be seen as a result of alpha 1 stimulation of Müllers muscle. Vasoconstriction of the nasopharyngeal and oral blood vessels may lead to a dryness of the nose and mouth. These can be decreased to some extent by digital nasolacrimal occlusion. These side effects are seen more commonly with apraclonidine. Minimal mydriasis may occur with brimonidine and apraclonidine. However, the effect is too small too cause a risk of angle closure. In case of clonidine miosis is seen in both the treated eye and the fellow eye. A concerning side effect is follicular conjunctivitis (especially of the lower lid) and periocular dermatitis. These are the most common

reasons for discontinuation of therapy. Brimonidine has lower rate of allergy as compared to apraclonidine. Use of purite instead of benzalkonium chloride and a drug concentration of 0.15% or 0.1% has shown lower allergy rates with brimonidine. These formulations are preferred to brimonidine-benzalkonium chloride (BAC) formulations due to better tolerability while maintaining similar efficacy.[48,49]

Other side effects include itching, hyperemia and photophobia. Anterior segment vasoconstriction has been noted with topical brimonidine 0.2%. This is presumably mediated via local extrajunctional alpha-2 receptors.

Systemic Side Effects

Systemic side effects of brimonidine include:

- **Sedation:** It is mediated by postsynaptic receptors located in the locus coeruleus, behind the blood-brain barrier.
- **Hypotension and Bradycardia:** They are thought to be related to both central and peripheral actions.[50] The production of hypotension as well as sedation by alpha-2 agonists has been shown to correlate well with their ability to cross the blood–brain barrier
- Transient dry nose and dry mouth occurs due to vasoconstriction
- Fatigue and drowsiness
- Bradycardia, hypotension and apnea are more commonly seen in elderly and very young. These are more with brimonidine and clonidine as these agents are lipophilic in contrast with apraclonidine which is lipophobic.
- There have been reports of bradycardia, hypotension, hypothermia, hypotonia, and apnea in infants after topical brimonidine. It should be used with great caution and not at all in children younger than 5 years

because of the potential for CNS depression.[51,52]

Clinical Indications

Long-term management of open angle glaucoma and ocular hypertension.

To prevent or treat IOP spikes in Laser procedures like:

- **Argon laser trabeculoplasty:** Post laser IOP spikes are due to the release of pigments, blood or cellular debris that is caught in the meshwork. Apraclonidine 0.5% one drop 30 minutes before and one drop immediately after procedure controls these spikes. Even a single drop after the procedure has a similar effect. Brimonidine 0.2% has an equivalent effect to apraclonidine.
- **Laser iridotomy:** Additionally, alpha 1 activity of apraclonidine decreases blood flow and thus decreasing bleeding especially in Nd:YAG iridotomies.
- **Nd:YAG Capsulotomies:** Prevents IOP spikes post Nd:YAG laser capsulotomies.

To treat acute pressure rises in: Postsurgical, traumatic, angle closure, inflammatory and neovascular glaucomas.

Brimonidine is classified by the US Food and Drug Administration as category B (presumed safety based on animal studies) in terms of safety during pregnancy (**Tables 1 and 2**). Thus Brimonidine may be relatively safe in pregnant women. However one must keep in mind to stop the drug during lactation as it is secreted in the breast milk and can cause serious side effects like CNS depression, apnea and hypotension in infants.

Contraindications

- *Infants and children:* Bradycardia, hypotension, hypothermia, hypotonia, and apnea has been reported

Table 1 Safety categories of glaucoma drugs in pregnancy

Category	Glaucoma medications
A	Applies to drugs for which adequate and well controlled human studies have failed to demonstrate a risk to the fetus.
B	Applies to drugs for which human fetal risk is relatively unlikely based on either negative animal studies and no adequate and well-controlled human studies, or positive animal studies and negative adequate and well controlled human studies.
B	Applies to drugs for which human fetal risk is unknown based on positive animal studies (or no animal studies) and no adequate and well controlled human studies.
D	Applies to drugs for which positive human evidence of fetal risk is available, but whose use in a pregnant women may be necessary.
X	Applies to drugs for which positive animal studies or positive human evidence of fetal risk is available and whose use in a pregnant woman is contraindicated.

Table 2 Drug toxicity classification in pregnancy

Category	Glaucoma medications
A	None
B	Brimonidine, Dipivefrin
C	Acetazolamide, Betaxolol, Carbachol, Carteolol, Dorzolamide, Echothiophate, Epinephrine, Glycerine, Latanoprost, Levobunolol, Mannitol, Methazolamide, Metipranolol, Physostigmine, Pilocarpine, Timolol, Urea
X	Demecarium

- CNS disorders
- Used in caution in patients with severe cardiovascular and cerebrovascular disease
- Raynuad's phenomenon or other peripheral circulatory abnormalities
- Since they decrease anterior segment circulation, so they are preferably avoided in anterior segment ischemic syndrome and severe diabetic retinopathy.

- *Patients on MAO inhibitors:* They potentiate the centrally mediated actions of MAO inhibitors, especially hypotension and may lead to cardiovascular collapse.

Future
Experimental evidence has demonstrated that brimonidine is a potential neuroprotective agent; however, clinical trials have not demonstrated efficacy in humans with glaucoma.

Clinical trials are underway evaluating a new technology that administers brimonidine in a sustained delivery system similar to its intravitreal 700 µg dexamethasone implant. Intravitreal brimonidine as an implant for prevention of retinal apoptosis is being explored in patients with geographic atrophy (GA) due to age-related macular degeneration (AMD) or retinitis pigmentosa.

REFERENCES

1. Wikberg-Matsson A, Uhlén S, Wikberg JE. Characterization of alpha (1)-adrenoceptor subtypes in the eye. Exp Eye Res 2000;70:51-60.
2. Robinson JC, Kaufman PL. Effects and interactions of epinephrine, norepinephrine, timolol, and betaxolol on outflow facility in the cynomolgus monkey. Am J Ophthalmol 1990;15;109:189-9.
3. Daniel J Totvnsend, Richard F Brubake. Immediate effect of epinephrine on aqueous formation in the normal human eye as measured by fluorophotometry. Invest Ophthalmol Vis Sci 1980;19:255-6.
4. Sears MI. The mechanism of action of adrenergic drugs in glaucoma. Invest Ophthalmol 1966;5:115.
5. Adamek R. New perspective in glaucoma therapy with epinephrine and epinephrine derivatives. Klin Monatsbl Augenheilkd 1980;176:978.
6. Kerr CR, Hass I, Drance SM, et al. Cardiovascular effects of epinephrine and dipivalyl epinephrine applied topically to the eye in patients with glaucoma. Br J Ophthalmol 1982;66:109.
7. Wei C-P, Anderson JA, Leopold I. Ocular absorption and metabolism of topically applied epinephrine and dipivalyl ester of epinephrine. Invest Ophthalmol Vis Sci 1978;17:315.
8. Anderson JA, Davis WL, Wei C-P. Site of ocular hydrolysis of a prodrug, dipivefrin, and a comparison of its ocular metabolism with that of the parent compound, epinephrine. Invest Ophthalmol Vis Sci 1980;19:817.
9. Yablonski ME, Shin DH, Kolker AE, et al. Dipivefrin use in patients with intolerance to topically applied epinephrine. Arch Ophthalmol 1977;95:2157.
10. Thomas JV, Epstein DL. Timolol and epinephrine in primary open angle

glaucoma: Transient additive effect. Arch Ophthalmol 1981;99:91.

11. Thomas JV, Epstein DL. Study of the additive effect of timolol and epinephrine in lowering intraocular pressure. Br J Ophthalmol 1981;65:596.

12. Goldberg I, Ashburn FS Jr., Palmberg PF, et al. Timolol and epinephrine; a clinical study of ocular interactions. Arch Ophthalmol 1980;98:484.

13. Keates EC, Stone RA. Safety and effectiveness of concomitant administration of dipivefrin and timolol maleate. Am J Ophthalmol 1981.

14. Bloom HR. Additive effect of betaxolol and epinephrine in primary open angle glaucoma. Arch Ophthalmol. 1986;104(8):1178-84.

15. Hyong PF, Rulo A, Greve E, Watson P, Alma A. The additive intraocular pressure-lowering effect of latanoprost in combined therapy with other ocular hypotensive agents. Surv Ophthalmol 1997;41Suppl 2:S93-8.

16. Reinecke RD, Kuwabara T. Corneal deposits secondary to topical epinephrine. Arch Ophthalmol 1963;70:170.

17. Green WR, Kaufer GJ, Dubroff S. Black cornea: a complication of topical use of epinephrine. Ophthalmologica 1976;154:88.

18. Donaldson DD. Epinephrine pigmentation of the cornea. Arch Ophthalmol 1967;78:74.

19. Barishak R, Romano A, Stein R. Obstruction of lacrimal sac caused by topical epinephrine. Ophthalmologica 1969;159:373.

20. Spaeth GL. Nasolacrimal duct obstruction caused by topical epinephrine. Arch Ophthalmol 1967;77:355.

21. AE, Becker B. Epinephrine maculopathy. Arch Ophthalmol 1968;79:552.

22. Michels RG, Maumenee AE. Cystoid macular edema associated with topically applied epinephrine in aphakic eyes. Am J Ophthalmol 1975;80:379.

23. Miyake K, Shirasawa E, Hikita M, et al. Synthesis of prostaglandin E in rabbit eyes with topically applied epinephrine. Invest Ophthalmol Vis Sci 1988;29:332.

24. Mehelas TJ, Kollarits CR, Martin WG. Cystoid macular edema presumably induced by dipivefrin hydrochloride (Propine). Am J Ophthalmol 1982;92:682.

25. Liesegang TJ. Bulbar conjunctival follicles associated with Dipivefrin therapy. Ophthalmology 1985;92:228-33.

26. Kerr CR, Hass I, Drance SM, Walters MB, Schulzer M. Cardiovascular effects of epinephrine and dipivalyl epinephrine applied topically to the eye in patients with glaucoma. Br J Ophthalmol 1982;66:109-14.

27. Lee DA, Topper JE, Brubaker RF. Effect of clonidine on aqueous humor flow in normal human eyes. Exp Eye Res 1984;38:239.

28. Toris CB, Camras CB, Yablonski ME. Acute versus chronic effects of brimonidine on aqueous humor dynamics in ocular hypertensive patients. Am J Ophthalmol 1999;128:8-14.

29. The peripheral and central neural actions of clonidine in normal and glaucomatous eyes. Invet ophthalmol V Sci 1978;17:149-58.

30. Toris CB, Gleason ML, Camras CB, Yablonski ME. Effects of apraclonidine on aqueous humor dynamics in human eyes. Ophthalmology 1995;102:456-61.

31. Burke J, Schwartz M. Preclinical evaluation of brimonidine. Surv Ophthalmol 1996;41(Suppl 1):S9–S18.

32. Toris CB, Gleason ML, Camras CB, Yablonski ME. Effects of brimonidine on aqueous humor dynamics in human eyes. Arch Ophthalmol 1995;113:1514-7.

33. Wheeler L, WoldeMussie E, Lai R. Role of alpha-2 agonists in neuroprotection. Surv Ophthalmol 2003;48 Suppl1:S47-51.

34. Lai RK, Chun T, Hasson D, et al. Alpha-2 adrenoceptor agonist protects retinal function after acute retinal ischemic injury in the rat. Vis Neurosci. 2002;19:175-85.

35. Dong CJ, Guo Y, Agey P, et al. Alpha2 adrenergic modulation of NMDA receptor function as a major mechanism of RGC protection in experimental glaucoma and retinal excitotoxicity. Invest Ophthalmol Vis Sci. 2008;49:4515-22.

36. Harrison R, Kaufmann CS. Effects of a topically administered solution on intraocular pressure and blood pressure in open-angle glaucoma. Arch Ophthalmol 1977;95:1368-73.

37. Hodapp E, Kolker AE, Kass MA, Goldberg I, Becker B, Gordon M. The effect of topical clonidine on intraocular pressure. Arch Ophthalmol 1981;99:1208-11.

38. Krupin T, Stank T, Feitl ME, Apraclonidine pretreatment decreased the acute intraocular pressure rise after laser trabeculoplasty or iridotomy. J Glaucoma 1992;1:79.

39. Robin AL. Short-term effects of unilateral 1% apraclonidine therapy. Arch Ophthalmol 1988;106:912-5.

40. Kitazawa Y, Taniguchi T, Sugiyama K. Use of apraclonidine to reduce acute intraocular pressure rise following Q-switched Nd:YAG laser iridotomy. Ophthalmic Surg 1989;20:49.

41. Sridhar Rao B, Badrinath SS. Efficacy and safety of apraclonidine in patients undergoing anterior segment laser surgery. Br J Ophthalmol 1989;73:884.

42. Cullom RD Jr. Schwartz LW. The effect of apraclonidine on the intraocular pressure of glaucoma patients following Nd:YAG laser posterior capsulotomy. Ophthalmic Surg 1993;24:623.

43. Katz LJ, Brimonidine study group. Brimonidine tartrate 0.2% twice daily vs. timolol 0.5% twice daily. 1-year results in glaucoma patients. Am J Ophthalmol 1999;127:20.

44. LeBlanc RP, Brimonidine study group 2. Twelve month results of an ongoing randomized trial comparing brimonidine tartrate 0.2% and timolol 0.5% given twice daily in patients with glaucoma or ocular hypertension. Ophthalmol 1998;105:1960.

45. Simmons ST. Alphagan/Trusopt Study Group. Efficacy of brimonidine 0.2% and dorzolamide 2% as adjunctive therapy to beta-blockers in adult patients with glaucoma or ocular hypertension. Clin Ther 2001;23(4): 604-19.

46. Robin AL. The role of alpha-agonists in glaucoma therapy. Curr Opin Ophthalmol 1997;8:42-9.

47. Walters TR. Development and use of brimonidine in treating acute and-chronic elevations of intraocular pressure: a review of safety, efficacy, dose response and dosing studies. Surv Ophthalmol 1996;41 Suppl 1:S19-26.

48. Arthur S, Cantor LB. Update on the role of alpha-agonists in glaucoma management. Exp Eye Res. 2011 Sep;93(3):271-83.

49. Katz LJ. Twelve-month evaluation of brimonidine-purite versus brimonidine in patients with glaucoma or ocular hypertension. J Glaucoma 2002;11:119-26.

50. Nordland JR, Pasquale LR, Robin AL, et al. The cardiovascular, pulmonary, and ocular hypotensive effects of 0.2% brimonidine. Arch Ophthalmol 1995;113:77-83.

51. Enyedi LB, Freedman SF. Safety and efficacy of brimonidine in children with glaucoma. J AAPOS 2001;5: 281-4.

52. Al-Shahwan S, Al-Torbak AA, Turkmani S, Al-Omran M, Al-Jadaan I, Edward DP. Side-effect profile of brimonidine tartrate in children. Ophthalmology 2005;112:2143.

PROSTAGLANDINS ANALOGUES

The effect of prostaglandins in the eye was first reported in 1985. The prostaglandin analogues and prostamides were added to the armamentarium of the antiglaucoma medications in 1994. The prostaglandin analogues include latanoprost, travoprost, tafluprost and unoprostone and the prostamides include bimatoprost.

They have been in use to lower the IOP for more than a decade and are a reasonable choice for the first line of therapy in many cases. Since their advent they have added significantly to our ability to manage glaucoma.

PHARMACOLOGY

Prostaglandins are produced in many tissues of the body including the ocular tissues. The precursor of prostaglandin synthesis is arachidonic acid. Arachidonic acid metabolism (arachidonic acid cascade) results in production of a class of agents termed as the eicosanoids, which include the prostaglandins, thromboxanes and leukotrienes **(Flowchart 1)**.[1]

Prostaglandin receptors are coupled with G protein and bind to specific prostaglandins. These receptors are distributed widely in ocular tissue, which accounts for the diverse biologic effects of prostaglandins on the eye. There are four subtypes of prostaglandin or prostanoid receptors: EP, FP, IP and TP and they are specific for prostaglandins PGD_2, PGE_2, PGF_{2alfa}, and PGI_2 or TXA_2 respectively.[2] In the eye the prostaglandins have an inflammatory and miotic effect. PGF_{2alfa} and its derivatives have an IOP lowering effect in humans. The clinical use of naturally occurring prostaglandins has not had a very successful effect in the eye as their use was associated with many ocular adverse effects.[3] Thus the PGF_{2alfa} analogues were developed. They have better tolerability and equal or improved efficacy when compared to their natural counterparts. These analogues include:

- **Isopropyl unoprostone:** It is a docosanoid derivative and has a low affinity for prostaglandin receptors.
- **Latanoprost:** It was the first commercially available PGA but second after unoprostone. It is the only one which needs to be administrated twice daily. It was first introduced in Japan in 1993.
- Travoprost.
- **Bimatoprost:** It is derived from cell membrane bound limits. It is derived from anandamide and not arachidonic acid. It has structural similarities to PGF_{2alfa} however it does not bind to the PGF_{2alfa} receptor. It is chemically related to prostamide F. The prostamide receptor has not been identified.
- **Tafluprost:** It is the latest addition to and is also available as a preservative free formulation.

MECHANISM OF ACTION[4-9]

The exact pathway, to lower IOP, after binding of the prostaglandins to FP receptors is not fully understood. The two possible *mechanisms* that are under consideration are: Relaxation of the ciliary muscle and remodeling of the extracellular matrix of the ciliary body.

The prostaglandin analogues reduce IOP by increasing the uveoscleral outflow. They stimulate enzymes which degrade and remodel the extracellular matrix of cells along the uveoscleral pathways. They trigger a cascade of tissue remodeling enzymes such as metalloproteinases and transcription factors. The collagen is degraded and the increase in uveoscleral outflow is due to re-structuring of the ciliary muscle with increased between the muscle bundles. Stimulation of the FP-receptor increases the amount of metalloproteinases (MMP) in the ciliary muscle and the change in collagen turnover results in loss of collagens. The induction of MMP exceeded the induction of TIMPs in the ciliary body which explains the effect on uveoscleral outflow. A maximal effect on IOP is seen after 8-12 hours. This promotes aqueous humor outflow via this pathway and reduces IOP. Most PG analogues act by this mechanism although via different receptors.

Unoprostone acts by a different mechanism. It opens maxi-K channels that reach an activation threshold only during depolarization and/or at high intracellular Ca^{2+} concentration. It

Flow chart 1 Arachidonic acid cascade

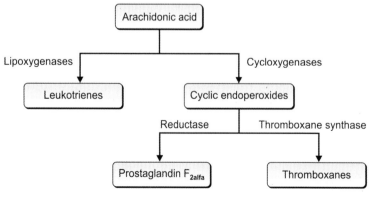

mainly increases conventional outflow following calcium dependent tissue contraction.

Because of the rapid onset of IOP lowering after administration, there has been some speculation that the PG analogues also exert an effect on the conventional outflow by changes in the trabecular meshwork. A relaxation of the contractile trabecular meshwork has been proposed. This effect on the trabecular route has been proposed but is not proven. FP receptors are present in ciliary body and trabecular meshwork. What is known from *in vitro* studies is the fact that intraocular calcium signaling pathways in human trabecular meshwork cells are affected by PG analogues. The direct effect on the conventional outflow pathway is currently under investigation. Clinical tonography cannot clearly separate between the two outflow routes, but the major effect is on uveoscleral flow. A combined IOP lowering effect may be postulated with increased outflow via the uveoscleral pathway as the major effect.[10]

Latanoprost, travoprost and tafluprost are all esterified pro-drugs and hydrolyzed by corneal esterases to their pharmacologically active free acids (carboxylic acid forms) when they pass through the cornea. Bimatoprost is a prodrug with an ethyl amide instead of an isopropyl ester on the alpha chain. It is partially hydrolyzed by amidase to its free acid. This free acid (17-phenyl-PGF_{2alfa}) is an effective FP receptor agonist. Once the prodrug is cleaved by the corneal enzymes the free form of the drug enters the anterior chamber and aqueous humor and activates the FP receptors in the ciliary body. It is also suggested that bimatoprost may directly permeate the sclera and act on the receptors in the ciliary body increasing the uveoscleral outflow. No short term escape or long term drift is seen with prostaglandin analogues.

Changes in the potency as well as side effects of the PG analogues are due to the difference in the molecule. The dosing is once daily expect for unoprostone which is given twice a day. Usually the drugs are prescribed at bedtime. The plasma half life is very brief and the peak concentration in plasma is less than 10^{-10} M. Thus the systemic side effects and contralateral IOP lowering is minimal. In van der Valk's meta-analysis, latanoprost reduced IOP by 28%–31% from baseline, travoprost by 29%–31%, and bimatoprost by 28%–33%.[11]

LATANOPROST

Latanoprost was approved for the treatment of glaucoma in 1996. It is rapidly hydrolyzed in the cornea, and its active metabolite, a latanoprost free acid reaches a peak aqueous humor level of 15-20 ng/ml 1-2 hours after topical administration. A low pH may enhance the penetration provided by a high concentration of BAK or buffers. In a dose of once a day in the evening, the IOP lowering effect starts after 3-4 hours of instillation and lasts for over 24 hours. The free acid (latanoprost acid) is metabolized rapidly in the liver by beta oxidation and finally eliminated through the feces and urine.

Compared to a standard twice a day dose of Timolol 0.5%, Latanoprost 0.005% at once daily dose produces more diurnal IOP reduction.[12] A decrease of 31% of morning IOP with latanoprost and 35% of evening IOP with latanoprost as compared to 27% of Timolol at 6 months has been observed.[13]

Latanoprost provides a more uniform around the clock IOP reduction.[14]

Greater rate of response, examined by percentage reduction in IOP, mm Hg IOP reduction, and achieving a designated IOP target, has been observed..[15,16]

26% of latanoprost treated eyes show an increase in treatment response when comparing the 3 month point with the 2 week point. This was only seen in 22% of Timolol treated cases.[17] It is also effective in combination with most of other antiglaucoma medications.

Latanoprost shows a minimal response in pediatric population and in patients with a higher baseline IOP at the start of therapy.[18,19] Studies are underway to explore its use in the pediatric population.

Latanoprost needs to be refrigerated during storage although currently generic preparations are available which do not require refrigeration.

UNOPROSTONE

This prodrug was approved by the FDA in 2000. It is a docosanoid whose base molecule is derived from docosahexaenoic acid, a substance found in the retina. It is an analogue of a pulmonary metabolite of PGF2 alpha.[20] Structurally it is similar to latanoprost with a substitution of a double bonded oxygen for one of the hydroxyl groups. However, it acts by a different mechanism as explained earlier in the chapter and the IOP lowering is less than other PG analogues.

It acts by mainly increasing the conventional outflow.[21] Its duration of action is shorter requiring a twice daily dosage. Unoprostone 0.15% lowers IOP by 3-4 mm Hg.[22] The side effect profile is similar to latanoprost. Comparison studies with timolol show it to be less effective IOP lower. Ocular side effects are mainly related to surface toxicity. Uveitis and iris hyperchromia are less common as compared to latanoprost. Currently it is available in Japan.

TRAVOPROST

Travoprost is an isopropyl ester of a potent PGF2 alpha agonist. It is also a prodrug and is hydrolyzed to the active agonist by the corneal and scleral esterases. It has a high affinity and selectivity for the FP receptors. This is because of the double bond at the carbon 13-14 position with a CF_3 side group on the carbon ring. This results in a prolonged hypotensive action but a higher incidence of hyperemia. The concentration used is 0.004% given preferably at bedtime. It has a better IOP lowering effect than timolol and a good diurnal control. It gives a 30 -33% decline in IOP from baseline as compared to 25% with Timolol.[23,24]

It shows similar IOP levels over a 24 hour period as latanoprost but a single dose may have a longer duration of action from a single dose. Some patients uncontrolled with latanoprost may improve if switched over to travoprost. Travoprost and bimatoprost.[25]

When given with other antiglaucoma medications it produces additional IOP lowering. The preservative used is BAK. Another formulation with the different preservative from BAK is also available. It contains ions and buffers similar to those used in artificial tears. On instillation in the eye, these come in contact with the positively charged ions present in the tear film and become inactive. It may be useful the patients with BAK toxicity or those on multiple medication.

BIMATOPROST

It is PGF2 alpha analogue where the carboxylic acid is replaced by a neutral ethylamide. Thus it is an ethylamide of 17 phenyl PGF2 alpha. It has been available since 2001. It has little direct effect on PGF2 alpha receptors. It is different from the above mentioned PG analogues in many aspects. Its mechanism of action is not clear. It is postulated that it is not converted to its free acid and enters the eye unchanged through the sclera and acts on the prostamide receptor. However studies have

found amidases within the corneal epithelium which hydrolyze the amide molecule. This may act on the same set of FP receptors. It increases aqueous outflow by both conventional and uveoscleral pathways. It is safe and superior to timolol.[26,27] When compared to latanoprost and travatan the IOP reduction is similar or better.[28,29] A statistically significant but clinically small advantage of bimatoprost over latanoprost and travoprost has been demonstrated by some investigator where as others have found no difference. It lowers IOP by 30% at once a day dosing. It appears to be slightly more effective than the other agents but with a concomitant increasing local side effects.

XLT group comparing three prostaglandin analogues found all 3 comparable in their ability to lower IOP. Non responders to latanoprost may have a better response with bimatoprost.[30] It is available in a concentration of 0.03%. This concentration which is higher than latanoprost or travoprost allows a better penetration of the drug through the cornea. It is given once at bedtime and shows a good control of diurnal fluctuations.

Side effect profile: More hyperemia is reported with bimatoprost 0.03%. This is due to its high affinity to PG EF receptors. However hyperemia may be less with a new formulation with 0.01% concentration. Increased periocular skin pigmentation is seen in 3-10%. It is due to increased transfer of melanosomes to basal keratocytes. No atypia or proliferation of melanocytes has been noted.

TAFLUPROST

Tafluprost is a PGF2 alpha derivative in which the 15-position hydroxyl group is substituted by 2 fluorine atoms. Because of this substitution, ketonization by 15-hydroxy-dehydrogenase (one of the major pathways involved in the metabolization of PGs) does not

occur as a result of which it is metabolized only through beta-oxidation of the alpha-chain of PG skeleton. Tafluprost has an affinity for the FP receptor that is about 12 times higher than that of latanoprost, and has almost no potential to bind to the other receptors. It is available in a concentration of 0.0015% and is used once daily at bedtime. It lowers IOP by increasing the aqueous outflow through the uveoscleral pathway. In a non inferiority trial, the magnitude of the IOP reduction with tafluprost and latanoprost treatment group after 4 week administration was 6.6 ± 2.5 mm Hg (27.6 ± 9.6%) and 6.2 ± 2.5 mm Hg (25.9 ± 9.7%), respectively.[31,32] The ophthalmic solution is preservative free and can be stored at room temperature.[33]

Its plasma concentration is low and is cleared rapidly from the circulatory system. Its active form (tafluprost acid), can be detected in plasma for up to one hour after topical administration, with a peak at 10 minutes.

FDA has approved tafluprost ophthalmic solution (Zioptan, Merck) 0.0015%, a preservative-free prostaglandin analog ophthalmic solution for reducing elevated intraocular pressure (IOP) in patients with open angle glaucoma. This was based on efficacy and safety results from 5 controlled clinical studies of up to 2 years in 905 patients using both preservative-containing and preservative-free formulations. Zioptan, dosed once-daily in the evening has been found to lower IOP at 3 and 6 months by 6 to 8 mm Hg and 5 to 8 mm Hg, respectively, from a baseline pressure of 23 to 26 mm Hg.

Ocular side effects: Common ocular side effects include conjunctival hyperemia, increased pigmentation of the iris, periorbital tissue (eyelid) and eyelashes. The preservative-free solution of tafluprost has reduced toxicity in human conjunctival epithelial cell lines when compared with other preserved prostaglandin analogues. Tafluprost may induce a lower incidence of iris and periocular skin pigmentation than latanoprost.

OVERVIEW OF IOP LOWERING EFFECT[34-40]

The peak and trough reductions of IOP for bimatoprost, travoprost and latanoprost range from 31-33% and 28-29% respectively. The diurnal and nocturnal IOP lowering of prostaglandin analogues has been found to be superior to other agents. Prostaglandins lower IOP to a greater extent than timolol in the nocturnal period as demonstrated in several 24 h studies.[37,38] Prostaglandin analogues lower IOP beyond 24 h thus compensating, to some extent, for patients missing occasional doses of medication.[39,40] Thus these medications are more 'forgiving'. No tachyphylaxis or long term drift is seen with these agents.

DOSAGE

Latanoprost (0.005%), Travoprost (0.004%), and Bimatoprost (0.03%), Tafluprost all administered at once a day dose at night **(Table 3)**. More frequent dosing of these agents results in a decrease in IOP lowering efficacy of the drug.

0.15% Unoprostone is of twice daily dosage.

Storage: Unopened bottles of latanoprost should be refrigerated at temperatures between 2°C and 8°C, whereas opened bottles can be stored safely at room temperature for up to 6 weeks. Generic formulations which can be kept at room temperature are available. Bimatoprost can be stored at temperatures between 15°C and 25°C. Travoprost can be safely stored between 2°C and 25°C for up to 6 weeks.

DRUG INTERACTIONS

- Additional 13–37% IOP reduction with Timolol. Hence fixed combinations of 0.005% latanoprost and 0.5% Timolol available.
- Additional 15% in IOP when latanoprost used in combination with carbonic anhydrase inhibitors.
- Combination of bimatoprost with brimonidine reduces IOP to a lower value than either drugs alone as well as more than latanoprost combined with timolol.
- Additive with pilocarpine. Some studies have found an IOP lowering effect when given in combination with pilocarpine. The order and timing of administration of pilocarpine and latanoprost is important and the combination is more effective a when the bedtime dose of pilocarpine is administered 1 hour after administration of latanoprost.[40a]
- Switching between different agents in the class is not of much use, though in some nonresponders to latanoprost, bimatoprost

successfully reduced IOP. The reason is not known.

CLINICAL INDICATIONS

Used as a first line treatment in primary open angle glaucoma and many secondary open angle glaucomas.

SIDE EFFECTS

Ocular Side Effects

The most commonly seen side effects include irritation, redness, blurring, pain, itching, watering, of vision, lid edema, blepharitis and allergy. Mild corneal epithelial erosions and a transient decrease in corneal sensitivity may be seen.

Conjunctival Hyperemia[41-44]

The conjunctival hyperemia which occurs during treatment with prostaglandin analogues may be due to the release of nitric oxide. The frequency of hyperemia varies between 5 and 15% The hyperemia rate is usually much higher in treatment naïve eyes or after a long washout period as compared to previously treated eye. In a majority of cases this hyperemia is minimal and a clear tendency for a time dependent decrease of severity is typical. Therefore, discontinuation of successful treatment with a PGF2 alpha analogue because of conjunctival hypheremia in the early days or weeks of the treatment is not recommended. In the short term, latanoprost induces significantly less hyperemia

Table 3 Dose and formulations of prostaglandin analogues

Name	*Bimatoprost*	*Latanoprost*	*Tafluprost*	*Travoprost*	*Unoprostone*
Concentration	0.03%	0.005%	0.0015%	0.004%	0.12%,0.15%
Preservative	BAK (0.005%) –	BAK (0.02%)/ Nil (BAK free with swollen micelle microemulsion or SMM technology)	Nil –	BAK (0.015%)/ Sofzia	BAK (0.1%) –
Dose	Once a day	Once a day	Once a day	Once a day	Twice a day

as compared to bimatoprost or travoprost. The following is the rate of hyperemia seen with the available agents (both preserved and unpreserved):

- Latanoprost: 5-15%
- Unoprostone: 10-25%
- Travoprost: 35-50%
- Bimatoprost: 5- 45%
- Tafluprost: 12%

Unoprostone is generally well tolerated but can produce punctuate keratopathy.

Increase of Iris Pigmentation[45-47]

This is an irreversible side effect of all PGF2 alpha analogue. It is seen in the first month of therapy and usually develops in the first year of treatment. It is caused by increased transcription and increased activity of tyrosinase in the iris stromal melanocytes and increase in melanin pigment within each melanocyte. It does not produce melanocyte proliferation and does not involve mitotic activity of the melanocytes. Eyes with mixed color irides containing brown areas are more susceptible to color change. The incidence iris color change varies between 1 and 3% after 6-12 months of travoprost therapy, 5-10% in latanoprost users and 1.1-1.5% in bimatoprost users.

Eyelash Changes[48,49]

Hypertrichosis, i.e. increase length, pigmentation and thickness of eyelashes along with darkening is seen commonly in all cases (**Figure 2**). It is more prominent with monocular use. Discontinuations of treatment results in reversal of eyelash pigmentation and hypertrichosis after spontaneous shedding of lashes. Rarely poliosis has been reported in chronic use of bimatoprost, latanoprost and travoprost.[50] Mechanism is by stimulation of the growth phase of the hair cycle in the dermal papilla. Bimatoprost, Travoprost produce significant increase in both hyperemia and eyelash changes as compare to latanoprost. All three produce iris color darkening at a similar frequency:

- Latanoprost: 0-25%
- Unoprostone: 0-25%
- Travoprost: 0.7-52%
- Bimatoprost: 3-36%

Few patients may complain as many prefer the long lashes due to cosmetic reasons. However, it can lead to complaints if unilateral.

Increased Periocular and Eyelid Skin Pigmentation

It is a reversible side effect of PGF2 alpha analogue medication not seen very commonly.[51-54] Skin hyperpigmentation occurs from increased melanogenesis and increased transfer of melanosomes to basal keratinocytes, with the absence of melanocyte proliferation and melanocyte atypia. It has been postulated that factors other than drug exposure (UV exposure, genetic factors, hormonal, method of drug application and pre-existing diseases with hyperpigmentation) may determine the degree of skin pigmentation which occurs.

Damage to Blood Aqueous Barrier

Recurrence of uveitis, cystoid macular edema or herpetic keratitis is seen rarely following treatment with PGF2 alpha analogues.[55-58] These side effects are usually seen in eyes susceptible to inflammation due to previous or low grade ongoing uveitis, herpetic keratitis or macula diseases complicated cataract, epiretinal membrane, retinal vein occlusion in the presence of missing or open posterior capsule.[59] All these side effects are reversible after discontinuation of therapy. They should be avoided or used cautiously in patients with multiple risk factors for CME. One should lookout for signs of inflammation and cystoid

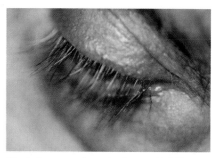

Fig. 2 Increased eye lash growth following use of prostaglandin analogues

macular edema in patients receiving PGs.

Rarely, reversible deepening of the lid sulcus[60] and iris cysts[61,62] (reversible) and poliosis[50] may be seen.

Systemic Side Effects

The amount of prostaglandins entering the circulation from the low doses of the ester used to lower IOP is a small fraction of the endogenous prostaglandins normally released from all the body tissues and therefore they have little clinical effect of cardiac and respiratory systems. Systemic side effects are rare. The active amount of PG analogue apply topically is 1000 fold less than the amount produced daily in the body. Latanoprost has a systemic half life of 17 minutes and is rapidly converted to its inactive metabolite in the liver and excreted in the urine. It does not produce contralateral IOP lowering. Headache, myalgias, flu like symptoms, abdominal cramps[63] and arthralgias are rare side effect. No cardio-vascular or respiratory changes are seen and they can be given safely in patients with asthma.[64] Pregnancy and lactation are contraindications for use of the topical PGF2 alpha analogues.[65,66]

Rare Side Effects

- Reversible deepening of the lid sulcus
- Iris cyst (reversible)
- Abdominal cramps

REFERENCES

1. Marrow JD, Roberts LJ II. Lipid-derived autacoids: eicosanoids and platelet-activating factor. In: Hardman JG, Limbird LE, eds. Goodman and Gilman's the pharmacological basis of therapeutics, 10th ed. New York: McGraw-Hill, 2001.

2. Cole man RA, Smith WL, Narumiya S. International Union of pharmacology classification of prostanoid receptors and their subtypes. Pharmacol Rev 1994;46:205.

3. Bito LZ, Stjernschantz J. The ocular effects of prostaglandins and other eicosanoids. New York, Alan R. Liss 1989.

4. Gabelt BT, Gottanka J, Lutjen-Drecoll E, et al. Aqueous humor dynamics and trabecular meshwork and anterior ciliary muscle morphologic changes with age in rhesus monkeys. Invest Ophthalmol Vis Sci 2003;44:2118.

5. Nilson SF, Sperber GO, Bill A. The effect of prostaglandin F2 alpha-1-isopropylester (PGF2-alpha-IE) on uveoscleral outflow. Prog Clin Biol Res 1989;312:429.

6. Tamm E, Ritting M, Lutjen-Drecoll E. Electron microscopy and immunohistochemical studies of the intraocular pressure lowering effect of prostaglandin F2 alpha. Fortschr Ophthalmol 1990;87:623.

7. Richter M, Krauss AH, Woodward DF, et al. Morphological changes in the anterior eye segment after long-term treatment with different receptor selective prostaglandin agonists and a prostamide. Invest Ophthalmol Vis Sci 2003;44:4419.

8. Toris CB, Camras CB, Yablonski ME: Effect of PhXA41, a new prostaglandin F2α analog, on aqueous humor dynamics in human eyes. Ophthalmology 1993,100:1297-304.

9. Lindsey JD, Kashiwagi K, Kashiwagi F, Weinreb RN: Prostaglandins alter extracellular matrix adjacent to human ciliary muscle cells in vitro. Invest Ophthalomol Vis Sci 1997,38:2214-23.

10. Toris CB, Gabelt BT, Kaufman PL. Update on the mechanism of action of topical prostaglandins for intraocular pressure reduction. Surv Ophthalmol 2008;53:S107-20.

11. van der Valk R, Webers CA, Schouten JS, Zeegers MP, Hendrikse F, Prins MH. Intraocular pressure-lowering effects of all commonly used glaucoma drugs: a meta-analysis of randomized clinical trials. Ophthalmology 2005;112:1177-85.

12. Watson P, Stjernschantz J. A six-month, randomized, double masked study comparing latanoprost with timolol in open angle glaucoma and ocular hypertension; the latanoprost study group. Ophthalmology 1996; 103:126.

13. Alm A, Stjernschantz J. Effects on intraocular pressure and side effects of 0.005% latanoprost applied once daily, evening or morning: a comparison with timolol. Scandinavian Latanoprost Study Group. Ophthalmology 1995;102:1743.

14. Racz P, Ruzsonyi MR, Nagy ZT, et al. Around-the-clock intraocular pressure reduction with once daily application of latanoprost by itself or in combination with timolol. Arch Ophthalmol 1996;114:268.

15. Hedman K, Alm A, Gross RL. Pooled-data analysis of three randomized, double-masked, Six month studies comparing intraocular pressure-reducing effects of latanoprost and timolol in patients with ocular hypertension. J Glaucoma 2003;12:463.

16. Camras CB. Comparison of latanoprost and timolol in patients with ocular hypertension and Glaucoma: a six month masked, multicenter trial in the United States. The United States Latanoprost Study Group. Ophthalmology 1996;103:138.

17. Camras CB, Hedman K. Rate of response to latanoprost or timolol in patients with ocular hypertension or glaucoma J Glaucoma 2003;12:466.

18. Enyedi LB, Freedman SF, Buckley EG. The effectiveness of latanoprost for the treatment of pediatric glaucoma. JAAPOS 1999;3:33.

19. Yang CB, Freedom SF, Myers JS, et al. Use of latanoprost in the treatment of glaucoma associated with Sturge-Weber syndrome. Am J Ophthalmol 1998;126:600.

20. Haria M, Spencer CM. Unoprostone (isopropyl unoprostone) Drugs Aging. 1996;9:213-8. discussion 219-20.

21. Toris CB, Zhan G, Camras CB. Increase in outflow facility with unoprostone treatment in ocular hypertensive patients. Arch Ophthalmol 2004;122: 1782-7.

22. Jampel HD, Bacharach J, Sheu WP, Wohl LG, Solish AM, Christie, Latanoprost/Unoprostone Study Group. Randomized clinical trial of latanoprost and unoprostone in patients with elevated intraocular pressure. Am J Ophthalmol 2002;134: 863-7.

23. Goldberg I, Cunha-Vaz J, Jakobsen JE, et al. Comparison of topical travoprost eye drops given once daily and timolol 0.5% given twice daily in patients with open angle glaucoma or ocular hypertension. J Glaucoma 2001;10:414.

24. Goldberg I, Cunha-Vaz J, Jakobsen JE, et al. Comparison of topical travoprost eye drops given once daily and timolol 0.5% given twice daily in patients with open-angle glaucoma or ocular hypertension. J Glaucoma 2001;10:414-22.

25. Eisenberg DL, Toris CB, Camras CB. Bimatoprost and travoprost: a review of recent studies of two new glaucoma drugs. Surv Ophthalmol 2002; 47(Suppl 1):S105-15.

26. Brandt J, Vandenburgh, AM, Chen K, et al. Comparison of once-or twice

daily bimatoprost with twice-daily timolol in patients with elevated IOP. Ophthalmology 2001;108:1023.

27. Sherwood M, Brandt J, for the Bimatoprost Study Groups 1 and 2. Six-month comparison of bimatoprost once-daily and twice-daily with timolol twice-daily in patients with elevated intraocular pressure. Surv Ophthalmol 2001;45(Suppl 4): S361-8.

28. Noecker RS, Dirks MS, Choplin NT, Bernstein P, Batoosingh AL, Whitcup SM, Bimatoprost/Latanoprost Study. A six-month randomized clinical trial comparing the intraocular pressure-lowering efficacy of bimatoprost and latanoprost in patients with ocular hypertension or glaucoma. Group. Am J Ophthalmol 2003;135(1):55-63.

29. Eisenberg DL, Toris CB, Camras CB. Bimatoprost and travoprost: a review of recent studies of two new glaucoma drugs. Surv Ophthalmol 2002; 47(Suppl 1):S105-15.

30. Gandolfi SA, Cimino L. Effect of bimatoprost on patients with primary open-angle glaucoma or ocular hypertension who are nonresponders to latanoprost. Ophthalmology 2003; 110:609-14.

31. Uusitalo HMT, Pillunat LE, Baudouin C, et al. Phase III, 24-month study investigating the efficacy and safety of tafluprost vs latanoprost in patients with open-angle glaucoma or ocular hypertension. Acta Ophthalmologica 2008;86:S243.

32. Kuwayama Y, Komemusi S. Phase III confirmatory study of 0.0015% DE-085 (Tafluprost) ophthalmic solution as compared to 0.005% Latanoprost ophthalmic solution in patients with open-angle glaucoma or ocular hypertension. Atarashii Ganka 2008; 25:1595-602.

33. Uusitalo H, Kaarniranta K, Ropo A. Pharmacokinetics, efficacy and safety profiles of preserved and preservative-free tafluprost in healthy volunteers. Acta Ophthalmol Suppl 2008;242:7-13.

34. Parrish RK, Palmberg P, Sheu WP; XLT Study Group. A comparison of latanoprost, bimatoprost, and travoprost in patients with elevated intraocular pressure: a 12-week, randomized, masked-evaluator multicenter study. Am J Ophthalmol 2003;135:688-703.

35. Gandolfi S, Simmons ST, Sturm R, Chen K, VanDenburgh AM, for the Bimatoprost Study Group 3. Three-month comparison of bimatoprost and latanoprost in patients with glaucoma and ocular hypertension. Adv Ther 2001;18:110-21.

36. Hylton C, Robin AL. Update on prostaglandin analogs. Curr Opin Ophthalmol 2003;14:65-9.

37. Liu JH, Medeiros FA, Rigby SL, Weinreb RN. Comparing diurnal and nocturnal effects of brinzolamide and timolol on intraocular pressure in patients receiving latanoprost monotherapy. Ophthalmology 2009;116:449-54.

38. Sit A, Asrani S. Effects of medications and surgery on intraocular pressure fluctuation. Surv Ophthalmol 2008;53: S45-55.

39. Dubiner HB, Sircy MD, Landry T, Bergamini MV, Silver LH, Darell Turner F, et al. Comparison of the diurnal ocular hypotensive efficacy of travoprost and latanoprost over a 44-hour period in patients with elevated intraocular pressure. Clin Ther 2004;26:84-91.

40. Sit A, Weinreb RN, Crowston J, Kripke D, Liu JH. Sustained effect of travoprost on diurnal and nocturnal intraocular pressure. Am J Ophthalmol 2006;141:1131-3.

40a. Kent AR, Vroman DT, Thomas TJ, Hebert RL, Crosson CE. Interaction of pilocarpine with latanoprost in patients with glaucoma and ocular hypertension. J Glaucoma 1999;8: 257-62.

41. Feldman RM. Conjunctival hyperemia and the use of topical prostaglandins in glaucoma and ocular hypertension. J Ocul Pharmacol Ther 2003;19:23-35.

42. Honrubia F, García-Sánchez J, Polo V, de la Casa JM, Soto J. Conjunctival hyperaemia with the use of latanoprost versus other prostaglandin analogues in patients with ocular hypertension or glaucoma: a meta-analysis of randomised clinical trials. Br J Ophthalmol 2009;93(3):316-21.

43. Kurtz S, Mann O. Incidence of hyperemia associated with bimatoprost treatment in naïve subjects and in subjects previously treated with latanoprost. Eur J Ophthalmol 2009; 19:400-3.

44. Li N, Chen XM, Zhou Y, Wei ML, Yao X. Travoprost compared with other prostaglandin analogues or timolol in patients with open-angle glaucoma or ocular hypertension: meta-analysis of randomized controlled trials. Clin Experiment Ophthalmol 2006;34:755-64.

45. Stjernschantz JW, Albert DM, Hu DN, Drago F, Wistrand PJ. Mechanism and clinical significance of prostaglandin-induced iris pigmentation. Surv Ophthalmol. 2002 Aug;47 Suppl 1:S162-75.

46. McCarey BE, Kapik BM, Kane FE. Low incidence of iris pigmentation and eyelash changes in 2 randomized clinical trials with unoprostone isopropyl 0.15%. Unoprostone Monotherapy Study Group. Ophthalmology 2004; 111:1480-8.

47. Higginbotham EJ, Schuman JS, Goldberg I, Gross RL, VanDenburgh AM, Chen K, Whitcup SM. One-year, randomized study comparing bimatoprost and timolol in glaucoma and ocular hypertension. Arch Ophthalmol 2002;120:1286-93.

48. Johnstone MA. Hypertrichosis and increased pigmentation of eyelashes and adjacent hair in the region of the ipsilateral eyelids of patients treated with unilateral topical latanoprost. Am J Ophthalmol 1997;124:544-7.

49. Hart J, Shafranov G. Hypertrichosis of vellus hairs of the malar region after unilateral treatment with bimatoprost. Am J Ophthalmol 2004;137:756-7.

50. Chen CS, Wells J, Craig JE. Topical prostaglandin F(2alpha) analog induced poliosis. Am J Ophthalmol 2004;137:965-6.

51. Kook MS, Lee K. Increased eyelid pigmentation associated with use of latanoprost. Am J Ophthalmol 2000;129:804-6.

52. Herndon LW, Williams RD, Asrani S, Wand M. Increased periocular pigmentation with ocular hypotensive lipid use in African Americans. Am J Ophthalmol 2003;135:713-5.

53. Wand M, Ritch R, Isbey EK, Zimmerman TJ. Latanoprost and periocular skin color changes. Arch Ophthalmol 2001;119:614-5.

54. Kapur R, Osmanovic S, Toyran S, Edward DP. Bimatoprost-induced periocular skin hyperpigmentation histopathological study. Arch Ophthalmol 2005;123:1541-6.

55. Aydin S, Ozcura F. Corneal oedema and acute anterior uveitis after two doses of travoprost. Acta Ophthalmologica Scandinavica, 2007;85:693-4.

56. Suominen S, Välimäki J. Bilateral anterior uveitis associated with travoprost. Acta Ophthalmologica Scandinavica 2006;84:275-6.

57. Wand M, Gaudio AR. Cystoid macular edema in the era of ocular hypotensive lipids. Am J Ophthalmol 2002; 133:403-5.

58. Kroll DM, Schuman JS. Reactivation of herpes simplex keratitis after initiating bimatoprost treatment of glaucoma. Am J Ophthalmol 2002;133:401-3.

59. Arcieri ES, Santana A, Rocha FN, Guapo GL, Costa VP. Blood-aqueous barrier changes after the use of prostaglandin analogues in patients with pseudophakia and aphakia: a 6-month randomized trial. Arch Ophthalmol 2005;123: 186-92.

60. Aihara M, Shirato S, Sakata R. Incidence of deepening of the upper eyelid sulcus after switching from latanoprost to bimatoprost. Jpn J Ophthalmol 2011;55:600-4.

61. Browning DJ, Perkins SL, Lark KK. Iris cyst secondary to latanoprost mimicking iris melanoma. Am J Ophthalmol 2003;135:419-21.

62. Krohn J, Hove VK. Recurring iris pigment epithelial cyst induced by topical prostaglandin F2 alpha analogues. Arch Ophthalmol 2008;126:867-8.

63. Lee YC. Abdominal cramp as an adverse effect of travoprost. Am J Ophthalmol 2005;139:202-3.

64. Hedner J, Everts B, Möller CS. Latanoprost and respiratory function in asthmatic patients: randomized, double-masked, placebo-controlled crossover evaluation. Arch Ophthalmol 1999;117:1305-9.

65. Coleman AL, Mosaed S, Kamal D. Medical Therapy in Pregnancy. J Glaucoma 2005;14:414-6.

66. Johnson SM, Martinez M, Freedman S. Management of glaucoma in pregnancy and lactation. Surv Ophthalmol 2001;45:449-54.

CARBONIC ANHYDRASE INHIBITORS

Carbonic anhydrase inhibitors (CAIs) are sulphonamide derivates which reduce IOP by decreasing aqueous humor production. They cause IOP reduction when administered by systemic or topical routes. Interestingly, they are the only agents available for both topical and systemic IOP lowering. Acetazolamide was first used in 1954 by Becker as an oral agent to reduce IOP. Both the topical and systemic CAIs have a *common mechanism of action* but *differ primarily in* the severity of side effects.

MECHANISM OF ACTION

Carbonic Anhydrase

Carbonic anhydrase (CA) is an enzyme responsible for the catalytic hydration of CO_2 and dehydration of H_2CO_3 in the ciliary epithelium.[1-6] This results in the formation of bicarbonate (HCO_3^-) and H^+ which is an important step in aqueous humor formation.

$$CO_2 + H_2O \xrightleftharpoons{CA} H_2CO_3 \xrightleftharpoons{} HCO_3^- + H^+$$

The bicarbonate produced in the above reaction is essential for active secretion of aqueous humor (AH). There are *14 isoenzyme* forms of CA encoded by their corresponding genes and having a *varied cellular distribution*. The *eye has four CA isoenzymes* CA1 to CA4. Two isozymes of CA (II & IV) are present in the ciliary pigmented epithelium. The *CA II isoform*, located in the ciliary processes of the human eyes, is the *main therapeutic target of CAIs*. Failure of CAIs to lower IOP is seen in eyes with CA type II deficiency.[7] CA II inhibition affects the ion transport involved in aqueous humor secretion.[8-12] CA inhibitors also alter the ocular blood flow and cause metabolic acidosis and have an adrenergic activity.[13,14] Inhibition of >99% of CA II isozyme in ciliary processes epithelium is required to achieve adequate IOP reduction.

Inhibition of Carbonic Anhydrase

The CA inhibitors (CAI) have an active moiety, which is identical to carbonic acid and complimentary to CA, which interferes with the function of the enzyme. The CAIs thus lower IOP by reducing aqueous humor formation.

Effect on IOP

Systemic acetazolamide: IOP decrease is seen within 30 minutes, peak drug action is seen at 1 hour and lasts for 6-8 hours. The washout time is 3 days for systemic CAIs.

Systemic CAIs lower IOP by about 30%.

Topical agents: Fluorophotometric studies show topical carbonic anhydrase inhibtors to decrease aqueous humor flow by 21% to 30% during the day. Unlike timolol they also reduce the already lowered production rate by an additional 24% at night. A combination of topical carbonic anhydrase inhibitors with timolol reduces the rate from 33% by timolol alone to 44% by the combination. Given as monotherapy, topical dorzolamide is less effective suppressing aqueous flow by only 17%.

> **Note** Acetazolamide is relatively nonselective, (acting on both CA II and IV isomers) as compared to the topical CAIs which have a special affinity for CA II. This may be responsible for the smaller IOP lowering effect of topical as compared to the systemic agents.

SYSTEMIC CARBONIC ANHYDRASE INHIBITORS

These include dichlorphenamide, ethoxzolamide, acetazolamide and methzolamide, commercially available oral carbonic anhydrase inhibitors include acetazolamide and methazolamide. Dichlorphenamide is also available but not used commonly.

Acetazolamide[14-19]

Acetazolamide is relatively nonselective, (acting on both CA II and IV isomers) as compared to the topical CAIs which have a special affinity for CA II. This may be responsible for the smaller IOP lowering effect of topical as compared to the systemic agents.

It is a frequently used agent. It has been shown to reduce intraocular pressure by 30%. It is supplied in 125 mg, 250 mg tablets and 500 mg sustained release capsules (SRC). Effective IOP reduction is achieved and the maximum dose which can be given is 250 mg four times a day and 500 mg of the sustained release capsules two times a day. Once a day SR capsules may be better tolerated, the effect lasting for 24 hours in many patients. Dose in infants is 5-10 mg/kg 6 hourly (flavored syrup). The serum half life of acetazolamide is 4 hours. It is not metabolized and is actively secreted by the renal tubules and then passively resorbed by nonionic diffusion. IOP reduction parallels the plasma level of the drug.

Acetazolamide binds to plasma proteins to the extent of 93% and most of it is excreted unmetabolized by the kidney. This is in contrast to methazolamide which is only 25% bound to the proteins and is therefore less limited by renal function.

The IOP begins to drop in 1-2 hours, returns to baseline in 4-12 hours. With the **sustained release capsule**, IOP begins to drop in 2-4 hours; is minimum IOP at 8 hours and reaches baseline in 12-24 hours. The peak effect is 2-4 hours and duration of action 8-12 hours.

Intravenous Dose
- 500 mg ampules
- Dissolved in 5-10 ml of distilled water
- I/V 250-500 mg
- IOP drops within minutes.

Methazolamide[20-22]
It is available in tablets of 25 mg, 50 mg. It has a plasma half life of 14 hours and is less bound to plasma proteins. Thus the required dose of 25-50 mg twice a day is less than acetazolamide. Methazolamide is less effective than acetazolamide in reducing IOP. However it is also less likely to cause side effects because of its pharmacodynamics. It is metabolized primarily in the liver in contrast to acetazolamide which is excreted unchanged through the kidney. The metabolism of methazolamide makes it a safer choice than acetazolamide for patients with advanced renal disease. Although methazolamide has been reported to cause urinary tract calculi most prefer methazolamide to acetazolamide in patients with a history of nephrolithiasis.
- IOP begins to drop in 1-2 hours
- IOP reaches back to baseline in 12-24 hours
- Peak effect is seen after 6-8 hours, duration of action is 10-18 hours.

Side Effects of Oral CAI[23-36]
The oral CAIs have a variety of systemic side effects (**Table 4**):
- Paraesthesias are the most common complaint and occur in 2/3 of patients but may diminish with time
- Anorexia and appetite loss is observed in half the patients. Fatigue, malaise and transient diarrhea have also been reported. Other less common side effects include confusion, nocturia, decreased libido and depression.
- Renal calculi (Nephrolithiasis) may result from decreased excretion of citrate and magnesium and the production of acholine urine. These are 10-15 times more common with systemic CAI.
- A significant potassium loss may occur if used for a prolonged time or in complication with other potassium depleting medications (thiazide diuretics steroids)
- Systemic acidosis associated with the oral CAIs can be a problem for patients using salicylates and those with hepatic, renal, adrenal, or pulmonary disease.
- *Sickle cell disease:* The induced metabolic acidosis may cause sickling of RBC in susceptible patients. This may be more pronounced in patients with traumatic glaucomas as the increased sickling could delay resolution of hyphemas, clogging of TM, compromising optic nerve circulation.
- Bilateral choroidal effusion with acute secondary angle closure has been reported with systemic acetazolamide.

Effect on Blood Flow
CAIs produce metabolic acidosis with a secondary vasodilatation and improvement in blood flow (systemic with oral and local with topical). There is a conflicting report from studies and no evidence based information suggesting any benefit with regard to ocular perfusion.

Life Threatening Complications
Though rare, blood dyscrasias and Steven Johnson syndrome are life threatening complications. The hematologic side effects can be fatal. Thrombocytopemia and agranulocytosis may occur within 6 weeks of therapy. These are reversible on withdrawing the drug. In patients on chronic systemic CAI use, monitoring blood counts with pretreatment counts and then 2 monthly can be done. However cost is an issue and some of the most

---

Paresthesias of fingers, toes and circumoral region – common side effect. Potassium depletion occurring during the initial phase of therapy because of increased urinary excretion is the explanation.

Serum electrolyte imbalance – metabolic acidosis as a result of bicarbonate depletion. Manifests as malaise, fatigue, weight loss, anorexia, depression and decreased libido.[24,25] Manage with alkali supplements with sodium bicarbonate or sodium acetate. Avoid CAI in cases with hepatic insufficiency, renal failure, adrenocortical insufficiency, hyperchloremic acidosis, depressed sodium or potassium levels, or severe pulmonary obstruction.[23]

Gastro-intestinal symptoms manifesting as vague abdominal discomfort, metallic taste, nausea and diarrhea. *Cause unknown.* Taking medication with meals usually helps.[24]

Renal calculi formation is typical to this class of drug. The mechanism is related to the reduce excretion of urinary citrate or magnesium,[21,26] as both are responsible to keep calcium salts in solution. Alkalinization of urine also predisposes to calcium precipitation.[27,28] Management might require a reduction in dose.

Rare but reported are cases with blood dyscrasias viz thrombocytopenia, agranulocytosis, aplastic anemia and neutropenia in patients receiving CAI therapy.[29-33] These serious adverse effect are idiosyncratic, non dose related and variable in onset. Agranulocytosis and TCP are acute in onset manifesting with acute bacterial infections and bleeding[34] are completely reversible on cessation of therapy. Aplastic anemia in contrast has a delayed, insidious onset and is frequently fatal. Monitoring blood cell counts are not cost effective so obtaining interval patient history and being vigilant for relevant hematological symptoms is important.

Dermatological side effects such as maculopapular and urticarial type of skin eruptions as well as Stevens-Johnson syndrome[35-36]

Table 4 Side effects of oral Carbonic Anhydrase Inhibitors (CAIs)

Systemic
General
Paresthesias of fingers, toes
Metallic taste in mouth
Carbonated beverages taste flat
Malaise
Weight loss
Headache
Central Nervous System
Depression
Loss of libido
Pulmonary
Respiratoy decompensation in patients with chronic obstructive pulmonary disease
Cardiovascular
Decreased blood pressure (mild)
Gastrointestinal
Nausea
Epigastric burning
Renal/Genitourinary
Nephrolithiasis (Calcium oxalate and calcium phosphate stones)
Urinary frequency (Usually a transient early complaint)
Renal Failure
Ocular
Induced Myopia (rare)
Bilateral secondary angle closure glaucoma
Serious side effects
Idiosyncrasy
Blood dyscrasias like thrombocytopenia, agranulocytosis, aplastic anemia, neutropenia

severe blood dyscrasias would not be prevented by this. Decision may be made on a case to case basis. Clinical history of bleeding and infections must be asked at each visit.

Indications of Systemic CAIs
- Acute reduction of IOP as in acute primary angle angle closure,

secondary glaucomas like phacolytic, phacomorphic, traumatic glaucoma
- To achieve corneal clarity in case of corneal edema by IOP reduction before laser procedures
- Following laser procedures to control IOP spikes
- Following surgery (for short term IOP control)
- Short term treatment before surgery
- Contraindications to topical therapy

Contraindications of Systemic CAI
- Sulphonamide hypersensitivity
- Adrenal insufficiency
- Hepatic cirrhosis
- Renal failure
- Chronic respiratory acidosis
- Hyperchloremic alkalosis
- Hyponatremia/hypokalemia
- Diabetic ketoacidosis/unstable diabetes
- Urolithiasis
- Sickle cell disease
- Pregnancy/lactation
- Concomitant use of aspirin/corticosteroids (requires special monitoring)
- Cardiac glycosides like digitalis as hypokalemia can be lethal in this situation

Drug Interactions
The drug interactions with other systemic agents are mostly due to the induced metabolic acidosis.

- Potentiating of effects of oral hypoglycemics
- Potentiating of effects of anticoagulants
- Partial blockage of anticholinestrases

Role in Other Ocular Conditions
Retinal pigment epithelium (RPE) is rich in carbonic anhydrase. So these agents are used for management of cystoid macular edema (CME) and pigmentary retinal dystrophy.

Nonocular Use
- Vertigo (reduce potassium concentration in endolymph)
- High altitude pulmonary and cerebral edema
- Metabolic acidosis increases ventilation, arterial oxygen tension and reduces fatigue, nausea
- *Papilledema:* Reduces rate of cerebrospinal fluid (CSF) formation

TOPICAL CARBONIC ANHYDRASE INHIBITORS
The numerous and significant side effects associated with the systemic CAI prompted a tremendous effort to search for topically acting CAI. Topical CAI available for clinical use are Dorzolamide and Brinzolamide **(Table 5)**.

Dorzolamide[37-43]
It is marketed as a 2% solution since 1995. Twice a day instillation reduces

Table 5 Topical carbonic anhydrase inhibitors

	Dorzolamide	*Brinzolamide*
Formulation	Solution	Suspension
Concentration	2%	1%
Dose	BD-TDS	BD-TDS
pH	5.6	7.5
Osmolality	----NA	300 mOsm/kg
BAK	0.0075%	0.01%
Site of ocular absorption	Cornea	Cornea
Washout period	1 week	1 week

IOP by 21 and 13% (peak and trough times) and 3 times a day dosing improves the trough effect. An eight hourly dose is recommended for monotherapy and 12 hourly dose for adjunct therapy. It has additive effects with both aqueous suppressants and aqueous outflow enhancing agents. Peak effects is seen after 3 hours. It is well tolerated in children less than 6 years as compared to oral acetazolamide. Its IOP lowering effect is maintained on long term use without any tachyphylaxis and it is reasonably well tolerated. In EGPS an IOP reduction of 15-22% was seen with dorzolamide at 5 years of follow up.

It is also available in fixed combination with timolol. Its ocular hypotensive effect is equivalent to the two agents used separately but simultaneously. This combination has been reported to be as effective as latanoprost. Dorzolamide may show a slightly better additively with latanoprost as compared to beta blockers or brimonidine.

Brinzolamide[44-52]

It is highly lipophilic and available since 1998 as a 1% suspension (in a carbomer) which shows good corneal penetration at a pH of 7.5. It has a prolonged duration of action due to increased contact time, reduced surface irritation as compared to its original solution form. Brinzolamide given thrice a day was found to be as effective as dorzolamide and timolol. The IOP reduction is between 15 and 22%. When added to timolol an additional 13-16% reduction is observed. Brinzolamide is also additive to latanoprost. Patients have less stinging and pain as compared to dorzolamide. However a higher rate of transient blurring of vision is noted with brinzolamide. It does not appear to alter corneal endothelial cell density or corneal thickness in patients with normal corneas.

In monotherapy IOP reduction reaches a peak at 2 hours after instillation with 16-22% reduction (12 hour trough reduction 13.2-18.9% in POAG and ocular hypertension). Efficacy is similar to betaxolol but less than PGA and timolol. Longterm IOP control is stable with no drift phenomenon.

Combination with other classes of drugs (beta blockers and prostaglandin analogues) are available. A combination with prostaglandin analogues is found to be effective as the PGA along with increasing uveoscleral outflow also increase the carbonic anhydrase (CA) activity in ciliary epithelium leading to a secondary increase in aqueous humor secretion. This action may be blocked by adjunctive CAIs.

Topical agents have a wider indications of use as compared to systemic. They are mainly used as an adjunct. They may be used as primary therapy in patients where other drugs are contraindicated.

Indications of Topical CAIs

- Mainly as a second line and adjunctive therapy
- Monotherapy (tid dose)
  - ❖ Contraindications to beta blockers
  - ❖ Side effects with prostaglandin analogues
  - ❖ Side effects with alpha agonists

Drawbacks of Monotherapy with CAIs

- Modest IOP reduction
- TID dose

> **Note** Topical carbonic anhydrase inhibitors are not likely to produce any additional IOP lowering in patients on a full dose of oral carbonic anhydrase inhibitors

SIDE EFFECTS OF TOPICAL CAIs

Ocular Side Effects of Topical CAIs

Minimal ocular adverse reactions, such as irritation immediately post instillation, bitter taste, transient blurred vision and occasional hypersensitivity reactions including periorbital dermatitis are seen. Increase in mean corneal thickness has been observed in eyes with compromised endothelial counts, but in healthy eyes this is not clinically significant

- Altered or metallic taste is seen in upto 25% patients.
- Periorbital dermatitis and allergic conjunctivitis.[53]
- Adverse effect on corneal endothelial cells by inhibition of CAII. This worsens the status of compromised corneas. This may not be reversible after withdrawl of drug.[54]
- Transient myopia, choroidal detachment and secondary angle closure glaucoma are infrequent side effects of all sulphonamide derivatives and have been seen with both topical and systemic CAIs.
- Marginal keratitis is a rare allergic complication of dorzolamide.

Systemic Side Effects of Topical CAIs

Although topical CAI are systemically absorbed their serum levels are relatively low. Thus they do not cause any significant change in electrolyte or/and balance. Dorzolamide and its metabolite are largely bound to RBC cholinesterase RBC CA is depressed to 21% of normal levels. This may be seen for months after the drug has been discontinued. However no systemic symptom has been attributed to it.

Other rare side effects include fatigue, urticaria, headache, dizziness or depression. Gastrointestinal discomfort may occur in the find few days.

Thrombocytopenia and Steven Johnson Syndrome may rarely occur.

Pregnancy and Lactation

Pregnancy is a relative contraindication and these drugs should to be used only if use justifies potential risk to fetus. Carbonic anhydrase inhibitors are excreted in the milk, and may influence the red blood cells in the newborn.

Children

Oral CAI have been reported to cause growth retardation due to metabolic acidosis in children. Although not as effective as oral acetazolamide, topical dorzolamide causes a significant IOP reduction in children with glaucoma.[55,56]

REFERENCES

1. Hewett-Emmett D. Evolution and distribution of the carbonic anhydrase gene families. EXS 2000;90:29.

2. Wistrand PJ. Carbonic anhydrase inhibition in ophthalmology. Carbonic anhydrases in cornea, lens, retina and lacrimal gland. EXS 2000;90:413.

3. Dobbs PC, Epstein DL, Anderson PJ. Identification of isoenzyme C as the principal carbonic anhydrase in human ciliary processes. Invest Ophthalmol Vis Sci 1979;18:867.

4. Lutjen-Drecoll E, Lonnerholm G, Eichhorn M. Carbonic anhydrase distribution in the human and monkey eye by light and electron microscopy. Graefes Arch Clin Exp Ophthalmol 1983;220:285.

5. Hageman GS, Zhu XL, Waheed A, et al. Localization of carbonic anhydrase IV in a specific capillary bed of the human eye. Proc Natl Acad Sci USA 1991;88:2716.

6. Kim CY, Whittington DA, Chang JS, et al. Structural aspects of isozyme selectivity in the binding of inhibitors to carbonic anhydrases II and IV. J Med Chem 2002;45:888.

7. Krupin T, Sly WS, Whyte MP, et al. Failure of acetazolamide to decrease intraocular pressure in patients with carbonic anhydrase II deficiency. Am J Ophthalmol 1985;99:396.

8. Berggren L. Direct observation of secretory pumping in vitro of the rabbit eye ciliary processes. Influence of ion milieu and carbonic anhydrase inhibition. Invest Ophthalmol 1964;19:266.

9. To CH, Do CW, Zamudio AC, et al. Model of ionic transport for bovine ciliary epithelium; effects of acetazolamide and HCO. Am J Physiol Cell Physiol 2001;280:C1521.

10. Maren TH. The rates of movement of Na^+, Cl^-, and HCO_3 from plasma to posterior chamber; effect of acetazolamide and relation to the treatment of glaucoma. Invest Ophthalmol 1976;15:356.

11. Holland MG, Gipson CC. Chloride ion transport in the isolated ciliary body, Invest Ophthalmol 1970;9:20.

12. McLaughlin CW, Zellhuber-McMillan S, Peart D, et al. Regional differences in ciliary epithelial cell transport properties. J Membr Biol 2001;182:213.

13. Civan MM. The eye's aqueous humor from secretion to glaucoma. San Diego, Academic Press, 1998.

14. Bietti G, Virno M, Pecori-Giraldi J, et al. Acetazolamide metabolic acidosis, and intraocular pressure. Am J Ophthalmol 1975;80:360.

15. Maus TL, Larsson LI, McLaren JW, et al. Comparison of dorzolamide and acetazolamide as suppressors of aqueous humors flow in humans. Arch Ophthalmol 1997;115:45.

16. McCannel CA, Heinrich SR, Brubaker RF. Acetazolamide but not timolol lowers aqueous humor flow in sleeping humans. Graefes Arch Clin Exp Ophthalmol 1992;230:518.

17. Dailey RA, Brubaker RF, Bourne WM. The effects of timolol maleate and acetazolamide on the rate of aqueous formation in normal human subjects. Am J Ophthalmol 1982;93:232.

18. Joyce PW, Mills KB, Richardson T, et al. Equivalence of conventional and sustained release oral dosage formulations of acetazolamide in primary open angle glaucoma. Br J Clin Pharmacol 1989;27:597.

19. Havener WH. Ocular pharmacology, 5th et al. St. Louis, CV Mosby 1983.

20. Maren TH, Haywood JR, Chapman SK, et al. The pharmacology of methazolamide in relation to the treatment of glaucoma. Invest Ophthalmol Vis Sci 1977;16:730.

21. Constant MA, Becker B. The effect of carbonic anhydrase inhibitors on urinary excretion of citrate by humans. Am J Ophthalmol 1960;49:929.

22. Becker B. Use of methazolamide (Neptazane) in the therapy of glaucoma: comparison with acetazolamide (Diamox). Am J Ophthalmol 1960;49:1307.

23. Block ER, Rostand RA. Carbonic anhydrase inhibition in glaucoma. Hazard or benefit for the chronic lung? Surv Ophthalmol 1978;23:169.

24. Epstein DL, Grant WM. Carbonic anhydrase inhibitors side effects: Serum chemical analysis. Arch Ophthalmol 1977;95:1378.

25. Wallace TR, Fraunfelder FT, Petursson GJ, et al. Decreased libido: a side effect of carbonic anhydrase inhibitor. Ann Ophthalmol 1979;11:1563.

26. Grant W, Leopold I, ed. Symposium on ocular therapy. St Louis: Mosby 1972:19(6).

27. Parthasarathi S, K Myint K, Singh G, Mon S, Sadasivam P, Dhillon B. Bilateral acetazolamide-induced choroidal effusion following cataract surgery. Eye 2007;21:870-2.

28. Kondo T, Sakaue E, Koyama S, et al. Urolithiasis during treatment of carbonic anhydrase inhibitors. Folia Ophthalmol Jpn 1968;19:576.

29. Wisch N, Fischbein FI, Siegel, et al. Aplastic anemia resulting from the use of carbonic anhydrase inhibitors. Am J Ophthalmol 1973;75:130.

30. Gangitano JL, Foster SH, Contro RM. Nonfatal methazolamide-induced aplastic anemia. Am J Ophthalmol 1978;86:138.

31. Werblin TP, Pollack IP, Liss RA. Blood dyscrasias in patients using methazolamide (Neptazane) for glaucoma. Ophthalmology 1980;87:350.

32. Fraundfelder FT, Meyer SM, Bagby GC Jr, et al. Hematologic reactions to carbonic anhydrase inhibitors. Am J Ophthalmol 1985;100:79.

33. Mogk LG, Cyrlin MN. Blood dyscrasias and carbonic anhydrase inhibitors. Ophthalmology 1988;95:768.

34. Zimran A, Beutler E. Can the risk of acetazolamide-induced aplastic anemia be decreased by periodic monitoring of blood cell counts? Am J Ophthalmol 1987;104:654.

35. Gandham SB, Spaeth GL, Di Leonardo M, et al. Methazolamide-induced skin eruptions. Arch Ophthalmol 1993;111:370.

36. Flach AJ, Smith RE, Fraunfelder FT. Stevens-Johnson syndrome associated with methazolamide treatment reported in two Japanese-American women. Ophthalmology 1995;102:1677.

37. Kitazawa Y, Azuma I, Iwata K, et al. Dorzolamide, a topical carbonic anhydrase inhibitor; a two week dose response study in patients with glaucoma or ocular hypertension. J Glaucoma 1994;3:275.

38. Lippa EA, Schuman JS, Higginbotham EJ, et al. MK-507 versus sezolamide: comparative efficacy of two topically active carbonic anhydrase inhibitors. Ophthalmology 1991;98:308.

39. Wilkerson M, Cyrlin M, Lippa EA, et al. Four-week safety and efficacy study of dorzolamide. A novel, active topical carbonic anhydrase inhibitor. Arch Ophthalmol 1993;111:1343.

40. Strahlman E, Tipping R, Vogel R. A six-week dose-response study of the ocular hypotensive effect of dorzolomide with a one-year extension. Dorzolamide dose-response study group. (Erratum Appears in Am J Ophthalmol 1996;122:928) Am J Ophthalmol 1996;122:1.

41. Strahlman ER, Vogel R, Tipping R, et al. The use of dorzolamide and pilocarpine as adjunctive therapy to timolol in patients with elevated intraocular pressure; the dorzolamide additivity study group. Ophthalmology 1996;103:1283.

42. Petounis A, Mylopoulos N, Kandarakis A, et al. Comparison of the additive intraocular pressure-lowering effect of latanoprost and dorzolamide when added to timolol in patients with open angle glaucoma or ocular hypertension: a randomized, open-label, multicenter study in Greece. J Glaucoma 2001;10:316.

43. Adamsons I, Clineschmidt C, Polis A, et al. The efficacy and safety of dorzolamide as adjunctive therapy to timolol maleate gellan solution in patients with elevated intraocular pressure: additivity study group. J Glaucoma 1998;7:253.

44. Silver LH. Dose-response evaluation of the ocular hypotensive effect of brinzolamide ophthalmic suspension (Azopt): brinzolomide dose-response study group. Surv Ophthalmol 2000; 44(suppl2):S147.

45. Sall K. The efficacy and safety of brinzolomide. 1% ophthalmic suspension (Azopt) as a primary therapy in patients with open angle glaucoma or ocular hypertension: brinzolomide primary therapy study group. Surv Ophthalmol 2000;44(suppl 2):S155.

46. Seong GJ, Lee JH, et al. Comparison of intraocular pressure-lowering efficacy and side effects of 2% dorzolamide and 1% brinzolamide. Ophthalmologica 2001;215:188.

47. Shin D. Adjunctive therapy with brinzolamide 1% ophthalmic suspension (Azopt) in patients with open angle glaucoma or ocular hypertension maintained on timolol therapy. Surv Ophthalmol 2000;44(suppl2):S163.

48. Michaud JE, Friren B. Comparison of topical brinzolamide 1% and dorzolamide 2% eye drops given twice daily in addition to timolol 0.5% in patients with primary open angle glaucoma or ocular hypertension. Am J Ophthalmol 2001;132:235.

49. Lippa EA, Aasved H, Airaksinen PJ, et al. Multiple-dose, dose-response relationship for the topical carbonic anhydrase inhibitor MK-927. Arch Ophthalmol 1991;109:46.

50. Martens-Lobenhoffer J, Banditt P. Clinical pharmacokinetics of dorzolamide. Clin Pharmacokinet 2002;41:197.

51. Barnebey H, Kwok SY. Patients acceptance of a switch from dorzolamide to brinzolamide for the treatment of glaucoma in a clinical practice setting. Clin Ther 2000;22:1204.

52. van der Valk R, Webers CA, Schouten JS, Zeegers MP, Hendrikse F, Prins MH. Intraocular pressure-lowering effects of all commonly used glaucoma drugs: a meta-analysis of randomized clinical trials. Ophthalmology 2005; 112:1177-85

53. Delaney YM, Salmon JF, Mossa F, Gee B, Beehne K, Powell S. Periorbital dermatitis as a side effect of topical dorzolamide. Br J Ophthalmol 2002;86:378-80.

54. Wirtitsch MG, Findl O, Heinzl H, Drexler W. Effect of dorzolamide hydrochloride on central corneal thickness in humans with cornea guttata. Arch Ophthalmol 2007;125:1345-50.

55. Futagi Y, Otani K, Abe J. Growth suppression in children receiving acetazolamide with antiepileptic drugs. Pediatr Neurol 1996;15:323-6.

56. Portellos M, Buckley EG, Freedman SF. Topical versus oral carbonic anhydrase inhibitor therapy for pediatric glaucoma. J AAPOS 1998;2:43-7.

HYPEROSMOTIC AGENTS

Hyperosmotic agents are systemic drugs used to achieve a rapid and transient reduction in IOP. They constitute a class of drugs that can be administered orally or intravenously to treat acute, significant elevations of intra ocular pressure not controlled by other antiglaucoma agents. Their mechanism of action is different from all other available antiglaucoma agents. They are invaluable for controlling IOP spikes when other agents fail. However, severe and even life threatening side effects contraindicate their use for chronic therapy.

Mechanisms of Action[1,2]
Reduction of Vitreous Volume
The systemic hyperosmotic agents reduce IOP by increasing the plasma osmolality as compared to the extravascular fluid. Osmolality of blood is increased by 20-30 mOsm/l. They penetrate blood aqueous barrier poorly. Since they penetrate very slowly into the vitreous which is avascular, water is drawn from the eye (mainly the vitreous), into the circulation via retinal and uveal blood vessels. The vitreous shrinks, leading to a decrease in IOP. The IOP reduction in glaucomatous eyes is more than that seen in normal eyes. The effect lasts until the osmotic gradient is established. This depends upon the molecular weight of the hyperosmotic agent. Sometimes a reversal of osmotic gradient may occur if the osmolality of the dehydrated vitreous becomes more than the plasma. It is also possible especially if the blood ocular barrier is not intact and the drug enters the vitreous leading to a rebound increase in IOP. The IOP lowering depends on:
- Ocular penetration
- Distribution in body fluids

- Molecular weight and concentration
- Dose
- Rate and route of administration
- Clearance rate
- Mechanism of diuresis

The duration of action of hyperosmotic agents depends upon their capacity for entering the eye. Glycerol, isosorbide and mannitol are large molecules that do not readily enter the eye and have a longer duration of action than drugs with smaller molecules that can enter the eye, like ethanol or urea. The onset of action ranges between 10 minutes and 1 hour. The duration is usually 4 to 8 hours. Glycerol and isosorbide have the fastest onset of action.

Hypothalamic-Neural Theory
A secondary mechanism involving osmoreceptors has been suggested and is supported by both animal and human studies. It is mediated through osmoreceptors in the hypothalamus in the CNS. These osmoreceptors may alter aqueous humor production via efferent fibers in the optic nerve.

This is supported by the fact that the decrease in IOP and increase in plasma osmolality does not always correlate. Moreover, small doses given I/V have been found to decrease IOP without affecting osmolality. Injection of hyperosmolar agents into the 3rd ventricle has also been found to alter IOP without affecting plasma osmolality. This theory is however disputed by other studies.

Patients should be instructed not to drink water or other fluids after administration of these agents as this may reduce their efficacy due to decrease in the osmotic gradient.

Indications
Hyperosmotic agents are used for the short term control of IOP and management of acute glaucoma. They are especially of use in managing transient IOP spikes, and for preoperative lowering of IOP. They reduce the risk of surgical decompression, choroidal effusion in predisposed eyes and in eyes with markedly elevated IOPs.

In an acute attack of angle closure, hyperosmotic agents can reduce the IOP to a level at which blood flow to the pupillary sphincter is high enough for pilocarpine to bring the pupil down and the iris out of the angle.

Hyperosmotic agents are used to treat acute IOP elevations in secondary glaucomas. In such situations they may help to avoid any glaucoma surgery or allow surgery in a more controlled situation.

Hyperosmotic agents may be used to treat post laser spikes in some cases.

Apart from reducing the IOP they also cause shrinkage of the vitreous allowing the lens to move posteriorly. This causes deepening of the anterior chamber and is useful in the management of Aqueous Misdirection Syndrome (AMS) and acute angle closure attack in addition to the IOP lowering effect.

The blood aqueous barrier is disrupted in inflamed eyes. Therefore hyperosmotic agents may be less capable or creating a gradient between the intraocular contents and the blood, and thus they may be less effective.

Since the mechanism of action of the agents is different from any other glaucoma medication their effective is additive to other antiglaucoma medications. They are generally used for short term and rapid onset of IOP lowering in cases with:
- Acute primary angle closure attack
- Secondary glaucoma
- Post laser IOP spikes

- Preoperative IOP lowering
- Traumatic hyphema
- Neovascular glaucoma (NVG)
- Aqueous misdirection (Malignant glaucoma)
- Topical use to reduce corneal edema.

ORAL HYPEROSMOTIC AGENTS

The advantage of oral agents is a more convenient outpatient administration and less systemic side effects. A variable gastrointestinal absorption of some agents like glycerol makes their effect less predictable. However their safety profile is better, they are less likely to produce volume load in borderline cardiac patients.

Glycerol or Glycerin

It was the first clinically used oral hyperosmotic agent.[3] It is administered orally as a liquid in a dose of: 1-1.5 g/kg or 2-3 ml/kg of body weight. It is available as a 50% solution in 0.9 saline containing 0.62 grams of glycerol/ml. The ocular hypotensive effect occurs fast, within 10 minutes of administration, peaks at 30 minutes-1 hour and lasts for 5 hours. It is distributed throughout the extracellular body fluid but has poor ocular penetration. This enhances the osmotic gradient effect, lowers the IOP and allows repeated administration. It is less effective in lowering the IOP as compared to the intravenous hyperosmotic agents due to variable absorption from the gastro intestinal tract (GIT).

Glycerol is also a component of body fat and is thus readily metabolized. This increases the safety profile and causes less diuresis. At the same time since it is metabolized to glucose, it can lead to hyperglycemia and glycosuria. This coupled with the caloric content of 4.32 kcal/g and the osmotic diuresis with resultant dehydration can cause problems with repeated administration in patients with diabetes. Thus it is contraindicated in diabetics.

Advantages

- It can be given on an outpatient basis
- Rapid onset of action

Disadvantages

- Unpalatable
- There is a high incidence of nausea and vomiting.
- The caloric value of glycerol and metabolites along with the osmotic dehydration
- It can lead to ketoacidosis in diabetic patients.

Isosorbide

It was first used in 1967.[4] It is rapidly and entirely absorbed from the GIT, not metabolized and does not cause hyperglycemia. It is not sweet and less likely to cause nausea. It is currently unavailable.

Ethanol

In high doses, ethanol decreases IOP by its hyperosmotic action and inhibition of antidiuretic hormone (ADH) in the CNS. Intoxication limits its clinical use.

INTRAVENOUS HYPEROSMOTIC AGENTS

These produce a faster and greater IOP reduction as compared to oral agents. These include mannitol and urea. Urea is less effective than mannitol and is rarely used.

Mannitol

It has been used as an agent to lower IOP since 1962.[5,6] It is stable as a 20% solution. However at lower temperatures it is soluble only upto 15% and crystals may form in the solution. Before using, the bottle must be inspected for the presence of crystals and the solution should be warmed to dissolve any crystals which may be present. A blood administration filter may be used in the I/V line to prevent the crystals from entering the blood stream.

Dosage

It is given in a dose of 1-2 g/kg body weight of a 20% solution intravenously in 45-60 min (60 drops/min). The ocular hypotensive effect starts in 15-30 minutes and reaches a peak at 30-60 minutes. The ocular hypotensive effect lasts for 6 hours. It should be given around 45 min-1 hour prior to surgery. Lower doses may be equally in effective in lowering IOP in some cases. Mannitol is not metabolized and is excreted unchanged in the urine. It penetrates the eye poorly and this improves its ability to lower the IOP. However it has certain disadvantages. These include:

Disadvantages

- Greater cellular dehydration
- Large volume of fluid required
- CNS dehydration especially in elderly
- Renal failure
- Patient with renal failure are unable to excrete the large fluid volume.
- Load on patient with congestive cardiac failure (CCF) due to increased blood volume.

SIDE EFFECTS OF HYPEROSMOTIC AGENTS

The dehydration of the extravascular space and the increased intravascular volume is responsible for the side effects of hyperosmotic agents **(Table 6)**. The increased vascular volume may strain the cardiac and renal system. This may well be tolerated by a healthy person but can be serious especially in elderly and patients with compromised or borderline cardiac, renal or hepatic function. Thus, these drugs should be used with caution in such patients. The most frequent side effects seen are headache, nausea and vomiting.

Headache occurs due to cerebral dehydration and decreased intracranial

Table 6 Side effects of hyperosmotic agents

Gastrointestinal	Renal/Genitourinary
• Nausea	• Diuresis
• Vomiting	• Loss of potassium
• Diarrhea	• Urinary retention
• Abdominal cramps	• Anuria
Cardiovascular	**Miscellaneous**
• Angina	• Arm pain
• Congestive heart failure	• Skin slough (Urea)
• Hypertension	• Dehydration
• Vascular overload	• Electrolyte imbalance
Pulmonary	• Thrombophlebitis
• Pulmonary edema	• Acidosis
Central Nervous System	• Diabetic Ketoacidosis (glycerol)
• Headache	• Hyperosmolar non-ketotic coma
• Backache	• Urticaria
• Confusion	• Laryngeal edema
• Disorientation	• Anaphylactic reaction
• Chills	• Hyphema
• Fever	• Suprachoroidal hemorrhage
• Subdural hematoma	• Blurred vision
• Subarachnoid and subdural hemorrhage	
• Seizure	

pressure. In a more severe form, the cerebral dehydration can cause confusion and disorientation. Shrinking of the brain can stretch vessels, leading to intracranial hemorrhage.

Nausea and vomiting are commonly seen with oral agents. Thus if at all, they should be with caution prior to surgery.

Diuresis is common and occurs due to the increased vascular volume as well as the effect of hyperosmotic agent itself. Thus anesthetized patients may require catheterization especially elderly patients with prostrate hypertrophy. When given preoperatively patients must be instructed to void before coming to the operating room.

They may precipitate **pulmonary edema and CCF** in patients with borderline cardiac and renal status. The side effects are dose related show minimum required dose must be given.

Renal failure is a contraindication for hyperosmotic use. The intravascular overload produced by the inability to excrete the large volume of fluid produces dilution and electrolyte imbalance in the form of hyponatremia and hypokalemia. This may lead to seizures or coma. The kidneys are also unable to excrete the hyperosmotic agent worsening the situation. The patients may require hemodialysis to prevent rapid neurological deterioration.

The conversion of glycerol into sugar can cause serious problems for **diabetic patients**, but it has the advantage of placing less strain on the renal system.

Intravenous administration of urea causes severe **local tissue necrosis**.

Thrombophlebitis has also been reported. In contrast extravasation of mannitol produces localized tissue swelling and thrombophlebitis is uncommon.

- Nausea and vomiting seen frequently with oral agents, presumably because of the heavy sweet taste. This is transient and can be minimized by serving it with lemon on ice.
- Diuresis is particularly problematic with IV agents and can lead to urinary retention in cases with enlarged prostate.
- Cardiovascular overload leading to CCF and pulmonary edema seen more in IV agents.
- Acidemia, anaphylactic reaction, backache, confusion and disorientation, diarrhea, giddiness seen more with IV agents.

Contd...

- Cerebral dehydration leading to stretch and subsequent rupture of the aqueous vein leading to life threatening subdural hematoma.

Contraindications

- Anuria
- Acute pulmonary edema
- Cardiovascular disorders
- Renal diseases

Topical Hyperosmotic Agents

Glycerol

Glycerol can be used as a diagnostic tool to clear corneal edema in eyes with epithelial edema. This can in turn permit visualization of the angle with gonioscopy. The effect is rapid and the cornea clears within 1-2 minutes of application. However it is short lasting and the dehydrating effect persists for 1-5 minutes.

Sodium Chloride

5% ointment and drops are available to chronically dehydrate corneas. The ointment has been shown to decrease stromal thickness upto 24%. A maximum effect is produced in 3-4 hours lasting for upto 7 hours. Blurring of vision, mild burning and irritation are common but minor side effects. The solution form has little effect on corneal thickness.

REFERENCES

1. Robbins R, Galin MA. Effect of osmotic agents on vitreous body. Arch Ophthalmol 1969;82:694-9.
2. Galin MA, Binkhorst RD, Kwitko ML. Ocular dehydration. Am J Ophthalmol 1968;66:233-5.
3. Virno M, Cantorre P, Bietti C, Bucci MG. Oral glycerol in ophthalmology: a valuable new method for the reduction of intra ocular pressure. Am J Ophthalmol 1963;55:1133-42.
4. Becker B, Kolker AE, Krupin T. Isosorbide, an oral hyperosmotic agent. Arch Ophthalmol 1967;78:147-50.
5. Weiss DI, Shaffer RN, Wise BL. Mannitol infusion to reduce intra ocular pressure. Arch Ophthalmol 1962;68:341-7.
6. Smith EW, Drance SM. Reduction of human intra ocular pressure with intravenous mannitol. Arch Ophthalmol 1962;68:734-7.

FIXED COMBINATIONS

One of the primary reasons for nonadherence in glaucoma is the inconvenience associated with eye drop instillation. In recent years the number and use of fixed combinations of IOP-lowering medications for treatment of glaucoma and ocular hypertension has grown substantially. The fixed combinations are important adjuncts to the armamentarium of available glaucoma therapies and offer critical options for patients who require more than one medication to control intraocular pressure. They are stable preparations of multiple active agents in a single bottle. Usually, fixed combinations contain 2 medications in a single bottle. Ideally a fixed combination should contain drugs that are safe and effective and that work well in combination with each other.

Advantages
This offers several advantages over concomitant use of the medications from separate bottles. These include:

- Increase in patient convenience that results from the use of fewer bottles
- Likely to lead to better adherence.
- No possibility of a washout effect
- No need to wait between instillation of the separate eye drops
- Daily exposure to preservatives be decreased
- Potential cost savings

Improving Adherence
One of the primary reasons for nonadherence in glaucoma is the inconvenience associated with eye drop instillation. There appears to be a closer relationship between adherence and the number of eye drops per day as compared to the number of medications. Fixed combinations reduce the burden of a complex glaucoma treatment regime and improve the patient's adherence to therapy. It is more convenient to instill 1 drop of a fixed combination than 2 drops from separate bottles of the component medications. Moreover less local side effects like ocular irritation, probably due to less exposure to preservatives may also improve compliance.

Therapeutic Effect
Some combinations may have a better IOP lowering effect when given as fixed combinations.

A substantial proportion of patients on multiple drops wait less than 3 minutes after taking an IOP-lowering medication before instilling a second medication. This results in a *washout effect* which can be avoided by using only 1 drop of a fixed combination. This indirectly increases the efficacy.

Ocular Surface Disorders
Ocular surface disease is significantly less common with fixed combination therapies as it decreases the exposure to preservatives. Exposure to BAK or other preservatives is significantly reduced as compared to patients on multiple unfixed medications. This reduces the chance of conjunctival inflammation and improves the chances of success of any future glaucoma surgery. Preservative free fixed combinations may be available in the near future.

Less Adverse Effects
Certain fixed combinations may have better safety profiles than their components monotherapy and in some cases may be better tolerated than the unfixed preparations. This can be due to a reduced exposure to preservatives and the presence of beta blocker (as in combination of Timolol and Brimonidine). A significantly lower incidence of treatment-related adverse events has been observed in patients treated with the fixed combination than in those treated with brimonidine alone.

Cost
Potential cost saving. The availability of generic fixed combinations is a potential advantage.

Limitations
Use as First Line of therapy
If a fixed combination is administered as a first line of treatment, the IOP lowering effect of the individual components cannot be confirmed. Nor can the side effect be attributed to one particular agent. This limits their use as first line agents in routine clinical practice. However, under certain circumstances they may be used as initial therapy. These include:

- More rapid IOP reduction in those patients presenting with either high pressure or advanced damage.
- A low target pressure. A reduction of greater than 30% in target pressure is not feasible with the currently available monotherapies. In such cases starting with a

fixed combination may be a better option.

- In patients where follow-up is an issue, a fixed combination as initial therapy may be used.

Efficacy

Although therapy is generally as efficacious as unfixed therapy, the IOP-lowering effect has not been quite as good as expected with some of the new fixed combinations, when compared with unfixed combinations of the same medicines. In such cases it is better to opt for unfixed therapy.

Advanced Glaucoma

In patients with advanced glaucoma where maximum reduction of pressure is essential, unfixed therapy may be the better option.

Flexibility

Fixed combinations provide a less flexible approach to patient care.

Limited Choice of Components

Most available fixed combinations currently contain timolol 0.5% solution, which may be risky if administered to elderly, patients with COPD and less efficacious in those who are already receiving beta-blocker therapy for other conditions.

Different Dosing Schedule

Enhanced reduction in pressure with some fixed combination may be less than originally anticipated. This could be due to timolol being used only once a day in prostaglandin and timolol fixed combination. The exact reasons are not clear. Moreover the dosing time for this combination is unclear. Unfixed combinations may have a small insignificant greater IOP reduction than the same medications. Dorzolamide and timolol combination compared to its individual components (Timolol 0.5% 2 times a day and Dorzolamide 3 times

a day) had a significantly reduced IOP reduction (0.7 mm Hg) at the morning trough.

CONCLUSION

Most studies involving fixed combinations include patients with ocular hypertension and primary open angle glaucoma. The applicability of these results to other glaucomas needs further investigations.

Currently, various studies comparing fixed with unfixed combinations do not take into account factors like enhanced adherence, improved convenience and reduced cost to patients. These factors form an important part of the clinical management of the patient and may translate to better IOP control.

> **Note** The treating clinician should consider the benefits of fixed versus unfixed therapy when switching uncontrolled patients to combination treatment or when initiating combination therapy.

43 | Laser Trabeculoplasty

Matthew C Willett, Todd E Woodruff, Deepak P Edward

ARGON LASER TRABECULOPLASTY

INTRODUCTION

The use of lasers to treat glaucoma was a subject of common research in the 1970's since the idea of noninvasively lowering intraocular pressure was highly appealing as an alternative to filtering surgery and glaucoma medications. However, early research with different lasers and techniques demonstrated poor long-term results.[1] In a paper by Wise and Witter in 1979, argon laser trabeculoplasty (ALT) was reported as an alternative to more invasive filtering surgery with minimal risks and high success rates.[1] Since then, many reports have outlined the technique, efficacy and utility of this procedure.

MECHANISM OF ACTION

In general, three different mechanisms of action of ALT have been postulated and studied; the mechanical, biologic (cellular), and repopulation theories.[2]

The mechanical theory suggests that the laser burns contract the trabecular meshwork resulting in the opening of Schlemm's canal.

The cellular theory suggests that laser photocoagulation causes a multitude of inflammatory and other biological reactions that result in increased outflow, whereas **the repopulation theory** states that ALT induces cell division and repopulation of the trabecular endothelial cells.

The Mechanical Theory

Wise and Witter's[1] initial hypothesis was that laser trabeculoplasty reduces IOP by increasing aqueous outflow. They calculated that as little as 1 percent contraction at each of the laser burns would reduce the trabecular ring diameter enough to open the intertrabecular spaces and widen Schlemm's canal. This was supported by the work of Rodrigues, et al[3] who

evaluated 22 trabeculectomy specimens from patients with prior ALT ranging from hours to one year prior to trabeculectomy. Using scanning and transmission electron microscopy, they observed early changes including "disruption of the trabecular beams, nuclear and cytoplasmic tissue debris, clusters of melanin pigment granules, fibrinous material, macrophages, and focal edema of corneal endothelial cells." Tissue excised at six months or later showed almost total obliteration of the trabecular beams as well as a membrane over the inner uveal meshwork at the burn sites. No evidence of trabecular puncture was noted. This refuted the premise that ALT disrupts the juxtacanalicular area, as histopathologic changes were limited to the inner portion of the TM. Wise and Witter agreed that the mechanism may lie in a circumferential contraction of the meshwork, causing opening of Schlemm's canal. Van der Zypen, however, postulated that focal scarring and contraction of the trabecular beams widened the adjacent intertrabecular spaces, thus increasing outflow facility independent of a circumferential affect.[4]

The Cellular Theory

Multiple arguments have been made against the mechanical theory. The most notable is that a decrease in pressure is observed with laser irradiation of the iris, ciliary body or cornea alone.[4] It is, therefore logical to speculate that mechanical change, atleast alone, is not the sole mechanism at play. Melamed and Epstein[5] performed ALT on monkey eyes and found support for the idea that it is the interburn areas that result in increased aqueous outflow. By using tracers they demonstrated a complete lack of flow at the area of laser burns, but increased labeling in the areas between spots. These areas showed juxtacanalicular herniations and vacuoles of the inner wall of Schlemm's canal. The authors theorized that stimulation of trabecular cells increased their biologic activity and resulted in removal of debris which is "clogging" the intertrabecular spaces. Some of these observations were supported by additional findings reported by Johnson[6] who evaluated 19-autopsy eyes that had undergone ALT during life. He found that the juxtacanalicular region expanded in eyes treated with ALT, with superimposed giant vacuoles partially filling Schlemm's canal. Although this finding was dependent on the type of fixation used, it was noted with significantly increased frequency in post ALT eyes compared to normal eyes and those with POAG who had not received laser treatment. He theorized that the opening of the trabecular lamellae between laser applications would result in increased aqueous flow, and that this increased flow, combined with the release of inflammatory factors caused the architectural changes in the juxtacanalicular trabecular meshwork.

Others have focused their research on the biologic effects of ALT. Parshley and associates[7] examined the effect of ALT on anterior segment organ cultures on stromelysin, a metalloproteinase that is thought to degrade trabecular proteoglycans. They observed a dramatic and sustained increase in stromelysin in the juxtacanalicular area, supporting their hypothesis that ALT induces biologic remodeling of the extracellular matrix, leading to increased aqueous outflow. Increase in other metalloproteinases, such as gelatinase 1, have also been reported.[4] Others have noted increased levels of prostaglandins, cytokines and macrophages following laser treatment, raising the possibility of their involvement in the therapeutic effect.[8,2]

The Repopulation Theory

Van Buskirk and Blysma[9,10] provided evidence suggesting that the principal factor in ALT might be the repopulation of cells in the trabeculum induced by ALT. Using organ-cultured trabecular meshwork subjected to ALT and then exposed to titrated thymidine, they demonstrated the incorporation of thymidine into trabecular cell DNA in the nonburned sites. This suggests that laser treatment stimulates the division of trabecular endothelial cells both inside and outside of the 180 degrees of treated area. Two weeks after laser exposure, these cells were noted to migrate from the region of Schwalbe's line to the area of the burns, possibly repopulating these areas. Masuyama's work on monkey eyes also argues against the mechanical theory, since ALT produced no change in the cross-sectional area of Schlemm's canal.

Whether through a mechanical or biologic mechanism, or a combination of both, there is general agreement that ALT lowers IOP by increasing outflow. Brubaker and Liesegang[11] showed a significant increase in the tonographic facility of outflow as well as a decreased apparent resistance to aqueous outflow following ALT. They also found a greater change in these parameters in patients who responded to ALT compared to nonresponders. Yablonski and associates[12] also evaluated outflow using fluorophotomteric and tonographic measurements, concluding the primary effect of ALT was to increase true outflow facility.

At this point, the exact mechanism of ALT remains elusive. Though studies show general agreement that it results in increased aqueous outflow, further study is needed to delineate the mechanism of action that leads to this result.

INDICATIONS

The utility of ALT was initially studied in patients with uncontrolled primary open-angle glaucoma. Additional studies found generally favorable responses in pigmentary glaucoma and pseudoexfoliation syndrome (XFS).

ALT was most often employed to prevent or postpone the need for more invasive filtering surgical procedures in patients who could not be controlled medically.

As more information regarding long-term results and safety became available, ALT was considered as a means to decrease patient medication load and as an initial treatment. The use of ALT as initial treatment was especially attractive in areas of the world where medication cost and availability are restrictive. Thomas and associates[13] treated 30 eyes with ALT as initial treatment. In an average follow-up period of over seven months, 83 percent of eyes avoided the need for further intervention. Rosenthal et al[14] treated 33 patients and found 55 percent of patients had successful lowering of

IOP (mean drop of 13 to 14 mm Hg) to levels negating the need to institute medical treatment, with a follow-up of six to eighteen months. The glaucoma laser trial (GLT) (described later in this chapter) evaluated initial treatment with ALT or timolol and found that the two were comparable.[15] With the advent of improved topical medications since the inception of ALT in the 1970s, however, using medication as a first line treatment is generally accepted in developed countries.

CONTRAINDICATIONS

Many forms of glaucoma respond less favorably to ALT. In some little response is noted, and in others ALT seems to worsen the disease. These include patients with uveitic glaucoma, iridocorneal endothelial syndrome (ICE) and those with developmental abnormalities of the trabecular meshwork; iridocorneal mesodermal dysgenesis, juvenile and congenital glaucoma.[16-18] Patients with congenital glaucoma generally show little to no response to ALT.[17] Thomas and associates[16] in a small series of three eyes with congenital glaucoma showed an average decrease in postoperative IOP of 3.3 mm Hg, and all patients underwent filtering surgery. Wilensky and Weinreb[18] reported no benefit of ALT in six eyes with juvenile glaucoma, and in two the IOP actually worsened.

Varying degrees of success have been reported with angle-recession glaucoma and angle-closure glaucoma, depending upon the amount of the angle involved. Pennebaker and Stewart[19] evaluated 50 eyes with varying anterior chamber anatomy and found reasonable effectiveness as long as the trabecular meshwork can be visualized.

TECHNIQUE

Since its inception, multiple studies have been done to determine the optimal technique for argon laser trabeculoplasty. In the original technique reported by Wise and Witter 100 burns were applied to 360 degrees of trabecular meshwork with laser settings of 0.1 second, 50 μm, and 1000 to 1500 mW.[1] Attempted modifications have included variations in power, time, extent, location of burns and mono vs. bichromatic laser.[20-26] The results of these studies have helped to minimize side effects and maximize intraocular pressure reduction.

Power Settings

A study by Rouhiainen and Teravirta compared power ranging from 0.1 to 1 W and found better results with 0.5 W or higher.[20] Rouhiainen et al[22] designed a study to evaluate laser power variations on the postoperative IOP elevation, as well as the overall effectiveness of the treatment. They randomized patients to 0.5, 0.7 and 0.9 W. There were no statistically significant differences in pressure lowering effect at one week between the groups. The mean postoperative IOP rise was lowest in the 0.5 W group and highest in the 0.9 W group. There was a statistically significant increase in immediate postoperative IOP in the 0.9 W group, and 75 percent of IOP spikes of 10 mm Hg or more were from the 0.9 W group. Rouhiainen also performed a trial comparing peripheral anterior synechiae formation using 0.5, 0.6, 0.7 and 0.8 W settings and found the only statistically significant increase in PAS was at 0.8 W.[27]

Duration

Blondeau et al[20] retrospectively compared duration of 0.2 to 0.1 seconds and found no significant differences in IOP or visual acuity. It is important to note that this study consisted of only 14 to 15 patients per group and a follow-up time of one week, making the results of limited clinical utility.

Hugkulstone conducted a similar study and found no difference in PAS formation or IOP lowering with evaluation up to 18 months.[28]

Number of Burns, Amount of Tissue Treated

Multiple studies have evaluated number of burns and amount of trabecular meshwork treated. Although, wise calculated that two sessions were not additive compared with full treatment at a single session, papers began to emerge evaluating a lower number of burns or dividing full treatment into multiple sessions.[29] Frenkel et al[21] compared either 50 burns to half of the trabecular meshwork or 35 burns to one-third and found no significant difference between groups. Weinreb et al[24] compared 50 burns over half to 100 burns over the entire trabecular meshwork and found no significant difference at 2 months. They did note a statistically significantly lower IOP at 2 months in eyes that did not have an IOP spike in the immediate postoperative period. They concluded that a 50 spot initial treatment was superior to 100 spots as it decreased the incidence of complications in the immediate postoperative period. The lack of benefit in treating the entire trabecular meshwork initially was also supported by Schwartz and associates.[26] Their study manipulated spot size, number of burns, extent of angle treated, and location of burns (anterior versus posterior trabecular meshwork). They found no differences except a smaller acute IOP rise in the anterior meshwork treatment group and a decreased effect if only 90 degrees was treated with 25 burns.

The acceptance of initially treating one-half of the trabecular meshwork led to several other studies. Klein and associates[25] evaluated a two stage approach, treating alternate 180 degree sections of the angle, separated by one month. They found that two-thirds of the total decrease in IOP occurred after a stage one treatment. They did find clinically useful decreases after stage two in some of the patients who showed little improvement in IOP after stage one. Their final recommendation was a single treatment of one-half of the trabecular meshwork. At one-month or more a second stage is used only if the IOP remains at an unacceptable level.

Grayson et al[23] postulated that because most people have more pigment in the inferior trabecular meshwork, the initial treatment should be done in that location to maximize effect. No differences were observed between the two groups, suggesting no advantage to location when partial treatment is performed.

Postoperative IOP Spikes

Most postoperative IOP spikes occur between three and four hours after treatment[30] and many studies have examined methods of preventing these IOP spikes. Rosenblatt and Luntz[31] studied the effect of technique on postoperative IOP spikes. They found further evidence that treatment with less than 0.81 W and anterior placement of laser burns was significantly associated with a lower risk of an IOP spike of greater than 10 mm Hg.

Multiple studies have evaluated a variety of glaucoma medications to minimize postoperative IOP spikes. These include alpha-adrenergic agonists, topical carbonic anhydrase inhibitors and pilocarpine. The **Brimonidine-ALT Study Group**[32] evaluated the combined results of 471 patients treated with brimonidine 0.5 percent before and/or after ALT, and found significantly lower postoperative IOP spikes with all regimens compared to vehicle alone. Rates of IOP rise greater than 10 mm Hg were 1 percent with brimonidine either before, or before and after, and 2 percent with

brimonidine used after treatment. Ren et al[33] compared prophylactic use of apraclonidine 1 percent to pilocarpine 4 percent in 228 patients undergoing ALT. While they found equivalent protection in both groups, they found a significantly improved response with one medication when the patient was on long-term use of the other medication. Dapling, Cunliffe and Longstaff[34] evaluated the postoperative pressure control of apraclonidine 1 percent and pilocarpine 4 percent alone and in combination. They reported a significant decrease in IOP spikes in the combination group compared to either agent alone. Only 8 percent of eyes in the combination group had a postoperative rise in IOP, and in all this was 1 mm Hg or less. None of the eyes in any group experienced an IOP rise greater than 10 mm Hg. In other studies, apraclonidine 1 percent and apraclonidine 0.5 percent were compared to brimonidine 0.2 percent and the results were equivalent.[35-37]

Carbonic anhydrase inhibitors have also shown effective prophylaxis in prevention of post ALT IOP spikes. Metcalfe and Etchells[38] evaluated oral acetazolamide 500 mg given one hour prior to ALT in a double-blind placebo-controlled trial of 100 eyes. It was found to have a significant protective effect, decreasing immediate IOP spikes from 92 percent in the placebo group to 18 percent. Incidence of IOP rise greater than 10 mm Hg was decreased from 30 to 0 percent. In one study, dorzolamide 2 percent showed prevention of post-ALT IOP spikes in 100 percent of patients treated.[39]

Various anti-inflammatory agents have been studied in patients undergoing ALT to decrease postoperative inflammation and PAS formation. Herbort and associates[40] evaluated post ALT inflammation in 53 eyes of patients with pseudoexfoliative or pigmentary glaucoma who received either diclofenac sodium

0.1 percent or placebo using a laser flare-cell meter (LFCM, Kowa FC-1000.) They choose these types of glaucoma based on previous work showing higher rates of postoperative inflammation compared to POAG.[41] In a double-blind study they found significantly less inflammation in the diclofenac group, ranging from 0 to 12 percent, compared to 52 to 64 percent for the placebo group (the range was based on the amount of measured flare they considered clinically relevant).

The Fluorometholone-Laser Trabeculoplasty Study Group evaluated 0.25 percent fluorometholone (given one day prior to and four times a day for six days after ALT) compared to placebo in a double-blind study.[42] They found that the fluorometholone group experienced significantly less inflammation compared to placebo. There was no difference in postoperative IOP spikes between the groups. The long-term results, with a mean average follow-up of over four years, showed no adverse outcome on the efficacy of ALT when fluorometholone was employed.[39,43]

Mittra and associates[30] evaluated the need for postoperative IOP monitoring. In a retrospective review of 407 ALT procedures with perioperative aproclonidine, they found that one day postoperative IOP elevations lacked predictive value for pressure elevation at one month, or for the eventual need for further therapy. They concluded that one day postoperative IOP checks were unnecessary.

In general, most practitioners now treat 180 degrees with 45 to 50 spots on the initial treatment.[28] Laser parameters typically used are a 50 μm spot size, duration of 0.1 seconds and intensity adjusted to cause mild blanching at the threshold of bubble formation. Patients are typically pretreated with a pressure lowering medication to prevent postoperative IOP spike, and then given a mild topical steroid or NSAID to use for the next four to six days after treatment.

EFFICACY

The utility of ALT has been evaluated in multiple settings **(Table 1)**. Many studies, especially those in the early development of ALT, focused on preventing or postponing filtering surgery in patients failing maximum medical therapy. Other studies looked at the effectiveness of ALT as initial treatment or to help patients decrease or eliminate topical medications.

In all studies, the ultimate "success" or "failure" of ALT treatment depended on the criteria used to quantify those terms. In the most basic sense, failure of ALT can be defined as an insufficient response necessitating the need for more invasive glaucoma surgery, principally trabeculectomy. The percentage of patients who successfully avoid filtering surgery after ALT depends on multiple factors, including, importantly, the length of follow-up of the particular study. A wide range of 'success' is seen in various studies, ranging from 10 to 94 percent.[16,17,44,45] Thomas and associates[16] found 87.5 percent of phakic patients avoided surgical intervention. Pollack and associates[46] followed 33 eyes of patients with POAG for 18 months and found 18 percent of eyes failed to have an adequate response to ALT and needed trabeculectomy.

As time progressed and long-term follow-up information became available, a decrease in efficacy of ALT was noted with time. This phenomenon is not unique to ALT, as the response to other interventions such as medication and surgery has been shown to decrease with time.[47] Fink and colleagues[48] followed patients up to 42 months and in their study defined success as IOP lower than baseline without progression of optic nerve cupping or visual field loss. The initial success rate was 75 percent, but it dropped to 45 percent at 42 months. There was a 23 percent reduction of IOP at three months, with the maximum reduction occurring at six to nine months. Grinich et al[45] found success rates of 79 percent at one year that dropped to 59 percent by three years. The 10-year results of AGIS showed a failure rate of 49.2 to 52.5 percent depending on race, but the difference between race was not statistically different.[49] Shingleton and colleagues[50] reported a 5-year failure rate on their series of 93 eyes to be 52 percent. A later paper from the same group reported a ten year Kaplan-Meier survival curve of 32 percent, while life-table analysis of the sixty eyes with POAG was similar at 31 percent.[51] They also noted that eyes with successful IOP control at 1 year had a chance of success at ten years of 42 percent. Other ten year reports

Table 1 ALT studies

Study	Study size	Treatment	Follow-up	Definition of success	IOP reduction	Response rate	Comments
Thomas and associates[5]	334 eyes	360° in 1 or 2 sessions	Up to 21 months	No filtering surgery	7.1 mm Hg	87.5%	
Pollack and associates[17]	33 eyes	360°	18 months	No filtering surgery	12 mm Hg	82%	
Fink and colleagues[13]	82 eyes	360°	42 months (mean 24.5 months)	IOP < 22 mm Hg and no progression	N/A	45%	
Grinich et al[22]	112 eyes	360° in 1 or 2 sessions	36 months	IOP < 22 mm Hg and no progression	N/A	79%-1 years 59%-3 years	No sustained difference between XFS and POAG
AGIS4	776 eyes		10 years			50%	
Shingleton and colleagues[23,24]	118 eyes	360°	60 months	IOP < 19 mm Hg, ↓ IOP 2 mm Hg and no progression	8.9 ± 5.2 mm Hg at 10 years	77%-1 years 32%-10 years	
Thomas and associates[19]	30 eyes	360°	7 months	No need for further intervention	10.1 mm Hg	83%	ALT as initial treatment
Glaucoma laser trial (GLT)[54]	271 patients	360° in 2 sessions	9 years	No filtering surgery	7-10 mm Hg	92%	ALT as initial treatment. May have received medication or retreatment during follow-up
Schultz et al[15]	19 patients	360°	12 months	Stable visual field	N/A	74%	

have cited failure rates from around 45 percent[29,47] to over 90 percent.[17]

Considering that all of the above results are based on eyes with significant disease refractory to medical treatment, such that the patients were suitable for filtering surgery, one may question whether a different failure rate would be observed in eyes treated by ALT at the time of initial diagnosis. As described previously, Rosenthal and associates[14] evaluated 33 eyes with primary open-angle glaucoma using ALT as the primary treatment. Only two eyes required filtering surgery. Thomas and associates[13] treated 30 eyes with ALT as initial treatment. In an average follow-up period of over seven months 83 percent of eyes avoided the need for further intervention.

The Glaucoma Laser Trial

The glaucoma laser trial (GLT) was a multicenter, randomized clinical trial that compared initial treatment of primary open-angle glaucoma with ALT versus 0.5 percent timolol.[15] At two years, eyes initially treated with ALT had an IOP 2 mm Hg lower than eyes initially treated with timolol. When followed for up to 9 years they found that initial treatment with ALT was atleast as beneficial as starting with timolol in terms of IOP control, visual field changes, change in cup to disc area and eventual need for filtering surgery. The rate of failure for each group, if defined as the need for filtering surgery, was 8 percent for the ALT group and 11 percent for the medication group. It is important to note that these were the initial treatment in each group, and after this point both groups were eligible for all treatments possible, i.e. patients initially treated with ALT may have later been placed on medication and vice versa.

EFFECT ON DIURNAL PRESSURE

Argon laser trabeculoplasty (ALT) has also been reported to have a favorable effect on glaucomatous diurnal curves. It has been reported that eyes with glaucoma have larger variations of IOP throughout the day, and that this variation can be linked to glaucoma damage independent of the mean IOP.[52] Greenidge et al[52] studied twenty-five patients for eight weeks after ALT and found mean IOP reduction of 22 percent, mean peak pressure decrease of 25 percent, mean pressure range decrease of 30 percent and decreased pressure fluctuations of 25 percent. Schultz et al[53] prospectively followed the visual fields of 19 patients after ALT and also found that decreased variance in IOP was associated with stability of visual fields. They reported a 74 percent success rate defined by a stable visual field for up to one year.

Mean Decrease in IOP

The reported mean decrease in IOP from baseline ranges from 4.9 to 10 mm Hg.[1,16,47,51] An important factor in the amount of pressure reduction resulting from ALT is the baseline IOP. Multiple studies have shown that the decrease in IOP, both in absolute and terms of percentage, is proportional to pretreatment IOP levels (i.e. eyes with higher baseline IOP experience greater decrease in IOP).[16,25,45,54-56] This includes eyes that were retreated.[57] AGIS,[58] however, reported that higher preintervention IOP's were associated with ALT failure, suggesting that although patients with higher IOP may experience greater reductions, this may not be sufficient to stabilize their disease. Sharpe and Simmons[56] studied 85 eyes with IOP below 20 mm Hg, for an average of 30 months, to observe the affect of ALT on patients with lower starting pressure. They noted 13 percent of eyes progressed to needing subsequent filtering surgery, a more frequent occurrence than seen in most studies involving higher starting IOPs.

Decrease in Number of Medications

The utility of ALT to allow patients to decrease the number of topical medications has been studied, as the benefit to both cost percentage and compliance would be a strong indication for ALT if it proved successful, especially in certain patient populations. Success rates range from around 30.4 percent[16] to 61 percent.[46] Vaidergorn and Susanna[59] studied 73 patients with well controlled glaucoma to see if ALT could allow patients to discontinue medications while maintaining adequate control of the disease. With a mean follow-up of over 16 months, 54.9 percent of patients had successfully discontinued at least one topical hypotensive medication without significant change in IOP compared to baseline.

Eyes with Previous Glaucoma Surgery

Few reports have addressed the use of ALT in patients with previous glaucoma surgery. The ability of patients treated with ALT to avoid additional glaucoma surgery in one such study was 56.6 percent.[16]

EFFECT OF PATIENT CHARACTERISTICS

Factors shown to influence the efficacy of argon laser trabeculoplasty include pretreatment IOP level (discussed above), lens status, type of glaucoma, patient age, race, and iris color.[8,16,17,47,49,53,58,60,61]

Lens Status

Outcomes of ALT are generally less favorable in aphakic patients compared to phakic or pseudophakic patients.[16,17] Thomas and associates[16] found 87.5 percent of phakic compared to 62.1 percent of aphakic eyes avoided surgical intervention. Schwartz, Wilson and Schwartz[61] analyzed the records of 63 aphakic and pseudophakic patients and found pseudophakic patients had a significantly superior response. They concluded that although 60 percent of aphakic patients had an unsuccessful treatment (with success defined by decrease in IOP of 3 mm Hg or more, final IOP less than 21 mm Hg and no need for further intervention) ALT should still be considered in this population as they are often older patients with multiple comorbidities.

Secondary Open-Angle Glaucoma

Few of the original studies on ALT focused on its effect in secondary forms of open-angle glaucoma. Robin and Pollack addressed this paucity of information in a pilot study of 55 eyes of 46 patients.[62] The forms of glaucoma included pigmentary (11 eyes), pseudoexfoliation (XFS) (4 eyes), angle-closure after iridotomy (4 eyes), phakic eyes after previous filtration surgery (7 eyes), aphakic eyes (6 eyes), aphakic eyes after previous filter (6 eyes), congenital glaucoma (4 eyes), uveitic glaucoma (8 eyes), angle-recession glaucoma (4 eyes), and Sturge-Weber syndrome (2 eyes.) In general, they found that 73 percent of patients had a response sufficient to avoid filtering surgery, 53 percent of which achieved IOP control with fewer medications. Looking at each individual disease category, pigmentary glaucoma patients had a postoperative IOP below 22 mm Hg in eight of eleven eyes. All patients with pseudoexfoliation avoided further surgery, as did all with previous angle-closure glaucoma followed by successful iridotomy, patients with Sturge-Weber and aphakic patients. Six of seven eyes with previous filter avoided additional filtering surgery. Of note, no statistically significant decrease in IOP was noted following ALT in patients with uveitic, angle-recession and congenital glaucoma.

Pseudoexfoliative and Pigmentary Glaucoma

Pseudoexfoliative and pigmentary glaucoma have been the subject of multiple other studies and have generally been found to demonstrate an excellent response to ALT.[29,45,47,55] Ritch, Pollack and Levene[63] retrospectively analyzed 32 eyes of patients with pigmentary glaucoma to determine the long-term response in this subset. Thirty four percent of eyes eventually required filtering surgery at an average of 12 months. Success rates, defined as IOP less than 21 mm Hg and lack of need for filtering surgery, were 80 percent at 1 year, dropping to 45 percent at 6 years. Interestingly, younger patients had a significantly higher success rate at 6 years by life-table analysis, when compared to older subjects. This is contrary to results normally seen in patients with primary open-angle glaucoma, in which younger patients generally show poorer responses to ALT.[29,45,64] The authors hypothesized that this is due, at least in part, to the location of pigment in different age groups in pigmentary glaucoma. They note that pigment in surgical specimens of younger patients is most dense in the uveoscleral and corneoscleral meshwork, contrasting to dense pigment primarily in the corneoscleral meshwork and external wall of Schlemm's canal in older patients. They postulated that it is the increased energy absorption by the cells surrounding Schlemm's canal in older patients which may adversely affect ALT results.

Lehto[65] reported long-term results on his series of nine patients with pigmentary glaucoma. In this small series, the initial pressure-lowering effect was 53 percent which decreased to 14 percent (4 mm Hg) over time. The failure rate as defined by need for filtering surgery was 11 percent (one patient) at the end of 5.5 years. It is important to note that three of the nine eyes in this series only received 180 degrees of treatment with ALT, and the author does not indicate if the failure patient received a second treatment. Also, the mean number of laser applications was 68.5 burns for 180 degrees and 143.3 burns for 360 degrees, which is higher than what is generally considered standard treatment.

Threlkeld et al[66] compared long-term results of ALT in 66 eyes with primary open-angle glaucoma (POAG) to 29 eyes with pseudoexfoliative glaucoma (XFS). They followed these patients for three years and compared results using three different measures of failure. Defining failure as need for glaucoma surgery, failure rates at 1 year were 9 percent for the POAG eyes and 8 percent for XFS eyes. By 3 years rates for both groups were 22 percent. Next, defining failure as need for glaucoma surgery or a third laser treatment, at 1 year failure rates were 11 percent for POAG and 8 percent for XFS, changing to 24 percent (POAG) and 39 percent (XFS) by year 3. The most encompassing failure mode was defined as glaucoma surgery, third laser treatment, 2 IOP measurements greater than 22 mm Hg, or IOP greater than 85 percent of baseline. One year failure rates were 40 percent (POAG) and 18 percent (XFS) and 3 year failure rates were 58 percent (POAG) and 47 percent (XFS.) The 3 year results were not statistically different by log-rank tests. The conclusion of this study was that although patients with XFS initially show a more favorable response to ALT than those with primary open-angle glaucoma, this response fades with time and approximates that of patients with POAG by 3 years. Grinich and associates[45] also found no significant difference in success and failure rates in XFS vs POAG at three years, and Shingleton and colleagues[51] found no significant difference up to ten years.

Sherwood and Svedbergh[54] reported on 55 eyes of patients with XFS. Success in their study was defined as a decrease in mean IOP of 20 percent and no 2 consecutive IOPs greater than 21 mm Hg. Thirty-eight percent received only 180 degrees of treatment, while the remainder received full treatment in a two stage approach separated by weeks. 74 percent of patients had a successful response at 1 year based on their criteria. Analysis of 24 hour diurnal curves showed an average decrease in peak IOP of 8.4 mm Hg corresponding to a 28 percent reduction from baseline, and a 34 percent decrease in the fluctuation of the pressure curve. Comparing patients with baseline mean IOP of less than 21 mm Hg to those greater than 21 mm Hg, success rates were 30 percent compared to 79 percent respectively. Exfoliation glaucoma does, therefore, demonstrate a greater response in patients with higher baseline IOP just as seen in other forms of glaucoma. An additional finding was that 16 percent of patients had a postoperative IOP spike of 10 mm Hg or greater, suggesting that patients with pseudoexfoliative glaucoma need closer monitoring in the initial hour following ALT.

Patient Age

Patient's age may affect the response to ALT. In general patients of younger age tend to respond less favorably, especially those less than 40 years old.[16,29,58] This is based on studies of primary open-angle glaucoma, but the opposite may be true in younger patients with pigmentary glaucoma as discussed elsewhere in this chapter. Safran and associates[64] found that 60 percent of eyes of patients with POAG under 40 years of age failed treatment with ALT and needed filtering surgery within two years. This was compared to only a 7 percent failure rate in eyes of older PAOG patients. In general, most believe that younger aged patients with POAG and uncontrolled pressures are unlikely to avoid filtering procedures. If ALT is offered to younger patients, they should be counseled on the need for frequent follow-up and likelihood of eventual failure.

Race

Differences in efficacy depending on race have been noted in several studies with conflicting results. Studies have shown that blacks have more advanced disease at initial diagnosis and greater frequency of blindness from the disease, raising the question as to whether glaucoma damage is more rapid in this subset or simply discovered later.[47,55,60]

The Advanced Glaucoma Intervention Study (AGIS) randomized eyes with uncontrolled primary open-angle glaucoma into two possible treatment sequences; ALT-trabeculectomy-trabeculectomy (ATT) or trabeculectomy-ALT-trabeculectomy (TAT).[49,58,60] These patients were then followed for up to ten years. The authors noted a statistically significant difference in response according to race. At four years of follow-up, the outcome in white patients favored the TAT sequence.[60] The opposite was found in black patients, with a more effective decrease in progression noted in the ATT sequence. Another consistent difference noted was that on average black patients were prescribed more medications. They concluded that ALT retards glaucoma progression more effectively in black patients than white patients. In a later report detailing 10 year follow-up information, initial ALT and initial trabeculectomy failed at rates that were equal between the races.[49,58] More importantly, though, visual acuities were worse in black patients having initial trabeculectomy compared to those having initial laser, and the difference persisted through the 10 years of the study. This result is not unexpected, since trabeculectomy is linked to cataract formation with resultant reduction in visual acuity. Since white patients, on average, had cataract surgery earlier that

black patients, it is problematic to draw comparisons between the visual acuity outcomes between the two races. White patients had less visual field loss in the TAT sequence compared to white patients in the ATT sequence after 1.5 years and subsequent follow-up of up to ten years.

Schwartz and colleagues[47] initially noted no difference in the results of ALT with regards to race in their series of 82 eyes. However, with long-term follow-up of up to 54 months they noted a decreased response to ALT in black patients. With success defined as stable visual field and nerve appearance, as well as decreased IOP of at least 3 mm Hg, they found that ALT was successful in 65 percent of white patients but only 32 percent of black patients. Congruent with this they found patients with blue irides did better than those with brown irides. Kaplan-Meier survival curves showed that the median time before reaching an IOP greater than 21 mm Hg was 12 months for black patients and 60 months for white patients.

Other studies have failed to show a difference of response in black compared to white patients. In Wise's original series, he noted excellent response of blacks and Native Americans to ALT.[44] Although the number of eyes of black patients was small, Thomas and associates[16] failed to find a racial difference in treatment response in their series. Krupin and associates[55] compared 2 year results of 68 black patients and 42 white patients and found no difference in average failure rate or IOP. They note that they only compared patients with primary open-angle glaucoma and excluded patients with pseudoexfoliative and pigmentary glaucoma, secondary forms of glaucoma which are more common in white patients and are known to respond favorably to ALT.

RETREATMENT

Multiple studies have evaluated the utility of repeat treatment with ALT. In all of the studies listed, retreatment was performed on eyes with previous favorable and sustained response to the initial 360 degree ALT treatment. Brown and associates[57] reported successful retreatment rates of 38 percent at six weeks, defined as obviating the need for further surgical intervention and with an average decrease in IOP of 10.2 mm Hg. Messner et al[67] found similar results of 36 percent at six weeks, which decreased to 21 percent by six months.

Grayson and colleagues[8] defined success by four criteria; IOP below 21 mm Hg or decreased 15 percent, no filtering procedure needed, no further ALT, no progression on disc exam or visual field testing. In their results they found 78 percent success at three months and 73 percent at 12 months. Of note, the initial treatment for the majority of these patients was 65 burns compared with the standard 100. They were retreated with approximately 50 burns. When the subgroup of patients with standard treatment was evaluated separately, a 43 percent success rate at 12 months was noted, which is closer to other studies. Jorizzo et al[68] reported 14 eyes that received retreatment of 40 to 50 burns per 180 degrees, and found that 73 percent experienced a significant decrease in IOP at one year (average reduction in IOP was 14 mm Hg for the 180 degree group and 12 mm Hg for the 360 degree group at six weeks.)

Another study by Richter and associates[69] found IOP control at 1 year of 33 percent, and only 14.5 percent at 1.75 years. Feldman and colleagues[70] followed 50 eyes of 44 patients until pressure control was lost. They found 21 percent of eyes maintained the desired response at one year but none

maintained an adequate pressure response for 5 years. They conclude that at best retreatment with ALT serves as a temporizing measure, and at worst delays definitive treatment until further damage has occurred.

A proposed mechanism for retreatment failure as well as late ALT failure is the formation of a membrane in the chamber angle after treatment. In a study of trabeculectomy specimens of 54 eyes previously treated with ALT and 64 control specimens, Koller and associates[71] found a significantly higher incidence of membranes in eyes treated with ALT. They also found that this was directly proportional to the number of 360 degree treatments.

In general, few would advocate additional ALT after a total of 360 degree treatment. With the advent of new medications, SLT, and better surgical techniques, better options are available and should be utilized in most instances.

COMPLICATIONS

Multiple complications have been reported with ALT. In considering these, it is important to note the initial studies were done using more energy than is typically used today. In addition, preoperative and postoperative medications were not always used, or inconsistently used, in early studies. As techniques and adjunctive medications have evolved, fewer and less frequent complication rates are encountered. Complications reported include:[16,31,71,72]

- Iritis
- Formation of peripheral anterior synechiae (PAS)
- Membrane formation in the chamber angle
- Postoperative IOP spikes
- Loss of the central island of vision secondary to IOP spikes.

The most worrisome complication of ALT is postoperative spikes in IOP. Using the original settings specified by Wise and Witter, the incidence of these spikes ranged from 36 percent[37] to 46 percent[52] and a postoperative IOP spike of 10 mm Hg or more was seen in 1.6 percent[61] to 33 percent.[55] In the AGIS report of 458 eyes that underwent ALT as first or second intervention, IOP spikes occurred in 3.3 percent.[58]

Risk factors for IOP spikes have been conflicting. Some studies showed transient increases in intraocular pressure were associated with moderate to heavy pigmentation of the trabecular meshwork.[15] Others have shown them to be associated with posterior placement of laser burns and energy over 0.8 watts.[31] Multiple studies evaluating prophylactic treatment with topical medications show reduced incidence of postoperative IOP spikes, with many reporting no IOP spikes greater than 5 to 10 mm Hg.[34-36,39]

The exact mechanism of the postoperative IOP spike is debatable. Multiple studies on both human and monkey eyes have reported immediate evaluation of ALT burns shows multiple areas of debris, pigment and architectural disruption, which may play a part in the postoperative IOP spikes.[17,73] Hollo and colleagues[74] found an immediate increase in aqueous humour endothelin 1 concentration in rabbits after ALT, which was associated with IOP spikes. This has been shown to cause increased IOP when given exogenously, suggesting this molecule may be the etiology of immediate post-ALT IOP spikes. No data from humans regarding the role of this molecule has yet been reported.

Iritis resulting from ALT is generally reported as mild and lasting less than one week.[16,58] Mermoud, Pittet and Herbort[41] reported inflammation patterns of 71 eyes after 180 degree ALT treatments, measured with a laser flare-cell meter (LFCM, Kowa FC-1000). They found that the anterior chamber inflammation peaked two days after treatment and was found in 49 percent of eyes. It was significantly more frequent in eyes with pigmentary glaucoma and with exfoliation syndrome compared with POAG. The authors note that the greater laser absorption in pigmentary glaucoma could be an explanation for the higher intensity and frequency of inflammation noted in this group, and that previous studies have demonstrated that patients with exfoliation syndrome also show a greater inflammatory reaction with all surgery. In each of the 17 eyes that had inflammation that was deemed significant enough to treat, the inflammation resolved completely with topical diclofenac sodium.

Peripheral anterior synechiae formation after ALT has been reported in 0.7[58] to 47.1 percent of patients.[16] Most of these are small peaked synechiae to the level of the scleral spur, with larger synechiae to the level of the trabecular meshwork present in 27 percent.[16] Even these larger PAS did not appear to alter the IOP response and success rates in some studies, though other studies have shown smaller IOP decreases in these eyes.[16] PAS formation was reported to be more frequent in brown iris color in one study, and found to have no relation in another.[15,72] Rouhiainen, Markku and Erkki[72] studied the correlation between laser burn location and energy used, and PAS formation. Of the 120 eyes that received ALT treatment the laser burns were directed either on the anterior or posterior border of the pigmented band and with laser power levels of 500, 600, 700 or 800 mW. They found that with 500 mW laser power and anterior burns no PAS developed. With 800 mW posterior burns 40 percent of eyes developed PAS. Significant differences were found between power groups, suggesting that PAS incidence increases as power settings increase. PAS were also significantly more frequent with posterior burns, which has been reported in other studies as well.[15]

Other reported complications include hemorrhage from the trabecular meshwork, which is rare, with a reported incidence of 2.3[16] to 5 percent.[44] No adverse affect on IOP was reported. Stürmer et al[75] reported on risk factors for trabeculectomy failure in young patients and found a significant deleterious relationship to previous ALT.

Conclusion

In the past 30 years, ALT has been accepted as a useful treatment for various forms of glaucoma. Its efficacy in postponing or negating the need for more invasive filtering surgeries is well documented. It has relatively few complications, especially compared to these more invasive procedures. Modifications of laser settings as well as adjunctive medications have given good long-term results in many patients. Even with the advent of new, safer, and more effective drugs in the ophthalmologist's armamentarium, ALT continues to be used and studied as an effective treatment for various forms of glaucoma.

SELECTIVE LASER TRABECULOPLASTY

INTRODUCTION

Despite the widespread popularity of ALT, the procedure has shortcomings, principal among them being the significant tissue disruption and coagulation damage caused by the laser. Some believed the biological events brought on by ALT may lead to membrane formation over the trabecular meshwork leading to late failures, and others suggested it may lead to an increased rate of bleb encapsulation in subsequent trabeculectomies.[76] Researchers continued to evaluate different wavelengths and techniques with the hope of finding an alternative that would be more efficacious and/or cause fewer complications when used for laser trabeculoplasty.

Studies began to emerge using the Nd:YAG laser. This laser, when compared to argon gas laser had the advantage of smaller size, longer operating life, and high electrical to optical efficiency.[77] Kwasniewska and associates,[78] in a 1993 report, evaluated 106 eyes treated with trabeculoplasty using a **continuous wave Nd:YAG laser**. Success was defined as reduction in IOP to 22 mm Hg or less without further laser or surgical intervention. Success rates at 6, 12 and 24 months were 83.3 percent, 78.7 and 71.5 percent respectively. They concluded that Nd:YAG laser trabeculoplasty was a safe and effective alternative to ALT. Latina and colleagues published the first results of a multicenter pilot study of trabeculoplasty using a **Q-switched 532-nm Nd:YAG laser** in 1998.[79] There are several proposed advantages of the Q-switched, frequency doubled Nd:YAG (532 nm) laser over a continuous wave or free running mode that has a wavelength of 1064 nm. Most importantly, the optical absorption by melanin increases with shorter wavelengths, thus the same effect can be achieved with a lower energy.[77] Additionally, based on Latina's previous work with Park, the very short exposure time of the Q-switched YAG resulted in the selective targeting of pigmented TM cells without causing as much thermal or collateral damage. **The more precise selection of the target tissue led to the name selective laser trabeculoplasty (SLT)**. Since then, multiple studies have been done to evaluate this new treatment modality.

MECHANISM OF ACTION

One of the principal arguments for SLT is that it causes little or no ultrastructural damage to the trabecular meshwork.[80] Latina and Park[81] experimented using Q-switched Nd:YAG and frequency-doubled Nd:YAG lasers, as well as other lasers, and found that selective cytotoxity and death of pigmented trabecular meshwork cells, without change to adjacent nonpigmented cells, could be achieved with pulse duration of 1 microsecond or less. The lack of structural change in eye subjected to SLT, which has a duration far less than 1 millisecond, leads to the question of its mechanism of action.

Despite the apparent lack of structural change in initial reports, the damaging effects of ALT and SLT are conflicting. Kramer and Noecker[82] studied the affect of ALT and SLT on human autopsy eyes using scanning and transmission electron microscopy. They found that ALT caused crater formation, coagulative damage, and disruption of the trabecular beams. Evaluation of the post-SLT eyes showed only cracking of intracytoplasmic pigment granules and disruption of the trabecular endothelial cells **(Figures 1A and B)** Cvenkel and co-workers,[83] using both light and transmission electron microscopy, evaluated the affect of SLT and ALT administered to eyes 1 to 5 days prior to planned enucleation. They found that both lasers caused splitting and fragmentation of the trabecular beams, but to a lesser extent in the SLT group. They also noted better preservation of long-spacing collagen with the SLT-treated eyes. The actual significance of these findings is currently unknown.

They suggested that SLT may work at the cellular level through phagocytosis by macrophages or stimulation of new healthy TM growth.

To date a definitive mechanism for SLT has not been clearly elucidated. Although reports of the amount of damage induced are conflicting, all show that it is less than that observed with ALT. Whether the mechanism is the same as that of ALT or through a different mechanism remains to be determined.

INDICATIONS

Selective laser trabeculoplasty (SLT) is indicated in the treatment of open-angle glaucoma, PXF and pigmentary glaucoma. It is considered safe and effective in patients previously treated with ALT.[79,84] It is also considered safe in forms of glaucoma which are relatively contraindicated for ALT, including juvenile and inflammatory glaucoma.[84,85]

Rubin et al[86] retrospectively reviewed the charts of 7 patients (7 eyes) on maximal medical therapy secondary to intravitreal steroid-induced elevated IOP who were treated with SLT. They noted a rapid decrease in IOP by three weeks, and five of seven patients were able to avoid further surgery after one or two SLT treatments.

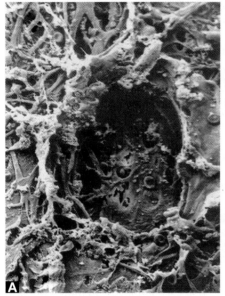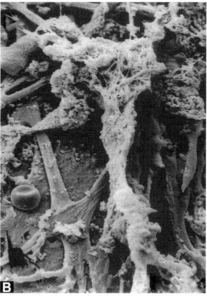

Figs 1A and B Argon laser trabeculoplasty, energy 0.7 mJ/pulse, 50 mm spot. (A) There is disruption of the rope-like components of the uveal meshwork portion of the trabecular meshwork, creating an ablation crater measuring 95 × 3 × 70 mm (arrows). There was scrolling, whitening, and bleb formation of the surrounding collagen, (original magnification, 3469); (B) Higher magnification shows there is scrolling, whitening, and bleb formation of the collagen indicative of coagulative damage, (original magnification, 31210). (Reproduced with permission from Ophthalmology, Vol 108, Kramer TR, Noecker RJ, Comparison of the morphologic changes after selective laser trabeculoplasty and argon laser trabeculoplasty in human eye bank eyes, 773-9, Copyright Elsevier)

CONTRAINDICATIONS

At this point, SLT is contraindicated in closed angle glaucoma. No contraindication to pigmentary glaucoma or heavily pigmented glaucoma exists, although such patients should be treated with caution as marked and sustained postoperative IOP spikes have been reported in some such cases.[76,90] No studies have been reported on congenital glaucoma or other forms of glaucoma with developmental abnormalities of the angle structures.

TECHNIQUE

The original technique outline by Latina et al[79] used a Coherent Selecta 7000 laser, a frequency-doubled Q-switched Nd:YAG laser emitting at 532 nm with a pulse duration of 3 nsec and a spot size of 400 μm. A Goldman

three-mirror goniolens was used with methylcellulose 1 percent after topical anesthetic. The helium-neon aiming beam was focused on the pigmented trabecular meshwork, and energy was set at 0.8 mJ for the first spot and then decreased or increased in 0.1 mJ increments to between 0.2 and 1.7 mJ until no visible affects on the TM or bubble formation was noted. Fifty adjacent but not overlapping laser spots were placed over 180 degrees. After treatment, prednisolone acetate 1 percent drops were administered and continued four times a day for five days. Postoperative IOP was measured at one and two hours and continued if an IOP rise greater than 5 mm Hg was noted.

In a later paper by Latina and Leon,[84] the desired endpoint is described as "tiny champagne bubbles" with 50 percent of laser spots. They also advocate

pretreatment with apraclonidine (0.5%) to prevent postoperative IOP spikes. As a result of studies showing that a post-SLT macrophage response may contribute to IOP lowering, they advocated either no postoperative anti-inflammatory medications or ketorlac tromethamine 0.4 percent or prednisolone acetate 1 percent three times a day for 3 to 4 days as reasonable treatment options. They also noted that patients with heavier pigment, as seen in pigmentary and pseudoexfoliative glaucoma amongst others, should be treated with lower energy to reduce IOP spikes.

Prasad and associates[87] retrospectively studied the efficacy of 180 and 360 degree SLT treatments as initial treatment in patients with OAG or OHT with a 6 to 24 month follow-up. No significant difference in baseline IOP was noted between the groups, but at two years patients had a mean IOP reduction of 28 percent in the 180 degree group and 35 percent in the 360 degree group. Other studies have supported the finding that a 360 degree treatment in one or two stages is more efficacious than 180 degree treatment alone.[76] Although, IOP fluctuation less than 3 mm Hg was not statistically different between the groups, IOP fluctuation less than 2 mm Hg was, and odds of achieving IOP fluctuation less than 2 mm Hg were 5.7 times greater in the 360 degree group with follow-up period of 6 to 24 months. The authors point out that IOP fluctuation has been identified as a possible independent risk factor for visual field loss.

George and colleagues[88] retrospectively studied the effect of overlapping SLT spots. SLT with overlapping spots was compared to nonoverlapping spots and ALT. SLT with nonoverlapping burns and ALT were found to be equivalent; however SLT with overlapping spots showed a significantly reduced efficacy.

Several studies have evaluated the difference in absolute pressure reduction between patients treated postoperatively with non-steroidal anti-inflammatory agents compared to topical steroid treatment. No statistical difference has been observed, suggesting the use of these medications to alleviate postoperative pain and inflammation has no deleterious effect on the results of treatment.[89,90]

EFFICACY

Studies have shown SLT to be effective as a primary treatment, in patients on maximal tolerated medical therapy to postpone or avoid filtering surgery, and to decrease patient dependence on topical medication. Average IOP reduction has been reported from 18 percent to 40 percent **(Table 2)**.[76,79]

In the initial report by Latina et al[79] 53 patients with uncontrolled open-angle glaucoma underwent SLT. These patients included a group with previous ALT and one without previous ALT. At 26 weeks the average decrease in baseline IOP for all eyes was 18.7 percent (4.6 mm Hg). Defining success as 3 mm Hg or more decrease in IOP from baseline, both groups showed 70 percent success. Kim and Moon[91] reported on sixteen eyes and found a 20 percent reduction in IOP at one year. Birt[92] compared SLT, SLT after ALT and ALT and reported one year decrease in IOP of 23 percent, 19.3 and 24 percent

respectively. There was no statistical difference between groups. Average reported decreases in IOP from baseline at one year range from around 4 to 5 mm Hg[91-93] to around 8 mm Hg.[89]

Nagar and Shah[86,93] evaluated the effect of SLT or latanoprost on the diurnal tension curves of forty patients with OAG or OHT. At six months the reduction in IOP fluctuation was 50 percent for SLT and 83 percent for latanoprost, which was a statistically significant difference. Of note is the fact that the SLT group had a statistically significant higher baseline IOP, and diurnal tension curves were not evaluated over 24 hour periods. McIlraith et al[89] studied one year results utilizing either SLT or latanaprost as an initial treatment for patients with OAG or OHT and found equivalent results between the two groups. IOP reduction was 31 percent in the SLT and 30.6 percent in the latanoprost group.

Other studies have evaluated not only the efficacy of SLT as initial treatment, but also the possible cost benefit ratio. Mao et al[90] used a cohort of 268 eyes to develop a prediction rule to estimate the probability of acceptable IOP reduction after SLT in OAG and OHT. Defining efficacy as a minimum postoperative IOP reduction of 20 percent or more at 6 months, they found SLT efficacy is positively associated with IOP elevation before treatment and negatively associated with maximum

IOP recorded. They theorized that the findings are related to the timing of SLT. The findings appear to result from the fact that in initial treatment, higher pressures were associated with a better chance of a 20 percent drop in IOP, but in eyes on maximum medical therapy, the opposite was true; higher IOPs were associated with less chance of lowering the IOP by 20 percent. They suggest that these findings support the premise that SLT is most efficacious as a primary therapy in treatment naïve eyes. Lee and Hutnik[94] evaluated the projected cost comparison of SLT versus hypotensive medication. If SLT was expected to be repeated every two years, a comparison to mono-, bi-, and tri-drug therapy produced a six year cost savings of $206.54, $1668.64 and $2992.67 per patient, respectively. If the above scenario was changed for repeat SLT every three years, the costs savings change to $580.52, $2040.82 and $3366.65 per patient, respectively. Other studies have been done which show 87 percent of patients treated with SLT were able to decrease drug usage by an average of 1.5 medications, measured at one year after trabeculoplasty.[76]

EFFECT OF PATIENT CHARACTERISTICS

Multiple studies show no difference in response to SLT based on differences in sex, race, diabetes, hypertension, previous treatment with ALT,

Table 2 SLT studies (Modified from paper by Barkana and Belkin[90])

Study	Study size	Treatment	Follow-up	Definition of success	IOP reduction	Response rate	Comments
Latina et al[77]	53 eyes	180°	26 weeks	↓IOP ≥ 3 mm Hg	5.8 mm Hg	70%	Equivalent in eyes with and without previous ALT
Nagar and Shah[86]	20 eyes	360°	6 months	20% ↓ IOP	6.2 mm Hg	75%	
McIlraith et al[81]	100 eyes	180°	12 months	20% ↓ IOP	8.3 mm Hg	83%	Treatment naive
Hodge et al[87]	72 eyes	180°	23.8 ± 4.88 months	20% ↓ IOP	5.8 mm Hg	60%	

DIODE LASER TRABECULOPLASTY

Diode laser trabeculoplasty (DLP) has been evaluated as a possible alternative to ALT. The major proposed advantage is the portable nature of these devices, making them ideal for practitioners with multiple satellite facilities as well as for use in remote areas of developing countries. Moriarty and colleagues[104] evaluated the effect of a 180 degree treatment to 25 eyes. After two years of follow-up they found a 7.9 mm Hg decrease in IOP, which is comparable to results reported with ALT. In contrast, Englert and collogues[105] noted significantly greater IOP reduction at 3 months comparing DLT to ALT. Eleven patients received ALT in one eye and DLT in the other eye. The IOP reduction at three months was 2.4 ± 16.9 percent in the DLP group and was 30 ± 16.5 percent in the ALT group. More recent studies have suggested that both ALT and DLP may be comparably effective.[106] McMillan et al[107] utilized scanning electron microscopy to evaluate cadaver eyes treated with DLT and ALT and found similar damage to the trabecular beams with both treatment types.

CONCLUSION

Despite all of the controversy surrounding laser trabeculoplasty, published data to date does not show the superiority of one treatment technique over the other. SLT has been shown to cause less structural damage than ALT in histopathologic specimens, but the clinical superiority and relevancy of this is yet to be determined. Efficacy in retreatment of eyes previously treated with ALT shows conflicting evidence in superiority of one modality over the other. The recent report of repeat SLT showing equivalent efficacy to primary SLT treatment is promising, but further studies and long-term reports will need to be done before declaring a significant advantage. Evaluating all of the data published thus far, the only conclusion is that SLT and ALT display similar efficacy and complications, and both treatments show utility in the treatment of glaucoma. DLP is another alternative due to its portable nature.

REFERENCES

1. Wise, JB, Witter SL. Argon laser therapy for open-angle glaucoma. A pilot study. Arch Ophthalmol 1979;97:319-22.

2. Stein, JD, Challa. Mechanisms of action and efficacy of argon laser trabeculoplasty and selective laser trabeculoplasty. Curr Opin Ophthalmol 2007;18:140-5.

3. Rodrigues MM, Spaeth GL, Donohoo P. Electron microscopy of argon laser therapy in phakic open-angle glaucoma. Ophthalmology 1982;89:98-210.

4. Pham H, et al. Argon laser trabeculoplasty versus selective laser trabeculoplasty. Surv Ophthalmol 2008;53:641-6.

5. Melamed S, Epstein DL. Alterations of aqueous humour outflow following argon laser trabeculoplasty in monkeys. Br J Ophthalmol 1987;71:776-81.

6. Johnson DH. Histologic findings after argon laser trabeculoplasty in glaucomatous eyes. Exp Eye Res 2007;85:557-62.

7. Parshley DE, et al. Laser trabeculoplasty induces stromelysin expression by trabecular juxtacanalicular cells. Invest Ophthalmol Vis Sci 1996;37:795-804.

8. Grayson DK, et al. Long-term reduction of intraocular pressure after repeat argon laser trabeculoplasty. Am J Ophthalmol 1988;106:312-21.

9. Bylsma SS, et al. Trabecular cell division after argon laser trabeculoplasty. Arch Ophthalmol 1988;106:544-7.

10. Van Buskirk EM. Pathophysiology of laser trabeculoplasty. Surv Ophthalmol 1989;33:264-72.

11. Brubaker RF, Liesegang TJ. Effect of trabecular photocoagulation on the aqueous humor dynamics of the human eye. Am J Ophthalmol 1983;96:139-47.

12. Yablonski ME, Cook DJ, Gray J. A fluorophotometric study of the effect of argon laser trabeculoplasty on aqueous humor dynamics. Am J Ophthalmol 1985;99:579-82.

13. Thomas JV, et al. Argon laser trabeculoplasty as initial therapy for glaucoma. Arch Ophthalmol 1984;102:702-3.

14. Rosenthal AR, Chaudhuri PR, Chiapella AP. Laser trabeculoplasty primary therapy in open-angle glaucoma. A preliminary report. Arch Ophthalmol 1984;102:699-701.

15. The glaucoma laser trial (GLT) and glaucoma laser trial follow-up study: 7. Results. Glaucoma Laser Trial Research Group. Am J Ophthalmol 1995;120:718-31.

16. Thomas JV, Simmons RJ, Belcher D 3rd. Argon laser trabeculoplasty in the presurgical glaucoma patient. Ophthalmology 1982;89:187-97.

17. Spaeth GL, Baez KA. Argon laser trabeculoplasty controls one third of cases of progressive, uncontrolled, open angle glaucoma for 5 years. Arch Ophthalmol 1992;110:491-4.

18. Wilensky JT, Weinreb RN. Early and late failures of argon laser trabeculoplasty. Arch Ophthalmol 1983;101:895-7.

19. Pennebaker GE, Stewart WC. Response of argon laser trabeculoplasty with varying anterior chamber anatomy. Ophthalmic Surg 1991;22:301-2.

20. Blondeau P, Roberge JF, Asselin Y. Long-term results of low power, long duration laser trabeculoplasty. Am J Ophthalmol 1987;104:339-42.

21. Frenkel RE, et al. Laser trabeculoplasty: how little is enough? Ophthalmic Surg Lasers 1997;28:900-4.

22. Rouhiainen HJ, Terasvirta ME, Tuovinen EJ. Laser power and post-operative intraocular pressure increase in argon laser trabeculoplasty. Arch Ophthalmol 1987;105:1352-4.

23. Grayson D, et al. Initial argon laser trabeculoplasty to the inferior vs superior half of trabecular meshwork. Arch Ophthalmol 1994;112:446-7.

24. Weinreb RN, et al. Influence of the number of laser burns administered on the early results of argon laser trabeculoplasty. Am J Ophthalmol 1983;95:287-92.

25. Klein HZ, Shields MB, Ernest JT. Two-stage argon laser trabeculoplasty in open-angle glaucoma. Am J Ophthalmol 1985;99:392-5.

26. Schwartz LW, et al. Variation of techniques on the results of argon laser trabeculoplasty. Ophthalmology 1983;90:781-4.

27. Rolim de Moura C, Paranhos Jr A, Wormald R. Laser trabeculoplasty for open angle glaucoma. Cochrane Database Syst Rev; 2007(4). p. CD003919.

28. Hugkulstone CE. Argon laser trabeculoplasty with standard and long duration. Acta Ophthalmol (Copenh) 1990;68:579-81.

29. Ticho U, Nesher R. Laser trabeculoplasty in glaucoma. Ten-year evaluation. Arch Ophthalmol 1989;107:844-6.

30. Mittra RA, Allingham RR, M.B. Shields MB. Follow-up of argon laser trabeculoplasty: is a day-one postoperative IOP check necessary? Ophthalmic Surg Lasers 1995;26:410-3.

31. Rosenblatt MA, Luntz MH. Intraocular pressure rise after argon laser trabeculoplasty. Br J Ophthalmol 1987;71:772-5.

32. Effect of brimonidine 0.5% on intraocular pressure spikes following 360% argon laser trabeculoplasty. The Brimonidine-ALT Study Group. Ophthalmic Surg Laser, 1995;26:404-9.

33. Ren J, et al. Efficacy of apraclonidine 1% versus pilocarpine 4% for prophylaxis of intraocular pressure spike after argon laser trabeculoplasty. Ophthalmology 1999;106:1135-9.

34. Dapling RB, Cunliffe IA, Longstaff S. Influence of apraclonidine and pilocarpine alone and in combination on post laser trabeculoplasty pressure rise. Br J Ophthalmol 1994;78:30-2.

35. Chevrier RL, et al. Apraclonidine 0.5% versus brimonidine 0.2% for the control of intraocular pressure elevation following anterior segment laser procedures. Ophthalmic Surg Lasers 1999;30:199-204.

36. Barnes SD, et al. Control of intraocular pressure elevations after argon laser trabeculoplasty: comparison of brimonidine 0.2% to apraclonidine 1.0%. Ophthalmology 1999;106:2033-7.

37. Chen TC, et al. Brimonidine 0.2% versus apraclonidine 0.5% for prevention of intraocular pressure elevations after anterior segment laser surgery. Ophthalmology 2001;108:1033-8.

38. Metcalfe TW, Etchells DE. Prevention of the immediate intraocular pressure rise following argon laser trabeculoplasty. Br J Ophthalmol 1989;73:612-6.

39. Hartenbaum D, et al. A randomized study of dorzolamide in the prevention of elevated intraocular pressure after anterior segment laser surgery. Dorzolamide Laser Study Group. J Glaucoma 1999;8:273-5.

40. Herbort CP, et al. Anti-inflammatory effect of diclofenac drops after argon laser trabeculoplasty. Arch Ophthalmol 1993;111:481-3.

41. Mermoud A, Pittet N, Herbort CP. Inflammation patterns after laser trabeculoplasty measured with the laser flare meter. Arch Ophthalmol 1992;110:368-70.

42. Shin DH, et al. Effect of topical anti-inflammatory treatment on the outcome of laser trabeculoplasty. The Fluorometholone-Laser Trabeculoplasty Study Group. Am J Ophthalmol 1996;122:349-54.

43. Kim YY, et al. Effect of topical anti-inflammatory treatment on the long-term outcome of laser trabeculoplasty. Fluorometholone-Laser Trabeculoplasty Study Group. Am J Ophthalmol 1998;126:721-3.

44. Wise JB. Long-term control of adult open angle glaucoma by argon laser treatment. Ophthalmology 1981;88:197-202.

45. Grinich NP, Van Buskirk EM, Samples JR. Three-year efficacy of argon laser trabeculoplasty. Ophthalmology 1987;94:858-61.

46. Pollack IP, Robin AL, Sax H. The effect of argon laser trabeculoplasty on the medical control of primary open-angle glaucoma. Ophthalmology 1983;90:785-9.

47. Schwartz AL, Love DC, Schwartz MA. Long-term follow-up of argon laser trabeculoplasty for uncontrolled open-angle glaucoma. Arch Ophthalmol 1985;103:482-4.

48. Fink AI, et al. Therapeutic limitations of argon laser trabeculoplasty. Br J Ophthalmol 1988;72:263-9.

49. Ederer F, et al. The Advanced Glaucoma Intervention Study (AGIS): 13. Comparison of treatment outcomes within race: 10-year results. Ophthalmology 2004;111:651-64.

50. Shingleton BJ, et al. Long-term efficacy of argon laser trabeculoplasty. Ophthalmology 1987;94:1513-8.

51. Shingleton BJ, et al. Long-term efficacy of argon laser trabeculoplasty. A 10-year follow-up study. Ophthalmology 1993;100:1324-9.

52. Greenidge KC, Spaeth GL, Fiol-Silva Z. Effect of argon laser trabeculoplasty on the glaucomatous diurnal curve. Ophthalmology 1983;90:800-4.

53. Schultz JS, et al. Intraocular pressure and visual field defects after argon laser trabeculoplasty in chronic open-angle glaucoma. Ophthalmology 1987;94:553-7.

54. Sherwood MB, Svedbergh B. Argon laser trabeculoplasty in exfoliation syndrome. Br J Ophthalmol 1985;69:886-90.

55. Krupin T, et al. Argon laser trabeculoplasty in black and white patients with primary open-angle glaucoma. Ophthalmology 1986;96:811-6.

56. Sharpe ED, Simmons RJ. Argon laser trabeculoplasty as a means of decreasing intraocular pressure from "normal" levels in glaucomatous eyes. Am J Ophthalmol 1985;99:704-7.

57. Brown SV, Thomas JV, Simmons RJ. Laser trabeculoplasty re-treatment. Am J Ophthalmol 1985;99:8-10.

58. The Advanced Glaucoma Intervention Study (AGIS): 11. Risk factors for failure of trabeculectomy and argon laser trabeculoplasty. Am J Ophthalmo 2002;134:481-98.

59. Vaidergorn PG, Susanna R Jr. Argon laser trabeculoplasty and reduction of ocular hypotensive medication used by glaucoma patients. Can J Ophthalmol 2006;41:44-50.

60. The Advanced Glaucoma Intervention Study (AGIS): 9. Comparison of glaucoma outcomes in black and white patients within treatment groups. Am J Ophthalmol 2001;132:311-20.

61. Schwartz AL, Wilson MC, Schwartz LW. Efficacy of argon laser trabeculoplasty in aphakic and pseudophakic eyes. Ophthalmic Surg Lasers 1997;28:215-8.

62. Robin AL, Pollack IP. Argon laser trabeculoplasty in secondary forms of open-angle glaucoma. Arch Ophthalmol 1983;101:382-4.

63. Ritch R, et al. Argon laser trabeculoplasty in pigmentary glaucoma. Ophthalmology 1993;100:909-13.

64. Safran MJ, Robin AL, Pollack IP. Argon laser trabeculoplasty in younger patients with primary open-angle glaucoma. Am J Ophthalmol 1984;97:292-5.

65. Lehto I. Long-term follow up of argon laser trabeculoplasty in pigmentary glaucoma. Ophthalmic Surg 1992;23:614-7.

66. Threlkeld AB, et al. Comparative study of the efficacy of argon laser trabeculoplasty for exfoliation and primary open-angle glaucoma. J Glaucoma 1996;5:311-6.

67. Messner D, et al. Repeat argon laser trabeculoplasty. Am J Ophthalmol 1987;103:113-5.

68. Jorizzo PA, Samples JR, Van Buskirk EM. The effect of repeat argon laser trabeculoplasty. Am J Ophthalmol 1988;106:682-5.

69. Richter CU, et al. Retreatment with argon laser trabeculoplasty. Ophthalmology 1987;94:1085-9.

70. Feldman RM, et al. Long-term efficacy of repeat argon laser trabeculoplasty. Ophthalmology 1991;98:1061-5.

71. Koller T, et al. Membrane formation in the chamber angle after failure of argon laser trabeculoplasty: analysis of risk factors. Br J Ophthalmol 2000;84:48-53.

72. Rouhiainen HJ, Terasvirta ME, Tuovinen EJ. Peripheral anterior synechiae formation after trabeculoplasty. Arch Ophthalmol 1988;106:189-91.

73. Melamed S, Pei J, Epstein DL. Short-term effect of argon laser trabeculoplasty in monkeys. Arch Ophthalmol 1985;103:1546-52.

74. Hollo G, Lakatos P, Vargha P. Immediate increase in aqueous humour endothelin 1 concentration and intra-ocular pressure after argon laser trabeculoplasty in the rabbit. Ophthalmologica 2000;214:292-5.

75. Sturmer J, Broadway DC, Hitchings RA. Young patient trabeculectomy. Assessment of risk factors for failure. Ophthalmology 1993;100:928-39.

76. Barkana Y, Belkin M. Selective laser trabeculoplasty. Surv Ophthalmol 2007;52:634-54.

77. Damji KF, et al. Selective laser trabeculoplasty v argon laser trabeculoplasty: a prospective randomised clinical trial. Br J Ophthalmo, 1999;83:718-22.

78. Kwasniewska S, et al. The efficacy of cw Nd:YAG laser trabeculoplasty. Ophthalmic Surg 1993; 24:304-8.

79. Latina MA, et al. Q-switched 532-nm Nd:YAG laser trabeculoplasty (selective laser trabeculoplasty): a multicenter, pilot, clinical study. Ophthalmolog, 1998;105:2082-8; discussion 2089-90.

80. Cioffi GA, Latina MA, Schwartz GF. Argon versus selective laser trabeculoplasty. J Glaucoma 2004;13:174-7.

81. Latina MA, Park C. Selective targeting of trabecular meshwork cells: in vitro studies of pulsed and CW laser interactions. Exp Eye Res 1995;60:359-71.

82. Kramer TR, Noecker RJ. Comparison of the morphologic changes after selective laser trabeculoplasty and argon laser trabeculoplasty in human eye bank eyes. Ophthalmology 2001;108:773-9.

83. Cvenkel B, et al. Acute ultrastructural changes of the trabecular meshwork after selective laser trabeculoplasty and low power argon laser trabeculoplasty. Lasers Surg Med 2003;33:204-8.

84. Latina MA, de Leon JM. Selective laser trabeculoplasty. Ophthalmol Clin North Am 2005;18:409-19,vi.

85. Latina MA, Tumbocon JA. Selective laser trabeculoplasty: a new

treatment option for open angle glaucoma. Curr Opin Ophthalmol 2002; 13:94-6.

86. Rubin, B, et al. The effect of selective laser trabeculoplasty on intraocular pressure in patients with intravitreal steroid-induced elevated intraocular pressure. J Glaucoma 2008;17:287-92.

87. Prasad N, et al. A comparison of the intervisit intraocular pressure fluctuation after 180 and 360 degrees of selective laser trabeculoplasty (SLT) as a primary therapy in primary open angle glaucoma and ocular hypertension. J Glaucoma 2009;18:157-60.

88. George MK, et al. Evaluation of a modified protocol for selective laser trabeculoplasty. J Glaucoma 2008;17:197-202.

89. McIlraith I, et al. Selective laser trabeculoplasty as initial and adjunctive treatment for open-angle glaucoma. J Glaucoma 2006;15:124-30.

90. Mao AJ, et al. Development of a prediction rule to estimate the probability of acceptable intraocular pressure reduction after selective laser trabeculoplasty in open-angle glaucoma and ocular hypertension. J Glaucoma 2008;17:449-54.

91. Kim YJ, Moon CS. One-year follow-up of laser trabeculoplasty using Q-switched frequency-doubled Nd: YAG laser of 523 nm wavelength. Ophthalmic Surg Lasers 2000;31:394-9.

92. Birt CM. Selective laser trabeculoplasty retreatment after prior argon laser trabeculoplasty: 1-year results. Can J Ophthalmol 2007;42:715-9.

93. Nagar ME, Luhishi E, Shah N. Intraocular pressure control and fluctuation: the effect of treatment with selective laser trabeculoplasty. Br J Ophthalmol 2009;93:497-501.

94. Lee R, Hutnik CM. Projected cost comparison of selective laser trabeculoplasty versus glaucoma medication in the Ontario Health Insurance Plan. Can J Ophthalmol 2006;41:449-56.

95. Hodge WG, et al. Baseline IOP predicts selective laser trabeculoplasty success at 1 year post-treatment: results from a randomised clinical trial. Br J Ophthalmol 2005;89:1157-60.

96. Juzych MS, et al. Comparison of long-term outcomes of selective laser trabeculoplasty versus argon laser trabeculoplasty in open-angle glaucoma. Ophthalmology 2004;111:1853-9.

97. Hong BK, et al. Repeat selective laser trabeculoplasty. J Glaucoma 2009;18:180-3.

98. Kim DY, Singh A. Severe iritis and choroidal effusion following selective laser trabeculoplasty. Ophthalmic Surg Lasers Imaging 2008;39:409-11.

99. Harasymowycz PJ, et al. Selective laser trabeculoplasty (SLT) complicated by intraocular pressure elevation in eyes with heavily pigmented trabecular meshworks. Am J Ophthalmol 2005;139:1110-3.

100. Realini T. Selective laser trabeculoplasty: a review. J Glaucoma 2008;17:497-502.

101. Damji KF, et al. Selective laser trabeculoplasty versus argon laser trabeculoplasty: results from a 1-year randomised clinical trial. Br J Ophthalmol 2006;90:1490-4.

102. Martinez-de-la-Casa JM, et al. Selective vs argon laser trabeculoplasty: hypotensive efficacy, anterior chamber inflammation, and postoperative pain. Eye 2004;18:498-502.

103. Girkin CA. Selective vs Argon laser trabeculoplasty: controversy in evolution. Am J Ophthalmol 2007;144:120-1.

104. Moriarty AP, et al. Long-term follow-up of diode laser trabeculoplasty for primary open-angle glaucoma and ocular hypertension. Ophthalmology 1993;100:1614-8.

105. Englert JA, et al. Argon vs diode laser trabeculoplasty. Am J Ophthalmol 1997;124:627-31.

106. Agarwal HC, et al. Comparative evaluation of diode laser trabeculoplasty vs frequency doubled Nd: YAG laser trabeculoplasty in primary open angle glaucoma. Eye 2006;20:1352-6.

107. McMillan TA, et al. Comparison of diode and argon laser trabeculoplasty in cadaver eyes. Invest Ophthalmol Vis Sci 1994;35:706-10.

## 44

Laser Iridotomy and Other Laser Procedures

R Ramakrishnan

LASER PROCEDURES IN GLAUCOMA

Lasers have achieved a widespread use in the management of glaucoma in conjunction with surgical procedures such as trabeculectomy. They various uses of lasers in glaucoma are:

- Laser iridotomy
- Iridoplasty
- Laser suturelysis
- Laser trabeculoplasty
- Laser bleb remodelling
- Closure of cyclodialysis cleft
- Laser synechiolysis
- Gonio photocoagulation
- Photomydriasis (Pupilloplasty)
- Laser assisted deep sclerectomy (LADS)
- Laser cyclophotocoagulation.

Laser trabeculoplasty and cyclophotocoagulation have been discussed in separate chapters. Some of the procedures are described in detail below.

LASER IRIDOTOMY

Laser iridotomy is an effective treatment for angle closure glaucoma (ACG) and also used as a prophylactic measure in the fellow eye of patients with acute angle closure. The complications of surgical iridectomy include hemorrhage, cataract, wound leak, and photophobia as well as the complications associated with retrobulbar anesthesia and any intraocular surgery. In 1956, Meyer Schwickerath used a photocoagulator to create a hole in the iris. Ever since the advent of lasers, laser iridotomy has replaced incisional iridotomy. The current popular lasers are Nd:YAG and argon lasers. Laser surgery has become the preferred method in almost all cases. Both argon laser and Nd:YAG laser are effective in relieving pupillary block. The argon laser dominated iridotomy procedures in the 1980s, but the Nd:YAG laser is now increasingly being favored. The only time an argon laser should be used is when bleeding is anticipated or when a Nd:YAG instrument unavailable.

Indications for Laser Peripheral Iridotomy

- Primary angle-closure glaucoma
- Acute angle-closure glaucoma
- Subacute (intermittent) angle-closure glaucoma
- Creeping (chronic) angle-closure glaucoma
- Plateau iris syndrome
- Combined mechanism glaucoma

- ❖ Open angle with narrow inlets that make application of laser trabeculoplasty burns difficult
- Fellow eye (Prophylactic)
  - ❖ Of patient with angle-closure glaucoma
  - ❖ Of patient with malignant glaucoma
- Malignant glaucoma/aqueous misdirection syndrome
- Pupillary block glaucoma
- Nanophthalmos
- Pigmentary glaucoma
- Incomplete surgical iridotomy.

Contraindications

- Corneal edema
- Excessively shallow anterior chamber or completely sealed angle
- When angle closure is not due to pupillary block (e.g. neovascular or ICE membrane)
- Patient on anticoagulants.

Patient preparation: Pilocarpine 2 percent is used for miosis. This helps to tighten the peripheral iris and also pulls it away from the cornea.

An alpha agonist is used 1 hour pre laser to blunt any IOP spike and also to decrease bleeding.

The procedure is performed under topical anesthesia using an Abraham lens or Wise iridotomy lens and a coupling agent.

Advantages of Lenses
- Improve visualization
- Minimize epithelial barriers by acting as heat sink
- Concentrates the energy into a smaller space
- Separates the lids and fixes the eye.

Preferred Site
- Peripheral as it avoids damage to the intraocular lens
- Peripheral site avoids lens damage
- Preferably superior nasal quadrant as it is covered by the lid
- Avoid 2 O' clock and 9 O' clock
- Thin peripheral area of iris. (Crypt)

Signs of Successful Completion
- Posterior iris movement and deepening of anterior chamber (AC)
- Cloud of pigment billowing forward
- Transillumination
- Visibility of anterior lens capsule
- Minimum size is 150 to 200 μ.

Technique
Pilocarpine and topical anesthetic are instilled.

Alpha-agonist can be considered along with pilocarpine to blunt

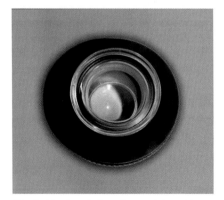

Fig. 1 Abraham's lens for peripheral laser iridotomy

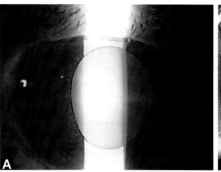
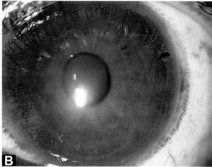

Figs 2A and B Peripheral laser iridotomy

postoperative pressure spikes. An anti-reflective-coated contact lens (e.g. CGI, Abraham or Wise lens) **(Figure 1)** prevents blinking, reduces eye movements, provides magnification, focuses the laser beam, and minimizes corneal burns during the procedure. The preferred site is usually between 11 and 1 O'clock positions, where it will be covered by the lid and it is best located at the base of an iris crypt to facilitate penetration **(Figures 2A and B)**. After the beam has been focused perfectly on the anterior iris surface the joystick is advanced very slightly so that the focus is in the iris stroma. Burns are applied until penetration is completely established by a gush of pigment-colored aqueous streaming through the iridotomy into the anterior chamber. If bleeding occurs pressure with the lens is applied to the eye (up to 60 sec).

The photo disruptive Nd:YAG laser 'punches' through the iris **(Figure 3)**. Thus, it simplifies technique for all eyes because iris pigment and iris density are less important factors and requires fewer pulses and less energy than an argon laser to create a patent iridotomy. In Q-switched mode energy applied is 5 to 7 mJ with a run of three bursts per activation, for a total power of 15 to 21 mJ per shot. It is usually possible to penetrate with one or, at the most, three bursts. Nd:YAG iridotomies tend to close less frequently and may minimize the risk of pupillary peaking caused by thermal contraction.

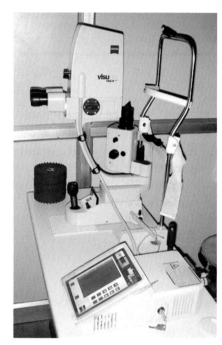

Fig. 3 Nd:YAG laser machine

However, Nd:YAG laser iridotomy has greater risk of posterior synechiae and hemorrhage (usually transient) than argon laser. Nd:YAG has also been used successfully for PI in cases of pigmentary glaucoma and pigment dispersion syndrome, reducing iris concavity and possibly relieving the relative pupillary block; however, care has to be taken for the rlsk of postoperative IOP spike.

The effect of the argon laser is primarily thermal and burns through the iris. Very dark and very light irides present technical difficulties. Using a condensing contact lens, the typical initial laser settings are 0.02 to 0.1 second of duration, 50 μm spot size, and 800 to 1000 MW of power. There are number of variations in technique and iris color dictates which technique is chosen. *Sequential argon lasers and Nd:YAG laser iridotomy* is used primarily in patients with bleeding diseases. Iridotomy is begun with the argon laser and completed with the Nd:YAG laser at 2 to 3 mJ. The semiconductor diode laser also has recently been used for peripheral iridotomy. Because argon laser has many desirable effects, including the ability to make stretch burns, make contraction burns, coagulate blood vessels, and thin the stroma, the combination of argon and Nd:YAG laser techniques for iridotomy may allow the advantages of both laser modes to be exploited.

Complications of Laser Peripheral Iridotomy

Complications	Argon	Nd:YAG
Ghost image	Occasionally	Common
Posterior synechiae	Routine unless preventive treatment used	Very rare
Corneal changes	Uncommon	Should not occur
Transient uveitis	Moderate	Mild
Persisting uveitis	Occasionally	Should not occur
Hyphema	Extremely rare	Occasionally
Postoperative IOP spike in eye without IOP problem	Occasionally	Very rare
Postoperative IOP spike in eye with pre-existing elevation of IOP on medications	Routine and severe	Common and may be severe
Transient blurring of vision	Mild	Very mild
Pupillary distortion	Not infrequent	Should not occur
Diplopia (a function of placement of peripheral iridotomy)		
Late closure quite eye	Occasionally common	Does not occur can occur
Eye with continuing inflammation		

Iritis: Laser iritodomy is usually followed by mild iritis. Postlaser topical corticosteroid drops may be prescribed to manage it.

Hyphema

Hyphema is more common after iridoplasty as compared to Nd:YAG PI. Temporary elevation of IOP by pressure with contact lens helps to control the bleeding. Bleeding may be more severe in patients of an anticoagulants. Thus a history must be taken prior to the procedure.

IOP Elevation

Elevations in IOP are seen in 17 to 27 percent patients following laser iridotomy. These can be prevented by using alpha agonists pre- and post-laser. The IOP should be measured 1 hour post laser and any spikes must be managed.

Corneal Endothelial and Stromal Damage

A corneal burn can occur if iris is near the cornea. It results in clouding and reduces the visibility. The amount of energy reaching the iris is also poorly focused.

When a corneal burn occurs, a new site may be chosen. If one wants to continue at the same site, the energy is decreased or exposure time is reduced.

Extensive burning can lead to presistant corneal edema.

Incomplete Laser Iridotomy
Late closure

Theoretically a 15 μ hole is adequate to restore aqueous flow. However, this has a tendency to get occluded by pigment or may close when the pupil is dilated. 150 to 200 μ is considered an adequate size.

Retinal and foveal burns have been reported with argon lasers.

Cataract

Localized whitening of the lens, i.e. a localized lens opacity, corresponding to the site of LPI can occur especially after argon laser LPI. Usually these opacities do not progress. Mild inflammation following LPI may also accelerate cataract formation.

PERIPHERAL IRIDOPLASTY

Defined as controlled heating and contraction with flattening of the surface of the peripheral iris. Argon laser peripheral iridoplasty (ALPI) involves placing laser burns of low power, large spot size, and long duration in the extreme periphery, to contract the iris stroma between the site of the burn and the angle.

Indications

- Primary angle closure glaucoma
- Acute (preliminary to iridectomy) corneal edema preventing adequate iridotomy
- Plateau iris
- Nanophthalmos
- Retraction of early, weak PAS
- Open angle glaucoma
  (As adjunct to laser trabeculoplasty in eyes with narrow entry to AC angle)

This procedure can be used to open the angle temporarily, or in other types of angle closure such as plateau iris syndrome and nanophthalmos. Argon laser iridoplasty is now used as an adjunct to laser trabeculoplasty and other outflow procedures. It is also useful in the treatment of medically uncontrollable acute ACG, to open the angle enough to permit safer peripheral laser iridotomy.

Procedure

The procedure is performed using topical anesthesia and an Abraham lens is used.

The laser is set to produce contraction burns on a maximally constricted iris with pilocarpine. Parameters are (200-500 μ spot size/0.5 sec/200-400 mW) 4 to 10 burns per quadrant are applied.

Complications

- Iritis
- Pupillary distortion (Rare)
- Corneal burns
- Hemorrhage (Rare)
- Lenticular opacity (Rare)
- Peripheral anterior synechiae
- Transient IOP spike.

LASER SUTURE LYSIS

One of the most significant advances in filtration surgery, the selective cutting of sutures after trabeculectomy, has had a profound effect on decreasing immediate postoperative hypotony

and its sequelae while maintaining the benefits of full-thickness surgery. The effective window for lysis of sutures without antimetabolites is 0 to 21 days, with effectiveness falling rapidly after 14 days. The use of antimetabolites such as 5-fluorouracil extends this greatly and sutures can be lysed with good effect up to 4 to 6 weeks postoperatively. The use of mitomycin-C deserves special mention. In general, an increased interval to suture lysis will decrease the chances of hypotony and also decrease the effect. Suture lysis after the use of mitomycin-C may be attempted in the face of a failed filter with good results. There are some limitations in that nylon sutures will depigment over time and will heat more slowly. Great care should be taken to avoid buttonhole formation during suture lysis after the use of mitomycin-C. The technique requires the use of a continuous-wave argon or quasi-continuous wave laser (frequency doubled Nd:YAG; 532 nm), argon dye (610 nm), krypton (647.1 nm) or diode (810 nm) laser. In a postoperative eye with any blood or hemoglobin present in the subconjunctival space, the most useful lasers are those that can emit 610 nm laser light or in the red spectrum, such as krypton. This wavelength (610 nm) is poorly absorbed by hemoglobin and decreases the possibility of a conjunctival buttonhole. If hemoglobin

is absent, there is some evidence that yellow (585 nm) or orange (610 nm) may limit conjunctival damage.

Patient Evaluation and Preparation

The number and the effect each scleral flap suture had at the time of surgery should be reviewed. Phenylephrine (2.5%) may be given to reduce congestion of the tissues before treatment. Three laser suture lysis lenses are in widest usage. All three lenses thin and blanch overlying tissues, allowing visualization of the sutures. All three lenses help hold the eyelid; the Hoskins and Ritch lenses have flanges for this purpose (**Figure 4A**). The Hoskins and Mandelkorn laser suture lysis lenses provide magnification and smaller spot sizes which effectively increase irradiance. This should be taken into account when selecting continuous-wave power and exposure duration. Care should be taken in handling the Hoskins lens, as the neck is somewhat fragile.

Procedure

Topical anesthetic agents are used. The patient is asked to look down and the iridectomy is used to locate the approximate area of the scleral flap. The continuous-wave power should start low (50 μ; 0.05–0.1 s, 400 mW). The laser spot should be focused on the suture to produce one long cut end which will lie flat (**Figure 4B**). After

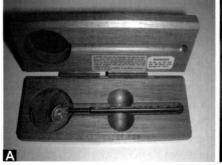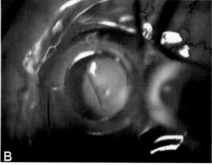

Figs 4A and B (A) Hoskins lens used for argon laser suture lysis.
(B) Argon laser suture lysis with Hoskins lens

successful lysis, the lysed suture ends will retract; occasionally the suture blanches but does not retract. This indicates that sufficient tension in the suture to cause retraction does not exist, and that no extra filtration can be gained by pursuing this suture. The one suture per session rule should be observed, especially when mitomycin-C has been used. Additional sutures may be cut after careful evaluation a few hours after the initial attempt.

Complications

Complications are mainly limited to small conjunctival buttonholes from the laser and hypotony with or without buttonhole formation. These may be treated with patching and with or without aqueous suppressants as the clinical situation dictates. If anti-metabolites have been used, the use of a McAllister contact lens without patching may be used to help close the conjunctival defect. This lens provides tamponade and may be tolerated for 1 to 2 weeks if needed. The use of aqueous suppressants is also an option with this lens. Bleb-related endophthalmitis is a continuous concern in any patient with a thin filtering bleb. The status of the scleral flap sutures should always be ascertained. If there appears to be an impending suture extrusion, this should be stopped by segmenting the suture or rounding the end.

## 45

History of Filtering Surgeries: Past, Present and Future

━━━ R Ramakrishnan ━━━

CHAPTER OUTLINE
- ❖ Iridectomy and Acute Glaucoma
- ❖ Full Thickness Filtration Surgeries
- ❖ Partial Thickness Filtration Surgeries
- ❖ Antifibrotic Agents
- ❖ Drainage Devices
- ❖ Nonpenetrating Glaucoma Surgeries
- ❖ Other Procedures

INTRODUCTION

The two conditions glaucoma and cataract were not differentiated until the time of Celsius (25BC–50AD) and later *Galen (131-210AD);* cataract was treatable, glaucoma was not. *AT Tabari* in 10th century was the first person who suggested an association between IOP and glaucoma followed by *Sams-ad-din* in the 14th century who described glaucoma as a migraine of eye or headache of the pupil. In the 19th century *Guthrie, Lawrence* and *Dondors* describe two separate condition with raised IOP; acute inflammatory syndrome and non congestive glaucoma.[1] Although an association between glaucoma and IOP was first suggested in 1962 by *Richard Bannister*, surgical attempt to treat glaucoma by lowering IOP developed only in the 19th century.[2]

The chronological history of various glaucoma filtering surgeries has been listed in **Table 1**.

EARLY PROCEDURES

Iridectomy and Acute glaucoma

Von Graefe in 1857 described the beneficial effect of an iridectomy in treating acute glaucoma but noted no improvement in cases of chronic glaucoma treated by the same method.

Simple Sclerotomy

Mackenzie in 1835 was the first to do an invasive procedure—sclerotomy. He later added a paracentesis.

Iridodesis

Because a paracentesis rapidly closed, *Critchett* in 1858 proposed drawing a piece of iris into the corneal wound to facilitate drainage by 'iris inclusion' or iridodesis. A broad needle was used to make a corneal incision at the limbus. The iris was drawn into the wound with a blunt hook and left with protruding part excised.

Louis de Wecker is regarded as father of glaucoma filtering surgery.

He was first to realize that it was scleral incision and not the excision of iris which was responsible for lowering of intraocular pressure. The goal of external filtration is to create new drainage pathway allowing aqueous to pass from anterior chamber into the subconjunctival space.

Filtration techniques can be classified as follows:

A. *Full thickness filtration surgeries:*
1. Sclerectomy
2. Iridencleisis
3. Trephination
4. Thermal sclerostomy
5. Laser sclerostomy
6. Internal sclerostomy.

Table 1 Chronological history of filtering operations

Date	Surgeon	Procedure
1830	Mackenzie	Sclerotomy
1857	Critchett	Iridencleisis
1869	Von Graefe	Filtering bleb
1869	Louis de Wecker	Anterior sclerotomy
1906	Lagrange	Sclerectoiridectomy
1906	Holth	Anterior lip sclerotomy
1907	Holth	Iridencleisis
1924	Preziosi	Thermal sclerostomy
1958	Scheie	Thermal sclerostomy with iridectomy
1962	Lliff and Hass	Posterior lip sclerectomy
1968	Carnis	Trabeculectomy

B. ***Partial thickness filtration surgeries:***
 1. Basic Trabeculectomy
 2. Modifications of Trabeculectomy
 3. Trabeculotomy.
C. ***Glaucoma drainage devices:***
 1. Setons
 2. Shunts and valves.
D. ***Nonpenetrating filtering surgeries:***
 1. Sinusotomy
 2. Ab externo trabeculectomy
 3. Deep sclerectomy
 4. Viscocanalostomy.

FULL THICKNESS FILTRATION SURGERIES

Anterior Sclerotomy

De Wecker in 1869-71 described the anterior sclerotomy with a *Graefe* type knife.[1] An incision and counter incision were made just behind the limbus with the knife drawn up toward the limbus as for a cataract incision but leaving the limbus intact. The goal was to form a filtering bleb but the incision soon closed. *De Wecker* added an iridectomy and *Dianoux* in 1905 proposed prolonged massage, neither of which was successful.

Small Flap Sclerotomy

In 1903, *Major Herbert* proposed a small flap sclerotomy where a small incision was made into the anterior chamber through the sclera behind and parallel to the limbus. A small limbus-based sclera flap was then raised and iris was incarcerated into the wound. There was no resection of scleral tissue.

Sclerecto-Iridectomy and Anterior-Lip Sclerectomy

Lagrange described a sclerectoiridectomy in 1906 in which a corneoscleral conjunctival flap was created with a *Graefe* knife. A sclerectomy of the anterior lip was done with scissors, followed by a basal iridectomy. No sutures were used. *O'Brian* in 1947 described 85 percent success with *Lagrange's* sclerectoiridectomy.

Posterior-Lip Sclerectomy

Iliff and *Haas* described a posterior-lip sclerectomy in 1962. Under a limbus-based conjunctival flap a 5 mm incision was made into the anterior chamber and a *Holth* scleral punch was used to make a scleral opening of 1 × 3 mm. An iridectomy was done. *Haas* in 1967 described an 85 percent success with posterior–lip sclerectomy, although complications included flat blebs, flat chambers, and choroidal detachments.

Iridencleisis

In 1908, *Holth*[3] described a procedure, beginning with a triangular 6 mm lance incision made in the conjunctiva 5 mm behind the limbus, the lance then being advanced into the anterior chamber at the limbus. A sector iridectomy was done with incarceration of one or both iris pillar into the scleral wound. No suture was used.

Posterior Trephination

Argyll-Robertson, one of the first to introduce the concept of producing a filtering scar by sclerectomy, proposed posterior trephining in 1876 at the junction of the pars plana and ciliary body.

Limbal Trephination

Elliot[4] in 1909 described a technique of limbal trephination as an easier operation. The operation was done under cocaine and adrenaline local anesthesia. However, if necessary a 'hypodermic of morphine' was used. A conjunctival flap was dissected either at the superior limbus or inferior limbus. *Elliot* noted that it was often easier to approach the inferior limbus of an eye of an anxious patient who tended to stay in upgaze. A trephine of 2 mm diameter was used. A strong miotic, eserine, was used at the end of each operation. Intraocular pressure was lowered in all cases. Subconjunctival filtration was noted to be 'very free'. No cases of 'septic accident' were described. The one complication *Elliot* mentioned was making the trephine hole too far posterior and entering the suprachoroidal space. If the bulging uveal tissue was excised vitreous may present.

Thermal Sclerostomy

Preziosi in 1924 proposed doing a thermal sclerostomy under a conjunctival flap. A galvano cautery was used in the absence of any knife incision to enter the anterior chamber, thereby creating a fistula.

Posterior–Lip Thermal Sclerostomy

Scheie[5] described a posterior–lip thermal sclerostomy in 1958. He had observed that application of an electric cautery for hemostasis of the posterior lip of an iridectomy incision produced inadvertent filtering blebs. The thinking of the time is illustrated in his introduction: '*the filtering cicatrice seemed to be best explained by slight retraction of the wound edges resulting from scleral shrinkage cause by the cautery.*' The fact the filtration occurred was surprising because many ophthalmic surgeons have cautioned against the use of cautery even for control of bleeding when performing a filtration operation.

The technique was done under local anesthesia. A limbus based conjunctival flap was raised. After initial cauterization of the sclera at the limbus a small scratch incision is made with the blade through the cauterized area 1 mm behind the limbus. Then cautery was progressively applied to the posterior lip of the incision, which was progressively deepened until the iris prolapsed through it. An iridectomy was done and the conjunctiva and Tenon's capsule were closed by 6.0 catgut in separate layers. No medication was instilled.

Scheie compared his thermal sclerostomy with iridencleisis and trephination. In a larger series of 111 eyes with open-angle glaucoma, the success rate of the *Scheie* procedure was 86 percent in controlling the IOP. The most frequent complication was flat or shallow anterior chamber. Hyphema occurred in 17 eyes, and hypotony in 20 eyes, but none had disc edema or loss of visual acuity. His success rate with iridencleisis was 83 percent in 141 eyes, with hypotony noted in just 3.5 percent. Delayed anterior chamber reformation occurred in seven eyes. *Leydhecker* found the success of *Eliott's* operations to be only about 60 percent; an unfavorable comparison with the 80 to 90 percent success of the *Scheie* procedure. **Throughout the 1960s and early 1970s, the *Scheie* procedure was one of the most frequently performed filtering procedures**.

Laser Sclerostomy

Laser sclerostomy is a filtering procedure that has not gained widespread popularity. Various techniques have been described either ab interno or ab externo, most of which were done with the THC:YAG (holmium) laser that creates a 200 µ diameter lumen (1/100th the surface area of *Elliot's* 2 mm trephine hole). Complications of this full–thickness procedure included more hypotony and flat or shallow anterior chambers than with the guarded filtration of trabeculectomy, as well as iris incarceration in the absence of an iridectomy.

Sinusotomy

Krasnov[6] published his sinusotomy or externalization of Schlemm's canal in the 1960s, assuming the site of obstruction to outflow was intrascleral beyond the outer wall of Schlemm's canal.

If the outer wall is opened leaving the inner wall intact, reduction of IOP should be obtained. A resection of a narrow 1.5 mm wide lamella of sclera directly over Schlemm's canal was made from the 10 to 2'o clock position. *Krasnov* said that care should be taken not to damage the inner wall of Schlemm's canal which is the trabecular zone. The moment of reaching Schlemm's canal is crucial in sinusotomy. If the diagnosis of intrascleral glaucoma should prove correct there is a constant flow of fluid through the undamaged trabecular meshwork. In cases of 'trabecular insufficiency' the site over Schlemm's canal will be more or less dry and a different surgical procedure should be used. This method consisted of removing a lamellar band of sclera and opening Schlemm's canal over 120 degree from 10 to 2 o' clock position, keeping inner wall of Schlemm's canal intact with overlying conjunctiva closed.

PARTIAL THICKNESS FILTERING PROCEDURES

Trabeculotomy

It is an alternative to goniotomy for surgical treatment of congenital and childhood glaucoma. In 1958 *Grant[7]* showed that approximately three-fourth of the resistance to outflow in enucleated human eyes could be eliminated by creating an opening between anterior chamber and the internal wall of Schlemm's canal. Trabeculotomy was performed to remove the possible obstruction to the aqueous outflow by congenital angle deformity.

Trabeculotomy ab externo was first described by *Burian, Allen and Harms*.[8] The main indications for the procedure were primary congenital glaucoma, failed goniotomy, combined cataract surgery and eyes with corneal haze. Following the induction of anesthesia the ophthalmic examination is repeated under anesthesia. A corneal

traction suture or superior rectus bridle suture can rotate the globe down, giving excellent exposure of the superior limbus, which can be very helpful for a limbus-based conjunctival flap. A conjuctival flap is made followed by a partial thickness triangular scleral flap. A central radial incision is made across scleral spur to cut the external wall of the Schlemm's canal and to avoid entering anterior chamber. The internal arm of trabeculotome is introduced into the canal and rotated into anterior chamber and rotation is continued until 75 percent of the probe arm length has entered the chamber. Then the rotation is reversed and instrument is withdrawn. The trabeculotome is then passed into canal on other side of radial incision and rotated into anterior chamber. In total, about 100 to 120 degree of trabecular meshwork is ruptured by this technique.

The scleral flap is closed with 10-0 nylon suture, one at apex and one on each lateral side of trabecular flap. The conjunctiva and tenon's capsule are closed with running suture of absorbable material.

The advantages are:

- Anatomically more
- Higher documented success rate
- Easier for well trained microsurgeons
- No visual distortion intraoperatively
- Less surgical trauma
- Possible in eyes with opaque corneas.

Trabeculectomy

Trabeculectomy first described by *Sugar[9]* in 1961 and popularized in late 1960s and 1970s as a means of avoiding the complication of full thickness procedure. In 1968, *Carnis[10]* reported good success in 17 eyes using microsurgical technique to perform a trabeculectomy under a sclera flap, which was hinged either posteriorly in the sclera or anteriorly at the limbus. After excision of Schlemm's canal and trabecular meshwork the flap was sutured in the place so as to be watertight.

Successful trabeculectomy surgery involves the reducing IOP and avoiding or managing complications. The success of trabeculectomy often depends upon appropriate and timely postoperative intervention to influence the functioning of the filter. Complete healing of epithelial and conjunctival wound with incomplete healing of the scleral wound is the goal of the procedure.

Filtering surgeries are the most popular operations for glaucoma with over a 100 years track record of success. Currently trabeculectomy, a guarded filtering surgery is the standard procedure whereby a sclerostomy is covered by a leaky scleral flap. By creating a fistula in the sclera at the limbus, the aqueous is rerouted into a potential space, the subconjunctival area **(Figure 1)**. If successful, there is the formation of an elevated conjunctival bleb, where the aqueous fluid gathers in a pocket prior to absorption into the surrounding blood vessels and lymphatics. Various modifications have been made in the technique to increase the success rate. These include use of antimetabolites, collagen implants, releasable sutures, laser suturelysis and anti-VEGF (anti vascular endothelial growth factor). As a result of the above, the success rate

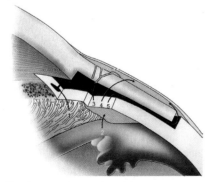

Fig. 1 Possible routes of aqueous humor flow associated with a trabeculectomy

of modern trabeculectomy in experienced hands is estimated between 60 and 100 percent depending on patient selection, definition of success and length of follow-up.

ANTIFIBROTIC AGENTS

The application of antifibrotic agents such as 5-Fluorouracil (5-FU) and Mitomycin C (MMC) resulted in greater success and lower IOP following trabeculectomy. However, serious postoperative complications can occur, and these agents must not be used indiscriminantly. Antifibrotic agents should be used with caution in primary trabeculectomies on young myopic patients because of an increased risk of hypotony.

5-Fluorouracil, a pyrimidine analogue, inhibits fibroblast proliferation and has proven useful in reducing scarring after filtering surgery. 5-Fluorouracil undergoes intracellular conversion to the active deoxynucleotide 5-fluoro-2'-deoxyuidine 5'-monophosphate which interferes with DNA synthesis through its action on thymidylate synthetase.

5-FU (50 mg/ml on a surgical sponge) may be used intraoperatively in a fashion similar to that described below for Mitomycin C. Regimens for postoperative administration vary according to the observed healing response. A total of 5 mg in 0.1 to 0.5 cc can be injected with relatively mild discomfort. The total dose can be titrated to the observed healing response and corneal toxicity. Complications such as corneal epithelial defects commonly occur and require discontinuation of 5-FU injections. The site of injection can be varied from 180 degree away to adjacent to the bleb.

Mitomycin-C is a naturally occurring antibiotic—antineoplastic compound that is derived from *Streptomyces caespitosus*. It acts as an alkylating agent after enzyme activation resulting in DNA crosslinking. Mitomycin-C is a potent

antifibrotic agent. It is most commonly administered intraoperatively by placing a surgical sponge soaked in MMC within the subconjunctival space in contact with sclera at the planned trabeculectomy site. Concentrations in current usage are typically between 0.2 and 0.4 mg/ml with duration of application from 1 to 4 minutes.

The results of trabeculectomy with antimetabolites were encouraging. Then as early postoperative complications related to wound leak, hypotony and late-onset complications associated with the bleb, antimetabolite use and failure began to emerge, surgeons looked for alternatives.

GLAUCOMA DRAINAGE DEVICES

These devices are designed to shunt aqueous from the anterior chamber into a subconjunctival reservoir. *Rollett* and *Moreau* in 1907 placed horse hair through corneal punctures in two cases of absolute glaucoma. *Zorab* used a silk loop through a keratome incision under the conjunctiva in a procedure he called aqueoplasty. Substances including gold leaf, platinum, various plastic rods and plates were placed in limbal wounds to act as wicks to keep a sclerostomy open. Results overall were poor. *Molteno*[11] was the first to report success with his episcleral plate joined to a plastic tube coming from the anterior chamber.

These drainage devices can be classified according to their mode of action.

- Translimbal aqueous drainage from anterior chamber to anterior subconjunctival space, e.g. Krupin-Denver valve.
- Translimbal aqueous drainage from anterior chamber into a posterior subtenon reservoir, e.g. Molteno, Schocket implant, Joseph valve, Long Krupin-Denver valve.
- Aqueous drainage from anterior chamber into the suprachoroidal space through a cyclodialysis cleft.

At the outset, aqueous drainage implants were not be used as a primary procedure in the surgical management of glaucoma. They were used for cases in which the prognosis for conventional filtering surgery was very poor (e.g. active neovascular glaucoma, active uveitis with secondary glaucoma, glaucoma associated with aphakia or pseudophakia and eyes with marked conjunctival scarring after penetrating keratoplasty, scleral buckling procedures, or trauma). They were also used in cases in which conventional glaucoma surgery had failed.

A brief description of the various types of available aqueous drainage implants.

1. ***Molteno implant:*** The Molteno implant consists of a silicone tube (outer diameter of 0.63 mm and inner diameter of 0.33 mm) that connects to the upper surface of a thin acrylic plate (13 mm in diameter), which acts as a collecting reservoir. The plate's surface is concave and fits easily to the contour of the sclera. The edge of the plate has a thickened rim (0.7 mm in height) that is performed to permit suturing of plate to sclera.

   The acrylic plate fits into the sclera surface between two rectus muscles. The plate promotes the formation of a vascular connective tissue that encapsulates the implant with formation of an aqueous—filled cavity with accumulation of aqueous drained from the anterior chamber. The bleb is stretched and distended with an increased surface area for flow either directly through connective tissue or into blood vessels.

2. ***Schocket implant:*** The Schocket implant shunts aqueous from the anterior chamber through a tube to the equatorial subtenon's collecting reservoir. In the Schocket implant the reservoir consists of an encircling no. 20 silicone band with its groove facing sclera. The silastic tube is inserted into the space between the inverted silicone band and episcleral through a side opening. Schocket and other investigators have reported a high success rate of IOP control in neovascular and other refractory glaucomas. It requires a 360 degree peritomy, suturing of an encircling band around the equator, and careful preoperative preparation of the silicon groove with side holes for the tube and suture securing it in place.

3. ***Krupin–Denver valve:*** The standard Krupin–Denver valve is a pressure sensitive, unidirectional valve implant consisting of an open supramid tube (outside diameter 0.58 mm and inner diameter of 0.38 mm) connected to a silastic tube with a slit valve. The valve has an opening pressure of 11 to 14 mm Hg and a closing pressure of 1 to 3 mm Hg lower. This valve mechanism should theoretically protects against extreme hypotony following implantation and allow constant pressure control by draining the anterior chamber at pressures higher than 14 mm Hg. The supramid tube is inserted into the anterior chamber at the limbus, whereas the silastic valve portion remains outside the eye. Supramid side arms provide stability to the implant and a means of fixating it to the sclera.

   The long-tube Krupin–Denver valve is a modification of the standard Krupin–Denver valve. The silastic tube is longer, extends posteriorly, and is fixated within the groove of a no. 220 silastic band. The band is sutured for 180 degree to sclera 11 mm behind the limbus.

4. ***White pump shunt:*** Consists of a silicone tube connected to a 16 to 18 ml balloon that has an outlet tube into the retrobulbar space. Digital massage or blinking activity pumps aqueous into and out of the balloon; thus a continuous flow of aqueous is maintained.

5. ***Joseph valve:*** The Joseph valve is a one-piece device consisting of a curved tube with a slit valve connected to a silicone rubber strap (surface area equals 800 mm sq) that is attached to 180 degree of the scleral circumference.

6. ***Baerveldt glaucoma implant:*** In 1992, George Baerveldt introduced a non valved drainage device made of silicone. It had a silicone tube which was attached to a silicone plate impregnated with barium. Initially, it was available in plates with surface areas of 3 sizes: 250, 350 and 500 mm square.

7. ***Ahmed glaucoma valve:*** In 1993, Mateen Ahmed developed a valved device ensuring a unidirectional flow of aqueous.

8. ***AADI:*** The Aurolab aqueous drainage implant has been developed by Aurolab in India. It is a non valved drainage device.

NONPENETRATING GLAUCOMA SURGERIES

Nonpenetrating filtering procedures reduce IOP by enhancing the natural aqueous outflow channels, while reducing outflow resistance located in the inner wall of the Schlemm's canal and the juxtacanalicular trabecular meshwork. They facilitate the aqueous egress through an intact Descemet's membrane. The advantages are the lack of sudden decompression of the eye, limited risk of hypotony, and the lack of need for an iridectomy. The eyes are relatively quiet, comfortable, and easy to manage with a low diffuse bleb postoperatively.

Besides obtaining adequate control of intraocular pressure, nonpenetrating glaucoma surgeries (NPGS) has two aims:

a. To create a Trabeculo-Descemet's window to allow a reproducible postoperative outflow resistance.

b. To promote the formation of an intrascleral bleb in order to reduce conjunctival bleb related complications.

Basic principle: With its small openings and tortuous flow pathways the JCT is considered to be the principle site of out flow resistance. Considering the histology of Schlemm's canal which is a channel oriented in a circumferential direction, with its large lumen, it is less likely to create a significant outflow resistance. In glaucomatous eyes, the trabecular meshwork expands into the lumen of the Schlemm's canal, leading to the subsequent narrowing of the lumen, this eventually increase the outflow resistance in raised intraocular pressure conditions. The goal of non penetrating glaucoma surgery is to improve the outflow facility but it retain some residual outflow resistance by maintaining a membrane between the anterior chamber and the scleral dissection. A great deal of interest has been directed towards the properties of the outflow resistance of this membrane before and after surgery. The various procedures include:

• Sinostomy
  (*Krasnov*)
• Ab externo trabeculectomy
  (*Edward Arenas, Colombia*)
• Viscocanalostomy
  (*Robert Stegman, South Africa*)
• Deep sclerectomy
  (*Mermoud, Switzerland*)
• Deep sclerectomy with collagen implant
• Laser assisted deep sclerectomy

• Excimer laser trabecular ablation (LTA)
  (*Arturo Maldonado-Bas, Argentina*)

Several techniques of nonpenetrating filtering surgeries based on the pioneer work of *Krasnov's* (1962) sinusotomy[5] have been described. Krasnov's Sinostomy has been discussed in detail earlier in the chapter.

Ab Externo Trabeculectomy

Zimmerman et al.[12] first described a nonpenetrating Ab externo trabeculectomy in 1984, where a deep sclerectomy was done with unroofing of Schlemm's canal, further removing the inner wall of Schlemm's canal and juxta canalicular trabeculum were removed, wound was then covered by a thin superficial scleral flap.

This technique was further modified, by removing the corneal stroma behind the anterior trabeculum and Descemets membrane, thereby increasing the aqueous outflow facility. This has been called **deep sclerectomy** and was first described by *Fyodrov* and *Kozlov* (1989). Later *Stegmann*[13] (1995) introduced viscocanalostomy.

The most common techniques used today are deep sclerectomy and viscocanalostomy.

Deep Sclerectomy

Deep sclerectomy is aimed to decrease the outflow resistance, in which, the internal wall of Schlemm's canal, juxtacanalicular meshwork, and the corneal stroma behind the anterior trabeculum and Descemets membrane is removed, without penetrating the anterior chamber, leaving behind a thin membrane known as trabeculo Descemets membrane or window. It acts as a guarded filter, where the Schlemm's canal is unroofed, and the aqueous drains. A CO_2 laser can

be used to make this window in laser assisted deep sclerectomy.

Viscocanalostomy

In viscocanalostomy, injection of high molecular weight viscoelastic ruptures the inner and outer walls of the schlemm's canal. These micro ruptures are likely to involve juxtacanalicular tissue and meshwork, facilitating the aqueous outflow. This probable mechanism was observed in various experimental studies done on human and animal eyes.

Canaloplasty

This modification of viscocanalostomy involves passing a suture 360 degrees around Schlemm's canal with the help of a lighted probe and tying it in place; the tension on the suture holds the canal open ("canaloplasty").[6]

NEW PROCEDURES

The **Glaukos iStent,** a titanium device placed inside the Schlemm's canal allows the aqueous humor to flow directly into the canal, bypassing the trabecular meshwork.[14] It is inserted via a clear corneal incision under topical anesthesia and has the advantage of being devoid of a bleb and associated complications. The **Gold Microshunt (GMS),** a biocompatible gold shunt implanted in the suprachoroidal space uses the eye's natural pressure differential (uveoscleral outflow) to divert the aqueous into the suprachoroidal space in a controlled fashion. It has the advantage of postoperative phototitration with a laser.[15] **The Ex-PRESS mini shunt**, a small stainless steel device is now most often implanted under a large partial thickness scleral flap. It lowers IOP effectively but has bleb related complications.[16] **Canaloplasty**, as explained before a variation of viscocanalostomy involves circumferential catheterization and viscodilatation of the entire length of the Schlemm's canal thus restoring the natural trabeculocanalicular outflow passage and effective lowering of the IOP in POAG.[17] An adjunct to the procedure involves placing a prolene suture in the canal. A canaloplasty microcatheter with an illuminated beacon tip has also been designed specifically to aid in the procedure. The illuminated tip enables trans scleral visualization of the advancing tip. *The trabectome* uses a microelectrocautery to ablate a strip of trabecular meshwork and the inner wall of Schlemm's canal with a focused electrosurgical pulse. This provides direct access of aqueous to outflow channels. Done in mostly in POAG, it provides a reasonable IOP reduction, a significant decrease in medications and can be combined with phacoemulsification.[18,19]

Lasers are also becoming increasingly popular with *Excimer Laser Trabeculostomy* being used to create small holes into inner wall of Schlemm's canal via anterior trabecular meshwork with minimal thermal effects and lack of coagulative damage. *Endocyclophotocoagulation (ECP)* involves photocoagulation of the ciliary processes under direct visualization and is usually combined with cataract surgery. Encouraging results have been reported in a study in Indian subjects with refractory glaucoma.[20]

CONCLUSION

In evaluating any new surgical procedure it wise to follow the word of Duke-Elder:[1] *Any operation devised for the relief of glaucoma should ideally be such as to preserve the function of the eye, maintain its tension in with in normal limits, and retain integrity of the globe.* The number of operations advocated from time to time is evidence that this ideal has never been attained.

REFERENCES

1. Duke-Elder S. System of Ophthalmology. London: Henry Kimpton 1969;11: 569-71.
2. Kronfeld P. The rise of the filter operations. Surv Ophthalmol 1972;17:168.
3. Holth S. Iridencleisis antiglaucomatous. Ann Oculist 1908;137:345-6.
4. Elloit RH. A preliminary note on a new operative procedure for the establishment of a filtering cicatrix in management of glaucoma. Ophthalmoscope 1909;7:804-6.
5. Scheie HG. Retraction of scleral wound edges as a fistulizing procedure for glaucoma. Am J Ophthalmol 1958;45:20-9.
6. Krasnow MW. Externalization of Schlemm's canal in glaucoma. Br J Ophthal 1968;52:157-61.
7. Grant WM. further studies on facility of flow through the trabecular meshwork. Arch Ophthalmol 1958;60:523.
8. Allen L, Burian HM. Trabeculotomy ab externo. Am J Ophthalmol 1962;53:19.
9. Sugar HS. The filtering operations a historical overview. Glaucoma 1981; 3:85.
10. Ciarns JE. Trabeculectomy, Preliminary report for a new method. Am J Ophthalmol 1968;66:673.
11. Malteno ACB. New implant for glaucoma clinical trail. Br J Ophthalmol 1971;53:606.
12. Zimmerman TJ, Kooner KS, Ford VJ, et al. Effectiveness of nonpenetrating trabeculectomy in aphakic patient with glaucoma. Ophthalmic Surg 1984;15: 44-50.
13. Stegmann RC. Viscocanalostomy: a new surgical technique for open angle glaucoma. An Inst Barraquer 1995;25: 225-32.
14. Spiegel D, Kobuch K. Trabecular meshwork bypass tube shunts: initial case series. Br J Ophthalmol 2002;86:1228-31.
15. Ozdamar A, Aras C, Karacorlu M. Suprachoroidal seton implantation in refractory glaucoma: a novel surgical technique. J Glaucoma 2003;12:354-9.
16. Maris PJ Jr, Ishida K, Netland PA. Comparison of trabeculectomy with Ex-PRESS miniature glaucoma device implanted under scleral flap. J Glaucoma 2007;16:14-9.
17. Shingeleton B, Tetz M, Korber N. Circumferential viscodilation and tensioning of Schlemm canal (canaloplasty) with temporal clear corneal phacoemulsification cataract surgery for open-angle glaucoma and visually significant cataract. J Cataract Refract Surg 2008;34:433-40.
18. Minckler D, Baerveldt G, Ramirez MA, Mosaed S, Wilson R, Shaarawy T, et al. Clinical results with the Trabectome, a novel surgical device for treatment of open-angle glaucoma. Trans Am Ophthalmol Soc 2006;104:40-50.
19. Godfrey DG, Fellman RL, Neelakantan A. Canal surgery in adult glaucomas. Curr Opin Ophthalmol 2009;20:116-21.
20. Murthy GJ, Murthy PR, Murthy KR, Kulkarni VV, Murthy KR. Indian J Ophthalmol 2009;57:127-32.

46 Wound Healing in Glaucoma Surgery and Role of Antimetabolites in Glaucoma Filtering Surgery

Nikhil S Choudhari, L Vijaya

CHAPTER OUTLINE
❖ Wound Healing in Glaucoma Surgery
❖ Failure of Glaucoma Filtering Surgery
❖ Antimetabolites and Glaucoma Filtering Surgery
❖ Developments in the Usage of Antimetabolites in Glaucoma Filtering Surgery
❖ Technique of Application of Antimetabolites
❖ Complications of Antimetabolite Use
❖ Recent Advances

INTRODUCTION

Trabeculectomy represents a delicate balance between maintaining the integrity of the eye and prevention of excess scarring that precludes aqueous filtration. Recent time has seen a significant improvement in the efficacy of antiglaucoma medications. However, it appears that improvements in medical therapy have resulted in an overall decrease in the number of lower risk filtering procedures. As a result, there has been a shift in the trabeculectomy case mix towards a higher risk. Understanding the healing response of the eye and its thoughtful modifications with the use of antimetabolites is cardinal to improve surgical success in the current era.

WOUND HEALING IN GLAUCOMA SURGERY

The surgical procedure in any tissue is followed by a complex wound healing process. The process attempts strong wound healing that is desirable. The glaucoma surgery is unique in the sense that an excessive wound healing can lead to filtration failure. The phases of wound healing applicable to the glaucoma filtering surgery[1] are described below.

Inflammatory Phase (First 4 Days)

Tissue trauma resulting from glaucoma filtering surgery leads to constriction of blood vessels and leakage of plasma proteins and blood cells to the extracellular space. This results in an accumulation of fibrinogen, fibronectin, and platelets. Owing to the effect of tissue factors like histamine, serotonin, prostaglandins, leukotrienes, and complement factors, a clot of fibrin, fibronectin, platelets, and trapped blood cells is formed.

Proliferative Phase (5–14 Days)

Inflammatory cells, including monocytes and macrophages, migrate into the clot. The macrophages release factors that stimulate fibroblast migration and proliferation. Most fibroblasts secrete procollagen, which in turn is transformed into collagen stabilized by mucopolysaccharides.

Angiogenesis and fibroblast proliferation result in granulation tissue.

Remodeling Phase (Begins at Day 5)

This is the last phase of wound healing that begins during the fibroblastic phase and can last for more than a year. During this phase, collagen matures

and the number of fibroblasts and blood vessels decreases. A dense collagenous subconjunctival scar is formed.

FAILURE OF GLAUCOMA FILTERING SURGERY

Failure of the glaucoma filtering surgery can occur at one or more of the following sites (**Figure 1**):

1. *Sclerostomy:* The sclerostomy can be obstructed by iris or vitreous.
2. *Scleral flap:* Healing of the scleral flap can cause filtration failure.
3. *Episclera:* Episcleral fibrosis at the external aperture of the scleros-

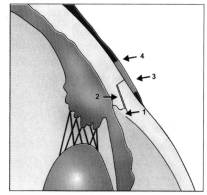

Fig. 1 Sites where failure of glaucoma filtering surgery is possible: 1. Sclerostomy; 2. Scleral flap; 3. Episclera; 4. Conjunctival bleb

tomy can prevent aqueous entering the subconjunctival space.

4. ***Conjunctival bleb:*** Encystment of the filtering bleb by the scar tissue can lead to trapping of the aqueous entering the subconjunctival space.

The common factor in most cases of filtration failure is excessive scarring in the subconjunctival space and this may be reduced using antimetabolite agents.[2] The use of multiple antiglaucoma medications can increase the number of preactivated conjunctival cells (macrophages, lymphocytes, mast cells and fibroblasts), thereby increasing the risk of bleb fibrosis. Administration of topical steroids prior to the filtering surgery is advocated if intensive glaucoma medication has been administered for longer periods.[3,4]

ANTIMETABOLITES AND GLAUCOMA FILTERING SURGERY

Indications for Antimetabolite Usage in Glaucoma Filtering Surgery[5]
Eyes with increased risk of scarring

Low-Risk
- No risk factors
- Long term use of topical medications (β-blockers/pilocarpine)
- African race.

Intermediate-Risk
- Young age
- Long term use of topical (adrenaline)
- Previous conjunctival surgery (cataract extraction, squint/retinal detachment surgery)
- Several low–risk factors.

High-Risk
- Aphakic glaucoma
- Neovascular glaucoma
- Chronic conjunctival inflammation.

- ***Inflammatory eye disease:*** Uveitis, ocular pemphigoid, Stevens – Johnson syndrome
- Previous failed trabeculectomy/tube
- Multiple risk factors.

Antimetabolites in Use
5 – Fluorouracil (5-FU)
Mechanism of action[6]
5-FU is a halogenated pyrimidine analogue. It decreases the biosynthesis of pyrimidine nucleotides by inhibiting thymidylate synthase, the enzyme that catalyzes the rate limiting step in DNA synthesis. This results in death of rapidly growing cells. Fluorouracil is much more lethal to logarithmically growing cells than to stationary cells. 5-FU is also incorporated into DNA or RNA leading to other cytotoxic actions including DNA strand breakage and a decrease in protein synthesis.

Drug availability
5-FU is available as a solution in the strength of 50 mg/ml. It can be administered intra or postoperatively.

Intraoperative use
- Administered on bare sclera on a sponge
- 25 or 50 mg/ml solution
- Time of exposure should be 3 to 5 minutes (shorter time has minimal effect)
- Rinse the surface thoroughly with balanced salt solution or normal saline after use.

Postoperative use
- Relative contraindication in the presence of corneal epithelial problem
- 5 mg injections (0.1 ml of 50 mg/ml undiluted solution)

- Adjacent to the bleb (but not into the bleb since pH of 9) or 180 degrees away from bleb
- Multiple injections possible.

Mitomycin C (MMC)
Mitomycin is an antibiotic isolated from *Streptomyces caespitosus.*

Mechanism of Action
MMC is activated *in vivo* to an alkylating agent. Binding to DNA leads to cross-linking and inhibition of DNA synthesis and function.[6] MMC can interfere with any phase in the cell cycle, and therefore is cell cycle phase-nonspecific. It also inhibits RNA and protein synthesis.[6] It is much more potent than 5-FU. *In vivo*, MMC produces long-term inhibition of fibroblast division, whereas inhibition after 5–FU exposure is temporary.[7,8] In cell culture experiments, 5-FU was toxic to fibroblasts but spared capillary endothelial cells whereas MMC was cytotoxic to both cell types.[9] These differences between the activity of MMC and 5-FU may account for the observed clinical differences in bleb morphology in eyes treated with them.

Drug Availability
MMC is available as powder in strengths of 2, 10 and 40 mg. Care must be taken while preparing the required strength of the drug (see below). It can be administered intra or postoperatively.

Intraoperative use
- ***Concentration:*** 0.1 to 0.5 mg/ml
- Administered on bare sclera on a sponge
- ***Duration of application:*** 1 to 5 minutes
- Avoid contact with cut edge of the conjunctival flap

- Rinse the surface thoroughly with balanced salt solution or normal saline after use.

Postoperative use
- **Concentration:** 0.02 mg/ml
- Adjacent (but not into) the bleb or 180 degrees away from bleb Multiple injections possible.

DEVELOPMENTS IN THE USAGE OF ANTIMETABOLITES IN GLAUCOMA FILTERING SURGERY

The use of antimetabolites was popularized by the work of Parrish and colleagues from Miami in the 1980s, after work on 5-FU for experimental proliferative vitreoretinopathy.[10] Experimental work in the laboratory lead to pilot trials, culminating in the **5-Fluorouracil filtration surgery study (FFSS)**.[11-13] In this trial, patients who had previous failed filtration surgery or cataract surgery were randomized to either postoperative 5-FU or no injections. Twenty eight (27%) of the 105 eyes in the 5-FU group and 54 (50%) of the 108 eyes in the standard filtration surgery group (no- 5-FU) were classified as failures, defined by reoperation for control of IOP during the first year or an IOP more than 21 mm Hg at the one year visit.[11] At 5 years, the failure rate dropped to 54 (51%) in the 5-FU treated group and 80 (74%) in the standard filtration surgery group.[13] This was a revolutionary result at the time for this difficult group of patients.

Although early findings were encouraging, long-term results have been less convincing. Suzuki et al[14] studied 87 high risk eyes (previous cataract surgery or failed glaucoma surgery) that underwent trabeculectomies augmented with postoperative 5-FU injections. Successful control of intraocular pressure (IOP) was defined as IOP less than 21 mm Hg or a reduction of 33 percent if the preoperative pressure was less than 21 mm Hg. Despite good control of IOP at 1 year, trabeculectomies showed a continued drift towards failure over time with success rates of 61 percent at 5 years, 44 percent at 10 years and 41 percent at 14 years.[14]

The use of an intraoperative application of MMC was another major innovation in the field. The technique was first used by Chen in 1981,[15] but did not gain wide spread popularity until the late 1980s and early 1990s. Subsequently, randomized trials showed an intraoperative application of MMC to be superior to post operative injections of 5-FU.[16-19] A single intraoperative application of MMC is also much more convenient than multiple subconjunctival 5-FU injections in the postoperative period. MMC-aided trabeculectomy was found to be successful in controlling IOP in darkly pigmented Indian population.[20]

Intraoperative 5-FU has been shown to be at least as effective as intraoperative MMC in controlling IOP of eyes undergoing *primary* trabeculectomy.[21-23] Till date, there is no report comparing intraoperative 5-FU versus MMC use in high risk glaucoma filtering surgeries. However, because MMC is more potent than 5-FU and has longer lasting effects on cultured fibroblasts, clinicians tend to prefer MMC over 5-FU in high-risk glaucoma filtering surgeries.

Handling of Antimetabolites

Antimetabolites are extremely toxic drugs. The patient and the operating room staff must be protected from exposure to these drugs while handling them. A number of countries have specific regulations or guidelines elating to the handling of these drugs. At minimum, a separate sterile work area should be used for mixing antimetabolites and the staff handling these drugs must wear protective gloves. Care must be taken while preparing the desired strengths of these agents so as not to cause back spray or aerosol formation.

Preparation Techniques

5-FU: 5-FU is available as a solution in the strength of 50 mg/ml. Usually the same strength is used for intraoperative use. It may be diluted to 25 mg/ml and used intraoperatively.

MMC: Mitomycin C is available as powder in strengths of 2, 10 and 40 mg. During operation, the drug is freshly reconstituted with distilled water or normal saline in concentrations of 0.1 – 0.5 mg/ml. The color of the reconstituted solution is light purple.

> **Note** A different color indicates ineffective drug that should be discarded. The solution, once reconstituted, can be used throughout the day for multiple surgeries but should be discarded at the end of the day.

A new formulation for single use, Mitosol has recently been approved by FDA (not yet marketed till the time of publishing this book). Each vial of Mitosol contains a sterile lyophilized mixture of 0.2 mg of mitomycin and 0.4 mg of mannitol in a 1:2 concentration ratio. When reconstituted with 1 ml of sterile water for injection, the solution contains 0.2 mg/mL mitomycin. Sponges provided within the Mitosol Kit are saturated with the solution, utilizing the entire reconstituted contents of the vial and used intraoperatively.

TECHNIQUE OF APPLICATION OF ANTIMETABOLITES

It is important to achieve a good hemostasis prior to antimetabolite application. The antimetabolites are strictly applied to the extraocular tissues.

Polyvinyl alcohol sponge is used for drug delivery to the subconjunctival space. The sponge is cut into several small pieces and soaked in the solution of the antimetabolites. Excess drug is squeezed out and then the sponges are applied directly over the bare sclera for the desired length of time. At the end of the application, the sponges are taken out and the area of application is thoroughly washed with balanced salt solution or normal saline. The soaked sponges must be disposed in an incinerator and the instruments used while application of the sponges must not be used in the surgery.

Improvements in the use of Intraoperative Antimetabolites (Figure 2)

Use of intraoperative MMC rapidly became popular principally because of its efficacy and ease of application. Unfortunately, problems with MMC became apparent and that gradually lead to the improvements in the use of intraoperative antimetabolites to reduce the incidence and severity of associated complications and also to enhance the surgical success rate as follows.

Judicious Use of Antimetabolites

Use weaker agents (intraoperative 5-FU) or lower concentrations of MMC in low risk eyes or in eyes at high risk of hypotony or other complications of antimetabolites.

Use of Nonfragmenting Sponge

Polyvinyl alcohol sponge should be preferred over methylcellulose sponge. Polyvinyl alcohol sponge is less friable after cutting than the cellulose sponge, and less likely to leave remnants behind after removal.[24]

Limiting Conjunctival Exposure to the Antimetabolites

The cut edge of the conjunctival flap should be protected from exposure to the antimetabolite to possibly avoid retardation of conjunctival flap healing. Significant bleb dysesthesia can result if the bleb forms in the interpalpebral space. Exposure of the nasal and temporal conjunctiva to the antimetabolite should be avoided.

Wide Area of Application of Antimetabolites

A wide area of antimetabolite application is more likely to produce a diffuse bleb with less thinning of the bleb roof. This can be achieved using multiple small sponges soaked in the antimetabolite over a wide area posterior to the site of the sclera flap. The type of conjunctival flap may have influence in this regard. The fornix-based conjunctival flap can allow wider posterior dissection (**Figure 3A**). Alternatively, a limbus-based flap can be used with the traditional single large sponge application of the antimetabolite (**Figure 3B**). There is some evidence that limbus-based flaps may be more likely to develop serious bleb-related complications and may develop these earlier than fornix-based flaps.[25] The higher rates of complications could be attributable to the differences in bleb morphology, with limbus-based flap cases more likely to develop cystic blebs.[25]

Treating Under Both Scleral Flap and Conjunctival Flap

Trabeculectomy failure primarily due to healing of the scleral flap is uncommon. Application of the antimetabolite prior to scleral flap dissection should, therefore treat the primary target tissue i.e. fibroblasts of the tenon's capsule and episclera. On the other hand, if a large surface area sclera flap is desired, a larger area of contact for scleral healing results and application of the antimetabolite both under the conjunctival as well as the scleral flap should be considered.

Improvements in the use of Postoperative 5-FU
Using Lower Dose Regimens

The original regimen of 21 injections of 5 mg of 5-FU given 180 degrees from the bleb as used in the FFSS[10-12] (twice a day for 1 week then once a day for 1 week) has now evolved, and most ophthalmologists give less than 10 injections with longer intervals in between injections. The lower dose regimens may reduce the incidence of corneal side effects of 5-FU.

Injections Given Closure to the Bleb Area

This may increase efficacy of the same dose of the drug. But the injection

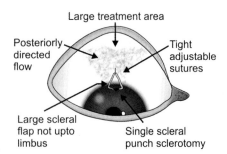

Fig. 2 Improvements in the use of intraoperative antimetabolites

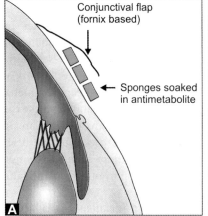 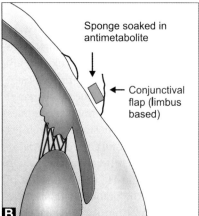

Figs 3A and B The influence of the fornix based (A) and limbus based. (B) Conjunctival flap on the effective area of application of antimetabolites

should never be injected into the bleb as the solution has a pH of 9.

Other Measures to Reduce Corneal Epitheliopathy

These include use of long subconjunctival needle track and use of small bore needle e.g. 30 gauge needles. In addition, prior injection of subconjunctival viscoelastic followed by injection of 5-FU on the far side of viscoelastic may prevent reflux of 5-FU in the tear film.[26]

Use in Conjunction with Intraoperative Antimetabolites

This can reduce postoperative need for 5-FU injections.

COMPLICATIONS OF ANTIMETABOLITE USE

Corneal epithelial toxicity

The most common side effect of postoperative 5-FU injections is corneal epithelial toxicity that is reported in over 50 percent of eyes. By adjusting the frequency of postoperative 5-FU subconjunctival injections according to the clinical response, Weinreb[27] has shown low rate (29%) of detectable changes in corneal epithelium.

Complications related to bleb morphology

The use of MMC is associated with thin, cystic, avascular conjunctival blebs. There have been numerous reports that associate this bleb morphology to ocular hypotony. Most eyes develop bleb avascularity within the first year after surgery.[28] Excessive filtration in the postoperative period seems to be the most important cause of ocular hypotony associated with optic disc edema, vascular tortuosity and macular chorioretinal folds with reduction in visual acuity. In their 5 year follow-up of 123 eyes that underwent trabeculectomy with MMC (0.25-0.5 mg/ml for

0.5 to 5 minutes), Bindlish et al[29] found a high incidence of ocular hypotony (IOP < 6 mm Hg) in 42.2 percent, and hypotony maculopathy in 8.9 percent of eyes. Young and myopic eyes are reportedly more prone to develop hypotony maculopathy due to longer axial length and thereby reduced scleral rigidity.[30]

Long-onset bleb leak is more common after trabeculectomy associated with MMC use than that with 5-FU use.[31] These late-onset bleb leaks are more commonly associated with endophthalmitis.[32] Inferior limbal trabeculectomy carries much higher risk of infection.[32] Patients with eyes undergoing glaucoma surgery with MMC and avascular blebs should be monitored indefinitely. Recent research suggest that a large surface area of antimetabolite application together with fornix-based conjunctival flaps leads to diffuse, posteriorly extended noncystic conjunctival blebs **(Figure 4)** with a reduction in bleb related complications.[25]

Aqueous hyposecretion due to toxicity of MMC may be another mechanism of ocular hypotony. Disruption of ciliary body epithelium beneath the site of MMC application has been shown in an enucleated human eye[33] and also in a rabbit model.[34,35]

Intraocular Toxicity of MMC

MMC has been shown to cause marked corneal endothelial loss, corneal stromal necrosis, anterior chamber reaction and hemorrhagic iris necrosis in animal studies.[35] Therefore, every precaution should be taken to avoid accidental exposure of intraocular tissues to MMC.

RECENT ADVANCES

Considering the potentially serious complications of the antimetabolites in current use, more physiological

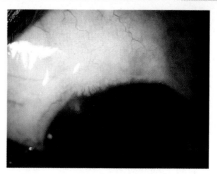

Fig. 4 A well functioning, diffuse bleb with microcysts

anti-scarring agents are under investigation. Of all the growth factors involved in the wound-healing cascade, transforming growth factor-beta (TGF-β) has been shown to be one of the most potent stimulators of conjunctival fibroblast proliferation. TGF-β2 is the most predominant mammalian isoforms in the eye. A recent phase III randomized, double-masked multicenter, placebo-controlled trial[36] has shown a comparable efficacy and safety profile of CAT-152 (lerdelimumab), a monoclonal antibody to TGF-β2, in preventing the progression of fibrosis in patient undergoing first-time trabeculectomy for primary open-angle or chronic angle-closure glaucoma.

SUMMARY

The current era is experiencing a shift towards higher risk trabeculectomy procedures. The success rate of glaucoma filtering surgery can be improved by a thoughtful use of antimetabolites. A judicious use of the available antimetabolite agents, increased surface of application and fornix based conjunctival incisions have led to a significant reduction in cystic blebs and long term complications such as endophthalmitis. Better methods of applying postoperative antimetabolite agents are also described. Research in the use of newer antiscarring agents is underway.

REFERENCES

1. Collignon NJ. Wound healing after glaucoma surgery: how to manage it? Bull Soc Belge Ophthalmol 2005;295: 55-9.

2. Madhavan HN, Rao SB, Vijaya L, et al. In vitro sensitivity of human Tenon's capsule fibroblasts to mitomycin C and its correlation with outcome of glaucoma filtration surgery. Ophthalmic Surg 1995;26:61-7.

3. Broadway DC, Grierson I, Sturmer J, et al. Reversal of topical antiglaucoma medication effects on the conjunctiva. Arch Ophthalmol 1996;114:262-7.

4. Khaw PT, Chang L, Wong TT, et al. Modulation of wound healing after glaucoma surgery. Curr Opin Ophthalmol 2001;12:143-8.

5. Broadway DC, Chang LP. Trabeculectomy, risk factors for failure and the preoperative state of the conjunctiva. J Glaucoma 2001;10:237-49.

6. Salmon SE, Sartorelli AC. Cancer chemotherapy, in Katzung BG (Ed): Basic and clinical pharmacology. Appleton-Lange 1998.pp.881-911.

7. Khaw PT, Doyle JW, Sherwood MB, et al. Prolonged localized tissue effects from 5-minute exposures to fluorouracil and mitomycin. Arch Ophthalmol 1993;111:263-7.

8. Khaw PT, Sherwood MB, Doyle JW, et al. Intraoperative and postoperative treatment with 5-Fluorouracil and mitomycin C: long term effects in vivo on subconjunctival and scleral fibroblasts. Int Ophthalmol 1992;16:381-5.

9. Smith S, Damore PA, Dreyer EB. Comparative toxicity of mitomycin C and 5-fluorouracil in vitro. Am J Ophthalmol 1994;118:332-7.

10. Blumenkranz M, Hernandez E, Ophir A, et al. 5-fluorouracil: new applications in complicated retinal detachment for an established antimetabolite. Ophthalmology 1984;91:122-30.

11. The fluorouracil filtering surgery study Group. Fluorouracil filtering surgery study one year follow up. Am J Ophthalmol 1989;108:625-35.

12. The fluorouracil filtering surgery study group: Three – year follow-up of the fluorouracil filtering surgery study. Am J ophthalmol 1993;115:82-93.

13. The fluorouracil filtering surgery study group: Five-year follow up of the fluorouracil filtering surgery study. Am J Ophthalmol 1996;121:349-66.

14. Suzuki R, Dickens CJ, Iwach AG, et al. Long-term follow-up of initially successful trabeculectomy with 5-fluorouracil injections. Ophthalmology 2002;109:1921-4.

15. Chen CW. Enhanced intraocular pressure controlling effectiveness of trabeculectomy by local application of mitomycin C. Trans Asia Pacif Acad Ophthalmol 1983;9:172-7.

16. Skuta GL, Beeson CC, Higginbotham EJ, et al. Intraoperative mitomycin versus postoperative 5-Fluorouracil in high-risk glaucoma filtering surgery. Ophthalmology 1992;99:438-44.

17. Kitazawa Y, Kawase K, Matsushita H, et al. Trabeculectomy with mitomycin. A comparative study with fluorouracil. Arch Ophthalmol 1991;109:1693-8.

18. Katz GJ, Higginbotham EJ, Lichter RR, et al. Mitomycin C versus 5-Fluorouracil in high risk glaucoma filtering surgery. Ophthalmology 1995;102:1263-9.

19. Akarsu C, Onol M, Hasaneisoglu B. Postoperative 5-fluorouracil versus intraoperative mitomycin C in high-risk glaucoma filtering surgery: extended followup. Clin Exp ophthalmol 2003;31:199-205.

20. Ramakrishnan R, Mochon J, Robin AL, et al. Safety and efficacy of mitomycin C trabeculectomy in southern India. A short-term pilot study. Ophthalmology 1993;100:1619-23.

21. Vijaya L, Mukhesh BN, Shantha B, et al. Comparison of low-dose intraoprative mitomycin-C vs 5-fluorouracil in primary glaucoma surgery: a pilot study. Ophthalmic Surg Lasers 2000; 31:24-30.

22. Singh K, Mehta K, Shaikh NM, et al. Trabeculectomy with intraoperative mitomycin C versus 5-fluorouracil. Prospective randomized clinical trial. Ophthalmology 2000;107:2305-9.

23. WuDunn D, Cantor LB, Palanca-Capistrano AM, et al. A prospective randomized trial comparing intraoperative 5-fluorouracil vs mitomycin C in primary trabeculectomy. Am J Ophthalmol 2002;134:521-8.

24. Pool TR, Gillespie IH, Kne G, et al. Microscopic fragmentation of ophthalmic surgical sponge spears used for delivery of antiproliferative agents in glaucoma filtering surgery. Br J Ophthalmol 2002;86:1448-9.

25. Wells AP, Cordeiro MF, Bunce C, et al. Cystic bleb formation and related complications in limbus-versus fornix based conjunctival flaps in pediatric and young adult trabeculectomy with mitomycin C. Ophthalmology 2003; 110:2192-7.

26. Khaw PT. Advances in glaucoma surgery: evolution of antimetabolite adjunctive therapy. Journal of glaucoma 2001;(Suppl 1):S81-4.

27. Weinreb RN. Adjusting the dose of 5-fluorouracil after filtration surgery to minimize side effects. Ophthalmology 1987;94:564-70.

28. Anand N, Arora S, Clowes M. Mitomycin C augmented glaucoma surgery: evolution of filtering bleb avascularity, transconjunctival oozing, and leaks. Br J Ophthalmol 2006;90:175-80.

29. Bindlish R, Condon GP, Schlosser JD, et al. Efficacy and safety of mitomycin-C in primary trabeculectomy: five-year followup. Ophthalmology 2002;109: 1336-42.

30. Fannin LA, Schiffman JC, Budenz DL. Risk factors for hypotony maculopathy Ophthalmology 2003;110:1185-91.

31. Greenfield DS, Liebmann JM, Jee J, et al. Late-onset bleb leaks after glaucoma filtering surgery. Arch Ophthalmol 1998;116:443-7.

32. Greenfield DS, Suner IJ, Miller MP, et al. Endophthalmitis after filtering surgery with mitomycin. Arch Ophthalmol 1996;114:943-9.

33. Nuyts RM, Felten PC, Pels E, et al. Histopathologic effects of mitomycin C after trabeculectomy in human glaucomatous eyes with persistent hypotony. Am J Ophthalmol 1994;118:225-37.

34. Mietz H, Addicks K, Diestelhorst M, et al. Extraocular application of mitomycin C in a rabbit model: cytotoxic effects on the ciliary body and epithelium. Ophthalmic Surg 1994; 25:240-4.

35. Morrow GL, Stein RM, Heathcote JG, et al. Ocular toxicity of mitomycin C and 5-fluorouracil in the rabbit. Can J Ophthalmol 1994;29:268-73.

36. CAT-152 0102 Trabeculectomy Study Group, Khaw P, Grehn F, Hollo G, et al. A phase III study of subconjunctival human anti-transforming growth factor beta (2) monoclonal antibody (CAT-152) to prevent scarring after first-time trabeculectomy. Ophthalmology 2007;114:1822-30.

47 Trabeculectomy—Surgical Techniques and Complications

P Sathyan, MS Sunil, R Ramakrishnan

CHAPTER OUTLINE
- Objectives of Glaucoma Surgery
- Principle of Glaucoma Surgery
- Preoperative Considerations
- Anesthesia
- Trabeculectomy: Surgical Technique
- Special Considerations
- Early Bleb Titration
- Complications of Glaucoma Filtering Surgery
- Management of the Leaking Bleb: An Overview

INTRODUCTION

An association between glaucoma and elevated intraocular pressure was first suggested in 1622 by Richard Bannister. However, surgical attempts to treat glaucoma by lowering intraocular pressure were developed only in the, 19th century. In 1830, Mac Kenzie described a sclerotomy and later a paracentesis, but found that both were only temporarily beneficial in lowering the intraocular pressure (IOP). In 1968, Cairns reported a microsurgical technique called trabeculectomy and it is still considered as the gold standard glaucoma filtering surgery. Cairns introduced a limbal based conjunctival flap (LBCF) technique and Luntz introduced a fornix based conjunctival flap technique (FBCF) in 1980. The technique for trabeculectomy has undergone many modifications since then and still continues to evolve.

OBJECTIVES OF GLAUCOMA SURGERY

Glaucoma therapy is aimed at protecting optic nerve and preserving visual function. Currently, IOP is the only modifiable risk factor which we can address. There is no universal treatment that is applicable to all type of

glaucomas. Despite advances in anti glaucoma medications a significant percent of patients still require surgical intervention. Hence, treatment has to be individualized on case by case basis. *Trabeculectomy* aims at excising the trabecular meshwork and creating a fistula through which aqueous humor drains from anterior chamber and accumulates in the subconjunctival space or subtenons' space forming a filtering bleb. The hallmark of functioning bleb are the subepithelial clear spaces representing microcystic accumulation of aqueous humor.

> **Note** The aim of surgery is to maintain useful vision and to avoid further glaucomatous damage by lowering intraocular pressure.

PRINCIPLE OF GLAUCOMA SURGERY

Ocular tissues are inherently equipped with a good healing response immediately after tissue injury. As a consequence of surgical trauma to conjunctiva and sclera, blood vessels are damaged and disrupted leading to sequence of tissue repair phenomenon. In most surgical procedures, it is desirable to enhance postoperative wound healing response. However, in

glaucoma filtering surgery wound healing can lead to episcleral fibroproliferation and histologically dense collagenous tissue with resulting filtering failure. To maximize the potential for successful outcome of trabeculectomy, it is desirable to selectively inhibit wound healing response in sclera and episcleral tissue while simultaneously leaving conjunctival wound healing intact.

PREOPERATIVE CONSIDERATIONS

The success of guarded filtration as an initial procedure in lowering intraocular pressure to 21 mm Hg or less is about 80 to 90 percent for chronic open-angle glaucoma and other open angle glaucomas like pseudoexfoliation glaucoma and pigmentary glaucoma.[1,2] A functional bleb, as mentioned earlier is the cornerstone of filtration surgery **(Figure 1)**.[1] Characteristics of the bleb depend on the operative technique, postoperative medications, patient's age, and the type of glaucoma.[1,3]

Preoperative Counseling
- Detailed information including the indication, type of surgery, its possible complications, need for regular

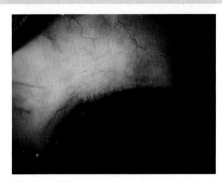

Fig. 1 A diffuse, moderately elevated well functioning bleb seen after trabeculectomy with a fornix-based conjunctival flap

follow-up should be explained in patients vernacular language.

- In order to avoid unrealistic expectations from the patient, they should be informed that this surgery aims at preserving the existing vision.

- Chances of snuff out phenomenon also should be explained in advanced cases of glaucoma.

Because cataract progression is a significant risk after filtration surgery, the patient should be warned that, although the surgery may be successful in halting glaucomatous progression, visual acuity may decrease. An informed consent should be obtained from the patient. Giving "informed consent" implies consenting after being informed of the risks of the procedure. Both the common, minor complications and the rarer, serious complications must be addressed. It must be clearly reminded that the basic goal is to preserve, not to improve vision.

Ocular Status

The location of the filtering fistula is partially determined by the configuration of the angle. In the presence of a narrow angle, especially with peripheral anterior synechiae (PAS), the excision of the internal corneoscleral block should be more anterior than usual to avoid the iris root and ciliary body. Conjunctiva that is scarred from previous surgery is difficult to dissect from

the underlying sclera; buttonholes in the flap may result. Thus, any area with adequately mobile conjunctiva should be selected for resurgery.

The following factors deserve attention preoperatively:

1. **Lids and adnexa:** Abnormal lid positions, lagophthalmos, blepharitis (including meibomian gland dysfunction) increases the risk of bleb dysesthesias, exposure and bleb infection.

2. **Conjunctiva:** Allergy and toxicity to medications results in follicular conjunctivitis, conjunctival cytological changes leading to dry eyes. Conjunctival hyperemia with evident filliform vessels, use of multiple medications for longer duration of time are the risk factors for failure. Conjunctival scarring postsurgery (e.g. pterygium surgery, prior ECCE, scleral buckling or pars plana vitrectomy) leaves behind minimal healthy conjunctiva for bleb survival.

3. **Cornea:** In cases of prior keratoplasty, trabeculectomy should be planned in such a way to avoid graft-host interface or peripheral anterior synechiae (PAS).

4. Uveitis to be treated aggressively prior to and after surgery.

5. **Refractive errors:** Myopic eyes are more likely to develop hypotony postoperatively and hyperopic eyes are more likely to develop malignant glaucoma in the postoperative period.

6. **Lens (Aphakia):** There is increased risk of suprachoroidal hemorrhage. Thin sclera and conjunctival scarring makes surgery difficult. Thorough anterior vitrectomy is a prerequisite.

Pseudophakia: Areas of conjunctival scarring and prior cataract incision should be avoided. There are less chances of developing postoperative shallow chamber in pseudophakic eyes.

Phakic eyes: They are more likely to develop shallow anterior chamber postoperatively.

Indications of Surgery

Surgery has been considered as second modality of therapy. However, even with recent advances in medical therapy compliance, adherence and adverse events are still the major concern.

Absolute Indications

1. Glaucoma not controlled on maximal medical therapy.

2. Rapid deterioration of vision with advanced glaucomatous damage is an indication of early surgery.

3. Disease progression despite good control of IOP indicating fluctuation in IOP as the probable cause. Filtering surgery reduces fluctuation in IOP better than medical therapy as shown by various studies.

4. Increase in intraocular pressure to a level considered likely to cause rapid worsening of the optic disc or visual field.

5. Glaucomas refractory to medical therapy like developmental glaucomas, uveitic glaucoma, angle recession glaucoma and steroid induced glaucoma.

6. Poor compliance.

Relative Indications

1. **Economic considerations:** In developing countries like India, where in cost and compliance are the major drawbacks for effective management of glaucoma, surgery at affordable cost may be considered as first choice.

2. Ocular or systemic side effects of antiglaucoma medications.

Preoperative Workup and Preparation

1. Thorough ophthalmic evaluation including IOP, visual fields and ONH evaluation is mandatory.

2. Complete systemic evaluation with respect to diabetes, hypertension,

cardiovascular diseases should be performed. In patients with cardiovascular disorders and stroke who are on antiplatelet drugs and anticoagulants these drugs should be stopped with the advise of the physician and appropriate remedial measures.

3. ***Tear film status and its evaluation:*** Medications which affect the ocular surface and disrupt the blood aqueous barrier like prostaglandin analogs, alpha agonists, pilocarpine and beta-receptor antagonists should be stopped 1 to 2 weeks prior to surgery. Preoperative short course of topical steroids helps in reducing the conjunctival inflammation. In one eyed patients, preoperative conjunctival culture sensitivity is preferable.

4. Prophylactic peripheral iridotomy in angle closure disease.

5. In case of resurgery, the original surgical site usually has significant conjunctival scarring and increased vascularity. It is often easier and more successful to reoperate at an adjacent area with less fibrosis. Conjunctival mobility should be checked pre operatively to plan the site of surgery.

Certain glaucoma medications may be stopped at least 72 hours before surgery, if possible. However, in some advanced cases none of the medications is stopped for fear of wiping out central fixation. *Pilocarpine* may be stopped at least 72 hours before as it promotes inflammation and break down of the blood-aqueous barrier and stimulates contraction of the pupillary sphincter and cillary muscle. Paralysis of these muscles is highly important after filtration surgery to help avoid posterior synechiae, pupillary block, and flat anterior chambers and malignant glaucoma. As mentioned earlier, *oral anticoagulants* such as dicoumarol, aspirin, and dipyridamole should be stopped to minimize a bleeding diathesis if there are no contraindications for stopping them. This should be done in consultation with the treating physician. If the intraocular pressure is greater than 30 mm Hg, or otherwise thought to be too high, an intravenous hyperosmotic agent such as mannitol may be administered at 0.5 to 1 mg/kg over 45 minutes, beginning at least 1 hour before surgery.

ANESTHESIA

Trabeculectomy may be done under retrobulbar, peribulbar, subtenon or topical anesthesia.

Hyaluronidase, an enzyme that breaks down hyaluronic acid—the polysaccharide matrix of tissue interstitial spaces is added to the anesthetic for the retrobulbar/peribulbar injection. Lyophilized 150 U of the solid material is dissolved in 30 ml of local anesthetic solution. It should not be used when greater chemosis is undesirable. A facial block can be administered to supplement (to weaken the orbicularis oculi) when retrobulbar block is used. A subtenons block can be used.

Subconjunctival anesthesia is less preferred as it may cause scarring due to hemorrhage and local tissue damage. Topical anesthesia supplemented with intracameral anesthesia has several advantages as it avoids conjunctival damage, chemosis, subconjunctival hemorrhage but with major limitation of lack of akinesia.

Adrenaline in anesthetic solutions is preferably avoided because of the vasoconstricting effect which may prove to be hazardous in glaucoma. The practice of placement of Honan balloon or super pinky should be used with caution or not at all in trabeculectomy because a seemingly insignificant elevation of intraocular pressure may be hazardous in advan-ced glaucoma.[4]

General anaesthesia (GA) is considered in pediatric age group, highly anxious patients or with suboptimal mental status. GA gives maximal control over systemic blood pressure and also IOP intraoperatively which favors good outcome.

Points to be Remembered

- Higher volume of local anesthetic with adrenaline can compromise ONH circulation either by volume or by vasoconstrictive effect of adrenaline especially in advanced glaucoma.
- Avoid compressive devices like super pinky or honans balloon in advanced glaucomas. Instead, a controlled gentle digital massage is sufficient.
- Inadequate anesthesia is not uncommon. Additional 1 to 2 cc of subtenon's anesthesia may be useful to reduce the pain and discomfort.
- Repeat blocks should preferably be avoided.

Pearls for a Good Outcome

- Good anesthesia and akinesia
- Minimal bleeding
- Low vitreous pressure
- Comfortable patient.

TRABECULECTOMY: SURGICAL TECHNIQUE

Surgical Exposure

After adequate anesthesia and akinesia, the eye to be operated is cross checked, painted and draped. An eye speculum designed to lower the pressure over the eyeball with an adjustable screw is beneficial. It is inserted and adjusted to avoid any pressure on the globe when the eyelids are kept open.

Superior Rectus Bridle Suture

A superior rectus traction suture helps to rotate the globe inferiorly to bring the superior bulbar conjunctiva into view. This gives good exposure superiorly for better dissection and maneuverability.

Technique: A muscle hook is used to infraduct the globe. Forceps may be avoided as it may cause conjunctival hemorrhage and button holing. 4-0 silk is used for bridle suture which is put 7 to 7.5 mm from the limbus **(Figure 2)**. A short and crisp bite should be taken to prevent button holing of conjunctiva which may cause postoperative leakage.

Complications of bridle suture
- Superior rectus hematoma
- Conjunctival button holing
- Disinsertion of the muscle
- Postoperative ptosis
- Globe perforation.

Corneal Traction Suture
Alternative to the bridle suture a corneal traction suture can also be used. It gives a good exposure superiorly.

Technique: 8-0 silk/nylon suture is used for corneal traction suture. It is placed 1 mm anterior to the limbus. The bite is 4 to 5 mm wide and at a depth of 2/3rd to 3/4th corneal thickness. It should not be too deep or too superficial to cause cheese wiring. Gentle and constant traction should be applied. Intermittent traction should be avoided which may cause cheese wiring.

It is preferred in pediatric glaucoma, soft eyeball, patients with narrow and deep sockets, thin sclera, high myopia, conjunctival arteriovenous malformations.

Conjunctival Flap
Either a fornix based or a limbal based conjunctival flap can be made using a Wescott or Vannas scissors and a nontoothed forceps. Neither type of conjunctival flap is superior to the other in terms of intraocular pressure reduction or ultimate success; but the character of the resulting bleb is different. A limbus based flap produces a more localized and elevated bleb with a 'ring of steel' while a fornix based flap produces a diffuse and more posterior bleb.

Limbus-based Flap
To make a limbal-based flap **(Figure 3)**, conjunctiva over the superior rectus insertion is held and elevated, putting the conjunctiva between the forceps and the superior rectus tendon on traction. A small opening is made through conjunctiva with sharp dissection and the incision is extended 8 mm from and parallel to the limbus. Tenon's capsule is incised 2 mm anterior to the conjunctival incision so as to avoid the anterior ciliary arteries near the superior rectus tendon insertion. While the conjunctival tenons flap is elevated by holding the tenons, blunt dissection is done until the limbal area is exposed. The corneoscleral sulcus should become clearly visible, with no fibres crossing it. The end point is a clear definition of the surgical limbus with the three zones of clear, blue and white limbal tissue.

Fornix-based Flap
To make a fornix based flap, disinsertion of the conjunctiva and tenon's capsule from limbus is performed with a Vannas or Wescott scissors Blunt tipped westcotts' tenotomy scissors is used for dissection **(Figures 4A and B)**. Initial opening is 2 mm wide at the preferred site of surgery and blades are insuinated under the tenons' capsule towards both sides and 7 to 8 mm posteriorly to create space for placing sponges soaked with antifibrotics. Tenonectomy should be avoided as far as possible when antifibrotics are used, but limited tenonectomy should

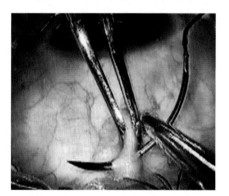

Fig. 2 Superior rectus bridle suture

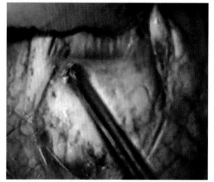

Fig. 3 Limbus-based conjunctival flap

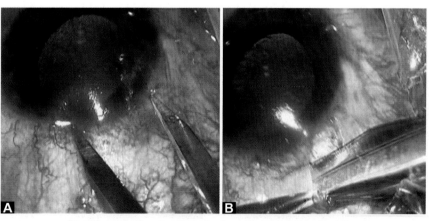

Figs 4A and B Construction of a fornix based conjunctival flap be done in young patients with very thick highly vascularized tenon's capsule which contributes to rapid healing. A fornix based conjunctival flap is easier to make and close with less chance of buttonholing. Disadvantages with fornix based flaps include difficulty in locating posterior sources of bleeding and the possibility of postoperative aqueous humor leakage at the limbus, especially if adjunctive antifibrotic therapy is used.

Hemostasis

Minimal adequate subconjunctival and episcleral hemostasis is essential to prevent healing responses triggered by the blood. It also facilitates meticulous dissection of the scleral flap. Unipolar or bipolar wet field cautery is ideal. Heat cautery is not preferred (**Figure 5**). Cauterization of the perforators which are marked by the loops of axenfeld should be avoided as it may cause ischemia of the anterior segment. Excess cautery over the scleral flap and cautery over sclera bed should be avoided as it leads to shrinkage and improper apposition of the edges during closure.

Application of Antifibrotic Agents

Antifibrotics can be applied either before or after fashioning the scleral groove of appropriate dimensions and depth, or underneath the sclera flap. Mitomycin C (MMC) is the most widely used primary antifibrotic (**Figures 6A and B**). MMC is used in the concentration varying from 0.2 to 0.4 mg/ml (0.02–0.04%) and for a duration varying between 1 and 4 minutes depending on the risk factors. 5-fluorouracil is most commonly used to augment the survival of the blebs postoperatively. Dose for intraoperative use is 25 to 50 mg/ml for a period of 5 min. Antifibrotics should be applied using Weckcell sponge cut into smaller bits spread over a larger area. Regular cotton tipped applicator soaked in MMC should be avoided as it may leave cotton fibers behind which results in high rate of postoperative complications like scleral necrosis. Conjunctiva and tenons' should be handled using nontoothed forceps while placing the sponges. Contact of the sponges with cut edges of conjunctiva should be avoided. Conjunctiva tends to retract over the sponges, hence it should be pulled and held pressed at the limbus for few seconds. After the time limit, sponges are removed and the area should be washed with adequate balanced salt solution (BSS) (atleast 20–30 cc). While flushing, tenons capsule should be lifted and pulled over limbus to form a pouch and saline should be injected forcefully.

The Scleral Flap

After the conjunctival flap is made bleeding vessels of the sclera are cauterized using light cautery. A partial thickness scleral flap is then fashioned. It may be triangular, quadrangular, rectangular or rhomboid in shape. Many surgeons prefer a triangular scleral flap of 4 by 4 mm with base at the limbus. Many glaucoma surgeons have reduced the size of the scleral flap in recent years (**Figures 7A to E**). The partial thickness scleral flap in combination with antifibrotic agents and postoperative laser suture lysis or releasable sutures, confers many of the advantages of a full-thickness procedure while retaining the safety and reduced complications of a guarded one.

While fixating the globe, the outline of the flap is incised to approximately one-half scleral depth with a sharp blade like Bard Parker blade no. 11 placed perpendicular to the globe. A diamond knife with preset depth can also be used. The flap is undermined with the lamellar dissection with crescent blade or with Bard Parker blade no. 15. The apex of the flap should be lifted after making the sclera groove. Using Castroviejo corneal suture forceps, the flap is lifted and with constant traction towards cornea and a lamellar plane is dissected. To get clean lamellar dissection, 2 to 3 small incisions are made with the blade tip at the left edge of the groove and then it is extended to the right edge of the flap.

The dissection is carried a little beyond blue gray zone but the edges of the flap should not extend beyond the blue gray zone. This is known to direct the flow posteriorly and prevent postoperative shallow chamber. The junction of the posterior border of blue gray zone and the sclera marks the external

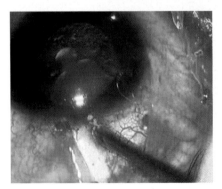

Fig. 5 Unipolar cautery for hemostasis

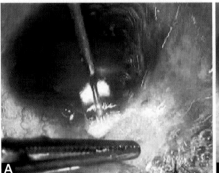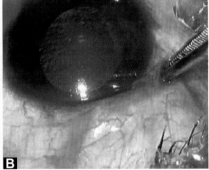

Figs 6 A and B Intraoperative application of Mitomycin C soaked sponges

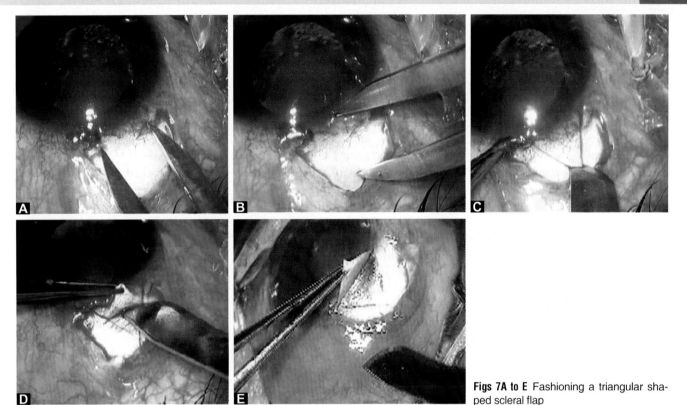

Figs 7A to E Fashioning a triangular shaped scleral flap

landmark of the sclera spur. Blue gray zone overlies the trabecular meshwork.

The dissection is then continued across the limbus to 1 to 2 mm into clear cornea **(Figure 7F)**. A crescent blade can also be used. In eyes with small anterior segments, or those with peripheral anterior synechiae, the scleral flap must be dissected further anteriorly. The scleral flap is best held with a nontoothed forceps to help avoid a perforation or tear. Keeping the area

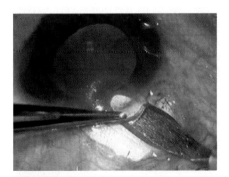

Fig. 7F The dissection is continued across the limbus to 1 to 2 mm into clear cornea

meticulously dry and using relatively high magnification help the surgeon raise the flap accurately and safely. Square, rectangular, triangular and semicircular shapes have been used for the scleral flap, but the shape has nothing to do with the success rate.

Paracentesis/Side Port

A corneal paracentesis is made before opening the globe. During paracentesis, superior rectus should be released and speculum should be loosened. It can be done on either side (right/left) at 3 o'clock or 9 o'clock position just anterior to limbal vessels based on the convenience of the surgeon. V-shaped lancet **(Figure 8)**, MVR blade or 26 gauge needle can be used to create the sideport. The entry into chamber should be tangential to the limbus and parallel to the iris plane in order to avoid inadvertent damage to iris and lens. The width of the sideport should be 0.5 to 0.6 mm (half the width

of 1 mm V-shaped lancet). In case of a preoperative shallow anterior chamber, it is advisable to make a small entry and then extend the incision rather than entering in one stroke. The lancet should be slowly withdrawn to facilitate controlled decompression of the globe. Larger sideport can give rise to aqueous leak and iris prolapse.

Advantages of the paracentesis

- In advanced glaucomas, paracentesis helps in controlled decom-

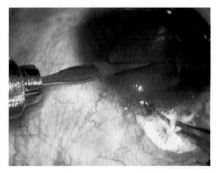

Fig. 8 Paracentesis

pression which inturn prevents "snuff out" phenomenon.

- It allows the anterior chamber to be reformed with viscoelastic or Ringer lactate solution as the need may be, in case the anterior chamber (AC) becomes shallow during the surgery.
- Titration of the bleb at the end of surgery can be done and a patent sclerostomy, with adequate aqueous flow can be ensured.
- In case of persistent shallow chamber during the postoperative period, AC reformation is facilitated through the sideport.

The Stoma/Ostium

Now using a 1 mm V-shaped lancet blade, the anterior chamber is entered through the clear cornea under the partial thickness scleral flap. Using the Kelly's punch, an internal block of tissue containing the trabecular meshwork is excised in 5 to 6 bites from the posterior lip of the incision. A smaller sclerostomy of 1.5 to 2 × 2 mm is adequate (**Figures 9A and B**). At least 1 mm of the scleral bed is left on either side of sclerostomy, so that when scleral flap is sutured the sclerostomy margins are not exposed. Care should be taken to avoid punching posterior to sclera spur (at the posterior edge of blue gray zone) to avoid damage to ciliary body.

Alternatively, the internal block excision can be done with two radial incisions with a sharp microblade or diamond knife put under the scleral flap. The tissue between the radial incisions is excised with Vannas scissors.

Peripheral Iridectomy

A peripheral iridectomy is then done. Iridectomy aims at preventing iris incarceration into sclerostomy. It is performed through the sclerostomy using either iridectomy forceps or Lims' forceps and vannas' scissors (**Figure 10**). Forceps should be angled vertically down to avoid too large an iridectomy with resultant glare and diplopia. Iris is cut keeping the scissors parallel to limbus, which gives a broad based iridectomy. Base of the iridectomy should be little wider than sclerostomy opening, so that possible iris incarceration in the sclerostomy wound can be avoided. Forceful pulling of the iris can cause iridodialysis and or lens damage. The iridectomy must be large enough to ensure that the edges of the iris do not occlude the trabeculectomy site.

Scleral Flap Suturing

The scleral flap is reapproximated to the scleral bed with interrupted (fixed sutured) or releasable 10-0 nylon sutures. The suturing technique has undergone various modifications in

order to increase the longevity of bleb function. Suturing has evolved through fixed sutures, releasable sutures and adjustable sutures to modulate the aqueous flow postoperatively.

Interrupted sutures

They are placed at both corners of the flap in the case of a rectangular flap. The posterior edge usually scars down postoperatively, eventually leaving only the anterior radial edges of the scleral flap leaking. Therefore, the posterior edge can be tightly apposed with a third suture. In the case of triangular flap, an apical suture and one suture in the middle of either sides of the flap are put (**Figure 11**). The needle should be passed through the partial thickness flap (1 mm from scleral flap edge) without the aid of forceps because a forceps may damage the flap. The needle is brought out 1 mm from the edge of the partial thickness intact sclera. The knot is adequately tightened by 2-1-1 throws. Knot is pulled away from the sclera flap and buried.

Interrupted suture knots are rotated onto the scleral side. It must be kept in mind that the technique of scleral flap suturing regulates the flow of aqueous. Apposition of scleral flap to the sclera bed offers resistance to aqueous flow through the sclerostomy. This resistance can be regulated by technique of suturing, suture position and

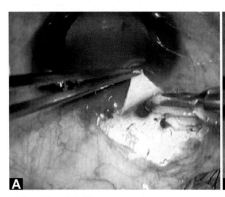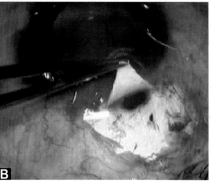

Figs 9A and B The trabeculectomy ostium is fashioned with a Kelly's descemet punch

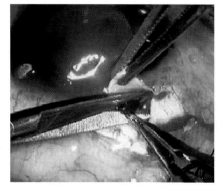

Fig. 10 Peripheral iridectomy

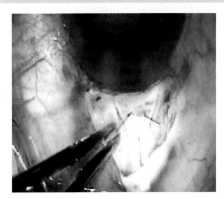

Fig. 11 Scleral flap sutures (fixed)

tension. When the scleral flap is poorly constructed and tied with loose sutures it results in postoperative hypotony. If the sutures are too tight the IOP is high postoperatively.

Releasable Sutures

Releasable sutures were introduced by Schaffer et al. but popularized by Cohen and Osher. This technique minimized the incidence of shallow anterior chamber and hypotony in early postoperative period with the advantage of releasing the suture once the wound and anterior chamber stabilize or when the IOP starts to rise **(Figures 12A and B)**.

For a triangular flap, 1 to 2 releasable sutures are adequate. Single releasable suture at the apex can be adequate when it is supplemented with 1 or 2 fixed flap sutures on either side of the sclera flap **(Figure 12C)**. Alternatively, one or both of the side sutures can be

put as a releasable ones. For a rectangular flap 1 to 2 releasable sutures can be supplemented with fixed flap sutures based on the titration of the bleb at the end of flap closure. Distal most sutures from the limbus are made releasable to direct the aqueous flow more posteriorly. Suture tightness is adjusted based on the egress of fluid from the scleral flap edges. Releasable sutures can be released within 10 to 14 days in nonaugmented trabeculectomy, but in cases of antifibrotic augmented surgery delayed release after 2 to 3 weeks would be beneficial as postsuture removal hypotony is more likely prior to 3 weeks. In cases where IOP remains well controlled sutures well buried may not necessarily be removed.

Technique of releasable sutures: 10-0 nylon suture is used for releasable sutures.

1. The first curvilinear bite is passed through partial corneal thickness 1 to 2 mm anterior and parallel to the limbus starting 4 to 5 mm to the perpendicular line passing through the apex of the flap, depending on right/left handed surgeon (right hand surgeon start from right side). Suture is passed for a length of 3 to 4 mm and taken out.

2. The second short vertical bite passes in line with the apex 1 to 2 mm anterior to limbus through

partial corneal thickness and comes out at the limbus.

3. The third bite is also vertical and is taken at the apex of the flap and out through the partial thickness of intact sclera posterior to the flap.

4. Needle end of the suture is held with tying forceps and four throws are taken on the needle holder and tied to suture segment lying on the scleral flap to make a slip knot. No additional throws or knots are applied over this. The tightness is adjusted based on the approximation of the flap edges and egress of the fluid. Needle end of the suture should be trimmed little away from the slip knot, but the suture end should not overly the limbus. The corneal end of the suture is cut flush with surface of the cornea to avoid leaving protruding end of the suture. These sutures can be released when required under topical anesthesia using slit lamp magnification. The exteriorized corneal loop is pulled out slowly and constantly till the slip knot is released with suture tying forceps.

Adjustable sutures

It is an alternative technique of scleral flap suturing. Specially designed forceps with smooth edges (Khaw adjustable suture forceps) is used to

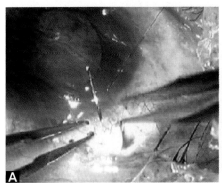
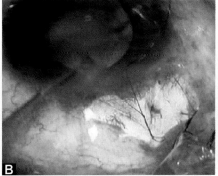
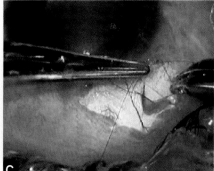

Figs 12A to C Technique of releasable suture

adjust the suture tension transconjunctivally in the postoperative period. The adjustable sutures allows gradual titration of IOP.

Anterior Chamber Reformation

Using a blunt, 30 gauge cannula, the anterior chamber is reformed with balanced salt solution through the paracentesis to determine whether a controlled leak is present around the scleral flap. Adequacy of filtration at the sides of the scleral flap is judged with cellulose sponges or cotton pledget. If the flow is excessive and the anterior chamber shallows, the slipknots are tightened and/or additional sutures are placed. If the leakage appears inadequate, and a firm globe by finger tension is present after reformation, the surgeon may loosen the slipknots or remove the permanent tight sutures and replace them with looser sutures, or apply cautery to the radial edges of the scleral flap or to the sclera adjacent to the scleral flap anteriorly, causing the wound to gape, or make small scleral flap incisions with Vannas scissors to relax the tension of the flap or as a last resort raise the scleral flap again and enlarge the internal ostium.

Conjunctival Flap Closure

After this, meticulous closure of the conjunctiva is done. For a limbal based flap 8-0 or 9-0 vicryl suture using an atraumatic is used to close the conjunctiva in a running, locking fashion incorporating tenon's in alternating bites (**Figures 13A and B**). It is preferable to separately close the tenons and the conjunctiva in two layers. With a fornix based conjunctival flap, a wing shaped closure using 8-0 or 9-0 vicryl or nylon is a good technique. In this the free conjunctival edge is made taut against the limbus preventing the leak through the edge. Two sutures are placed at either end of the conjunctival incision. The initial conjunctival opening which is wider is anchored to the limbus with 2-3 bites (purse string suture). The first bite starts from the intact limbal conjunctival end with the partial thickness scleral bite and passes through the anterior most cut end of the conjunctiva, and the second and third bite approximates the two cut edges of the conjunctiva. The knot is tied with 2-1-1 throws and tightened. The other end is anchored at the limbus with partial thickness scleral bite and single suture making sure the conjunctival edge is taut and flush with the limbus in order to avoid postoperative leak from the conjunctival edge. Any relaxing incisions are also closed tightly. The tapered vascular needle produces an opening in the conjunctiva which is only as large as the suture material limiting the leak around it.

Bleb Titration

At the end of the surgery, titration is done through the sideport with 26 gauge hyprodissection cannula with balanced salt solution. Mild to moderate elevation of the bleb ensures patency of sclerostomy and adequate tightness of scleral flap sutures (**Figure 14**). In addition, water tightness of conjunctival closure is also checked. Balanced salt solution is then injected through the paracentesis with a 30 guage blunt cannula to deepen the anterior chamber and elevate the bleb.

One drop of atropine eye drops and one drop of steroid-antibiotic eye drops are instilled at the completion of surgery. This will accomplish dilatation of pupil, before postoperative inflammation can stimulate muscle spasm.

> **Note** If a periocular injection of antibiotic or steroid is needed, it should be given in inferior fornix away from bulbar conjunctiva, because retrograde flow of the injected material into the anterior chamber may be possible, with potential corneal toxicity.

Early Postoperative Period

Topical medications used in the immediate postoperative period include cycloplegics, corticosteroids, and antibiotics. Cycloplegics paralyze the ciliary muscle and tightens the zonular-iris-lens diaphragm and maximally deepens the anterior chamber. It also

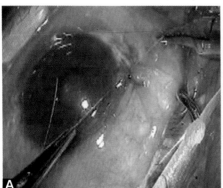
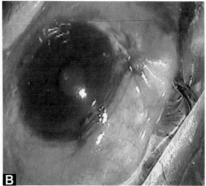

Figs 13A and B The conjunctival flap is sutured with 8-0 Vicryl

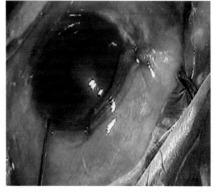

Fig. 14 Anterior chamber is reformed with BSS through the paracentesis

maintains the blood aqueous barrier, thereby limiting proteinaceous exudation and cellular infiltration into the anterior chamber. It also gives symptomatic relief from pain of postoperative ciliary spasm.[4] Generally, atropine is used as the cyclopegic agent because of its long action and its potential to reduce the risk of postoperative malignant glaucoma. A broad-spectrum antibiotic may be used for about 1 to 2 weeks as theoretical prophylaxis against bleb infection and endophthalmitis. If there is corneal toxicity from 5-fluorouracil (5-FU), topical antibiotics are used at a reduced frequency until it has cleared.

Postoperative follow-up and Assessment

The first 10 postoperative days are vital for ascertaining the adequacy and extent of filtration. Any critical modifications, are made at this time.

The following parameters should be assessed

1. **Bleb:** Look for the extent and height, vascularity, and possible wound leaks. Subconjunctival 5-fluorouracil can be given.
2. **Anteior chamber:** Look for any hyphema or hypopyon. Assess anterior chamber depth. A shallow postoperative anterior chamber can be graded follows:
   - *Grade 1:* Peripheral corneal-iris touch
   - *Grade 2:* Corneal-iris touch up to the pupillary margin
   - *Grade 3:* Lens-cornea apposition.
3. **Cornea:** Look for clarity, epithelial erosion, edema.
4. Intraocular pressure should be determined.
5. The fundus should be examined for presence of choroidal detachment or suprachoroidal hemorrhage.
6. **Optic disc and macula:** Decompression retinopathy can occur postoperatively.

7. Ocular massage, argon laser suture lysis or release of releasable suture can be done in this period.

SPECIAL CONSIDERATIONS

Some special considerations in glaucoma filtering surgery are as follows:

Angle Closure Glaucoma

In cases of angle closure glaucoma and other cases predisposed to flat anterior chamber it is better to make the scleral flap thicker than usual and suture it more securely. It is essential to ensure that the anterior chamber remains well formed when filled with balanced salt solution.

Antifibrotic Agents

The use of intraoperative mitomycin C (MMC) and 5-fluorouracil (5-FU) has greatly improved the results of filtration surgery in less favorable cases like young patients, eyes with previous failed filtration surgery, aphakic and pseudophakia eyes, and eyes with neovascular glaucoma or active uveitis. Although 5-FU is less effective than MMC in developing successful filtering blebs, the long-term side effects of 5-FU also are less serious than those of MMC.[5,6]

5-Fluorouracil

With 5-FU there are two major methods of application: postoperative subconjunctival injection and intraoperative application. Initially, 5-FU was used as an adjunct to glaucoma surgery by subconjunctival administration during the postoperative period. The initial dosage, 5 mg twice daily for the first week and daily for the second week after surgery was associated with significant side effects, most of which were related to the cornea. A good response with fewer injections (five to ten injections over a 2-week interval after surgery) has been found. The eye is examined carefully after surgery to verify that there is no conjunctival wound leak. Only

if the Seidel test is negative, then the injections may be given. 5 to 10 injections are then given over the following 2 weeks.

Method of Application of 5-FU

Postoperative: 0.1 ml (5 mg) of 5-FU is directly withdrawn from the vial (50 mg/ml) into a tuberculin syringe. The needle is removed and replaced with a short, sharp, disposable 30-gauge needle. Thorough conjunctival anesthesia should be attained with topical 4 percent Xylocaine or proparacaine. The patient is seated comfortably at the slit-lamp, and under topical anesthesia the injection is placed in the subconjunctival tissue in the inferior cul-de-sac. The farther the needle can be introduced under the conjunctiva, the more likely the 5-FU will not leak from the puncture site. Leakage is the major cause for corneal complications related to the subconjunctival injection of 5-FU. 5-FU can also be administered intraoperatively with sponges in a manner similar to that used for MMC.

Intraoperative: Major advantages of the intraoperative use of 5-FU include its ease of administration. Intraoperative administration may not be as effective as postoperative injections. It is preferable to use a limbus-based conjunctival flap when 5-FU is given intraoperatively. A fluid-retaining sponge (polyvinyl or mersel) is fashioned to approximatetly 2 to 3 mm long and wide and about 0.5 mm thick. This is soaked in undiluted 5-FU and placed on the sclera so that the tenon's capsule is in contact with the sponge, and the sponge is left in position for 5 minutes. The eye is irrigated with 5 to 15 ml of balanced salt solution, which is absorbed with gauze pads placed around the eye. Some surgeons prefer to make either the scleral flap grooves or the entire scleral flap dissection before applying the 5-FU. The scleral flap should be at least one-third scleral thickness because thinner flaps tend to leak excessively, predisposing to flat anterior chambers.

Mitomycin C

Mitomycin C applied intraoperatively was the first antifibrotic agent used to increase the success of filtration surgery. MMC is more potent than 5-FU[7] **(Figures 15A and B)**. The application of MMC is very similar to that of 5-FU. Concentrations of 0.2 to 0.5 mg/ml for 2 to 5 minutes have been used. The ideal concentration and contact time has not been determined. Higher concentrations and longer duration are associated with greater effect but with a greater likelihood of complications, like a very thin avascular bleb and postoperative hypotony.[8,9] Most surgeons currently use a concentration of 0.2 or 0.4 mg/ml for 2 to 3 minutes.

Method of Application of MMC

MMC-soaked sponge (Mersel or polyvinyl) is placed on the intact scleral surface before dissecting the scleral flap. This technique may reduce the penetration of the drug to the ciliary body, where it can cause prolonged postoperative hypotony and prevents drug entry into the anterior chamber where it may cause endothelial toxicity. The conjunctiva and tenon's capsule is draped over the sponge, making sure that the cut edge does not come in contact with it. The surgical site is irrigated with 15 to 30 ml of balanced salt solution, which is collected on gauze pads. The remainder of the trabeculectomy is performed as described previously, with special attention given to creating a tight closure of the scleral flap, in order to maintain a formed anterior chamber, and performing a watertight conjunctival closure using a tapered needle.

EARLY BLEB TITRATION
Digital Massage

Digital ocular massage lowers intraocular pressure, causing early adhesions to break and force more aqueous to flow through the sclerostomy site, establishing an increased flow rate via the larger bleb. The surgeon or patient can either press firmly through the lower lid against the cornea for 5 to 10 seconds or push with two fingers on either side of the filtration bleb with the eye in down-gaze. Another technique is to apply focal pressure on the conjunctiva overlying the radial edge of the scleral flap using a moistened cotton-tipped applicator, it deforms the edge of the trabeculectomy flap rather than markedly elevating

intraocular pressure. Early scar formation is broken by the misalignment of the flap edge. Iris incarceration in the sclerostomy, hyphema, bleb rupture, or dehiscence of an incisional wound can occur with digital massage.

Postoperative Suture Release

Although guarded filtration surgery decreases the incidence of postoperative flat anterior chambers, other complications can occur, such as hypotony due to excessive filtration or elevated intraocular pressure from a tightly closed scleral flap. Postoperative release of the sutures promotes aqueous humor flow through the sclerostomy and around the edges of the scleral flap when intraocular pressure is too high. Through suture release, the scleral flap can elevate, lowering the IOP. Early postoperative titration of bleb function can be achieved with argon laser suture lysis or with the use of releasable scleral flap sutures.

Argon Laser Suture Lysis

Laser suture lysis is performed under topical anesthesia. A Hoskin's lens is positioned over the flap to flatten the conjunctival bleb, enabling a clear view of the nylon suture. **(Figure 16A)**. In addition, the lens helps to blanch the conjunctiva, to open up the lids, provides magnification and fixes the globe. The sutures are always lysed one at a time. Best time for suture lysis is 4 to 6 weeks trabeculectomy with antimetabolites. A power setting of 200 to 400 mW at 0.05 to 0.1 second duration and a 50 to 100 um spot size is used to lyse the suture. This should result in immediate reduction of intraocular pressure and elevation of the bleb. Digital message or focal pressure on the edge of the scleral flap may be required for the elevation of the bleb if it does not occur spontaneously after suture lysis. Complications specific to argon laser suture lysis include difficulty in identifying the suture because

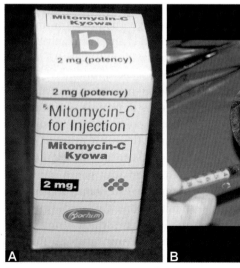
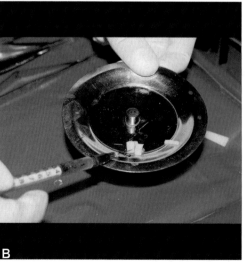

Figs 15A and B Mitomycin MMC soaked sponges are used for intraoperative application

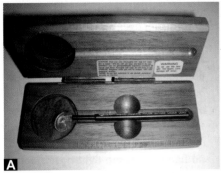 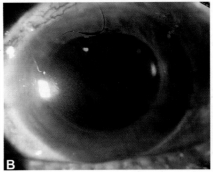 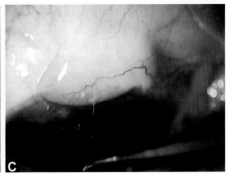

Figs 16A to C (A) Hoskins lens used for argon laser suturelysis (ALS); (B) Releasable suture (arrow); (C) The releasable suture can be released postoperatively to lower the IOP

of overlying edema of the conjunctiva or tenon's capsule. Argon laser suture lysis should not be performed if subconjunctival blood surrounds the suture as the blood will absorb the laser energy, resulting in a conjunctival buttonhole.

Releasable Sutures

The advantages of controlling early postoperative bleb function led to the surgical application of scleral flap sutures that could be released at the slit-lamp (releasable sutures) **(Figures 16B and C)**. One technique has already been explained earlier in the text. In to one of the techniques technique, a mattress-type scleral flap suture is externalized with the knot on the cornea. These sutures may be cut easily with a microblade. Removing a suture, digital message, and focal pressure on the edge of the scleral flap all have the same goals. Fibrosis of the scleral flap usually occurs within 2 to 3 weeks after surgery. So suture lysis or suture release may not be effective after 3 weeks. However, late suture lysis may be effective especially if intraoperative antimetabolites have been used.

Filtration Surgery Combined with Cataract Extraction

Routine extracapsular cataract surgery with sutures or manual small incision cataract surgery or phacoemulsification can be combined with trabeculectomy. When it is combined with phacoemulsification it can be at single site (i.e. both trabeculectomy and cataract surgery are done through superior site) or two sites (i.e. temporal clear corneal phacoemulsification is combined with superior trabeculectomy). In combined surgery at single site, a fornix based conjunctival flap is better as it does not interfere with visibility for phacoemulsification unlike a limbal based flap (Discussed in detail in a separate chapter).

COMPLICATIONS OF GLAUCOMA FILTERING SURGERY

Trabeculectomy is also fraught with complications like any other surgery, even higher than modern cataract surgery. They can vary from trivial to vision threatening. Complications of trabeculectomy can be classified as:

Intraoperative complications
- Conjunctival flap related complications
- Sclera flap related complications
- Intraoperative bleeding
- Vitreous loss
- Lens injury
- Suprachoroidal hemorrhage.

Early postoperative complications: (within 3 months postoperatively)
- Shallow anterior chamber
  - ❖ With hypotony
  - ❖ With high IOP

- Normal anterior chamber depth
  - ❖ With hypotony
  - ❖ With high IOP
- Hyphema
- Decompression retinopathy
- Hypotonous maculopathy
- Wipe out phenomenon
- Infection.

Late postoperative complications: (after 3 months postoperatively)
- Late leakage of the filtering bleb
- Failure of the filtering bleb
- Blebitis and bleb related endophthalmitis
- Cataract formation
- Dysesthetic bleb (overhanging blebs, painful blebs)
- Hypotony and associated maculopathy
- Ptosis
- Strabismus.

Complications Related to Anesthesia

Anesthesia for glaucoma surgery should minimize the risk of further compromise of optic nerve function. General anesthesia should be avoided whenever possible. The trauma of extubation and the occasional coughing and vomiting associated with general anesthesia can lead to postoperative suprachorodial hemorrhage and shallow anterior chamber. Currently, general anesthesia is indicated for children and for adults who cannot cooperate. In children, diagnostic evaluation and therapeutic procedures require general anesthesia.

Retrobulbar or peribulbar injections have several potential disadvantages for glaucomatous eyes. For example, extravasation of anesthesia into the lids may limit exposure of the conjunctival fornix. Although this is not typically a problem in cataract surgery, the creation of a limbus based flap for glaucoma surgery becomes difficult. A sudden increase in orbital pressure from injection of anesthetic or retrobulbar hemorrhage may result in compromised optic nerve blood flow and may worsen existing damage. Topical anesthesia supplemented with subtenons infiltration as necessary provides adequate anesthesia with a minimum of risk. Adrenaline (vasoconstricting agents) should be avoided because of the potential for circulatory compromise in eyes with advanced glaucomatous optic neuropathy. Anticoagulants and antiplatelet drugs including aspirin, should be discontinued before surgery if possible. If retrobulbar hemorrhage occurs and intraocular pressure rises significantly with a tense orbit, optic nerve compression may ensue. An immediate lateral canthotomy should be performed and mannitol should be given intravenously. The surgery should be postponed until the hemorrhage resolves, usually within 2 to 3 weeks and repeat retrobulbar injection should be avoided.

Intraoperative Complications
Conjunctival Flap Related Complications
Conjunctival tears and buttonholes can occur during conjunctival incision, tenons dissection, especially with the use of toothed forceps or excess traction over the conjunctival edge. These complications can be worsened by adjuvant use antifibrotics and scarred conjunctiva due to previous surgeries. Conjunctival shrinkage is seen more commonly with long-term exposure of conjunctiva to antiglaucoma medications and preservatives.

Long-term visual outcome and intraocular pressure control after trabeculectomy are similar when fornix or limbus based conjunctival flaps are used. Limbus based flaps offer the advantages of ease of watertight closure and ability to perform earlier suture lysis and digital compression. They are technically more difficult and take longer to create than fornix based flaps. One of the most frequent causes of wound-related problems with limbus based flaps is failure to make the initial incision adequately posterior. Fornix based conjunctival flaps provide better visualization of limbal anatomy during surgery and decrease the risk of accidental conjunctival buttonholing. Watertight closure, however, is more difficult to obtain. Incorporation of the anterior edge of tenon's capsule into the wound enhances the likelihood of creating a watertight incision while closing the limbus based flap, as does closure with running or mattress sutures.

Careful handling of the conjunctiva is critical. Toothed forceps should never be used on the conjunctiva. Blunt scissors should be utilized for dissection. Scarred conjunctiva needs to be manipulated with added care. Rectus muscle traction sutures may buttonhole the conjunctiva, damage the muscle, and cause bleeding from the anterior ciliary arteries. Alternatively, a 6-0 to 8-0 traction suture may be placed mid thickness through clear cornea, approximately 1 mm anterior to the conjunctival insertion may be used. An additional advantage of this suture is that it can be used to move the eye in any direction during surgery to provide maximal exposure and minimal stretch on and inadvertent tearing of the conjunctiva.

At the conclusion of surgery, fluorescein dye should be applied to the conjunctival surface and the bleb formed by anterior chamber irrigation to aid in the detection of previously unrecognized buttonhole defects or wound leaks. Focal pressure on the sclera adjacent to the scleral flap may facilitate bleb formation if the scleral flap sutures are tight or if blood or viscoelastic are occluding the ostium. Buttonholes and wound leaks are readily appreciated under these conditions. A buttonhole detected intraoperatively should be closed. Immediately before buttonhole closure, the conjunctival incision line should be gently reapposed to the limbus in fornix based cases and to the posterior conjunctival incision line in limbus based cases. Tenon's capsule, if present, should be incorporated into the buttonhole during closure to provide additional support. The location of the conjunctival tear determines the method of repair. If a large buttonhole is noted during early stages of a filtration operation, it is best to select a new site. If the buttonhole is located in the center of the conjunctival flap or further posteriorly, a purse-string suture with 10-0 nylon can be attempted either internally on the undersurface of the conjunctiva or externally if the flap has already been reapproximated. A tapered atraumatic needle should be used to avoid creating a larger conjunctival defect. The most common location for a buttonhole is near the limbus, where it may be either oversewn with adjacent conjunctiva, sutured directly to the cornea or sclera, closed as purse string, or sealed with application of a tissue patch. If a conjunctival dialysis occurs at the limbus during the dissection of a limbus based flap, a buried mattress suture can be used for repair. Alternatively, a small buttonhole at this location can be repaired by creating a conjunctival peritomy and excising the buttonhole. The corneal epithelium in this area should be removed and the conjunctiva sutured to the cornea with mattress sutures. If a buttonhole is detected before the intraoperative application of 5-fluoroucil (5-FU) or mitomycin C, consideration should be given to repair the defect and judiciously using these drugs.[10]

Most early, limbal postoperative wound leaks seal spontaneously without intervention in the absence of adjunctive antifibrosis therapy. However, an increased rate of anterior chamber shallowing resulting from conjunctival wound leaks in cases with fornix based flaps has been reported.

Scleral Flap Related Complications

The scleral flap can be either too thin or too thick. Thicker flaps lead to underfiltration. Thinner flaps with adjuvant use of antifibrotics are prone to tearing, buttonholing and avulsion. A buttonhole in a thin flap is sealed with a plug of tenon's capsule, donor sclera or dura matter graft. Sometimes a new scleral flap may need to be raised. If the scleral flap is too thick, anterior chamber can be entered prematurely. If there is a premature entry due to a thick scleral flap more superficial scleral lamellae should be dissected to advance the sclera flap into clear cornea. Minimal cautery only should be used to avoid gaping of the edges of the sclera flap which may cause excessive filtration.

Flap shrinkage can occur with excess cautery. Accidental amputation of flap can occur during flap dissection, during peripheral iridectomy or during vitrectomy in case of vitreous loss and while suturing of the flap.

If the flap tears and the buttonholes are large and occur during wound construction the site should be changed. However, minor tear after sclerostomy can be repaired with 10-0 nylon sutures. In case of flap shrinkage, additional sutures may be required to reduced the excess aqueous flow.

Descemets Detachment

Small scrolls of Descemet's membrane may be detached at the limbal wound or at the paracentesis track site which is inconsequential. It can be repositioned by injecting an air bubble into the anterior chamber.

Shallow Anterior Chamber

Every attempt is done to prevent intraoperative shallowing of the anterior chamber,[11] either by using viscoelastic material or preplaced sclera flap sutures. However, the viscoelastic[12] may impede aqueous flow across a tightly closed scleral lip. It may also tamponade a surgical wound and may mask a potential wound leak.

Intraoperative Bleeding
Hyphema

Intraoperative anterior chamber hemorrhage most commonly occurs at the time of iridectomy. Bleeding can occur from conjunctival dissection, episcleral and perforating vessels, from sclerostomy site or after iridectomy (involving ciliary body). Bleeding occurs from cut radial iris vessels or from a traumatized greater arterial circle within the ciliary body and is best treated with light compression, as most iris root ciliary body bleeding will spontaneously stop within minutes. The scleral flap should be held open while the pulsatile bleeding continues to allow the blood to exit the eye. This and gentle irrigation will keep the anterior chamber from filling with blood. The scleral flap must not be sutured until all bleeding has stopped, as this often leads to postoperative blockage of the internal ostium by the clotted blood. Persistent bleeding also may be treated with viscoelastic or air tamponade.

Certain precautions help in preventing intraoperative bleeding. These include preoperative stoppage of systemic antiplatelet and anticoagulant drugs under the treating physicians' guidance. Gentle handling of the ocular tissues with adequate wetfield cautery is useful for smooth sailing during surgery. Bleeding from sclerostomy can occur due to more posterior punching of the tissue and hence, care should be taken to punch till the blue white junction and not exceeding beyond it.

Suprachoroidal Hemorrhage

A suprachoroidal hemorrhage can occur at the time of surgery or in the first few postoperative days, generally within the first 48 hours.[13] The main risk factors for delayed choroidal hemorrhage include prolonged hypotony and ciliochoroidal effusion. If an intraoperative choroidal hemorrhage is suspected, the wound should be closed immediately. Shallowing of anterior chamber and dark expansion of choroid are signs of suprachoroidal hemorrhage. The anterior chamber should be reformed with air or a viscoelastic agent. Watertight closure may be difficult if the internal ostium has already been made. Posterior sclerotomies have been recommended to drain the hemorrhage and allow anterior chamber reformation. However, they are rarely needed or helpful at the time of the initial surgical complication. Furthermore, the immediate concern is closure of the incision. Once the eye has been closed, intravenous mannitol can be used to lower the intraocular pressure and stabilize the eye. The prognosis for recovery of vision is good as long as the eye can be closed without loss of uvea or retina. Drainage of the hemorrhage may be necessary later.

Avoiding prolonged hypotony is the best method of decreasing the risk of suprachoroidal hemorrhage. This goal can be achieved by preplacing scleral flap sutures to minimize the duration of intraoperative hypotony and tighter scleral flap suture closure with postoperative suture lysis or releasable sutures in high-risk eyes. Other factors which help in prevention are preoperative well controlled IOP, preplaced scleral flap sutures, controlled decompression of the globe, injection of viscoelastic in AC before entering into AC, use of punch instead of block excision and in case surgery under of general anesthesia hyperventilation during GA causing vasoconstriction can prevent overt SCH.

Iridectomy Related Complications

These incude a large iridectomy, iridodialysis or inadvertent cyclodialysis cleft.

Vitreous Loss and Lens Injury

Vitreous loss and lens injury occur when lens zonular complex is inadvertently damaged during iridectomy PI, the risk increases in cases of angle closure glaucoma or sudden decompression of globe with anterior shifting of iris lens diaphragm. Management includes avoiding posterior sclerostomy and basal peripheral iridectomy. Anterior vitrectomy should be done to avoid blockage of the ostium with vitreous.

Early Postoperative Complications
Elevated IOP

Early, undetected increase in pressure after trabulectomy could result in further visual field loss or loss of central fixation and could account for the so-called 'snuff out/wipe out' phenomenon described following filtration surgery. Very high pressures occur more commonly in eyes receiving sodium hyaluronate to reform the anterior chamber.[12] Other potential causes of an early postoperative intraocular pressure rise include malignant glaucoma, pupillary block, choroidal hemorrhage, tight scleral flap sutures and blockage of the internal ostium by an incompletely excised Descemet's membrane, iris root, ciliary

processes, vitreous, lens capsule, blood or fibrin.[4]

Gonioscopy is mandatory to assess the patency of the internal ostium and should be performed with a lens of diameter smaller than the cornea to avoid accidental conjunctival or bleb injury. If the internal ostium is free of obstruction, gentle digital pressure to the globe or to the edge of the scleral flap is often sufficient to relieve the blockage. On the other hand, blockage of the internal ostium by iris, vitreous, cillary body, lens, or membranes often requires laser or incisional surgery to prevent filtration failure.

Complications Due to Scleral Flap Suture Release

Laser suture lysis and releasable sutures add to the safety of trabeculectomy by permitting titration of postoperative intraocular pressure to avoid hypotony and shallow anterior chamber. The advantage of laser sutures lysis is that the suture ends remain buried beneath the conjunctiva, whereas releasable sutures remain exteriorized and may protrude for an extended period of time if they do not need to be released. Laser suture lysis should be performed with as little conjunctival manipulation and laser energy as possible. A Hoskins suture lysis lens under topical anesthesia can be used. One suture should be cut at a time to minimize the risk of hypotony. Cautious digital massage or pressure to the edge of the scleral flap following suture lysis often helps to elevate the bleb if it does not do so spontaneously. Suture lysis should be completed within 2 to 3 weeks for trabeculectomy without antifibrotic agents, The window period is longer for trabeculectomy with antifibrotic agents.

Wound Leak

Although best detected and treated intraoperatively, conjunctival breaks

or suture track leaks may develop or be detected postoperatively. Patients with these problems generally fall into two categories: *those with flat or nonexistent blebs and those with elevated blebs.* The most important factor in deciding whether repair is necessary is the appearance of the bleb rather than the specific intraocular pressure. If the bleb is flat, intervention is indicated, particularly if the bleb is injected. The presence of anterior chamber shallowing and hypotony also strongly suggest the need for intervention.

Simple patching may facilitate leak closure. Contact lenses of appropriate size may help promote re-epithelialization. Noninvasive methods of increasing intraocular pressure by compressing the scleral flap when excessive flow is present include symblepharon rings and Simmons' tamponade shells. Buttonholes and wounds leaks are more problematic when they occur in eyes receiving adjunctive antifibrosis therapy. Most leaks seal spontaneously or with mechanical pressure. Wound leaks or dehiscence after mitomycin C therapy may be more difficult to treat.

Shallow AC with Low IOP

Causes of postoperative shallowing of the anterior chamber may be divided based on the anatomic appearance of the eye and the intraocular pressure. Low IOP and a flat or shallow anterior chamber may be due to overfiltration **(Figures 17A and B)**, ciliochoroidal detachment with reduced aqueous production, a cyclodialysis cleft, or a wound leak. The absence of bleb formation is consistent with wound leakage or buttonhole, until proven otherwise. If the chamber is shallow but the pressure is elevated or too high aqueous misdirection syndrome (malignant glaucoma) may be present.

The grading system commonly used to note anterior chamber depth (in a shallow AC) is as follows:

Grade 1: Peripheral iris-cornea touch
Grade 2: Iris sphincter-cornea touch
Grade 3: Lens-cornea or vitreous-cornea touch.

Grade 1 flat chambers usually reform spontaneously. The type and timing of treatment of grade 2 chambers are not clear. In some cases, observation may be sufficient; in others, the surgeon may simply reform the anterior chamber with air or a viscoelastic agent, to keep it formed until the ciliary body and choroid reattach and aqueous production is re-established. Air may predispose to cataract formation and is not recommended in phakic eyes. Lens-cornea touch requires immediate correction. It is associated with a significant risk of corneal endothelial cell loss and decompensation, cataract, bleb failure, and formation of anterior and posterior synechiae, as compared to eyes with anterior chamber shallowing without lens-cornea touch. It is better to inject a viscoelastic agent initially and if this does not work, choroidal drainage can be performed.

Bleb Leak

Early wound dehiscence when limbus based conjunctival flaps are utilized and retraction of the flap in fornix based cases (wound leak) are the most serious wound related complications and generally require immediate surgical repair, particularly if any edge of the scleral flap should become exposed **(Figures 18A and B)**. Definitive therapy for an early postsurgical conjunctival wound leak is suturing closure with nonabsorbable suture on an atramautic needle.

The trend toward tighter scleral flap sutures and sequential suture release has decreased the incidence and degree of postoperative anterior chamber shallowing and hypotony. Excessive aqueous flow due to loose scleral flap sutures (over filtration) is best managed by external tamponade rather than surgical correction, as the inflammation associated with repeat surgery may lead to bleb failure.

Conservative therapy is often the best approach to the patient with a shallow anterior chamber, as most will reform spontaneously, even if the course of shallowing is prolonged. Topical steroids, cycloplegics are given. Suppression of inflammation and cyclitis limits the extent of aqueous hyposecretion contributing to hypotony and anterior chamber shallowing. Although bleb leaks often seal spontaneously, large diameter contact lenses are available for posterior suture track leaks and conjunctival buttonholes.

Overfiltration

Overfiltration leads to hypotony. The anterior chamber may be shallow or of normal depth. A large and diffuse bleb is present. Wound leak is absent and Siedel's test is negative.

Overfiltration occasionally may respond to patching, usually with an attempt at focal compression over the region of excessive aqueous flow through the upper lid. One of the best methods of tamponade with minimal patient discomfort is the use of a symblepharon ring. The Simmons' tamponade shell provides greater pressure but is less well tolerated.

Reformation of a shallow anterior chamber can be done with balanced salt solution, air, viscoelastic agents, or expandable gases. Other techniques to decrease the filtration include compression sutures, autologous blood injection into the bleb, cryo or laser application to reduce the size of the bleb. Surgical revision may be required in some cases.

Ciliochoroidal Detachment

Ciliochoroidal detachment is more common after full-thickness surgery than trabeculectomy **(Figure 19)**. The detachment is usually transient resolving with the administration of topical, and systemic corticosteroids. Prophylactic sclerotomy may prevent the development of ciliochoroidal effusion in predisposed eyes, such as those with elevated episcleral venous pressure and nanophthalmos. Surgical drainage is usually unnecessary unless there is a cornea lens touch with shallowing of the anterior chamber or in kissing choroidals to allow continued aqueous drainage.

Shallow AC with Elevated IOP

The differential diagnosis **(Table 1)** includes pupillary block (rare when an iridectomy is present), choroidal hemorrhage (may be detected with ophthalmoscopy or ultrasonography), annular choroidal detachment with anterior rotation of the ciliary body

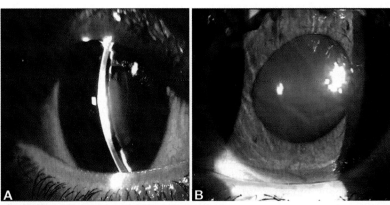

Figs 17A and B Postoperative hypotony with a shallow anterior chamber and DM folds due to an over filtering bleb

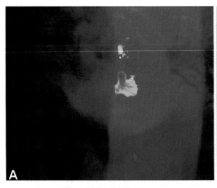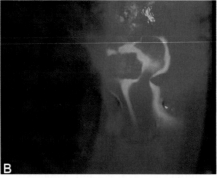

Figs 18A and B Postoperative wound leak. A positive Siedel's test

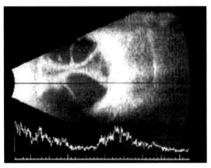

Fig. 19 Picture of a B-scan ultrasonogram showing choroidal detachment (kissing choroids) following trabeculectomy

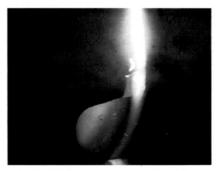

Fig. 20 Aqueowwus misdirection

Table 1 Differential diagnosis of shallow AC with elevated IOP

	Pupillary block	*Suprachoroidal hemorrhage*	*Aqueous misdirection*
Nature of AC shallow-ing	Iris bombe	Diffuse	Diffuse
Siedel test	Siedel's negative	Siedel's negative	Siedel's negative
IOP	Normal to high	Normal to high	Normal to high
Fundus	Normal	Dark choroidal elevation	Normal
Treatment	Laser iridotomy	Observation, if large, needs drainage when echography shows liquefaction of blood	Mydriatic/cycloplegic, drugs, osmotic drugs. Aqueous suppressants, YAG hyaloidotoy, diode CPC, vitreous tap or viter-ectomy

causing angle closure and malignant glaucoma (aqueous misdirection; ciliary block).

Aqueous Misdirection Syndrome

In aqueous misdirection, posterior pooling of aqueous humor either within or behind the vitreous causes forward movement of the lens-iris or hyaloid-iris diaphragm, resulting in a flat anterior chamber with an elevated pressure **(Figure 20)**.

It occurs due to posterior misdirection of aqueous into vitreous cavity. Smaller eyes with reduced axial length, nanophthalmos, eyes with angle closure glaucoma are more prone to develop aqueous misdirection due to restricted anterior flow by anteriorly rotated iris processes and intact hyaloid phase.

Prevention: It can be prevented by prophylactic sclerotomies in nanophthalmos, prophylactic iridotomy in eyes with angle closure and preoperative good IOP control with hyperosmotic agents. Tight scleral flap closure and combining cataract extraction with trabeculectomy debulks the lens and prevents flat AC.

Management (Table 2): Medical treatment of aqueous misdirection is successful in most cases. Atropine 1 percent, a topical beta-blocker, and systemic administration of a hyperosmotic and a carbonic anhydrase inhibitor may be used. A patent iridotomy is ensured and Nd:YAG anterior hyaloidotomy is done.

When medical management is not successful, pars plana vitrectomy with or without a lensectomy (in phakic patients) must be performed in combination with the vitrectomy. Distruption of the anterior hyaloid face is important.

Pupillary Block

Pupillary block may occur when PI is not patent (lamellar PI/obstructed by fibrin, blood or vitreous).

Management includes medical treatment to lower the IOP, laser peripheral iridotomy and mydriatics to break the posterior synechiae along with topical steroids will break the attack.

Normal Anterior Chamber Depth with High IOP

Causes of a high IOP post-trabeculectomy with a normal anterior chamber depth include obstruction of the ostium by blood, fibrin, vitreous, iris/ciliary processes, tight scleral flap sutures, failing bleb and steroid induced IOP response. Usually the bleb is low or flat.

Table 2 Management of aqueous misdirection syndrome

Initial management with mydriatics/ cycloplegics and IOP lowering agents
↓
Nd:YAG laser hyaloidotomy through peripheral iridectomy and through the peripheral capsule
↓
In phakic eyes vitrectomy can be combined with catract extraction and IOL implantation in pseudophakic eyes vitrectomy with posterior capsulotomy is needed

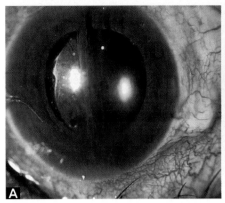 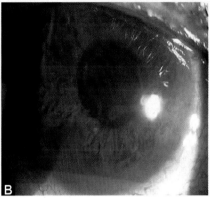

Figs 21A and B Postoperative hyphema

Management: Gonioscopy should be performed to ensure patency of the ostium. Nd:YAG laser can be used to disrupt any fibrin, vitreous or iris blocking the ostium. In cases where flap sutures are tight ocular massage or suture release helps in reducing the IOP. Failing bleb can be managed by increasing the topical steroids (*per se* may increase IOP in steroid responders), ocular massage, postoperative augmentation with antimetabolites and needling of the bleb.

Hyphema

Postoperative hyphemas may range from a mild trickle of blood from the ostium to total hyphema (**Figures 21A and B**). Small hyphemas may be observed in the early postoperative period. They are usually self-limiting and clear within 24 to 48 hours after surgery. Only rarely is surgical intervention required in the form of AC wash in cases of subtotal to total hyphema, when risk of corneal blood staining exists.

Loss of Fixation

Loss of central fixation may occur after apparently uncomplicated glaucoma surgery. Most recent studies report a risk of less than 1 to 2 percent. This phenomenon typically occurs in eyes with advanced glaucomatous damage with split fixation or visual field loss within 5 degrees of fixation. The risk of *"snuff-out"* after surgery is low

for patients with a sparing of central fixation.[14]

To minimize the risk of loss of central fixation in susceptible eyes, sub-tenons anesthesia should be given rather than retrobulbar injections. Epinephrine, which may affect optic nerve circulation, should not be administered with the anesthetic. Postoperative IOP spikes should be avoided and strict postoperative IOP monitoring with prevention and prompt management of IOP spikes is recommended.

Retinal Complications

Decompression retinopathy due to a sudden decompression of the eye with raised IOP may manifest as retinal, subretinal and occasionally as suprachoroidal hemorrhage. This is due to a sudden and large decrease in IOP causing a transient increase in retinal and choroidal blood flow. The most common appearance is that mimicking central retinal vein occlusion. *Hypotonic maculopathy* occurs in those with chronic hypotony. This is characterized by choroidal folds in macular area, macular thickening and disc swelling.

Acute Postoperative Endophthalmitis

Acute postoperative endophthalmitis occurs in less than 0.1 percent patients after trabeculectomy where povidone

–iodine is used preoperatively for bacterial prophylaxis.

Late Postoperative Complications
Filtration Failure

Filtration failure is the most common late postoperative complication. It is due to wound healing responses along the path of aqueous outflow. It can be due to:

- Significant subconjunctival fibroblast proliferation
- Healing response with synthesis of collagen and other extracellular matrix in the area of trabeculectomy.

Recognizing failure is particularly important during the first 2 weeks after surgery when the healing process is most active. Depth of the anterior chamber, appearance of the bleb, gonioscopic appearance of the internal ostium and the response to digital pressure to the globe facilitate recognition of filtration failure, which may be classified by anatomic location (internal or external) and temporally (early or late in the postoperative period).

External Factors

Appearance of the bleb is the most important postoperative feature and this feature tends to change over time. Congestion and vascularization of the bleb indicate the presence of inflammation and they are poor prognostic signs **(Figures 22A and B)**. Their presence in the postoperative period is often the first indication that the bleb may fail. Injection and vascularization typically occur before any elevation of intraocular pressure. Subsequently, the bleb undergoes progressive loculation leading to bleb encapsulation.

Gonioscopy allows direct visualization of the internal ostium. *Digital compression* is extremely important in helping to determine the location of the obstruction to aqueous flow. In a failing bleb, compression may result in either elevation of the bleb (focal or diffuse) or a resistance to elevation. If compression fails to elevate the bleb and the internal ostium is free of obstruction, the obstruction at the level of the external ostium. Transient bleb formation with lowering of the intraocular pressure suggests the presence of tight scleral flap sutures or loculation.

Internal Factors
Blockage of Internal Ostium
Blockage of internal ostium is usually due to obstruction of the internal ostium by incarceration of iris, vitreous, ciliary body, ciliary processes, lens, blood or fibrin. Late blockage of the internal ostium may be produced by fibrovascular membrane in neovascular glaucoma, fibrous tissue in fibrous ingrowth, epithelium in epithelial downgrowth or corneal endothelium and Descemet's membrane in the iridocornealendothelial syndrome. Iris or ciliary process pigment epithelium of iris or ciliary body may proliferate and block the internal ostium. Carefully inspecting the wound intraoperatively and keeping the excised tissue block as far anterior as possible will avoid most of these postoperative bleb failure problems. Internal ostium should be inspected in all cases of postoperative bleb failure using gonioscopy and if the incarceration is present, it

should be removed early otherwise these eye require resumption of medical therapy or repeat trabeculectomy. Argon and Nd:YAG lasers have been used to successfully open internally blocked sclerostomy sites.

Blockage of External Ostium
Blockage of external ostium by increased external resistance at the *Conjuctiva-Tenon's capsule-Episcleral interface* is the major cause of failure of filtration surgery. This external blockage results in an initial failure to establish an adequate filtration bleb. Inadequate aqueous flow through the fistula due to aqueous hyposecretion or tight scleral flap sutures contribute to this process by allowing the conjunctiva to remain in contact with the episclera. Subsequent vascularization, leukocytic infiltration, connective tissue proliferation and the formation of granulation tissue limit subconjunctival aqueous flow. Late failure is most commonly due to scarring at the *Conjunctiva-Tenon's capsule-Episcleral interface.*

Bleb needling re-establishes free flow of aqueous from AC to subconjunctival bleb space. It breaks the adhesions formed between conjunctiva and scleral flap and/or from scleral flap to scleral bed. Bleb needling can be performed at any time from early postoperative weeks to years after surgery. Prior to bleb needling site of reduced outflow has to be identified by slit lamp examination and gonioscopy. If the ostium is obstructed, it should be dealt accordingly.

Bleb needling can be performed under slit lamp, using magnifying loupes or operating microscope.

All the above methods need strict aseptic measures (with povidone iodine and antibiotic eye drops) and appropriate anesthesia prior to the procedure.

Slit-lamp needling: Bleb should be easily accessible and the patient should

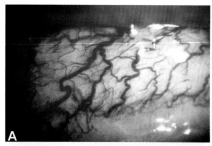
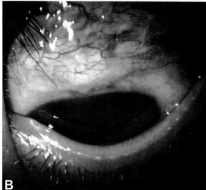

Figs 22A and B A failed bleb. Note the vascularization with the cork screw vessels

be able to maintain the head and eye positions as requested. Needles used are 25 to 27 gauge bent at 60 degree angle. The needle is introduced into subconjunctival space 5 to 10 mm distal to the scleral flap area (to avoid bleb leak close to filtration site). Needle is advanced towards the area of revision, to and fro movements are made through the scar tissue (bevel facing anteriorly) to ensure enough space for aqueous filtration. If this is not successful in raising the bleb, then attempts should be made to cut the scleral flap edge and lift the scleral flap with needle. Needle has to be advanced under the flap through the ostium into AC.

Antimetabolite usage with needling – both 5-FU and MMC can be used for needling. 5-FU is used in the concentration of (0.1 ml of 50 mg/ml or 0.2 ml of 25 mg/ml). It is injected near the intended site of revision, or away from the site to minimize chances of its entrance into the AC. MMC is used in the concentration ranging from 0.004 mg/ml to 0.4 mg/ml similar to that of 5-FU.

Encapsulated Bleb (Tenon Cyst)

Bleb encapsulation (Tenon cyst) develops in approximately 10 to 28 percent of eyes after filtering surgery, typically during the first 8 postoperative weeks **(Figures 23A and B)**. The incidence was higher after filtering surgery for congenital and juvenile glaucoma. Risk factors for the development of tenons cyst include secondary glaucoma, prolonged use of topical antiglaucoma medications, prior ALT, younger individuals and tendency for keloid formation. Histopathology reveals dense subconjuctival connective tissue, few cells and no cellular lining. Bleb encapsulation may be accompanied by progressive conjunctival hyperemia. Typical appearance is loculation, thickening of the subconjunctival connective tissue and elevated intraocular pressure. The bleb will be dome like and firm although the overlying conjunctiva may be mobile leading on to uncontrolled intraocular pressure. In most cases, the pressure decreases within 2 to 4 months with the use of aqueous suppressants. The decrease in aqueous production and intraocular pressure associated with medical therapy allows for remodeling of the cyst wall and eventually improves aqueous flow across it. After resolution, the antiglaucoma therapy may be reduced or stopped.

Treatment of Encapsulated Blebs

Many encapsulated blebs, particularly those that are only partially loculated, may resolve spontaneously or respond to intensive topical steroid therapy or digital compression. The various techniques include:

Digital compression

Pressure to the edge of the scleral flap under direct visualization with a moistened cotton-tipped applicator or with the surgeon's finger through the upper lid may cause a momentary gape between the edge of the scleral

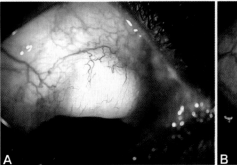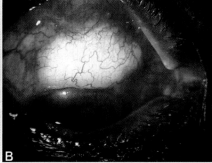

Figs 23A and B Tenon cyst

flap and the scleral bed establishing a bleb as the aqueous is forced to flow through the ostium. But iris incarceration resulting in filtration failure can occur.

Needling

If resolution does not occur and a cyst is present needling can be done. Needling is the procedure that allows the surgeon to create an opening(s) in the wall of an encapsulated bleb or raise a flattened bleb at the slit-lamp or in the operating room via subconjunctival manipulation with a small-gauge needle. The technique involves elevation of the conjunctiva off the surface of the globe with balanced salt solution or anesthetic with a small-gauge needle. The underlying episcleral/tenon's capsule scarring is then incised with the needle. If this does not succeed in restoring filtration, the edge of the scleral flap may be elevated.

Surgical revision

If the final pressure is not low enough to permit preservation of the remaining visual field or if medical therapy is insufficient to control the intraocular pressure elevation, surgical revision with adjunctive antifibrosis agents is warranted. In some cases excision of the tenon's cyst *in toto* is required.

Vision Loss Despite Controlling IOP

Progressive visual field loss may be related to inadequate lowering of intraocular pressure, continued glaucomatous optic neuropathy due to a vascular process unrelated to intraocular pressure-induced mechanical stress, or changes in optic nerve head blood flow and physiology during surgery or due to steroid-induced elevation of intraocular pressure after trabeculectomy has been reported.[14]

Cataract

The administration of topical and systemic corticosteroids may increase the rate of cataract formation and progression. There is also a strong correlation with flat anterior chamber. Other causes may be hypotony, postoperative inflammation, lens corneal touch, lens trauma, and intraoperative use of MMC.

Late Bleb Leaks

Treatment of late leaking filtering bleb is difficult and the options include patching, oversized bandage contact lenses, trichloroacetic acid application, focal cautery, cryotherapy, cautery, tamponade shells or rings. Aqueous suppressants reduce flow and permit surface epithelialization. Patching with donor sclera, injection of autologous blood into the bleb and surgical revision are other options.

Chronic Hypotony

The incidence of chronic postoperative hypotony is higher after full-thickness procedures and 5-FU/MMC augmented trabeculectomy as compared to trabeculectomy without adjunctive antifibrosis therapy. Mild hypotony (intraocular pressure <10 mm Hg but >6 mm Hg) does not significantly reduce vision. Interestingly, many eyes with chronic hypotony do not develop visual compromise.

Hypotony Maculopathy is characterized by low IOP (<6 mm Hg) with sudden drop in visual acuity. Fundus showed typical disc edema, choroidal folds and macular edema. This is more common in young myopes, pigmentary glaucoma and with use of mitomycin C.

Aim of the therapy is to decrease excessive aqueous flow and eliminate ciliochoroidal effusion. Cryoapplication, cauterization, photocoagulation, injection of autologous blood, compression sutures (**Figure 24**) and trichloroacetic acid all have been used to shrink blebs. Bleb revision is often required but frequently results in less successful filtration. Hypotony leads to transudation of fluid into the potential space between the sclera and uveal tissues. When hypotony is present it is often difficult to ascertain whether the hypotony caused the ciliochoroidal detachment, or vice versa. Late hypotony and ciliochoroidal detachment can develop after aqueous suppressant therapy in previously filtered eyes.

Bleb Related Endophthalmitis

The cumulative incidence of bleb-related endophthalmitis after filtration surgery range from 0.2 to 9.6 percent.[15] With the advent of antifibrosis agents, the late bleb-related endophthalmitis rate is increasing. The infection is due to migration of bacteria through the bleb wall, as opposed to early postoperative endophthalmitis, which results from entry of organisms into the eye at the time of surgery.

A milky-white appearing infected bleb is characteristic of bleb-related endophthalmitis. A purulent hypopyon may be present (**Figures 25A to E**).

In most cases the infection starts in the bleb and spreads into the anterior chamber. Later it spreads into the vitreous, causing a full-blown endophthalmitis. Thin-walled, cystic blebs and chronic bleb leaks appear to be risk factors for this complication. The most commonly involved organisms include staphylococcal and streptococcal species. Bleb related endophthalmitis has been reported after contact lens wear in the presence of inadvertent filtering blebs. If the infection is confined to the anterior segment, topical and periocular injections of antibiotics may suffice. A vitreous tap also should be performed if a hypopyon is present or if there is any indication of vitreous involvement by ophthalmoscopy, slit-lamp biomicroscopy or ultrasonography. After the antibiotics have been used for 12 to 24 hours, topical steroids should be initiated to prevent scarring and preserve the filtration site. If the vitreous is involved, intravitreal antibiotics are injected after taking samples for microbiological analysis. A vitrectomy is advisable to debulk the organisms, endotoxins and debris.

Corneal Complications

Corneal surface problems are common after the use of antifibrotic agents. Anterior migration of the bleb (**Figures 26A to E**) onto the cornea may result in tear film abnormalities with secondary dellen formation, ocular surface irregularities, induced astigmatism, etc. In case of bleb migration of the cornea producing cosmetic problem or discomfort (bleb dysesthesia), excision of the corneal portion of the bleb after it has been reflected with an iris spatula usually suffices. The conjunctival edge may have to be closed with 10-0 nylon sutures.

The most frequently encountered complication is corneal surface

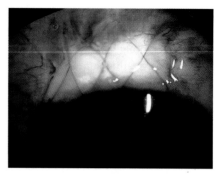

Fig. 24 Compression sutures for an overfiltering bleb

toxicity related to the effect of 5-FU on the constantly dividing cells of the corneal epithelium. At high total doses epitheliopathy may last longer than 4 weeks after cessation of the drug in otherwise healthy corneas. Other reversible corneal complications attributed to 5-FU include filamentary keratitis, dellen, keratinization, and corneal epithelial iron lines.

Corneal epithelial pigment lines (striate melanokeratosis), related to an ingrowth of pigment containing limbal stem cells are more commonly seen in black or darkly pigmented patients and usually resolve after several months without any permanent sequelae. Herpes simplex keratitis, bacterial corneal ulcers, corneal keratinization and scaring and infectious crystalline keratopathy secondary to streptococcus viridans have been reported. Mitomycin C is extremely toxic to intraocular contents.

Releasable Suture Related Complications

• **Wind shield wiper keratopathy:** Occurs due to rubbing of the suture end on the cornea with lid movements when the suture is out of the corneal track. It appears as wedge shaped keratopathy around the loose end of the suture (**Figure 27**). It resolves with release of suture or trimming of the suture.

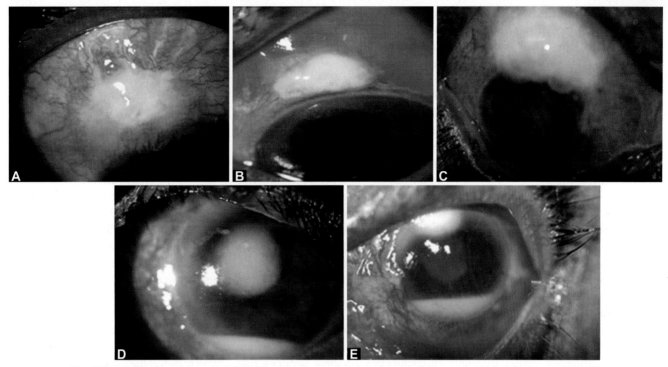

Figs 25A to E Blebitis and endophthalmitis following trabeculectomy. Various stages and clinical presentations

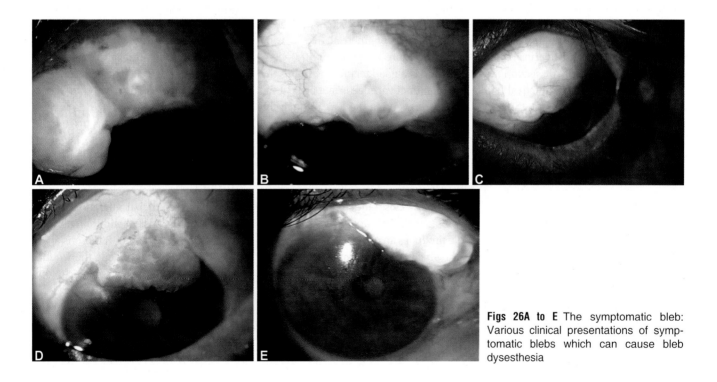

Figs 26A to E The symptomatic bleb: Various clinical presentations of symptomatic blebs which can cause bleb dysesthesia

- Persistent track left behind after suture trimming or removing the suture may predispose to bleb infection.
- During suture removal, the suture may break before the slip knot is released. It should be supplemented with laser suture lysis if need be.
- The complications include—epithelial abrasion/epithelial defect, subconjunctival bleed.
- If the removal is delayed then the exteriorized end of suture gets deeply buried under corneal epithelium. Such sutures may be left in place rather than to risk the deep corneal dissection.

Ptosis and Strabismus

Causes: Superior blocks, superior rectus bridle suture, accidental damage to superior rectus during dissection of limbal based conjunctival flap, and toxicity to superior rectus muscle with posteriorly placed MMC sponges.

Prevention: Corneal traction suture can be used instead of superior rectus bridle suture, careful dissection in cases of limbal based conjunctival flap and minimizing traction on the eye avoids damage to elevator complex.

Treatment: Conservative treatment as most cases settle spontaneously, but

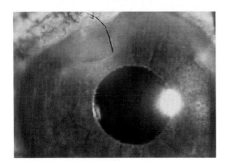

Fig. 27 Windshield wiper syndrome due to releasable suture

sometimes surgical correction may be required in nonresolving cases associated with diplopia or for cosmetic reasons.

MANAGEMENT OF THE LEAKING BLEB: AN OVERVIEW

Leaking blebs can result in hypotony and shallowing of the anterior chamber resulting in maculopathy, suprachoroidal hemorrhage, peripheral anterior synechiae, cataract, endophthalmitis, etc. Bleb leak may be seen as high as 40 percent in immediate postoperative period especially in cases where antibifrotic agents are used. Majority of such leaks are transient.

Prevention

It is of utmost importance to prevent a bleb leak by careful tissue handling of conjunctiva. Minimal handling that too with only nontoothed forceps and blunt scissors is mandatory. Meticulous conjunctival closure is necessary to prevent leak at the incision site. With a fornix based conjunctival flap, a wing shaped closure using 9-0 or 10-0 vicryl or nylon is a good technique. In this the free conjunctival edge is taut against the limbus preventing the leak through the edge. For limbal based flaps 9-0 vicryl suture using a vascular needle is used to close the conjunctiva in a running, locking fashion incorporating tenon's fascia in alternating bites. Some surgeons separately close the tenon's and the conjunctiva. The tapered vascular needle produces an opening in the conjunctiva which is only as large as the suture material limiting the leak around it.

If antimetabolites are used, care should be taken to avoid.

Argon laser suture lysis can itself produce bleb leaks due to mechanical injury by contact lens and also by

the laser itself as it is absorbed from subconjunctival space. Lower energy settings may be necessary for suturolysis in cases of blebs where antimetabolites are used.

Management

Conjunctival Buttonholes

Any conjunctival buttonhole should be sutured with a 10-0 nylon or non absorbable suture on a tapered vascular needle. Conjunctiva anterior to the anterior lip of the buttonhole is penetrated and the needle is passed across the defect to come out through the posterior lip. This is done without the use of forceps as the use of forceps may enlarge the buttonhole contact between the antimetabolite and the edge of the conjunctiva. If the leak is large enough, bleb revision combined with scleral patch graft is the ideal option.

Treatment of Postoperative Bleb Leaks

Aqueous suppressants can decrease aqueous humor production enough to reduce the flow through the leak, there by facilitating epithelial proliferation across the defect and closure of the opening. Along with aqueous suppressants pressure patching is also useful. Another technique is placement of a large diameter (14-24 mm) contact lens, so that the contact lens completely covers the area of leakage. Contact lens should be kept for at least one week to facilitate epithelial migration, but it always carries a risk of endophthalmitis. A symblepharon ring or Simmons shell may be used to tamponade the wound leak, but they are less tolerated by the patient.

Cyanoacrylate glue may be used to close a conjunctival opening.[16] For this the surrounding tissue is dried and a drop of cyanoacrylate is placed over the defect. A soft contact lens is then applied over the glue to decrease patient discomfort. A commercial fibrin adhesive, *Tissel* has been used to close a bleb leak. This glue is applied simultaneously with thrombin to form a fibrin clot at the site of application. The procedure is performed under operating microscope, using topical anesthesia. The field must be dry during the application because fibrin will not adhere to wet tissue. Injection of autologous blood to create inflammation, originally described for the treatment of hypotony, has been applied successfully for leaking blebs.

Bleb leaks that occur weeks to months after surgery often require surgical management. If the leak persists despite the conservative management, the conjunctival wound can be closed with a 9-0 or 10-0 nylon with a tapered vascular needle. If the bleb is thin walled such a suturing technique may not be advisable because it could tear the tissue edge and can cause a large leak. Surgical revision of the bleb using free conjunctival grafts, scleral patch grafts, rotational conjunctival-tenon's flap is necessary if suturing is not effective. Another approach is excising the entire cystic and leaking area of the bleb and then undermining the surrounding conjunctiva and Tenon's posterior to the surgical site. The conjunctiva is then advanced and

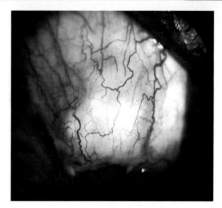

Fig. 28 Scleral patch graft

sutured in place at the limbus. A scleral patch graft **(Figure 28)** can also be used. Relaxing incisions may be given in posterior conjunctiva.

REFERENCES

1. Addicks EM, et al. Histologic characteristics of filtering blebs in glaucomatous eyes, Arch Ophthalmol 1983;101:795.

2. Ainsworth JR, Jay JL. Cost analysis of early trabeculectomy versus conventional management in primary open angle glaucoma. Eye 1991;5:322.

3. Allen RC, et al. Filtration surgery in the teatment of neovascular glaucoma. Ophthalmology 1982;89:1181.

4. Benedikt OP. Drainage mechanism after filtration, Glaucoma 1979;1:71.

5. Bellows AR, Johnstone MA. Surgical management of chronic glaucoma in aphakia. Ophthalmology 1983;90:807.

6. Bansal RK, Gupta A. 5-fluorouracil for trabeculectomy in patients under the age of 40 years. Ophthalmic Surg 1992;23:278.

7. Bank A, Allingham RR. Application of mitomycin-C during filtering surgery. Am J Ophthalmol 1993;116:377.

8. Ramakrishnan R, Michon J, Robin AL, Krishnadas R. Safety and efficacy of mitomycin C trabeculectomy in southern India. A short-term pilot study. Ophthalmology 1993;100:1619-23.

9. Robin AL, Ramakrishnan R, Krishnadas R, et al. A long-term dose-response study of mitomycin in glaucoma filtration surgery. Arch Ophthalmol 1997;115:969-73.

10. Ball SF. Concentration change and activity of fluorouracil in the external segment of the eye after subconjunctival injection. Arch Ophthalmol 1989;107:1276.

11. Batterbury M, Wishart PK. Is high initial aqueous outflow of benefit in trabeculectomy? Eye 1993;7:109.

12. Alpar JJ. Sodium hyaluronate in glaucoma surgery. Ophthalmic Surg 1986;17:724.

13. Ariano ML, Ball SF. Delayed nonexpulsive suprachoroidal hemorrhage after Trabeculectomy. Ophthalmic Surg 1987;18:661.

14. Agarwal SP, Hendeles S. Risk of sudden vision loss following trabeculectomy in advanced primary open angle glaucoma. Br J Ophthal 1986;70:97.

15. Aschkenzi I, et al. Risk factors associated with late infection of filtering blebs and Endophthalmitis. Ophthalmic Surg 1991;22:570.

16. Aminlari A, Sassani JW. Tissue adhesive for closure of wound leak in filtering operations. Glaucoma 1989;11:86.

48

Collagen Implants in Glaucoma Filtering Surgery

Ashish Kumar, R Ramakrishnan

CHAPTER OUTLINE

- Composition and Safety
- Mechanism of Action
- Efficacy
- Indications
- Technique
- Postoperative Course and Appearance of the Bleb

Driven largely by the surgeons' desire to lower IOP more safely and efficiently than by standard trabeculectomy with antimetabolites, an exciting period of innovation in glaucoma surgery is underway. Since a long time, ophthalmologists have used antimetabolites such as mitomycin C (MMC) and 5-fluorouracil, tissue plasminogen activator and corticosteroids to modulate wound healing in glaucoma filtering surgery. Unfortunately, the application of antifibrotics to inhibit fibroblasts during or after trabeculectomy usually increases the success rate but induces some severe early and late complications, including wound leakage, corneal toxicity and hypotony maculopathy, bleb leaks, blebitis, and endophthalmitis. Histopathological examination of blebs after filtering surgery with these agents reveals irregularities in the conjunctival epithelium, breaks in the basement membrane, and hypocellularity of conjunctiva and subconjunctival tissue. Resultant avascular thinning of the layers of the conjunctiva decreases the defence mechanism and leads to an increased risk of bleb infection and endophthalmitis. The use of collagen matrix in glaucoma filtering surgery is a recent development in modulating wound healing. Collagen implants can increase the efficacy of trabeculectomy without the need for antifibrotic agents like mitomycin C.

COMPOSITION AND SAFETY

The source of collagen matrix is porcine. The lyophilized porcine collagen is extracted from porcine skin with special pathogen free (SPF) certification. This artificial porcine extracellular matrix is made of **atelocollagen** cross-linked with glycosaminoglycan. Collagen from mammals is highly homologous; the difference between porcine, bovine or even human is very less.

The quality from the material source to the finished product is closely monitored. The collagen source comes with a certificate of origin and hygiene. The manufacturing process is certified by **ISO 9001 and ISO 13485** and has passed biocompatibility testing in accordance with **ISO 10993** Biological Evaluation of Medical Devices. However, human source has contagious disease risk and bovine mainly has BSE concern. The manufacturers claim that additional potential concerns such as viruses, BSE, bacteria, and pyrogens have been addressed thoroughly in the manufacturing process control, which includes quality control testing, validations, and risk analyses.

MECHANISM OF ACTION

Scar formation over the trabecular flap and subconjunctival space is the common cause of bleb failure. Collagen implants are **not inhibitors or antifibrotic agents**. Ologen™ is composed of 3-D collagen–glycosaminoglycan copolymers, which form a porous structure. Instead of using antifibrotic agents, the porous structure provides a scaffold for fibroblasts to grow randomly, which could reduce scar formation effectively. The collagen matrix itself can function like a reservoir to absorb the aqueous humor. It also provides pressure on the scleral flap to create controlled drainage in the subconjunctival space. The collagen matrix is biodegraded around 90 to 180 days depending on the postoperative medication(s), stress, tissue site, predetermined intrinsic inflammatory and remodeling mechanisms.

This phenomenon can effectively reduce the scar formation without the complications of antifibrotic agents. The normalized wound healing also helps produce functional bleb formation.

EFFICACY

The efficacy of collagen matrix has been demonstrated in animal models.[1-3] Chen et al performed standard trabeculectomy on 17 rabbits, with their left eye receiving the collagen matrix implant and their right eye serving as surgical controls. During the first few days, the postoperative reduction in IOP (15%) was equal in both groups. Pressure had decreased to 55 percent below baseline values at day 28 in the treated eyes but had returned to preoperative levels by day 21 in the control eyes. Histological examination showed a prominent bleb in the treated eyes compared with scarring and limited bleb formation in the control eyes.[2]

INDICATIONS

Glaucoma Surgery

- Trabeculectomy
- Deep sclerectomy
- Bleb revision.

Other Indications

- Strabismus surgery
- Ocular surface reconstruction
- Oculoplastic surgery
- Grafts donor sites
- Pterygium excision
- Subconjunctival scar revision.

TECHNIQUE

Ologen currently comes in two sizes for glaucoma filtering surgery: 6×2 mm and 12×1 mm. The numbers 6 and 12 refer to the diameter of the round implant, **(Figures 1A to C)** and the numbers 2 and 1 refer to its thickness. Both sizes of the device have been used with good success. It also comes in a variety of shapes: round, donut, cylinder, rectangular.

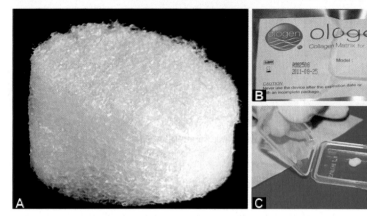

Figs 1A to C (A) Collagen implant; (B and C) Collagen implant (ologen)

Guarded filtering surgery is performed based on the surgeon's preferred technique. One can make either a limbus **(Figure 2)** or a fornix-based conjunctival incision **(Figures 3A to C)**. The main surgical challenge is in the closure of the scleral flap. After tying the sutures, the collagen matrix is placed over the scleral flap. No suture is required to secure the implant, and as soon as it touches the sclera, it absorbs aqueous and moulds to the scleral tissue. **The Collagen matrix does not need to be presoaked or prepared in any way**.

With trabeculectomy, many surgeons may prefer to place several tight sutures to prevent early hypotony. The Ologen can be implanted on the top of the scleral flap and suture the and the sutures may be tied loosely in order to encourage aqueous flow.

The larger version can be placed through a 4 mm limbal incision with fornix-based conjunctival flap. The process requires some manipulation. The implant has to be folded slightly for insertion and then teased flat. The 6×2 mm device is much easier to place over the scleral flap with a small limbal incision because of the implant's greater thickness and smaller diameter, but it can be more difficult than with the larger implant to visualize the sutures for laser suture lysis during the

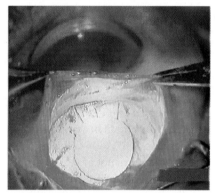

Fig. 2 Trabeculectomy with collagen implant (limbus-based flap)

postoperative period. With a limbus-based conjunctival flap, no manipulation is required at all because of the large exposure afforded by the larger posterior wound in the fornix. Both sizes of the implant can be used with either type of conjunctival wound depending upon the surgeon's comfort and experience over time. After the collagen matrix's placement, the surgeon closes the conjunctiva in his or her usual meticulous fashion to ensure that the wound is watertight.

POSTOPERATIVE COURSE AND APPEARANCE OF THE BLEB

During first few weeks it is difficult to visualize the sutures through the collagen matrix making argon laser suture lysis difficult. One way to circumvent this

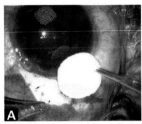 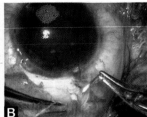 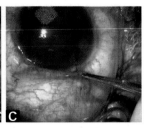

Figs 3A to C Trabeculectomy with Collagen implant (Fornix-based flap)

problem is to place the collagen matrix on the posterior edge of the flap. The sutures can be seen through the implant if pressed firmly with a suture lysis lens.

Another option is to use releasable sutures to close the scleral flap.

It should be kept in mind that the collagen matrix helps to limit hypotony through a tamponading effect over the scleral flap. The presence of the collagen matrix under the conjunctiva has been observed even 2-5 months after surgery. The implant becomes thin as it biodegrades.

The blebs are not avascular even 4 to 6 months postoperatively. Patients usually maintain low IOPs without medication, just like patients who have received intraoperative MMC.

Advantages

Although collagen matrix is more expensive than MMC, it offers several advantages.

- The collagen matrix helps to limit hypotony through a tamponading effect over the scleral flap. Unlike MMC, postoperative hypotony has not been observed as significant complication
- Modulates wound healing without producing thin, avascular blebs. As a result there is less risk of complications associated with these types of blebs.
- **Decreased surgical time:** Not using antimetabolites saves a significant amount of time intraoperatively, each case is at

least 2-5 minutes shorter. This is significant on a high-volume surgical day.

- **No special handling precautions:** Unlike an antimetabolite, no special handling and disposing precautions are required.
- The collagen matrix is not a teratogen like MMC.

Disadvantages

Laser suture lysis is difficult as the sutures are covered by the implant and not clearly visible. The 12×1 mm implant appears to have reduced the problem. This thinner implant can be more difficult to place than the 2×6 mm collagen matrix careful dissection of the posterior space under tenon's capsule is necessary.

CONCLUSION

Collagen matrix has been found to be safe and effective in the short-term, and it may help to reduce MMC related complications and, improve efficiency. Clearly, a prospective, randomized trial comparing MMC with collagen matrix is warranted.

REFERENCES

1. Zelefsky JR, Hsu WC, Ritch R. Biode-gradable collagen matrix implant for trabeculectomy. Expert Rev Ophthalmology 2008;3:613-7.

2. Chen HS, Ritch R, Krupin T, Hsu WC. Control of filtering bleb structure through tissue bioengineering: an animal model. Invest Ophthalmol Vis Sci 2006;47(12):5310-4.

3. Hsu WC, Ritch R, Krupin T, Chen HS. Tissue bioengineering for surgical bleb defects: an animal study. Graefes Arch Clin Exp Ophthalmol 2008; 246(5):709-17.

## 49

Dysfunctional Filtering Blebs

Anup Das, Mohideen Abdul Kader

CHAPTER OUTLINE

INTRODUCTION

Glaucoma filtration surgery is aimed to lower intraocular pressure (IOP) by creating a fistula between inner compartments of the eye and subconjunctival space, i.e. filtering bleb. However, improvement in IOP control after guarded filtration procedures is associated with high frequency of bleb related complication like bleb leaks, flat anterior chamber, hypotony, encapsulation. Though the techniques to improve the function of filtering blebs and to treat postoperative complication have progressed over past decade, still close monitoring and appropriate interventions in time may decrease the incidence of dysfunctional bleb.[1]

FEATURES OF FILTERING BLEBS

The appearance of the bleb after trabeculectomy is the hallmark and an indicator of how effective the filtering procedure is.[2] A filtering bleb can be described according to the following morphological features:

1. Elevation
2. Vascularization
3. Thickness of wall
4. Extent in clock hours
5. Localized or diffuse
6. Presence or absence of microcysts.

In a retrospective study, Pitch G et al. standardized morphological criteria to classify developing filtering bleb **(Table 1)**. They used the following parameters:[3]

1. Presence or absence of microcyst at 3 sectors of filtering bleb **(Figure 1)**.
2. Quality of conjunctival vessels compared with standard photograph (+ to +++) **(Figures 2A and B)**.
3. Shape of conjunctival vessels compared with standard photographs **(Figure 3)**.
4. Presence or absence of encapsulation (Yes or no) **(Figure 4)**.
5. Height of the filtering blebs compared with standard photographs (+ to +++) **(Figure 5)**.

Table 1 Morphological criteria to classify developing filtering bleb

Favorable bleb development	Unfavorable bleb development
Microcysts of the conjunctiva	Increased vascularization
Paucity of vessels	Cork Screw vessels
Diffuse bleb	Encapsulated bleb
Moderate elevation of the bleb	High dome appearance

Thus a bleb can undergo any modification and can assume any one of the following forms over time: (According to the classification of Migdal and Hitchings):[4]

1. Type I bleb (very low IOP, elevated bleb)
   - Thin, polycystic
   - Transconjunctival flow of aqueous
   - Good filtration
2. Type II bleb (Ideal bleb) (low IOP, elevated bleb)
   - Thin, diffuse
   - Relatively avascular
   - Microcysts
   - Indicate good filtration
3. Type III bleb (High IOP, low localized bleb)
   - Flat with no microcystic spaces
   - Surface contain engorged blood vessels
   - Nonfiltering
4. Type IV encapsulated bleb (High IOP, Tenon's cyst)
   - Localized, highly elevated
   - Dome-shaped, firm
   - Cyst like cavity of hypertrophied Tenon's capsule

- ❖ Surface-engorged blood vessels
- ❖ Time—2 to 8 weeks postoperative period
- ❖ Associated dellen formation.

Other bleb classification and grading systems include Moorfields and IBAGS. Shingelton et al.[5] described certain early warning sign of failing filtration and corelated the bleb appearance to the level of IOP. A framework for categorizing failing filter using IOP and bleb characteristics is shown in **Table 2**.

Usually elevated, large, thin, avascular filtering blebs are associated with better IOP control than the low blebs with thick, vascularized walls.

AN OVERVIEW OF FACTORS AFFECTING GROSS MORPHOLOGY AND FUNCTION OF A FILTERING BLEB[6,7]

- Previous scarring and increased wound healing response may lead to bleb failure.
- Full thickness procedures produce more thin walled bleb than trabeculectomy.
- Limbus based conjunctival flap are associated with more cystic blebs.
- Thin, cystic blebs are more common with the use of antimetabolites like mitomycin C (MMC) and 5- fluorouracil (5FU).
- Prolonged postoperative steroid therapy is associated with thin blebs.
- Patients on multiple topical antiglaucoma medications preoperatively have more chances of scarring.

Histopathologic Observation

A good functioning bleb has the following histological findings:[8]
1. Normal epithelium
2. Subepithelial connective tissue—thin, loosely arranged and has clear channel like spaces 50 to 200 μ diameter corresponding to microcyst.

Analysis of the histopathology of an avascular bleb (post trabeculectomy with MMC) shows:
1. Irregular epithelium
2. Numerous microcyst
3. Largely acellular spaces in subepithelium
4. Cytoplasmic vacuoles in epithelium with necrotic nuclear material in superficial epithelial cells.

Addick's et al.[9] described a failed filtering bleb as having:
1. Normal epithelium
2. Dense collagenous connective tissue in subepithelium
3. Increased inflammatory response in conjunctival dermis and Tenon's capsule.

Hichings and Gierson[10] observed that in an encapsulated bleb the capsule consisted of amorphorous basement like material wide spacing collagen and elastic fibers.

Broadway et al.[11] showed the effect of topical antiglaucoma medication on conjunctival epithelium and effect on conjunctiva after reversal of therapy. They observed an increase in the number of conjunctival inflammatory cells (macrophages, lymphocytes, mast cells and fibroblasts) after multiple drug therapy. Use of topical fluorometholone (1%) and stopping the antiglaucoma medication prior to trabeculectomy lead to 81 percent success as compared with 50 percent without pretreatment with steroids.

DYSFUNCTIONAL BLEB AND RELATED PROBLEMS

Patterns of filtration failure may be classified as:
1. **High IOP, low bleb**
   - ❖ External subconjunctival fibrosis
   - ❖ Internal sclerectomy obstruction
2. **High IOP, dome like bleb**
   - ❖ Encapsulated bleb or Tenons cyst
2. **Low IOP, flat bleb**
   - ❖ Bleb leak
3. **Low IOP, elevated bleb**
   - ❖ Overfiltration
   - ❖ Hypotony.

THE OVERFILTERING BLEB AND HYPOTONY[12]

Predisposing Factors

Decreased aqueous production due to:
- Inflammation
- Cilio-choroidal detachment
- Retinal detachment
- Inadvertent use of aqueous suppressants.

Increased aqueous outflow due to:
- Bleb leak
- Overfiltration following use of 5FU, MMC (**Figure 1**).

Clinical Findings
a. IOP < 6 mm Hg
b. Shallow anterior chamber
   - ❖ Grade 1—Peripheral iridocorneal apposition with central formed AC
   - ❖ Grade 2—Pupillary - border-corneal apposition without lenticular touch
   - ❖ Grade 3—Central lens corneal touch.
c. Bleb—Avascular, Siedel's test negative.

Table 2 Causes of failing filter

High IOP	Low IOP
Low Bleb – Subconjunctival fibrosis – Closure of Internal sclerectomy ostium	**Flat Bleb** – Bleb Leak
High Bleb – Encapsulated bleb (Tenon's cyst)	**Elevated Bleb** – Overfiltration – Antimetabolites related hypotony

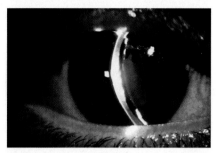

Fig. 1 Hypotony in the early postoperative period following trabeculectomy with mitomycin C. Note the shallow anterior chamber and the folds in the Descemet's membrane

d. Persistent loss of vision, cystoid macular edema (CME), optic disc edema.

Management

a. *Conservative:* Grade I or II flat anterior chamber (FAC) is managed conservatively. Restriction of physical activity is recommended. This is especially important in patients with aphakia and vitrectomized eyes as the risk of suprachoridal hemorrhage is high.

  ❖ Tamponade–Pressure patching, large bandage contact lens, Simmon's shell, symblepharon ring
  ❖ Topical and Systemic steroids
  ❖ Cycloplegics.

  Usually grade I flat anterior chamber (FAC) resolves with conservative management, Grade II FAC may need AC reformation with viscoelastics (Healon-5, Healon GV), air, nonexpansile mixture of SF6 or c3f8 in air.

b. *Surgical management:* Grade III FAC requires surgical intervention as it is an emergency procedures. choroidal drainage is done along with AC reformation by air, viscoelastics or non expansile gases. Various modalities of treatment to manage the overfiltering bleb are:

  i. *Chemical irritants:* 0.25-1 percent silver nitrate or 50 percent trichloro acetic acid is applied topically, which induces chemical conjunctival burn and subsequent inflammation and wound healing.

  ii. *Autologous subconjunctival blood:* Approximately 0.1 to 0.5 ml of autologous blood is injected into the bleb and ensured to enter into AC to be effective. The complications include elevated IOP, bleb failure, temporary reduction in visual acuity.

  iii. *Cryotherapy:* A 2 to 5 application of cryotherapy with –50ºC to 60ºC for 10 to 30 second duration is applied over lateral border of filtrating bleb initially. More than one session may be needed to achieve the desired goal.

  iv. *Diathermy and cauterization:* This procedure is not preferred because of increase risk of perforation of bleb. The mechanism is to induce cicatrization and shrinkage of bleb by inducing inflammation.

  v. *Argon laser:* Under topical anesthesia, the conjunctiva is painted with Rose Bengal or methelene blue dye. Laser power of 300 to 500, spot size 200 to 500 μ, Duration 0.25 is used to produce visible shrinkage of bleb surface with approximately 100 burns.

  vi. *Nd:YAG thermal laser:* Under retrobulbar/peribulbar anesthesia 30 to 40 spots of power 3 to 4 continuous wave Nd:YAG laser is placed over the entire bleb in a grid pattern. measured by observing whitening and wrinkling of conjunctival epithelium.

Other techniques includes:
  ❖ Resuturing of scleral flap
  ❖ Scleral patch graft with conjunctival advancement
  ❖ Scleral flap revision.

BLEB LEAK[13,14]
Predisposing Factors

a. Early bleb leak is due to inadverant button hole in conjunctiva, or wound leak through conjunctival incision **(Figure 2A)**.

b. *Late bleb leak:* This is more commonly seen after antimetabolite augmented trabeculectomy or after full thickness filtering procedures.

Clinical Findings

a. IOP < 6 mm Hg
b. Shallow AC
c. Bleb-flat, Siedel's test positive **(Figure 2B)**
d. Decreased vision, striate keratopathy, choroidal detachments, chances of endophthalmitis.

Management

a. *Intraoperative precautions:*
  ❖ Careful conjunctival dissection
  ❖ Avoidance of toothed forceps
  ❖ Meticulous flap closure
  ❖ Avoidance of contact between MMC and conjunctival wound edges and copious irrigation.

b. *Managing early bleb leaks:*
  ❖ *Conservative:*
    ♦ Decrease dose of steroids
    ♦ Tight pad and bandage, BCL, collagen shields
    ♦ Irritants like aminoglycoside drops
    ♦ Systemic aqueous suppressants (acetazolamide).
  ❖ *Surgical and laser:*
    ♦ Argon laser (500 μ, 0.1 sec) treatment of the area
    ♦ Suturing (mattress or purse string) the leak with 10-0 nylon
    ♦ Sliding and rotational conjunctival and Tenons flap graft, free conjunctival grafts or scleral patch graft—if the above measurs fails.

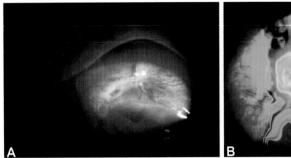
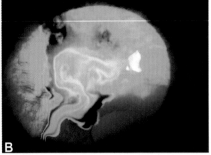

Figs 2A and B (A) Bleb leak due to conjunctival button hole; (B) Positive Siedel's test

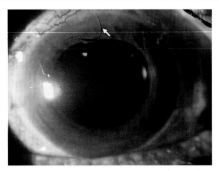

Fig. 3 Releasable suture

❖ *Others:*
  ◆ Cyanoacrylate and fibrin tissue glue
  ◆ Autologous blood injection into the bleb.
c. ***Managing late bleb leaks***
  ❖ Sliding and rotational conjunctival and Tenon's flap graft
  ❖ Free conjunctival grafts
  ❖ Scleral patch grafts.

FAILING AND FAILED BLEBS[15,16]

Failing and failed blebs are those associated with inadequate IOP control and impending or established obstruction of aqueous outflow. They may be classified as:

Early Failed Blebs

This includes bleb of less than 1 month duration, associated with high IOP and low hyperemic bleb. Causes may be due to internal obstruction by blood, fibrinous clot, vitreous, iris or incompletely excised Descemet's membrane or scleral tissue or fibroblastic tissue, sub-conjunctival and episcleral fibrosis, tight scleral flap.

Prevention and Management

a. Use of intraoperative antimetabolites (5 FU/MMC).
b. Increase the dose topical corticosteroids.
c. Treat the cause, e.g. blocked ostium.
d. ***Digital ocular massage and compression:*** Digital ocular compression can be applied to the inferior sclera or cornea through the inferior eyelid or to the sclera posterior to the scleral flap through the superior eyelid. Focal compression is applied with a moistened cotton tip at the edge of the scleral flap.
d. ***Suturelysis:*** It is performed within the first 2 weeks after the surgery without antimetabolite; with metabolites pressure reduction till 3 months after surgery has been reported. In late postoperative period fibrosis of the scleral flap may negate any beneficial effect of this procedure. Laser suturelysis can be performed with argon, krypton or diode laser. Argon laser parameters are 50 μm spot size, 0.1 second exposure time and 200 to 500 mW of power. It should be performed in a conservative stepwise manner. Usually only one suture is cut at a time to avoid over filtration and a flat anterior chamber.
e. ***Releasable sutures:*** Releasing releasable sutures **(Figure 3)** are equally effective as laser suture lysis.
f. ***Tissue plasminogen activator:*** tPA (up to 25 mg) can be injected into the anterior chamber after paracentesis of an equivalent volume (0.1 ml), or subconjunctivally.
g. ***Laser internal bleb revision:*** The laser disrupts the tissue responsible for the obstruction, opening the sclerostomy. If a pigmented tissue is responsible for the obstruction (i.e. iris), the argon laser may also be successful.

Late Failed Blebs

This refers to those blebs with history of good bleb functions and adequate control of IOP postoperatively for at least 1 month but later failed **(Figure 4)**. Pathogenesis is increased resistance to aqueous flow at the level of subconjunctival space, the scleral flap, or the sclerostomy.

Here subconjunctival and episcleral fibrosis are the most common types of filtration failure. Internal closure of the sclerostomy is less common. Usually associated warning signs of failing filtration like bleb vascularization, bleb inflammation and bleb thickening.

Management

The management of late failing blebs depends primarily on the site of aqueous resistance, which determines failure of filtering blebs:

a. ***Subconjunctival and episcleral fibrosis:*** External approach like – by Nd:YAG laser or bleb needling.
b. ***In cases with obstruction of the sclerostomy:*** An internal revision by Nd:YAG laser or argon laser can be tried.
c. In failed cases, repeat trabeculectomy is done or a glaucoma drainage device is implanted.

BLEB ENCAPSULATION (TENON'S CYST)[17]

The frequency of encapsulated blebs in trabeculectomies without antimetabolites ranges from 8.3 to 28 percent.

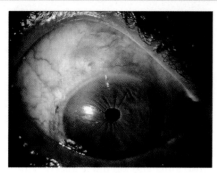

Fig. 4 Failed bleb

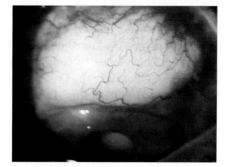

Fig. 5 Encapsulated bleb

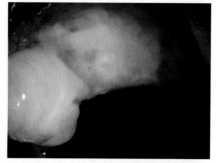

Fig. 6 Symptomatic bleb (Bleb Dysesthesia)

Predisposing factors include:
- Males
- Glove powder
- Prior treatment with sympathomimetics
- Prior ALT
- Prior surgery
- Young age
- Black race.

This type of bleb commonly appears within 2 to 4 weeks after surgery. They are usually localized, high, and tense, with vascular engorgement of the overlying conjunctiva and a thick connective tissue **(Figure 5)**.

Prevention and Management

a. Use of intraoperative antimetabolites in high-risk cases.

b. Increasing doses of topical steroids.

c. Subconjunctival 5 FU (5 mg/0.1 ml), 90° to 180° away from the bleb for 2 to 3 weeks.

d. Digital ocular compression.

e. Topical aqueous suppressants.

f. Needling with 5 FU.

g. Surgical excision of fibrous tissue.

The long-term prognosis for IOP control in eyes that develop encapsulated blebs is relatively good. About 90 percent achieve pressures of 21 mm Hg or less, after 1 year of follow-up, although medical therapy is often required.

SYMPTOMATIC BLEB/BLEB DYSESTHESIA

Filtering blebs usually are asymptomatic or reasonably well tolerated. Most patients are aware of a conjunctival "blister"; however, others have various degrees of discomfort. Symptoms are frequent in nasal or large blebs or when there is extension into cornea **(Figure 6)**. Common complications include superficial punctuate keratopathy, difficulty with blinking, tear film abnormalities with secondary Dellen formation or ocular surface irregularities, foreign-body sensation, and induced astigmatism.

Management includes: Frequent use of artificial tears is the recommended initial treatment for symptomatic blebs and problems related to irregular tear distribution. If the problems persist, surgical bleb excision or conjunctival flap reinforcement is the primary treatment for large blebs. Although the results of surgery are generally good, there is the possibility of bleb failure. More conservative methods to shrink blebs include cryotherapy, Nd:YAG laser thermotherapy, argon laser, diathermy, and cauterization.

BLEBITIS AND ENDOPHTHALMITIS

Late bleb infections may occur in at least 1 percent of eyes with successful filtering operations, and are more common with thin, avascular blebs. Blebitis is recognized by marked conjunctival injection surrounding a thin, sometimes leaking bleb.

The bleb itself contains a cellular reaction that ranges from layered cells to a chalk white appearance. Other signs and symptoms include blurred vision, mucoid discharge, and pain. Unless treated promptly with fortified antibiotics, endophthalmitis may result with potential loss of the eye.

Bleb related endophthalmitis **(Figure 7)** is best managed in conjunction with a vitreoretinal surgeon because vitrectomy and intraocular antibiotic injection may be indicated. Patients with filtration blebs should be warned of this complication and always told to seek care immediately if any symptoms of bleb infection develop.

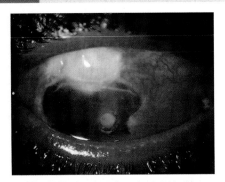

Fig. 7 Bleb-related endophthalmitis

CONCLUSION

The desired outcome of glaucoma filtering surgery is a functioning bleb formation, adequate IOP control and preservation of vision. The use of antimetabolites has helped improve IOP control but it is associated with a higher rate of bleb related complication. Achieving these goals can be a daunting task but fortunately, a number of treatments have been developed that can make their attainment relatively straightforward. An understanding of the timing and phases of the wound healing process, combined with thorough risk-factor assessment and careful postoperative examination of the bleb will greatly aid the glaucoma surgeon in timely and appropriate interventions to maximize function and longevity of the trabeculectomy bleb.

REFERENCES

1. A Azuara-blano, Katz LJ. Dysfunctional filtering blebs survey of Ophthalmlogy; 1998.pp.93-126.

2. Sugar HS. The course of change in size of successful filtering cicatrices. Am J Ophthalmol 1960;49:795-800.

3. Picht G. Classification of filtering blebs in Trabeculectomy: biomicroscopy and functionality. Current opinion in ophthalmol 1998;9:2-8.

4. Migdal C, Hitching R. The developing bleb: effect of topical antiprostaglandins on the outcomes of glaucoma fistulising surgery. Br J Ophthalmol 1983;67(10):655-60.

5. Shingeloton B. Management of failing glaucoma filter.Ophthalmic Surg 1996;27:445-51.

6. Spaeth GL. A prospective, controlled study to compare the Scheie procedure with Watson's trabeculectomy. Ophthalmic Surg 1980;11:688-94.

7. Costa VP, Moster MR, Wilson RP, et al. Effects of topical mitomycin C on primary trabeculectomies and combined procedures. Br J Ophthalmol 1993;77:693-7.

8. Shields MB, Scroggs MW, Sloop CM, Simmons RB. Clinical and histopathologic observations concerning hypotony after trabeculectomy with adjunctive mitomycin C. Am J Ophthalmol 1993;116:673-83.

9. Addicks EM. Histologic characteristics of filtering blebs in glaucomatous eyes 1983;101:795-8.

10. Hitchings RA, Grierson I. Clinicopathological correlation in eyes with failed fistulizing surgery. Trans Ophthalmol Soc UK 1983;103:84-8.

11. Broadway DC. Adverse effects of topical AGM. The outcome of filtering surgery. Arch ophth 1994;112:1437-45.

12. Liebmann JM, Ritch R. Complications of glaucoma surgery. In: Ritch R, Shields MB, Krupin T (Eds). The Glaucomas. St Louis: Mosby; 1996.pp.1715-6.

13. Zacharia PT, Deppermann SR, Schuman JS. Ocular hypotony after trabeculectomy with mitomycin C. Am J Ophthalmol 1993;116:314-26.

14. Stewart WC, Shields MB. Management of anterior chamber depth after trabeculectomy. Am J Ophthalmol 1988;106:41-4.

15. Cohen JS, Shaffer RN, Heterington J Jr, Hoskins HD Jr. Revision of filtration surgery. Arch Ophthalmol 1977;95:1612-5.

16. Scott DR, Quigley HA. Medical management of a high bleb phase after trabeculectomies. Ophthalmology 1988;95:1169-73.

17. Sherwood MB, Spaeth GL, Simmons ST, et al. Cysts of Tenon's capsule following filtration surgery. Medical management. Arch Ophthalmol 1987;105:1517-21.

## 50

Cataract and Glaucoma

Amy Parminder, Timothea Ryan, Bradford Shingleton

INTRODUCTION

Cataract and glaucoma frequently coexist particularly in an aging population and, therefore, present a unique challenge to the ophthalmologist. While certain management issues are unique to either cataract or glaucoma alone, the presence of either disease impacts significantly on the management of the other. This chapter will review current issues in glaucoma and cataract management including special circumstances.

CATARACT ASSESSMENT

The primary concern in cataract assessment is the determination of whether the patient has a visually significant cataract. This determination is made by grading of the lens opacity and assessment of functional status including *activities of daily living (ADL)*. Other causes of visual impairment should be excluded including retinal and optic nerve disease as well as ocular surface disease. The evaluation of the cataract can be made challenging by the presence of miotic pupils particularly in patients with pseudoexfoliation and longstanding miotic therapy.

Assessment should be made through a maximally dilated pupil and may include ancillary testing such as brightness acuity, contrast sensitivity and glare testing. Occasionally a cataract may be too dense and may preclude a view of the posterior segment. Under these circumstances, evaluation should include B-scan ultrasound.

GLAUCOMA ASSESSMENT

Determination of the type and extent of glaucoma damage is often made challenging in the presence of cataract due to the inability to view the optic nerve and alteration in visual field testing. Cataract can also infrequently be the cause of glaucoma, for example, phacomorphic and phacolytic glaucoma. Glaucoma and elevated intraocular pressure (IOP) as well as the treatment of glaucoma in the form of topical antiglaucoma therapy and laser and surgical therapy can contribute to cataract formation and progression.[1]

Early postoperative IOP elevation can occur in postcataract surgery patients with glaucoma particularly with the use of intraoperative viscoelastics. Glaucomatous eyes have compromised trabecular meshwork and reduced outflow facility resulting in lower tolerance to viscoelastics, inflammation and debris. The ability to manage IOP elevation in a postcataract patient, especially one with coexisting glaucoma, must be taken into account in the surgical decision-making process. Factors that affect treatment include the patient's ability to tolerate antiglaucoma medications, effectivity of pressure lowering medications, drug allergies, and predisposing medical conditions that would preclude treatment with specific drugs.

The increased risks of surgery in glaucomatous eyes are in part due to miotic pupils, posterior synechiae, peripheral anterior synechiae, zonular weakness and dehiscence, and an increased risk of suprachoroidal hemorrhage. Other risk factors are due to conditions that coexist with glaucoma, such as nanophthalmos, high hyperopia, myopia, exfoliation (XFS), and diabetes. Previous surgery with scarring or a pre-existing bleb makes glaucoma surgery more challenging. The toxic effect of medications on conjunctiva, medication compliance, and allergy affect surgical planning and outcomes.

There may be an increased risk of cystoid macular edema (CME) with BAK (benzalkonium) preserved eye-drops.

In a patient with coexisting cataract and glaucoma, the surgical decision must be made whether to treat glaucoma first or cataract in a staged procedure, to perform a combined procedure or to perform a single procedure treating either the glaucoma or cataract alone. The advantages and disadvantages of each approach must be considered and then customized.

SURGICAL MANAGEMENT
Cataract Surgery Alone

Cataract surgery alone may suffice in eyes with little or no glaucoma damage or in eyes with well-controlled glaucoma on minimal medications. Small incision phacoemulsification surgery has a small but statistically significant IOP lowering effect in normal eyes, glaucoma suspects, and glaucomatous eyes which extends one to five years postoperatively.[2-4] This IOP reduction may be greatest in eyes with relatively narrower angles and higher preoperative IOP.[5] Glaucoma surgery can still be successful at a later time if needed, particularly if conjunctiva is not violated superiorly.

Glaucoma Surgery First, Cataract Surgery Later

Glaucoma surgery alone is favored in patients with little or no coexisting cataract. Cataract can progress after trabeculectomy and the success of the filtration surgery may be compromised by subsequent cataract surgery. Glaucoma surgery first and cataract surgery later is favored in eyes with active inflammation (uveitic glaucoma) or anterior segment neovascularization (neovascular glaucoma) when the IOP is uncontrolled and IOL implantation is contraindicated at that time.

Combined Cataract and Glaucoma Surgery

Multiple options exist for the type of glaucoma surgery combined with cataract extraction **(Box 1)**. The most common is phacoemulsification with posterior chamber intraocular lens combined with trabeculectomy **(Figures 1 and 2)**.

Combined surgery has the advantage of treating both diseases with a single surgical intervention and IOP reduction tends to be greater than with cataract surgery alone. Disadvantages include increased surgery time which can increase surgical risk. More intensive postoperative care is also required. Against-the-rule-astigmatism can be exacerbated with larger superior incisions, larger sclerostomies, particularly block dissections and antimetabolite use.

Indications: Combined surgery should be considered when in the presence of a visually significant cataract more than three medications are required for IOP control or if the patient is intolerant or allergic to glaucoma medications. The presence of significant cupping or visual field loss might warrant a concomitant glaucoma procedure as the optic nerve is less able to tolerate perioperative IOP rise. Other factors favoring combined surgery include: monocular patient, and the presence of other risk factors for glaucoma including XFS, pigment dispersion syndrome and angle recession.

Special circumstances may warrant *deferral of cataract surgery* such as active uveitis, neovascular glaucoma and acute angle closure glaucoma.

Preoperative preparation of the glaucoma patient for cataract surgery is similar to the standard cataract surgery patient with some modifications. Topical antibiotics and nonsteroidal anti-inflammatory eyedrops three days prior to surgery is recommended. Miotics should be discontinued one week before surgery and

Box 1
Options for combined cataract and glaucoma surgery
• Standard trabeculectomy with and without antimetabolites (5-fluorouracil and mitomycin C)
• Endocyclophotocoagulation (ECP)
• External cyclophotocoagulation (CPC)
• Deep sclerectomy
• Viscocanalostomy
• Canaloplasty
• Trabectome®
• Express shunt
• Glaucoma drainage devices

a dilation regimen should be added with nonsteroidal anti-inflammatory drops if pupilloplasty is anticipated. Prostaglandin analogs may also be discontinued as postoperative CME is a matter of concern. Consider cessation of anticoagulation in high-risk eyes.

Special Circumstances
Miotic Pupils

Miotic pupils are not an uncommon finding in glaucoma patients as many older patients have been on long-term miotic therapy. Older patients and patients with PXF do not dilate well. Excessive iris manipulation may also lead to intraoperative miosis.

Intraoperative floppy iris syndrome (IFIS): Flomax® (Tamsulosin) is a selective alpha1-blocking agent used for benign prostatic hypertrophy in males and for urinary hesitancy in females. The alpha1 receptor is present in iris dilator smooth muscle. The IFIS or intraoperative floppy-iris syndrome patients manifest fluttering and billowing of iris stroma due to normal fluid movement, iris prolapse through the cornea incisions, and progressive pupil constriction.[6-8]

Discontinuing may improve but not eliminate IFIS and may even occur years after alpha blockers are discontinued.

The goal in small pupil management is to have adequate visualization

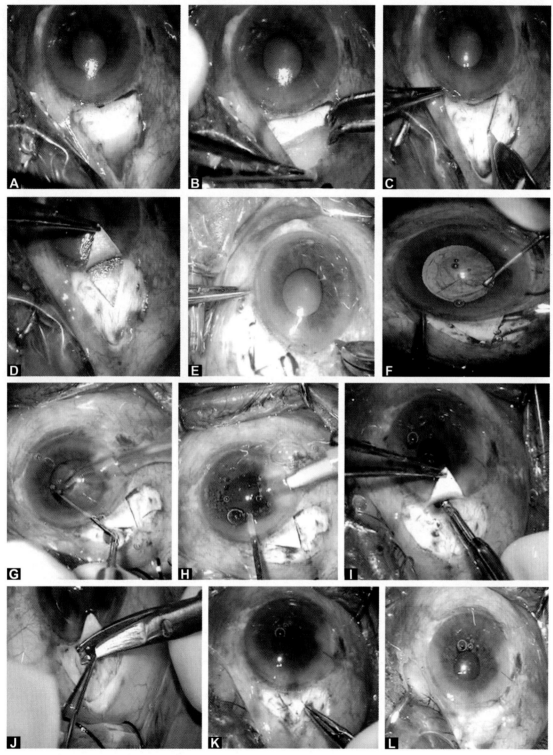

Figs 1A to L Steps of two site combined cataract and glaucoma surgery: (A) The conjunctival incision is made adjacent to the limbus for the fornix based conjunctival flap; (B) After minimal cautery a sponge soaked in mitomycin C is applied on the sclera; (C and D) A triangular scleral flap by lamellar dissection up to the limbus; (E) A clear corneal tunnel incision is made temporally; (F) CCC is performed; (G) Phacoemulsification is done (temporal clear corneal); (H) A foldable intraocular lens is implanted; (I) Anterior chamber is entered with a keratome and a sclerostomy is fashioned using a scleral Kelly Descemet's punch; (J) A basal iridectomy is done; (K) The scleral flap is sutured using 3 10-0 nylon sutures; (L) Conjunctiva is sutured with 8-0/9-0 Vicryl

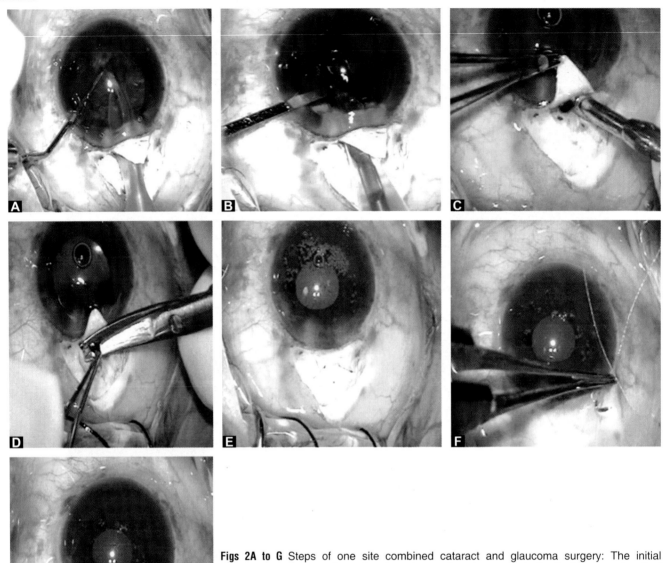

Figs 2A to G Steps of one site combined cataract and glaucoma surgery: The initial steps are same as the twin site phacotrabeculectomy. A fornix base conjunctival flap is fashioned and after light electrocautery a sponge soaked in mitomycin C is applied. After irrigating it with plenty of fluid a triangular partial thickness scleral flap is fashioned. Capsulorhexis is done and the anterior chamber is entered: (A) Phacoemulsification is done through the same site; (B) A foldable intraocular lens is implanted; (C) A sclerostomy is fashioned using a scleral Kelly Descemet's punch; (D) A basal iridectomy is done; (E) The scleral flap is sutured using 3 10-0 nylon sutures; (F and G) Conjunctiva is sutured with 8-0/9-0 Vicryl

by achieving adequate pupil size (4-5 mm), with preservation of normal pupil contour and reactivity. Excessive intraoperative iris manipulation should be avoided. Epinephrine in the infusion bottle is often helpful. Stripping of peripupillary membranes with sweeping and release of synechiae and aspiration of pigment on the anterior capsule can be performed. Frequently, the above technique in combination with viscoelastic pupil expansion is all that is required to perform safe phacoemulsification.

Bimanual iris stretch with a pair of Kuglen hooks or mechanical pupil dilators often eliminates the need for scissor sphincterotomies, but should be avoided in potential IFIS patients. Self-retaining pupil expanders such as the Malyugin Ring (Microsurgical Technology, Redmond, WA) can also be used. Self-retaining iris retractors requiring additional paracentesis incisions are also helpful. Pupil expanders and retractors are particularly helpful for IFIS.

Exfoliation Glaucoma

The complication rate in eyes with exfoliation glaucoma is greater than in normal eyes (3-5.8%) due primarily to zonular dehiscence and small pupil.[9-11] Preoperative assessment is critical for surgical planning. Anterior chamber depth asymmetry, phacodonesis, visibility of the lens equator on eccentric gaze, decentered nucleus on primary gaze, changes in contour of the lens periphery and an axial depth of less than 2.5 corneal thickness are all important findings indicating zonular weakness. Intraoperative clues that might suggest zonular weakness include limited nucleus rotation, anterior chamber depth instability, dramatic anteroposterior lens position shift and a "pseudoelastic" capsule.

Intraoperative surgical techniques might include a posterior incision if zonular weakness is anticipated. A larger, intact capsulorhexis is helpful, particularly if considering a capsule tension ring or segment (CTR, CTS) which distributes centrifugal force circumferentially to oppose capsule constriction and zonule separation. Hydrodissection is important to gain free rotation of the nucleus within the capsular bag so that aspiration forces are not transmitted to the capsule fornices during phacoemulsification.

The IOL decentration can occur with all types of intraocular lenses. Foldable acrylic lenses may reduce anterior capsule contraction. An all polymethylmethacrylate lens is more resistant to postoperative IOL shift and a large optic is more forgiving if decentration should occur. Capsular bag fixation is optimal since it reduces pigment dispersion and potential for UGH syndrome.

Nanophthalmos/High Hyperopia with Shallow Anterior Chamber

Nanophthalmos and high hyperopia patients frequently have a high lens/eye volume ratio with small corneas, thick sclera and miotic, fixed pupils. Preoperative preparation may include mannitol and use of a small volume anesthetic block with compression. Associated findings include small, deep set orbits with tight lids. Modification of surgical technique involves use of prophylactic sclerotomies, a temporal, anteriorly placed clear cornea incision to avoid iris prolapse and use of a highly retentive OVD such as Healon V to flatten the iris contour. Vitreous aspiration or pars plana vitrectomy can be particularly helpful to increase anterior chamber depth. Iris retractors and goniosynechialysis may be required. Accurate IOL calculation should be performed with up-to-date software, such as Holladay 2 or Hoffer Q. Piggyback IOL's may be required. Two silicone lenses without square edges or 2 PMMA lenses have the lowest risk of interlenticular opacification in Piggyback IOL situations. These hyperopic eyes are more susceptible to aqueous misdirection.

TECHNIQUES FOR COMBINED SURGERY
One Site Approach: Combined Cataract and Trabeculectomy Surgery via a Single Incision

A single incision approach (Figures 2A to G) to combined surgery is simple, safe, fast, and effective. This approach, however, is potentially less comfortable for the temporal cataract surgeon. Overall, it is important for the surgeon to choose his or her best operation, whichever minimizes manipulation and is most atraumatic to tissues.

Technique

For any filtration surgery combined with phacoemulsification, a paracentesis is mandatory for testing filter outflow and for performing two-handed phacoemulsification. Minimizing the size of the superior conjunctival flap spares virgin conjunctiva for repeat filtration, if needed. Small incision foldable IOL phacoemulsification minimizes the extent of conjunctival manipulation. A corneal traction suture is especially helpful with limbal-based conjunctival flaps.

During conjunctival flap dissection it is important to minimize manipulation of tissues with use of nontoothed or cellulose sponges for flap retraction, and maintenence of meticulous hemostasis with underwater unipolar diathermy. Limbal-based and fornix-based conjunctival flaps have similar results in reduction of IOP, bleb development, visual outcomes, and reduction of glaucoma medications.[12] Limbal-based flaps are associated with less bleb leaks and permit earlier laser suture lysis (LSL), digital pressure, and 5-FU injections postoperatively. However, limbal-based trabeculectomy is more tedious than fornix-based, requiring more time to complete and may be associated with a higher rate of encapsulated blebs and anterior localized blebs.

To create a limbal-based conjunctival flap, an incision is made at least 10 mm posterior to the limbus. A relatively thin dissection is desirable with separation of conjunctiva and Tenon's plane. Dissection is carried forward to the anterior reflection of the conjunctiva using a #15 Bard-Parker blade, a Tooke knife, or iris spatula as needed.

A fornix-based conjunctival flap is a particularly useful approach for scarred conjunctiva. This approach is faster than the limbal-based technique, but may be associated with more anterior leaks, which can compromise bleb development if not treated.

Tenon's fascia should be excised at this stage only if it is exuberant. Excision may also be helpful in uveitic eyes with a high propensity to scar. Excision of Tenon's should be minimized if an intraoperative antimetabolite is utilized.

After conjunctival flap dissection is complete, an antimetabolite can be applied for a pre-specified length of time. Mitomycin C is a commonly used antimetabolite that is an antibiotic derivative of *Streptomyces caespitosus*. Mitomycin C inhibits DNA replication by inhibiting mitosis and protein synthesis. It also inhibits fibroblast proliferation. The effect of mitomycin is localized to the treated area. It is approximately 125 times more potent than 5-fluorouracil (5-FU). The antimetabolite should be applied topically underneath the conjunctiva prior to entering the anterior chamber.

To apply mitomycin, a cut cellulose or Gel foam sponge is saturated with the antimetabolite. The dosage is **0.2 to 0.5 mg/ml**. Many surgeons advocate a broad zone of application. The duration of application varies from **1 to 5 minutes,** with a trend towards shorter application time. The cut edge of conjunctiva should be kept away from the mitomycin-soaked sponge.

The major benefit of using mitomycin is that a lower IOP is achieved. An alternative to mitomycin is 5-fluorouracil (5-FU). The dosage of this antimetabolite is 50 mg/ml and it is applied for 5 minutes intraoperatively. Jampel[13] found a questionable effect of this medication and Chang found a 31% reduction of IOP.[14] Antimetabolite pledgets can be applied before or after scleral flap mobilization; we favor before mobilization.

Next, a 1/3 to 1/2 thickness scleral flap and sclerotomy are made. The base of the flap should equal the size required for IOL implantation. Generally, we perform the sclerectomy after IOL implantation. We favor closing the scleral flap with interrupted 10-0 nylon. **A longer suture pass facilitates postoperative laser suture lysis (LSL).** In assessing how tight to close the scleral flap, one should strive for slow spontaneous aqueous flow under the flap with

Pearls
- Nontoothed forceps for minimal tissue trauma
- Minimal excision of Tenon's if antimetabolite is used
- Keep the cut edge of the conjunctiva away from the mitomycin C soaked pledget
- Tight flap closure in high-risk cases
- Longer flap sutures facilitate LSL

maintenance of anterior chamber depth. Tighter flap closure is beneficial in eyes at higher risk for postoperative bleeding. Horizontal mattress flap compression sutures may be used to reduce the risk of hypotony in antimetabolite-enhanced combined procedures.[15]

Releasable scleral flap sutures are another consideration. Multiple techniques have been described but all are effective in reducing postoperative hypotony.[16-18] The timing of when to release the suture is similar to LSL. Placing releasable sutures requires more time, and again, there can be astigmatism issues involved. After the scleral flap and sclerotomy portion of the procedure are complete, attention is turned to conjunctival closure. It is wise to utilize nontoothed forceps to protect the tissues from excessive trauma. Frequently used sutures for closure of a limbal-based flap include 9-0 Vicryl (Ethicon BV-100), 10-0 nylon (Ethicon BV-75), or 10-0 Biosorb (Alcon P-3). These all have thin, tapered, vascular needles. Some ophthalmologists prefer a layered closure of first Tenon's capsule, then conjunctiva.

To close a fornix-based conjunctival flap, wing sutures can be placed using 10-0 nylon on a regular needle or 8-0/9-0 Vicryl. Alternatively, the flap can be closed with 9-0 nylon (Ethicon VAS 100), 9-0 Vicryl, or 10-0 Vicryl with a standard limbal remnant running suture closure technique. The **Wise technique** is a third technique which uses 9-0 nylon (Ethicon VAS 100) and is good for scarred conjunctiva.[19] For wing suture

closure, first denude the limbal corneal epithelium with light cautery. Strive for a broad apposition of conjunctiva to cornea well anterior to the scleral flap. A single, imbricating wing suture is often adequate. The advantage to this technique is that is minimizes sutures at the sclerectomy thereby reducing inflammation. The disadvantage is that there can be wound leaks and anterior bleb migration.

For a running suture closure utilizing a residual remnant of conjunctiva, it is important to confirm adequate tension of the running suture. This technique minimizes leaks and anterior migration of the bleb. It has the disadvantage of having sutures near the sclerectomy, which may increase inflammation. After conjunctival closure, it is important to test filtration and bleb elevation via the paracentesis. Topical 2 percent fluorescein can be used to test for leaks.

Corneal relaxing incisions can be made intra- or postoperatively to correct astigmatism if desired. Caution is indicated when correcting for astigmatism in combined surgery and should only be performed if the surgeon documents a stable scleral mobilization technique. Rectangular scleral flaps with mitomycin application and tight 10-0 nylon sutures may be associated with initial with-the-rule astigmatism and later against-the-rule astigmatism drift.

Results: Single Incision Surgery

The results of combined surgery via a single incision are very promising. One-year follow-up of this procedure with no mitomycin showed a mean decrease in IOP of 5 mm Hg.[20] Greater than 75 percent of these patients had a decreased medication requirement. The IOP reduction was sustained at 3 years but there were increased medication requirements. In another study, phacotrabeculectomy with mitomycin resulted in a mean IOP decrease of 8 mm Hg at 30 months postoperative with a significant decrease in number of medications.[21] When comparing single site surgery and a fornix-based conjunctiva flap with 2-site phacotrabeculectomy surgery and a limbus-based flap, both were similarly effective in lowering IOP and reducing the number of glaucoma medications at 3 year follow-up.[22]

Combined Cataract and Trabeculectomy Surgery via Separate Incisions (Two Site Approach)

Separation of the incisions for combined cataract and trabeculectomy surgery is felt by some ophthalmologists to enhance development of effective filtration. This technique also permits phacoemulsification from a temporal position that is most comfortable for many cataract surgeons (Figures 1A to L). Making separate incisions permits a simple, safe, and effective procedure. One disadvantage is that combined surgery via two sites takes longer than surgery via a single incision.

For the two-incision technique, phacoemulsification is performed first from a temporal clear cornea approach. A foldable IOL to allow for a small incision is preferred. Placing a buried 10-0 nylon suture to close the wound allows early digital pressure in the postoperative phase and also minimizes the chance of inadvertent intraocular seepage of antimetabolite into the eye during trabeculectomy.

For the second component of the procedure, trabeculectomy is performed from a superior approach. A conjunctival flap of surgeon preference is formed (either fornix-based or limbal based). An antimetabolite, if indicated, is used at this stage. Next, standard trabeculectomy is performed.

A combined procedure via separate incisions yields equivalent to better IOP control than single-site procedures

and may require less glaucoma medications postoperatively.[13] Another study showed equal IOP reduction, visual improvement, and medication reduction between single-site versus two-site combined procedures.[23] The two-site procedure can induce a small amount of with-the-rule astigmatism, being advantageous for patients with against-the-rule astigmatism.

In conclusion, choosing to perform combined cataract and trabeculectomy via two sites is a matter of surgeon preference because there are no overwhelming advantages to this technique compared to single-site surgery.

Combined Surgery Utilizing Other Types of Glaucoma Procedures

Combining **phacoemulsification with a tube/shunt** placed at a site remote from the limbus is another option for combined surgery. All types of implants are possible (e.g. Molteno, Baerveldt, Ahmed, and Krupin). The Express® mini-shunt is an implant placed underneath a scleral flap that shunts aqueous to a site near the limbus. This procedure is very similar to standard trabeculectomy and can readily be combined with cataract surgery.

Ciliary body endoscopic cyclophotocoagulation (ECP) is another option for combined surgery.[24] Chronic postoperative inflammation which is characteristic of all external cycloablative therapies can occur; however, such inflammation appears to be much less with ECP. The technique to perform combined phacoemulsification and ECP begins with standard phacoemulsification through a clear cornea or scleral tunnel incision. Next, viscoelastic is injected into the anterior chamber and posterior chamber. The ECP console is used to gain direct visualization of the ciliary processes (CP). Energy delivery is titrated with the foot pedal, with the effect proportional to both time and distance from the CP

with whitening and shrinkage of the CP as a treatment endpoint. There should be no popping or bubble formation which means too much energy is being used. After treatment of 270 degrees of angle, viscoelastic is removed.

Uram and Gayton report excellent results with ECP.[24,25] Berke et al showed a more modest IOP reduction.[26] Their group studied 626 eyes with a mean follow-up of 3 years. With combined phacoemulsification and ECP there was a 2 mm Hg decrease of IOP and a 50% reduction of medication usage. This result was compared to phacoemulsification alone, which showed no significant reduction in IOP and no reduction in medication. The phaco-ECP group showed a 2 mm Hg reduction in IOP (1.8 with phacoemulsification alone), and an 80 percent reduction in medication (14% with phacoemulsification alone). Fifty-four percent of patients required no medications after surgery (10% with phacoemulsification alone). They did not stratify based on preoperative IOP. The studies above reported no chronic inflammation, no increased rate of cystoid macular edema, and no occurrence of phthisis.

The advantages to ECP when combined with trabeculectomy include its simplicity, lack of bleb formation, sustained reduction in medication requirements, and rapid recovery time. One disadvantage of this procedure includes the need for special equipment, which is expensive. The ECP may not be indicated for advanced glaucoma, as it often causes only a modest reduction in IOP.

Deep sclerectomy procedures can be combined with phacoemulsification.

Viscocanalostomy, described by Stegmann,[27] yielded a 4.3 mm Hg reduction of IOP at one year and a 3.6 mm Hg reduction in IOP at three years.[28] This was superior to phacoemulsification alone. Shoji found a similar reduction in IOP of 3 mm Hg at two years in normal-tension glaucoma eyes, and this was also superior to phacoemulsification alone.[29] Kobayashi showed that mitomycin phacotrabeculectomy results were equal to phacoviscocanalostomy results at 1 year.[30]

Canaloplasty with a Schlemm's canal tension suture yielded a mean IOP reduction of 8 mm Hg at one year with a significant reduction in glaucoma medication requirement (GMR).[31,32]

Additional deep sclerectomy procedures that can be combined with phacoemulsification include wick procedures with collagen wick (aquaflow), hyaluronic acid implant (Sourdille),[33] lens or sclera.[34] These can be done with or without an antimetabolite. All these deep sclerectomy procedures can be performed with a clear corneal phaco or phaco underneath a scleral flap superiorly.

The **Glaukos ab interno shunt** into Schlemm's canal is a newer procedure described by Craven (American Academy of Ophthalmology poster 2007). This procedure resulted in a 4.4 mm Hg reduction in IOP at one year (18.3%) with a 1.4 mean decrease in GMR.

Excimer laser trabeculotomy (ELT): Berlin, Neuhann, and others described excimer laser trabeculotomy, ab interno (ELT).[35-37] The trabectome®, as described by Francis (American Academy of Ophthalmology poster 2007), resulted in a 22 percent mean reduction in IOP and a GMR reduction from 3 to 1.5 at 6 months.

Additional procedures include the Brown deep sclerectomy with Eye Pass bidirectional glaucoma tube shunt, ab interno quadrantic trabeculectomy, trabeculotomy as described by Neuhann, Gimbel and others.[37,38] Endoscopic erbium:YAG laser goniopuncture resulted in a 30 percent reduction in IOP at 1 and 3 years with a significant reduction in IOP requirements.[39]

Other procedures described include an internal tube shunt into the suprachoroidal space, a Gold implant (Solx, Inc., Waltham, Ma), a clear corneal technique reverse-hinge trabeculectomy (Langerman),[40] goniosynechialysis for angle closure glaucoma, Holmium laser sclerostomy described by Terry and others,[41] and cyclodialysis described by Montgomery and Gills,[42] Shields and Simmons.[43] This latter procedure was mainly used in the ICCE and ECCE eras.

TWO-STAGE SURGERY: GLAUCOMA PROCEDURE FIRST, CATARACT SECOND

When performing filtering surgery prior to and separate from cataract surgery it is advisable to create the bleb superior to superonasal. This permits easier future access for the subsequent cataract operation. Filtering surgery with antimetabolite is favored because there may be less compromise to the filter with future cataract surgery and cataract progression is not a concern with these agents. A tube-shunt procedure or other nonfiltering glaucoma surgery can also be undertaken prior to subsequent cataract surgery.

The AGIS study showed that trabeculectomy increases the risk of cataract formation by 78 percent.[44] This risk is higher if there is increased inflammation or a flat anterior chamber at the time of the trabeculectomy. An evidence-based review also found that glaucoma surgery is strongly associated with increased incidence and progression of cataract.[45] One study reported a 24 percent rate of cataract extraction after trabeculectomy in young patients (mean 43.7 years) with a mean follow-up time was 26 months.[46]

With subsequent cataract surgery after glaucoma surgery the same considerations apply as with cataract surgery alone. Additionally, it is important to be aware of possible low endothelial cell counts. It is most

favorable to wait as long as possible for cataract extraction after glaucoma surgery, preferably at least 3 to 6 months. A Honan balloon or external pressure should not be utilized preoperatively. A functioning filtering bleb should not be touched during surgery – consider placing viscoelastic on and in the bleb for protection.

The favored location for cataract surgery after filtering surgery is temporal (90 degrees away from the bleb). A clear cornea or scleral tunnel incision can be constructed from this location. Less ideal options include a superior clear cornea incision adjacent to the bleb or a clear cornea incision anterior to the bleb. The anterior incision is beneficial because there is no conjunctival manipulation but creates a more difficult phacoemulsification and nuclear expression; it may also increase astigmatism.

Suturing the cataract wound permits earlier digital pressure postoperatively, if necessary, but no stitches are required as with any clear cornea or scleral tunnel incision. At the conclusion of the case, confirm that the sclerectomy is patent and that the bleb is elevated. Consider using trypan blue to determine this and performing an internal/external revision of the bleb if an obstruction is present.

Topical mitomycin C application to the bleb is an option at the time of cataract surgery but efficacy in reducing IOP remains to be determined.

Postoperatively, vigorous topical steroids and nonsteriodal anti-inflammatory eyedrops are recommended

---

Pearls
- Wait at least 3-6 months for cataract extraction after glaucoma surgery
- Avoid external pressure
- Leave the functioning filtering bleb untouched
- Suturing the cataract wound permits early bleb manipulation

and supplemental 5-FU as needed. A bleb needling for bleb compromise may be required after cataract surgery with or without 5-FU or mitomycin.

Results of Glaucoma Procedure First, Cataract Second

The results of 58 eyes that underwent phacoemulsification after filtering surgery showed a slight increase in IOP (1.9 mm Hg), improved vision, and stable glaucoma medication requirements at 1 year postoperatively.[47] Clear cornea and scleral tunnel incision approaches yielded equivalent results. The IOP increased 2 mm Hg (from approximately 12 to 14 mm Hg) at one year on average.

Factors Associated with Bleb Compromise

Factors that may be associated with increased bleb compromise are a preoperative IOP greater than 10 mm Hg, increased iris manipulation during cataract surgery, age less than 50, a postoperative IOP spike, pre-existing uveitis, and cataract surgery within 6 months of filter surgery.[48,49]

Decision-making for Cataract Surgery in the Presence of a Filtering Bleb

Many factors go into planning cataract surgery after glaucoma surgery has taken place.

If the *IOP is too high* preoperative, consider adding internal/external revision of the bleb at the time of clear-cornea phacoemulsification with or without antimetabolite. Another option is to refilter at a new site, place a tube-shunt, perform ECP or external diode, or proceed with another nonfiltering glaucoma procedure simultaneous to phacoemulsification. The decision process is based on the bleb and conjunctiva status. If the IOP

is acceptable, give vigorous topical steroids postoperatively to minimize inflammation, consider 5-FU supplementation, and watch for a postoperative IOP spike.

If the eye has a *low IOP,* certain aspects of the phacoemulsification may be more difficult. These include paracentesis, capsulorhexis, and nuclear cracking. Corneal striae form readily, limiting the intraocular view. Techniques to minimize these problems include viscoelastic use and use of a diamond knife to make the incisions. Proper incision size is very crucial in a soft eye. In eyes with hypotony it is also difficult to calculate the IOL power because the axial length may be shorter (up to 3 mm) than the normal state/fellow eye. Cataract surgery can lead to increased IOP, resulting in an increased axial length. This axial length is still shorter than the prefilter eye with normal or high IOP and normal axial length. One strategy is to base the IOL calculation on an axial length approximately midway between the presumed prehypotony axial length and the actual hypotony axial length. Immersion ultrasound measurements are most accurate in these cases.

IOP elevation after cataract surgery alone may be enough to reduce hypotony maculopathy changes. Autologous blood injection is an option to be considered at the time of phacoemulsification to limit bleb function. Another method to raise IOP at the time of phacoemulsification is to revise the bleb using a pericardium graft or horizontal mattress compression sutures as described by Palmberg.[15]

Glaucoma Surgery in the Pseudophakic Eye

The state of the conjunctiva, capsule, and vitreous are critical for decision-making

in the face of glaucoma surgery after a cataract operation. Various procedures are possible in the pseudophakic eye: filters, non-penetrating surgery, tube-shunts, cyclophotocoagulation, and many others. The results of 52 filters in pseudophakic eyes with a minimum of 1-year follow-up (mean 3 years) showed stable vision and a decrease in IOP from a mean of 25 mm Hg preoperative to 13 mm Hg postoperative.[50] The mean number of medications used preoperatively was 3.3, which decreased to 1.0 postoperatively. *The results of trabeculectomy in eyes with virgin conjunctiva are not significantly different from eyes with previously manipulated conjunctiva, assuming that the conjunctiva is reasonably mobile.*

If YAG capsulotomy is needed in a patient with glaucoma, 1/5 of patients have a postlaser IOP rise of greater than 5 mm Hg. Three percent of patients have a postlaser spike of greater than 10 mm Hg.[51] These pressure spikes tend to occur within the first hour after YAG.

Postoperative Care for Cataract and Filter Surgery Combinations

Multiple adjuncts are available to the ophthalmologist for managing IOP postoperatively. Compression at the edge of the flap (*the Traverso maneuver*) can facilitate aqueous egress and bleb development if used early in the postoperative phase. *Laser suture lysis* (LSL) can increase the flow through a tight scleral flap. If no mitomycin is used intraoperatively, LSL can be performed from postoperative day 3 to 10. It is best to delay LSL for 2 weeks, if possible, when mitomycin is used during surgery to minimize the chance of hypotony. The beneficial effect of LSL in mitomycin treated eyes can be seen even if used months after surgery. To perform LSL, use an Argon, Krypton, or

Diode laser with a 50-micron spot size, 250 to 1000 mw power and 0.1 seconds, duration. A Hoskins or 4-mirror Zeiss lens is used to compress the conjunctiva and blanch the overlying vessels. Longer sutures are easier to cut than shorter sutures. Immediate compression at the edge of the scleral flap at the completion of the laser procedure is often helpful. The timing to release releasable sutures is the same as for LSL of interrupted flap sutures.

Bleb leak: A large diameter (14-24 mm) contact lens tamponade can be used if a bleb leak develops. As mentioned previously, leaks are more commonly seen with fornix-based conjunctival flaps than with limbus-based flaps. Bleb leaks may seriously compromise bleb development and must be treated.

Bleb failure: Supplemental 5-FU can be helpful in salvaging a bleb if signs of failure appear. These signs include injection over the bleb, hemorrhage, vascularization, thickening, or localization. The 5-FU works by inhibiting fibroblast proliferation. A 0.1 ml dose with a concentration of 50 mg/ml is injected subconjunctivally 180 degrees away from the bleb. Injections can be moved toward the bleb with passage of time. These injections can be coupled with *needling of the bleb* directly at the level of the scleral flap to break adhesions, or above the flap if an episcleral cap is present (Lederer/ Mardelli technique).[52] Needling can be performed at the slit lamp in a cooperative patient with or without 5-FU or mitomycin. A *surgical revision* in the operating room can also be performed (internal or external bleb revision).

> **Pearls**
> Keep the vial of 5-FU away from light to preserve its potency

To prepare for a 5-FU injection topical proparacaine is given. The medication is drawn into a 1 cc syringe and a 30-gauge needle is attached. The number of injections given is titrated to clinical response. The 5-FU should be withheld if a conjunctival wound leak or large corneal epithelial defect is present. Superficial punctate keratitis is common and is not a contraindication to the continued use of 5-FU. The 5-FU should be used in conjunction with frequent topical steroids and digital pressure, as needed. Be sure to keep the vial of 5-FU away from light to preserve its potency.

Tenon's cyst (encapsulated bleb) development is important to recognize and treat in a timely fashion. The key time for diagnosis is 1 to 4 weeks postoperative. It is critical to treat encapsulation associated with elevated IOP. Possible treatment options include digital pressure by the patient, medical therapy including glaucoma medications, topical steroids, 5-FU, and needling. Surgical revision in the operating room is a further option if the treatments above fail.

Hypotony is a common postoperative complication and is highly associated with intraoperative use of mitomycin and postoperative avascular blebs. Hypotony may lead to CME, disc edema, and hypotony maculopathy. It occurs less often in combined procedures than in primary filters. The treatment includes closing any leaks that are present first, then autologous subconjunctival blood injection, laser, cryo, or surgical bleb revisions. Surgical options include suturing the scleral flap more securely, using conjunctival compression sutures, using a patch graft over the scleral flap, excising a devitalized bleb, and performing posterior segment surgery (such as to drain choroidal effusions).

HISTORY AND NEW FRONTIERS

The modern era of cataract and glaucoma surgery began in the 1970s when *ICCE plus a filter or cyclodialysis* were performed. It was preferable at that time to perform the filter first. In the 1980s *ECCE and trabeculectomy* became more common. Factors that helped modernize these procedures to where we are today include the development of viscoelastic agents, advancements in IOL design, and the advent of LSL and releasable suture techniques. In the 1990s *phacotrabeculectomy* became more common, associated with the ongoing advancements of small incision phacoemulsification with foldable IOL implants and antimetabolites. Starting in 2000, we gained a greater appreciation of the potential to separate these versus simultaneous surgery. We learned the effect phacoemulsification has on IOP, both before and after filtering surgery. Our appreciation and modernization of *non-penetrating deep sclerectomy* procedures and other approaches to Schlemm's canal have greatly evolved in this modern era.

New frontiers in the field of cataract and glaucoma surgery include implanting IOL's through smaller incisions, a field-enhancing IOLs, and medical implants that are neuroprotective, neuroregenerative, and IOP-lowering. Investigation into continuously measuring IOP via an IOL is being conducted. We are looking towards improved antimetabolites, the use of anti-VEGF agents to control bleb vascularity, and photodynamic therapy of the conjunctiva to modify fibroblast proliferation. Many glaucoma and cataract specialists feel the most important challenge to tackle in the future is the development of effective nonfilter based surgical procedures to reduce bleb-associated problems.

REFERENCES

1. Chandrasekaran S, Cumming RG, Rochtchina E, Mitchell P. Associations between elevated intraocular pressure and glaucoma, use of glaucoma medications, and 5-year incident cataract: the Blue Mountains Eye Study. Ophthalmology 2006;113:417-24.

2. Shingleton BJ, Gamell LS, O'Donoghue MW, Baylus SL, King R. Long-term changes in intraocular pressure after clear corneal phacoemulsification: Normal patients versus glaucoma suspect and glaucoma patients. J Cat Refract Surg 1999;25:885-90.

3. Shingleton BJ, Wadhwani RA, O'Donoghue MW, Baylus SL, Hoey H. Evaluation of intraocular pressure in the immediate post-operative period following phacoemulsification. J Cat Refract Surg 2001;27:524-7.

4. Shingleton BJ, Pasternack JJ, Hung JW, O'Donoghue MW. Three and five-year changes in intraocular pressures after clear cornea phacoemulsification in open angle glaucoma patients, glaucoma suspects and normal patients. J Glaucoma 2006;15:494-8.

5. Issa SA, Pacheco J, Mahmood U, Nolan J, Beatty S. A novel index for predicting intraocular pressure reduction following cataract surgery. Br J Ophthalmol 2005;89:543-6.

6. Bendel RE, Phillips MB. Preoperative use of atropine to prevent intraoperative floppy-iris syndrome in patients taking tamsulosin. J Cat Refract Surg 2006;32:1603-5.

7. Chang DF, Campbell JR. Intraoperative floppy iris syndrome associated with tamsulosin. J Cat Refract Surg 2005;31:664-73.

8. Chang DF, Osher RH, Wang L, Koch DD. Prospective multicenter evaluation of cataract surgery in patients taking Tamsulosin (Flomax). Ophthalmology 2007;114:957-64.

9. Shingleton BJ, Heltzer J, O'Donoghue MW. Outcomes of phacoemulsification in patients with and without pseudoexfoliation syndrome. J Cat Refract Surg 2003;29:1080-6.

10. Shingleton BJ. Phacoemulsification and the small pupil. In: Crandall A, Masket S (Eds.) Cataract Surgery. London: Martin Donitz; 1995.pp.223-30.

11. Shingleton BJ, Nguyen BK, Eagan EF, Nagao K, O'Donoghue MW. Pseudo-exfoliation and cataract surgery in 1000 patients: a single surgeon series. Outcomes of phacoemulsification in fellow eyes of patients with unilateral pseudoexfoliation. J Cat Refract Surg (in press).

12. Shingleton BJ, Chaudhry IM, O'Donoghue MW, Baylus SL, King RJ, Chaudhary MB. Phacotrabeculectomy: Limbus-based versus Fornix-based conjunctival flaps in fellow eyes. Ophthalmology 1999;106:1152-5.

13. Friedman DS, Jampel HD, Lubomski LH, Kemper JH, Quigley H, Congdon N, Levkovitch-Verbin H, Robinson KA, Bass EB. Surgical strategies for coexisting glaucoma and cataract. An evidence-based update. Ophthalmology 2002;109:1902-15.

14. Chang L, Thiagarajam M, Moseley M, Woodruff S, Bentley C, Khaw PT, Bloom P. Intraocular pressure outcome in primary 5 FU phacotrabeculectomies compared to 5 FU trabeculectomies. J Glaucoma 2006;15:475-81.

15. Palmberg PF, Zacchei A. Compression sutures—A new treatment for leaking or painful filtering blebs. [ARVO abstract] Invest Ophthalmol Vis Sci 1996;37:S444.

16. Johnstone MA, Wellington DP, Zcil CJ. A releasable scleral-flap tamponade suture for guarded filtration surgery. Arch Ophthalmol 1993;111:398-403.

17. Cohen JS, Osher RH. Releasable suture in filtering and combined surgery. Ophthalmol Clin North Am 1988;1:187-97.

18. Wilson RP. Technical advances in filtration surgery. In: McAllister JA, Wilson RP (Eds). Glaucoma. Boston, Butterworths; 1986.pp.243-50.

19. Wise JB. Mitomycin-compatible suture technique for fornix-based conjunctival flaps in glaucoma filtration surgery. Arch Ophthalmol 1993;111:992-7.

20. Shingleton BJ, Kalina P. Combined phacoemulsification, intraocular lens implantation and trabeculectomy with modified scleral tunnel and single-stitch closure. J Cat Refract Surg 1995; 21:528-32.

21. Jin GLC, Crandall AS, Jones JJ. Phacotrabeculectomy: assessment of outcomes and surgical improvements. J Cat Refract Surg 2007;33:1201-8.

22. Cotran PR, Roh S, McGwin G. Randomized comparison of 1-site and 2-site phacotrabeculectomy with 3-year follow-up. Ophthalmology 2008;115:447-54.

23. Shingleton BJ, Price RS, O'Donoghue MW. Comparison of 1-site vs. 2-site phacotrabeculectomies. J Cat Refract Surg 2006;32:799-802.

24. Uram M. Ophthalmic laser microendoscope endophotocoagulation. Ophthalmology 1992;99:1829-32.

25. Gayton JL, Van Der Karr MA, Sanders V. Combined cataract and glaucoma surgery: Trabeculectomy vs endoscopic laser cycloablation. J Cat Refract Surg 1999;25:1214-9.

26. Berke SA, Cohen AJ, Sturm RJ, Caronia RM, Nelson DB. Endoscopic cyclophotocoagulation (ECP) and phacoemulsification in the treatment of medically controlled open angle glaucoma. J Glaucoma 2000;9:1.

27. Stegmann R, Pienarr A, Miller D. Viscocanalostomy for open-angle glaucoma in black African patients. J Cat Refract Surg 1999;25:316-22.

28. Park M, Tanito M, Nishikawa M, Hayeshi K, Chihera E. Combined viscocanalostomy and cataract surgery

compared with cataract surgery in Japanese patients with glaucoma. J Glaucoma 2004;13:55-61.

29. Shoji T, Tanito M, Takahashi H, Park M, Hayashi K, Sakurai Y, Nishikawa S, Chihara E. Phacoviscocanalostomy requiring cataract surgery only in patients with coexisting normal-tension glaucoma: Midterm outcomes. J Cat Refract Surg 2007; 33:1209-16.

30. Kobayashi H, Kobayashi K. Randomized comparison of the intraocular pressure-lowering effect of phacoviscocanalostomy and phacotrabeculectomy. Ophthalmology 2007;114:905-14.

31. Shingleton BJ, Tetz M, Korber N. Circumferential viscodilation and tensioning of Schlemm's canal (canaloplasty) combined with temporal clear corneal phacoemulsification cataract surgery for the treatment of open-angle glaucoma and visually significant cataract – one-year results. J Cat Refract Surg 2008;34:433-40.

32. Lewis RA, VonWolff K, Tatz M, Korber N, Kearney JR, Shingleton BJ, Samuelson TW. Canaloplasty: circumferential viscodilation and tensioning of Schlemm's canal using a flexible microcatheter for the treatment of open-angle glaucoma in adults. Interim clinical study analysis. J Cat Refract Surg 2007;33:1217-26.

33. Sourdille P, Santiago PY, Villain F, Yamamichi M, Tahi H, Parel JM, Ducournau Y. Reticulated hyaluronic acid implant in nonperforating trabecular surgery. J Cat Refract Surg 1999;25:332-9.

34. Anwar M, El-Sayyed F, el-Maghraby A. Lens capsule inclusion in trabeculectomy with cataract extraction. J Cat Refract Surg 1997;23:1103-8.

35. Berlin MS, Ahn R. Perspectives on new laser techniques in managing glaucoma. Ophthalmol Clin North Am 1995;8:341-63.

36. Berlin, MS. ELT, Excimer laser trabeculostomy. Ocular Surgery News 2001; 19:348-9.

37. Neuhann T, Scharrer A, Haefliger E. Excimer laser trabecula ablation ab interno (ELT) in the treatment of open-angle glaucoma. Ophthalmo-Chirurgie 2001;13:53-8.

38. Gimbel HV, Anderson Pennu EE, Ferensowicz M. Combined cataract surgery, intraocular lens implantation and viscocanalostomy. J Cat Refract Surg 1999;25:1370-5.

39. Feltgen N, Mueller H, Ott B, Frenz M, Funk J. Combined endoscopic erbium:YAG laser goniopuncture and cataract surgery. J Cat Refract Surg 2003;29:2155-62.

40. Langerman DW. Architectural design of a self-sealing corneal tunnel, single-hinge incision. J Cat Refract Surg1994; 20:84-8.

41. Terry S. Combined no-stitch phaco-emulsification cataract extraction with foldable silicone intraocular lens implantation and holmium laser sclerostomy followed by 5-FU injections. Ophthalmic Surg 1992;23: 218-9.

42. Montgomery D, Gills JP. Extracapsular cataract extraction, lens implantation and cyclodialysis. Ophthalmic Surg 1980;11:343-7.

43. Shields MB, Simmons RJ. Combined cyclodiaysis and cataract extraction. Ophthalmic Surg 1976;7:62-73.

44. The AGIS Investigators. The advanced glaucoma intervention study, 8: Risk of cataract formation after trabeculectomy. Arch Ophthalmol 2001;199: 1771-80.

45. Hylton C, et al. Cataract after glaucoma filtration surgery. Am J Ophthalmol 2003;135:231-2.

46. Adelman RA, Branner SC, Afshar NA, Grosskreutz CL. Cataract formation after initial trabeculectomy in young patients. Ophthalmology 2003;110: 625-9.

47. Shingleton BJ, O'Donoghue MW, Hall PE. Results of phacoemulsification in eyes with preexisting glaucoma filters. J Cat Refract Surg 2003;29: 1093-6.

48. Chen PP, Weaver YK, Budenz DL, Feuer WJ, Parrish RK II. Trabeculectomy function after cataract extraction. Ophthalmology 1996; 105:1928-35.

49. Rebolleda G, Munoz-Negrete FJ. Phacoemulsification in eyes with functioning filtering blebs: a prospective study. Ophthalmology 2002;109:2248-55.

50. Shingleton BJ, Alfano C, O'Donoghue MW, Riviera J. The efficacy of glaucoma filtration surgery in pseudophakic patients with or without conjunctival scarring. J Cat Refract Surg 2004; 30:2504-9.

51. Barnes EA, Murdoch IE, Subramanian S, Cahili A, Kehoe B, Behrend M. Neodymium: Yttrium–Aluminum–Garnet capsulotomy and intraocular pressure in pseudophakic patients with glaucoma. Ophthalmology 2004; 111:1393-7.

52. Lederer CM Jr. Combined cataract extraction with intraocular lens implant and mitomycin augmented trabeculectomy. Ophthalmology 1996;103: 1025-34.

51 Managing Cataract and Glaucoma in Developing World—Manual Small Incision Cataract Surgery Combined with Trabeculectomy (MSICS-Trab)

R Venkatesh, R Ramakrishnan

CHAPTER OUTLINE
- ❖ Why Combined Surgery?
- ❖ Combined Surgery
- ❖ Surgical Technique for Manual Small Incision Cataract Surgery Combined with Trabeculectomy (MSICS-Trab)
- ❖ Postoperative protocol

INTRODUCTION

There is a strong inter-relation between surgical management of glaucoma and cataract. We know that performing cataract surgery alone can lower the intraocular pressure, by about 4 to 6 mm Hg. Both glaucoma and cataract are diseases whose prevalence increases with advancing age. People living in developing countries have the highest risk of developing blindness from glaucoma.[1] In some parts of East Asia; angle closure glaucoma predominates, whereas in most sections of the Indian subcontinent, Africa, and in Hispanic populations, open angle forms are more common.[2] Treatments for glaucoma vary depending on the type of glaucoma and the setting. Glaucoma filtration surgery also has a higher risk of inducing operable cataracts, especially with the addition of antimetabolites such as mitomycin-C or if shallow anterior chambers or persistent choroidal detachments occur.[3]

WHY COMBINED SURGERY?

Patients usually perceive the benefits of cataract surgery through increased vision leading to a betterment of their quality of life. The advent of small incision cataract surgery and intraocular lens implantation has greatly increased patients' satisfaction with surgical interventions. In contradiction, most perceive a worsening of their well-being after glaucoma surgery due to invariable loss of a few lines of visual acuity. In a developed nation, this concept may be possible to convey to a patient, but in a developing nation, the magnitude of this negative social marketing may increase many fold and even convince an entire village not to come for routine eye care as they may perceive that the doctors are bad, taking away good vision rather than restoring lost vision. Thus balancing the benefits of surgery with the risk of cataract formation is dependent on the social and economic setting in which glaucoma occurs.

Access to eye care is important, and as most tertiary care ophthalmology services are in urban centres people often have to travel far to receive good quality services. Access and distance to health care are critical factors associated with utilization of services as well as compliances in developing countries.[4] Good quality care for cataract is definitely available but the quality can vary greatly depending upon the location. Good surgical treatment for glaucoma in the developing world is much less readily available and most disease remain undetected.[5,6] This in part is due to an emphasis on training to detect and treat cataracts primarily which is the leading cause of reversible visual disability, and the relative lack of specialized glaucoma training. Drugs for glaucoma are also relatively expensive, difficult to obtain, and the quality of the generics may vary. Staffing and equipment for glaucoma care is limited. Thus persistence with medical therapy is low and inclination to perform surgery before medical treatment is much higher, in contrast to the developed world, where surgery is performed later.

Cataracts are the most common cause of surgically reversible blindness worldwide, and cataract formation as a complication of trabeculectomy adds to the burden of preventable sight loss. People are less likely to return for further surgery if they do not perceive a benefit, especially if treatment for glaucoma makes their vision worse. The high cost of present methods for glaucoma screening is a barrier to the identification of people at high-risk for glaucoma blindness. In essence, surgery has the potential to fulfil many features of an ideal approach to reduce IOP compared with medications. It can lower the IOP to low teens, achieve long-term IOP reduction, minimize IOP fluctuations, lower the long-term cost, and minimize systemic side effects. The major drawback, though, are the potentially devastating, but rare, ocular side effects such as endophthalmitis, suprachoroidal hemorrhage, and corneal decompensation.

COMBINED SURGERY

Trabeculectomy combined with cataract surgery is considered safe and effective in the management of cataract associated with glaucoma. It prevents early intraocular pressure (IOP) spikes responsible for visual field "wipe out" in eyes with advanced glaucoma undergoing cataract surgery and provides beneficial visual rehabilitation with long-term IOP control.[7]

The use of **phacoemulsification** and wound-healing modulators has improved the results of combined cataract and glaucoma surgery with intraocular lens implantation (glaucoma triple surgery). Reports suggest that IOP control is superior to standard extra capsular cataract surgery combined with filtering surgery.[8,9] Smaller wounds in eyes undergoing phacoemulsification have several advantages in addition to IOP control. These include less surgically induced astigmatism, earlier visual rehabilitation, and a decreased hospital stay.[10] The advantage of phacoemulsification is related to the smaller incision. But phacoemulsification has a relatively steep learning curve and is costly in terms of fixed and consumable equipment. Phacoemulsification requires constant power, good maintenance, and immediate service of the instruments or hand pieces. It is technically more difficult and carries a higher risk of complications in brunescent hard cataracts that typically occur more frequently in underserved populations.[11]

Extracapsular cataract extraction (ECCE) may be associated with problems related to wound suturing and greater astigmatism.

Manual small incision cataract surgery (MSICS) is an inexpensive alternative to phacoemulsification; it also achieves better uncorrected visual acuity compared to ECCE.[12] With MSICS, high-volume and cost-effective surgery is possible without compromising quality.[13] Randomized controlled trails have proved the safety and efficacy of MSICS compared with phacoemulsification in terms of visual recovery as well as intraoperative complications, depending on the surgical expertise.[14,15] With MSICS, any type of cataract can be tackled with ease and the time of surgery is not altered by the density of cataract in contrast to phacoemulsification. In the developing world, patients come later for surgery with more advanced cataracts. They often assume that loss of vision is a normal consequence of aging, are unable to come for routine eye care, or do not have the support system to easily bring them in for cataract surgery. The difference in the prevalence of advanced cataracts can be seen in multiple studies[16] and they often visit the hospital through outreach eye camps and they are also opportunistically found to simultaneously have elevated intraocular pressure and compromised optic nerves. We therefore need a cost-effective highly productive surgical technique to tackle both cataract and glaucoma. If a manual small-incision technique is used for the cataract surgery, the small-incision advantage should theoretically still be applicable for performing a combined surgery. And such a technique is called **manual small incision cataract surgery combined with trabeculectomy (MSICS-Trab)**. Mittal et al. found manual small incision cataract surgery combined with mitomycin-C augmented trabeculectomy to be safe and of equal efficacy as combined phacotrabeculectomy in terms of IOP control, compliations and visual rehabilitation.[17]

SURGICAL TECHNIQUE FOR MSCIS COMBINED WITH TRABECULECTOMY (MSICS-TRAB)

Anesthesia

MSICS-Trab surgery is performed under local anesthesia with either retrobulbar and facial block, or a peribulbar block.

Bridle Suture

A 4-0 silk bridle suture is placed beneath the tendon of the superior rectus muscle to create a superior tunnel. Advantages of a superior rectus bridle suture are as follows:

It helps to maneuver the globe and to fix it during the steps of surgery like tunneling and suturing.

More importantly it provides a counter traction force during procedures like nucleus removal and epinucleus delivery, thereby making these procedures easier and less traumatic.

Conjunctival Flap and Scleral Dissection

Initial incision: A fornix based conjunctival flap at the limbus with a chord length of approximately 6.5 mm is made (**Figure 1**). After Tenon's capsule is carefully dissected, light cautery is applied. Mitomycin-C, 0.4 to 0.5 mg/ml is applied to a broad area on a cellulose sponge for approximately 3 minutes and then copiously irrigated with balanced salt solution. A one-third to half-thickness limbus parallel external scleral groove, of around 6 to 6.5 mm in width is made 3 mm from the surgical limbus (**Figures 2 and 3**).

Sclerocorneal tunneling: The actual tunneling is done by gentle wriggling and swiping moment of the bevel up crescent blade along the tunnel. The posterior margin of the incision may be held and slightly elevated and the crescent blade wiggled back and forth gradually coming closer to the limbus. It should be uniform in thickness and extend up to 1.5 mm into the clear cornea along the entire width of the incision. This maneuver will prevent the tearing of the wound lips. During tunneling forward one should raise the tip and depress the heel of the blade to prevent premature entry into the anterior chamber.

Creating a side port entry: One side port entry is usually made using a 15 degrees super blade at the 10 o'clock position and perpendicular to the tunnel in the clear cornea adjacent to the limbus. It is useful for:

i. Injection of viscoelastics to prevent the keratome from accidentally injuring the anterior lens capsule

ii. To form the anterior chamber at the end of the procedure, so as to insure that the rate of fluid leaving the flap is not too great which could cause a flat chamber.

iii. To aspirate residual subincisional superior cortex at the end of irrigation and aspiration.

Internal corneal incision: This is done using a sharp 3.2 mm angled keratome. The heel of the keratome is raised until the blade becomes parallel to the iris plane resulting in a dimple on the corneal surface. The keratome is then advanced anteriorly in the same plane until the anterior chamber is entered and the internal wound is visualized as a straight line (**Figure 4**). During extension of the incision, care should be taken to keep it in the same plane. The anterior chamber is totally reformed with viscoelastics hydroxyl propyl methyl cellulose (HPMC) before extending the incision.

Capsulotomy

One of the significant advantages of MSICS over phacoemulsification is that the former can be performed with any form of capsulotomy; continuous curvilinear capsulorhexis (CCC) may be the ideal choice in view of good centration of the IOL. The diameter of the CCC is determined by the anticipated size of the endonucleus and it should have a minimum diameter of 5 mm to enable easy prolapse of the endonucleus into the anterior chamber. If the CCC created is smaller than desired, it is safer to make relaxing incisions and convert it to canopener capsulotomy. Capsular staining with 0.1 ml of 0.06 percent trypan blue is helpful in cases with white and dense brown nuclei where a good red reflex is not visible. The capsular staining helps in making the difficult step of nucleus prolapse through an intact capsulorhexis safe and effortless, because the dye stained capsular rim is distinctly visible all throughout the surgery. In fact, in cases of brown and black cataracts with much denser and larger

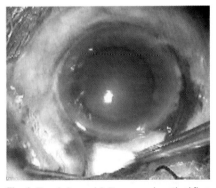

Fig. 1 Fornix based 6.5 mm conjunctival flap

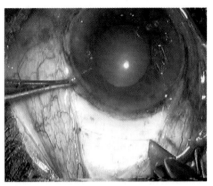

Fig. 2 Construction of a partial thickness limbus parallel external scleral groove of around 6–6.5 mm in width made 3 mm from the surgical limbus

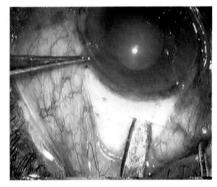

Fig. 3 Wriggling and swiping moment of the bevel up crescent blade along the tunnel in either direction

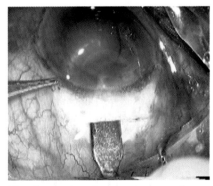

Fig. 4 Anterior chamber entry using a bevelled down 3.2 mm keratome with internal wound visualized as a straight line

nuclei, a can opener capsulotomy is preferred, as it may facilitate a more effortless prolapse of the hard nucleus into the anterior chamber. Multiple confluent small tears (approximately 15 to 20 punctures per quadrant) are preferred to avoid capsular tags.

Hydroprocedures

Hydrodissection is performed after removal of the viscoelastics in the anterior chamber, using a 27 gauge bent tip cannula attached to a syringe filled with balanced salt solution (BSS). In the presence of a capsulorhexis, this procedure is completed in one smooth step by very gently injecting the fluid beneath the anterior capsular rim. A fluid wave is appreciated when fluid is injected in the right plane. Tenting up the edge of the anterior capsulorhexis and injecting fluid ensures cortical cleaving hydrodissection. In the presence of a can opener capsulotomy, small amounts of fluid can be injected in multiple quadrants so as to "unshackle" the nucleus from the confines of the cortex. At the end, a complete hydrodissection should be confirmed by ability to freely rotate the endonucleus within the capsular bag. Rotation of the nucleus also polishes the epithelial cells from the equator and may play a role in reducing posterior capsular opacification rates.

Prolapse of Nucleus into the Anterior Chamber

Hydroprolapse: Hydrodissection is usually done at 9 or 3 o'clock position and the fluid wave is allowed to continue without decompressing the bag (as opposed to phacoemulsification), until one part of the equator of nucleus is forced out of the capsulorhexis. The purpose of continued injection of fluid is to slowly and gently increase the hydrostatic pressure within the bag to slowly prolapse

the nucleus. Once part of the equator is anterior to the capsulorhexis, the hydroprolapse is stopped. Viscoelastic is slowly injected beneath the exposed equatorial region. Then a Sinskey hook is introduced through the scleral tunnel and the nucleus is rotated in a tire rolling fashion either clockwise or anticlockwise to elevate the entire nucleus into the anterior chamber.

Mechanical method: In cases where it is difficult to prolapse the nucleus following hydrodissection and in cases of white or hard cataracts, the mechanical method can be used. The nucleus may be hard and bulky in brown and white cataracts. Hence it is difficult to prolapse a pole out of the capsular bag by mere hydrostatic pressure created during hydrodissection. Also, the posterior capsule in such cases is thinned making it easier for it to give way (posterior capsular tear and nucleus drop) if hydrostatic pressure builds within the capsule during forceful hydrodissection (intraoperative capsular block syndrome). The nucleus can be levered out of the bag using a Sinskey hook even without hydroprocedures if the nuclear attachment is found to be almost non-existent with the cortex. In hypermature morgagnian cataracts with liquefied milky cortex, it is worthwhile to wash away certain amount of milky cortical matter using a Simcoe cannula through a small opening created in the anterior lens capsule. This enables to reduce intralenticular pressure and provides easy access to freely rotate the nucleus within the capsular bag before prolapsing the nucleus. In cases with compromised zonules, a second instrument (cyclodialysis spatula) is passed between the hooked nuclear pole and the posterior capsule through a side port and the nucleus is rotated out using the support provided by the second instrument, reducing stress on the zonules.

Nucleus Extraction

Once the nucleus is prolapsed into the anterior chamber, it can be extracted through the tunnel by one of the following techniques:
- Irrigating Vectis technique
- Phacosandwich technique
- Modified Blumenthal technique
- Fish Hook technique.

Irrigating Vectis technique: This technique is a combination of mechanical and hydrostatic forces to express the nucleus. After the nucleus is prolapsed into the anterior chamber, viscoelastics are liberally but gently injected, first above and then below the nucleus. The upper layer shields the corneal endothelium, while the lower layer pushes the posterior capsule and iris diaphragm posteriorly. This maneuver creates adequate space in the anterior chamber for atraumatic nuclear delivery. A good superior rectus bridle suture is necessary for the success of this step. The bridle suture is held loosely in one hand. After checking the patency of the ports, the vectis is now inserted beneath the nucleus with concave side up with the fellow hand. If it is an immature cataract, one will be able to see the margins of the vectis under the nucleus in place.

As the superior rectus bridle suture is pulled tighter, the irrigating vectis is slowly withdrawn without irrigating, until the superior pole of the nucleus is engaged in the tunnel. Irrigation is then started and the vectis is slowly withdrawn, while pressing down the posterior scleral lip till the entire nucleus is expressed out of the section **(Figure 5)**. The force of irrigation has to be reduced when the maximum diameter of the nucleus just crosses the inner lip of the tunnel to help prevent the nucleus from being forcibly expelled with consequent sudden anterior chamber decompression and shallowing of anterior chamber.

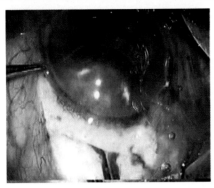

Fig. 5 Irrigating vectis under the nucleus with the nucleus engaged in the width of the tunnel. The nucleus is thus expressed out of the tunnel

Phacosandwich Technique

This technique is employed in cases with hard nucleus, as sandwiching the nucleus with the help of two instruments can help us to deliver the nucleus without enlarging the tunnel. In this technique, a Sinskey hook is used in addition to the vectis to sandwich the nucleus. The nucleus should be sufficiently dense to prevent cheese wiring of the two instruments engaging it. The key requisite is that the anterior chamber must be adequately filled with viscoelastics to avoid endothelial damage by the second instrument and also make sufficient space for sliding the vectis beneath the nucleus. A curved vectis measuring approximately 4 mm at its greatest width and 8 mm in length is then introduced underneath the nucleus. The vectis should be allowed to find its own plane and this should not require any force for positioning. Once the vectis is placed beneath the nucleus, the Sinskey hook is carefully introduced and placed on top of the nucleus, sandwiching it between the vectis and the Sinskey hook. The tip of the Sinskey hook is placed beyond (inferiorly) the central portion of the lens to get a better grip using a two - handed technique. With the Sinskey hook in the dominant hand and vectis in the other, the nucleus is sandwiched

and extracted, being slowly pulled towards the wound. While extracting the nucleus, an assistant should pull the superior rectus suture, and at the same time should pull the globe down by grasping the conjunctiva at 6 o'clock position near the limbus with the help of the toothed forceps. The outer portion of the nucleus, the epinucleus and a portion of the cortex will be sheared off in this technique and can be removed with the irrigating vectis after nucleus delivery.

Modified Blumenthal technique: This technique differs in that it requires an *"anterior chamber maintainer"*. This is a hollow tube with 0.9 mm outer diameter and 0.65 mm inner diameter which is attached to a BSS bottle, suspended approximately 50 to 60 cm above the patient's eye.

Two small beveled entries are made in the cornea, one is 1.5 mm long, placed between 5 and 7 o'clock position for connecting the anterior chamber maintainer. The other port is 1 mm wide, placed at 11 o'clock position for the entry of various instruments. The fluid flow from anterior chamber maintainer is stopped during the capsulotomy. The bottle height is maintained at 50 to 60 cm from the patient's head. After a good hydrodissection, the nucleus is prolapsed into anterior chamber with mechanical snudging. Free nucleus in a deep anterior chamber is ready for being propelled out by the hydropressure generated by anterior chamber maintainer system.

A plastic glide 3 to 4 mm wide, 0.3 mm thick and 3 cm long is inserted under the nucleus, one-third to half width nucleus distance. Now the bottle height is raised between 60 to 70 cm and slight pressure is applied over the lens glide on the scleral side. Intermittent pressure will engage more and more nucleus out of the tunnel's mouth. Subsequently, few more taps to

open the scleral tunnel valve with the glide will enable the epinucleus and cortex to flow out of anterior chamber.

Fish Hook technique: After making the scleral tunnel of adequate length, a side port opening is made with 15° blade and anterior chamber is filled with viscoelastics. The anterior chamber is entered with a slit knife, and extended. A linear capsulotomy or a envelope type of capsulotomy is made, In a linear or envelop capsulotomy, a linear incision is made into the anterior lens capsule using a bent 26G needle from 2 to 10 o' clock extending till the pupillary margin (well dilated). Then Vannas scissors are used to cut either end in a curvilinear fashion towards 6 o' clock. The capsular flaps thus created on either side are joined using Utrata's capsule holding forceps. After a thorough hydrodissection, anterior chamber is filled with viscoelastics and only the superior pole of the nucleus is brought into the anterior chamber. Viscoelastics are injected both in front and behind the nucleus again. A 30G needle with its tip modified as a fish hook is entered into the anterior chamber with sideways tilt to prevent endothelial injury. It is then maneuvered behind the nucleus to hook the undersurface of the nucleus. Viscoelastics can be reinjected if there is difficulty in traversing the fish hook. Once the nucleus is hooked, it is slided out with slight pressure by the hook on the posterior lip of the tunnel. The nucleus is thus delivered without performing extensive maneuvers in the anterior chamber.

Epinucleus Removal, Cortex Aspiration and IOL Implantation

After the extraction of endonucleus from the anterior chamber, a mixture of epinucleus and viscoelastics materials remain in the anterior chamber. It is easier to remove this mixture with the help of an irrigating vectis. It can be removed by either of the following methods:

i. It can be flipped out of the bag by introducing the Simcoe cannula under the anterior capsular rim and lifting out the epinucleus in toto into the anterior chamber. The prolapsed epinucleus can then be extracted by depressing the inferior scleral lip with the Simcoe cannula and pulling the superior rectus bridle suture at the same time.

ii. The epinucleus can also be manipulated using viscodissection. A significant amount of epinucleus can be retained within the bag, especially in cases of soft cataracts with corticocapsular adhesions. It becomes difficult to find a cleavage plane between the capsule and the epinucleus. Resistant epinuclear plates can be quite unnerving for the surgeon. If such a scenario arises, viscoelastics material can be injected under the capsular rim, between the capsule and epinucleus and the latter is lifted out of the bag into the anterior chamber and extracted through the tunnel.

The rest of the cortical matter can then be aspirated using a Simcoe cannula. As the size of the wound is at least 6 mm, it is preferable to place a 6 mm optic rigid three piece PMMA IOL, if a can opener capsulotomy has been made. In case, a capsulorhexis has been performed then a single piece lens can be implanted in the bag. **(Figure 6)**.

Trabeculectomy

The trabeculectomy is then performed after the nucleus and cortex is removed by excising a block of 2 mm by 1 mm trabecular tissue from the posterior lip of the scleral tunnel incision using a Kelly's descemet's membrane punch (cutting backwards)

(Figures 7 and 8). The goal is to excise a block with at least 1.0 mm overlap by the scleral flap. Through the punched window a peripheral iridectomy is performed **(Figures 9 and 10)**. The scleral tunnel is well approximated and closed with two interrupted, 10-0 nylon sutures on either side of the punched area, until there is a good approximation of the anterior and posterior scleral flaps **(Figure 11)**. Releasable sutures can also be used to approximate the scleral tunnel. The conjunctival flap is closed with 8-0 braided dyed (violet) polyglactin (Vicryl®) suture in a watertight manner **(Figure 12)**. The patency of trabeculectomy is tested by injecting ringer's lactate through the side port.

POSTOPERATIVE PROTOCOL

Postoperatively, the patient is put on tapering course of antibiotic steroid eye drops for a period of six weeks.

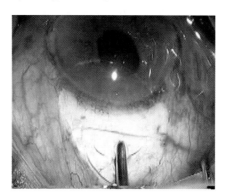

Fig. 6 Insertion of PCIOL

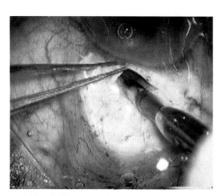

Fig. 7 Punching in progress in the posterior lip of the scleral tunnel

A cycloplegic is given twice daily for a period of two weeks and nonsteroidal anti-inflammatory drugs four times daily for four weeks in order to prevent cystoid macular edema. The preoperative antiglaucoma drugs if any are discontinued in the immediate postoperative period. Thereafter, the patient is followed up at 3 monthly intervals for 1 year, then every 6 monthly as a preferred practice pattern.

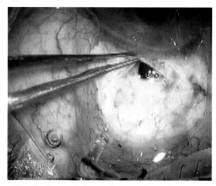

Fig. 8 Completion of punching of ostium

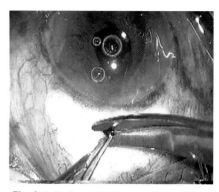

Fig. 9 Initiation of iridectomy through the punched area

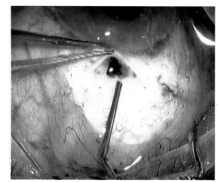

Fig. 10 Completion of iridectomy

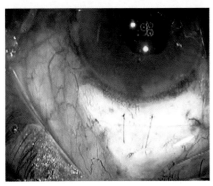

Fig. 11 Good tight closure of scleral tunnel with two 10-0 nylon suture on either side of the punched site

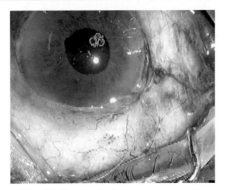

Fig. 12 Conjuntival wing sutures with 8-0 Vicryl

Unpublished data on retrospective analysis of mitomycin-C augmented trabeculectomy combined with single

site MSICS show that a significant reduction in IOP levels (16.59 +/- 4.01 mm Hg) was observed at 6th month

follow-up (p=0.035) compared to preoperative IOP (30.4 +/- 10.3 mm Hg), irrespective of the type of glaucoma. Subgroup analysis showed that there was a significant difference in IOP levels of chronic angle closure glaucoma group compared to secondary open angle glaucoma (pseudoexfoliation, pigmentary glaucoma) group (p=0.015) at 6 months follow-up. However, no statistically significant difference was observed in the IOP comparisons between primary open angle glaucoma and chronic angle closure glaucoma groups or primary open angle glaucoma and secondary open angle glaucoma groups.

REFERENCES

1. Chen PP. Risk factors for blindness from glaucoma. Curr Opin Ophthalmol 2004; 15:107-11.
2. Thomas R, Chandra Sekhar G, Kumar RS. Glaucoma management in developing countries: medical, laser, and surgical options for glaucoma management in countries with limited resources. Curr Opin Ophthalmol 2004;15:127-31.
3. Robin AL, Ramakrishnan R, Krishnadas R, Smith SD, Katz JD, Selvaraj S, Skuta GL, Bhatnagar R. A long-term Dose Response Study of Mitomycin-C in Glacuoma Filtration Surgery. Arch Ophthalmol 1997;115:969-74.
4. Lee BW, Sathyan P, John RK, Singh K, Robin AL. Predictors of Barriers Associated with Poor Follow-up in Patients with Glaucoma in South India, Arch Ophthalmol, in press.
5. Nirmalan PK, Katz J, Robin A L, Krishnadas R, Ramakrishnan R, Thulasiraj R D, Tielsch J. Utilisation of eye care services in rural south India: the Aravind Comprehensive Eye Survey. Br J Ophthalmol 2004;88: 1237-41.
6. Robin AL, Nirmalan PK, Krishnadas R, Ramakrishnan R, Katz J, Tielsch J, Thulasiraj RD. The utilization of eye care services by persons with

glaucoma in rural south India. Trans Am Ophthalmol Soc; 2004.pp.47-56.
7. Hopkins JJ, Apel A, Trope GE, et al. Early intraocular pressure after phacoemulsification combined with trabeculectomy. Ophthalmic Surg Lasers 1998;29:273-9.
8. Carlson DW, Alward WL, Barad JP, et al. A randomized study of mitomycin augmentation in combined phacoemulsification and trabeculectomy. Ophthalmology 1997;104:719-24.
9. Kosmin AS, Wishart PK, Ridges PJ. Long-term intraocular pressure control after cataract extraction with trabeculectomy: phacoemulsification versus extracapsular technique. J Cataract Refract Surg 1998;24:249-55.
10. Chia WL, Goldberg I. Comparison of extracapsular and phacoemulsification cataract extraction techniques when combined with intra-ocular lens placement and trabeculectomy: short-term results. Aust N Z J Ophthalmol 1998;26: 19-27.
11. Bourne RR, Minassian DC, Dart JK, Rosen P, Kaushal S, Wingate N. Effect of cataract surgery on the corneal endothelium: modern phacoemulsification compared with extracapsular cataract surgery. Ophthalmol 2004;111:679-85.

12. Muralikrishnan R, Venkatesh R, Prajna VN, Frick KD. Economic cost of cataract surgery procedures in an established eye care centre in Southern India. Ophthalmic Epidemiol 2004;11:369-80.
13. Venkatesh R, Muralikrishnan R, Balent LC, Prakash SK, Prajna NV. Outcomes of high volume cataract surgeries in a developing country. Br J Ophthalmol 2005;89:1079-83.
14. Gogate P, Deshpande M, and Nirmalan PK. Why Do Phacoemulsification? Manual Small-Incision Cataract Surgery Is Almost as Effective, but Less Expensive. Ophthalmology 2007;114:965-8.
15. Ruit S, Tabin G, Chang D, Bajracharya L, et al. A Prospective Trial of Phacoemulsification versus Manual Sutureless Small-Incision Extracapsular Cataract Surgery in Nepal. Am J Ophthalmol 2006;143:32-8.
16. Ruit S, Robin AL, Pokhrel RP, Sharma A, DeFaller J. Extracapsular cataract extraction in Nepal: 2-year outcome. Arch Ophthalmol 1991;109:1761-3.
17. Mittal S, Mittal A, Ramakrishnan R. Safety and efficacy of manual small-incision cataract surgery combined with trabeculectomy: Comparison with Phacotrabeculectomy. Asian Journal Ophthalmol 2008;10:221-9.

52 | Glaucoma Drainage Devices

Mona Khurana, R Ramakrishnan

DEFINITION

Glaucoma drainage devices create an alternate pathway from the anterior chamber channeling the aqueous out of the eye to a subconjunctival bleb.

HISTORY

Interestingly it all started with a horse hair in 1906 when Rollet and Moreau[1] used a horse hair as a wick through a paracentesis to drain a hypopyon from the anterior chamber. Subsequently, Zorab in 1912 performed 'aqueoplasty' using a silk loop as a seton to drain aqueous humor translimbally from the anterior chamber to the subconjunctival space.[2] Following this a variety of materials were used including metals (like gold, tantalum, platinum and stainless steel), suture materials, glass rods, cartilage, lacrimal canalicular tissue and silicone strips. Vail[3] placed a silk thread in a track from the vitreous cavity to the subconjunctival space. These early devices were setons or stents used to maintain the patency of a fistula. The success of these procedures was limited by progressive inflammation and fibrosis around the implanted material, migration, conjunctival erosion and infection.

Tube shunts were used to drain aqueous from the anterior chamber to the distant sites like lacrimal sac,[4] angular vein, superficial temporal vein,[5] vortex vein[6] and conjunctival cul de sac.[7] Complications like erosion of extraocular part, reverse flow (blood and tears) and risk of endophthalmitis limited their clinical use. Tubes inserted at the limbus into the anterior chamber seemed to offer the advantage of maintaining a patent conduit for the flow of aqueous into the subconjunctival space.[8] However, the encapsulation of the external tube led to failure.

In 1969, Molteno was the first to introduce the concept of implants.[9] This consisted of a tube connected to a distal end plate. His initial design consisted of a short acrylic tube attached to a thin acrylic plate. The plate was sutured to the sclera near the limbus and the tube was introduced into the anterior chamber. Since the plate was near the limbus it resulted in an anterior bleb which was associated with complications like plate exposure, tube erosion, scar formation and subsequent failure. So he introduced the concept of long tube and plate in which the fluid was drained away from the source to increase the success rate.[10] This resulted in a larger posterior bleb.

All the currently available devices are based on this concept. Further modifications have been made in this design involving basically two aspects: an increase in surface area and the concept of a valve to provide resistance to outflow.

Theodore Krupin (1976) introduced a glaucoma drainage device with a unidirectional and pressure sensitive slit valve.[11] This valve offered resistance to outflow and prevented early hypotony. In 1993, Marteen Ahmed introduced the Ahmed glaucoma valve (AGV) which had a valve designed to open at an IOP of 8 mm Hg.

To increase the surface area, Molteno introduced the double plate implant. In 1992, George Baerveldt introduced the Baerveldt implant. It consisted of a non-valved silicone tube attached to a large Barium impregnated silicone plate.

TYPES OF GLAUCOMA DRAINAGE DEVICES (GDDs)

Basically GDDs can be classified into 3 groups:

1. ***Setons (Latin word for bristle):*** It is a non hollow linear shaft which allows drainage either by bulk flow by preventing apposition or by means of surface tension along material (wick like action). Setons have no internal mechanism.
2. ***Shunts:*** They are passive tubular structures incapable of influencing anterograde or retrograde flow. They allow a bidirectional flow.
3. ***Valves:*** They are designed for a pressure—sensitive unidirectional flow of aqueous with set internal flow resistance.

GDDs can also be classified as nonrestrictive or restrictive devices **(Table 1)**.

MECHANISM OF ACTION

The basic design of all GDDs is a tube that shunts aqueous humor from the anterior or posterior chamber to a plate located in the equatorial region of the globe. The plates are made of biocompatible material to which fibroblasts cannot adhere. Over a period of time, a fibrous capsular forms over the plate of the drainage device. This forms a bleb which is different from that of a trabeculectomy bleb. The aqueous drains from the anterior chamber and pools into the space between the plate and the surrounding fibrous capsule. Histologicaly, the wall of the bleb consists of microcysts and a fibrous capsule. The aqueous diffuses passively through the capsule. This fibrous

Table 1 Types of drainage devices

Non restrictive	Restrictive
• Molteno	• Krupin valve with disc
• Baerveldt	• Ahmed
• Schocket	• Joseph
	• Optimed
	• White pump shunt

capsule offers the major resistance to aqueous flow. Its thickness and surface area are important determinants of resistance to aqueous flow. The surface area of the capsule depends up on the size of the end plate. Consequently increasing the surface area of the plate increases the area of the capsule formed. This leads to increased diffusion of aqueous although there is an upper limit beyond which it may not improve outflow.

Thickness of the capsule: The longterm success of any glaucoma drainage device appears to be limited by the fibrous reaction around the endplate. In the initial 1 month following the surgery, a collagen inner capsule surrounded by a granulomatous reaction is formed. Over the next 4 months the granulomatous reaction resolves and the collagen stroma become less complex. Finally the bleb consists of an inner collagen like lamellae and outer connective tissue with microcysts spaces. This initial period may be responsible for the hypertensive phase which resolves once the inflammatory reaction subsides. Increased aqueous levels of TGF beta in the incoming 'glaucomatous aqueous' may also contribute a low grade inflammation and prolong this phase.[12-14] Bleb failure occurs due to increased thickness of the fibrous capsule. One of the mechanisms may be movement of implant plate against the scleral surface resulting in low grade inflammation.

INDICATIONS OF GDDs

At the outset, GDDs were used to treat refractory glaucomas. These consist of glaucomas which do not respond to medical or surgical treatment and require re-surgery. Generally they were used when trabeculectomy (or multiple trabeculectomies) had failed to control the IOP or when it was unlikely to succeed. However, with time these devices gained popularity

due to improvements in design, material and surgical technique. The lack of bleb related complications associated with trabeculectomy added to their advantage. GDDs appear to be as successful as trabeculectomy with antifibrotic agents in eyes that had undergone prior conjunctival surgery. They are preferable in neovascular glaucoma, iridocorneal endothelial syndrome (ICE syndrome) and developmental glaucomas where a trabeculectomy is likely to fail. Success has been reported in eyes which have undergone surgeries like cataract extraction (pseudophakic/aphakic), penetrating keratoplasty and vitreo retinal surgeries. They may also be the procedure of choice in cases where surgery is indicated for concomitant glaucoma and other ocular disorders like vitreo retinal disorders. They are indicated in eyes with scarred conjunctiva due to previous multiple surgeries, Steven Johnson syndrome , cicatricial pemphigoid and other ocular surface disorders. They have also been used to manage glaucoma associated with keratoprothesis.

Currently owing to the encouraging results of clinical trials, the spectrum of indications continues to expand **(Table 2)**. They may either be used after failed glaucoma filtering procedures or where a filtering procedure is likely to fail. Their role as a primary procedure in aphakic and pseudophakic eyes has been shown by the Tube versus Trabeculectomy Study (TVT). It is discussed later in the chapter. The role as a primary procedure is currently being evaluated by ongoing studies. The decision for implanting a GDD needs to be based on a case to case basis.

IMPLANT DESIGNS

The desired features of an ideal implant are listed in **Table 3**. As explained earlier, the basic design of all implants

Table 2 Indications for glaucoma drainage devices

- Refractory glaucoma
- High-risk of failure of trabeculectomy
- NVG
- ICE syndrome
- Aniridia
- Post-traumatic glaucoma
- Young patients
- Glaucoma in aphakic/pseudophakic
- Uveitic glaucoma
- Glaucoma following PKP and vitreo-retinal surgery
- Conjunctival scarring
  - Multiple surgeries
  - Ocular surface diseases
  - Chemical burns
  - Steven-Johnson syndrome
  - Cicatricial pemphigoid
- Previously failed glaucoma surgery
- Eyes with scleral thinning
- Patients with history of blebitis or bleb-related endophthalmitis
- Pediatric glaucoma (refractory)

Table 3 Properties of an ideal implant

- The devices should made up of non-reactive synthetic materials which do not induce foreign body reaction
- A more posterior shunting of aqueous to an equatorial sub-tenon's device
- These devices should establish a potential space around which the drained aqueous can pool and be sequestered for incremental absorption
- The devices should made up of a tube attached to an equatorial plate of greater height than the plate thus preventing collapse of the conjunctiva and subsequent blockage of posterior exit of tube with conjunctiva

consists of a long tube connected to an end plate based on the Molteno's model. The various models differ with respect to:

- Size
- Shape
- Material
- Open tube or flow restriction/valves.

Size and Shape

The ideal size of the end plate is still not known. It is believed that an increase in size of the end plate leads to a lower

Table 4 Some common types of GDD

Type	Material (End-plate)	Size	Type of device
Ahmed glaucoma valve	Polypropylene	96 mm² (S1)	Valved
		184 mm² (S2)	
	Silicone	364 mm² (B1)	
		96 mm² (FP8)	
		184 mm² (FP7)	
		364 mm² (F×1)	
Baerveldt's shunt	Silicone	250 mm²	Non-valved
		350 mm²	
Krupin	Silastic	183 mm²	Valved
Molteno	Silicone	134 mm²	Non-valved
		268 mm²	

IOP and better success rate. To achieve this either the size of the single plate can be increased (e.g. Baerveldt) or another plate can be attached to the single plate by a silicone tube (e.g. AGV and Molteno double plate). The percentage reduction of mean postoperative IOP may be influenced by the size of the end-plate, but only to a certain point. Beyond this, other factors such as the degree of encapsulation around the endplate influence the final intraocular pressure.

Materials

Materials influence the amount of inflammation and the thickness of the capsule. Flexible plates cause less inflammation as compared to rigid ones. Thus a thinner capsule results which offers less resistance to outflow of aqueous.

Open Tube or Flow Restriction Valves

GDDs can be classified according to presence or absence of a flow restriction mechanism into non-valved and valved.

The devices currently used in clinical practice are listed in **Table 4**.

NONVALVED IMPLANTS
Molteno Implant

The original design introduced by Molteno in 1969 consisted of a single round acrylic plate 8.4 mm in diameter. The long tube and posterior plate model has a larger polypropylene plate 13 mm in diameter with a surface area of 134 mm² resulting in the formation of a large posterior bleb. There is a thickened perforated rim to allow suturing to the sclera. The silicone tube is 0.63 mm in external diameter and 0.30 mm in internal diameter and opens on the convex upper surface **(Figure 1A)**.

Currently many variations of the Molteno implant (IOP, Inc., Costa Mesa, California; Molteno Ophthalmic Limited, Dunedin, New Zealand) are available. To increase the surface area a double plate model was introduced with an additional plate of 13 mm plate

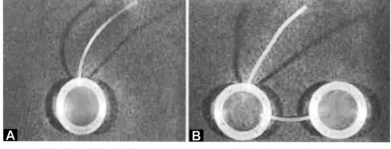

Figs 1A and B (A) Molteno single plate; (B) Molteno double plate

Table 5 Molteno drainage implant

Single plate	Double plate	Dual-chambered (Molteno 3)

• Silicone translimbal tube 8–10 mm
• Episcleral acrylic plate:
  – Curvature—13 mm
  – Surface area—135 mm²
  – Suture holes—2
	• Additional second 13 mm plate connected to primary plate by 10 mm silicone tube entering 90° away from primary intracameral tube
	• Secondary plate sutured to episcleral
	• Surface area 270 mm²
		• Designed to prevent post-operative hypotony and over-filtration
		• V-chamber
		  GL-Single plate 230 mm²
		  GS-Single plate 175 mm²
		  Plate thickness—0.4 mm
		  Maximum height of ridge—1.5 mm
		  Tube diameter—0.34 mm (internal)
		  — 0.54 mm (external)

connected to the primary plate by 10 mm silicone tube entering 90° away from primary intracameral tube. This increased the surface area to 268 mm² **(Figure 1B)**. It is positioned under the superior rectus. Both right and left versions are available. A pediatric size is available with an 8 mm plate. The dual chamber Molteno implant has a ridge on the upper surface of the end plate to reduce postoperative hypotony. It has a V-chamber **(Table 5)**. This ridge divides the upper space into two and an area of 10.5 mm² around the opening of the silicone tube.

The Molteno 3 has a larger, thinner, more flexible plate with an oval subsidiary ridge on its upper surface. This design allows the implant to sit snugly between and slightly beneath the adjacent extraocular muscles. When covered by Tenon's tissue the subsidiary ridge of the implant and the overlying Tenon's tissue together form a self-cleaning 'biological valve' which cannot become blocked by exudate or blood clot. This biological valve reduces postoperative hypotony by restricting the drainage of aqueous to the small primary drainage area until the IOP rises sufficiently to lift the tissues and allow drainage of aqueous over the entire plate. This modification results in a thinner bleb capsule, a lower final IOP and less need for post-operative hypotensive agents.

Baerveldt's Implant

The **Baerveldt's** implant (Advanced Medical Optics, Inc., Santa Ana, California) consist of a Barium impregnated soft silicone end-plate with a surface area of either 250 mm² (20 × 13 mm), 350 mm² (32 × 14 mm) and 425 mm² (36 × 17.5 mm). It is a non resistive implant which is placed beneath two adjacent recti muscles. Fenestrations in the plate allow growth of fibrous bands reducing the height of the bleb. These were introduced to decrease the incidence of diplopia seen due to the high bleb formed with the previous model **(Figures 2A and B)**. The Pars Plana Model allows the tube to be placed in the posterior chamber. A Hoffman elbow prevents the kinking of the tube in the pars plana model.

Schocket Tube Shunt

This consists of a silicone tube which extends from the anterior chamber to the grooved portion of a 360° encircling silicone band similar to that used in RD surgeries. The tube is 0.64 mm in external diameter and 0.3 mm in internal diameter. It is secured with non absorbable sutures to prevent slippage. A smaller diameter tubing may reduce the incidence of hypotony. The capsule around the band functions as a reservoir for aqueous drainage.[15,16] It can be modified in the following ways:

- Band: 360 degree #20 (surface area 300 mm² or #220 silicone band)
- 90° beneath the 2 recti.
- Insertion of tube into pre-existing equatorial encirclage band after retinal surgery.

VALVED/RESTRICTIVE IMPLANTS
Krupin Valve[17,18]

This was a restrictive GDD designed to overcome the problem of early postoperative hypotony.[11] Its oval end plate is made of silicone and has a surface area of 183 mm². The distal end of tube contains horizontal and vertical slits which work as a unidirectional valve with an opening pressure of 9 to 11 mm Hg. The outflow tube in the earliest model was small, ending 2 to 3 mm posterior to the limbus resulting in a bleb in the inter palpaebral fissure with a high failure rate. Subsequent models consisted of a longer tube.

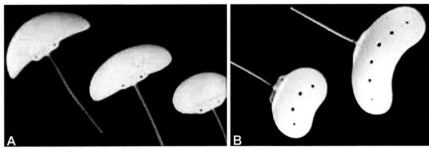

Figs 2A and B Baerveldt shunt (A) Without fenestrations; (B) With fenestrations

Ahmed Glaucoma Valve (AGV)

The AGV (New World Medical, Inc., Rancho Cucamonga, California) consists of a pear or scarab shaped end-plate made of poly propylene or silicone. The plate model has fenestrations or eyelets for suturing **(Figure 3)**.

Available versions include models with a polyproylene end plate (S_2, S_3, B1), models with a silicone end-plate (FP7, FP8, FX1) and a double plate model: FX1. The surface area of the end-plate is 96 mm² (S_3 and FP8) in the pediatric model, 184 mm² (S2, FP7) in the single plate and 364 mm² (B1 and FX1) in the double plate. In addition models for pars plana insertion are also available.

The AGV has a valve mechanism which opens at a pressure of 8 mm Hg. The valve consists of silicone elastomer which separates at an IOP of 8 to 12 mm Hg. A specially designed trapezoidal chamber creates a venturi effect reducing aqueous flow through the device (according to the Bernoulli equation of hydrodynamic principle). An increased exit velocity of aqueous through a smaller outlet port as compared to the inlet reduces friction and helps in evacuating aqueous from the valve. Elastic membranes help to regulate the flow at all times by changing their shape and the tension on them helps in reducing hypotony. Care should be taken not to damage the chamber during insertion of the valve.

It allows the IOP to be lowered from the first postoperative day without causing hypotony. The smaller size of the AGV allows it to be placed easily in one quadrant without affecting ocular motility. Valved devices prevent early postoperative hypotony. Non valved devices may produce lower IOPs but need a flow restrictive techniques to prevent early postoperative hypotony.

Optimed Glaucoma Pressure Regulator

It consists of PMMA matrix of conductive resistors. It is made up of multiple microtubules providing a pressure gradient. The tubules connect to an anterior chamber silicone tube 0.38 mm in internal diameter and 0.76 mm in external diameter. The models vary with respect to the length of the passageway. The aqueous flow occurs through a capillary action when pressure in the eye is more than 10 mm Hg. The device has a surface area of 18 mm² **(Figure 4)**.

White Pump Shunt

It is a one piece silicone implant consisting of a silicone tube, anchoring struts and a reservoir bound by two unidirectional valves and an outlet tube. One end is inserted into the anterior chamber while the other end is connected to a 16 to 18 mm balloon which has an outlet into the retrobulbar space. The distal end of tube contains two unidirectional valves which opens at a pressure below 5 to 15 mm Hg minimizing hypotony and prevent reflux of aqueous. Digital massage or blinking activity pumps aqueous into and out of balloon.

Joseph's One-Piece Tube and Drainage Device

It consists of a curved 180° equatorial plate and a curved sialistic tube which is inserted into the anterior chamber. A unidirectional slit valve is present in the tube near the plate.

OTHER GDDs
Eye Pass

Eye pass consists of two flexible silastic tubes joined in a Y configuration **(Figure 5)**. The two arms of the Y are inserted into Schlemm's canal, and the stem of the Y is inserted into the anterior chamber. Results were not very encouraging and currently it is not available.

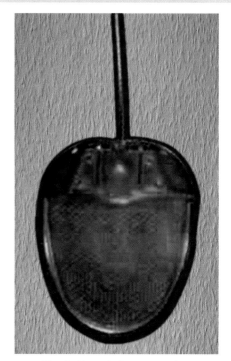

Fig. 3 Ahmed glaucoma valve

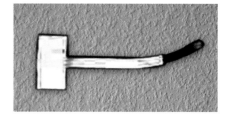

Fig. 4 Optimed valve

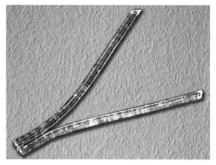

Fig. 5 Eye pass glaucoma implant

Express™ Glaucoma Filtration Device (Optonol Ltd, Neve Ilan, Israel)

It is a non valved stainless steel device about 3 mm long (2.96 for R 50 and 2.64 for model P 50) with an external diameter of 400 μ and internal diameter of 50 μ. Some models come in an internal diameter of 200 microns also (P 200). It has a flange at its proximal end that prevents it from being implanted too deeply. It is available in a variety of designs. A spur behind its tip prevents it from extrusion. The external plate of this device is 1 mm* 1 mm. The scleral flap is made slightly thicker. and the device is inserted just anterior to the scleral spur after making an entry with a 27 guage needle. A special injector is used to insert this mini shunt. The key step in insertion is that it enters the eye with the spur facing the long axis of the entry point (at 90 degrees). It is then rotated into its final position. The external pate must be flush with the sclera before closing the scleral flap. Currently it is inserted into the anterior chamber under a partial thickness rectangular scleral flap without any peripheral iridectomy **(Figures 6A and B)**. Studies comparing it with trabeculectomy are underway and long-term results are awaited. It is mainly used in eyes with open angle glaucoma with fairly deep anterior chambers. The lower incidence of early postoperative hypotony as compared to trabeculectomy may be attributed to the small lumen size of 50 microns. The commonest complication encountered is tube blockage which can be treated by laser.

GMS Gold Shunt

It is made of 24 karat gold and consists of 3 parts: in the anterior chamber, intrascleral and suprachoroidal. The GMS gold shunt is a controlled cyclodialysis implant or a trabeculo supra choroidal shunt. It connects the anterior chamber to the suprachoroidal space. It is an attempt to control and titrate the traditional cyclodialysis procedure. Aqueous drains into the suprachoroidal space. The implant is a thin, elongated, wafer like and cruciform shaped with corrugated surface channels and holes in the horizontal limb. Two plates or leaflets are fused together concealing

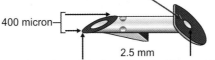

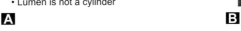

- A 3 mm long, 400 micron diameter (27 gauge) tube
- Made of implantable stainless steel
- Blunt needle-like tip
- Additional side holes prevent iris plugging
- Lumen is not a cylinder

A   **B**

Figs 6A and B (A) Express mini shunt; (B) Positioning of express mini shunt. Conjunctival incision 1–2 mm behind limbus, preparatory hole with 27 gauge needle, slide in implant on the introducer

channels connecting the anterior and posterior opening. It comes as 2 models of different weight and channel size (XGS5 AND XGS 10). Gold is inert and biocompatible. The head of the implant sits in the anterior chamber, and the tail sits in the suprachoroidal space. Fluid passes through and around the shunt into the suprachoroidal space. No bleb is formed. The Deep Light Glaucoma Treatment System includes a titanium sapphire laser and a phototitrable gold microshunt.

Aurolab Aqueous Drainage Implant (AADI)

It is a low cost, non resistant tube device based on Baerveldt implant. It reduces intraocular pressure by draining aqueous from anterior chamber into subconjunctival space formed around base of the implant. AADI is a non-valved aqueous shunt **(Figure 7)** made of Nusil permanent implant silicone elastomer which has passed tissue culture cytotoxicity testing.

The surface area of the AADI end plate is 350 millimeter square and the silicone tube length is 32 millimeter. The AADI may be inserted through a 100 degree conjunctival incision. The lateral wings of the AADI are designed for positioning under the rectus muscles. The end plate is positioned between the rectus muscles and is attached to the sclera about 10 millimeters posterior to the limbus with non absorbable sutures through the fixation

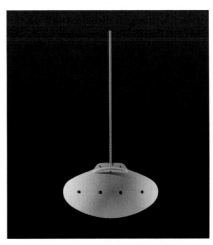

Fig. 7 Aurolab Aqueous Drainage Device (AADI)

holes of the implant. Temporary tube occlusion is accomplished by ligating it with 7 zero vicryl suture. The absorbable suture reliably lyses 4 to 6 weeks postoperatively causing spontaneous opening of the tube. A 23 gauge needle is used to make an entry incision into the anterior chamber at the posterior limbus parallel to the iris plane. The tube is inserted through the needle track, proper positioning of the tube anterior to the iris and posterior to the cornea should be confirmed. The limbal portion of the tube is covered with a donor scleral/corneal patch graft. Lower postoperative IOP is expected with capsules that are thinner and have large surface areas. The capsule surface area is directly related to the size of the end plate. Therefore, an implant with a larger endplate produces a larger surface area of encapsulation and greater IOP reduction.

The end-plate of the AADI has fenestrations that allow growth of fibrous bands reducing the profile of the bleb.

The low profile of the AADI makes it particularly suitable for infero-nasal placement as a majority of the patients posted for a drainage implant surgery have a history of one or two failed filters. Currently studies are underway to evaluate its safety and efficacy in reducing the intraocular pressure and preventing further damage to optic nerve and functional visual field loss in advanced refractory glaucoma.

SURGICAL TECHNIQUE

The basic surgical technique is similar for all GDDs **(Figure 8)**. They differ in respect to:

- Size of the conjunctival incision
- Methods of flow restriction
- Anterior chamber or pars plana insertion of the tube.

Preoperative Evaluation

A careful preoperative assessment and planning regarding placement of the GDD is essential for successful and uneventful surgery. Anatomy of the anterior segment should be evaluated thoroughly. The lens status and the presence of vitreous in the anterior chamber should be determined. Location of PAS should be determined on gonioscopy. Any excessive area of conjunctival scarring and any pre-existing explant from a previous retinal surgery must be noted. All these factors determine the type, position and success of the procedure. These can be listed as:

- Corneal status and clarity
- Anterior chamber depth
- Lens status
- Presence/absence of vitreous in the anterior chamber

- Gonioscopic examination of the angle of anterior chamber
- Site of peripheral anterior synechiae
- Pre-existing explants
- Silicone oil in the anterior chamber
- Areas of extensive conjunctival scarring.

The procedure is generally performed under peribulbar or retrobulbar anesthesia. A superior rectus bridle suture is passed. Corneal traction sutures can be placed for better exposure.

Conjunctival Incision

The superior temporal quadrant is the preferred site in most cases.[19,20] The advantages are: a better surgical exposure and less chance of motility disturbances.[21] In some situations it may the required to place it supero nasally or in the inferior quadrant. Inferior quadrant placement may be required in eyes with silicone oil in the anterior chamber (silicone oil induced glaucoma) or when other quadrants are not available or in case of a second GDD.

> Superior nasal quadrant implants are associated with increased incidence of motility disorders.

A fornix based flap is dissected with a size ranging from 90° to 180° depending upon the size of the implant. A relaxing incision may improve exposure. The conjunctiva and Tenons are dissected from the sclera. The blood vessels may be cauterized using light cautery.

Implant Preparation

- Priming of valves (AGV)
- Restriction of lumen in nonrestrictive devices.

Priming the Valves

Krupin: It needs to the irrigated with BSS to confirm that the valve slits allow flow.

AGV: BSS must be injected through the free end of the silicone tube using a 30 gauge cannula. This breaks the surface tension between the 2 silicone sheets so that the valve can function. Care should be taken not to inject the fluid too forcefully **(Figures 8A to M)**.

Restriction of Lumen

In case of non-valved devices the aqueous flow needs to be restricted until the fibrous capsule forms over the endplate. This minimizes the chance of early postoperative hypotony. A single or two stage technique may be used. This can be achieved by:

Two stage implantation

The plate is placed subconjunctivaly without inserting the tube into the anterior chamber. Once the fibrous capsule has formed after 4-6 weeks, the tube is inserted in to the anterior chamber.

Single Staged

Alternatively, the preferred technique is the occlusion of the tube by a variety of procedures before inserting it in to the anterior chamber. Once the fibrous capsule forms in 4-6 weeks, the suture dissolves/is removed/lysed allowing aqueous to drain into the capsule. Various techniques include:

- Ligation of tube with polyglactin suture near the tube plate junction. Closure may be confirmed by irrigating the BSS through the tube. This prevents flow of aqueous in the early postoperative period. Aqueous flow is established at a later stage when the suture loses its tensile strength.
- Occluding the lumen of the tube with a nylon or polypropylene suture (4-0) (Ripcord sutures). The suture end is placed subconjunctivally near the inferior limbus to aid in subsequent removal.
- 10-0 polypropylene suture to ligate the near the tube tip. This may be

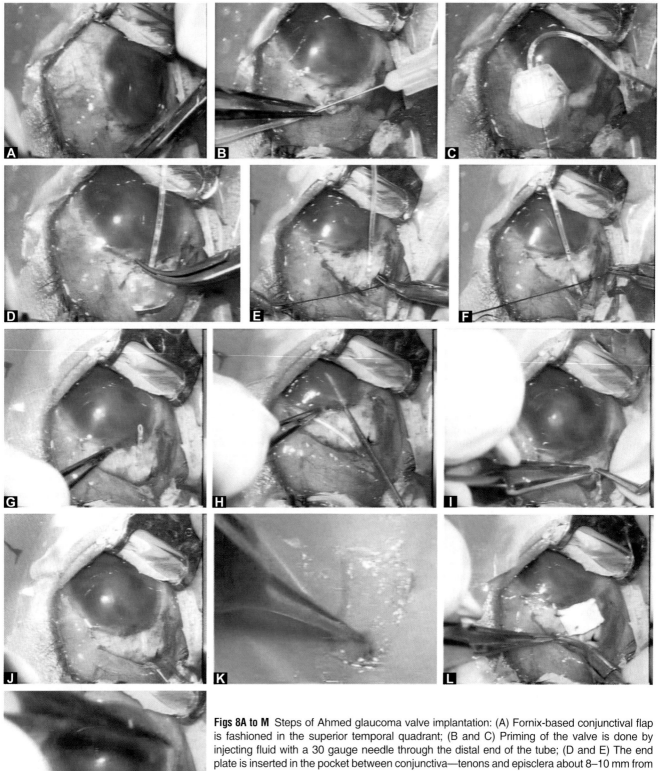

Figs 8A to M Steps of Ahmed glaucoma valve implantation: (A) Fornix-based conjunctival flap is fashioned in the superior temporal quadrant; (B and C) Priming of the valve is done by injecting fluid with a 30 gauge needle through the distal end of the tube; (D and E) The end plate is inserted in the pocket between conjunctiva—tenons and episclera about 8–10 mm from the limbus. It is sutured with a nonabsorbable suture; (F) The tube is sutured to the episclera with a loosely tied nonabsorbable suture; (G) The tube is trimmed with a 30 degree bevel up; (H) The track for the tube is made with a 23 gauge needle just posterior to the limbus. The needle must be kept parallel to the iris; (I and J) The tube is inserted into the anterior chamber through the track made with a 23 gauge needle; (K and L) The tube is covered with a scleral patch graft; (M) Conjunctival closure lysed by argon laser at a later stage. Argon laser suturolysis at a later stage can be done.

Some surgeons prefer to make small perforation or slits in the tube for some initial drainage.

Attachment of End Plate

A pocket is created by blunt dissection between the tenons and the episclera. The end plate is tucked into this subtenons space and sutured into position with 8-0 silk or 9-0 prolene suture about 8 to 10 mm from the limbus. This prevents both anterior or posterior migration of the end plate. Larger-sized implants like Baerveldt or double plate ones need to the tucked under the recti muscles. A Schoket type drainage device needs more extensive dissection depending upon the size of the band. Implants with plates larger in the anterior posterior direction should not be placed too posteriorly to prevent optic nerve damage. A distance no more than 8 mm from the limbus is advisable. The sclera is thin in the equatorial region and care should be taken to avoid perforation.

Insertion of the Tube

The tube is cut with a bevel of around 30^0 to facilitate insertion. The length should be to allow 2 to 3 mm segment to extend into the anterior chamber from its site of entry. An entry is made into the anterior chamber with a 23 needle gauge needle at the posterior limbus. The needle should be kept parallel to the iris plane. The tube is inserted through the track with forceps (non toothed or specially designed). It should be inserted bevel up and positioned in the anterior chamber without touching the cornea or the iris. A track made with a 23 gauge needle creates a water tight seal preventing hypotony due to leakage around the tube. Viscodilation of the canal may be helpful in tube insertion.

Patch Graft

Its function is to reinforce the limbus tissue and stabilize the tube. It prevents conjunctival erosion and exposure of the tube. Materials used include:
- Sclera (less likely to dissolve)
- Cornea (for cosmetic purposes)
- Pericardium and Dura are also used.
- Some surgeons prefer to make a partial thickness scleral flap or tunnel. However, there is a risk of erosion.

The graft is placed with its anterior edge at the original conjunctival insertion covering most of the anterior part of the tube and scleral fistula. It is anchored to the episclera using the non absorbable sutures (8–0).

Conjunctival Closure

Meticulous conjunctival closure is required to prevent retraction or dehiscence erosion, occlusion, fibrous in growth. It can be done in the following ways:

Fornix based flap: Anchoring sutures
Limbus based flap: Sutured in two layers
Relaxing: Any relaxing incisions are sutured in two layers.

Use of Antimetabolites

Some surgeons apply mitomycin-C in the quadrant where the GDD is to be placed. The general consensus is that antimetabolites do not offer any added advantage.[22]

SPECIAL SITUATIONS
Cornea

Following GDD implantation in post penetrating keratoplasty (PKP) eyes corneal decompensation can occur resulting in graft failure.[23-26] The cause of the decompensation is multifactorial:
- Previous surgeries (multiple) and pre-existing endothelial loss
- Prolonged use of antiglaucoma medications with preservatives

- Tube related endothelial cell loss (rate of 2 cells/sq mm/month)[27]
- Direct tube corneal touch
- Suturing of eye.

Another situation which one may encounter is:

PKP in eyes with pre-existing tubes:
- These eyes may require revision with placement of the tube away from endothelium.
- Suture placement across anterior chamber to direct the tube away from the cornea can also be tried
- Alternatively pars plana insertion of the tube combined with vitrectomy can be done to avoid rejection of the graft.[28]

> Anterior segment fibrosis may occur due to increase levels of TGF beta in the anterior chamber due to retrograde flow from the bleb causing low grade inflammation. This is seen more commonly in non-valved devices due to retrograde aqueous flow.

Neovascular Glaucoma (NVG)

GDD usually are the first choice in such cases. The tube should be placed in the anterior chamber in such a away so as to prevent occlusion eye progressive fibrosis and to avoid neovascular tissue at the angle. Anti VEGF agents may be used to prevent intraoperative bleeding. In eyes with NVG, the success of glaucoma drainage devices decreases with time due to underlying progression of the retinal disease. Mermoud et al. reported a success rate 62.5 percent at 1 year, 52.9 percent at 2 years, 43.1 percent at 3 years, 30 percent at 4 years and 10.3 percent at 5 years.[29]

Pre-existing Scleral Buckle

Both conjunctival scarring and the presence of a Buckle present a special challenge for a GDD implantation in eyes post retinal detachment surgery. A silicone tube may be introduced into the pre-existing fibrous capsule around the scleral buckle. Tube ligation is not required as the capsule is already present. Alternatively, a smaller Baerveldt can be placed underneath, behind or over the buckle or its wings may be trimmed to decrease its size.

Silicone Oil Filled Eyes

The plate may be placed in the inferior inferonasal or inferotemporal quadrant. This reduces the loss of silicone oil through the tube. Polypropylene implants may be a better option.

COMPLICATIONS

They can be divided into intraoperative, early and late postoperative[30-43] **(Table 6)**. Most can be classified as tube or plate related.

Intraoperative Complications

The prevalence of intraoperative complications is similar to trabeculectomy. During the surgery, there may be problems with tube insertion. A large needle track may lead to leakage around the tube whereas a narrow track will cause difficultly in tube insertion. A 23 g needle (external diameter 0.6 mm) is ideal for making the entry track. Tube insertion in thin sclera can pose a problem. Proper selection of a site where the sclera is thicker must be done is such cases. It may also be inserted through the ciliary sulcus behind the iris in pseudophakic eyes. In such cases, it

should be longer to prevent blockage by the iris.

While anchoring the end plate to the sclera, scleral perforation may occur. Care should be taken to visualize the needle throughout its course in the sclera. In case of perforation, retinal cryopexy should be done along with a prompt retinal consultation to rule out or manage retinal detatchment.

Other intraoperative complications include hyphema especially in NVG where there may be new vessels at the point of tube entry. Vitreous prolapse may occur during the procedure and may cause tube obstruction. Intraoperative suprachoroidal hemorrhage is rare, occurring in eyes with very high IOP preoperatively. It can be prevented by preoperative IV mannitol and slow decompression of the eye intraoperatively. An AC maintainer can also be used.

Postoperative Complications
Hypotony

Hypotony and choroidal effusions in the postoperative course with implants is a serious complication.[33,34] It is more commonly seen with nonvalved implants. Until the fibrous capsule has developed around the external plate to regulate aqueous flow, nonvalved tube implants offer very low resistance to flow resulting in hypotony and its

sequelae. The best way to prevent this potential complication is by temporarily obstructing the tube lumen by using the various techniques described earlier in the chapter. Hypotony can also result from overfiltration, the leakage around the tube in both valved and non-valved implants. If early postoperative hypotony is associated with a flat anterior chamber a viscoelastic is injected into the anterior chamber along with topical and oral Steroids and cycloplegic eye drops. If the flat chamber and hypotony reoccur, then removal of the tube from the anterior chamber is recommended to prevent corneal decompensation with planning to reposition the tube into the anterior chamber with in the next few days. Large choroidal detachments may need surgical drainage.

Hypotony is treated by treating the cause. Visual loss from hypotony maculopathy, extreme shallowing of the anterior chamber and severe choroidal detachment may even warrant removal of the implant or a permanent occlusion of the proximal tube or removal of the tube from the anterior chamber, which permanently removes the effect of the entire implant. Permanent ligation of the tube to the distal plate of double plate Molteno implant, has the advantage of reducing, but not completely eliminating the effect of the implant.

Elevated Intraocular Pressure

Drainage implant procedures can also be complicated by elevated IOP in either the early or late postoperative period.

Hypertensive Phase

Early hypotony may be followed by a hypertensive phase, which is characterized by a transient IOP elevation associated with the formation of the capsule. During this phase (which starts 4-6 weeks after surgery), the

Table 6 Complications of glaucoma drainage devices

Intraoperative	Early postoperative	Late complications
• Oversized anterior chamber entry	• Pupillary block	• Increased IOP
• Scleral perforation	• Hypotony	• Hypotony
• Ciliary body bleeding	• Hyphema	• Tube migration
• Vitreous loss	• Inflammation	• Implant erosion, Plate extrusion
• Injury to lens	• Tube obstruction	• Corneal decompensation
• Injury to endothelium	• Increased IOP	• Cataract
• Descemet's membrane stripping	• Aqueous misdirection	• Endophthalmitis
• Iris damage		• Ocular motility disturbances, diplopia
• Conjunctival button hole		• Tube blockage
• Muscle disinsertion		
• Kinking of tube		

edema disappears and fibrous tissue develops in the deepest layers of the bleb. During the first 1 to 4 weeks of this phase, the bleb wall becomes congested, causing the IOP elevation. Congestion and inflammation subsequently subside, with IOP reduction and stabilization over the next 3 to 6 months. The hypertensive phase is common following implantation of the Ahmed valve, occurring 30-82 percent of patients. It is comparatively less with the silicone model (FP7) as compared to the polypropylene (S2) plate implant. Aqueous suppressants can be used to both decrease the IOP during this phase. It also facilitates remodeling of the capsule by decreasing the inflow of the glaucomatous aqueous which is proinflammatory.

Tube Obstruction

The inner diameter of the tube is quite narrow and thus prone to blockade. Elevated IOP in the early postoperative period may occur due to obstruction of the tube by fibrin, blood, iris, vitreous membranes, or silicone oil **(Figures 9 and 10)**. Site of blockage is usually at the ostium in the anterior chamber. Other causes could be kinking of the tube. Neodymium-yttrium aluminum garnet laser membranectomy can be used for reopening blocked glaucoma tube shunts and maintaining the patency. Other techniques to open the occluded tube include irrigation of the

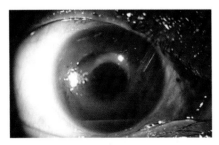

Fig. 9 Hyphema following AGV implantation

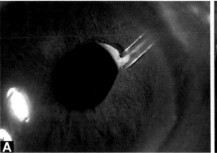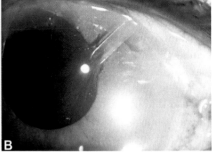

Figs 10A and B (A) Tube occluded with cortex; (B) Vitreous

tube with balanced salt solution using a 30 gauge cannula through a paracentesis incision, and intracameral injection of tissue plasminogen activator to dissolve a fibrin clot. The tube may also need to be repositioned when it is blocked.

Steroid Response

Steroid response can result in an increased IOP and must be ruled out.

Bleb Failure

Late IOP elevation, especially when the intraocular potion of the tube appears to be patent, is usually due to an excessively thick fibrous capsule. Fluid aspiration from the bleb or needling revision with antimetabolites can improve function of the encapsulated drainage implant. It is more successful when the implant has a larger surface area, although the risk for severe complications, including endophthalmitis, exists.

When needling is unsuccessful after a few attempts, it may be beneficial to remove a portion of the encapsulated bleb beneath the conjunctiva. When all the above fail, a new GDD may be implanted in another quadrant.[35]

It should be differentiated from a steroid response that can be seen in eyes on topical corticosteroids therapy despite the presence of a functioning drainage implant.

Migration, Extrusion and Erosion of the Implant

Tube retraction and tube migration

Tube migration may occur after implantation of GDDs over a period of time. Shifting of the implant plate along the scleral surface with eye movements may cause the tube to retract. If the tube is not adequately secured to the sclera it may migrate posteriorly out of the anterior chamber or even erode through the cornea. Anterior migration of the tube can occur due to the dislocation of the external plate. This may require repositioning of the tube and securing it to the sclera with additional 9 to 0 prolene sutures. Extrusion of the implant may be common in children. As the eye grows the tube may require repositioning of the tube from the original site. If the tube retracts out of the anterior chamber, tube extenders may be used.[36]

Avulsion of an implant after blunt trauma may force the tube against the cornea, causing corneal melting and requiring explantation of the implant and possibly corneal grafting.

Erosion of the silicone tube through the overlying conjunctiva is a recognized complication of the aqueous shunts **(Figures 11A to C)**. It can be focal or a frank plate extrusion. A partial thickness scleral flap does not prevent erosion of the tube. The tube and fistula site should be covered with preserved sclera, dura, fascialata or pericardium.

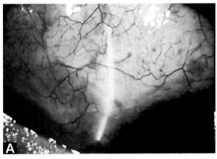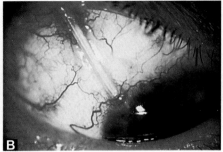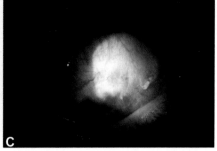

Figs 11A to C (A) Eroded patch graft with conjunctival thinning; (B) Tube erosion; (C) Tube retraction

Note If a scleral graft is too thick, it may elevate the limbal conjunctiva enough to produce dellen formation. Conversely, a thin scleral patch graft may predispose the tube to erosion.

Management

Due to poor tissue integrity repair is difficult. Patch graft with mobilization of the adjacent conjunctiva should be done at the earliest to reduce the risk of hypoyony and endophthalmitis. Removal followed by a new GDD in another quadrant is another option.

Endophthalmitis

Recurrent *propionibacterium acnes* endophthalmitis has been reported after Molteno tube revision, based on a positive culture of anterior chamber needle aspirate.

Removal of the glaucoma drainage implant in case of endophthalmitis may be necessary to remove the contaminated foreign body. Early postoperative endophthalmitis, following placement of an implant, may be successfully treated by immediate removal of the implant and surgical management of the infection.

Endophthalmitis may also occur in the late postoperative course.[37] Exposure of the implant seems to be a major risk factor for these infections. Surgical revision with a patch graft in all cases in which there is an exposed tube is indicated to prevent this potentially devastating complication **(Figures 10A and B)**.

Corneal Decompensation

In patients with pre-existing corneal endothelial cell dysfunction and in post penetrating keratoplasty patients corneal decompensation **(Figure 12)** may occur due to multiple mechanism.[38]

• Tube corneal touch leads to focal endothelial cell loss.
• Mechanical rubbing of tube against the corneal endothelium
• Disruption of blood aqueous barrier.

Hypotony may cause corneal edema and should be distinguished from corneal decompensation.

Prevention: The tube should be placed as posterior as possible. Pars plana insertion of the tube may be done in vitrectomized eyes using a Hoffman elbow available with Baerveldt and an adjustable pars plana clip available with the Ahmed valve. The site of insertion should be covered by a patch graft.

Cataract

Localized lens opacities may occur in phakic eyes with a tube implant due to tube lens touch.

Diplopia and Strabismus

Development of strabismus after GDD implantation can be due to the following mechanisms:

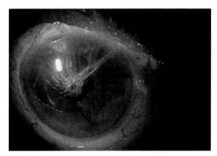

Fig. 12 Corneal decompensation due to tube corneal touch

• Stretching of rectus muscle away from the globe by the bleb capsule
• Posterior fibrosis of extraocular muscles by scar tissue from the bleb capsule. (More likely in implants placed near or beneath the recti) The Baerveldt shunt has fenestrations to allow fibrous tissue to growth through and limit the bleb height.[39]
• Adherence to orbital fat
• Scarring or tucking of the extraocular muscle. Tucking of the superior oblique muscle tendon in case of superior nasal quadrant placement can lead to a Pseudo Brown's syndrome[20,21,40]
• Diplopia may decrease or disappear over time as the inflammation and ocular edema subside. Diplopia in downgaze is particularly disturbing. Prism spectacles can be used to manage any residual diplopia. Rarely squint surgery or removal of implant. Surgical

correction is difficult and may jeopardize bleb function.

Aqueous Misdirection Syndrome

Aqueous misdirection syndrome is uncommon implantation of GDDs.[41] If occurs patient presents with a normal or high IOP with axial shallowing of the anterior chamber. Conservative management can be done. In case it fails, surgical management is required.

Suprachoroidal hemorrhage

There is a risk of development of supra choroidal hemorrhage in the early postoperative period especially in the first few days.[42] Factors predisposing factors include: hypotony, elderly patients, hypertension and choroidal effusion.[35]

SUCCESS

The GDDs are mostly used in complicated cases. Success rates vary according to the type of glaucoma. Success depends on multiple factors **(Table 7)**. Of all the indications, the success rates are for NVG over time are the lowest.

Type of device: The overall success rate in terms of IOP control and in preserving the vision among the glaucoma drainage devices appears similar in cases with intractable glaucoma.[43-48] The percentage reduction in the IOP among the groups is similar.

Table 7 Prognostic factors for success of GDD

• Tube patency
• Bleb development
• Capsule porosity
• Type of glaucoma
– Better after failed filtration surgery in POAG, PACG
– Poor with NVG, uveitic, pediatric glaucoma.

Role of size: In a prospective study, When comparing the 350 mm^2 vs 500 mm^2 Baerveldt implant no statistical difference in the overall surgical success rate or intraocular pressure control at 18 months.[49] This finding may indicate that there is a maximum useful end-plate surface area beyond which there is minimal improvement in the IOP control.

The success rate of GDDs decreases at the rate of 10 percent per year leading to a 50 percent failure rate at 5 years.[50]

Complications and the Type of GDD

The design of the glaucoma drainage device influences the incidence of the postoperative complications, especially early postoperative hypotony and diplopia. The Ahmed valve and the Krupin valve have lower incidence of early postoperative hypotony compared to the Molteno when inserted without an outflow restricting modification. The incidence of diplopia was highest with the Baerveldt implant and is probably related to the insertion of the wings of the end plate underneath the recti muscles, leading to subsequent scar tissue formation and muscle imbalance. It may be due to the height of the bleb or due to the adhesions to the recti muscles as the Baerveldt endplate is inserted under the muscle belly.[49]

The Ahmed Baerveldt Comparison study (ABC) is an ongoing multicenter, randomized, prospective clinical trial comparing the AGV(FP7) and the Baerveldt 350 mm^2.[51] Prelimanary results reveal that the Baerveldt group required more surgical interventions postoperatively. Although the average IOP after 1 year was slightly higher in patients who received an AGV, there

were fewer early and serious postoperative complications associated with the use of the AGV than the BGI.

Some studies report an IOP control comparable to trabeculectomy while others claim a higher success rate with trabeculectomy. GDDs only infrequently achieve IOPs in the low teens in contrast to trabeculectomy with antimetabolites. Thus when the target IOP is low, a trabeculectomy is preferable. The Tube Versus Trabeculectomy (TVT) Study was designed to prospectively compare the safety and efficacy of tube shunt surgery (Baerveldt 350 mm^2) and trabeculectomy with mitomycin-C (MMC) in eyes with prior ocular surgery.[52,53] While the tube group had a higher overall success rate after 5 years, the rates of complete success were not statistically different between treatment groups. There was a trend towards a higher incidence of hyphema in the trabeculectomy group and persistent diplopia and tube erosion in the tube group. Serious complications were comparable between the two groups. Both procedures were associated with similar IOP reduction and use of supplemental medical therapy at 5 years. Additional glaucoma surgery was needed more frequently after trabeculectomy with MMC than tube shunt placement. The results of the TVT study suggested the need to compare the safety and efficacy of tube shunt surgery and trabeculectomy with MMC in patients at low-risk of surgical failure, including eyes without previous ocular surgery. **The Primary Tube Versus Trabeculectomy (PTVT) Study** is an ongoing multicenter randomized clinical trial comparing the safety and efficacy of tube shunt surgery using a 350 mm^2 Baerveldt glaucoma implant to trabeculectomy with MMC (0.4 mg/ml for 2 minutes) as the initial surgical procedure in patients with glaucoma considered at low-risk for failure.

CONCLUSION

Traditionally, GDDs have been used in eyes which are not good candidates for trabeculectomy. Thus GDDs have been a 'second option'. Ongoing studies and various modifications in technique and design have influenced this role and patients who are good candidates for trabeculectomy are being considered for GDD implantation. The most common devices used currently are the AGV and the Baerveldt. Both have their own advantages and disadvantages. Research is ongoing to create a device which offers a predictable resistance to aqueous outflow resulting in the desired amount of outflow immediately after implantation with stability in the early post- operative period. While studies indicate similar success rates in trabeculectomy with antimetabolites the surgeon is faced with a new set of complications after GDD implantation. Results of long-term studies will add valuable insights. Currently their use depends on the individual case and the surgeon's comfort and experience with the procedure.

REFERENCES

1. Rollet M, Moreau M. Traitement de le hypopyon par le drainage capillaire de la chambre anterieure. Rev Gen Ophthalmol 1906;25:481.

2. Zorab A. The reduction of tension in chronic glaucoma Ophthalmoscope 1912;10:258.

3. Vail D. Retained silk thread or 'seton' drainage from the vitreous chamber to Tenon's lymph channel for the relief of glaucoma. Ophthal Rec Chicago 1915;24:184.

4. Mascati N. A new surgical approach for the control of a class of glaucomas. Int Surg 1967;47:10.

5. Rajah -Sivayoham I. Camero venous shunt for secondary glaucoma following orbital venous obstruction. Br J Ophthalmol 1968;52:483.

6. Lee PF, Wong WT. Aqueous venous shunt for glaucoma: report on 15 cases. Ann Ophthalmol 1974;6:1083.

7. Camras C. Valved tube shunt from the anterior chamber to the external ocular surface for use in refractory glaucoma. Invest Ophthalmol Vis Sci 1992;33S:949.

8. Honrubia FM, Grijalbo MP, Gomez ML, et al. Surgical treatment of neovascular glaucoma. Trans Am Ophthalmol Soc (UK) 1979;99:89.

9. Molteno ACB. New implant for glaucoma clinical trial Br J Ophthalmol 1969;53:606.

10. Molteno ACB, Straughan JL, Ancker E. Long tube implants in the management of glaucoma. S Afr Med J 1976;50: 1062.

11. Krupin T, Podos SM, Becker B, et al. Valve implants in filtering surgery. Am J Ophthalmol 1976;81:232-5.

12. Freedman J. Supra-Tenon's placement of single plate Molteno implant. Poster 5th international glaucoma symposium, Cape Town, South Africa 2005.

13. Epstein E. Fibrosis response to aqueous. Its relationship to glaucoma in black patients. Br J Ophthalmol 1959; 43:641-7.

14. Tripathi RC, Li J, Chan WF, et al. Aqueous in glaucomatous eyes contains an increased level of TGF-beta 2. Exp Eye Res 1994;59:723-7.

15. Schocket SS, Nirankari VS, Lakkhanpal V, et al. Anterior chamber tube shunt to an encircling band in the treatment of neovascular glaucoma. Ophthalmology 1982;89:1188.

16. Schocket S. Investigations of the reason for success and failure in the anterior shunt to the encircling band procedure in the treatment of refractory glaucoma. Trans Am Ophthalmol Soc 1986;84:743.

17. Krupin T, Kaufman P, Mandell A, et al. Filtering valve implant surgery for eyes with neovascular glaucoma. Am J Ophthalmol 1980;89:338.

18. Krupin T, Kaufman P, Mandell AI, et al. Long-term results of valve implants in filtering surgery for eyes with neovascular glaucoma. Am J Ophthalmol 1983;95:775.

19. Smith SL, Starita RJ, Fellman RL, et al. Early clinical experience with the Baerveldt 350 mm^2 glaucoma implant and associated extraocular muscle imbalance. Ophthalmology 1993;100:914-8.

20. Prata JA Jr, Minckler DS, Green RL. Pseudo-Brown's syndrome as a complication of glaucoma drainage implant surgery. Ophthalmic surg 1993;24:608-11.

21. Ball SF, Ellis GS Jr, Herrington RG, et al. Brown's superior oblique tendon syndrome after Baerveldt glaucoma implant. Arch Ophthalmol 1992;110: 1368.

22. Minckler D, Vedula SS, Li T, Mathew M, et al. Aqueous shunts for glaucoma. Cochrane Database Syst Rev 2006;2: CD004918.

23. Arroyave CP, Scott IU, Fantes FE, et al. Corneal graft survial and intraocular pressure control after penetrating keratoplast and glaucoma drainage device implantation. Ophthalmology 2001;108:1050-8.

24. Kirkness CM, Moshegov C. Post keratoplasty glaucoma. Eye 1988;2(S1):19-26.

25. Rapuano C, et al. Results of alloplastic tube shunt procedures before, during

or after penetrating keratoplasty Cornea 1995;14:26.

26. Ayyala R. Penetrating keratoplasty and glaucoma. Surv Ophthalmol 2000; 45:91.

27. McDermott ML, Swendris RP, Shin DH, et al. Corneal endothelial cell counts after Molteno implantation. Am J Ophthalmol 1993;115:93-6.

28. Smiddy WE, Rubsamen PE, Grajewski A. Vitrectomy for pars plana placement of a glaucoma seton. Ophthalmic surg 1994;25:532-5.

29. Mermoud A, Salmon JF, Alexander P, et al. Molteno tube implantation for neovascular glaucoma. Long-term results and factors influencing outcome. Ophthalmology 1993;100:897-902.

30. Sidoti PA, Minckler DS, Baerveldt G, et al. Epithelial ingrowth and glaucoma implants. Ophthalmology 1994; 101:872.

31. Sariksan SR. Tube shunt complications and their prevention. Curr Opin Ophthalmol 2009;20:126-30.

32. Law SK, Kalenak JW, Connor TB, et al. Retinal complications after aqueous shunt surgical procedures for glaucoma. Arch Ophthalmol 1996;114:1473.

33. Singh Kuldev, William E Smiddy, Andrew G Lee, et al. Persistent choroidal effusion. Ophthalmology review: a case study approach. 2001, Thieme: New York.

34. WuDunn D, Ryser D, Cantor LB. Surgical drainage of choroidal effusion following glaucoma surgery. J glaucoma 2005;14:103-8.

35. Shah AA, WuDunn D, Cantor LB. Shunt revision versus additional tube shunt implantation after failed tube shunt surgery in refractory glaucoma. Am J Ophthalmol 2000; 129:455.

36. Smith MF, Doyle JW. Results of another modality for extending glaucoma drainage tubes. J glaucoma 1999;8:310.

37. Gedde SJ, Scott IU, Tabandeh H, et al. Late endophthalmitis associated with glaucoma drainage implants. Ophthalmology 2001;108:1323-7.

38. Lee RK, Fantes F. Surgical management of patients with combined glaucoma and corneal transplant surgery. Curr Opin Ophthalmol 2003;14:95-9.

39. Smith SL, Starita RJ, Fellman RL, et al. Early clinical experience with Baerveldt 350 mm^2 glaucoma implant and associated extraocular muscle imbalance. Ophthalmology 1993;100:914.

40. Christmann LM, Wilson ME. Motility disturbances after Molteno implants. J Pediatr Ophthalmol Strabismus 1992; 29:44-8.

41. Greenfield DS, Tello C, Budenz DL, et al. Aqueous misdirection after glaucoma drainage device implantation. Ophthalmology 1999;106:1035-40.

42. Nguyen QH, Budenz DL, Parrish RK 2nd. Complications of Baerveldt glaucoma implants. Arch Ophthalmol 1998; 116:571-5.

43. Ayyala RS, Zurakowski D, Monshizadeh R, et al. Comparison of double plate Molteno and Ahmed of glaucoma valve in patients with advanced uncontrolled glaucoma. Ophthalmic Surg Lasers 2002;33:94.

44. Taglia DP, Perkins TW, Gangnon R, et al. Comparison of the Ahmed glaucoma valve, the Krupin eye valve with disk, and the double plate Molteno implant. J Glaucoma 2002; 347:347.

45. Wang JC, See JL, Chew PT. Experience with the use of Baerveldt and Ahmed glaucoma drainage implants in an Asian population. Ophthalmology 2004;111:1383.

46. Syed HM, Law SK, Nam SH, et al. Baerveldt-350 implant versus Ahmed valve for refractory glaucoma: a case controlled comparison. J Glaucoma 2004;13:38.

47. Tsai JC, Johnson CC, Dietrich MS. The Ahmed shunt versus the Baerveldt shunt for refractory glaucoma: a single surgeon comparison of outcome. Ophthalmology 2003;110:1814.

48. Hong CH, Arosemena A, Zurakowski D, et al. Glaucoma drainage devices: a systematic literature review and current controversies. Surv Ophthalmol 2005; 50:48-60.

49. Lloyd MA, Baerveldt G, Fellenbaum PS, et al. Intermediate- term results of a randomized clinical trial of the 350- versus the 500-mm^2 Baerveldt implant. Ophthalmology 1994;101: 1456-63.

50. Mills RP, Reynolds A, Emond MJ, Barlow WE, et al. Long-term survival of Molteno glaucoma drainage devices. Ophthalmology 1996; 103:299-305.

51. Budenz DL, Barton K, Feur WJ, et al. For the Ahmed Baerveldt Study Group. Treatment Outcomes in the Ahmed Baerveldt Comparison Study after One Year of Follow-up. Ophthalmology 2011;118: 443-52.

52. Gedde SJ, Schiffman JC, Feuer WJ, Herndon LW, Brandt JD, Budenz DL. Three years follow up of Tube Versus Trabeculectomy Study. Am J Ophthalmol 2009;148:670-84.

53. Gedde SJ, Schiffman JC, Feuer WJ, Herndon LW, Brandt JD, Budenz DL. Treatment Outcomes in the Tube Versus Trabeculectomy (TVT) Study After Five Years of Follow-up. Am J Ophthalmol 2012;153:789-803.

53 | From Deep Sclerectomy to Canaloplasty Re-establish the Natural Outflow in Patients with Chronic Open-Angle Glaucoma

Gabor B Scharioth

CHAPTER OUTLINE

INTRODUCTION

Glaucoma is an optic neuropathy in which the optic nerve is damaged with typical loss of nerve fibers and increasing cupping of the optic disc, leading to progressive, irreversible loss of vision. It is often, but not always, associated with increased pressure of the fluid in the eye. The nerve damage involves loss of retinal ganglion cells in a characteristic pattern.

There are many different subtypes of glaucoma but they can all be considered a type of optic neuropathy. Raised intraocular pressure (IOP) is a significant risk factor for developing glaucoma. Untreated glaucoma leads to permanent damage of the optic nerve and resultant visual field loss, which can progress to blindness.

Glaucoma has been nicknamed the "sneak robber of sight" because the loss of vision normally occurs gradually over a long period of time and is often only recognized when the disease is quite advanced. Once lost, this damaged visual field cannot be recovered.

MAGNITUDE OF GLAUCOMA

Worldwide, it is the second leading cause of blindness and affects approximately 66 million people in the world. In some countries, e.g. United States of America where approximately 1,00,000 people are totally blind and approximately 3,00,000 are blind in one eye from glaucoma, it is the leading cause of blindness. Glaucoma affects 1 in 200 people aged fifty and younger, and 1 in 10 over the age of eighty.[1-4]

TYPES OF GLAUCOMA

Glaucoma can be divided roughly into two main categories, 'open angle' and 'closed angle' glaucoma. Open-angle Glaucoma accounts for 90 percent of glaucoma cases in the United States and Europe. It is painless and does not have acute attacks. The only signs are gradually progressive visual field loss, and optic nerve changes (increased cup-to-disc ratio on fundoscopic exam). Closed-angle Glaucoma accounts for <10 percent of glaucoma cases in the United States and Europe, but as much as half of glaucoma cases in other nations (particularly Asian countries). About 10 percent of patients with closed angles present with acute angle closure crisis characterized by sudden ocular pain, seeing halos around lights, red eye, very high intraocular pressure (>30 mm Hg), nausea and vomiting, sudden decreased vision, and a fixed, mid-dilated pupil. Acute angle closure is an ophthalmologic emergency.

RISK FACTORS

The major risk factor for most glaucomas and focus of treatment is increased intraocular pressure. Intraocular pressure is a function of production of aqueous humor by the ciliary processes of the eye and its drainage through the trabecular meshwork. Aqueous humor flows from the ciliary processes into the posterior chamber, bounded posteriorly by the lens and the zonules of Zinn and anteriorly by the iris. It then flows through the pupil of the iris into the anterior chamber, bounded posteriorly by the iris and anteriorly by the cornea. From here the trabecular meshwork drains aqueous humor via Schlemm's canal into scleral plexuses and general blood circulation. In open angle glaucoma there is reduced flow through the trabecular meshwork and/or the Schlemm´s canal; in angle closure glaucoma, the iris is pushed forward against the trabecular meshwork, blocking fluid from escaping.

The inconsistent relationship of glaucomatous optic neuropathy with ocular hypertension has provoked hypotheses and studies on anatomic structure, eye development, nerve compression trauma, optic nerve blood flow, excitatory neurotransmitter, trophic factor, retinal ganglion cell/axon degeneration, glial support cell, immune, and aging mechanisms of neuron loss.

But lowering intraocular pressure is the only proven means to slow or halt disease progression in studies of those at high risk of developing glaucoma Ocular Hypertension Treatment Study (OHTS),[5] those with early to moderate glaucoma Collaborative Initial Glaucoma Treatment Study and Early Manifest Glaucoma Trial (EMGT)[6-8] and those with more advanced glaucoma Collaborative Initial Normal-Tension Glaucoma Study[9,10] and Advanced Glaucoma Intervention Study (AGIS).[11] Across all randomized, controlled trials, lowering IOP by at least 18 percent (mean) from baseline resulted in at least a 40 percent reduction in rates of worsening of glaucoma over 5 years. These studies confirm that a pathophysiological basis for glaucoma is elevated IOP.

If the condition is detected early enough it is possible to arrest the development or slow the progression with medical and surgical means.

ANTIGLAUCOMA SURGERY

First successful antiglaucomatous sur- gery was performed by German ophthalmologist Albrecht von Graefe in 1852. This was a peripheral iridectomy, which was only successful in acute angle closure glaucoma. In the following one hundred years various surgical techniques addressed open angle glaucoma problematic. Since early 1970 trabeculectomy described by Sugar, Cairns and later Fotinopoulos became the standard of care in open-angle glaucoma surgery.[12-14] This widely used procedure involves a surgically formed pathway for aqueous humor between the anterior chamber and the subconjunctival space to lower intraocular pressure in treatment of glaucoma. Main goal is the formation of a functioning filtering bleb. This is a relatively unphysiological approach. Scleral as well as conjunctival scarring lead to the introduction of antimetabolites as adjunctive for filtering bleb depending glaucoma surgeries.

Numerous intraoperative and postoperative complications have been cited following trabeculectomy.[15-19] These include hypotony, maculopathy, blebitis/endophthlamitis, hyphema, suprachoroidal hemorrhage or effusions, encapsulation of the bleb with resultant IOP elevation, loss of visual acuity, and increased risk for cataract formation. In addition, intensive postoperative care, including bleb massage, laser suturolysis, release of releasable sutures, needling, or 5-fluorouracil injections, may be needed to achieve primary success. Recently several authors reported relatively high failure rate of trabeculectomy after long-term follow-up.

All this led surgeons to search for a more physiological and bleb independent surgical approach in IOP lowering glaucoma surgery. Surgical treatment of the natural aqueous outflow system, including Schlemm´s canal, to restore normal function and IOP control without penetration of the intraocular space has long been the interest in the study of open-angle glaucoma as an alternative to penetrating and bleb dependent methods.[20,21]

In 1964 Krasnov published his first report on sinusotomy. This operation consisted of removing a lamellar band of the sclera, opening the Schlemm´s canal over 120 degrees from 10 to 2 o´clock. The inner wall of Schlemm´s canal was untouched and then the conjunctiva was closed. Krasnov believed that the aqueous outflow resistance in the majority of primary open-angle glaucoma was situated at the level of the scleral drainage veins and not in the trabeculum.[22,23] In the same year Walker published a paper about surgery of the Schlemm´s canal.[24] Other authors also reported on nonpenetrating filtering surgery, leaving in place the trabeculum and the inner wall of Schlemm´s canal.[25-28] Sinusotomy was relatively safer then full-thickness surgery with almost no postoperative complications. But this procedure became never popular because it was a difficult operation. It needed a surgical microscope at a time when this was not readily available. Moreover, the surgical results were not convincing.[29-34]

NONPENETRATING FILTERING SURGERY

Deep Sclerectomy and Viscocanalostomy

Several techniques of nonpenetrating filtering glaucoma surgery based on Krasnov´s sinusotomy have been described. Nonpenetrating trabeculectomy was proposed by Zimmermann in 1984[35] and Arenas[36] first published the term ab-externo trabeculectomy in 1991. Fyodorov stressed on removing the corneal stroma behind the anterior trabeculum and Descemet´s membrane and term this deep sclerectomy.[37]

Deep sclerectomy is aimed to decrease the outflow resistance, in which the internal wall of Schlemm's canal, juxtacanalicular meshwork and the corneal stroma behind the anterior trabeculum and Descemet's membrane is removed, without penetrating the anterior chamber, leaving behind a thin Descemet's membrane. This membrane is known as trabeculo-Descemet's membrane or window. Deep sclerectomy then acts as a guarded filter, where Schlemm's canal is unroofed, and the aqueous drains through the "trabeculo-Descemet's window".

Stegmann et al described a variant of nonpenetrating glaucoma surgery termed it viscocanalostomy to emphasize the importance of injecting high-viscosity sodium hyaluronate (Healon GV) into the Schlemm's canal and the surgically created ostia as well into the sclerectomy site under the superficial scleral flap.[38] The injection of high molecular weight viscoelastic probably ruptures the inner and outer walls of the Schlemm's canal, these microruptures are likely to involve juxtacanalicular tissue and meshwork, facilitating the aqueous facility. This probable mechanism was observed in various experimental studies done on human and animal eyes. Hence, this technique functions as a gentle trabeculectomy, which provides aqueous to bypass the abnormal resistance.

Further development of nonpenetrating approaches included the use of implants at the surgical site in the late 1990s and early 2000s.[39-41] These implants were either absorbable (i.e. SK Gel, AquaFlow, HealaFlow) or non-absorbable (T-Flux). We compared SK-Gel versus T-Flux in different patients with and without combined phacoemulsification. Deep sclerectomy was performed with a relatively good success rate and with no difference between both implants.[42,43] Most surgeons prefer to close the scleral flap loose to induce subconjunctival filtration in contrast to a watertight closure in viscocanalostomy, which could be named the first bleb independent

nonpenetrating glaucoma surgery. Although these nonpenetrating surgical procedures for glaucoma effectively reduced IOP and lowered the incidence of postoperative complications compared with penetrating procedures such as trabeculectomy, comparative clinical studies indicates that IOP decreases more significantly with trabeculectomy, especially when used in conjunction with antimetabolites.[44-50]

Canaloplasty

Cannulation of Schlemm's canal with a silk suture was described in 1960 for partial trabeculotomy.[51] A modified technique using a 6 × 0 polypropylene suture was later used for 360 degree trabeculotomy for treatment of congenital glaucoma.[52] All previous nonpenetrating glaucoma surgeries were able to reach two to three clock hours of Schlemm's canal while a procedure treating the entire canal should be theoretically more effective. We reported a technique using the 6 × 0 polypropylene suture for catheterization of the entire Schlemm's canal and while withdrawing the suture a 10 × 0 polypropylene suture is installed in the canal and finally knotted under tension.[53] This is a very difficult and time consuming technique with a relatively high risk of mispassage of the 6 × 0 polypropylene suture into the anterior chamber or suprachoroidal space. Recent advances in technology have allowed surgeons to use a flexible microcatheter to access the entire length of Schlemm's canal more atraumatically. This technique is called canaloplasty and seems to be the logical evolution to viscocanalostomy.[54,55] In our results with canaloplasty in 72 eyes with open angle glaucoma and no previous glaucoma surgery complete success rate after 12 months was 86 percent and regarding a target pressure of 18 mm Hg qualified success rate was 90.4 percent.[56]

Principal Surgical Techniques for Deep Sclerectomy and Viscocanalostomy

The conjunctiva may be opened either at the fornix or at the limbus. A 5 × 5 mm rectangular or parabolic shaped scleral flap **(Figure 1)** is performed including one-third of the scleral thickness (about 300 µm, depending on the total scleral thickness in the particular case). To be able to reach the Descemet´s membrane later during the dissection of the deeper scleral flap, the superficial scleral flap has to be prepared 1 to 1.5 mm anteriorly into the perilimbal clear cornea. The initial incision is made with a no.11 stainless steel blade (e.g. 15° slit knife for paracentesis) or a diamond knife. The flap dissection is done with a ruby blade or a bevel-up crescent knife **(Figures 2 and 3)** (i.e. 1 mm ultrasharp minidisc knife, Grieshaber Alcon, USA).

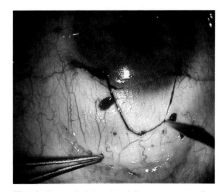

Fig. 1 Superficial scleral flap, note no diathermy of episcleral vessels is performed

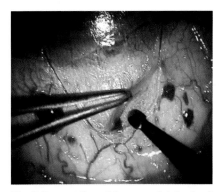

Fig. 2 Preparation of the superficial scleral flap with a Mini-Crescent knife

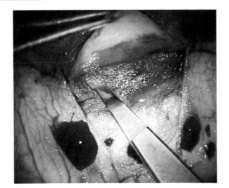

Fig. 3 Dissecting the superficial scleral flap into the clear cornea

Next, deep sclerokeratectomy is performed by making a slightly smaller second flap then the superficial one (**Figure 4**), leaving a step of sclera at the sides allowing for a tighter closure of the superficial flap in case of an intraoperative perforation of the trabeculo-Descemet's membrane or intended watertight closure for visco-canalostomy/canaloplasty. Then the deep scleral flap is dissected towards the cornea using ruby knife or crescent stainless steel knife. This dissection has to be made down to a depth very close to the choroids/ciliary body and carefully carried anteriorly keeping the level of dissection as constant as possible. In case of opening of the suprachoroidal space dissection is continued just a few scleral fibers above. The change of the direction of the scleral fibers to a limbus-parallel bundle indicates the scleral spur. Just behind this the Schlemm's canal is opened and unroofed (**Figure 5**). Care is taken to dissect the ostia of Schlemm's canal clearly, because it is believed that this reduces the risk of collapse and scarring of these surgical ostia.

A paracentesis/side port incision is made. It is used to reduce intraocular pressure to very low level. This maneuver reduces the risk of perforation of the trabeculo-Descemet's-membrane. The dissection is carried forward to expose a small segment of the Descemet's membrane, creating a trabeculo-descemetic window of about 1 to 1.5 mm (**Figure 6**). The corneal stroma can be separated from the Descemet's membrane by blunt dissection, i.e. with a sponge while the edges of the deep scleral flap are cut towards the cornea with the knife. In some cases the adhesion of Descemet's membrane to the stroma is more tight. In these cases a blunt spatula or the Mini-Crescent knife could be used with sweeping like limbus parallel motion to release these adhesions. This part of the surgery is quite challenging because there is a high risk of perforation of the anterior chamber.

The deep sclerocorneal flap is then removed by cutting in the clear corneal part with a delicate small and very sharp scissor (i.e. Vannas or Galand scissor) (**Figure 7**). At this stage of the procedure, there should be percolation of aqueous through the remaining membrane. This can be checked also by applicating fluorescein to the surgical area (s.c. Rentsch-Seidel test). The amount of percolation is checked while drying the surgical area with a sponge. To increase the outflow facility the inner wall of the Schlemm's canal is peeled partially including the endothelium and the juxtacanalicular trabecular meshwork. A special designed forceps or an ordinary capsulorhexis forceps can be used. Occasionally the inner wall of the Schlemm's canal is fibrosed and an initial radial cut is necessary to be able to start the peeling. In the next step of the surgery ophthalmic visco-surgical device (OVD) is injected in

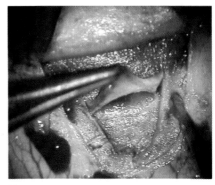

Fig. 5 Opening of the Schlemm's canal, note the color difference in the scleral bed indicating the right depth of preparation

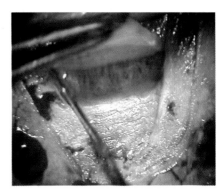

Fig. 6 Enlarging the descemetic window for optimal exposition of the trabeculo-descemetic membrane, note the percolation of aqueous humor without perforation of the membrane, iris is visible through the intact membrane

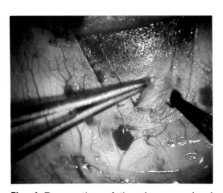

Fig. 4 Preparation of the deeper scleral flap using a Mini-Crescent knife, note the smaller size of the deeper scleral flap

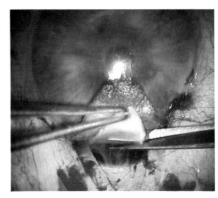

Fig. 7 Deep sclerectomy – dissection of the deeper scleral flap with Vannas scissors

the surgical ostia of Schlemm´s canal (This is known as **Viscocanalostomy**) **(Figure 8)**. To keep the intrascleral space (scleral lake) created patent, an implant or OVD may be used. The superficial scleral flap is then repositioned and sutured with 10 × 0 nylon or absorbable sutures. The superficial scleral flap is sutured loose **(bleb dependend deep sclerectomy)** for creating a subconjunctival filtering bleb or as watertight **(Figure 9)** as possible **(bleb independent viscocanalostomy)** for forcing internal filtration into the Schlemm´s canal and then into the collector channels.

Deep Sclerotomy Implants

To avoid secondary collapse of the scleral lake due to adhesion of the superficial scleral flap or contact of descemetic window, a space-maintainer implant is placed in the surgical created scleral bed. In deep sclerectomy we have used over the past decade SK-Gel (Coreal, France) and T-Flux (Zeiss Meditech, Germany, fomer produced by Ioltech, France).

SK-Gel, that has been used in deep sclerectomy to maintan the scleral lake is a reticulated hyaluronic acid implant of 500 μm thickness **(Figure 10)**. It was available into sizes 3.5 × 3 mm and 4.5 × 3 mm, while the first one was designed for watertight closure the second was partially left outside the superficial scleral flap to increase the subconjunctival filtration. To provide watertight closure we use the smaller model. The material is biocompatible and absorbable over a long period of several months, occasional years. The advantage of this implant is that it occupies a large volume in the filtration area without swelling while allowing for a sufficient circulation of the aqueous humor and does not require suture fixation.

A hydrophilic acrylic non-absorbable implant (T-Flux implant, IOL Tech Laboratories, France, now Zeiss Meditec, Germany), has been used

to maintain the scleral lake and to prevent collapse of the surgical ostia of Schlemm´s canal **(Figure 11)**. It is a T-shaped implant with a 4 mm arm length, 2.75 mm body height, and 0.1 to 0.3 mm thickness. Each arm is inserted into the surgical ostia of Schlemm´s canal and the design facilitates drainage into the Schlemm´s canal. The implant is either secured with a 10 × 0 nylon suture in the foot´s hole or the shape of the deep sclerectomy is adapted to the implant design to stabilize it in the scleral bed. A second hole in the anterior part of the T-Flux implant is designed to facilitate a goniopuncture (Nd:YAG laser descemetotomy) to the descemetic window to increase outflow postoperatively.

Canaloplasty

A new procedure called canaloplasty was introduced to overcome some of the problems associated with the previous procedures. The idea of implanting a fine tensioning suture into the Schlemm´s canal to enlarge the entire 360 degree of Schlemm´s canal should theoretically:

- Widen the intertrabecular spaces,
- Prevent collapse of the canal, the surgical ostia and the descemetic window,
- Prevent herniation of the inner wall into the ostia of collector channels,

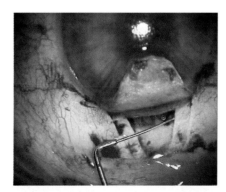

Fig. 8 Viscocanalostomy with injection of OVD into the ostia of Schlemm´s canal with a special cannula

- Keep the entire Schlemm´s canal open and make collector channels away from the surgical site available for drainage.

From March 2008 a microcatheter (iTrack, iScience, USA) for a canaloplasty became commercially available. This device has a 200 μm diameter shaft

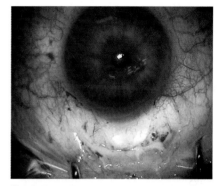

Fig. 9 Watertight closure of the superficial scleral flap with 5-7 interrupted sutures (10 x 0 absorbable suture)

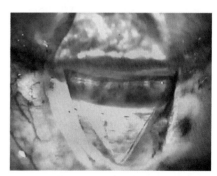

Fig. 10 SK-Gel in deep sclerectomy placed in the scleral bed

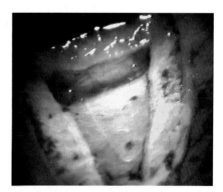

Fig. 11 T-Flux positioned in scleral bed, note both arms are implanted in the surgical ostia of Schlemm´s canal

with a atraumatic distal tip approximately 250 µm in diameter (**Figure 12**). The device incorporated an optical fiber to provide an illuminated beacon tip to assist in surgical guidance. The illuminated tip was seen trans-sclerally during catheterization of Schlemm's canal to identify the location of the distal tip of the microcatheter. The microcatheter has a lumen of about 70 µm with a proximal Luer lock connector through which an OVD (e.g. Healon GV) or dye (e.g. tryptane blue, indocyanin green, fluorescein) could be delivered.

The new Glaucolight (DORC, The Netherlands) is thinner and has an outer diameter of just 150 µm with a blunt atraumatic tip (**Figure 13**). The light source is already adapted and can be placed in the sterile operating area. The Glaucolight can be slightly bent at its end by the surgeon to reduced the risk of mispassage (e.g. into ostia of larger collector channel) during catheterization.

A special forceps is used to manipulate the microcatheter and place the tip into the surgically created ostia of Schlemm's canal (**Figure 14**). The microcatheter is advanced 12 o'clock hours within the canal while the surgeon observes the location of the beacon tip through the sclera (**Figures 15 to 17**).

After the catheterization of the entire canal length with the microcatheter and with the distal tip exposed at the surgical site, a 10 × 0 polypropylene suture is tied to the distal tip and the microcatheter withdrawn, pulling the suture into the canal (**Figures 18 and 19**). The suture is cut from the microcatheter and then tied in a loop, encircling the inner wall of the canal using a slip knot or a locked four throw knot (**Figure 20**). To reduce risk of rupture of Descemet membrane and to facilitate a more effective tensioning of the 10 × 0 polypropylene suture the IOP is previously lowered through a paracentesis.

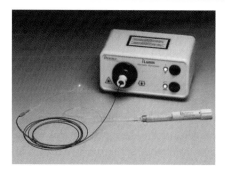

Fig. 12 Track (iScience, USA) attached to external light source (iLumin, iScience, USA) to illuminate the tip of the fiber, special syringe for delivering OVD

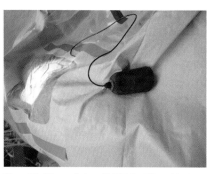

Fig. 13 Glaucolight (DORC, The Netherlands) with integrated battery powered LED light source and clip, attached to the sterile patients cover just next to the surgical area, pressing at sensor of the sterile case for illuminating the fiber tip

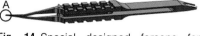

Fig. 14 Special designed forceps for marking the superficial scleral flap and for atraumatic and more controlled manipulation of the catheter (DORC, The Netherlands)

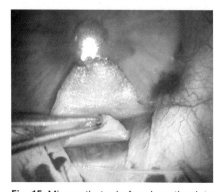

Fig. 15 Microcatheter before insertion into the Schlemm's canal

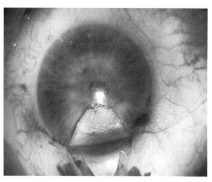

Fig. 16 Red spot indicating the position of the microcatheter at 5 o'clock position in the Schlemm's canal

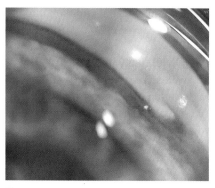

Fig. 17 Intraoperative gonioscopic few with illuminated tip of the microcatheter (red dot) in the Schlemm's canal, note the heavily pigmented trabecular meshwork in this eye

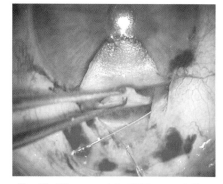

Fig. 18 After complete 360° cannulation of the Schlemm's canal

The superficial scleral flap is repositioned and tightly closed with five to seven single absorbable sutures (i.e. 10 × 0 Vicryl, Ethicon). Now OVD is gently injected under the scleral flap to reduce

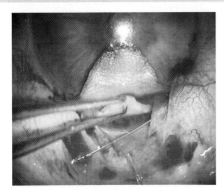

Fig. 19 10 x 0 Prolene tensioning suture is fixed to the microcatheter

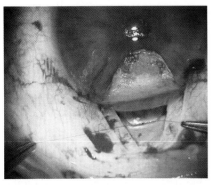

Fig. 20 After withdrawing of the microcatheter the suture is cut off and knotted under tension to pull the inner wall of Schlemm´s canal and the Descemet's window towards the anterior chamber to prevent failure of the surgery due to collapse of these structures

the risk of bleeding into the sclerectomy site and to prevent scarring in this area. Anterior chamber is refilled with balanced salt solution to normal or slightly elevated IOP and conjunctiva is repositioned and fixed with two to four single absorbable sutures.

Whether additional injection of OVD into the entire canal is necessary is unclear. We could prove that the procedure did work without the use of iTrack catheter and circumferential injection of OVD.

Aqueous Humor Dynamics after Nonpenetrating Glaucoma Surgery

The goal of nonpenetrating glaucoma surgery is to improve the natural out

flow facility but it retain some residual outflow resistance by maintaining a membrane between the anterior chamber and the scleral dissection. There is probably an increased uveoscleral outflow through the thin remaining scleral layer in the bed of the deep sclerectomy. Aqueous humor may reach from the scleral space to the Schlemm's canal back and is subsequently drained out by the aqueous veins. Experiments in animal models revealed that there is development of new aqueous drainage veins in the scleral space, few days after deep sclerectomy. In successful human deep sclerectomy cases this intrascleral bleb was evidenced by ultrasound biomicroscopy studies, a great deal of interest has been directed towards the properties of this outflow resistance of the membrane before and after surgery has been calculated. In viscocanalostomy the microruptures after high molecular weight viscoelastic involving juxtacanalicular tissue and meshwork facilitate the aqueous outflow.

Aims of nonpenetrating glaucoma surgery
- To create a trabeculo-Descemet's window to allow a reproducible postoperative outflow resistance
- To promote the formation of an intrascleral bleb in order to reduce conjunctival bleb related complications.

Contraindications
Absolute contraindication
    Neovascular glaucoma
Relative contraindication
    Narrow angle glaucoma
    Post argon laser trabeculoplasty
    Angle recession glaucoma

POSTOPERATIVE FOLLOW-UP

The first-two days are vital for judging the outcome of surgery. Most recommended follow-up regimen is to examine the patient on 1st and 3rd postoperative day, followed by weekly examination for one month,

monthly examination for the next 6 months and then after every 6 months. Complicated cases need more frequent review, so follow-up schedule can be made accordingly.

Follow-up Evaluation
- Bleb is assessed for its extent, height, vascularity, cysts and possible wound leaks
- Anterior chamber examination for hyphema, hypopyon and depth
- Corneal examination for its clarity or epithelial erosion
- Intraocular pressure
- Fundus examination: to rule out choroidal detachment, suprachoroidal hemorrhage
- Optic nerve head and macula
- Ultrasound biomicroscopy can be done, if required to assess the surgical site.

COMPLICATIONS OF NON-PENETRATING GLAUCOMA SURGERY
Intraoperative Complications
Prolapse of Descemet's Membrane
Descemet's membrane can prolapse while advancing the deeper scleral flap into the cornea which eventually leads to the perforation of membrane. Prophylactic paracentesis is therefore made to decompress the globe thereby avoiding this complication.

Perforation of Trabeculo-Descemet's Membrane
The perforation usually occurs in the thinnest position either at the level of anterior trabecular meshwork or at the Descemet's membrane level. A small perforation may lead to a larger tear formation, which may eventually lead to iris prolapse. Smaller perforation without iris prolapse can be left as it and overlying scleral flap is tightly sutured with 10-0 nylon suture.

Slightly larger perforation where iris prolapse is suspected, high molecular weight viscoelastic is injected and deep scleral flap is sutured with a collagen graft, which physically seals the hole. The superficial scleral flap is then closed tight. Some larger perforation may need a peripheral iridectomy, or the nonpenetrating glaucoma surgery has to be converted into conventional filtering surgery.

Hemorrhage

Intraoperative bleeding may occur from uveal tissue during flap formation or during deep scleral flap excision. Bleeding at any stage can lead to fibroblast formation, which should be minimized by use of local vasoconstrictor and wet field cautery. Intraocular hemorrhage is not so common, if at all it occurs it may arise from uveal or retinal vessel especially in cases where preoperative intraocular pressure was higher and postoperative intraocular pressure drops below 3 to 4 mm Hg.

Blood reflex from Schlemm's canal ostia may occur when episcleral venous pressure is higher than the intraocular pressure. In such cases high molecular weight viscoelastic is injected into the anterior chamber to artificially raise the intraocular pressure.

EARLY POSTOPERATIVE COMPLICATIONS

Wound Leak

It has to be confirmed by positive Seidel's test. Usually it stops leaking by itself after discontinuation of steroid therapy. If not then resuturing is to be considered.

Hyphema

It occurs in the form of microhyphema either originating from iris vessel or leak of red blood cells through the trabeculo–Descemet's membrane. A small hyphema does not require any treatment.

Choroidal Detachment

So far average incidence of choroidal detachment is 2.5 percent according to various studies. It not only occurs due to low postoperative intraocular pressure but also due to direct aqueous humor passage from the scleral space, since there is a very thin scleral layer is remaining in place after deep sclerectomy. For shallow detachments cycloplegics and anti-inflammatory medications (steroids or nonsteroidal) are the treatment of choice. Large detachment may require suprachoroidal fluid drainage.

Hypotony

Hypotony is described as intraocular pressure of 5 mm Hg or less on first postoperative day. According to some investigators early hypotony is a good indicator of good surgical dissection.

LATE POSTOPERATIVE COMPLICATIONS

Fibrosis of Conjunctival Bleb

The incidence conjunctival bleb fibrosis in nonpenetrating glaucoma surgery has been reported by many investigators. Due to the presence of intrascleral bleb in this surgery, intraocular pressure remains adequate in most of the cases, and no intervention is generally required. Some authors believe in giving 5-FU injection or topical anti-inflammatory drops to prevent further scarring.

Raised Intraocular Pressure

Late or intermediate onset of raised intraocular pressure may occur due to long-term use of steroid or subconjunctival fibrosis. Most of such cases require goniopuncture by Nd:YAG laser to lower the outflow resistance. If this technique fails, one may need additional antiglaucoma medications or repeat surgery.

Late Rupture of Descemet's Membrane

This may occur due to gradual, progressive rise of pressure. The proposed mechanism is that there is progressive collection of aqueous humor in the intrascleral bleb, and this aqueous humor causes backward pressure towards the Descemet's membrane, which may eventually lead to perforation and iris prolapse. Such cases where iris blocks the aqueous outflow, surgical intervention should be considered.

CONCLUSION

The results of our retrospective analysis confirm the results of other studies, in that in open-angle glaucoma a deep sclerectomy with implantation of a device in combination with phacoemulsification lowers IOP in a clinically relevant way over a long period.

The effect seems to be independent from the absorbable or nonabsorbable property of the implant, while the risks of a combined surgery are few when performed by an experienced surgeon.

Canaloplasty is a new very effective bleb independent intraocular pressure lowering procedure with a very low complication rate. Longer follow up is need to understand the long-term success rate and effects of the tensioning suture on intraocular tissue.

The commercially available catheter for canaloplasty (Glaucolight, DORC and iTrack, iScience, USA) reduceces surgical time and improves safety of the procedure. The procedure was successful even without injection of ophthalmic viscosurgical device throughout the entire Schlemm´s canal.

Nonpenetrating bleb independent glaucoma surgery is possible, has a very low complication rate and could lead to re-establishing the natural outflow in patients with open-angle glaucoma.

Nonpenetrating glaucoma surgery	
Advantages	**Disadvantages**

• No bleb related complications
  – Less chance of bleb leak – early or late
  – Less chance of blebitis, endophthalmitis
  – Contact lens wear less likely to be problematic
  – Bleb dysthesis rare
• Reduced risk of prolonged hypotony
• No sudden decompression of anterior chamber
• Less chances of
  – Suprachoroidal hemorrhage
  – Serous choroidal detachments
• Less intraocular inflammation
• No need for iridectomy
• Less chance of intraocular bleeding
• Fewer postoperative visits
• Conjunctiva is spared for future glaucoma surgery
• More rapid visual rehabilitation postoperatively
	• Technically more difficult
	• Long learning curve
	• Long operating time
	• Requires specialized instruments
	• Cost of instruments
	• About 10 percent have actual perforation into anterior chamber requiring iridectomy
	• Intraocular pressure less likely to be lowered sufficiently in advanced glaucoma
	• Pressure lowering may not last as long
	• Frequent goniopuncture required in more than 50 percent patients
	• Can be performed only in a limited category of glaucomas

REFERENCES

1. Quigley HA. The number of persons with glaucoma world-wide. Br J Ophthalmol 1996;80:389-93.

2. Pizzarello L, Abiose A, Ffytche T, et al. Vision 2020: The Right to Sight: a global initiative to eliminate avoidable blindness. Arch Ophthalmol 2004;122(4):615-20.

3. Congdon N, O´Colmain B, Klaver CC, et al. Causes and prevalence of visual impairment among adults in the United States 2004;122 (4);477-85.

4. Friedman DS, Wolfs RC, O´Colmain BJ, et al. Prevalence of open-angle glaucoma among adults in the United States. Arch Ophthalmol 2004;122(4):532-8.

5. Kass MA, Heuer DK, Higginbotham EJ, et al. The Ocular Hypertension Treatment Study: a randomized trial determines that topical ocular hypotensive medication delays or prevents the onset of primary open-angle glaucoma. Arch Ophthalmol 2002;120(6):701-13, discussion 829-30.

6. Lichter PR, Musch DC, Gillespie BW, et al. Interim clinical outcomes in the Collaborative Initial Glaucoma Treatment Study comparing initial treatment randomized to medical or surgery. Ophthalmology 2001;108 (11):1943-53.

7. Heijl A, Leske MC, Bengtsson B, et al. Reduction of intraocular pressure and glaucoma progression: results from the Early Manifest Glaucoma Trial. Arch Ophthalmol 2002;120 (10):1268-79.

8. Leske MC, Heijl A, Hussein M, et al. Factors for glaucoma progression and the effect of treatment: the Early Manifest Glaucoma Trial. Arch Ophthalmol 2003;121:48-56.

9. Collaborative Initial Normal-Tension Glaucoma Study Group. Comparision of glaucomatous progression between untreated patients with normal-tension glaucoma and patients with therapeutically reduced intraocular pressures. Am J Ophthalmol 1998;126:487-97.

10. Collaborative Initial Normal-Tension Glaucoma Study Group. The effectiveness of intraocular pressure reduction in the treatment of normal-tension glaucoma. Am J Ophthalmol 1998;126:498-505.

11. AGIS (Advanced Glaucoma Intervention Study) Investigators. The Advanced Glaucoma Intervention Study (AGIS): 7. The relationship between control of intraocular pressure and visual field detoriation. Am J Ophthalmol 2000;130 (4):429-40.

12. Sugar HS. Experimental trabeculectomy in glaucoma. Am J Ophthalmol 1961;51:623.

13. Cairns JE. Trabeculectomy. Preliminary report of a new method. Am J Ophthalmol 1968;66(4):673-9.

14. Fronimopoulus J, Lambrou N, Pelekis N, Christakis C. Elliot´s trepanation with scleral cover (procedure for protecting the fistula in Elliot´s trepanation with a lamellar sclleral cover). Klin Monbl Augenheilkd. 1970;156 (1):1-8.

15. Jones E, Clarke J, Khaw PT. Recent advances in trabeculectomy technique. Curr Opin Ophthalmol 2005; 16:107-13.

16. Mac I, Soltau JB. Glaucoma-filtering bleb infections. Curr Opin Ophthalmol 2003;14:91-4.

17. Borisuth NSC, Phillips B, Krupin T. The risk of glaucoma filtration surgery. Curr Opin Ophthalmol 1999;10:112-6.

18. Ophir A. Encapsulated filtering bleb; a selective review–new deductions. Eye 1992;6:348-52.

19. Gedde SJ, Herndon LW, Brandt JD, et al. Surgical complications in the tube versus trabeculectomy study during the first year of follow-up. Am J Ophthalmol 2007;143:23-31.

20. Ellingsen BA, Grant WM. Trabeculotomy and sinusotomy in enucleated human eyes. Invest Ophthalmol 1972;11:21-8.

21. Johnstone MA, Grant WM. Microsurgery of Schlemm's canal and the human aqueous outflow systeme. Am J Ophthalmol 1973;76:906-17.

22. Krasnov MM. (Sinusotomy in glaucoma). Vestn Oftalmol 1964;77:37-41.

23. Krasnov MM. Externalization of Schlemm's canal (sinusotomy) in glaucoma. Br J Ophthalmol 1968; 52:157-61.

24. Walker WM, Kanagasundaram CR. Surgery of the canal of Schlemm. Trans Ophthalmol Soc UK 1964;84:427-42.

25. Aasved H. Trabeculotomy, trabeculectomy and sinusotomy – some clinical results. Acta Ophthalmol 1973;120 (Suppl):33-8.

26. Artamonov VP. (Effectiveness of subscleral sinusotomy in glaucoma). Vestn Oftalmol; 1980.pp.5-8.

27. Babushkin AE, Baltabaev FR. (Modification of sinusotomy). Vestn Oftalmol 1991;107:7-9.

28. Smelovskii AS. (Sinusotomy, its modification and possible combination with other operations). Vestn Oftalmol 1967;80:31-6.

29. Krasnov MM. Symposium: microsurgery of the outflow channels. Sinusotomy. Foundations, results, prospects. Trans Am Acad Ophthalmol Otolayngol 1972;76:368-74.

30. Postic S, Stankov-Tomic M. Krasnov's sinusotomy in chronic simple glaucoma. Bull Mem Soc Fr Ophthalmol 1967;80:716-26.

31. Remky H. Extended sinusectomy (trabeculectomy with cyclodialisis effect). Late results and analysis of failures. Klin Monatsbl Augenheilkd. 1986;188:278-82.

32. Rosengren B. Sinusotomy according to Krasnov. Ophthalmol Soc UK. 1966;86:261-9.

33. Surer JL. Experimental ocular sinusotomy, some technical difficulties. J Am Osteopath Assoc 1972;71:716-22.

34. Vlk J. Krasnov's sinusotomy in the treatment of chronic glaucoma. Cesk Oftalmol 1974;30:345-7.

35. Zimmerman TJ, Kooner KS, Ford VJ, et al. Trabeculectomy vs. nonpenetrating trabeculectomy: a retrospective study of two procedures in phakic patients with glaucoma. Ophthalmic Surg 1984;15:734-40.

36. Arenas E. Trabeculectomy ab externo. Highlights Ophthalmol 1991;19:59-66.

37. Fyodorov SN, Ioffe DI, Ronkina TI. Deep sclerectomy: technique and mechanism of a new antiglaucomatous procedure. Glaucoma 1984;6: 281-3.

38. Stegmann R, Pinenaar A, Miller D. Viscocanalostomy for open-angle glaucoma in black African patients. J Cataract Refract Surg 1999; 25:316-22.

39. Sourdille P, Santiago P-Y, Villain F, et al. Reticulated hyaluronic acid implant in nonperforating trabecular surgery. J Cararact Refract Surg 1999; 25:332-9.

40. Ambresin A, Shaarawy T, Mermoud A. Deep sclerectomy with collagen implant in one eye compared with trabeculectomy in the other eye of the same patient. J Glaucoma 2002; 11:214-20.

41. Sanchez E, Schnyder CC, Sickenberg M, et al. Deep sclerectomy: results with and without collagen implant. Int Ophthalmol 1996/97;20:157-16.

42. Wiermann A, Zeitz O, Jochim E, Matthiessen L, Wagenfeld P, Galambos G, Scharioth G, Mathiessen N, Klemm K. A comparison between absorbable and non-absorbable scleral implants in deep sclerectomy (T-Flux and SK-Gel). Opthalmologe 2007;104(5):409-14.

43. Schreyger F, Scharioth GB, Baatz H. SK-Gel implant versus T-Flux implant in the contralateral eye in deep sclerectomy with phacoemulsification: Long-term follow-up. The Open Ophthalmology Journal 2008;2:57-61.

44. O´Bart DPS, Shiew M, Edmunds B. A randomized, prospective study comparing trabeculectomy with viscocanalostomy with adjunctive antimetabolite usage for the management of open angle glaucoma uncontrolled by medical therapy. Br J Ophthlamol 2004;88:1012-7.

45. Yalvac IS, Sahin M, Eksioglu U. Primary viscocanalostomy versus trabeculectomy for primary open-angle glaucoma; three years prospective randomized clinical trial. J Cataract Refract Surg 2004;30:2050-7.

46. Carassa RG, Bettin P, Fiori M, Brancato R. Viscocanalostomy versus trabeculectomy in white adults affected by open-angle glaucoma; a 2-year randomized, controlled trial. Ophthalmology 2003; 110:882-7.

47. Kobayashi H, Kobayashi K, Okinami S. A comparison of the intraocular pressure-lowering effect and safety of viscocanalostomy and trabeculectomy with mitomycin C in bilateral open-angle glaucoma. Graefes Arch Clin Exp Ophthalmol 2003;241:359-66.

48. Cillino S, Di Pace F, Casuccio A, Lodato G. Deep sclerectomy versus punch trabeculectomy: effect of low dose mitomycin C. Ophthalmologica 2005;219:281-6.

49. Lüke C, Dietlein TS, Jacobi PC, et al. A prospective randomized trial of viscocanalostomy versus trabeculectomy in open-angle glaucoma: a 1-year follow-up study. J Glaucoma 2002;11: 294-9.

50. Goldsmith JA, Ahmed IK, Cradall AS. Nonpenetrating glaucoma surgery. Ophthalmol Clin North Am 2005; 18(3):443-60.

51. Smith R. A new technique for opening the canal of Schlemm. Br J Ophthalmol 1960;44:370-3.

52. Beck AD, Lynch MG. 360° trabeculotomy for primary congenital glaucoma. Arch Ophthalomol 1995;113: 1200-2.

53. Scharioth GB. Cartheterless Viscocanaloplasty, 6th Congress of Romanian Society of Ophthalmology 2007, Sinaia, Romania. and 3rd International Meeting on Innovative Glaucoma Surgery, Recklinghausen, Germany.

54. Lewis RA, von Wolff K, Tetz M, et al. Canaloplasty: circumferential viscodilation and tensioning of Schlemm´s canal using a flexible microcatheter for the treatment of open-angle glaucoma in adults: interim clinical study analysis. J Cataract Refract Surg 2007; 33:1217-26.

55. Lewis RA, von Wolff K, Tetz M, et al. Canaloplasty: circumferential viscodilation and tensioning of Schlemm´s canal using a flexible microcatheter for the treatment of open-angle glaucoma in adults: Two-year interim clinical study results. J Cataract Refract Surg 2009; 35:814-23.

56. Scharioth GB. "The management of advanced glaucoma with penetrating and nonpenetrating techniques" and "Canaloplasty" presented at XXVIII Congress of the European Society of Cataract and Refractive Surgeons, 2010, Paris, France.

54 Cyclodestructive Procedure

R Ramakrishnan

Management of intractable glaucoma is still a challenging situation in the field of glaucoma management. In these conditions destroying a portion of ciliary body has been a strategy used for decades.[1,2] This helps to control glaucoma by reducing the secretion of aqueous humor from the ciliary body. Cyclodestructive procedures using cautery were generally replaced by cyclocryotherapy in the early 1960. Many procedures were tried to ablate the ciliary body. Newer techniques provide the opportunity to expand the indications of this procedure to patients who have good visual potential. More recently many procedures have been tried to achieve good control of IOP with fewer complications and less postoperative pain. The various cyclodestructive procedure are:

- Diathermy (Weve 1933)[3]
- Beta irradiations[4]
- Cycloelectrolysis[5]
- Cyclocryotherapy
- Therapeutic ultrasound
- Laser cycloablations.

Weve reported the use of diathermy in 1933. The modified penetrating diathermy was introduced by Vogt[6] in 1936. This procedure was abandoned following low success rate and significant hypotony as reported by Walton and Grant.[7] Beta irradiations did not become popular because of their cataractogenic property. Cycloelectrolysis did not demonstrate any advantages over diathermy and, therefore, never gained acceptance.

INDICATIONS

Cycloablative procedures are generally reserved for patients who have a poor visual prognosis and a for conventional filtering surgery. The various indications include:

- Refractory ocular pain in absolute glaucoma
- Uncontrolled IOP despite maximum tolerated medical therapy
- Multiple failed filtrations or shunt surgery
- Cases with severely scarred conjunctiva and poor visual prognosis

- Neovascular glaucoma
- Aphakia and pseudophakic glaucoma
- Glaucoma following penetrating keratoplasty (PKP)
- Traumatic glaucoma
- Glaucoma following vitreo retinal surgery
- Secondary glaucoma due to chronic uveitis
- Congenital glaucoma (multiple failed procedures).

CONTRAINDICATIONS

- Thin sclera
- Limbal deformation
- Scleritis
- Phakic eyes with good vision.

CYCLOCRYOTHERAPY

Bietti in 1950 proposed this technique by which IOP is reduced by freezing the ciliary body.[8] This procedure is ideal for pain relief in those patients with limited visual potential. Even though it was very effective in controlling the IOP its continued use has been limited by higher rate of complications such as severe pain, severe inflammation, visual loss, phthisis bulbi.

In fact Krupin et al.[9] reported 34 percent phthisis bulbi and a 58 percent incidence of visual loss in eyes with neovascular glaucoma. Although most surgeons do laser photocoagulation, cyclocryotherapy is still useful for selected cases because the procedure is easily and rapidly performed as an out patient procedure. It is equally effective, requires less costly equipment and is readily performed in various settings.

Goal

The goal of this procedure is to destroy the ciliary process epithelium by freezing it with a cryoprobe through the intact conjunctiva and sclera. The extent of area treated can be adjusted based on the amount of hypotensive response required. Usually 120 to 180 degrees of cyclo destruction is required. Higginbotham et al evaluated the effects of graded cyclocryotherapy on IOP, aqueous humor flow rate and permeability of the blood aqueous barrier in cats, suggesting that this treatment can be titrated to some extent.[10]

This procedure is usually done under retrobulbar anesthesia. A large sized retina cryo probe is used. Typically the procedure involves freezing the ciliary body to a temperature of –80°C for to 60 seconds. Generally 180° of the ciliary body is treated.

ULTRASOUND

Therapeutic ultrasound is an attractive method of cycloablation which requires specialized instruments that deliver focused ultrasound energy to the ciliary body while the eye is immersed in a water bath.

The ultimate results of both cyclo-cryo therapy and therapeutic ultrasound are almost similar. In addition the cost of this equipment is very high and it carries high-risk of scleral thinning.

LASER CYCLOABLATION

Laser Cyclophotocoagulation

The basic principle is that laser energy is applied to destroy the ciliary epithelium stroma and vascular supply in order to reduce aqueous humor production and lower the IOP. It is a procedure by which laser energy is used to destroy the ciliary epithelium, stroma and vascular supply. Cycloablation was first tried with Xenon arc laser in 1961 by Weeker et al.[11] Later Beckman et al reported the use of Ruby laser in 1972 and then the neodymium laser in 1973.[12] Later in 1980 Fankhauser used thermal mode Nd:YAG laser (1064 nm) to destroy ciliaryl epithelium through transcleral route. Diode laser with a

wavelength of 810 nm can also be used to do this procedure. The various lasers used include:

- Semiconductor diode laser (810 nm)
- Nd:YAG (1064 nm)
- Krypton laser
- Diode laser, a solid state laser is currently preferred due to its compact size, low maintenance and better absorption by uveal melanin.

The various routes of delivery include:

- Noncontact
- Contact
- Transpupillary
- Endocyclophotocoagulation.

Noncontact Method

This is performed using the thermal mode Nd:YAG laser under retrobulbar anesthesia through slit-lamp. A tangential beam of laser is projected 1.0 to 1.5 mm posterior to the limbus,

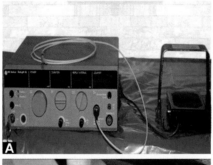
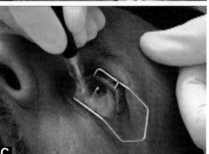
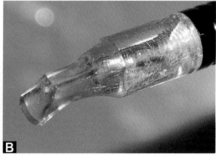

Figs 1A to C (A) Diode laser machine; (B) G probe; (C) Diode laser cyclophotocoagulation (DLCP) being done with G probe

maximum defocusing and an energy level of 8 joules. The success rate ranges from 45 to 86 percent.[12] Generally 3 to 9 o'clock meridians are avoided to prevent damage the long posterior ciliary arteries. Here 30 to 40 applications are directed at the limbus. A specialized contact lens may be useful to help control eye movements, compress the conjunctiva and assist in placing laser application.

Contact Method

Brancato et al. were the first to evaluate the contact method of Nd:YAG laser cycloablation. This technique destroys the ciliary epithelium in a more focused fashion than noncontact currently the Diode laser is used. The G-probe is placed directly on the conjunctiva (after a retro or peribulbar block) placed 0.5 to 1 mm from the and held perpendicular to the sclera (**Figures 1A to C**). Optimal parameter have been noted to be for the Nd:YAG laser. With the Diode laser the settings are: 1600 to 2000 for 2000 ms with POP sound in 50 percent of the burns. We prefer to use lesser energy and a longer duration. The intraocular pressure reduction was almost similar between cyclocryotherapy and Nd:YAG cyclophotocoagulation.

The procedure is done under peribulbar or retrobulbar anesthesia. Postoperatively all antiglaucoma medicines are continued. Pilocarpine and prostaglandin analogs are avoided. Cycloplegics, topical steroids and analgesics are also prescribed.

ENDOCYCLOPHOTOCOAGULATION

Endocyclophotocoagulation is currently under clinical study. Endoscopic probe and laser delivery fiber is introduced via a limbal clear corneal incision and cycloablation is done under direct visualization. It may be more useful for glaucoma in aphakia and pseudophakia or in combination with phacoemulsification.

Transpupillary Cyclophotocoagulation: Lee[13] reported the application of argon laser through a well-dilated pupil via a slit lamp delivery system a technique known as transpupillary cyclophotocoagulation.

COMPLICATIONS OF CYCLODESTRUCTIVE PROCEDURES
- Severe pain
- Hypotony and phthisis bulbi
- Decrease in vision
- Severe intraocular inflammation (Acute and Chronic)
- Rise in intraocular pressure
- Vitreous hemorrhage
- Corneal decompensation
- Retinal or choroidal detachment
- Scleral thinning
- Cataract in phakic patients
- Hyphema
- Vitritis
- Aqueous misdirection
- Corneal decompensation
- Retinal or choroidal detachment
- Sympathetic ophthalmia.

REFERENCES

1. Schuman J. Cycloablation in Albert DM Jacobie: Principles and practice of Ophthalmology, 2nd edn; 2000. pp.3013-23.
2. Gaasterland DE. The magnificent light. Evolution of laser surgery for glaucoma. Van Buskirk EM, Shields MB; 1997.pp.293-307.
3. Weve HJM. Zentralbl Ophthalmol 1933. pp.29:562.
4. Haik GM. Beta irradiation in glaucoma AJO 1948;31:945-52.
5. Berens C. Cycloelectrolysis for glaucoma. Trans Am Ophthalmol Soc 1949;47:364.
6. Vogt A. Klin Montatsbl Augenheilkd 1936;97:672.
7. Walton DS, Grant WM. Penetrating cyclodiathermy. Arch Ophthal 1970; 83:47-8.
8. Bietti, et al. Surgical intervention on the ciliary body. JAMA 1950;142:889-97.
9. Krupin T, et al. Cyclocryotherapy in neovascular glaucoma. Am J Ophthalmol 1978;86:24-6.
10. Higginbotham EJ. Effects of cyclocryotherapy on aqueous humor dynamics in cats. Arch Ophthal 1988;106: 396-403.
11. Weeker R, et al. Effects of photocoagulation of ciliary body upon ocular tension. Am J Ophthalmol 1961;52: 156-63.
12. Beckman, et al. Nd:YAG cyclophotocoagulation. Arch Ophthalmol 1973; 90:27-8.
13. Lee, et al. Argan laser photocoagulation of the ciliary process in Aphakic glaucoma. Arch of Ophthalmol 1979; 97:2135-8.

PART 5

Glaucoma—Future

55 | Neuroprotection in Glaucoma

Suresh Puthalath, R Ramakrishnan

CHAPTER OUTLINE

INTRODUCTION

Glaucoma, as we now know, is not a disease of intraocular pressure (IOP) alone. Traditionally, glaucoma was viewed as a disease of elevated IOP, in which visual loss could be prevented by lowering the pressure. Today, however, glaucoma is viewed as an optic nerve disease in which IOP is currently the most important modifiable risk factor. Although lowering IOP has been linked with the prevention of visual loss in may patients it has not been effective for all patients. Progression of disease despite a significant lowering of IOP has been demonstrated in all of the major, randomized clinical glaucoma trials, including the Advanced Glaucoma Intervention Study (AGIS) and the Collaborative Normal Tension glaucoma Study.[1,2] Recent studies have suggested that glaucoma is caused by multiple factors that ultimately lead to apoptotic death of retinal ganglion cells (RGCs) and subsequent optic nerve head atrophy.

Glaucoma is not just an anterior optic neuropathy, but is also chronic and involves the retinal ganglion cell axon. In general, most optic neuropathies involve the axons and do not affect the cell bodies directly. A wealth of evidence exists that glaucoma is primarily an axonal disease. The sites of damage, changes in the lamina cribrosa, and disc hemorrhages all suggests that the major stresses are at the neuroretinal rim (NRR).[3-5]

CURRENT CONCEPTS IN NEUROPROTECTION

Currently, the treatment of glaucoma is based on alleviating the most important modifiable risk factor, elevated IOP. However, this does not address the other potential causes of neuropathy, nor does it prevent the secondary loss of neurons due to released toxic factors. Therefore, neuroprotection has been proposed as an adjunctive therapeutic strategy for enhancing the survival and function of the RGC regardless of the cause of the glaucomatous neuropathy, Weinreb and Levin[6] have described neuroprotection in glaucoma as "a therapeutic paradigm for slowing or preventing the death of RGCs and thus maintaining physiologic function of the axons". Independent of cause, neuroprotection is aimed at blocking destructive events or enhancing survival mechanisms of the RGCs or optic nerve fibers.

WHAT IS NEUROPROTECTION?

Neuroprotection (NP) refers to the ability to prevent loss or to decrease the rate of loss of retinal ganglion cells with appropriate therapy to preserve a minimum critical number of retinal ganglion cells hence preventing loss of visual function. The term neuroprotection refers to protection of healthy but vulnerable neurons in the vicinity of dead cells/dying cells which are at risk of injury even after removal of primary insult. Glaucomatous optic neuropathy is a chronic disease manifesting as characteristic changes at the optic nerve head. Loss of retinal ganglion cells (RGC) is a characteristic hallmark of glaucomatous eyes. A variety of stimuli can trigger RGC death by primary neuronal injury which leads to release of number of factors, which secondarily damage the adjacent cells.

Flow chart 1 The Levels of Neuroprotection

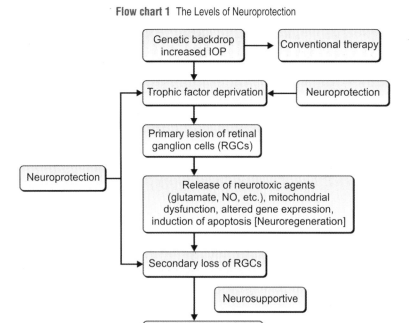

Table 1 Possible Pathological Mechanisms Leading to RGC Death

Primary Insults (Neural Damage)	Secondary Mechanisms (Deprivation of trophic factors)	
Mechanical	Excitotoxicity (Glutamate)	released
Ischemic-change in micro circulation at ONH	Nitric oxide	neuro toxic
Genetic metabolic	Free radicals	agents

The term **secondary degeneration** has been applied to progressive neuropathy that spreads to adjacent areas beyond the initially injured neuron site. The aim of therapeutic neuro protection is to protect these initially injured neurons from secondary degeneration. The neuronal damage is supposed to be driven by toxic factors like glutamate, NMDA, excitotoxins, free radicals and nitric oxide. These factors are released by primary insults and they trigger a series of events which finally lead to apoptosis. The functional damage to the nervous tissue continues to progress even after the primary cause has been removed. This may be the reason why some glaucoma patients continue to exhibit progressive neuropathy even after an offending factor such as high IOP has been controlled.

Biochemical Theory: Mechanism for Cellular Damage

Excitotoxic Hypothesis and Glutamate: The term *excitotoxic* was coined to describe dual action of specific amino acid—glutmate and aspartate. These are the normal neurotransmitters in the retina which can accumulate in excess, leading to toxic levels due to lack of proper regulation by the surrounding Muller cells (glial cells) resulting in RGC death.

NMDA and Glutamate Binding

Excitotoxicity of RGCs is mediated by over stimulation of a glutamate receptor, N-Methyl, D-aspirate (NMDA)

which has two agonist binding sites: One for glutamate and other for glycine. After the release of glutamate at injury site, Na^+ enters the cell. There is concomitant entry of Cl^- and H_2O, causing cellular swelling. This occurs in the acute phase of neuronal trauma. Depending on the severity of insult the cell may recover or proceed to further loss of function and cell death. In the delayed phase there is cellular influx of calcium and once the calcium homeostasis is altered a variety of abnormal biochemical reaction ensured. There is release of cytotoxic enzymes like protease, endonuclease and lipases that destroy the cell membrane. Free radicals accumulate and further disturb the essential metabolic function of cells.

Oxygen Free Radicals

These are oxygen containing molecules that carry one or more unpaired electron and react with the lipid, nucleic acid and proteins. These are produced after ischemic injury during the reperfusion phase. Free radicals are supposed to be involved in glaucoma and other chronic neuro degenerative diseases.

Nitric Oxide

Intracellular mediator of nitric acid in plasma and aqueous humor is cyclic Guanosine Monophosphate (cGMP). The level of cGMP is found to be lower in NTG. Significantly low levels of cGMP in plasma suggest a disorder of endothelium dependent vasoregulation. This might interfere with optic nerve head blood supply and play role in the determination of optic nerve damage. The final common pathway in ganglion cell death is apoptosis which can be initiated by pathological events like ischemia.

Nitric oxide (NO) systhase has three isoforms which are NOS1, NOS2, NOS3.

- NOS1 is present in retina
- NOS2 is absent in normal people and occasionally present in glaucoma
- NOS3 is a vasodilator and has neuroprotective action.

APOPTOSIS

Apoptosis is a *genetically programmed active` process of cell death* (cell suicide) characterized by chromatin concentration, intracellular fragmentation, membrane enclosed cellular fragments of 180 bp (apoptotic bodies) and phagocytosis by surrounding tissue without any associated inflammation. These DNA fragments can be stained by TUNEL procedure.

Mechanism of Apoptosis

Apoptosis may be triggered by a combination of biochemical factors produced as an end result of increased intraocular pressure and decreased perfusion. The predominant factors responsible for triggering apoptosis are decrease in neurotrophic factors especially brain derived neurotrophic factors (BDNF) due to axoplasmic stasis and an increase in toxic excitatory compounds such as glutamate.

A large number of compounds are under evaluation as potential neuroprotective agent for glaucoma therapy.

CURRENT APPROACHES IN NEUROPROTECTIVE INTERVENTION

1. Controlling the expression of apoptotic control genes.
2. Supplying RGC with neurotrophic factors.
3. Blocking apoptosis pharmacologically with drugs inhibiting different stages of cell death.
4. Enhancing the body's protective responses.

These can be achieved by Drug Therapy or Gene Therapy

Neuroprotection aims at blocking the primary and secondary degenerative events or even enhancing bodies protective mechanisms. It acts as a prophylaxis and should be present, at the time of injury and aimed at healthy ganglion cells. The primary destructive event is more likely to be repetitive. So treatment should be on a long-term basis aimed at blocking secondary degenerative mechanism.

POTENTIAL NEUROPROTECTIVE COMPOUNDS FOR GLAUCOMA THERAPY

- Alpha-2 adrenergic agonists
- Direct apoptosis inhibitors
- Free radicals scavengers
- Neurotrophins
- Nitric oxide inhibitors
- NMDA – Gated channel blockers
- Voltage – Gated calcium channel blockers
- Kynurenic acid and citicoline as endogenous neuroprotective substance
- Long-term *in vivo* drug delivery system
- Ocular gene therapy.

Some of these factors are discussed in detail.

Brimonidine and its NP Characteristics (0.2%)[7-9]

Brimonidine provides increased neuronal survival by increasing the expression of cellular survival factors. There is up regulation of the receptors of neuronal factors – basic fibroblasts growth factors (bFGF) and increased retinal bFGF

Flow chart 3 Achieving Neuroprotection (NP Strategy)

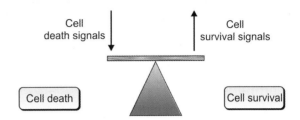

Flow chart 2 Mechanism of RGC damage

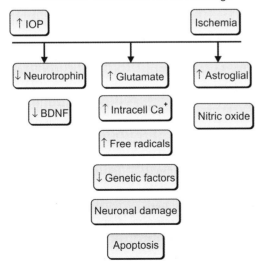

expression and increased bcl-2 and bcl-x gene expression. These:

1. Rescue retinal RGC from ischemic induced cell death.
2. Preserve retrograde axonal transport in surviving retinal ganglion cells and protect against ischemia induced degeneration.[10]

Neurotrophic support: Development and maintenance of RGC is regulated by neurotrophins.

- BDNF-LGB

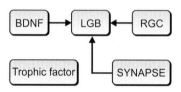

Ciliary Neurotrophic Factors

Recently transgenic technique used to deliver BDNF to retina – (a*deno associated viral vectors*) – may become a therapeutic reality.

Kynurenic Acid

It is a tryptophane metabolite which has neuroprotective activity *in vitro* and *in vivo*. The action is explained by the following properties:

- Endogenous competitive antagonism at the glycine binding site of the NMDA receptor.
- Non-competitive antagonism of acetylcholine at nicotinic receptors.

NMDA Gated Channel Blockers

High concentration of glutamate in the vitreous of glaucoma patients has been reported. Drugs that inhibit NMDA gated channel—*Memantine* approved by US for treatment in Alzheimer's under trial for glaucoma. Currently, memantine is an agent that shows potential for a NP benefit in a range of neurodegenerative disease. Safety and efficacy of memantine as a treatment option for glaucoma is yet to be established. Memantine is

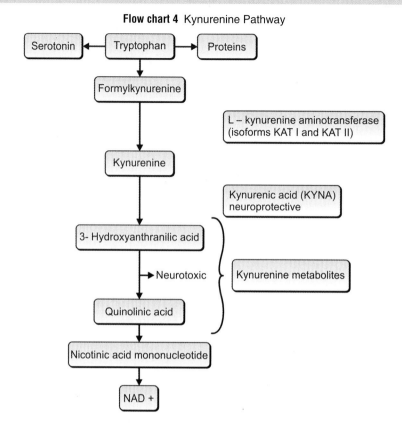

Flow chart 4 Kynurenine Pathway

a low affinity NMDA receptor antagonist that works by blocking the action of glutamate. It is approved in Alzheimer's disease.[11,12]

Voltage – Gated Channel Blockers

In ischemia/reperfusion injuries, calcium over load is a terminal event. Any agent which can decrease this influx can alleviate the events associated with cell damage. *Betaxolol* has shown effect as cal-cium channel blocker in retinal vessels. Dextromethorphan, flupirtine, memantine, MK- 801 all decrease calcium influx by inhibiting NMDA receptor.

Ginkgo Biloba Extract

An extract from the leafs of Ginkgo Biloba tree is used as dietary supplement for potential beneficial effect in vascular insufficiency and Alzheimer's disease. It is under trial in glaucoma.

WHERE ARE WE TODAY?

Results from *in vivo* and *in vitro* studies suggested that excitotoxicity is a major mechanism of RGC death.

Medications

Ongoing multicentric trials in humans with memantine have been promising. *Riluzole*, a drug used in amyotrophic lateral sclerosis (ALS) is also under trial in glaucoma neuroprotection.

Immuno Protection by Vaccination

An experiment study in rat has proven that neuroprotective vaccines can be tried in glaucoma. These vaccines are:

1. Myelin binding protein (MBP)
2. Glatiramer acetate (Cop-1).

The trials with MBP are not promising since it has the potential to cause complete paralysis of the body and experimental autoimmune uveitis. Cop-1 is a synthetic co-polymer which is under trial. It does not have complications like MBP.

FUTURE TRENDS

Gene therapy: In ocular gene therapy viral vectors mainly *adeno associated virus* (AAV) is used to deliver genes with neuroprotective substances directly to their location of action: RGC. With antisense strategies it is possible to selectively inhibit some genes responsible for increased ganglion cell loss. The *adeno associated virus* is a suitable vector system for the retina.[13]

Other Modalities

- Prevention of apoptosis by introduction of small molecule drug designed to turn of the expression of apoptosis related gene.
- As injectable molecules targeted towards modulators of apoptosis.
- Stem cell implantation.

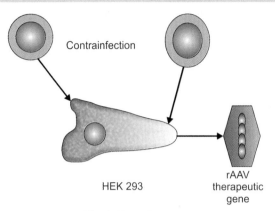

Fig. 1 Gene therapy

CONCLUSION

Irrespective of the involved mechanism in retinal ganglion cell death, neuroprotection is not likely to replace the current treatment of glaucoma in entirely as blocking apoptosis does not affect the (primary) stimulus causing the retinal ganglion cells to die. Blocking cell death, however, only relieves the retinal ganglion cells of the initial period of stress, allowing them to recover if the primary cause like a raised IOP is reduced and controlled. In the coming years blocking apoptosis of retinal ganglion cells, used in conjunction with conventional therapies would be the treatment of choice in the management of glaucoma.

REFERENCES

1. The AGIS Investigators. The advanced glaucoma intervention study, 6: effect of cataract on visual field and visual acuity. The AGIS Investigators. The Advanced Glaucoma Intervention Study (AGIS): 1. Study design and methods and baseline characteristics of study patients. Control Clin Trials 1994;15:299-325.

2. Collaborative Normal-Tension Glaucoma Study Group. The effectiveness of intraocular pressure reduction in the treatment of normal-tension glaucoma. Collaborative Normal – Tension Glaucoma Study Group. Am J Ophthalmol 1998;126:498-505.

3. Quigley HA, Nickells RW, Kerrigan LA, et al. Retinal ganglion cell death in experimental glaucoma and after axotomy occurs by apoptosis. Invest Ophthalmol Vis Sci 1995;36:774-86.

4. Tatton WG. Apoptotic mechanisms in neurodegeneration. Possible relevance to glaucoma. Survey of Ophthalmology 1999;9 (Suppl 1):S22-9.

5. Mittag TW, Danias J, Pohorence G, et al. Retinal damage after 3 to 4 months of elevated intraocular pressure in a rat glaucoma model. Invest Ophthalmol Vis Sci 2000;41:3451-9.

6. Weinreb RN, Levin LA. Is neuroprotection a viable therapy for glaucoma? Arch Ophthalmol 1999;117:1540-4.

7. Lafuente MP, Villegas, Mayor ME, et al. Neuroprotective effects of brimonidine against transient ischemia induced-retinal ganglion cell death: A dose response in vivo study. Exp Eye Res 2002;74:181-9.

8. Chalmers-Redman RM, Elstner MD, Mammen M, Tatton W: Alpha-2 adrenergic receptor activation by brimonidine reduces neuronal apoptosis by inducing new protein synthesis that maintains mitochondrial pore closure. Exp Eye Res 71:Abst385.

9. Kent A, Nussdorf J, Fellows D, Small D, David R. Vitreous concentration of topically applied brimonidine tartrate 0.2 percent. Ophthalmology 2001;108:784-7.

10. Collaborative Normal–Tension Glaucoma Study Group. Comparison of glaucomatous progression between untreated patients with normal – tension glaucoma and patients with therapeutically reduced intraocular pressures. Collaborative Normal – Tension Glaucoma Study Group. Am J Ophthalmol 1998;126:487-97.

11. WoldeMussie E, Yoles E, Schwartz M, et al. Neuroprotective effect of memantine in different retinal injury models in rats. J Glaucoma 2002;11:474-80.

12. Yucel YH, Gupta N, Zhang Q, et al. Memantine protects neurons from shrinkage in the lateral geniculate nucleus in experimental glaucoma. Arch Ophthalmol 2005;112:376-85.

13. Research group neuroprotection, dept of pathology of vision and neuro ophthalmology, university eye Hospital Tuebingen.

56 | Medical Management of Glaucoma— the Future

CHAPTER OUTLINE

- ❖ Prostaglandin Analogues
- ❖ Preservatives and Antiglaucoma Drugs
- ❖ Rho-Kinase Inhibitors
- ❖ Steroids – Different Approaches
- ❖ Neuroprotection in Glaucoma
- ❖ Anti-VEGF
- ❖ Other Agents – in Clinical Development
- ❖ Drug Delivery Systems
- ❖ Future of Nanomedicine in Vision Research
- ❖ Gene Therapy in Glaucoma

INTRODUCTION

Management of glaucoma is still a challenging problem in the field of ophthalmology. Till date many newer class of drugs are available to control intraocular pressure. Each has its our advantages and disadvantages. Research is going on to find out new formulations of existing drugs with varying concentration, preservatives and delivery system. Many formulations have also been tried to treat glaucoma with non intraocular pressure (IOP) lowering mechanism.

PROSTAGLANDIN ANALOGUES

Currently prostaglandin group of drugs and fixed combination of various drugs have revolutionized the management of glaucoma. Even though they have good intraocular pressure lowering effect, their use is limited by their side effects, cost, availability and storage. There is a new formulation of PGF2 analogues along with nitric oxide donating properties PF-03187207 under phase 2 trials. Now various studies are going

on around the world to find out the efficacy and safety of Latanoprost in children and angle closure glaucoma. A new PG analog AR 102 which has 150 fold greater potency at FP receptor than latanoprost is under clinical trial. In preclinical studies, the drug has shown greater efficacy and longer duration of action than latnoprost and better tolerability than Travoprost.

PRESERVATIVES AND ANTIGLAUCOMA DRUGS

Benzalkonium chloride (BAK) is the commonly used preservative in most of the topical antiglaucoma drugs. The BAK is basically a detergent. It prevents bacterial contamination and enhances corneal penetration. But it is toxic to corneal and trabecular cells and also thought to be one of the factor causing bleb failure. In addition it causes ocular surface disorders by altering the conjunctival cytology especially goblet cells. Preservative free drugs with stabilised oxychloro complex (SOC), HPMC methyl paraben, propyl paraben are

currently available. These drug formulations are available as single dose unims and minims.

Benzalkonium chloride is used in varying concentration ranging from 0.04 percent in latoprost to 0.004 percent in betagan. The concentration of BAK in Travatan is 0.015 percent, in Brimonindine Timolol combination 0.005 percent, Alphagan-P 0.005 percent, Ganfort 0.005 percent and Dorzolamide 0.008 percent. Purite is used as drug presevative in Lumigan 0.005 percent and in Alphagan-Z 0.005 percent.

Bctablockers are now available without preservative with SOC and HPMC. Timolol is not stable in formulations preserved with the gentler preservative purite. A preservative free prostaglandin, i.e. Tafluprost is available in Japan and Europe since 2008. BAK free Travatan-Z with borate, Zinc, Propylene glycol and sorbital is also available.

RHO-KINASE (ROCK) INHIBITORS

Rho-kinase is an enzyme that phosphorylates cytoskeletal regulatory proteins and many play an important role in increasing the aqueous out flow. Various formulations of Rho-kinase inhibitors like SNJ 1656, topical K-115, DE104 ophthalmic solutions are under phase I clinical trails.

STEROIDS – DIFFERENT APPROACHES

Various newer steroid formulations are available without typical corticosteroid ocular hypertensive effect. Anecortave acetate which is an angiostatic steroid was originally, approved for posterior juxta scleral injection in wet ARMD. Accidently with anterior subtenons injection, the IOP lowered to a considerable level. A study by Robin et al had shown that anterior juxtascleral injection of Anecortave acetate shows a considerable reductions in intraocular pressure in eyes with primary open angle glaucoma. But the efficacy is not longlasting. Repeated injection may be needed to control intraocular pressure.

They suggested that further additional studies are required to establish better efficacy, safety, optimal dosing, frequency, mechanism of action and potential additive to other intraocular pressure lowering therapies. In another studies by the same author in steroid induced glaucoma, Anecortave acetate lowered intraocular pressure substantially in some eyes with medically uncontrolled cases. But later studies based on data analysis and input from a panel of experts suggested that the IOP reduction and response rate provided by even the highest dose were not sufficient to support this novel approaches. So, this drug was discontinued in the usage of glaucoma.

NEUROPROTECTION IN GLAUCOMA

Various neuroprotective drug formulation have been tried in glaucoma and other neurological disorders. Some of the important forms are memantine, SRT 501, TGF beta shield, Beta amyloid inhibitors and epigallocatechin galleate. The phase 3 clinical trial examining the safety and efficacy of oral memantine as a treatment for glaucoma has shown that the progression of disease was significantly lower in patients receiving the higher dose of memantine compared to patients receiving lower dose of memantine. But there was no significant benefit compared patients receiving placebo. Therefore, the study failed to meet its primary endpoint.

ANTI-VEGF

Various anti-VEGF agents have been tried in neovascular glaucoma. Intravitreal and intracameral injection of Bevacizumab (Avastin) have shown a dramatic regression of neovascular glaucoma and neovascularization of the iris. Some cases may require repeat injection. Avastin is also being studied as subconjuntival injections for the prevention of bleb failure.

OTHER AGENTS – IN CLINICAL DEVELOPMENT

Studies are going on to find out the efficacy of selective muscarinic compound, Angiotensin II antagonist like olemesartan, serotonin receptor antagonist like Biovitrum, etc. Newer calcium channel blockers like Lomerizine is found increase the blood flow in optic nerve head.

DRUG DELIVERY SYSTEMS

Newer methods of drug delivery by nanoparticles, micro beads, microneedles, ocuscrts are being studied and found to be more effective with lesser amount of drug and better and greater bioavailability of drug in the targeted tissue with minimal systemic absorption and side effects.

Routes other than topical like transscleral, intravitreal, suprachoroidal route are being studied. Newer techniques like Iontophoresis, electrophoresis, photoacoustic delivery are under study.

FUTURE OF NANOMEDICINE IN VISION RESEARCH

Research is going on to use nanotechnology in drug delivery, immunomodulation, DNA repair, imaging, retinal neuroprosthesis. It is also being tried to repair the injured tissue. Nanoneuro knitting is a technique by which injured neuronal axons are repaired. Here there is a peptide nanofiber scaffold for brain repair and axon regeneration with functional return of vision occurs. It has been found that self-assembling peptide nanofiber-scaffold creates a permissive environment for axons to regenerate through acute injury site and "Knit" axon processes together.

Dendrimers, a combination of drugs that act in synergy was found to be effective in stopping surgical scar tissue formation in the eye after glaucoma surgery.

GENE THERAPY IN GLAUCOMA

The potential strategies on which gene therapy has been studied are IOP lowering, Neuroprotection and Wound healing in glaucoma surgery for prevention of scarring of trabeculectomy site.

The potential vectors for gene therapy are either non viral or viral. The non viral are:

- Naked DNA
- Interfering RNA – SIRNA and SH RNA
- Physical methods like electroporation i.e. local application of electrical pulses after DNA injection
- Chemical – Cationic lipids (Liposomes).

Viral

- HIV
- Adenoviral
- AAV
- Lentiviral.

Summary of Strategies used in Glaucoma Gene Therapy

Genes Studies	Target Genes, Proteins, Mechanisms	Target Tissues	Main Cellular and Molecular Changes Induced In Vitro or In Vivo	Outcome Expected
DN Rho	Inhibiting Rho	TM	Reduction of actin and focal adhesions in cultured TM cells; loss of intercellular adhesions in cultured SC cells	Increased conventional outflow
C3	Inactivating Rho by rebosylation	TM	Cell rounding; disruption of actin and loss of cellular adhesions in cultured HTM cells	Increased conventional outflow
DNRK	Inhibiting Rho-kinase	TM	Cell rounding; cell-cell detachment; reduction of actin, focal adhesion and myosin light chain phosphorylation in cultured TM cells	Increased conventional outflow
Caldesmon	Inhibiting actin-tropomyosin activating myosin MgATPase	TM	Formation of unique curvy actin networks and disruption of focal adhesions in cultured HTM cells	Increased conventional outflow
MMPs	Disrupting MMP/TIMP balance	TM/CM	Degrading the ECM	Increased uveoscleral, conventional outflow
PG synthase genes	Increasing MMP expression	CM	Upregulation of MMP expression acting to degrade ECM	Increased uveoscleral, conventional outflow
Specific siRNAs	Silencing gene expression	TM/Retina	Suppression of target genes (e.g. myocilin)	E.g. increased outflow, decreased AHF, neuroprotection
Bcl-2	Protecting the integrity of the mitochondrial membrane	Retina	RGG cells remained morphologically intact and survived	Neuroprotection
BIRC4	Inhibiting caspase	Retina	Increased optic nerve axon survival	Neuroprotection
BDNF	Neuroprotection	Retina	Increased neuromal survival	Neuroprotection
TrkB	BDNF receptor mediating	Retina	Increased neuromal survival	Neuroprotection
ERK	Neuroprotective activity of extracellular factors, including neurotrophins	Retina	Increased RGG survival	Neuroprotection
MEK1	The upstream activator of ERK1/2	Retina	Increased RGG survival	Neuroprotection
CNTF	Neuroprotection	Retina	Increased RGG survival	Neuroprotection
TNF-alpha	Inhibiting TNF-alpha	Retina	Increased RGG survival	Neuroprotection
p21	Regulating cell cycle and preventing proliferation of fibroblasts	Conjunctiva	Decreased fibroproliferation	Prevention of wound healing in filtering surgery

Clinical Implications – Examples

Gene directed therapy

Researchers used a virally administered gene to treat dogs with a form of Leber's congenital amaurosis (LCA) caused by a mutation in the same gene, RPE65, that can cause LCA and blindness in human children.

Several months after treatment, the dogs functional vision had been restored, and their electroretinograms were almost normal.

The National Eye Institute is sponsoring a phase I clinical trial of gene therapy for LCA.

There is a genetic basis to response to beta-blockers, and we also know that patients who have myocilin juvenile glaucoma are unresponsive to all medication therapies and require surgical therapy.

Index

Page numbers followed by *f* refer to figure and *t* refer to table